CONTENTS

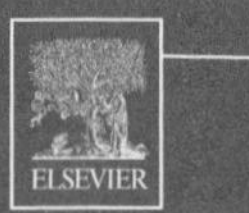

evolve

To access your Learning Resources, visit:
http://evolve.elsevier.com/criticalcaredrug/

Evolve® Resources for ***Mosby's Critical Care Drug Reference*** include the following:

- **200 Continually Updated Online Drug Monographs**
  Continually updated drug monographs from Gold Standard Clinical Pharmacology™ provide up-to-date information on 200 drugs commonly used in the critical care setting, expanding and updating the coverage provided in the book.

- **12 Interactive Drug Calculators**
  IV Time Calculator
  Body Surface Area Calculator
  Pediatric Dose Based on Body Surface Area Calculator
  IV Dose Rate Calculator
  PO Dosage Calculator: Capsule
  PO Dosage Calculator: Liquid
  PO Dosage Calculator: Tablet
  IV Dosage Calculator: Push
  IV Dosage Calculator: Infusion of a Dose per Patient Weight
  IV Dosage Calculator: Infusion of a Dose
  IV Dosage Calculator: Infusion of a Volume
  IV Dosage Calculator: Infusion of a Volume with Calibrated Tubing

- **WebLinks**
  A dynamic resource that lets you link to hundreds of websites covering drug information and related pharmacology. WebLinks are regularly updated, with new ones added as they develop.

- **Appendices**
  Nine appendices include information on pregnancy categories, poison antidotes, gastric decontamination, controlled drugs, dialysis, medication administration, dosage calculation, and more.

http://evolve.elsevier.com/criticalcaredrug/

MOSBY'S CRITICAL CARE DRUG REFERENCE

MOSBY'S
CRITICAL CARE DRUG REFERENCE

Marianne Saunorus Baird, RN, MN
Clinical Nurse Specialist
Saint Joseph's Hospital
Atlanta, Georgia

With

Christopher Bridgers, PharmD
Clinical Pharmacist
Saint Joseph's Hospital
Atlanta, Georgia

Paul Schmidt, RPh, BCPS
Pharmaceutical Care Pharmacist
Saint Joseph's Hospital
Atlanta, Georgia

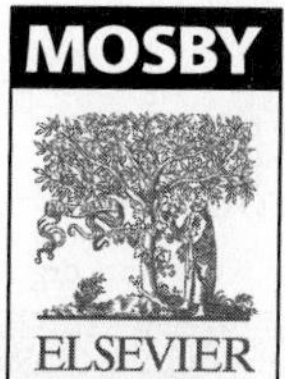

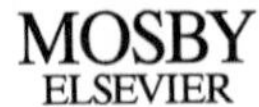

11830 Westline Industrial Drive
St. Louis, Missouri 63146

MOSBY'S CRITICAL CARE DRUG REFERENCE ISBN: 978-0-323-03167-7

Notice

Knowledge and best practice in this field are constantly changing. As new research and experience broaden our knowledge, changes in practice, treatment, and drug therapy may become necessary or appropriate. Readers are advised to check the most current information provided (i) on procedures featured or (ii) by the manufacturer of each product to be administered, to verify the recommended dose or formula, the method and duration of administration, and contraindications. It is the responsibility of the practitioner, relying on their own experience and knowledge of the patient, to make diagnoses, to determine dosages and the best treatment for each individual patient, and to take all appropriate safety precautions. To the fullest extent of the law, neither the Publisher nor the Author assumes any liability for any injury and/or damage to persons or property arising out of or related to any use of the material contained in this book.

The Publisher

Library of Congress Control Number: 2007928837

Acquisitions Editor: Lee Henderson
Developmental Editor: Rae Robertson
Publishing Services Manager: Melissa Lastarria
Senior Project Manager: Joy Moore
Design Direction: Karen O'Keefe Owens

Printed in the United States of America

Last digit is the print number: 9 8 7 6 5 4 3 2 1

I dedicate this book to my family, friends, and co-workers, who have provided me with the incredible support and understanding needed to undertake this project. Without the infusion of energy from those around me, I would not have been able to persevere.

PREFACE

Mosby's Critical Care Drug Reference is a comprehensive drug reference designed for all levels of clinicians in the critical care environment. Critical care physicians, advanced-practice nurses, and staff nurses alike require quick access to key information about medication management. Side effects or serious adverse effects must be readily identified, but they can easily be missed in the process of differential diagnosis. Numerous hospital admissions have resulted from mismanagement of medications by patients or inadvertent prescribing errors resulting from patients being attended by multiple, unrelated practitioners. As the acuity of hospitalized patients continues to increase and additional medications are introduced into the drug armamentarium, it is increasingly important to recognize interactions and serious adverse reactions, as well as the point at which it becomes necessary to adjust dosages because of organ dysfunction. This book includes specific information related to hemodynamics and the use of vasoactive and other medications for life support, and it provides expanded information about complications of many routinely used medications that may go unrecognized. Patients who are not critically ill can become critically ill because of medication mismanagement. This reference will assist in identifying possible medication-related symptoms to facilitate prompt and effective patient management in the critical care setting.

Experienced and novice critical care practitioners alike will benefit from the specialized information provided in this reference. The drugs are presented in such a way that the clinician can quickly discern key points for each medication. For additional information, the Critical Care Considerations section of each monograph provides details related to patient assessment, possible side effects, and serious reactions. Content about the effects of hemodialysis, peritoneal dialysis, and high-permeability hemodialysis is included as appropriate to assist with the timing of dosage adjustments. Information on the symptoms and management of overdose/toxicity—not readily available in other references—is provided, along with information related to the impact of renal replacement therapies.

The book is organized in two main parts. Part 1 contains drug monographs that include mechanism of action, available forms, indications and dosages, contraindications, interactions, diagnostic test effects, and side effects. A Critical Care Considerations section in each monograph includes information on administration and handling, precautions, serious adverse reactions, recognition/management of overdose and toxicity, and how the drug is affected by various methods of renal replacement therapy or dialysis. A special icon—⚑—is used to indicate High Alert drugs that pose increased danger to patients if used improperly. "Tall Man" lettering (e.g., methylPREDNISolone) is used where appropriate to differentiate drugs with look-alike/sound-alike names. Drugs in Part 1 are listed alphabetically by generic name. Convenient alphabetical thumb tabs assist in locating information quickly. The index in the back of the book assists in identifying drugs by trade name as well.

Many drugs not appearing in Part 1 of the book are included in the comparative drug tables located in Part 2. Drugs appearing in these tables are also cross-referenced in Part 1. The tables allow the clinician to quickly identify drugs in the same drug category.

An Evolve website is provided as an adjunct to the book and as a means to keep the content current. Twelve drug dosage calculators assist with dosage calculation, and regularly updated WebLinks link to hundreds of websites covering drug information and related pharmacology. Nine appendices offer additional information on pregnancy categories, poison antidotes, gastric decontamination, controlled drugs, dialysis, medication administration and calculation, and more.

Marianne Saunorus Baird, RN, MN

ACKNOWLEDGMENTS

I would like to acknowledge my devoted Elsevier editors, Lee Henderson and Rae Robertson, whose guidance has proven invaluable to me throughout this process. We learned much from each other. I would also like to acknowledge my co-writers, Paul Schmidt and Christopher Bridgers, for devoting countless hours to researching, writing, and reviewing the information.

CONTENTS

MOSBY'S
CRITICAL CARE DRUG REFERENCE

abacavir sulfate

See HIV Medications (p. 961)

abciximab

ab-siks'-ih-mab

Classes

Chemical: glycoprotein (GP) IIb/IIIa inhibitor

Therapeutic: antiplatelet agent

Pregnancy Category: C

Trade Names

Prescription: ReoPro

CLINICAL PHARMACOLOGY

Mechanism of Action

A GP IIb/IIIa receptor inhibitor that rapidly inhibits platelet aggregation by preventing the binding of fibrinogen to GP IIb/IIIa receptor sites on platelets. Therapeutic effect: Prevents closure of coronary arteries following percutaneous coronary intervention (PCI). Prevents acute cardiac ischemic complications.

PHARMACOKINETICS

Rapidly cleared from plasma. Initial-phase half-life is less than 10 min; second-phase half-life is 30 min. Platelet function generally returns within 48 hr.

AVAILABILITY

Injection: 2 mg/mL (5-mL vial).

INDICATIONS AND DOSAGE

PCI

IV Bolus

Adults: 0.25 mg/kg 10-60 min before angioplasty or atherectomy, then 12-hr IV infusion of 0.125 mcg/kg/min. Maximum: 10 mcg/min.

PCI (unstable angina)

IV Bolus

Adults: 0.25 mg/kg, followed by 18- to 24-hr infusion of 10 mcg/min, ending 1 hr after procedure.

CONTRAINDICATIONS

Active internal bleeding, arteriovenous malformation or aneurysm, cerebrovascular accident (CVA) with residual neurologic defect, history of CVA (within the past 2 yr), or oral anticoagulant use within the past 7 days unless prothrombin time is less than 1.2 times control, history of vasculitis, hypersensitivity to murine proteins, intracranial neoplasm, prior IV dextran use before or during percutaneous transluminal coronary angioplasty (PTCA), recent surgery or trauma (within the past 6 weeks), recent GI or GU bleeding (within the past 6 weeks or less), thrombocytopenia (less than 100,000 cells/microliters), and severe uncontrolled hypertension.

INTERACTIONS

Drug: **Anticoagulants, including heparin:** May increase risk of hemorrhage. **Platelet aggregation inhibitors (such as aspirin, dextran):** May increase risk of bleeding. **Thrombolytic agents (such as alteplase, reteplase, tenecteplase):** May increase risk of bleeding. Herbal: None known. Food: None known.

DIAGNOSTIC TEST EFFECTS

Increases activated clotting time (ACT), aPTT, and prothrombin time. Decreases platelet count.

IV INCOMPATIBILITIES

Administer in separate line; no other medication should be added to infusion solution.

SIDE-EFFECTS

Frequent: Nausea (14%), hypotension (14%), minor bleeding (4%-17%), back pain (18%). Occasional: Vomiting (7%), thrombocytopenia (<100,000 cells/mm^3) (2.5%-6%), major bleeding (1.1%-14%). Rare (3%): Confusion, dizziness, pain, peripheral edema, urinary tract infection

CRITICAL CARE CONSIDERATIONS

ADMINISTRATION/HANDLING

IV ALERT

- **Storage:** Store vials in refrigerator.
- **Preparation:** Solution normally appears clear and colorless. Do not shake. Discard any unused portion or any preparation that contains opaque particles.
- **Filtering:** For bolus injection and continuous infusion, use a sterile, nonpyrogenic, low-protein-binding 0.2- or 0.22-micron filter. The continuous infusion may be filtered either during drug preparation or at the time of administration.
- **Dilution:** Withdraw the desired dose and dilute in 250 mL of 0.9% NaCl or D_5W (for example, 10 mg in 250 mL equals a concentration of 40 mcg/mL).
- **Bolus dose:** The bolus dose may be given undiluted.
- **Separate IV:** Give in separate IV line; do not add other medications to infusion.

PRECAUTIONS

HEALTH-RELATED

- **Bleeding risk:** Use abciximab cautiously in patients who have had a PTCA within 12 hr of the onset of symptoms of acute MI, a prolonged PTCA (greater than 70 min), a failed PTCA, or are receiving aspirin, heparin, or thrombolytics because they are at increased risk for bleeding.

AGE-RELATED

- **Children:** Safety and efficacy of abciximab have not been established in children.
- **Elderly:** There is an increased risk of bleeding; use with caution.

PREGNANCY/LACTATION-RELATED

- Pregnancy category C; not recommended for use during pregnancy unless absolutely necessary; excretion into breast milk unknown; use caution in nursing mothers.

MONITORING

- **Baseline assessment:** Assess for risk of bleeding, check the insertion site and the distal pulse of the affected limb while the femoral artery sheath is in place.
- **Baseline lab work:** CBC, platelet count, prothrombin time, ACT, and aPTT. Consider type and screen in case of need for blood transfusion.
- **Ongoing lab work:** Monitor heparin anticoagulation (aPTT or ACT) and prothrombin time closely. Check platelet count and prothrombin time 2 to 4 hr after bolus dose, and 24 hr after treatment or before discharge, whichever is first.
- **Neurologic signs:** Monitor for changes in level of consciousness or behavior; intracranial hemorrhage may occur. Stop the drug immediately for unexpected neurological changes.
- **Heparin therapy:** Discontinue heparin 4 hr before the arterial sheath is removed. Stop abciximab and heparin infusion if serious bleeding uncontrolled by pressure occurs.
- **Femoral artery sheath in place:** Maintain complete bed rest with head of bed elevated at 30 degrees. Maintain affected limb in straight position.
- **Following sheath removal:** Apply femoral pressure for 30 min, either manually or mechanically, then apply a pressure dressing. If arterial closure device is not used, maintain bed rest for 6 to 8 hr after the sheath is removed or the drug is discontinued, whichever is later. Check site and distal pulse routinely for 6 hr after the femoral artery sheath has been removed.
- **Bleeding precautions:** Minimize blood draws, catheter placements, intubations, and numerous injections. Avoid IM injections and venipunctures. Avoid using indwelling urinary catheters and nasogastric tubes. Handle patients carefully and as infrequently as possible to prevent bleeding. Gently remove dressings and tape.
- **Bleeding:** Assess skin for ecchymosis and petechiae. Assess for GI, GU, and retroperitoneal bleeding, and for bleeding at all puncture sites. Determine the amount of female patients' menstrual discharge and monitor for any increase. Assess urine for hematuria. Monitor for any new or expanding hematomas.
- **Hemorrhage:** Assess for hypotension, tachycardia, abdominal or back pain, and severe headache.
- **Patient education:** Instruct patients to use an electric razor and a soft toothbrush to prevent bleeding. Instruct patients to report promptly black or red stool, coffee-ground emesis, red or dark urine, or red-speckled mucus from cough.

SERIOUS ADVERSE REACTIONS

- **Bleeding:** Major bleeding complications including intracranial hemorrhage may occur. If complications occur, stop the infusion immediately. Perform labwork to assess platelet count, prothrombin time, INR (international normalized ratio), and aPTT. May require transfusion of packed red blood cells.
- **Hypersensitivity reaction:** May occur, including analphylaxis. Manage with epinephrine, dopamine, theophyllines (aminophylline), antihistamines (diphenhydramine/Benadryl), and corticosteroids (hydrocortisone).
- **Cardiac:** Atrial fibrillation or flutter, bradycardia, ventricular tachycardia, complete atrioventricular block occur occasionally; pulmonary edema.

OVERDOSE/TOXICITY

- **Thrombocytopenia:** May be related to abciximab or additive effects of all medications which may lower platelet count, including heparin, sulfonamides, quinine, quinidine, thiazides, and phenytoin. Evaluate if medication interaction is present. Platelet transfusion may be needed.
- **Hypotension:** Vasopressors, including dopamine or norepinephrine, may be needed. If severe and patient nears arrest, manage

according to Advanced Cardiac Life Support guidelines.
- **GI decontamination:** No specific recommendations.

ANTIDOTE/DIALYSIS
- **Antidote:** No specific recommendations.
- **Dialysis:** Abciximab is unlikely to be removed using hemodialysis or peritoneal dialysis. No data are available on removal using high-permeability hemodialysis.

acarbose 

ay'-car-bose

Classes
Chemical: α-amylase inhibitor, α-glucosidase inhibitor
Therapeutic: antidiabetic, hypoglycemic

Pregnancy Category: B

Trade Names
Prescription: Glucobay ♣, Precose

Do not confuse Precose with PreCare.

CLINICAL PHARMACOLOGY
Mechanism of Action
An α-glucosidase inhibitor that inhibits breakdown of complex carbohydrates. This delays glucose absorption and results in a smaller rise in blood glucose concentration after meals. **Therapeutic Effect:** Lowers postprandial hyperglycemia.

PHARMACOKINETICS
Low absorption (less than 2%) within the GI tract. Extensive metabolism in the intestinal wall. Degraded in the intestine by bacterial and digestive enzymes. Excreted in feces and urine. **Half-life:** 2 hr.

AVAILABILITY
Tablets: 25 mg, 50 mg, 100 mg.

INDICATIONS AND DOSAGE
Diabetes mellitus
PO
Adults, Elderly: Initially, 25 mg three times per day with first bite of each main meal. May increase at 4- to 8-wk intervals. Maximum: For patients weighing more than 60 kg, 100 mg three times per day; for patients weighing 60 kg or less, 50 mg three times per day.

CONTRAINDICATIONS
Chronic intestinal diseases associated with marked disorders of digestion or absorption, cirrhosis, colonic ulceration, conditions that may deteriorate as a result of increased gas formation in the intestine, diabetic ketoacidosis, hypersensitivity to acarbose, inflammatory bowel disease, partial intestinal obstruction, or predisposition to intestinal obstruction.

INTERACTIONS
Drug: Beta-blockers: May increase the risk of hypoglycemia, hyperglycemia, or hypertension. **Digestive enzymes, intestinal absorbents (such as charcoal):** Reduces effects of acarbose. **Digoxin:** Acarbose decreases bioavailability of digoxin and lowers digoxin levels. **Fluoroquinolones:** May cause changes in blood glucose and increase the risk of hypoglycemia or hyperglycemia. **Sulfonylureas:** May increase the risk of hypoglycemia. **Warfarin:** May increase the risk of bleeding. **Herbal: Bitter melon, eucalyptus, fenugreek, ginseng, guar gum, St. John's wort:** May increase the risk of hypoglycemia. **Glucosamine, licorice:** May decrease the effectiveness of acarbose. **Food:** None known.

DIAGNOSTIC TEST EFFECTS
May increase AST (SGOT) and ALT (SGPT) levels (14%).

SIDE-EFFECTS
Side effects diminish in frequency and intensity over time. **Frequent:** Transient GI disturbances: flatulence (77%), diarrhea (33%), abdominal pain (21%)

CRITICAL CARE CONSIDERATIONS

ADMINISTRATION/HANDLING
PO ALERT
- Give acarbose with the first bite of each main meal.

PRECAUTIONS
HEALTH-RELATED
- Use acarbose cautiously in patients with fever or infection and those post-operative or post-trauma because the stress response induced by these conditions may cause loss of glycemic control.

AGE-RELATED
- **Children:** Safety and efficacy of acarbose have not been established in children.
- **Elderly:** Hypoglycemia may be difficult to recognize in the elderly. Age-related renal impairment may increase sensitivity to the glucose-lowering effect of acarbose.

PREGNANCY/LACTATION-RELATED

- Pregnancy category B: not recommended for use during pregnancy; hyperglycemia during pregnancy may require insulin therapy; excreted into breast milk in rats; no human data are available.

MONITORING

- **Baseline assessment:** Height, weight; assess diet and exercise patterns.
- **Baseline labwork:** Biochemical profile including blood glucose and liver function studies, hemoglobin A_{1C}.
- **Hyperglycemia management:** Acarbose may be discontinued if insulin infusion is required to control hyperglycemia. Drug may be resumed once glucose is controlled, vital signs stabilize, and patient is eating. Insulin infusion is recommended to manage hyperglycemia during critical illness.
- **Therapeutic effects:** Monitor for decreased blood glucose.
- **Hypoglycemia:** Monitor for anxiety, cool or clammy skin, diplopia, dizziness, headache, hunger, numbness, tachycardia, and tremors.
- **Hyperglycemia:** Monitor for deep rapid breathing, poor vision, fatigue, nausea, polydipsia, polyphagia, polyuria, and vomiting.
- **Changing glucose requirements:** Manage conditions that alter glucose requirements, including fever, increased activity or stress, or a surgical procedure.
- **Patient education:** Advise patients not to skip or delay meals. Instruct to consult a physician when glucose demands are altered (such as with fever, heavy physical activity, infection, stress, trauma). Encourage patients to avoid alcoholic beverages, and alert them that consistent carbohydrate diet, exercise, good personal hygiene (including foot care), not smoking, and weight control are essential parts of therapy.

SERIOUS ADVERSE REACTIONS

- Less than 1% severe GI distress.

OVERDOSE/TOXICITY

- **Hypoglycemia:** Will not cause hypoglycemia unless combined with other antidiabetic agents that lower blood glucose: insulin, sulfonylureas, meglitinides, and biguanides.
- **GI symptoms:** May cause GI symptoms similar to lactose intolerance, including bloating and flatulence.
- **GI decontamination:** No specific recommendations.

ANTIDOTE/DIALYSIS

- **Antidote:** No specific recommendations.
- **Dialysis:** No data are available on removal of acarbose using hemodialysis, high-permeability hemodialysis, or peritoneal dialysis.

acebutolol hydrochloride ⚑

See Beta-Adrenergic Blockers (p. 943)

acetaminophen

a-seat-a-mee'-noe-fen

Classes

Chemical: para-aminophenol derivative
Therapeutic: antipyretic, nonnarcotic analgesic

Pregnancy Category: B

Trade Names

Over the Counter: Abenol ♣, Acephen, Apacet, Arthritis Pain Formula, Aspirin Free Pain Relief, Feverall, Genapap, Liquiprin, Neopap, Panadol, Tapanol Tempra, Tempra ♣, Tylenol

Combinations

Prescription: With butalbital (Phrenilin); with butalbital and caffeine (Fioricet, Esgic, Isocet); with butalbital, caffeine, and codeine (Amaphen, Fioricet w/codeine); with codeine (Tylenol, Phenaphen No. 2, 3, 4); with dichloralphenazone and isometheptene (Midrin, Midchlor); with hydrocodone (Vicodin, Lorcet, Lortab); with oxycodone (Percocet, Roxicet, Tylox); with pentazocine (Talacen); with propoxyphene (Wygesic, Darvocet-N).
Over the Counter: With pamabrom + pyrilamine (Midol PMS, Pamprin); with antihistamine and decongestant (Actifed Plus, Drixoral Cold & Flu, Benadryl Sinus, Sine-Off, Sinarest); with decongestant, antihistamine, dextromethorphan (Nyquil).

Do not confuse with Fiorinal, Hycodan, Indocin, Percodan, or Tuinal.

CLINICAL PHARMACOLOGY

Mechanism of Action

A central analgesic for which the exact mechanism is unknown but appears to inhibit prostaglandin synthesis in the CNS and, to a lesser extent, block pain impulses through peripheral action. Acetaminophen acts centrally on the hypothalamic heat-regulating center, producing peripheral vasodilation (heat loss, skin erythema, sweating). **Therapeutic Effect:** Results in antipyresis. Produces analgesic effect. Results in antipyresis.

PHARMACOKINETICS

Route	Onset	Peak	Duration
PO	15-30 min	1-2 hr	4-6 hr

Rapidly, completely absorbed from the GI tract; rectal absorption variable (30%-40%). Protein binding: 10%-30%, increasing up to 50% with overdose. Widely distributed to most body tissues. Metabolized in liver; excreted in urine. Removed by hemodialysis. **Half-life:** 2-4 hr (half-life is increased in those with liver disease, elderly, neonates; decreased in children).

AVAILABILITY

Caplet (Genapap, Tylenol): 500 mg.
Caplet, extended release (Mapap, Tylenol Arthritis Pain): 650 mg.
Capsule (Mapap): 500 mg.
Elixir: 160 mg/5 mL.
Liquid, oral (Tylenol Extra Strength): 500 mg/15 mL.
Solution, oral drops (Genapap Infant): 80 mg/0.8 mL.
Suppository, rectal (Feverall): 80 mg; **Acephen, Feverall:** 120 mg, 325 mg, 650 mg.
Tablet (Genapap, Mapap, Tylenol): 325 mg, 500 mg.
Tablet, chewable (Genapap, Mapap, Tylenol): 80 mg.

INDICATIONS AND DOSAGE

Analgesia and antipyresis

PO

Adults, Elderly: 325-650 mg every 4-6 hr or 1 g 3-4 times/day. Maximum: 4 g/day. **Children under 12 yr:** 10-15 mg/kg/dose every 4-6 hr as needed. Maximum: 5 doses/24 hr or 2.6 g/24 hr. **Neonates:** 10-15 mg/kg/dose every 6-8 hr as needed.

Rectal

Adults: 650 mg every 4-6 hr. Maximum: six doses/24 hr. **Children 6-11 yr:** 325 mg every 4-6 hr as needed. **Neonates:** 10-15 mg/kg/dose every 6-8 hr as needed.

Dosage in renal impairment

Creatinine Clearance	Frequency
10-50 mL/min	Every 6 hr
Less than 10 mL/min	Every 8 hr

CONTRAINDICATIONS

Hypersensitivity to acetominophen, liver disease, or viral hepatitis, all of which increase the risk of hepatotoxicity.

INTERACTIONS

Drug: Alcohol (chronic use), hepatotoxic medications (e.g., phenytoin), liver enzyme inducers (e.g., cimetidine): May increase risk of hepatotoxicity with prolonged high dose or single toxic dose. **Warfarin:** May increase the risk of bleeding with regular use. **Herbal: St. John's wort:** May decrease acetominophen levels. **Food:** None known.

DIAGNOSTIC TEST EFFECTS

May increase serum bilirubin, prothrombin time (may indicate hepatotoxicity), AST (SGOT), and ALT (SGPT). Therapeutic serum level: 10-30 mcg/mL; toxic serum level: greater than 200 mcg/mL at 4 hr or 50 mcg/mL at 12 hr after ingestion.

SIDE-EFFECTS

Rare: Hypersensitivity reaction.

CRITICAL CARE CONSIDERATIONS

ADMINISTRATION/HANDLING

DOSING ALERT

- Children may receive repeat doses four to five times per day to a maximum of five doses in 24 hr.

PO ALERT

- Give acetaminophen without regard to meals.
- Tablets may be crushed.

RECTAL ALERT

- Moisten suppository with cold water before inserting high into the rectum.

PRECAUTIONS

HEALTH-RELATED

- Use cautiously in patients with G6PD deficiency or sensitivity to acetaminophen.
- **Liver disease:** Consider using another medication for control of fever or pain.
- **Slow respirations:** If respirations are 12/min or lower (20/min or lower in children), withhold the medication and contact the physician.
- **Fever lasting more than 3 days:** Monitor for severe or recurrent pain or high, continuous fever, which may indicate a serious illness.

AGE-RELATED

- **Children:** Use acetaminophen cautiously in children under 2 yr; oral use for more than 5 days in children may prompt toxicity. Children may repeat doses a maximum of five doses in 24 hr.
- **Elderly:** Use cautiously for more than 10 days to help minimize the chance of toxicity; adults follow similar dosage guidelines.

PREGNANCY/LACTATION-RELATED

- Pregnancy category B; did not cause fetal harm in animal studies; low concentrations in breast milk (1%-2% of maternal dose); compatible with breast-feeding.

MONITORING

- **Baseline assessment:** Obtain baseline vital signs to assess for fever. Assess onset, type, location, and duration of pain before acetaminophen is given for analgesia.
- **Lab work:** Biochemical profile including liver function (AST [SGOT], ALT [SGPT], alkaline phosphatase, bilirubin) tests.
- **Dose regularly to control pain:** The effect of the medication is reduced if full pain response recurs before the next dose.
- **Therapeutic effect:** Assess for relief of pain or fever.
- **Suspected overdose:** Monitor serum levels and assess for end organ damage (serum electrolytes, liver enzymes, bilirubin, prothrombin time, coagulation studies, CBC, protein, amylase).
- **Serum levels:** Therapeutic level is 10 to 30 mcg/mL. Toxic level is greater than 200 mcg/mL.

SERIOUS ADVERSE REACTIONS

- **Cardiac:** Hepatic damage may cause cardiac complications including dysrhythmias, ischemia, and injury (chest pain, pressure, ST depression or elevation, T wave inversion, nausea, and vomiting).
- **Respiratory:** Bronchospasms (wheezing with difficulty breathing) and tachypnea may occur as a side effect to the antidote acetylcysteine.
- **Neurologic:** Coma and seizures.
- **Renal:** Acute tubular necrosis with renal failure is seen in some cases but often resolves. Renal failure may be seen with acute liver failure.
- **Associated findings:** Hypophosphatemia, metabolic acidosis, hypothermia, hypoglycemia, thrombocytopenia, and hemorrhagic pancreatitis.

OVERDOSE/TOXICITY

- **Very common overdose:** One of the most commonly seen overdoses and the leading cause of acute liver failure; may result in permanent liver damage.
- **Toxicity:** Acetaminophen (paracetamol) toxicity is the primary serious reaction.
- **Early signs and symptoms of acetaminophen toxicity:** Anorexia, nausea, diaphoresis, and generalized weakness within the first 12 to 24 hr.
- **Acute liver failure–related hepatic encephalopathy:** Considered the hallmark sign of liver failure; begins with slurred speech, slight tremor, progressive somnolence, or increasing drowsiness; progressing to inappropriate behavior, marked confusion, and, finally, coma, with no response to painful stimuli.
- **Hepatocellular necrosis:** Later sign of toxicity with vomiting, right upper quadrant pain, elevated liver function tests 24-36 hr after ingestion
- **Cardiac and respiratory monitoring:** Monitor and support the cardiac and respiratory systems if overdose is suspected; use supplemental oxygen, consider intubation and mechanical ventilation if acute respiratory failure ensues, monitor serial 12-lead ECGs, and continuously monitor ECG for bradycardia or ventricular dysrhythmias.
- **GI decontamination:** Gastric lavage and ipecac are used only if less than 1 hr has elapsed. Administration of activated charcoal and N-acetylcysteine (NAC) should not be delayed to give ipecac and perform lavage.

ANTIDOTE/DIALYSIS

- **Antidote to acetaminophen toxicity:** N-AC.
- **Acetylcysteine and charcoal:** A combination of activated charcoal and N-acetylcysteine (Mucomyst, NAC) administered orally or via a gastric tube.
- **Dialysis:** Acetaminophen is removed by hemodialysis, is likely to be removed by high-permeability hemodialysis, and is not removed by peritoneal dialysis. Acetaminophen is cleared more than 90% hepatic and only 1%-4% renal.

*acetaZOLAMIDE

a-seat-a-zole'-a-mide

Classes

Chemical: carbonic anhydrase inhibitor, sulfonamide derivative

Therapeutic: anticonvulsant, antiglaucoma agent, diuretic

Pregnancy Category: C

Trade Names

Prescription: Dazamide, Diamox, Diamox Sequels

Do not confuse with *acetoHEXAMIDE.

CLINICAL PHARMACOLOGY

Mechanism of Action

A carbonic anhydrase inhibitor that reduces formation of hydrogen and bicarbonate ions from carbon dioxide and water by inhibiting, in proximal renal tubule, the enzyme carbonic anhydrase, thereby promoting renal excretion of sodium, potassium, bicarbonate, and water. Ocular: Reduces rate of aqueous humor formation, lowers intraocular pressure. **Therapeutic Effect:** Produces anticonvulsant activity.

PHARMACOKINETICS

Rapidly absorbed. Protein binding: 70%-90%. Widely distributed throughout body tissues including erythrocytes, kidneys, and blood-brain barrier. Not metabolized. Excreted unchanged in urine. Removed by hemodialysis. **Half-life:** 4-8 hr.

AVAILABILITY

Capsules, sustained release: 500 mg (Diamox Sequels).
Powder for reconstitution: 500 mg.
Tablets: 125 mg, 250 mg (Diamox).

INDICATIONS AND DOSAGE

Acute angle-closure glaucoma (open angle)

PO

Adults: 250 mg every 4 hr. Extended release 500 mg every 12 hr given in morning and evening.

Primary open-angle glaucoma

PO

Adults: 250 mg four times daily, maximum dose 1 g daily. Extended release 500 mg every 12 hr.

IV

Adults: 250 mg every 4 hr.

PO

Children: 8-30 mg/kg/day or 300-900 mg/m^2/daily divided in every-8-hr doses.

IV

Children: 20-40 mg/kg/day divided into every-6-hr doses (maximum 1 g/day).

Secondary glaucoma

PO

Adults: Extended release 500 mg PO every 12 hr.

Edema

IV

Adults: 250-375 mg (5 mg/kg) once daily given in the morning. Greater diuretic action may be attained by skipping a day of treatment rather than increasing dosage. Failure to produce diuresis may result from overdose or too frequent administration. **Children:** 5 mg/kg or 150 mg/m^2 once daily.

Epilepsy

PO

Adults: 8-30 mg/kg/day; optimum dose 375-1000 mg daily. **Children:** 8-30 mg/kg/day or 300-900 mg/m^2/day divided into every-6-8-hr doses (maximum 1 g daily).

Acute mountain sickness (treatment and prophylaxis)

PO

Adults: 1000 mg/day in divided doses. If possible, begin 24-48 hr before ascent; continue at least 48 hr at high altitude. **Adults:** Extended release: 500-1000 mg once daily.

Dosage in renal impairment

Creatinine Clearance	Dosage Interval
10-50 mL/min	Every 12 hr
Less than 10 mL/min	Avoid use

OFF-LABEL USES

Urine alkalinization, respiratory stimulant in chronic obstructive pulmonary disease.

CONTRAINDICATIONS

Severe renal disease, adrenal insufficiency, hypochloremic acidosis, hypersensitivity to *acetaZOLAMIDE or to any component of the formulation, severe hepatic disease, and hyponatremia/hypokalemia.

INTERACTIONS

Drug: Amphetamines: May increase effects and toxicity of amphetamines. ***CycloSPORINE:** May increase *cycloSPORINE trough concentrations and possible neprotoxicity and neurotoxicity. **Lithium:** May increase or decrease lithium levels. **Phenytoin:** May increase serum concentrations of phenytoin. **Quinidine:** May decrease urinary excretion of quinidine and increase

possibility of quinidine toxicity. **Salicylates:** May increase risk of *acetaZOLAMIDE accumulation and toxicity, including CNS depression and metabolic acidosis; may also cause salicylate toxicity. **Herbal:** None known. **Food:** None known.

DIAGNOSTIC TEST EFFECTS

May increase ammonia, bilirubin, glucose, chloride, uric acid, calcium. May decrease bicarbonate, potassium.

IV INCOMPATIBILITIES

No drug incompatibilities reported.

IV COMPATIBILITIES

Cimetidine (Tagament), procaine, ranitidine (Zantac), dextran.

SIDE-EFFECTS

Frequent: Unusual tiredness/weakness, diarrhea, increased urination quantity and or frequency, decreased appetite/weight, altered taste (metallic), nausea, vomiting, numbness in extremities, lips, mouth. **Occasional:** Depression, drowsiness. **Rare:** Headache, photosensitivity, confusion, tinnitus, severe muscle weakness, loss of taste.

CRITICAL CARE CONSIDERATIONS

ADMINISTRATION/HANDLING

IV ALERT

- **IV push dilution:** Dilute 500 mg in at least 5 mL D_5W. Minimum volume is 5 mL D_5W. Maximum concentration is 100 mg/mL.
- **IV push administration:** 100-500 mg/min. Maximum rate is 500 mg/min.
- **IV infusion dilution:** Reconstitute with at least 5 mL of sterile water to provide a solution containing no more than 100 mg/mL. Dilute further in at least 50 mL of either D_5W or 0.9% NaCl.
- **IV administration:** 4-8 hr for IV infusions.
- **Stability:** 5 days at room temperature and 44 days under refrigeration. Use within 24 hr of dilution.

PO ALERT

- Give *acetaZOLAMIDE without regard to food.
- Do not crush, chew, or swallow contents of long-acting capsules.

IM ALERT

- IM injection is not recommended because of pain secondary to the alkaline pH.

PRECAUTIONS

HEALTH-RELATED

- Use *acetaZOLAMIDE cautiously in patients with a history of hypercalcemia, diabetes mellitus, gout, digitalized patients, respiratory disease including pulmonary edema, and obstructive pulmonary disease and in those with sensitivity to sulfonamides.

AGE-RELATED

- **Children:** No age-related precautions have been noted.
- **Elderly:** Age-related renal impairment may prompt dosage reduction.

PREGNANCY/LACTATION-RELATED

- Pregnancy category C; premature delivery and congenital anomalies in humans; teratogenic (defects of the limbs) in mice, rats, hamsters, and rabbits; not recommended for nursing mothers.

MONITORING

- **Baseline assessment with glaucoma:** Assess affected pupil for dilation, response to light.
- **Baseline assessment with epilepsy:** Obtain history of seizure disorder—length, intensity, duration of seizure, presence of aura, LOC.
- **Baseline assessment with metabolic alkalosis:** Assess arterial blood gases for pH, HCO_3, and CO_2, and for cause of metabolic alkalosis.
- **Baseline assessment for edema/congestive heart failure:** Assess for pattern of weight gain/edema. Some edema may be drug induced.
- **Baseline lab work:** CBC, platelet count; arterial blood gas analysis if using to correct metabolic alkalosis; urine pH if used for urinary alkalinization when acidic medications such as phenobarbital, salicylates, or lithium are being taken.
- **Ongoing lab work:** Potassium, serum bicarbonate, serum electrolytes, and CBC with differential; blood glucose in diabetic patients. *AcetaZOLAMIDE may cause hyperglycemia. Urine pH in patients receiving acidic medications.
- **Possible acidosis:** Monitor for headache, lethargy progressing to drowsiness, CNS depression, Kussmaul respirations indicative of acidosis.
- **ECG monitoring for hypokalemia-induced dysrhythmias:** Assess for ventricular dysrhythmias, especially in patients receiving steroids or digitalis.

- **Hyperglycemia:** Monitor blood glucose in diabetics receiving insulin or oral hypoglycemic agents because *acetaZOLAMIDE may interfere with these drugs.
- **Glaucoma:** Monitor for reduction in intraocular pressure if used for glaucoma.
- **Epilepsy:** Assess for a decrease in the frequency or intensity of seizures.
- **Patient education:** Instruct patients to report any presence of tingling or tremor in hands or feet, unusual bleeding/bruising, unexplained fever, sore throat, or flank pain. *AcetaZOLAMIDE may cause drowsiness. Warn patients to avoid performing tasks that require mental alertness or motor skills until response to the drug is known.

SERIOUS ADVERSE REACTIONS

- **Metabolic acidosis:** Long-term therapy may result in acidotic state.
- **Bone marrow depression:** Aplastic anemia, thrombocytopenia, thrombocytopenic purpura, leukopenia, agranulocytosis, and hemolytic anemia.
- **Hypersensitivity:** Reactions include Stevens–Johnson syndrome.

OVERDOSE/TOXICITY

- **Nephrotoxicity/hepatotoxicity:** Occurs occasionally; manifested as dark urine/stools, pain in lower back, jaundice, dysuria, crystalluria, and renal colic/calculi.
- **Symptoms:** Hypokalemia-induced lethal cardiac dysrhythmias; metabolic acidosis, which may potentiate salicylate toxicity (anorexia, tachypnea, lethargy, coma, death); and hyponatremia (muscle weakness, confusion, paresthesias).
- **Management:** Supportive care for allergic/sensitivity reaction including endotracheal intubation, mechanical ventilation, support of blood pressure with IV fluids and vasopressors, and support of other failing organs if needed.
- **GI decontamination:** No specific recommendations.

ANTIDOTE/DIALYSIS

- **Antidote:** No recommendations.
- **Dialysis:** *AcetaZOLAMIDE is removed by hemodialysis. No definitive data is available on removal using high-permeability hemodialysis or peritoneal dialysis.

*acetoHEXAMIDE

See Antidiabetics (p. 911)

acetylcysteine

a-se-teel-sis'-tay-een

Classes

Chemical: amino acid, L-cysteine
Therapeutic: antidote, acetaminophen, mucolytic

Pregnancy Category: B

Trade Names

Prescription: Acetadote, Mucomyst, Parvolex ♣

Do not confuse acetylcysteine with acetylcholine.

CLINICAL PHARMACOLOGY

Mechanism of Action

An intratracheal respiratory inhalant that splits the linkage of mucoproteins, reducing the viscosity of pulmonary secretions. Therapeutic Effect: Facilitates the removal of pulmonary secretions by coughing, postural drainage, and mechanical means. Protects against acetaminophen overdose–induced hepatotoxicity.

PHARMACOKINETICS

Protein binding: 83% (injection). Rapidly and extensively metabolized in liver. Deacetylated by the liver to cysteine and subsequently metabolized. Excreted in urine. Half-life: 5.6 hr (injection).

AVAILABILITY

Injection (Acedote): 20% (200 mg/mL).
Inhalation Solution (Mucomyst): 10% (100 mg/mL), 20% (200 mg/mL).

INDICATIONS AND DOSAGE

Adjunctive treatment of viscid mucus secretions from chronic bronchopulmonary disease and for pulmonary complications of cystic fibrosis

Nebulization

Alert: Bronchodilators should be given 15 min before acetylcysteine. **Adults, Elderly: Children:** 3-5 mL (20% solution) three to four times per day or 6-10 mL (10% solution) three to four times per day. Range: 1-10 mL (20% solution) every 2-6 hr or 2-20 mL (10% solution) every 2-6 hr. **Infants:** 1-2 mL (20%) or 2-4 mL (10%) three to four times per day.

Treatment of viscid mucus secretions in patients with a tracheostomy

Intratracheal

Adults, Children: 1-2 mL of 10% or 20% solution instilled into tracheostomy every 1-4 hr.

A

Acetaminophen overdose
PO (Oral solution 5%)
Adults, Elderly, Children: Loading dose of 140 mg/kg, followed in 4 hr by maintenance dose of 70 mg/kg every 4 hr for 17 additional doses (unless acetaminophen assay reveals nontoxic level). Repeat dose if emesis occurs within 1 hr of administration. Continue until all doses are given, even if acetaminophen plasma level drops below toxic range.
IV
Adults, Elderly, Children: 150 mg/kg in 200 mL D_5W infused over 60 min, then 50 mg/kg in 500 mL D_5W infused over 4 hr, then 100 mg/kg in 1000 mL D_5W infused over 16 hr. See administration and handling.
Prevention of renal damage from dyes used during certain diagnostic tests
PO (Oral solution 5%)
Adults, Elderly: 600 mg twice per day for four doses starting the day before the procedure.

OFF-LABEL USES

Prevention of renal damage from dyes given during certain diagnostic tests (such as CT scans) or therapeutic procedures (e.g., angioplasty).

CONTRAINDICATIONS

Hypersensitivity to acetylcysteine.

INTERACTIONS

Drug: **Carbamazepine:** May increase the risk of subtherapeutic carbamazepine levels. **Nitroglycerin:** May enhance hypotension and nitroglycerin-induced headache. Herbal: None known. Food: None known.

DIAGNOSTIC TEST EFFECTS

None known.

SIDE-EFFECTS

Frequent: **Inhalation:** Stickiness on face, transient unpleasant odor. Occasional: **Inhalation:** Increased bronchial secretions, throat irritation, nausea, vomiting, rhinorrhea. Rare: **Inhalation:** Rash **Oral:** Facial edema, bronchospasm, wheezing

CRITICAL CARE CONSIDERATIONS

ADMINISTRATION/HANDLING

GENERAL ALERT

- **Discoloration:** Light purple discoloration of solution in opened bottles sometimes occurs but does not change the safety or the effectiveness of acetylcysteine.

PO ALERT

- **Oral solution:** To create the oral solution, dilute 20% solution with water or soft drink to create a 5% concentration. Use within 1 hr.
- Acetylcysteine solution has a foul odor similar to rotten eggs.
- If patients experience persistent vomiting with administration, inserting a nasojejunal tube may be done to administer the medication.

IV ALERT

- **Antidote and preventive infusions:** Give three infusions of different strengths: first dose (150 mg/kg) in 200 mL D_5W and infused over 60 min; second dose (50 mg/kg) in 500 mL D_5W and infused over 4 hr; third dose (100 mg/kg) in 1000 mL D_5W and infused over 16 hr.

INHALATION ALERT

- May administer either undiluted or diluted with 0.9% NaCl.
- When administering the solution by nebulizer, avoid using equipment that contains copper, iron, or rubber; the drug will react with these materials on contact.

PRECAUTIONS

HEALTH-RELATED

- Use acetylcysteine cautiously in patients with bronchial asthma and in debilitated patients with severe respiratory insufficiency.
- If bronchospasm progresses when treating an asthmatic patient, the medication should be discontinued immediately.

AGE-RELATED

- **Elderly:** Use cautiously in the elderly.

PREGNANCY/LACTATION-RELATED

- Pregnancy category B; did not cause fetal harm in animal studies; no well-controlled studies in breast-feeding women.

MONITORING

- **Baseline assessment:** Assess respiratory rate, depth, and rhythm before and during treatment to determine baseline respiratory status if drug is used as a mucolytic.
- **Bronchospasms:** If bronchospasm occurs, discontinue treatment. Administer a bronchodilator as needed.
- **Secretions:** Check the color, consistency, and amount of sputum. Increased amount

of liquified bronchial secretions may occur following treatment and must be cleared to maintain patent airway.
- **Hydration:** Provide PO or IV fluids to maintain adequate hydration.
- **Pulmonary hygiene:** Assist patients with coughing and deep-breathing techniques.
- **Use as an antidote-preventive:** If used as an antidote (such as for acetaminophen overdose and to counteract the nephrotoxic effects of radiographic contrast media), monitor for signs and symptoms associated with anticipated end-organ damage for the overdose drug or contrast media.
- **Patient education:** Inform patients that a disagreeable odor may emanate from the solution during initial administration, but that it disappears quickly.

SERIOUS ADVERSE REACTIONS

- Large doses may produce severe nausea and vomiting.
- Rash, urticaria, and pruritis may occur following initial injection within the first 2 hr, especially if infusion was given at a rapid rate.

OVERDOSE/TOXICITY

- **Respiratory:** Unusual breathing difficulties, respiratory failure.
- **Neurologic:** Somnolence, ataxia, seizures.
- **IV infusion:** If patients experience anaphylaxis while receiving infusion over 15 min for use as an antidote, slow the rate of infusion to finish over 1 hr.
- **Manage symptoms:** Symptoms should be managed according to standard management protocols for each symptom.
- **GI decontamination:** No specific recommendations.

ANTIDOTE/DIALYSIS

- **Antidote:** Although acetylcysteine is often used as an antidote, there is no clear "antidote for the antidote."
- **Dialysis:** No data are available on removal of acetylcysteine by hemodialysis, high-permeability hemodialysis, or peritoneal dialysis.

acyclovir

ay-sye'-kloe-veer

Classes

Chemical: acyclic purine nucleoside analog
Therapeutic: antiviral

Pregnancy Category: B

Trade Names

Prescription: Zovirax, Zovirax Topical

Do not confuse with Zostrix or Zyvox.

CLINICAL PHARMACOLOGY

Mechanism of Action

A synthetic nucleoside that converts to acyclovir triphosphate, becoming part of the DNA chain. **Therapeutic Effect:** Interferes with DNA synthesis and viral replication. Virustatic.

PHARMACOKINETICS

Poorly absorbed from the GI tract (10%-20%); minimal absorption following topical application. Protein binding: 9%-36%. Widely distributed. Partially metabolized in liver. Excreted primarily in urine. Removed by hemodialysis. **Half-life:** 2.5 hr (increased in impaired renal function).

AVAILABILITY

Capsules: 200 mg.
Tablets: 400 mg, 800 mg.
Injection Solution: 50 mg/mL.
Oral Suspension: 200 mg/5 mL.
Powder for Injection: 500 mg, 1000 mg.
Ointment: 5%.

INDICATIONS AND DOSAGE

Genital herpes (initial episode)

IV

Adults, Elderly, Children 12 yr and older: 5 mg/kg every 8 hr for 5 days.

PO

Adults, Elderly, Children 12 yr and older: 200 mg every 4 hr (or 5 times per day) for 10 days.

Topical

Adults, Elderly, Children 12 yr and older: Apply every 3 hr (or 6 times per day) for 7 days.

Genital herpes (recurrent)

PO (Less than six episodes per year)

Adults, Elderly, Children 12 yr and older: 200 mg every 4 hr (or 5 times per day) for 5 days.

PO (6 episodes or more per year)

Adults, Elderly, Children 12 yr and older: 400 mg 2 times per day or 200 mg 3-5 times per day for up to 12 mo.

Herpes simplex mucocutaneous

IV

Adults, Elderly, Children 12 yr and older: 5 mg/kg/dose every 8 hr for 7 days. **Children younger than 12 yr:** 10 mg/kg every 8 hr for 7 days.

Herpes simplex neonatal

IV

Children younger than 4 mo: 10 mg/kg every 8 hr for 10 days.

Herpes simplex encephalitis

IV

Adults, Elderly, Children 12 yr and older: 10 mg/kg every 8 hr for 10 days. **Children 3 mo-12 yr:** 20 mg/kg every 8 hr for 10 days.

Herpes zoster (caused by varicella)

IV

Adults, Elderly, Children 12 yr and older: 10 mg/kg every 8 hr for 7 days. **Children younger than 12 yr:** 20 mg/kg every 8 hr for 7 days.

Herpes zoster (shingles)

PO

Adults, Elderly, Children 12 yr and older: 800 mg every 4 hr (or 5 times per day) for 7-10 days.

Topical

Adults, Elderly: Apply to affected area 3-6 times per day for 7 days.

Varicella (chickenpox)

PO

Adults, Elderly, Children older than 12 yr or children 2-12 yr, weighing 40 kg or more: 800 mg 4 times per day for 5 days. **Children 2-12 yr, weighing less than 40 kg:** 20 mg/kg 4 times per day for 5 days. Maximum: 800 mg/dose. **Children younger than 2 yr:** 80 mg/kg/day.

Dosage in renal impairment

Dosage and frequency are modified based on severity of infection and degree of renal impairment.

PO, Normal dose 200 mg every 4 hr

Creatinine clearance greater than 10 mL/min: Give usual dose and at normal interval, 200 mg every 4 hr.

Creatinine clearance 10 mL/min and less: 200 mg every 12 hr.

PO, Normal dose 400 mg every 12 hr

Creatinine clearance greater than 10 mL/min: Give usual dose and at normal interval, 400 mg every 12 hr.

Creatinine clearance 10 mL/min and less: 200 mg every 12 hr.

PO, Normal dose 800 mg every 4 hr

Creatinine clearance greater than 25 mL/min: Give usual dose and at normal interval, 800 mg every 4 hr.

Creatinine clearance 10-25 mL/min: 800 mg every 8 hr.

Creatinine clearance less than 10 mL/min: 800 mg every 12 hr.

IV

Creatinine Clearance	Dosage %	Dosage Interval
Greater than 50 mL/min	100	8 hr
25-50 mL/min	100	12 hr
10-24 mL/min	100	24 hr
Less than 10 mL/min	50	24 hr

OFF-LABEL USES

Oral, parenteral: Prophylaxis of herpes simplex and herpes zoster infections, infectious mononucleosis.

Topical: Treatment adjunct for herpes zoster infections.

CONTRAINDICATIONS

Use in neonates when acyclovir is reconstituted with bacteriostatic water containing benzyl alcohol, hypersensitivity to acyclovir.

INTERACTIONS

Drug: **Nephrotoxic medications (such as aminoglycosides):** May increase the nephrotoxicity of acyclovir. **Probenecid:** May increase acyclovir half-life. **Varicella virus vaccine:** May decrease varicella virus vaccine effectiveness. Herbal: None known. Food: None known.

DIAGNOSTIC TEST EFFECTS

May increase BUN and serum creatinine concentrations.

IV INCOMPATIBILITIES

Aztreonam (Azactam), cefepime (Maxipime), diltiazem (Cardizem), *DOBUTamine (Dobutrex), *DOPamine (Intropin), levofloxacin (Levaquin), meropenem (Merrem IV), ondansetron (Zofran), piperacillin and tazobactam (Zosyn), total parenteral nutrition (TPN).

IV COMPATIBILITIES

Allopurinol (Alloprim), amikacin (Amikin), ampicillin, cefazolin (Ancef), cefotaxime (Claforan), ceftazidime (Fortaz), ceftriaxone (Rocephin), cimetidine (Tagamet), clindamycin (Cleocin), famotidine (Pepcid), fluconazole (Diflucan), gentamicin, heparin, hydromorphone (Dilaudid), imipenem (Primaxin), lorazepam (Ativan), magnesium sulfate, *methylPREDNISolone (SoluMedrol), metoclopramide (Reglan), metronidazole (Flagyl), morphine, multivitamins, potassium chloride, propofol (Diprivan), ranitidine (Zantac), vancomycin

SIDE-EFFECTS

Frequent: Parenteral (greater than 100%): Phlebitis or inflammation at IV site, lightheadedness
Topical (28%): Burning, stinging **Occasional: Oral (12%-6%):** Malaise, nausea, lightheadedness
Parenteral (3%): Pruritus, rash, urticaria
Topical (4%): Pruritus. **Rare: Oral (3%-1%):** Vomiting, rash, diarrhea, headache
Parenteral (2%-1%): Confusion, hallucinations, seizures, tremors
Topical (less than 1%): Rash

CRITICAL CARE CONSIDERATIONS

ADMINISTRATION/HANDLING

PO ALERT

- Give acyclovir without regard to food.
- Do not crush or break capsules.
- Store capsules at room temperature.

IV ALERT

- **Storage/stability:** Store vials at room temperature. Solutions of 50 mg/mL will remain stable for 12 hr at room temperature; they may form precipitate when refrigerated. Potency is not affected by precipitate or redissolution.
- **IV stability:** IV infusion (piggyback) will remain stable for 24 hr at room temperature. Yellow discoloration does not affect potency.
- **Initial reconstitution:** Add 10 mL of sterile water for injection to each 500-mg vial (50 mg/mL). Do not use bacteriostatic water for injection containing benzyl alcohol or parabens because this will cause a precipitate to form. Shake well until the solution is clear.
- **Final dilution:** Further dilute with at least 100 mL of D_5W or 0.9% NaCl. The final concentration should be less than or equal to 7 mg/mL.
- **Slow infusion:** Infuse the drug over at least 1 hr because renal tubular damage may occur with too-rapid administration.
- **Hydration:** Hydrate adequately during the infusion and for 2 hr afterward.

TOPICAL ALERT

- Avoid eye contact with the ointment or cream.
- Use a finger cot or rubber glove to prevent autoinoculation.

PRECAUTIONS

HEALTH-RELATED

- Use acyclovir cautiously in patients with dehydration, fluid and electrolyte imbalances, neurologic abnormalities, or hepatic impairment.
- **Renal impairment:** Use with great caution in patients with renal insufficiency, especially when using nephrotoxic agents concurrently.

AGE-RELATED

- **Children:** Safety and efficacy of acyclovir have not been established in children under 2 yr (under 1 yr for IV use); 10 mg/kg and 20 mg/kg doses in children from 3 mo to 16 yr achieved concentrations similar to those in adults receiving 5 mg/kg to 10 mg/kg.
- **Elderly:** Age-related renal impairment may require a dosage adjustment in the elderly. Effectiveness is similar to younger adults.

PREGNANCY/LACTATION-RELATED

- Pregnancy category B; has not caused harm in animal studies; excreted into breast milk; compatible with breast-feeding.

MONITORING

- **Baseline assessment:** Assess history of herpes simplex, zoster, or varicella. Determine history of allergies, particularly to acyclovir. Assess herpes simplex lesions before treatment to compare baseline lesions with those after treatment.
- **Lab work:** Biochemical profile including renal function studies (BUN, creatinine).
- **Hydration:** Provide adequate fluids during therapy to avoid precipitation in renal tubules (crystal formation), which can lead to renal failure.
- **Phlebitis:** Assess the IV site for signs and symptoms of phlebitis, including heat, pain, and red streaking over the vein.
- **Respiratory assessment:** Monitor respiratory rate, depth, and regularity.
- **Isolation:** Be sure to maintain appropriate isolation precautions in patients with chickenpox and disseminated herpes zoster.
- **Comfort measures:** Provide analgesics and comfort measures for discomfort related to lesions, especially in elderly and children.
- **Timely dosing:** Space doses evenly around the clock.
- **Patient education:** Inform patients that acyclovir does not permanently cure genital herpes. Caution patients with genital

A

herpes to avoid sexual intercourse while lesions are visible to prevent infecting partners. Advise patients not to touch lesions to prevent spreading the infection to new sites. Instruct patients to continue taking acyclovir for the full course of treatment as prescribed. Instruct patients to use a finger cot or rubber glove when applying the ointment. Encourage female patients to have a pap smear at least annually because of the increased risk of cervical cancer in women with genital herpes.

SERIOUS ADVERSE REACTIONS

- **Renal failure:** Rapid parenteral administration, excessively high doses, or fluid and electrolyte imbalance may produce renal failure.
- **Signs/symptoms of renal failure:** Abdominal pain, decreased urination, decreased appetite, increased thirst, nausea, and vomiting.
- *Toxicity has not been reported with oral or topical use.*

OVERDOSE/TOXICITY

- **Neurologic:** Headache, agitation, ataxia, confusion, dizziness, hallucination, paresthesia, psychosis, visual abnormalities.
- **Renal:** Hematuria, decreased urination, anuria, increased thirst, nausea, vomiting, decreased appetite.
- **Other symptoms:** Hypotension, diarrhea, vomiting, hives, rash, anemia, leukopenia, thrombocytopenia, elevated liver enzymes.
- **Hydration to prevent renal failure:** Adequate hydration is indicated to prevent precipitation of acyclovir in the renal tubules.
- **GI decontamination:** Use of activated charcoal may be considered in patients who have ingested large amounts of oral acyclovir, but typically this is not a drug of abuse.

ANTIDOTE/DIALYSIS

- **Antidote:** No specific recommendations.
- **Dialysis:** Acyclovir is removed by hemodialysis and is likely to be removed by high-permeability hemodialysis. It is not removed by peritoneal dialysis.

adalimumab

See Immunologics (p. 968)

adefovir dipivoxil

See Antivirals (p. 937)

adenosine

ah-den'-oh-seen

Classes

Chemical: endogenous nucleoside
Therapeutic: antidysrhythmic

Pregnancy Category: C

Trade Names

Prescription: Adenocard, Adenojec, Adenoscan, My-O-Den

CLINICAL PHARMACOLOGY

Mechanism of Action

A cardiac agent that slows impulse formation in the sinoatrial (SA) node and conduction time through the atrioventricular (AV) node. Adenosine also acts as a diagnostic aid in myocardial perfusion imaging or stress echocardiography. **Therapeutic Effect:** Depresses left ventricular function and restores normal sinus rhythm.

PHARMACOKINETICS

Rapidly cleared from the circulation via cellular uptake, primarily by erythrocytes and vascular endothelial cells. Extensively distributed and rapidly metabolized either via phosphorylation to adenosine monophosphate by adenosine kinase or via deamination to inosine by adenosine deaminase in the cytosol. **Half-life:** 10 seconds.

AVAILABILITY

Injection (Adenocard): 3 mg/mL in 2-mL, 4-mL syringes.
Injection (Adenoscan): 3 mg/mL in 20-mL, 30-mL vials.

INDICATIONS AND DOSAGE

Paroxysmal supraventricular tachycardia (PSVT)

Rapid IV bolus

Adults, Elderly, Children weighing 50 kg and more: Initially, 6 mg given over 1-2 sec. If first dose does not convert within 1-2 min, give 12 mg; may repeat 12-mg dose in 1-2 min if no response has occurred.
Children weighing less than 50 kg: Initially 0.05-0.10 mg/kg (maximum: 12 mg). IV every 2-5 min to a maximum of 0.25-0.3 mg/kg (maximum 30 mg).

Diagnostic testing

IV infusion

Adults: 140 mcg/kg/min for 6 min.

CONTRAINDICATIONS

Atrial fibrillation or flutter, second- or third-degree AV block, or sick sinus syndrome (with functioning pacemaker), ventricular tachycardia, hypersensitivity to adenosine.

INTERACTIONS

Drug: Carbamazepine: May increase degree of heart block caused by adenosine. **Dipyridamole:** May increase effect of adenosine. **Methylxanthines (e.g., caffeine, theophylline):** May decrease effect of adenosine. **Herbal:** None known. **Food:** None known.

DIAGNOSTIC TEST EFFECTS

None known.

IV INCOMPATIBILITIES

Any drug or solution other than 0.9% NaCl or D_5W.

SIDE-EFFECTS

Frequent (18%-12%): Facial flushing, dyspnea (12%), headache (18%), lightheadedness (12%). **Occasional (7%-2%):** Nausea (3%), chest pressure (7%). **Rare (less than or equal to 1%):** Numbness or tingling in arms; dizziness; diaphoresis; hypotension; palpitations; chest, jaw, or neck pain

CRITICAL CARE CONSIDERATIONS

ADMINISTRATION/HANDLING

IV ALERT

- Solution may be stored at room temperature and normally appears clear.
- Crystallization occurs if solution is refrigerated. If crystallization occurs, dissolve crystals by warming to room temperature. Discard unused portion.
- ***Administer undiluted very rapidly over 1 to 2 sec directly into vein, or if using an IV line, use the port closest to the insertion site.*** If the IV line is infusing fluid other than 0.9% NaCl, flush the line first before administering adenosine.
- ***Follow the rapid bolus injection with a rapid 0.9% NaCl flush.***

PRECAUTIONS

HEALTH-RELATED

- **Bronchospasms:** Adenosine may prompt bronchospasms in asthmatics (a relative contraindication), or other patients with bronchospastic or bronchoconstrictive disease.
- **Heart block:** Use adenosine cautiously in patients with heart block unless a cardiac pacemaker is in place.
- **Atrial fibrillation, atrial flutter, ventricular tachycardia:** Adenosine is ineffective in managing these dysrhythmias.
- **Decrease dosage:** Decrease dosage in patients on dipyradimole (Persantine) or carbamazepine (Tegretol) to avoid potentiating adenosine or causing a higher degree of heart block.
- **Increase dosage:** Consider increasing dosage in patients taking methylxanthines (e.g., theophyllines, caffeine, or caffeine-containing medications). Methylxanthines antagonize effects of adenosine.

AGE-RELATED

- **Children:** Although safety has not been established in patients under age 18 yr, adenosine has been used to convert paroxysmal supraventricular tachycardia (PSVT) in neonates, infants, children, and adolescents.
- **Elderly:** May have increased sensitivity with diminished heart function.

PREGNANCY/LACTATION-RELATED

- Pregnancy category C; no well-controlled studies in pregnant women; fetal effects unlikely.

MONITORING

- **Baseline assessment:** Assess vital signs including pulse oximetry before treatment.
- **Baseline diagnostic tests:** Twelve-lead ECG should be used to diagnose the tachycardia. Patients with atrial fibrillation or flutter and those with ventricular tachycardia require alternate management strategies per Advanced Cardiac Life Support (ACLS) guidelines.
- **Valsalva maneuver:** May be used before adenosine for managing tachycardia.
- **Rapid injection key to effectiveness:** Adenosine must reach systemic circulation to be effective. Follow administration technique carefully, or adenosine may not convert a controllable rhythm because of poor injection technique.
- **Rhythm changes:** If neither a few seconds of heart block nor asystole are seen after several IV bolus doses and the tachycardia fails to resolve, refer to ACLS guidelines for further management using amiodarone, beta-blockers, calcium channel blockers, synchronized cardioversion, and/or other strategies.
- **Continuous cardiac monitoring:** Implement continuous cardiac monitoring and document events associated with dysrhythmias.

- **Pulses:** Evaluate for change in apical and peripheral pulse rates, rhythm, and quality. Assess BP when changes are noted.
- **Reassessment:** Compare ongoing cardiac assessments to the baseline assessment before medication administration.
- **Hypoxemia:** Monitor for hypoxemia, which may signal heart failure using pulse oximetry (SpO_2). Assess respiratory rate, rhythm, and work of breathing. Compare current readings to what is considered normal for each patient.
- **Pharmacologic stress testing (Adenoscan [unlabeled]):** Monitor ECG continuously, vital signs frequently, and obtain images when infusion is complete; redistribution images should follow 3-4 hr later.
- **Fluid retention:** Monitor intake and output; assess for fluid retention, which may indicate impending heart failure secondary to the dysrhythmia.
- **Electrolytes:** Check serum electrolyte levels; hypokalemia may prompt tachycardias including ventricular tachycardia.
- **Patient education:** Advise patients to report unusual signs or symptoms, including chest pain, chest pounding or palpitations, or difficulty breathing or shortness of breath. Explain that facial flushing, headache, and nausea may occur during medication administration and that these symptoms will resolve.

SERIOUS ADVERSE REACTIONS

- Persistent dysrhythmias, bronchospasms, myocardial infarction, pulmonary edema, third-degree heart block, asystole requiring resuscitation.
- May produce short-lasting heart block and/or asystole, which resolves spontaneously after several seconds.

OVERDOSE/TOXICITY

- **Pharmacologic stress testing (off label):** If used as an infusion as part of pharmacologic stress testing (adenosine stress test), decrease infusion rate and if symptomatic dysrhythmia persists, discontinue infusion.
- Manage symptoms with accepted treatment guidelines for specific symptoms. Patients may be refractory to atropine, so other agents may be used to increase heart rate according to ACLS guidelines. Epinephrine infusion may help to relieve bronchospasms.
- **GI decontamination:** No specific recommendations.

ANTIDOTE/DIALYSIS

- **Antidote:** Aminophylline slow infusion may be used for persistent symptomatic dysrhythmias, which create hemodynamic instability; acts as a competitive antagonist to adenosine.
- **Dialysis:** Adenosine is unlikely to be removed by hemodialysis or peritoneal dialysis. No data are available on removal by high-permeability hemodialysis.

albuterol

al-byoo'-ter-ole

Classes

Chemical: sympathomimetic amine, β_2-adrenergic agonist
Therapeutic: antiasthmatic, bronchodilator

Pregnancy Category: C

Trade Names

Prescription: Accuneb, Airomir ✤, Proventil, Proventil-HFA, Proventil Repetabs, Ventolin, Ventolin HFA, Ventolin Rotacaps, Volmax, Vospire

Combinations

Prescription: with ipratropium (Combivent)

Do not confuse albuterol with Albutein or atenolol, or Proventil with Prinivil.

CLINICAL PHARMACOLOGY

Mechanism of Action

A sympathomimetic that stimulates β_2-adrenergic receptors in the lungs, resulting in relaxation of bronchial smooth muscle. **Therapeutic Effect:** Relieves bronchospasm and reduces airway resistance.

PHARMACOKINETICS

Route	Onset	Peak	Duration
PO	15-30 min	2-3 hr	4-6 hr
PO (extended-release)	30 min	2-4 hr	12 hr
Inhalation	5-15 min	0.5-2 hr	3-4 hr

Rapidly well absorbed from the GI tract; gradually absorbed from the bronchi after inhalation. Metabolized in the liver. Primarily excreted in urine. **Half-life:** 3.7-5 hr (PO); 3.8 hr (inhalation).

AVAILABILITY

Syrup: 2 mg/5 mL.
Tablets (Proventil, Ventolin): 2 mg, 4 mg.
Tablets (extended release): 4 mg (Proventil Repetabs, Volmax, VoSpire ER), 8 mg (Volmax, VoSpire ER).

Inhalation aerosol (Proventil, Ventolin): 90 mcg/spray.
Inhalation solution (AccuNeb): 0.75 mg/3 mL (0.63 mg/3 mL albuterol), 1.5 mg/3 mL (1.25 mg/3 mL albuterol).
Inhalation solution: 0.083% (Proventil), 0.5% (Proventil, Ventolin).
Inhalation capsule: 200 mcg.

INDICATIONS AND DOSAGE

Acute bronchospasm

Inhalation

Adults, Elderly, Children older than 12 yr: 4-8 puffs every 20 min up to 4 hr, then every 1-4 hr as needed. **Children 12 yr and younger:** 4-8 puffs every 20 min for 3 doses, then every 1-4 hr as needed

Nebulization

Adults, Elderly, Children older than 12 yr: 2.5-5 mg every 20 min for three doses, then 2.5-10 mg every 1-4 hr or 10-15 mg/hr continuously. **Children 12 yr and younger:** 0.15 mg/kg every 20 min for three doses (minimum: 2.5 mg), then 0.15-0.3 mg/kg every 1-4 hr as needed.

Bronchospasm

PO

Adults, Children older than 12 yr: 2-4 mg 3-4 times per day. Maximum: 8 mg 4 times per day **Elderly:** 2 mg 3-4 times per day. Maximum: 8 mg 4 times per day. **Children 6-12 yr:** 2 mg 3-4 times per day. Maximum: 24 mg/day. **Children 2-5 yr:** 0.1-0.2 mg/kg/dose 3 times per day. Maximum: 12 mg/day.

PO (Extended-Release)

Adults, Children older than 12 yr: 4-8 mg every 12 hr.

Nebulization

Adults, Elderly, Children older than 12 yr: 2.5 mg 3-4 times per day over 5-15 min. **Children 12 yr and younger:** 0.05 mg/kg every 4-6 hr. Minimum: 1.25 mg/dose. Maximum: 2.5 mg/dose.

Chronic bronchospasm

Inhalation

Adults, Elderly, Children 4 yr and older: 1-2 puffs every 4-6 hr. Maximum: 12 puffs per day.

Exercise-induced bronchospasm

Inhalation

Adults, Elderly, Children older than 12 yr: 2 puffs 15-30 min before exercise. **Children 12 yr and younger:** 1-2 puffs 5 min before exercise.

CONTRAINDICATIONS

History of hypersensitivity to albuterol or other sympathomimetics

INTERACTIONS

Drug: **Atomoxetine:** Increases heart rate and blood pressure. **Beta-blockers:** Antagonize effects of albuterol. **Digoxin:** May decrease digoxin levels. **MAOIs, tricyclic antidepressants:** May potentiate cardiovascular effects. **Cytochrome P450 enzyme metabolism:** Induces CYP3A4; drugs including carbamazepine, nafcillin, phenobarbital, and phenytoin may decrease the effects of albuterol. **Herbal:** None known. **Food:** None known.

DIAGNOSTIC TEST EFFECTS

May increase blood glucose level. May decrease serum potassium level.

SIDE-EFFECTS

Frequent: Headache (18%); nausea (4%); restlessness, nervousness, tremors (20%); dizziness (less than 7%); throat dryness and irritation, pharyngitis (less than 6%); BP changes including hypertension (5%-3%); heartburn, transient wheezing (less than 5%). **Occasional (3%-2%):** Insomnia, asthenia, altered taste
Inhalation: Dry, irritated mouth or throat; cough; bronchial irritation. **Rare:** Somnolence, diarrhea, dry mouth, flushing, diaphoresis, anorexia

CRITICAL CARE CONSIDERATIONS

ADMINISTRATION/HANDLING

PO ALERT

- Give albuterol without regard to food.
- Do not crush or break extended-release tablets.

INHALATION ALERT

- Shake container well before inhalation.
- Wait 2 min before inhaling the second dose to allow for deeper bronchial penetration.
- Rinse the mouth with water immediately after inhalation to prevent mouth and throat dryness.

NEBULIZATION ALERT

- Dilute 0.5 mL of 0.5% solution to a final volume of 3 mL with 0.9% NaCl to provide 2.5 mg.
- Administer over 5 to 15 min.
- The nebulizer should be used with compressed air or oxygen (O_2) at a rate of 6-10 L/min.

PRECAUTIONS

HEALTH-RELATED

- Use albuterol cautiously in patients with cardiovascular disease, diabetes mellitus, hypertension, or hyperthyroidism because it is a stimulant. Stimulants create stress, which may prompt increased myocardial oxygen consumption from tachycardia and increased BP, increased metabolic rate, and hyperglycemia.

AGE-RELATED

- **Children:** Safety and efficacy of albuterol have not been established in children less than 2 yr (syrup) or less than 6 yr (tablets).
- **Elderly:** Elderly may be more prone to tremors and tachycardia because of increased sensitivity to sympathomimetics.

PREGNANCY/LACTATION-RELATED

- Pregnancy category C; no well-controlled studies in pregnant women; excretion into breast milk unknown

MONITORING

- **Baseline assessment:** Assess pattern of bronchospasms; monitor pattern of dosing needed to maintain stability. Asthma can deteriorate over a period of hours or days, requiring reevaluation by the physician. Antiinflammatory corticosteroids may be required when asthma destabilizes.
- **Lab work:** ABGs to assess respiratory status, serum potassium levels. Hypokalemia may prompt tachycardia or ventricular dysrhythmias.
- **Bronchospasms:** Auscultate breath sounds for wheezing (indicates bronchoconstriction) and crackles (indicates pulmonary edema).
- **Respiratory distress:** Monitor for tachypnea, increased work of breathing, and change in respiratory pattern.
- **Hypoxemia:** Consider use of continuous or intermittent pulse oximetry to monitor oxygen saturation for hypoxemia.
- **Cardiac ischemia:** Monitor 12-lead ECG for signs of ischemia (ST depression) or myocardial infarction (ST elevation).
- **Pulse changes:** Monitor for tachycardia and for thready or irregular pulse.
- **Hydration:** Encourage patients to drink plenty of fluids to decrease the thickness of lung secretions.
- **Agitation:** Assess baseline behavior because albuterol prompts agitation and nervousness.
- **Emotional support:** Patients may become anxious because of difficulty breathing or the sympathomimetic response to the drug.
- **Avoid stimulants:** Avoid providing caffeinated products such as cocoa, cola, coffee, and tea.
- **Patient education:** Teach patients how to use an inhaler properly when nebulized treatments are transitioned including how to keep the inhaler clean. Consider use of a spacer if patients have difficulty with timing of inhalation. Instruct patients to rinse the mouth with water immediately after inhalation to prevent mouth and throat dryness.
- ***Advise patients to take no more than two inhalations at any one time because excessive use may decrease the drug's effectiveness or produce paradoxic bronchoconstriction.***

SERIOUS ADVERSE REACTIONS

- **Cardiac and hemodynamic instability:** Excessive sympathomimetic stimulation may produce palpitations, extrasystole, tachycardia, chest pain, a slight increase in BP followed by a substantial decrease, chills, diaphoresis, and blanching of skin.
- **Paradoxic bronchoconstriction:** Too frequent or excessive use may lead to decreased bronchodilating effectiveness and severe paradoxic bronchoconstriction.
- **Rashes/skin lesions:** Erythema multiforme and Stevens–Johnson syndrome have been reported in children.

OVERDOSE/TOXICITY

- **Unintentional overdose:** Most common in children and responds to management of symptoms—generally nausea, vomiting, and tachycardia.
- **Neurologic:** Nervousness, tremors, headache, sleeplessness, weakness, and dizziness.
- **Respiratory:** Severe bronchospasms.
- **Cardiovascular:** Tachycardia, palpitations, chest discomfort, flushing; ECG changes including prolonged QT interval, ST-segment depression, and increased BP.
- **Other symptoms:** Nausea, vomiting, muscle cramps.
- **Management:** Supportive care; provide symptom management while allowing the patient to eliminate the drug. Hypokalemia may ensue. Careful potassium replacement may be indicated.
- **GI decontamination:** No special recommendations.

ANTIDOTE/DIALYSIS

- **Antidote:** May consider use of beta-adrenergic blocking agents such as esmolol, metoprolol, or labetalol if deemed appropriate to manage tachycardia and hypertension but must be used cautiously to avoid bronchoconstriction; should be used if the patient remains hemodynamically unstable.

- **Dialysis:** Albuterol is unlikely to be removed by hemodialysis (insufficient evidence) or peritoneal dialysis. Insufficient data are available on removal by high-permeability hemodialysis.

alefacept

See Immunologics (p. 968)

alfentamine

See Opioid Analgesics (p. 980)

alfuzosin hydrochloride

ale-fyoo-zoe'-sin hye-droe-klor'-ide

Classes
Chemical: quinazoline
Therapeutic: α_1-adrenergic blocker

Pregnancy Category: B

Trade Names
Prescription: Uroxatral, Xatral

CLINICAL PHARMACOLOGY

Mechanism of Action
An α_1 antagonist that targets receptors around bladder neck and prostate capsule. **Therapeutic Effect:** Relaxes smooth muscle and improves urinary flow and symptoms of prostatic hyperplasia.

PHARMACOKINETICS

Rapidly absorbed and widely distributed. Protein binding: 90%. Extensively metabolized in the liver. Primarily excreted in feces. **Half-life:** 10 hr.

AVAILABILITY

Tablets (Extended-Release): 10 mg.

INDICATIONS AND DOSAGE

Benign prostatic hyperplasia
PO
Adults: 10 mg once per day, approximately 30 min after same meal each day.

CONTRAINDICATIONS

Moderate to severe hepatic disease, concomitant use of ketoconazole, itraconazole, ritonavir; hypersensitivity to alfuzosin

INTERACTIONS

Drug: Cimetidine: May increase alfuzosin blood concentration. **Ketoconazole, itraconazole, ritonavir:** May increase alfuzosin serum levels. **Other alpha-blockers, such as doxazosin, prazosin, tamsulosin, and terazosin:** May increase the alpha-blockade effects of both drugs. **Herbal:** None known. **Food:** Take with food.

DIAGNOSTIC TEST EFFECTS

None known.

SIDE-EFFECTS

Frequent (6%): Dizziness. **Occasional (3%-4%):** Fatigue, headache. **Rare (2%):** Nausea, dyspepsia (e.g., heartburn and epigastric discomfort), diarrhea, orthostatic hypotension, tachycardia, drowsiness

CRITICAL CARE CONSIDERATIONS

ADMINISTRATION/HANDLING

PO ALERT

- Give alfuzosin after the same meal each day.
- Extended-release tablets should not be crushed or chewed.

PRECAUTIONS

HEALTH-RELATED

- Use alfuzosin cautiously in patients with coronary artery disease, hepatic impairment, or orthostatic hypotension.
- **General anesthesia:** Use cautiously in patients under general anesthesia.

AGE-RELATED

- **Children:** Alfuzosin is not indicated for use in children.
- **Elderly:** No age-related precautions have been noted.

PREGNANCY/LACTATION-RELATED

- Pregnancy category B, but not indicated for use in women.

MONITORING

- **Baseline assessment:** Determine sensitivity to alfuzosin as well as other alpha-blockers, including doxazosin, prazosin, tamsulosin, and terazosin to avoid hypersensitivity reaction.
- **Lab work:** Biochemical profile including liver function (AST [SGOT], ALT [SGPT], alkaline phosphatase, bilirubin) tests.
- **Therapeutic effect:** Improved urinary flow, less dysuria.

- **Orthostatic hypotension:** Ambulate patients slowly and evaluate for dizziness; seen most commonly during first days of therapy.
- **Patient education:** When alfuzosin will be used outside the hospital, caution patients to avoid performing tasks that require mental alertness or motor skills until response to the drug is known. Teach patients not to chew or crush extended-release tablets and to take medication after the same meal daily. Instruct patients to report headaches promptly; may indicate that hypotension is present.

SERIOUS ADVERSE REACTIONS
- **Chest discomfort:** Ischemic chest pain may occur (rarely) due to hypotension.
- **Priapism:** Sustained, painful erection that does not resolve following orgasm or ejaculation. Can lead to permanent impotence if not appropriately managed.
- **Hypotension:** Patients may be very sensitive to alpha-adrenergic blockade.

OVERDOSE/TOXICITY
- **Symptoms:** Syncope, hypotension, loss of consciousness, possible tachycardia.
- **Management:** Place patients flat and elevate legs; treat hypotension according to current accepted standard of care.
- **GI decontamination:** No specific recommendations.

ANTIDOTE/DIALYSIS
- **Antidote:** No specific recommendations.
- **Dialysis:** Alfuzosin is unlikely to be removed by hemodialysis, high-permeability hemodialysis, or peritoneal dialysis.

allopurinol

al-oh-pure'-i-nole

Classes
Chemical: hypoxanthine isomer, xanthine oxidase inhibitor
Therapeutic: antigout agent

Pregnancy Category: C

Trade Names
Prescription: Aloprim, Apo-Allopurinol ♣, Zyloprim

Do not confuse with ZORprin.

CLINICAL PHARMACOLOGY
Mechanism of Action
A xanthine oxidase inhibitor that decreases uric acid production by inhibiting xanthine oxidase, an enzyme. **Therapeutic Effect:** Reduces uric acid concentrations in both serum and urine.

PHARMACOKINETICS

Route	Onset	Peak	Duration
PO/IV	2-3 days	7-10 days	2 wk

Well absorbed from the GI tract. Widely distributed. Metabolized in the liver to active metabolite. Excreted primarily in urine. Removed by hemodialysis. **Half-life:** 1-3 hr; metabolite, 18-30 hr.

AVAILABILITY
Tablets (Zyloprim): 100 mg, 300 mg.
Powder for Injection (Aloprim): 500 mg.

INDICATIONS AND DOSAGE
Chronic gouty arthritis
PO
Adults, Children older than 10 yr: Initially, 100 mg/day; may increase by 100 mg/day at weekly intervals. Maximum: 800 mg/day. Maintenance: 100-200 mg 2-3 times per day or 300 mg/day.
Prevention of uric acid nephropathy during chemotherapy
PO
Adults: Initially, 600-800 mg/day starting 2-3 days before initiation of chemotherapy or radiation therapy. **Children 6-10 yr:** 100 mg 3 times per day or 300 mg once per day. **Children less than 6 yr:** 50 mg 3 times per day.
IV
Adults: 200-400 mg/m^2/day beginning 24-48 hr before initiation of chemotherapy. **Children:** 200 mg/m^2/day. Maximum: 600 mg/day.
Alert: Maintenance dosage is based on serum uric acid levels. Discontinue following the period of tumor regression.
Prevention of uric acid calculi
PO
Adults: 100-200 mg 1-4 times per day or 300 mg once per day.
Recurrent calcium oxalate calculi
PO
Adults: 200-300 mg/day **Elderly:** Initially 100 mg/day, gradually increased until optimal uric acid level is reached.
Dosage in renal impairment
Dosage is modified based on creatinine clearance.

Creatinine Clearance	Dosage Adjustment
10-20 mL/min	200 mg/day
3-9 mL/min	100 mg/day
Less than 3 mL/min	100 mg at extended intervals

OFF-LABEL USES
In mouthwash following fluorouracil therapy to prevent stomatitis

CONTRAINDICATIONS
Hypersensitivity to allopurinol

INTERACTIONS
Drug: **Angiotensin-converting enzyme (ACE) inhibitors:** May cause hypersensitivity reactions. **Amoxicillin, ampicillin:** May increase incidence of rash. **Azathioprine, mercaptopurine:** May increase therapeutic effect and toxicity of azathioprine and mercaptopurine. Reduce azathioprine dose by one third or one fourth. **Oral anticoagulants:** May increase anticoagulant effect. **Thiazide diuretics:** Toxicity and risk of hypersensitivity are increased. Herbal: None known. Food: **Ethanol:** May decrease allopurinol effectiveness.

DIAGNOSTIC TEST EFFECTS
May increase BUN, serum creatinine, serum alkaline phosphatase, AST (SGOT), and ALT (SGPT) levels.

IV INCOMPATIBILITIES
Amikacin (Amikin), carmustine (BiCNU), cefotaxime (Claforan), *chlorproMAZINE (Thorazine), cimetidine (Tagamet), clindamycin (Cleocin), cytarabine (Ara-C), dacarbazine (DTIC), *diphenhydrAMINE (Benadryl), *DOXOrubicin (Adriamycin), doxycycline (Vibramycin), droperidol (Inapsine), fludarabine (Fludara), gentamicin (Garamycin), haloperidol (Haldol), *hydrOXYzine (Vistaril), idarubicin (Idamycin), imipenem-cilastatin (Primaxin), meperidine (Demerol), *methylPREDNISolone (Solu-Medrol), metoclopramide (Reglan), ondansetron (Zofran), prochlorperazine (Compazine), promethazine (Phenergan), streptozocin (Zanosar), tobramycin (Nebcin), vinorelbine (Navelbine)

IV COMPATIBILITIES
Bumetanide (Bumex), calcium gluconate, furosemide (Lasix), heparin, hydromorphone (Dilaudid), lorazepam (Ativan), morphine, potassium chloride

SIDE-EFFECTS
Occasional: **Oral:** Somnolence, unusual hair loss, rash, nausea, vomiting; **IV:** Rash, nausea, vomiting. Rare: Diarrhea, headache, Stevens–Johnson syndrome

CRITICAL CARE CONSIDERATIONS

ADMINISTRATION/HANDLING

PO ALERT
- May give allopurinol with or immediately after meals or milk.
- Ensure patients drink at least 10 to 12 8-ounce glasses of fluid each day. Provide IV hydration if patients are unable to consume PO fluids.
- **Dosage:** Administer dosages greater than 300 mg/day in divided doses.

IV ALERT
- **Vial storage:** Store vials at room temperature.
- **Reconstituted solution storage:** Store at room temperature; give within 10 hr. Do not use if precipitate forms or solution is discolored.
- **Dilution:** Reconstitute 500-mg vial with 25 mL sterile water for injection; produces a clear, almost colorless solution (concentration of 20 mg/mL).
- **Further dilution for intermittent IV infusion:** Further dilute with 0.9% NaCl or D_5W (19 mL of added diluent yields 1 mg/mL, 9 mL yields 2 mg/mL, and 2.3 mL yields maximum concentration of 6 mg/mL).
- **Infusion:** Infuse over 30 to 60 min.

PRECAUTIONS

HEALTH-RELATED
- Use allopurinol cautiously in patients with heart failure, diabetes mellitus, hypertension, or impaired renal or hepatic function.

AGE-RELATED
- **Children:** No age-related precautions; use in children is generally limited to those with a malignancy or inborn errors of purine metabolism.
- **Elderly:** May require reduced dose due to age-related renal, liver, and cardiac disease.

PREGNANCY/LACTATION-RELATED
- Pregnancy category C; allopurinol and oxypurinol have been found in the milk of a mother who was receiving allopurinol.

MONITORING

- **Baseline assessment:** Assess joint mobility, tenderness, pain, and swelling.
- **Baseline lab work:** CBC, hepatic enzymes, chemical profile including BUN/creatinine, and serum uric acid level.
- **Ongoing lab work:** Monitor chemical profile for renal insufficieny, hepatic enzymes for hepatitis/hepatic insufficiency, CBC for bone marrow depression, uric acid level for reduction (desired effect).
- **Concommitant warfarin:** Assess for bleeding and monitor prothrombin time/INR because allopurinol may prolong the half-life of warfarin (Coumadin).
- **Sensitivity:** Discontinue allopurinol immediately if rash or other evidence of allergic reaction appears to avoid early onset exfoliative dermatitis or purpuric lesions. Occurrence of hypersensitivity is increased in renal insufficient patients receiving thiazide diuretics (cholothiazide/Diuril).
- **Hydration:** Encourage high fluid intake (3000 mL/day). Monitor intake and output. Urine output should be at least 2000 mL/day. Examine urine for cloudiness and unusual color and odor, which may indicate renal calculi, glomerulonephritis, or pyelonephritis are developing.
- **Therapeutic response:** Assess for improved joint range of motion and reduced redness, swelling, and tenderness. An increase in gout attacks is sometimes seen during early allopurinol therapy.
- **Patient education:** Explain that it may take 1 wk or more for full therapeutic effect to be evident. When taking allopurinol outside the hospital, patients must maintain the same aggressive hydration. Warn patients to avoid tasks requiring mental alertness or motor skills until response to the drug is known.

SERIOUS ADVERSE REACTIONS

- **Rash:** Severe hypersensitivity/allergic reaction may follow appearance of rash.
- **GI effects:** Severe diarrhea, increased alkaline phosphatase/AST (SGOT)/ALT (SGPT).

OVERDOSE/TOXICITY

- **Allergic reaction:** Pruritic maculopapular rash possibly accompanied by malaise, fever, chills, joint pain, nausea, and vomiting is a toxic reaction.
- **Organ failure:** Bone marrow depression, hepatic toxicity, peripheral neuritis, and acute renal failure occur rarely.
- **Management:** Discontinue allopurinol immediately. Allergic reactions may require epinephrine, *diphenhydrAMINE (Benadryl), corticosteroids (hydrocortisone), endotracheal intubation, and mechanical ventilation. Rare cardiac arrest has been reported, which is managed by Advanced Cardiac Life Support (ACLS) guidelines.
- **GI decontamination:** No specific recommendations.

ANTIDOTE/DIALYSIS

- **Antidote:** No specific recommendations.
- **Dialysis:** Allopurinol is removed by hemodialysis and peritoneal dialysis and is likely to be removed by high-permeability hemodialysis. Allopurinol dose should be reduced in renal failure and renal-insufficient patients. Patients should receive 100 mg following hemodialysis on dialysis days. Removal may not immediately relieve toxic effects.

almotriptan maleate

See Triptans (p. 984)

alosetron hydrochloride

al-ohs'-eh-tron hye-droe-klor'-ide

Classes

Chemical: selective 5-HT_3 receptor antagonist

Therapeutic: antidiarrheal

Pregnancy Category: B

Trade Names

Prescription: Lotronex

Do not confuse Lotronex with Lovenox.

CLINICAL PHARMACOLOGY

Mechanism of Action

A serotonin (5-HT_3) receptor antagonist that mediates abdominal pain, bloating, nausea, vomiting, peristalsis, and secretory reflexes. **Therapeutic Effect:** Alleviates diarrhea, reduces gastric pain.

PHARMACOKINETICS

Rapidly absorbed after PO administration. Extensively metabolized in liver. Excreted primarily in urine (75%) and, to a lesser extent, in feces. **Half-life:** 1.5 hr.

AVAILABILITY

Tablets: 0.5 mg, 1 mg.

INDICATIONS AND DOSAGE

Irritable bowel syndrome

PO

Adults (women older than 18 yr): 0.5 mg twice per day for 4 wk, then increase to 1 mg twice per day. Maximum: 2 mg/day.

OFF-LABEL USES

Treatment of carcinoid diarrhea, irritable bowel syndrome in men.

CONTRAINDICATIONS

Breast-feeding; constipation; diverticulitis (active or history of); GI bleeding, obstruction, or perforation; history ischemic colitis, ulcerative colitis, or Crohn's disease; thrombophlebitis, concomitant administration with fluvoxamine, patients unable to understand or comply with "patient-physician agreement"; hypersensitivity to alosetron.

INTERACTIONS

Drug: **Amiodarone, ciprofloxacin, ketoconazole, norfloxacin, ofloxacin:** Increase alosetron effects. **Fluvoxamine:** Concomitant use is contraindicated. **Fluconazole, gemfibrozil, pioglitazone, NSAIDs, sulfonamides:** Increase alosetron effects. Herbal: **St. John's wort:** May increase alosetron blood concentration. Food: **All foods:** May decrease the absorption or delay the peak blood concentration of alosetron.

DIAGNOSTIC TEST EFFECTS

May increase serum alkaline phosphatase, bilirubin, ALT (SGPT), and AST (SGOT) levels.

SIDE-EFFECTS

Frequent (28%): Constipation. Occasional (10%-2%): Nausea (6%), GI or abdominal discomfort or pain (7%), dyspepsia, flatulence (6%). Rare: Sedation, abnormal dreams, anxiety

CRITICAL CARE CONSIDERATIONS

ADMINISTRATION/HANDLING

PO ALERT

- May give alosetron without regard to food, but it has been associated with delayed absorption and delayed peak action in some patients when taken with meals.

PRECAUTIONS

HEALTH-RELATED

- Use alosetron cautiously in patients with hepatic function impairment.
- **Males:** Alosetron is indicated for use in women only but has been used off-label in men for irritable bowel syndrome and carcinoid diarrhea; safety and efficacy have not been established in men.

AGE-RELATED

- **Children:** Safety and efficacy of alosetron have not been established in children younger than 12 yr.
- **Elderly:** No age-related precautions have been noted.

PREGNANCY/LACTATION-RELATED

- Pregnancy category B; no adequate well-controlled studies in pregnant women have been done; animal studies have not shown harm to the fetus; it is unknown if alosetron is excreted in breast milk.

MONITORING

- **Baseline GI assessment:** Determine history of abdominal distress, abdominal pain or discomfort, bloating, blood in stools, and diarrhea.
- **Lab work:** Biochemical profile including liver function tests (AST [SGOT], ALT [SGPT], bilirubin, alkaline phosphatase).
- **Baseline hydration assessment:** Assess skin turgor, urinary status, and mucous membranes for dryness to determine baseline hydration status.
- **Hydration:** Encourage patients to maintain adequate IV/PO fluid intake.
- **Bowel function:** Monitor pattern of daily bowel activity and stool consistency. Auscultate bowel sounds for peristalsis.
- **Therapeutic effect:** Evaluate for a decrease in GI signs and symptoms.
- **Ongoing bowel monitoring:** Urgency and diarrhea may be reduced within 1 wk of treatment, but alosetron's full therapeutic effects may not occur for up to 4 wk. Monitor for bloody diarrhea, severe constipation, or a sudden worsening of stomach pain, which may indicate the drug is ineffective or ischemic colitis is present.
- **Patient education:** Inform patients that persistent constipation may require interruption of treatment or drug management.

SERIOUS ADVERSE REACTIONS

- Acute ischemic colitis and serious complications of constipation have resulted in the need for blood transfusions and surgery.

OVERDOSE/TOXICITY

- Severe gastrointestinal distress including gastric pain, GI bleeding, and diarrhea.
- **Management:** Should be managed according to accepted standards for care of colitis or constipation. Ensure patients are well hydrated using IV fluids.
- **GI decontamination:** No specific recommendations.

ANTIDOTE/DIALYSIS

- **Antidote:** No specific recommendations.
- **Dialysis:** No data are available regarding removal of alosetron using hemodialysis, high-permeability hemodialysis, or peritoneal dialysis.

alprazolam

al-pray'-zoe-lam

DEA Schedule: IV

Classes

Chemical: benzodiazepine
Therapeutic: anxiolytic

Pregnancy Category: D

Trade Names

Prescription: Apo-Alpraz ♣, Niravam, Xanax, Xanax TS ♣, Xanax XR

Do not confuse alprazolam with lorazepam or Xanax with Tenex or Zantac.

CLINICAL PHARMACOLOGY

Mechanism of Action

A benzodiazepine that enhances the action of the inhibitory neurotransmitter gamma-aminobutyric acid in the brain. Therapeutic Effect: Produces anxiolytic effect from its CNS depressant action.

PHARMACOKINETICS

Well absorbed from GI tract. Protein binding: 80%. Metabolized in the liver. Primarily excreted in urine. Minimal removal by hemodialysis. Half-life: 11-16 hr.

AVAILABILITY

Oral solution (alprazolam Intensol): 1 mg/mL, 0.5 mg/5 mL.
Tablets (Xanax): 0.25 mg, 0.5 mg, 1 mg, 2 mg.
Tablets (extended release [Xanax XR]): 0.5 mg, 1 mg, 2 mg, 3 mg.
Tablets (orally disintegrating [Niravam]): 0.25 mg, 0.5 mg, 1 mg, 2 mg.

INDICATIONS AND DOSAGE

Anxiety disorders

PO (immediate release)

Adults: Initially, 0.25–0.5 mg 3 times per day. May titrate every 3-4 days. Maximum: 4 mg/day in divided doses. **Elderly, Debilitated patients, Patients with hepatic disease or low serum albumin:** Initially, 0.25 mg 2-3 times per day. Gradually increase to optimum therapeutic response.

PO (orally disintegrating)

Adults: 0.25-0.5 mg 3 times per day. Maximum: 4 mg/day in divided doses.

Anxiety with depression

PO

Adults: 2.5-3 mg/day in divided doses.

Panic disorder

PO (immediate release)

Adults: Initially, 0.5 mg 3 times per day. May increase at 3- to 4-day intervals. Range: 5-6 mg/day. Maximum: 10 mg/day. **Elderly:** Initially, 0.125-0.25 mg twice per day. May increase in 0.125-mg increments until desired effect attained.

PO (extended release)

Alert: To switch from immediate-release to extended-release form, give total daily dose (immediate-release) as a single daily dose of extended-release form. **Adults:** Initially, 0.5-1 mg once per day. May titrate at 3- to 4-day intervals. Range: 3-6 mg/day. Maximum: 10 mg/day. **Elderly:** Initially, 0.5 mg once daily.

PO (orally disintegrating)

Adults: Initially, 0.5 mg 3 times per day. May increase at 3- to 4-day intervals. Range: 5-6 mg/day. Maximum: 10 mg/day.

Premenstrual syndrome

PO

Adults: 0.25 mg 3 times per day.

OFF-LABEL USES

Management of premenstrual syndrome symptoms (mood disturbances, insomnia, and cramps), irritable bowel syndrome, treatment of agoraphobia, posttraumatic stress disorder, tremors, ethanol withdrawal, anxiety in children.

CONTRAINDICATIONS

Acute alcohol intoxication with depressed vital signs, acute angle-closure glaucoma, concurrent use of itraconazole or ketoconazole, myasthenia gravis, severe COPD

INTERACTIONS

Drug: Alcohol, other CNS depressants: Potentiate effects of alprazolam and may increase sedation. **Fluvoxamine, itraconazole, ketoconazole, nefazodone:** May inhibit metabolism and increase serum concentrations of alprazolam. **Herbal: Kava kava, valerian:** May increase CNS depressant effect of alprazolam. **St. John's wort:** May reduce effectiveness of alprazolam. **Food: Grapefruit, grapefruit juice:** May inhibit alprazolam's metabolism.

DIAGNOSTIC TEST EFFECTS

None known.

SIDE-EFFECTS

Frequent: Ataxia; light-headedness; transient, mild somnolence; slurred speech (particularly in elderly or debilitated patients), dry mouth. **Occasional:** Confusion, depression, blurred vision, constipation, diarrhea, headache, nausea. **Rare:** Behavioral problems such as anger, impaired memory, paradoxic reactions such as insomnia, nervousness, or irritability

CRITICAL CARE CONSIDERATIONS

ADMINISTRATION/HANDLING

PO ALERT

- Give alprazolam without regard to food.
- Crush tablets as needed.

EXTENDED RELEASE ALERT

- Administer once per day.
- Swallow tablets whole. Do not break, chew, or crush tablets.

PRECAUTIONS

HEALTH-RELATED

- Use alprazolam cautiously if impaired renal or hepatic function is present.

AGE-RELATED

- **Children:** Safety and efficacy of alprazolam have not been established in children younger than 18 yr.
- **Elderly:** Expect to give elderly patients small doses initially and to increase dosage gradually to avoid excessive sedation or ataxia.

PREGNANCY/LACTATION-RELATED

- Pregnancy category D; children born of a mother receiving benzodiazepines may be at risk for withdrawal symptoms; neonatal flaccidity and respiratory problems have been reported; chronic administration of diazepam to nursing mothers has been reported to cause infants to become lethargic and lose weight; alprazolam may have a similar effect

MONITORING

- **Baseline assessment:** Evaluate history of anxiety.
- **Lab work:** Biochemical profile including renal (BUN, creatinine) and liver function (AST [SGOT], ALT [SGPT], alkaline phosphatase, bilirubin) tests.
- **Therapeutic effect:** Evaluate for the desired therapeutic response, including a calm facial expression and decreased insomnia and restlessness.
- **Paradoxic CNS reactions:** Assess patients for paradoxic CNS reactions such as agitation, tension, and trembling, particularly early in therapy.
- **Autonomic responses:** Monitor for cold, clammy hands and diaphoresis.
- **Drowsiness:** Note drowsiness, which usually disappears with continued therapy.
- **Emotional support:** Offer emotional support to the anxious patient to further lessen anxiety.
- **Do not withdraw abruptly:** To avoid rebound agitation, alprazolam should not be withdrawn abruptly after long-term therapy.
- **Dry mouth:** Provide sour hard candy, gum, or sips of water for relief.
- **Patient education:** Encourage patients to stop smoking because smoking reduces alprazolam's effectiveness. Instruct patients to change positions slowly—from recumbent to sitting before standing—to prevent dizziness. If using the medication long term, caution patients to avoid tasks that require mental alertness or motor skills until response to the drug is known. Urge female patients on long-term therapy to use effective contraception during therapy and to notify the physician immediately of pregnancy or possible pregnancy to monitor for withdrawal symptoms in the patient and avoid harm to the fetus.
- **Long term use:** Evaluate patients' other medications, including OTC drugs, with the physician and/or pharmacist to avoid medication interactions.

SERIOUS ADVERSE REACTIONS

- **Rapid withdrawal:** Abrupt or too rapid withdrawal may result in pronounced restlessness, irritability, insomnia, hand

tremors, abdominal and muscle cramps, diaphoresis, vomiting, and seizures.
- Blood dyscrasias have been reported rarely.

OVERDOSE/TOXICITY
- **Neurologic:** Somnolence, confusion, slurred speech, diminished reflexes, and coma.
- **Cardiovascular:** Hypotension, tachycardia.
- **Respiratory:** Respiratory arrest.
- **Renal:** Renal failure due to rhabdomyolysis.
- **Associated findings:** Hypothermia.
- **Hemodynamic support:** Manage severe supraventricular tachycardia and hypotension according to Advanced Cardiac Life Support (ACLS) guidelines. Manage hypotension with fluids followed by vasopressor infusion with dopamine or norepinephrine (Levophed) if needed to maintain blood pressure.
- **Prevent respiratory complications:** Implement preventive strategies such as pulse oximetry to monitor for hypoxemia, oral airway or endotracheal intubation to maintain patent airway, and nasogastric tube to low suction to prevent aspiration.
- **Prevent seizures to help avoid rhabdomyolysis:** Consider use of phenytoin to prevent seizures. Seizures and muscle breakdown cause protein to precipitate in the kidneys, leading to rhabdomyolysis and renal failure.
- **Hypothermia:** Use a warming blanket to manage hypothermia if indicated.
- **GI decontamination:** Ipecac is used to induce vomiting if less than 60 min since ingestion or gastric lavage if within the same time frame. Activated charcoal is used to bind with the substance in the stomach.

ANTIDOTE/DIALYSIS
- **Antidote:** Flumazenil (Romazicon) reverses the sedative and respiratory depressant effects. Use flumazenil with caution if the patient has overdosed on multiple medications or is dependent on alprazolam. Flumazenil may prompt seizures in alprazolam-dependent patients and cause dysrhythmias in patients who also have high levels of cyclic (tricyclic) antidepressants. Repeat doses of flumazenil may be needed because the duration of action of alprazolam exceeds that of flumazenil.
- **Dialysis:** Alprazolam is not removed by hemodialysis, is not likely to be removed by peritoneal dialysis, and no data are available on removal using high-permeability hemodialysis.

alprostadil (prostaglandin E_1, PGE_1)

al-pros'-ta-dil

Classes
Chemical: prostaglandin E1
Therapeutic: antiimpotence agent, patent ductus arteriosus

Pregnancy Category: C

Trade Names
Prescription: Caverject, Edex, Muse, Prostin VR ♣, Prostin VR Pediatric

CLINICAL PHARMACOLOGY
Mechanism of Action

A prostaglandin that directly affects vascular and ductus arteriosus smooth muscle and relaxes trabecular smooth muscle. **Therapeutic Effect:** Causes vasodilation; dilates cavernosal arteries, allowing blood flow to and entrapment in the lacunar spaces of the penis.

PHARMACOKINETICS
Absorption occurs from the urethral lining when inserted as a urethral suppository. Protein binding: 81%-99% (injection). Rapidly metabolized. Excreted in urine and lung. **Half-life:** 5-10 min (injection).

AVAILABILITY
Injection (Prostin VR Pediatric): 500 mcg/mL.
Powder for injection (Caverject, Edex): 10 mcg, 20 mcg, 40 mcg.
Urethral pellet (Muse): 125 mcg, 250 mcg, 500 mcg, 1000 mcg.

INDICATIONS AND DOSAGE
Maintain patency of ductus arteriosus
IV infusion (continuous)
Neonates: Initially, 0.05-0.1 mcg/kg/min. Maintenance: 0.01-0.4 mcg/kg/min. Maximum: 0.4 mcg/kg/min.
Impotence
Pellet, intracavernosal
Adults: Dosage is individualized.

OFF-LABEL USES
Gangrene, pain due to severe peripheral arterial occlusive disease, treatment of pulmonary hypertension in infants, children.

CONTRAINDICATIONS

Conditions predisposing to anatomic deformation of penis, hyaline membrane disease, penile implants, priapism or conditions predisposing patients to priapism (sickle cell anemia, leukemia), respiratory distress syndrome, pregnancy, hypersensitivity to alprostadil.

INTERACTIONS

Drug: Anticoagulants, including heparin, thrombolytics: May increase risk of bleeding. **Sympathomimetics:** May decrease effect of alprostadil. **Vasodilators:** May increase risk of hypotension. **Herbal:** None known. **Food:** None known.

DIAGNOSTIC TEST EFFECTS

May increase blood bilirubin levels. May decrease glucose, serum calcium, and serum potassium levels.

IV INCOMPATIBILITIES

No information available.

SIDE-EFFECTS

Frequent: Intracavernosal: Penile pain (37%); prolonged erection, hypertension, localized pain, penile fibrosis, injection-site hematoma or ecchymosis, headache, respiratory infection, flulike symptoms (1%-4%)
Intraurethral: Penile pain (36%); urethral pain or burning, testicular pain, urethral bleeding, headache, dizziness, respiratory infection, flulike symptoms (3%)
Systemic: Fever, flushing, bradycardia, hypotension, tachycardia, diarrhea (1%-2%). **Occasional:** Intracavernosal: Hypotension, pelvic pain, back pain, dizziness, cough, nasal congestion (less than 1%)
Intraurethral: Fainting, sinusitis, back and pelvic pain (less than 3%)
Systemic: Anxiety, lethargy, myalgia, dysrhythmias, respiratory depression, anemia, bleeding, hematuria (less than 1%)

CRITICAL CARE CONSIDERATIONS

ADMINISTRATION/HANDLING

INTERCAVERNOSAL DOSAGE ALERT (FOR ERECTILE DYSFUNCTION)

Doses greater than 40 mcg (Edex) or 60 mcg (Caverject) are not recommended.

- Urethral pellet
- **Storage:** Refrigerate pellet unless used within 14 days.

IV ALERT (FOR PATENT DUCTUS ARTERIOSUS)

Give by continuous IV infusion or through umbilical artery catheter placed at ductal opening.

- **Storage:** Store the parenteral form in the refrigerator.
- **Dilution:** Dilute alprostadil before administration. Prepare a fresh dose every 24 hr and discard unused portions.
- **Continuous IV infusion:** Prepare by diluting 1 mL alprostadil, containing 500 mcg, with D_5W or 0.9% NaCl to yield a solution containing 2-20 mcg/mL. Diluting volumes can range from 25 to 250 mL, depending on the patient and the available infusion device.
- Infuse the lowest possible dose over the shortest possible time.
- Decrease the infusion rate immediately if a significant decrease in arterial pressure is noted via auscultation, Doppler transducer, or umbilical artery catheter.
- Discontinue the infusion immediately if signs and symptoms of overdose, such as apnea and bradycardia, occur.

PRECAUTIONS

HEALTH-RELATED

- **Hyaline membrane disease:** Not indicated for respiratory distress syndrome in children.
- **Priapism:** Use alprostadil cautiously in patients prone to priapism, such as those having leukemia, multiple myeloma, polycythemia, sickle cell disease, or with anatomic defects of the penis, including Peyronie's disease.
- **Bleeding potential:** Use cautiously in patients with coagulation defects, severe hepatic disease with coagulation defects, and thrombocytopenia.
- **Penile implants:** Patients with penile implants should not be treated with alprostadil.
- **Activity intolerance:** Should not be used in men for whom sexual activity is inadvisable.

AGE-RELATED

- **Neonates:** When used in neonates to maintain patent ductus until corrective or palliative surgery can be provided, may cause gastric outlet obstruction secondary to antral hyperplasia related to duration of the therapy and cumulative dose of the drug.

- **Poor response in neonates:** Response is poorer in infants with pO_2 values of less than 40 mmHg or those more than 4 days old.

PREGNANCY/LACTATION-RELATED

- Pregnancy category C.

MONITORING

PATIENTS MAINTAINING PATENT DUCTUS ARTERIOSUS

- **Baseline assessment:** Assess hemodynamic status and bleeding potential; monitor for respiratory distress.
- **Pediatric intensive care:** Treatment should be rendered by trained pediatric critical care practitioners.
- **Apnea:** Monitor for apnea which occurs in 10%-12% of patients; especially if less than 2 kg.
- **Arterial pressure:** Monitor arterial pressure for hypotension by auscultation, Doppler transducer, or umbilical artery catheter. Decrease the infusion rate immediately if a significant decrease in arterial pressure occurs.
- **Cardiac monitoring:** Maintain continuous cardiac monitoring.
- **Cardiopulmonary assessment:** Frequently assess heart sounds, femoral pulse (to monitor lower extremity circulation), respiratory status, BP, ABG values, and temperature.
- **Apnea and bradycardia:** If apnea or bradycardia occurs, discontinue infusion immediately and notify the physician.
- **Patient education:** Explain to parents the purpose of maintaining the patent ductus arteriosus for infants with pulmonary atresia, pulmonary stenosis, tricuspid atresia, tetralogy of Fallot, interruption of the aortic arch, coarctation of the aorta, or transposition of the great vessels.

PATIENTS WITH ERECTILE DYSFUNCTION OR IMPOTENCE

- **Onset of action:** Inform patients that their erection should occur within 2-5 min of administration.
- **Prolonged action:** Advise patients to notify the physician if their erection lasts longer than 4 hr or becomes painful.
- Warn patients with impotence not to use alprostadil if female sexual partners are pregnant unless a condom barrier is being used.

SERIOUS ADVERSE REACTIONS

- **Neurologic:** Cerebral bleeding, hypothermia, hyperirritability, hyperextension of the neck, seizures.
- **Cardiac:** Cardiac arrest occurs rarely.
- **Other symptoms:** Disseminated intravascular coagulation (DIC) and sepsis occur rarely.

OVERDOSE/TOXICITY

- **Respiratory:** Apnea, respiratory arrest.
- **Cardiovascular:** Bradycardia, cardiac arrest.
- **Associated findings:** Flushing of the face and arms.
- **Stop infusion:** Infusion should be stopped if serious reactions occur.
- **Manage arrest:** Manage respiratory and cardiac arrest according to Pediatric Advanced Life Support (PALS) guidelines for neonates.
- **Manage symptoms:** Symptoms must be managed on a case-by-case basis in critically ill neonates; supportive care for all body systems is rendered using accepted treatment guidelines.
- **Low probability of problems with erectile dysfunction:** Patients with erectile dysfunction are highly unlikely to experience toxicity or overdose.
- **GI decontamination:** No specific recommendations.

ANTIDOTE/DIALYSIS

- **Antidote:** No specific recommendations.
- **Dialysis:** Alprostadil is unlikely to be removed by hemodialysis and is not removed using high-permeability hemodialysis; no data are available on removal using peritoneal dialysis.

alteplase, recombinant 

al-teep'-lase

Classes

Chemical: tissue plasminogen activator (tPA)
Therapeutic: thrombolytic

Pregnancy Category: C

Trade Names

Prescription: Activase, Activase rt-PA ♣, Cathflo Activase

Do not confuse alteplase or Activase with Altace.

CLINICAL PHARMACOLOGY

Mechanism of Action

A tissue plasminogen activator that acts as a thrombolytic by binding to the fibrin in a thrombus and converting entrapped plasminogen to plasmin. This process initiates fibrinolysis. **Therapeutic Effect:** Degrades fibrin clots, fibrinogen, and other plasma proteins.

PHARMACOKINETICS

Rapidly metabolized in the liver. Primarily excreted in urine. Half-life: 35 min.

AVAILABILITY

Powder for Injection: 2 mg (Cathflo Activase), 50 mg (Activase), 100 mg (Activase).

INDICATIONS AND DOSAGE

Acute MI

IV Infusion

Adults weighing greater than 67 kg: 100 mg over 90 min, starting with 15-mg bolus over 1-2 min, then 50 mg over 30 min, then 35 mg over 60 min. Or a 3-hr infusion, giving 60 mg over first hr (6-10 mg as bolus over 1-2 min), 20 mg over second hr, and 20 mg over third hr. **Adults weighing 67 kg or less:** 1.25 mg/kg (total dose), starting with 15-mg bolus over 1-2 min, then 0.75 mg/kg over 30 min (maximum: 50 mg), then 0.5 mg/kg over 60 min (maximum: 35 mg). Or 3-hr infusion of 1.25 mg/kg giving 60% of dose over first hr (6%-10% as 1- to 2-min bolus), 20% over second hr, and 20% over third hr.

Acute pulmonary emboli

IV Infusion

Adults: 100 mg over 2 hr. Institute or reinstitute heparin near end or immediately after infusion when aPTT or thrombin time (TT) returns to twice normal or less.

Acute ischemic stroke

IV Infusion

Adults: 0.9 mg/kg over 60 min (load with 0.09 mg/kg [10% of 0.9 mg/kg dose] as IV bolus over 1 min). **Alert:** Dose must be given within the first 3 hr of the onset of symptoms.

Central venous catheter clearance

IV

Adults, Elderly: 2 mg; may repeat after 2 hr.

OFF-LABEL USES

Acute peripheral occlusive disease, basilar artery occlusion, cerebral infarction, deep vein thrombosis, femoropopliteal artery occlusion, mesenteric or subclavian vein occlusion, pleural effusion (parapneumonic)

CONTRAINDICATIONS

For use with pulmonary embolism (PE) and acute MI: Active internal bleeding, AV malformation or aneurysm, bleeding diathesis, intracranial neoplasm, intracranial or intraspinal surgery or trauma, recent (within past 2 mo) cerebrovascular accident, severe uncontrolled hypertension

For use with stroke: Intracranial or subarachnoid hemorrhage (or history of same), recent intraspinal or intracranial surgery, prolonged chest compressions, suspected aortic dissection, serious head trauma or previous stroke, seizure at time of stroke, active internal bleeding, intracranial neoplasm, arteriovenous malformation or aneurysm, known bleeding diathesis (including current use of anticoagulants) or INR greater than 1.7, administration of heparin within 48 hr preceding onset of stroke, elevated aPTT or low platelet count (less than 100,000/mm^3) at time of presentation, uncontrolled hypertension at time of presentation (systolic greater than 185 mmHg or diastolic greater than 110 mmHg), hypoglycemia (less than 50 mg/dL) or hyperglycemia (greater than 400 mg/dL)

INTERACTIONS

Drug: **Anticoagulants, enoxaparin, heparin, dalteparin:** May increase risk of hemorrhage. **Heparin:** Contraindicated when treating stroke; may use with acute MI and PE. **Platelet aggregation inhibitors, including aspirin, NSAIDs, ticlopidine:** May increase risk of bleeding. Herbal: The following may increase the risk of bleeding: Arnica, astragalus, bilberry, black currant, cat's claw, chaparral, dong quai, evening primrose, fenugreek, feverfew, garlic, ginger, ginkgo biloba, kava kava, licorice, tan-shen. Food: None known.

DIAGNOSTIC TEST EFFECTS

Decreases plasminogen and fibrinogen levels during infusion, which decreases clotting time (and confirms the presence of lysis). Decreases Hgb and Hct.

IV INCOMPATIBILITIES

*DOBUTamine (Dobutrex), *DOPamine (Intropin), heparin, nitroglycerin

IV COMPATIBILITIES

Lidocaine, metoprolol (Lopressor), morphine, nitroglycerin, propranolol (Inderal)

SIDE-EFFECTS

Frequent: Superficial bleeding at puncture sites, decreased BP. Occasional: Allergic reaction, such as rash or wheezing; bruising

CRITICAL CARE CONSIDERATIONS

ADMINISTRATION/HANDLING

SYSTEMIC IV ALERT

- **Storage:** Store vials at room temperature.

- **Preparation:** Reconstitute immediately before use with sterile water for injection.
- **Concentration:** Reconstitute 100-mg vial with 100 mL sterile water for injection (50-mg vial with 50 mL sterile water for injection) without preservative to provide a concentration of 1 mg/mL. May dilute further with equal volume D_5W or 0.9% NaCl to provide a concentration of 0.5 mg/mL.
- **Avoid shaking vial:** Gently swirl or slowly invert vial; avoid excessive agitation.
- **Color:** After reconstitution, solution normally appears colorless to pale yellow.
- **Stability:** Solution is stable for 8 hr after reconstitution. Discard unused portion.
- **Infusion pump:** Give by IV infusion via infusion pump. (See individual dosages above.)
- **Minor bleeding:** If minor bleeding occurs at the puncture site, apply pressure for 30 sec; if unrelieved, apply a pressure dressing.
- **Hemorrhage:** If uncontrolled hemorrhage occurs, discontinue the infusion immediately. Slowing the rate of infusion may worsen the hemorrhage.

CATHFLO ACTIVASE ALERT

- **Declotting a catheter:** Avoid undue pressure when injecting alteplase into the catheter because the catheter can rupture or expel a clot into circulation.
- **Storage:** Refrigerate unopened vials. Protect from light during extended storage.
- **Preparation:** Reconstitution immediately before use is recommended.
- **Stability:** Solution may be used up to 8 hr after reconstitution if refrigerated at 2°C to 30°C.

PRECAUTIONS

HEALTH-RELATED

- **Use cautiously in patients with risk of bleeding:** Recent (within past 10 days) major surgery or GI bleeding, organ biopsy, trauma, cerebrovascular disease, or cardiopulmonary resuscitation; in patients with diabetic retinopathy, endocarditis, left heart thrombus, occluded AV cannula or graft at infected site, severe hepatic or renal disease, or thrombophlebitis.

AGE-RELATED

- **Children:** Safety and efficacy of alteplase have not been established in children.
- **Elderly:** Use cautiously in the elderly. There is an increased risk of bleeding. Patients must be carefully selected and monitored.

PREGNANCY/LACTATION-RELATED

- Pregnancy category C; for stroke patients, alteplase is contraindicated for pregnant and breast-feeding women; unknown if excreted in breast milk.

MONITORING

PATIENTS WITH MI, PULMONARY EMBOLISM, OR ISCHEMIC STROKE

- **Baseline assessment:** Obtain baseline apical and peripheral pulse rates, BP, and record weight so that weight-based heparin dosage calculations can be done later as needed. Assess risk of bleeding for recent surgeries, trauma, stroke, poor blood glucose control, heart disease, kidney and liver disease.
- **Baseline diagnostic tests:** If alteplase is used to manage MI, evaluate 12-lead ECG, serum creatine kinase, and creatine kinase myocardial band (CK-MB) concentrations, and electrolyte levels. For stroke, a CT brain scan must be done to differentiate between hemorrhagic and ischemic stroke.
- **Lab work for all patients:** Assess for risk of bleeding before starting therapy with complete blood count and coagulation studies including thrombin time, aPTT, prothrombin time, and fibrinogen level. Biochemical profile including blood glucose for stroke patients; patients should be screened for liver and renal disease (BUN, creatinine, AST [SGOT], ALT [SGPT], bilirubin, alkaline phosphatase).
- **Ongoing lab work:** Monitor aPTT per facility protocol.
- **IV access:** Ensure three functional, large IV lines are in place before initiating infusion to avoid having to start an IV when patients are anticoagulated and prone to bleeding for injection sites.
- **Transfusion:** Expect to obtain a blood sample for blood type; screen and hold.
- **Myocardial infarction:** Ensure oxygen, aspirin, and nitroglycerin are received as appropriate before starting alteplase. Nitroglycerin infusion may continue.
- **Cardiac and pulse oximetry monitoring:** Perform continuous cardiac and pulse oximetry monitoring and assess for dysrhythmias in MI, pulmonary embolism, and ischemic stroke patients. Oxygen administration is recommended.
- **Vital signs:** Check BP, pulses, respiratory rate, and breath sounds every 15 min until stable; then check hourly to ensure

patients are not hypotensive, tachypneic, and tachycardic.

- **Relief of symptoms:** Monitor for relief of chest pain, shortness of breath, and improved neurologic status; notify physician if it continues or if condition deteriorates. Note symptoms' location, type, and intensity.
- **Bleeding risk:** Assess for bleeding, including overt blood and blood in body substances. Avoid procedures that may increase risk of bleeding such as IM injections or invasive procedures. Advise patients to report immediately signs of bleeding such as oozing from cuts or gums, hemoptysis, or hematuria.
- **Potential for intracranial bleeding:** Assess neurologic status frequently because the drug may cause intracranial hemorrhage.

PATIENTS WITH CLOTTED IV OR OTHER CENTRAL VENOUS ACCESS DEVICES (CVADs)

- Ensure appropriate volume of alteplase is inserted into clotted device by reading the volume of the device's lumen printed on the hub at the insertion site.
- Once alteplase has dwelled for the prescribed number of hours, aspirate medication before trying to flush the line to avoid systemically dosing the patient with alteplase.
- Restoration of CVAD function is assessed by the ability to withdraw blood.

SERIOUS ADVERSE REACTIONS

- **Hemorrhage:** Severe internal hemorrhage may occur. No incidence of intracranial hemorrhage has been reported with Cathflo Activase, but other bleeding events have been reported.
- **Reperfusion dysrhythmias:** Lysis of coronary thrombi may produce reperfusion-related atrial or ventricular dysrhythmias.
- **Use in stroke:** Alteplase is used to manage ischemic stroke but can cause hemorrhagic stroke.

OVERDOSE/TOXICITY

- **Bleeding:** If neurologic status deteriorates or if there is other hemorrhage, stop the infusion immediately. If bleeding is outside the cranium, blood transfusions should be given to replace lost red blood cells.
- **Management:** Replace clotting factors with cryoprecipitate and fresh frozen plasma to replace clotting factors depleted by plasmin. Replacing platelets should be considered if bleeding time is abnormal or dilutional thrombocytopenia occurs following massive blood transfusions for bleeding.
- **GI decontamination:** No specific recommendations.

ANTIDOTE/DIALYSIS

- **Antidote:** Consider antifibrinolytic agents (aminocaproic acid [Amicar] or tranexamic acid [Cyklocapron]) if transfusion therapy does not control bleeding.
- **Dialysis:** Alteplase is unlikely to be removed by hemodialysis and peritoneal dialysis. No data are available on removal by high-permeability hemodialysis.

aluminum hydroxide

a-loo'-mi-num hye-drox'-ide

Classes

Chemical: phosphate binder

Therapeutic: antacid; antidote; protectant, topical

Pregnancy Category: C

Trade Names

Over the Counter: Alternagel, Amphojel ♣, Basaljel ♣

CLINICAL PHARMACOLOGY

Mechanism of Action

An antacid that reduces gastric acid by binding with phosphate in the intestine and is then excreted as aluminum carbonate in feces; decreased serum phosphate levels may result in increased absorption of calcium. The drug also has astringent and adsorbent properties. **Therapeutic Effect:** Neutralizes or increases gastric pH; reduces phosphate levels in urine, preventing formation of phosphate urinary calculi; reduces the serum phosphate level; decreases the fluidity of stools.

PHARMACOKINETICS

Small amounts are absorbed from the intestine. Excreted in urine.

AVAILABILITY

Suspension: 320 mg/5 mL, 600 mg/5 mL (Alternagel only).

INDICATIONS AND DOSAGE

Antacid

PO

Adults, Elderly: 600-1200 mg between meals and at bedtime.

Hyperphosphatemia

PO

Adults, Elderly: Initially, 300-600 mg 3 times per day with meals. **Children:** Initially, 50-150 mg/kg/day in divided doses every 4-6 hr. Titrate to maintain serum phosphorus within normal range.

CONTRAINDICATIONS

People allergic to aluminum, intestinal obstruction

INTERACTIONS

Drug: **Iron preparations, isoniazid, ketoconazole, quinolones, tetracyclines, *cycloSPORINE, allopurinol, corticosteroids, mycophenalate, phenytoin, phenothiazines:** Decreases absorption of these drugs. **Methenamine:** May decrease effects of the methenamine. **Salicylate:** May increase salicylate excretion. Herbal: None known. Food: None known.

DIAGNOSTIC TEST EFFECTS

May increase the serum gastrin level and systemic and urinary pH. May decrease the serum phosphate level.

SIDE-EFFECTS

Frequent: Chalky taste, mild constipation, abdominal cramps. Occasional: Nausea, vomiting, speckling or whitish discoloration of stools

CRITICAL CARE CONSIDERATIONS

ADMINISTRATION/HANDLING

PO ALERT

- The usual dose of aluminum hydroxide is 30-60 mL.
- Administer aluminum hydroxide 1-3 hr after meals and at bedtime.
- Expect the dosage to be individualized based on the antacid's neutralizing capacity.
- Instruct patients to chew chewable tablets (combination forms) thoroughly before swallowing and then to drink a glass of water or milk.
- Shake the suspension well before use.

PRECAUTIONS

HEALTH-RELATED

- Use cautiously in patients with Alzheimer's disease, chronic diarrhea, constipation, dehydration, fecal impaction, fluid restrictions, gastric outlet obstruction, GI or rectal bleeding, impaired renal function, or symptoms of appendicitis.
- Prolonged use in renal failure patients may worsen dialysis osteomalacia and may cause encephalopathy related to elevated levels of aluminum.

AGE-RELATED

- **Children:** Aluminum hydroxide is contraindicated for children aged 6 yr or younger.
- **Elderly:** Use aluminum hydroxide cautiously in elderly patients.

PREGNANCY/LACTATION-RELATED

- Pregnancy category C (considered safe except for chronic, high-dose use).

MONITORING

- **Baseline assessment:** Assess for history of gastric acidity or heartburn.
- **Lab work:** Monitor serum aluminum, calcium, phosphate, and uric acid levels.
- **Withhold other medications:** Do not give other oral drugs within 1 to 2 hr of antacid administration.
- **Constipation:** Assess pattern of daily bowel activity and stool consistency.
- **Hydration:** Provide fluids to promote better elimination.
- **Response to drug:** Evaluate and document relief from gastric distress.
- **Patient education:** Instruct patients to chew chewable tablets (combination forms) thoroughly before swallowing and then to drink a glass of water or milk. Inform patients that stool discoloration may occur but will resolve when the drug is discontinued.

SERIOUS ADVERSE REACTIONS

- **Bowel obstruction:** Prolonged constipation may result in intestinal obstruction.
- **Bone destruction:** Excessive or chronic use may produce hypophosphatemia manifested as anorexia, malaise, muscle weakness, or bone pain, which may result in osteomalacia and osteoporosis.
- **Kidney stones:** Prolonged use may produce urinary calculi.

OVERDOSE/TOXICITY

- **Toxicity:** Toxic encephalopathy and worsening of dialysis osteomalacia may result from high levels of aluminum.
- **Signs of toxicity:** Constipation, colickly abdominal pain, anorexia, nausea, GI irritation, skin problems.
- **Aluminum level:** Plasma aluminum level should be obtained if toxicity is suspected.
- **GI decontamination:** No specific recommendations.

ANTIDOTE/DIALYSIS

- **Antidote:** Calcium disodium edentate (EDTA) is the main drug used to bind aluminum using chelation therapy, which facilitates excretion of aluminum in the urine. Should be used with caution for patients with renal insufficiency. Other medications used with lesser aluminum binding effects include tetracycline and deferoxamine.
- **Dialysis:** Hemodialysis does not remove aluminum well because it is bound to albumin and transferrin. There are no data on removal using high-permeability hemodialysis or peritoneal dialysis.

amantadine hydrochloride

See Antivirals (p. 937)

amikacin sulfate

am-i-kay'-sin sul'-fate

Classes
Chemical: aminoglycoside
Therapeutic: antibiotic

Pregnancy Category: D

Trade Names
Prescription: Amikin

Do not confuse amikacin or Amikin with Amicar.

CLINICAL PHARMACOLOGY

Mechanism of Action

An aminoglycoside antibiotic that irreversibly binds to protein on bacterial ribosomes. **Therapeutic Effect:** Interferes with protein synthesis of susceptible microorganisms.

PHARMACOKINETICS

Rapid, complete absorption after IM administration. Protein binding: 0%-10%. Widely distributed (does not cross the blood-brain barrier, low concentrations in cerebrospinal fluid). Excreted unchanged in urine. Removed by hemodialysis. **Half-life:** 2-4 hr (increased in impaired renal function and neonates; decreased in cystic fibrosis and burn or febrile patients).

AVAILABILITY

Injection: 50 mg/mL (Amikin Pediatric), 62.5 mg/mL (Amikin), 250 mg/mL (Amikin).

INDICATIONS AND DOSAGE

Moderate to severe infections

IV, IM

Adults, Elderly: 15 mg/kg/day in divided doses every 8-12 hr. Maximum 1.5 g/day. **Children, Infants:** 15-22.5 mg/kg/day in divided doses every 8 hr. Maximum 1.5 g/day. **Neonates:** 7.5-10 mg/kg/dose every 8-24 hr.

Dosage in renal impairment

Dosage and frequency are modified based on the degree of renal impairment and serum drug concentration. After a loading dose of 5-7.5 mg/kg, the maintenance dose and frequency are based on serum creatinine levels and creatinine clearance.

CONTRAINDICATIONS

Hypersensitivity to amikacin, other aminoglycosides (cross-sensitivity), or their components.

INTERACTIONS

Drug: Nephrotoxic medications, other aminoglycosides, ototoxic medications: May increase the risk of nephrotoxicity or ototoxicity. **Neuromuscular blockers:** May enhance neuromuscular blockade. **Herbal:** None known. **Food:** None known.

DIAGNOSTIC TEST EFFECTS

May increase serum bilirubin, BUN, serum creatinine, serum LDH, AST (SGOT), and ALT (SGPT), levels. May decrease serum calcium, magnesium, potassium, and sodium concentrations. Therapeutic peak serum level is greater than 30 mcg/mL; toxic trough serum level is greater than 10 mcg/mL.

IV INCOMPATIBILITIES

Amphotericin, ampicillin, cefazolin (Ancef), heparin, propofol (Diprivan)

IV COMPATIBILITIES

Amiodarone (Cordarone), aztreonam (Azactam), calcium gluconate, cefepime (Maxipime), cimetidine (Tagamet), ciprofloxacin (Cipro), clindamycin (Cleocin), diltiazem (Cardizem), enalapril (Vasotec), esmolol (BreviBloc), fluconazole (Diflucan), furosemide (Lasix), levofloxacin (Levaquin), lorazepam (Ativan), magnesium sulfate, midazolam (Versed), morphine, ondansetron (Zofran), potassium chloride, ranitidine (Zantac), total parenteral nutrition (TPN), vancomycin

SIDE-EFFECTS

Frequent: IM: Pain, induration
IV: Phlebitis, thrombophlebitis. **Occasional:** Hypersensitivity reactions (rash, fever, urticaria, pruritus), nephrotoxicity. **Rare:** Neuromuscular blockade (difficulty breathing, drowsiness, weakness), ototoxicity (auditory and vestibular).

CRITICAL CARE CONSIDERATIONS

ADMINISTRATION/HANDLING

DOSING ALERT

- **Dosing:** Space amikacin doses evenly around the clock.
- Drug dosage is based on ideal body weight.
- Peak and trough serum levels are determined periodically to maintain desired serum concentrations and minimize the risk of amikacin toxicity.

IV ALERT

- **Storage:** Store vials at room temperature.
- Solutions normally appear clear but may become pale yellow; the yellow color does not affect the drug's potency. Discard the solution if a precipitate forms or dark discoloration occurs.
- **Stability:** Intermittent IV infusion (piggyback) is stable for 24 hr at room temperature.
- **Dilution:** Dilute each 500 mg with 100 mL of 0.9% NaCl or D_5W.
- **Infusion:** Infuse over 30-60 min for adults and older children. Infuse over 60-120 min for infants and young children.

IM ALERT

- Give deep IM injections slowly to minimize patient discomfort. Injections administered into the gluteus maximus are less painful than those given in the lateral aspect of the thigh.

PRECAUTIONS

HEALTH-RELATED

- **Neurologic diseases:** Use amikacin cautiously in patients with eighth cranial nerve (vestibulocochlear nerve) impairment, myasthenia gravis, or Parkinson's disease.
- **Renal insufficiency:** Amikacin is excreted via glomerular filtration. Use with extreme caution in renal impaired patients.

AGE-RELATED

- **Children:** Use with extreme caution in neonates and premature infants who may be more susceptible to amikacin toxicity because of their immature renal function.
- **Elderly:** Elderly patients are at increased risk for amikacin toxicity, including ototoxicity because of age-related renal impairment. Half-life is prolonged. Consider less toxic alternative medications.

PREGNANCY/LACTATION-RELATED

- Pregnancy category C; although fetal ototoxicity has occurred after in utero exposure to other aminoglycosides, eighth cranial nerve toxicity has not been reported with amikacin; excreted into breast milk in low concentrations; poor oral bioavailability reduces potential for ototoxicity for the infant

MONITORING

- **Baseline assessment:** Determine history of allergies, especially to aminoglycosides and sulfites.
- **Lab work:** Monitor urinalysis results to detect casts, RBCs, WBCs, and decreased specific gravity. Monitor peak and trough serum amikacin levels. Steady-state drug levels are reached in 10 to 15 hr. Inform patients that laboratory tests are an essential part of therapy.
- **Peak/trough levels:** Assess drug levels. Therapeutic peak level is 20-30 mcg/mL; therapeutic trough level is 1-9 mcg/mL. Toxic peak level is greater than 35 mcg/mL; toxic trough level is greater than 10 mcg/mL (adult) and greater than 5 ng/mL (child).
- **Hydration:** Correct dehydration before beginning aminoglycoside therapy. Monitor intake and output to maintain hydration.
- **Potential for hearing loss:** Establish baseline hearing acuity before beginning therapy. Be alert for ototoxic side effects.
- **Identify infecting organism:** Obtain a specimen for culture and sensitivity testing before giving the first dose. Therapy may begin before test results are known.
- **Neurotoxic side effects:** Monitor for neurotoxic side effects including hearing, visual, balance, or urinary problems, even if they start after therapy is completed.
- **IM administration:** Assess for pain and induration at the IM injection site. Warn the patient that IM injection may cause discomfort. Evaluate the IV infusion site for

signs and symptoms of phlebitis, such as heat, pain, and red streaking over the vein.
- **Rash:** Inspect the skin for a rash.
- **Superinfection with fungus:** Be alert for signs and symptoms of superinfection, particularly changes in the oral mucosa, diarrhea, and genital or anal pruritus.
- **Potential for respiratory depression:** In patients with neuromuscular disorders, assess the respiratory response carefully.
- **Patient education:** Explain to patients the importance of receiving the full course of amikacin treatment. Caution patients not to take any other drugs without first discussing with the prescriber.

SERIOUS ADVERSE REACTIONS
- Aminoglycoside toxicity is possible at normal trough levels; half-life is 1.9-2.8 hr.
- If minor side effects persist or major symptoms appear, discontinue amikacin.
- Monitor fluid balance, creatinine clearance, and plasma levels carefully.
- Dosage should be reduced in chronic renal failure patients.

OVERDOSE/TOXICITY
- **Nephrotoxicity:** Increased thirst, decreased appetite, nausea, vomiting, increased BUN and serum creatinine levels, decreased creatinine clearance, albuminuria.
- **Neurotoxicity:** Manifested as muscle twitching, visual disturbances, tingling, seizures, and neuromuscular blockade.
- **Ototoxicity:** Tinnitus, dizziness, and loss of hearing.
- **Management:** Complexation with ticarcillin may be as effective as hemodialysis. Consider exchange transfusion in newborns.
- **GI decontamination:** No specific recommendations.

ANTIDOTE/DIALYSIS
- **Antidote:** Neuromuscular blockade using calcium salts or neostigmine may reverse symptoms.
- **Dialysis:** Amikacin is removed by hemodialysis and peritoneal dialysis and is likely to be removed by high-permeability hemodialysis.

amiloride hydrochloride
See Diuretics (p. 956)

aminocaproic acid
a-mee-noe-ka-proe'-ik as'-id

Classes
Chemical: monoaminocarboxylic acid, synthetic
Therapeutic: hemostatic

Pregnancy Category: C

Trade Names
Prescription: Amicar

Do not confuse Amicar with amikacin or Amikin.

CLINICAL PHARMACOLOGY
Mechanism of Action
A systemic hemostatic that acts as an antifibrinolytic and antihemorrhagic by inhibiting the activation of plasminogen activator substances. **Therapeutic Effect:** Prevents formation of fibrin clots.

PHARMACOKINETICS
Rapidly absorbed following PO administration. Does not appear to bind to plasma protein. Excreted rapidly in urine, mostly unchanged. **Half-life:** 2 hr.

AVAILABILITY
Syrup: 250 mg/mL.
Tablets: 500 mg.
Injection: 250 mg/mL.

INDICATIONS AND DOSAGE
Acute bleeding
PO, IV Infusion
Adults, Elderly: 4-5 g over first hr; then 1-1.25 g/hr. Continue for 8 hr or until bleeding is controlled. Maximum: 30 g/24 hr. **Children:** 100-200 mg/kg for 1 hr, then 33.3 mg/kg/hr; 100 mg/kg every 6 hr PO or IV.
Dosage in renal impairment
Decrease dose to 25% of normal.

OFF-LABEL USES
Control of bleeding in thrombocytopenia, control of oral bleeding in congenital and acquired coagulation disorders, prevention of recurrence of subarachnoid hemorrhage, prevention of hemorrhage in hemophiliacs following dental surgery, treatment of traumatic hyphema

CONTRAINDICATIONS
Evidence of active intravascular clotting process, disseminated intravascular coagulation without concurrent heparin therapy, hematuria

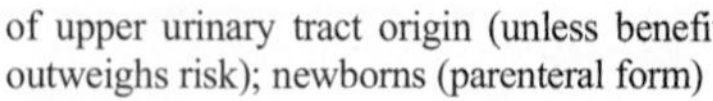

of upper urinary tract origin (unless benefit outweighs risk); newborns (parenteral form)

INTERACTIONS

Drug: Antiinhibitor coagulant complex, tretinoin: may increase the risk of thrombosis. **Herbal:** None known. **Food:** None known.

DIAGNOSTIC TEST EFFECTS

May elevate serum potassium level.

IV INCOMPATIBILITIES

Sodium lactate

SIDE-EFFECTS

Occasional: Nausea, diarrhea, cramps, decreased urination, decreased BP, dizziness, headache, muscle fatigue and weakness, myopathy, bloodshot eyes

CRITICAL CARE CONSIDERATIONS

ADMINISTRATION/HANDLING

PO ALERT

- Store tablets in a tight container. Protect syrup from freezing.
- Syrup may be given as an oral rinse for the control of bleeding during dental and oral surgery in hemophilic patients.

IV ALERT

- Do not give aminocaproic acid by direct injection.
- **Dilution:** Dilute each 1 g in up to 50 mL 0.9% NaCl, D_5W, Ringer's solution, or sterile water for injection. Do not use sterile water for injection in patients with subarachnoid hemorrhage.
- **IV infusion:** Give only by IV infusion. Infuse 5 g or less over the first hr in 250 mL of solution. Give each succeeding 1 g over 1 hr in 50 to 100 mL of solution. Too rapid infusion may produce dysrhythmias, including bradycardia.

PRECAUTIONS

HEALTH-RELATED

- Use aminocaproic acid cautiously in patients with hyperfibrinolysis or impaired cardiac, hepatic, or renal function.
- Administer a reduced dose if there is cardiac, renal, or hepatic impairment.

AGE-RELATED

- **Children:** Safety has not been established in children; no documented evidence of adverse effects.
- **Elderly:** Cautious use is advised due to risk of age-related renal impairment that may require dosage reduction.

PREGNANCY/LACTATION-RELATED

- Pregnancy category C; excretion in milk unknown; use caution in nursing mothers

MONITORING

- **Baseline assessment:** Obtain vital signs and assess neurologic status before and regularly during therapy. Monitor for hypotension before and during the infusion.
- **Baseline lab work:** CBC including platelet count; biochemical profile including renal and liver function tests and CPK; clotting studies (prothrombin time, aPTT, bleeding time, and disseminated intravascular coagulation [DIC] profile, as appropriate for diagnosis).
- **Ongoing lab work:** Monitor for increased serum creatine kinase (CPK) and AST (SGOT) levels daily to determine development of a skeletal myopathy.
- **Myopathy:** Assess for development of severe and continuous muscular pain or weakness, which may indicate myopathy.
- **Bleeding:** Monitor for hypotension and tachycardia, abdominal or back pain, hematuria, and severe headache indicative of hemorrhage. Check for ecchymoses, excessive bleeding from minor cuts or scratches, and petechiae; monitor female patients for increased menstrual flow; evaluate the gums for erythema and gingival bleeding.
- **Clotting:** Monitor for signs of clotting including symptoms of stroke, MI, peripheral arterial occlusion, acute renal failure, pulmonary embolus, bowel infarction.
- **Patient education:** Instruct patients to report red or dark urine, black or red stool, coffee-ground vomitus, blood-tinged mucus from cough, or any signs of abnormal bleeding and/or clotting. Patients should also promptly report muscle pain or weakness to a health care provider.

SERIOUS ADVERSE REACTIONS

- **Too rapid IV administration:** Produces tinnitus, rash, dysrhythmias, unusual fatigue, and weakness.
- **Grand mal seizure:** Rarely occurs, generally preceded by weakness, dizziness, and headache.

OVERDOSE/TOXICITY

- **Symptoms:** Muscle weakness, thrombophlebitis, thrombus formation, thromboembolism resulting in possible stroke, acute MI, pulmonary embolism, or loss

of perfusion to extremities or abdominal organs.
- **Management:** Immediate discontinuation of aminocaproic acid.
- **GI decontamination:** No specific recommendations.

ANTIDOTE/DIALYSIS
- **Antidote:** No specific antidote recommended because patients are often being treated for overactivity of the fibrinolytic system.
- **Dialysis:** Aminocaproic acid is removed by hemodialysis and peritoneal dialysis. No data are available on removal by high-permeability hemodialysis.

amiodarone hydrochloride

a-mee'-oh-da-rone hye-droe-klor'-ide

Classes
Chemical: iodinated benzofuran derivative
Therapeutic: antidysrhythmic, class III

Pregnancy Category: D

Trade Names
Prescription: Cordarone, Cordarone IV, Pacerone

Do not confuse amiodarone with amiloride or Cordarone with Cardura.

CLINICAL PHARMACOLOGY
Mechanism of Action
A cardiac agent that prolongs duration of myocardial cell action potential and refractory period by acting directly on all cardiac tissue. Decreases AV and sinus node function. **Therapeutic Effect:** Suppresses dysrhythmias.

PHARMACOKINETICS

Route	Onset	Peak	Duration
PO	3 days-3 wk	1 wk-5 mo	7-50 days after discontinuation

Slowly, variably absorbed from GI tract. Protein binding: 96%. Extensively metabolized in the liver to active metabolite. Excreted via bile; not removed by hemodialysis. **Half-life:** 26-107 days; metabolite, 61 days.

AVAILABILITY
Tablets: 100 mg (Pacerone), 200 mg (Cordarone, Pacerone), 300 mg, 400 mg (Pacerone).
Injection (Cordarone IV): 50 mg/mL.

INDICATIONS AND DOSAGE
Life-threatening recurrent ventricular fibrillation or hemodynamically unstable ventricular tachycardia
PO
Adults, Elderly: Initially, 800-1600 mg/day in 1-2 divided doses for 1-3 wk. After dysrhythmia is controlled or side effects occur, reduce to 600-800 mg/day for about 4 wk. Maintenance: 200-600 mg/day **Children:** Initially, 10-20 mg/kg/day in 1-2 doses for 4-14 days, then 5 mg/kg/day for several wk. Maintenance: 2.5 mg/kg/day or lowest effective maintenance dose for 5 of 7 days/wk.
IV Infusion
Adults: Initially, 1050 mg over 24 hr; 150 mg over 10 min, then 360 mg over 6 hr; then 540 mg over 18 hr. May continue at 0.5 mg/min for up to 2-3 wk regardless of age or renal or left ventricular function.

OFF-LABEL USES
Control of hemodynamically stable ventricular tachycardia, control of rapid ventricular rate due to accessory pathway conduction in preexcited atrial dysrhythmias, conversion of atrial fibrillation to normal sinus rhythm, in cardiac arrest with persistent ventricular tachycardia or ventricular fibrillation, paroxysmal supraventricular tachycardia, polymorphic ventricular tachycardia or wide complex tachycardia of uncertain origin, prevention of postoperative atrial fibrillation

CONTRAINDICATIONS
Bradycardia-induced syncope (except in the presence of a pacemaker), second- and third-degree AV block, severe hepatic disease, severe sinus-node dysfunction, pregnancy, hypersensitivity to amiodarone

INTERACTIONS
Drug: Antidysrhythmics, fluoroquinolones, macrolides, haloperidol: May increase cardiac effects. **Antiretrovirals:** Use is contraindicated with amprenavir, indinavir, nelfinavir, ritonavir, saquinavir, tipranavir. **Beta-blockers:** May increase effect of beta-blockers. **Digoxin, fosphenytoin, phenytoin:** May increase drug concentration and risk of toxicity of digoxin, fosphenytoin, and phenytoin. **Fluroquinolones (grepafloxacin, sparafloxacin):** Use is contraindicated. **HMG-CoA reductase inhibitors:** Concurrent use of amiodarone with lovastatin or simvastatin is not recommended. **Warfarin:** Increased risk of hemorrhage. **Ziprasidone:** Use is contraindicated. **Herbal:** St. John's wort, ephedra, dong quai **Food:** Grapefruit juice increases amiodarone effects.

DIAGNOSTIC TEST EFFECTS

May increase antinuclear antibody titers and AST (SGOT), ALT (SGPT), and serum alkaline phosphatase levels. May cause changes in ECG and thyroid function test results. Therapeutic serum level is 0.5-2.5 mcg/mL; toxic serum level has not been established.

IV INCOMPATIBILITIES

Aminophylline (theophylline), cefazolin (Ancef), heparin, sodium bicarbonate

IV COMPATIBILITIES

Dobutamine (Dobutrex), dopamine (Intropin), furosemide (Lasix), insulin (regular), labetalol (Normodyne), lidocaine, midazolam (Versed), morphine, nitroglycerin, norepinephrine (Levophed), phenylephrine (Neo-Synephrine), potassium chloride, vancomycin

SIDE-EFFECTS

Expected: Corneal microdeposits are noted in almost all patients treated for more than 6 mo (can lead to blurry vision), photosensitivity. **Frequent (greater than 3%): Parenteral:** Hypotension, nausea, fever, bradycardia. **Oral:** Constipation, cough, headache, decreased appetite, fever, malaise, nausea, vomiting, paresthesias, muscular incoordination, pulmonary fibrosis (2%-7%), visual disturbances/halos around lights (2%-9%). **Occasional (less than 3%): Oral:** Bitter or metallic taste; decreased libido; dizziness; facial flushing; blue-gray coloring of skin (face, arms, and neck); blurred vision; bradycardia; asymptomatic corneal deposits. **Rare (less than 1%): Oral:** Rash, vision loss, blindness, pulmonary fibrosis

CRITICAL CARE CONSIDERATIONS

ADMINISTRATION/HANDLING

DOSAGE ALERT

- Because the half-life of amiodarone is 28 days, if the patient experiences side effects or signs of toxicity, symptoms may persist for weeks.

PO ALERT

- Give amiodarone with meals to reduce GI distress.
- Tablets may be crushed if necessary.

IV ALERT

- **Storage:** Store at room temperature.
- **Cardiac arrest (unlabelled) (pulseless ventricular tachycardia or ventricular fibrillation):** Loading dose (up to 300 mg or 5 mg/kg) or supplemental boluses may be given undiluted.
- **Dilution:** Use glass or polyolefin containers for dilution.
- **Dilute loading dose:** 150 mg in 100 mL D_5W to yield a solution of 1.5 mg/mL.
- **Dilute maintenance dose:** 900 mg in 500 mL D_5W to yield a solution of 1.8 mg/mL. Solutions greater than 3 mg/mL can cause peripheral vein phlebitis.
- **Stability:** Use solutions held in PVC containers within 2 hr of dilution. Use solutions held in glass or polyolefin containers within 24 hr of dilution.
- **Light:** The solution does not need protection from light during administration.
- **Central venous catheter preferred:** Give amiodarone through a CVC if possible, using an inline filter.
- **Dosing:** Give a bolus of 150 mg over 10 min (15 mg/min) not to exceed 30 mg/min; then 360 mg over 6 hr (1 mg/min); then 540 mg at a rate of 0.5 mg/min over 18 hr. For infusions lasting longer than 1 hr, drug concentration should not exceed 2 mg/mL unless a CVC is used.

PRECAUTIONS

HEALTH-RELATED

- Use amiodarone cautiously in patients with thyroid disease, significant visual impairment, restrictive lung disease, cardiomyopathy, left ventricular dysfunction, AV heart block, and liver disease as it may worsen these conditions.
- **Hypokalemia and hypomagnesemia:** Should be corrected before use to reduce the chance of lethal dysrhythmias.
- **Ritonavir (Norvir):** Amiodarone should not be administered to patients taking ritonavir.
- **Ibutilide (Corvert):** Amiodarone should not be administered to patients taking ibutilide.

AGE-RELATED

- **Infants and neonates:** A manufacturer's warning has been issued citing potentially fatal or developmental side effects in infants and neonates.
- **Children:** Safety and efficacy of amiodarone have not been established in children.
- **Elderly:** Elderly may be more sensitive to amiodarone's effects on thyroid function and are more likely to have pulmonary toxicity and have increased incidence of ataxia or other neurotoxic effects. The half-life can be doubled (up to 47 days) in the elderly.

A

PREGNANCY/LACTATION-RELATED

- Pregnancy category D; due to a very long $t_{1/2}$, amiodarone should be discontinued several months before conception to avoid early gestational exposure, reserve for refractory dysrhythmias; newborns exposed to amiodarone should have TFTs; excreted into breast milk; contains high proportions of iodine; breast-feeding not recommended.

MONITORING

- **Baseline assessment:** Assess history of management of dysrhythmias and any breathing difficulties. Hypotension is common with initial dosing and bradycardia may occur. Assess vital signs immediately before giving amiodarone. Withhold medication and notify the physician if the apical or radial pulse rate is less than 60 beats/min or systolic BP is less than 90 mmHg.
- **Baseline diagnostic tests:** Chest X-ray, ECG, and pulmonary function tests because the drug can cause pulmonary fibrosis.
- **Baseline lab work:** Biochemical profile including liver enzyme levels (AST [SGOT], ALT [SGPT], and serum alkaline phosphatase).
- **Ongoing lab work:** Amiodarone blood level. Serum alkaline phosphatase, AST (SGOT) and ALT (SGPT) levels, hepatic and thyroid function tests for evidence of toxicity. Reduce dosage or discontinue amiodarone if toxicity is evident or liver enzyme levels are elevated per physician orders.
- **Therapeutic blood level:** 0.5 to 2.5 mcg/mL; amiodarone's toxic level has not been established.
- **Pulmonary toxicity:** Assess for respiratory distress, progressively worsening cough, dyspnea, and activity intolerance if amiodarone has been used at high doses or before admission. Discontinue or reduce the dosage of amiodarone if toxicity occurs per physician orders.
- **Thyroid disease assessment:** Dosage may need adjustment or an alternative medication may be warranted to avoid exacerbation of thyroid problems.
- **Baseline hyperthyroidism:** Assess for difficulty breathing, exophthalmos, eyelid edema, frequent urination, fever, dry skin, and weight loss.
- **Baseline hypothyroidism:** Assess for cool, pale skin, lethargy, night cramps, periorbital edema, and edema of the hands and feet.
- **Pulse:** Assess for bradycardia, irregular rhythm, and quality.
- **ECG:** Amiodarone can cause torsades de pointes. Monitor for changes such as widening of the QRS complex and prolonged PR and QT intervals. Obtain a 12-lead ECG if significant interval changes are noted.
- **Nausea and vomiting:** Manage per accepted standards.
- **Possible bluish discoloration of the skin and cornea:** Assess patients receiving amiodarone for longer than 2 mo for this side effect. Inform patients the bluish discoloration gradually disappears after amiodarone is discontinued.
- **Patient education:** Instruct not to discontinue amiodarone abruptly. Explain that compliance with the prescribed therapy is essential to control dysrhythmias. Do not take amiodarone with grapefruit juice, which causes increased plasma concentrations of amiodarone. Teach patients to monitor their pulse before taking amiodarone, to report shortness of breath or cough, to limit exposure to sunlight to protect against photosensitivity. Advise patients to report any vision changes to a health care provider immediately. Recommend ophthalmic exams every 6 mo.

SERIOUS ADVERSE REACTIONS

- **Cardiac:** Hypotension (common), cardiogenic shock, congestive heart failure.
- **Dysrhythmias:** Amiodarone prolongs the QT interval, may worsen existing dysrhythmias or produce new dysrhythmias (proarrhythmia) including torsades de pointes.
- **Pulmonary:** Pulmonary toxicity may begin with progressive dyspnea and cough with crackles, decreased breath sounds, pleurisy, heart failure, or hepatotoxicity.
- **Hepatotoxicity:** Elevated liver enzymes (ALT [SGPT], AST [SGOT], GGT), which can lead to liver failure.
- **Thyroid dysfunction:** Exacerbation of hypothyroidism or hyperthyroidism.
- **Hematologic:** Neutropenia, pancytopenia, aplastic anemia, hemolytic anemia.

OVERDOSE/TOXICITY

- **Pulmonary toxicity:** Alveolitis, pulmonary fibrosis, pneumonitis, acute respiratory distress syndrome.
- **Severe lethal dysrhythmias:** Prolonged QT interval leading to torsades de pointes, bradycardia, or progressive AV heart block. Infusion rate should be stopped if lethal dysrhythmias occur.

- **Cardiac pacemaker:** Transcutaneous pacing device should be available for patients with bradycardia or heart block. Atrial overdrive pacing may be needed to stabilize cardiac rhythm.
- **Dysrhythmias:** Should be managed according to Advanced Cardiac Life Support (ACLS) guidelines.
- **Management:** For torsades de pointes, stop all cardiac drugs (antidysrhythmic agents, digoxin) and cardioactive drugs such as phenothiazines and antidepressants. Potassium and magnesium should be normalized if levels are abnormal. Vasopressors such as norepinephrine or dopamine may be needed to manage hypotension along with fluid volume expansion.
- **28-day half-life:** Toxic effects remain for a prolonged period of time.
- **GI decontamination:** No specific recommendations.

ANTIDOTE/DIALYSIS

- **Antidote:** No specific recommendations.
- **Dialysis:** Amiodarone is not removed by hemodialysis and peritoneal dialysis. No data are available on removal using high-permeability hemodialysis.

amitriptyline hydrochloride

a-mee-trip′-ti-leen hye-droe-klor′-ide

Classes

Chemical: dibenzocycloheptene derivative, tertiary amine

Therapeutic: antidepressant, tricyclic, antineurologic, anxiolytic

Pregnancy Category: C

Trade Names

Prescription: Apo-Amitriptyline ♣, Elavil, Levate ♣

Combinations

Prescription: with chlordiazepoxide (Limbitrol); with perphenazine (Triavil)

Do not confuse amitriptyline with aminophylline or nortriptyline, or Elavil with Equanil or Mellaril.

CLINICAL PHARMACOLOGY

Mechanism of Action

A tricyclic antidepressant that blocks the reuptake of neurotransmitters, including norepinephrine and serotonin, at presynaptic membranes, thus increasing their availability at postsynaptic receptor sites. Also has strong anticholinergic activity. **Therapeutic Effect:** Relieves depression.

PHARMACOKINETICS

Rapidly and well absorbed from the GI tract. Protein binding: 90%. Undergoes first-pass metabolism in the liver. Primarily excreted in urine. Minimal removal by hemodialysis. **Half-life:** 10-26 hr.

AVAILABILITY

Tablets (Elavil): 10 mg, 25 mg, 50 mg, 75 mg, 100 mg, 150 mg.

INDICATIONS AND DOSAGE

Depression

PO

Adults: 50-150 mg/day as a single dose at bedtime or in divided doses. May gradually increase up to 300 mg/day. Titrate to lowest effective dosage. **Elderly:** Initially, 10-25 mg at bedtime. May increase by 10-25 mg at weekly intervals. Range: 25-150 mg/day. **Children 6-12 yr:** 1-5 mg/kg/day in 2 divided doses.

Pain management

PO

Adults, Elderly: 25-100 mg at bedtime.

OFF-LABEL USES

Relief of neuropathic pain, such as that experienced by patients with diabetic neuropathy or postherpetic neuralgia; treatment of anxiety, bulimia nervosa, migraine, nocturnal enuresis, panic disorder, peptic ulcer

CONTRAINDICATIONS

Acute recovery period after MI, use within 14 days of MAOIs, hypersensitivity to amitriptyline

INTERACTIONS

Drug: **Antithyroid agents:** May increase the risk of agranulocytosis. **Cimetidine, valproic acid:** May increase amitriptyline blood concentration and risk of toxicity. **Clonidine, guanadrel:** May decrease the effects of these drugs. **CNS depressants (including alcohol, anticonvulsants, barbiturates, phenothiazines, and sedative-hypnotics):** May increase CNS and respiratory depression and the hypotensive effects of amitriptyline. **MAOIs:** May increase the risk of neuroleptic malignant syndrome, seizures, hypertensive crisis, and hyperpyresis. **Phenothiazines:** May increase the sedative and anticholinergic effects of amitriptyline. **Sympathomimetics:** May increase the risk of cardiac effects. **Herbal:** None known. **Food:** None known.

DIAGNOSTIC TEST EFFECTS

May alter blood glucose levels and ECG readings. Therapeutic serum drug level is 120-250 ng/mL; toxic serum drug level is greater than 500 ng/mL.

SIDE-EFFECTS

Frequent: Dizziness, somnolence, dry mouth, orthostatic hypotension, headache, increased appetite, weight gain, nausea, unusual fatigue, unpleasant taste. **Occasional**: Blurred vision, confusion, constipation, hallucinations, delayed micturition, eye pain, dysrhythmias, fine muscle tremors, parkinsonian syndrome, anxiety, diarrhea, diaphoresis, heartburn, insomnia. **Rare**: Hypersensitivity, alopecia, tinnitus, breast enlargement, photosensitivity

CRITICAL CARE CONSIDERATIONS

ADMINISTRATION/HANDLING

DOSING ALERT

- Make sure at least 14 days elapse between the use of MAOIs and amitriptyline.

PO ALERT

- Give amitriptyline tablets with food or milk if GI distress occurs.

PRECAUTIONS

HEALTH-RELATED

- Use amitriptyline cautiously in patients with cardiovascular disease, diabetes mellitus, glaucoma, hiatal hernia, history of seizures, history of urine retention or urinary obstruction, hyperthyroidism, increased IOP, hepatic or renal disease, benign prostatic hyperplasia, or schizophrenia.

AGE-RELATED

- **Children:** More sensitive to an acute overdose and are at increased risk for amitriptyline toxicity. Only off-label uses are not recommended for children under 12 yr.
- **Elderly:** More sensitive to the drug's anticholinergic effects and are at increased risk for amitriptyline toxicity.

PREGNANCY/LACTATION-RELATED

- Pregnancy category C; excreted into breast milk; effect on nursing infant unknown but may be of concern.

MONITORING

- **Baseline assessment:** Observe and document appearance, behavior, interest in the environment, mood, and sleep pattern.
- **Lab work:** CBC and blood chemistry profile before and periodically during therapy, especially with long-term use.
- **Suicide:** Closely supervise patients at risk for suicide during early therapy. As depression lessens, energy level improves, increasing the likelihood of suicide attempts.
- **Therapeutic response:** Assess appearance, behavior, level of interest, mood, and sleep pattern to determine amitriptyline's therapeutic effect.
- **Side effects:** Monitor BP and pulse rate to detect dysrhythmias and hypotension.
- **Abrupt withdrawal:** Caution patients not to discontinue amitriptyline abruptly.
- **Therapeutic effect:** Inform patients that amitriptyline's full therapeutic effect may be noted in 2-4 wk.
- **Patient education:** Warn patients to avoid tasks that require alertness or motor skills until response to the drug is known. Advise changing positions slowly to prevent dizziness. Inform patients that a tolerance will develop to the drug's hypotensive and sedative effects during early therapy. Inform patients that sensitivity to sunlight may develop, making it easy to get sunburned. Urge patients to report any visual disturbances. Suggest sipping tepid water or chewing sugarless gum to relieve dry mouth.

SERIOUS ADVERSE REACTIONS

- **Abrupt withdrawal:** Abrupt discontinuation after prolonged therapy may produce headache, malaise, nausea, vomiting, and vivid dreams.
- Blood dyscrasias and cholestatic jaundice occur rarely.

OVERDOSE/TOXICITY

- **Cardiac:** Dysrhythmias, fatigue, dyspnea.
- **Dysrhythmias/ECG changes:** Sinus tachycardia, prolonged PR interval, prolonged QT interval, widened QRS complex greater than 100 msec, right axis deviation (positive deflection) of terminal QRS complex in lead AVR greater than 3 mm.
- **Neurologic:** Seizures, severe somnolence, hallucinations, agitation, weakness, fever.
- **Antimuscarinic effects:** Dilated pupils, blurred vision, tachycardia, hyperthermia, hypertension, decreased oral and bronchial secretions, dry skin, ileus, urinary retention, increased muscle tone, and tremor.

A

- **Toxicity:** Symptoms occur within the first 2 hr of ingestion or not at all. Should be screened by ECG and serum and/or urine TCA levels.
- **Management:** Ventilator-driven hyperventilation with IV saline to raise pH to 7.50 to 7.55 to induce respiratory alkalosis. Sodium bicarbonate IV infusion with initial bolus of 1-2 meq/kg until clinical improvement is noted or blood pH is 7.50-7.55 (induced metabolic alkalosis). Higher blood pH may be deleterious. IV potassium supplementation may be needed to correct hypokalemia that results from use of bicarbonate infusion. IV fluid infusion is used to manage hypotension. Vasopressors are used only when patients do not respond to fluid therapy. Seizures may respond spontaneously; if persistent, benzodiazepines (lorazepam, diazepam) may be used. Phenobarbital or propofol may be used if other medications fail.
- **GI decontamination:** Activated charcoal binds TCAs effectively and, if used, should be given in one dose within the first few hours of ingestion. The risks of using ipecac to induce vomiting outweighs the benefits. Adding gastric lavage to activated charcoal may enhance removal effects if done within the first hour of ingestion.

ANTIDOTE/DIALYSIS

- **Antidote:** No specific recommendations.
- **Dialysis:** Amitriptyline is not removed using hemodialysis and peritoneal dialysis. No data are available on removal using high-permeability hemodialysis.

amlodipine besylate

am-loe'-di-peen be'-si-late

Classes

Chemical: dihydropyridine
Therapeutic: antianginal, antihypertensive, calcium channel blocker

Pregnancy Category: C

Trade Names

Prescription: Norvasc

Combinations

Prescription: with atorvastatin (Caduet); with benazepril (Lotrel)

Do not confuse amlodipine with amiloride or Norvasc with Navane or Vascor.

CLINICAL PHARMACOLOGY

Mechanism of Action

A calcium channel blocker that inhibits calcium movement across cardiac and vascular smooth-muscle cell membranes. **Therapeutic Effect:** Relieves angina by dilating coronary arteries, peripheral arteries, and arterioles. Decreases total peripheral vascular resistance and BP by vasodilation.

PHARMACOKINETICS

Route	Onset	Peak	Duration
PO	0.5-1 hr	6-12 hr	24 hr

Slowly absorbed from the GI tract. Protein binding: 93%. Undergoes first-pass metabolism in the liver. Excreted primarily in urine. Not removed by hemodialysis. **Half-life:** 30-50 hr (increased in the elderly and those with liver cirrhosis).

AVAILABILITY

Tablets: 2.5 mg, 5 mg, 10 mg.

INDICATIONS AND DOSAGE

Hypertension

PO

Adults: Initially, 5 mg/day as a single dose. Increase dose by 2.5-mg increments every 7-14 days. Maximum: 10 mg/day. **Small-frame, fragile, elderly:** Initially, 2.5 mg/day as a single dose. **Children 6-17 yr:** 2.5-5 mg/day.

Angina (chronic stable or vasospastic)

PO

Adults: 5-10 mg/day as a single dose. **Elderly, Patients with hepatic insufficiency:** 5 mg/day as a single dose.

Dosage in hepatic impairment

Adults, Elderly: hypertension, 2.5 mg/day; Angina, 5 mg/day.

CONTRAINDICATIONS

Severe hypotension

INTERACTIONS

Drug: None known. **Food:** **Grapefruit, grapefruit juice:** May increase amlodipine blood concentration and hypotensive effects. **Herbal:** None known.

DIAGNOSTIC TEST EFFECTS

None known.

SIDE-EFFECTS

Frequent (greater than 5%): Peripheral edema, headache, flushing. **Occasional (less than 5%):** Dizziness, palpitations, nausea, unusual fatigue or weakness (asthenia). **Rare (less than 1%):** Chest pain, bradycardia, orthostatic hypotension.

CRITICAL CARE CONSIDERATIONS

ADMINISTRATION/HANDLING

PO ALERT

- Increase amlodipine dosage slowly over 7-14 days in accordance with patient response.
- Avoid giving amlodipine with grapefruit juice, which may increase amlodipine blood concentration.
- Amlodipine may be given without regard to food.

PRECAUTIONS

HEALTH-RELATED

- Use amlodipine cautiously in patients with aortic stenosis, heart failure, and impaired hepatic function.
- Cannot be used effectively to stop the effects of withdrawal of beta-blockers.

AGE-RELATED

- **Children:** Safety and efficacy of amlodipine have not been established in children under 6 yr.
- **Elderly:** Are more sensitive to amlodipine's hypotensive effects and half-life may be increased in the elderly.

PREGNANCY/LACTATION-RELATED

- Pregnancy category C; unknown if excreted into milk; use caution in nursing mothers.

MONITORING

- **Baseline assessment:** Assess BP and heart rate.
- **Baseline lab work:** Renal and hepatic function test results.
- **Hypotension:** If systolic BP is less than 90 mmHg, withhold amlodipine and discuss further BP management with other members of the health care team. Patients may report dizziness when hypotensive.
- **Chest discomfort/angina:** Monitor for patterns of chest discomfort.
- **Therapeutic effect:** Assess relief of chest discomfort and control of hypertension.
- **Edema:** Assess skin for flushing and peripheral edema, especially behind the medial malleolus and the sacral area, which is a side effect that sometimes warrants discontinuation of the drug.
- **Neurologic:** Monitor for weakness or headache.
- **Drug discontinuation:** Provide alternate antihypertensive if amlodipine is discontinued.
- **Patient education:** When using amlodipine outside the hospital, caution against abrupt discontinuation. Compliance with therapy is essential to control hypertension. Warn patients to avoid tasks that require alertness and motor skills until response to the drug is known. Urge patients to avoid drinking grapefruit juice while taking amlodipine.

SERIOUS ADVERSE REACTIONS

- **Cardiovascular:** Severe hypotension with reflex tachycardia, ventricular tachycardia, and atrial fibrillation.
- **Hepatic failure:** Half-life of amlodipine can increase to 56 hr in patients with liver failure because the drug is heavily metabolized in the liver.
- **Neurologic:** Rarely fatigue, headache, weakness, numbness, myalgias, arthralgias, tingling.
- **Gastrointestinal:** Vomiting and rarely GI hemorrhage.

OVERDOSE/TOXICITY

- **Symptoms:** May produce excessive peripheral vasodilation, flushing, and marked hypotension with reflex tachy-cardia.
- **Acute respiratory distress syndrome:** Has been reported with calcium channel blocker overdose, but this has not been well studied.
- **Acute liver injury:** Liver failure has been reported in rare cases.
- **Rhabdomyolysis with acute renal failure:** Has been reported.
- **Dysrhythmias:** Amlodipine lacks the detrimental effect on AV conduction seen with overdoses of other calcium channel blocking agents. Heart block and bradycardia are not likely.
- **Manage hypotension:** Use of antidotes and/or vasopressors may help resolve hypotension. Cardiac pacing can be used if the patient is bradycardic; slow heart rate is unlikely with amlodipine.
- **GI decontamination:** Oral activated charcoal may be effective if the patient presents within 1 hr of ingestion. Ipecac should not be used if the patient is unable to protect their airway. Whole bowel irrigation has not been proven effective in reducing calcium channel blocking agent absorption.

ANTIDOTE/DIALYSIS

- **Antidote:** Calcium is the antidote of choice. Use of calcium chloride may be preferable because it contains approximately three times the calcium concentration compared with calcium gluconate. Glucagon may be helpful in managing hypotension. Insulin/glucose increases myocardial contractility to help increase cardiac output, which may help to increase blood pressure.
- **Dialysis:** Amlodipine is not removed by hemodialysis, is unlikely to be removed using high permeability hemodialysis. No data are available on removal using peritoneal dialysis.

amobarbital sodium

am-oh-bar'-bi-tal soe'-dee-um

DEA Schedule: II

Classes
Chemical: barbituric acid derivative
Therapeutic: sedative/hypnotic

Pregnancy Category: D

Trade Names
Prescription: Amytal sodium

Combinations
Prescription: with secobarbital (Tuinal)

CLINICAL PHARMACOLOGY

Mechanism of Action

A barbiturate that depresses the sensory cortex, decreases motor activity, and alters cerebellar function. **Therapeutic Effect:** Produces drowsiness, sedation, and hypnosis.

PHARMACOKINETICS

Protein binding: 60%. Metabolized in liver primarily by the hepatic microsomal enzyme system. Primarily excreted in urine. **Half-life:** 16-40 hr.

AVAILABILITY

Powder for injection: 500 mg (amytal sodium).

INDICATIONS AND DOSAGE

Hypnotic

IM/IV

Adults, Children older than 6 yr: 65-200 mg at bedtime. **IM:** Administer deeply into a large muscle. Do not use more than 5 mL at any single site (may cause tissue damage). Maximum: 500 mg. **IV:** Use only when IM administration is not feasible. Administer by slow IV injection. Maximum: 50 mg/min in adults. **Children younger than 6 yr:** 2 to 3 mg/kg/dose IM.

Preanesthetic

IM/IV

Adults, Children older than 6 yr: 65-500 mg at bedtime.

Sedative

IV

Adults: 30-50 mg given 2 or 3 times/day.

OFF-LABEL USES

Anticonvulsant

CONTRAINDICATIONS

History of manifest or latent porphyria, marked liver dysfunction, marked respiratory disease in which dyspnea or obstruction is evident, and hypersensitivity to amobarbital products, use with voriconazole.

INTERACTIONS

Drug: **Anticoagulants, steroids:** May decrease the effects of anticoagulants and steroids. **Anticonvulsants, barbiturates, benzodiazepines, valproic acid:** May increase the metabolism of anticonvulsants, barbiturates, benzodiazepines, and valproic acid. **Central nervous system (CNS) depressants:** May increase respiratory depression and hypotension. **Corticosteroids, doxycline, griseofulvin:** May decrease the effect of corticosteroids, doxycycline, and griseofulvin. **MAOIs:** May cause convulsions and hypertensive crises. **Voriconazole:** Use is contraindicated; amobarbital significantly decreases serum levels of voriconazole. **Herbal:** **Valerian:** May increase central nervous system (CNS) depression. **St. John's Wort:** May decrease the effects of amobarbital sodium. **Food:** **Ethanol:** May increase central nervous system (CNS) depression. Food may decrease the rate of absorption.

DIAGNOSTIC TEST EFFECTS

May falsely elevate phenobarbital levels when measured with EMIT(R) system.

IV INCOMPATIBILITIES

Atracurium (Tracrium), cefazolin (Ancef), cephalothin, *chlorproMAZINE (Thorazine), cimetidine (Tagamet), clindamycin (Cleocin), codeine, *dimenhyDRINATE (Dramamine), *diphenhydrAMINE (Benadryl), droperidol (Inapsine), hydrocortisone, *hydrOXYzine (Atarax, Vistaril), insulin, isoproterenol (Isuprel), levorphanol (Levo-Dromaron), meperidine (Demerol), metaraminol (Aramine), methadone (Dolophine, Methadose), methyldopa (Aldomet), methylphenidate (Concerta, Ritalin), morphine (Avinza, Kadian, Roxanol), norepinephrine (Levophed), oxytetracycline (Terramycin), pancuronium (Pavulon), penicillin G (Bicillin), pentazocine (Talwin), phytonadione (AquaMEPHYTON, Mephyton), procaine (Novocain), prochlorperazine (Compazine), propiomazine (Largon), streptomycin, succinylcholine (Anectine), tetracycline (Sumycin), vancomycin (Vancocin)

IV COMPATIBILITIES

Amikacin, aminophylline, sodium bicarbonate

SIDE-EFFECTS

Frequent: Somnolence, headache, confusion, dizziness. **Occasional:** Nausea, vomiting, visual abnormalities (e.g., spots before eyes), difficulty focusing, blurred vision, dry mouth or pharynx, tongue irritation, water retention, increased sweating, constipation, or diarrhea

CRITICAL CARE CONSIDERATIONS

ADMINISTRATION/HANDLING

IV ALERT

- **Dilution:** Each 125 mg must be diluted with a maximum of 1.25 mL of sterile water for injection to make a 10% solution.
- **Opened vials:** Vials should not be left opened for more than 30 min before it is injected.
- **Injection:** Rate of IV injection should not exceed 50 mg/min to prevent sleep or sudden respiratory depression.
- **Storage:** Store at room temperature.

PRECAUTIONS

HEALTH-RELATED

- Use cautiously in patients with impaired cardiac, liver, or renal function.

AGE-RELATED

- **Children:** Behavioral changes are more likely to occur.
- **Elderly:** Behavioral changes are more likely to occur.

PREGNANCY/LACTATION-RELATED

- Pregnancy category D; small amount excreted in breast milk; use caution in nursing mothers

MONITORING

- **Baseline assessment:** Assess vital signs. Obtain history of allergies.
- **Lab work:** Biochemical profile including liver function (AST [SGOT], ALT [SGPT], alkaline phosphatase, bilirubin) studies.
- **Promote relaxation:** Provide an environment conducive to sleep.
- **Sedation:** Monitor level of sedation.
- **Oversedation:** Monitor for hypotension, bradycardia, decreasing respiratory rate, which may lead to respiratory depression.
- **Patient education:** Warn patients to avoid tasks that require mental alertness or motor skills until response to the drug is known. Explain that drug dependence or tolerance may occur with prolonged use of high dosages.

SERIOUS ADVERSE REACTIONS

- Tolerance may occur with repeated use. (See overdose/toxicity.)

OVERDOSE/TOXICITY

- **Symptoms:** Severe respiratory depression, skeletal muscle flaccidity, bronchospasm, heart failure, hypotension or hypertension, dysrhythmias, hypothermia, clammy skin, cyanosis, coma, and circulatory collapse. Patients may develop rhabdomyolysis.
- **Neurologic findings in severe overdose:** Mimics brain death with nonreactive pupils, loss of other brainstem reflexes, absent deep tendon reflexes. EEG may be isoelectric.
- **Management:** Supportive care, focusing on airway and ventilatory management. BP should be supported with IV fluids and vasopressors if IV fluids do not correct hypotension. Forced diuresis is not recommended. Vigorous rewarming for hypothermia. Any given dose may have a much stronger effect on a first-time user than a long-term user who has developed tolerance. Chronic users will develop withdrawal within 24 hr of abstaining from amobarbital.
- **GI decontamination:** No specific recommendations.

ANTIDOTE/DIALYSIS

- **Antidote:** No specific recommendations.
- **Dialysis:** Hemodialysis or hemoperfusion may help to remove amobarbital.

amoxapine

See Antidepressants (p. 906)

amoxicillin

a-mox-i-sil'-in

Classes

Chemical: penicillin derivative, aminopenicillin

Therapeutic: antibiotic

Pregnancy Category: B

Trade Names

Prescription: Amoxicot, Amoxil, Amoxil Pediatric Drops, Biomox, DisperMox, Moxilin, Novamoxin ♣, Polymox, Trimox, Wymox)

Do not confuse amoxicillin with amoxapine or DisperMox with Diamox or Trimox with Tylox.

CLINICAL PHARMACOLOGY

Mechanism of Action

A penicillin that inhibits bacterial cell wall synthesis. **Therapeutic Effect:** Bactericidal in susceptible microorganisms.

PHARMACOKINETICS

Well absorbed from the GI tract. Protein binding: 20%. Partially metabolized in the liver. Primarily excreted in urine. Removed by hemodialysis. **Half-life:** 1-1.3 hr (increased in impaired renal function).

AVAILABILITY

Capsules: 250 mg (Amoxil, Biomox, Trimox, Wymox), 500 mg (Amoxil, Biomox, Trimox).

Powder for reconstitution: 50 mg/mL (Amoxil Pediatric Drops, Trimox), 125 mg/5 mL (Amoxil, Trimox), 200 mg/5 mL (Amoxil), 250 mg/5 mL (Amoxil, Biomox, Trimox), 400 mg/mL (Amoxil).

Tablets (Amoxil): 500 mg, 875 mg.

Tablets (chewable [Amoxil]): 125 mg, 200 mg, 250 mg, 400 mg.

Tablets for oral suspension (DisperMox): 200 mg, 400 mg.

INDICATIONS AND DOSAGE

Susceptible infections

PO

Adults, Elderly: 250-500 mg every 8 hr or 500-875 mg every 12 hr. **Children older than 3 mo:** 25-50 mg/kg/day in two to three divided doses. **Children 3 mo and younger:** 20-30 mg/kg/day in two to three divided doses.

Lower respiratory tract infection

PO

Adults, Elderly: 500 mg every 8 hr or 875 mg every 12 hr.

Helicobacter pylori infection

PO

Adults, Elderly: 1 g twice per day in combination with clarithromycin and lansoprazole for 14 days.

Otitis media

PO

Children: 80-90 mg/kg/day in two to three divided doses.

Gonorrhea

PO

Adults, Elderly: 3 g as a single dose.

Endocarditis prophylaxis

PO

Adults, Elderly: 2 g 1 hr before procedure.
Children: 50 mg/kg 1 hr before procedure. Maximum: 2 g.

Dosage in renal impairment

Dosage interval is modified based on creatinine clearance.

Creatinine clearance 10-30 mL/min. Usual dose every 12 hr (250-500 mg).

Creatinine clearance less than 10 mL/min. Usual dose every 24 hr (250-500 mg).

OFF-LABEL USES

Treatment of Lyme disease and typhoid fever

CONTRAINDICATIONS

Hypersensitivity to any penicillin, infectious mononucleosis

INTERACTIONS

Drug: **Allopurinol:** May increase incidence of rash. **Oral contraceptives:** May decrease effectiveness of oral contraceptives. **Probenecid:** May increase amoxicillin blood concentration and risk of toxicity.
Herbal: None known. **Food:** None known.

DIAGNOSTIC TEST EFFECTS

May increase BUN and serum LDH, bilirubin, creatinine, AST (SGOT), and ALT (SGPT) levels. May cause a positive Coombs' test.

SIDE-EFFECTS

Frequent: GI disturbances (mild diarrhea, nausea, or vomiting), headache, oral or vaginal candidiasis. **Occasional:** Generalized rash, urticaria

CRITICAL CARE CONSIDERATIONS

ADMINISTRATION/HANDLING

PO ALERT

- Store tablets at room temperature.
- After reconstitution, the oral solution is stable for 14 days either at room temperature or refrigerated.
- Give amoxicillin without regard to food.
- Instruct patients to chew or crush chewable tablets thoroughly before swallowing.

PRECAUTIONS

HEALTH-RELATED

- ***Do not use in patients allergic to penicillin to avoid anaphylaxis.***
- Use amoxicillin cautiously in patients with antibiotic-associated colitis or a history of allergies, especially to cephalosporins.

AGE-RELATED

- **Neonates/young infants:** Immature renal function in neonates and young infants may delay renal excretion of amoxicillin.
- **Children:** Amoxicillin may lead to allergic sensitization, candidiasis, diarrhea, and skin rash in infants.
- **Elderly:** Age-related renal impairment may require a dosage adjustment in the elderly.

PREGNANCY/LACTATION-RELATED

- Pregnancy category B; excreted into breast milk in low concentrations; no adverse effects have been observed, but potential exists for modification of bowel flora and allergy/sensitization in nursing infant.

MONITORING

- **Baseline assessment:** Determine history of allergies, especially to cephalosporins or penicillins, before starting therapy.
- **Lab work:** Biochemical profile including renal function (BUN, creatinine) studies.
- **Penicillin allergy/reaction:** Withhold amoxicillin and promptly notify the physician if the patient experiences a rash or diarrhea. Although a rash is a common side effect of amoxicillin, it may also indicate hypersensitivity.
- **Colitis:** Severe diarrhea with abdominal pain, blood or mucous in stools, and fever may indicate antibiotic-associated colitis.
- **Nausea/vomiting:** Manage with standard measures. Provide IV hydration if severe symptoms occur. Consider use of another antibiotic.
- **Superinfection:** Be alert for signs and symptoms of superinfection, including anal or genital pruritus, black hairy tongue, diarrhea, increased fever, sore throat, ulceration or changes of oral mucosa, and vomiting.
- **Evenly space dosing:** Administer doses evenly around the clock.
- **Patient education:** Instruct patients to continue taking amoxicillin for the full course of treatment, to take the drug with meals if GI upset occurs, and to chew or crush the chewable tablets thoroughly before swallowing. Instruct patients to report diarrhea, rash, or other new symptoms promptly to a health care provider.

SERIOUS ADVERSE REACTIONS

- **Colitis:** Antibiotic-associated colitis, pseudomembranous colitis or *clostridium difficile* colitis, and other superinfections may result from altered bacterial balance.
- **Anaphylaxis:** Severe hypersensitivity reactions, including anaphylaxis and acute interstitial nephritis, occur in penicillin-sensitive patients.
- **Hematologic:** Anemia, hemolytic anemia, thrombocytopenia, leukopenia, agranulocytosis, eosinophilia, thrombocytopenic purpura.
- **Central nervous system:** Reversible hyperactivity, agitation, anxiety, seizures, behavioral changes, dizziness.

OVERDOSE/TOXICITY

- **Gastrointestinal:** Nausea, vomiting, diarrhea. Severe diarrhea with abdominal pain, blood or mucous in stool, and fever may indicate antibiotic-associated colitis.
- **Hepatic/liver:** Elevated liver enzymes (AST [SGOT], ALT [SGPT]), confusion, altered behavior.
- **Renal/kidneys:** Rare interstitial nephritis is indicative of hypersensitivity.
- **GI decontamination:** No specific recommendations.

ANTIDOTE/DIALYSIS

- **Antidote:** No specific recommendations. Discontinuing amoxicillin generally resolves adverse effects.
- **Dialysis:** Amoxicillin is removed by hemodialysis and is likely to be removed by high-permeability hemodialysis. It is not removed by peritoneal dialysis.

A

amoxicillin/clavulanate potassium

a-mox-i-sill'-in clav-u-lan'-ate

Classes

Chemical: penicillin derivative, aminopenicillin; β-lactamase inhibitor (clavulanate)
Therapeutic: antibiotic

Pregnancy Category: B

Trade Names

Prescription: Augmentin, Augmentin ES 600, Augmentin XR, Clavulin ♣

Do not confuse amoxicillin with amoxapine.

CLINICAL PHARMACOLOGY

Mechanism of Action

Amoxicillin inhibits bacterial cell wall synthesis, while clavulanate inhibits bacterial beta-lactamase. Therapeutic Effect: Amoxicillin is bactericidal in susceptible microorganisms. Clavulanate protects amoxicillin from enzymatic degradation.

PHARMACOKINETICS

Well absorbed from the GI tract. Protein binding: 20%. Partially metabolized in the liver. Primarily excreted in urine. Removed by hemodialysis. Half-life: 1–1.3 hr (increased in impaired renal function).

AVAILABILITY

Powder for oral suspension (Augmentin): 31.25 mg/5 mL-125 mg, 28.5 mg/5 mL-200 mg, 62.5 mg/5 mL-250 mg, 57 mg/5 mL-400 mg, 42.9 mg/5 mL-600 mg.
Tablets (Augmentin): 125 mg-250 mg, 125 mg-500 mg, 125 mg-875 mg.
Tablets (extended release [Augmentin XR]): 62.5 mg-1000 mg.
Tablets (chewable [Augmentin]): 31.25 mg-125 mg, 28.5 mg-200 mg, 62.5 mg-250 mg, 57 mg-400 mg.

INDICATIONS AND DOSAGE

Mild to moderate infections

PO

Adults, Elderly: 500 mg every 12 hr or 250 mg every 8 hr.

Severe infections, respiratory tract infections

PO

Adults, Elderly: 875 mg every 12 hr or 500 mg every 8 hr.

Community-acquired pneumonia, sinusitis

PO

Adults, Elderly: 2 g (extended-release tablets) every 12 hr for 7-10 days.

Sinusitis

PO

Adults, Elderly: 2 g (extended-release tablets) every 12 hr for 7-10 days. **Children weighing 40 kg and less:** 25-45 mg/kg/day (200 or 400 mg/5 mL powder or 200 or 400 mg chewable tablets) in two divided doses or 20-40 mg/kg/day (125 or 250 mg/5 mL powder or 125 or 250 mg chewable tablets) in three divided doses.

Otitis media

PO

Children: 90 mg/kg/day (600 mg/5 mL suspension) in divided doses every 12 hr for 10 days.

Usual neonate dosage

PO

Neonates, Children younger than 3 mo: 30 mg/kg/day (125 mg/5 mL suspension) in divided doses every 12 hr.

Dosage in renal impairment

Dosage and frequency are modified based on creatinine clearance.

All-ages: Creatinine clearance 10-30 mL/min, 250-500 mg every 12 hr. **All-ages:** Creatinine clearance 10 mL/min, 250-500 mg every 24 hr.

OFF-LABEL USES

Treatment of bronchitis and chancroid

CONTRAINDICATIONS

Hypersensitivity to any penicillins, infectious mononucleosis, history of cholestatic jaundice

INTERACTIONS

Drug: **Allopurinol:** May increase incidence of rash. **Oral contraceptives:** May decrease effects of oral contraceptives. **Probenecid:** May increase amoxicillin and clavulanate blood concentration and risk of toxicity. Herbal: None known. Food: None known.

DIAGNOSTIC TEST EFFECTS

May increase serum AST (SGOT) and ALT (SGPT) levels. May cause a positive Coombs' test.

SIDE-EFFECTS

Frequent: GI disturbances (mild diarrhea, nausea, vomiting), headache, oral or vaginal candidiasis. Occasional: Generalized rash, urticaria

A

CRITICAL CARE CONSIDERATIONS

ADMINISTRATION/HANDLING

DOSAGE ALERT

- Drug dosage is expressed in terms of amoxicillin. An alternative dosage is 500-875 mg twice daily for adults and 200-400 mg twice daily for children.

PO ALERT

- Store tablets at room temperature.
- After reconstitution, the oral solution is stable for 14 days either at room temperature or refrigerated.
- Give without regard to meals.
- Instruct patients to chew or crush chewable tablets thoroughly before swallowing.

PRECAUTIONS

HEALTH-RELATED

- ***Do not use in patients allergic to penicillin to avoid anaphylaxis.***
- Do not use in patients with mononucleosis to avoid erythematous skin rash.
- Use amoxicillin and clavulanate cautiously in patients with antibiotic-associated colitis or a history of allergies, especially to cephalosporins.
- Use with caution in patients with hepatic dysfunction/liver disease.

AGE-RELATED

- **Neonates/young infants:** Immature renal function in neonates and young infants may delay renal excretion of amoxicillin and clavulanate.
- **Children:** Amoxicillin and clavulanate may lead to allergic sensitization, candidiasis, diarrhea, and skin rash in infants.
- **Elderly:** Age-related renal impairment may require a dosage adjustment in the elderly.

PREGNANCY/LACTATION-RELATED

- Pregnancy category B; excreted into breast milk in low concentrations; no adverse effects have been observed.

MONITORING

- **Baseline assessment:** Determine history of allergies, especially to cephalosporins or penicillins, before starting therapy.
- **Lab work:** Biochemical profile including renal (BUN, creatinine) and liver function (AST [SGOT], ALT [SGPT], bilirubin, alkaline phosphatase) studies.
- **Penicillin allergy/reaction:** Withhold amoxicillin and promptly notify the physician if patients experience a rash or diarrhea. Although rash is a common side effect of amoxicillin, it may also indicate hypersensitivity.
- **Colitis:** Severe diarrhea with abdominal pain, blood or mucous in stools, and fever may indicate antibiotic-associated colitis.
- **Nausea/vomiting:** Manage with standard measures. Provide IV hydration if severe symptoms occur. Consider use of another antibiotic.
- **Superinfection:** Be alert for signs and symptoms of superinfection, including anal or genital pruritus, black hairy tongue, diarrhea, increased fever, sore throat, ulceration or changes of oral mucosa, and vomiting.
- **Evenly space dosing:** Administer doses evenly around the clock.
- **Patient education:** Instruct patients to continue taking amoxicillin for the full course of treatment, to take the drug with meals if GI upset occurs, and to chew or crush the chewable tablets thoroughly before swallowing. Instruct patients to report diarrhea, rash, or other new symptoms promptly to a health care provider.

SERIOUS ADVERSE REACTIONS

- **Colitis:** Antibiotic-associated colitis, pseudomembranous colitis or *Clostridium difficile* colitis, and other superinfections may result from altered bacterial balance.
- **Anaphylaxis:** Severe hypersensitivity reactions, including anaphylaxis and acute interstitial nephritis, occur in penicillin-sensitive patients.
- **Hematologic:** Anemia, hemolytic anemia, thrombocytopenia, leukopenia, agranulocytosis, eosinophilia, thrombocytopenic purpura.
- **Central nervous system:** Reversible hyperactivity, agitation, anxiety, seizures, behavioral changes, dizziness.

OVERDOSE/TOXICITY

- **Gastrointestinal:** Nausea, vomiting, diarrhea. Severe diarrhea with abdominal pain, blood or mucous in stool, and fever may indicate antibiotic-associated colitis.
- **Hepatic/liver:** Elevated liver enzymes (AST [SGOT], ALT [SGPT]), confusion, altered behavior.
- **Renal/kidneys:** Rare interstitial nephritis is indicative of hypersensitivity.
- **GI decontamination:** No specific recommendations.

A

ANTIDOTE/DIALYSIS

- **Antidote:** No specific recommendations. Discontinuing amoxicillin generally resolves adverse effects.
- **Dialysis:** Amoxicillin is removed by hemodialysis and is likely to be removed by high-permeability hemodialysis. It is not removed by peritoneal dialysis.

amphotericin B

am-foe-ter'-i-sin bee

Classes

Chemical: antifungal polyene antibiotic
Therapeutic: antifungal agent, parenteral

Pregnancy Category: B

Trade Names

Prescription: Abelcet, AmBisome, Amphocin, Amphotec, Fungizone, Fungizone for Tissue Culture

CLINICAL PHARMACOLOGY

Mechanism of Action

An antifungal and antiprotozoal that is generally fungistatic but may become fungicidal with high dosages or very susceptible microorganisms. This drug binds to sterols in the fungal cell membrane. **Therapeutic Effect:** Increases fungal cell-membrane permeability, allowing loss of potassium and other cellular components.

PHARMACOKINETICS

Protein binding: 90%. Widely distributed. Metabolic fate unknown. Cleared by nonrenal pathways. Minimal removal by hemodialysis. Amphotec and Abelcet are not dialyzable. **Half-life:** Fungizone, 24 hr (increased in neonates and children); Amphotec, 26-28 hr; Abelcet, 7.2 days; AmBisome, 100-153 hr.

AVAILABILITY

Cream, lotion, ointment (Fungizone): 3%.
Injection (powder for reconstitution): 50 mg (AmBisome, Amphocin, Amphotec, Fungizone), 100 mg (Amphotec).
Injection (suspension [Abelcet]): 5 mg/mL.

INDICATIONS AND DOSAGE

Cryptococcosis; blastomycosis; systemic candidiasis; disseminated forms of moniliasis, coccidioidomycosis, and histoplasmosis; zygomycosis; sporotrichosis; aspergillosis

IV Infusion (Fungizone)

Adults, Elderly: Dosage based on patient tolerance and severity of infection. Initially, 1-mg test dose is given over 20-30 min. If test dose is tolerated, 5-mg dose may be given the same day. If test dose is tolerated, 0.25 mg/kg is given on same day and 0.5 mg/kg on second day; then dosage is increased until desired daily dose reached. Total daily dose: 1 mg/kg/day up to 1.5 mg/kg every other day. Maximum: 1.5 mg/kg/day. **Children:** Test dose of 0.1 mg/kg/dose (maximum 1 mg) is infused over 30-60 min. If test dose is tolerated, initial dose of 0.4 mg/kg may be given on same day; dosage is then increased in 0.25-mg/kg increments as needed. Maintenance dose: 0.25-1 mg/kg/day.

Invasive fungal infections unresponsive to or intolerant of Fungizone

IV Infusion (Abelcet)

Adults, Children: 2.5-5 mg/kg/day as a single infusion.

Empiric treatment of fungal infections in patients with febrile neutropenia; aspergillosis, candidiasis, or cryptococcosis in patients with renal impairment and those who have experienced toxicity or treatment failure with Fungizone

IV Infusion (AmBisome)

Adults, Children: 3-5 mg/kg over 2 hr daily.

Invasive aspergillosis in patients with renal impairment and those who have experienced toxicity or treatment failure with Fungizone

IV Infusion (Amphotec)

Adults, Children: 3-4 mg/kg per day over 2-4 hr. Maximum: 7.5 mg/kg/day.

Cutaneous and mucocutaneous infections caused by *Candida albicans*, such as paronychia, oral thrush, perlche, diaper rash, and intertriginous candidiasis

Topical

Adults, Elderly, Children: Apply liberally to affected area and rub in 2-4 times per day.

OFF-LABEL USES

Febrile neutropenia, meningoencephalitis, paracoccidioidomycosis

CONTRAINDICATIONS

Hypersensitivity to amphotericin B or sulfites

INTERACTIONS

Drug: Bone marrow depressants: May increase the risk of anemia. **Digoxin:** May increase the risk of digoxin toxicity from hypokalemia. **Nephrotoxic medications:** May increase the risk of nephrotoxicity. **Steroids:** May cause severe hypokalemia. **Herbal:** None known. **Food:** None known.

DIAGNOSTIC TEST EFFECTS

May increase BUN, serum alkaline phosphatase, serum creatinine, serum AST (SGOT), and ALT (SGPT) levels. May decrease serum calcium, magnesium, and potassium levels.

IV INCOMPATIBILITIES

Abelcet, Ambisome, Amphotec: Do not mix with any other drug, diluent, or solution. Fungizone: Allopurinol (Aloprim), amifostine (Ethyol), aztreonam (Azactam), calcium gluconate, cefepime (Maxipime), cimetidine (Tagamet), ciprofloxacin (Cipro), docetaxel (Taxotere), *DOPamine (Intropin), *DOXOrubicin (Adriamycin), enalapril (Vasotec), etoposide (VP-16), filgrastim (Neupogen), fluconazole (Diflucan), fludarabine (Fludara), foscarnet (Foscavir), gemcitabine (Gemzar), magnesium sulfate, meropenem (Merrem IV), ondansetron (Zofran), paclitaxel (Taxol), piperacillin and tazobactam (Zosyn), potassium chloride, propofol (Diprivan), total parenteral nutrition (TPN), vinorelbine (Navelbine)

IV COMPATIBILITIES

None known; do not mix with other medications or electrolytes.

SIDE-EFFECTS

Frequent (greater than 10%): **Abelcet:** Chills, fever, increased serum creatinine level, multiple organ failure
Ambisome: Hypokalemia, hypomagnesemia, hyperglycemia, hypocalcemia, edema, abdominal pain, back pain, chills, chest pain, hypotension, diarrhea, nausea, vomiting, headache, fever, rigors, insomnia, dyspnea, epistaxis, increased hepatic or renal function test results
Amphotec: Chills, fever, hypotension, tachycardia, increased serum creatinine level, hypokalemia, bilirubinemia
Fungizone: Fever, chills, headache, anemia, hypokalemia, hypomagnesemia, anorexia, malaise, generalized pain, nephrotoxicity
Topical: Local irritation, dry skin. Rare: **Topical:** Rash

CRITICAL CARE CONSIDERATIONS

ADMINISTRATION/HANDLING

IV ALERT (ALL FORMS)

- **High risk for reactions:** Obtain orders for drugs to reduce the risk or severity of adverse reactions during IV therapy (fever, chills, hypotension, nausea, vomiting) such as antiemetics, antihistamines, antipyretics, small doses of corticosteroids, and agents to prevent shaking chills.
- **Test dose:** A small test dose is recommended before starting the infusion.
- **Strict asepsis:** Observe strict aseptic technique during reconstitution because no bacteriostatic agent or preservative is present in the diluent.
- **Thrombophlebitis:** The potential for thrombophlebitis may be decreased by using pediatric scalp vein needles or by adding dilute heparin solution, as prescribed.
- **Slow intravenous infusion:** Amphotericin B should be administered by slow IV infusion; solution concentration varies with each form of the medication.
- **Do not dilute with saline:** Do not dilute with saline solutions or mix with other electrolytes. Use plain dextrose 5% solution for dilution.

IV ALERT (ABELCET)

- **Storage/stability:** Refrigerate unreconstituted Abelcet solution. Reconstituted Abelcet solution is stable for 48 hr if refrigerated and for 6 hr at room temperature.
- **Preparation:** Shake Abelcet 20-mL (100-mg) vial gently until contents are dissolved. Withdraw required dose using the 5-micron filter needle supplied by the manufacturer.
- **Final concentration:** Dilute each 1 mL (5 mg) of Abelcet in 4 mL of D_5W to yield a final concentration of 1 mg/mL.
- **Slow IV infusion:** Infuse Abelcet over 2 hr by slow IV infusion. Shake the contents if the infusion exceeds 2 hr.

IV ALERT (AMBISOME)

- **Storage/stability:** Refrigerate unreconstituted Ambisome solution. Reconstituted Ambisome solution of 4 mg/mL is stable for 24 hr; reconstituted solution of 1-2 mg/mL is stable for 6 hr.
- **Initial concentration:** Reconstitute each 50-mg vial of Ambisome with 12 mL sterile water for injection to provide a concentration of 4 mg/mL.
- **Final concentration:** Shake the Ambisome vial vigorously for 30 sec. Then withdraw the required dose and empty the syringe contents through a 5-micron filter into an infusion of D_5W to provide final concentration of 1-2 mg/mL.
- **Slow IV infusion:** Infuse Ambisome over 2 hr by slow IV infusion.

IV ALERT (AMPHOTEC)

- **Storage/stability:** Store unreconstituted Amphotec solution at room temperature. Reconstituted Amphotec solution is stable for 24 hr.
- **Initial concentration:** Add 10 mL of sterile water for injection to each 50-mg vial of Amphotec to provide a concentration of 5 mg/mL. Shake the vial gently.
- **Final concentration:** Further dilute Amphotec only with D_5W, using the specific amount recommended by the manufacturer, to provide a concentration of 0.16-0.83 mg/mL.
- **Slow IV infusion:** Infuse Amphotec over 2-4 hr by slow IV infusion.

IV ALERT (FUNGIZONE)

- **Storage/stability:** Refrigerate unreconstituted Fungizone solution. Reconstituted Fungizone solution is stable for 24 hr at room temperature or for 7 days if refrigerated. Diluted solution less than or equal to 0.1 mg/mL should be used promptly. Do not use the solution if it is cloudy or contains a precipitate.
- **Initial concentration:** Rapidly inject 10 mL of sterile water for injection into each 50-mg vial of Fungizone to provide a concentration of 5 mg/mL. Immediately shake the vial until the solution is clear.
- **Final concentration:** Further dilute each 1 mg of Fungizone in at least 10 mL of D_5W to provide a concentration of 0.1 mg/mL.
- **Slow IV infusion:** Infuse Fungizone over 2-6 hr by slow IV infusion.

PRECAUTIONS

HEALTH-RELATED

- Use amphotericin B cautiously in patients with renal impairment and in those receiving antineoplastic therapy, including leukocyte transfusions, which may result in pulmonary toxicity. Amphotericin B is prescribed only for progressive, potentially fatal fungal infections.
- **Renal failure:** Dose should be reduced for patients with renal failure.
- **Nephrotoxicity:** Conventional amphotericin B (Fungizone) is more nephrotoxic than the amphotericin B complexes Abelcet, AmBisome, and Amphotec.
- **Blood glucose:** Glucose should be well controlled before beginning the infusion.

AGE-RELATED

- **Children:** Safety and efficacy of amphotericin B have not been established in children. Therefore, expect to use the smallest dose necessary to achieve optimal results.
- **Elderly:** No age-related precautions have been noted for the elderly. Consider age-related impaired organ functions.

PREGNANCY/LACTATION-RELATED

- Pregnancy category B.

MONITORING

- **Baseline assessment:** Before giving amphotericin B, obtain history of allergies, especially to amphotericin B and sulfites.
- **Lab work:** Before and daily during therapy CBC, serum potassium and magnesium levels, and renal and liver function tests should be taken.
- **Altered lab results:** Include hypomagnesemia, hypo- and hyperkalemia, hypocalcemia, liver function tests (elevated AST [SGOT], ALT [SGPT], GGT, bilirubin, and alkaline phosphatase), and renal function tests (elevated BUN and creatinine).
- **Reduce nephrotoxicity:** Other nephrotoxic medications should be avoided, if possible.
- **Premedication:** Obtain premedication orders to reduce the adverse reactions of IV therapy.
- **Adverse reactions:** Adverse reactions include abdominal pain, anorexia, chills, fever, nausea, vomiting, and tremors. If adverse reactions occur, slow the infusion rate and give prescribed drugs to provide symptomatic relief. For patients with a severe reaction and those without orders for symptomatic relief, stop the infusion and notify the physician.
- **Monitor for reactions:** Monitor BP, pulse, respirations, and temperature twice every 15 min, then every 30 min for the first 4 hr of the infusion to assess for adverse reactions.
- **Phlebitis:** Evaluate the IV site for signs of phlebitis (heat, pain, and red streaking over the vein). Thrombophlebitis is common and is sometimes relieved by adding heparin 1000 units to each infusion.
- **Skin reactions:** Assess the skin for burning, irritation, or pruritus.
- **Monitor renal function:** Monitor intake and output and renal function test results to assess for nephrotoxicity.
- **Therapeutic effect:** Prolonged amphotericin B therapy over weeks or months is usually necessary to achieve the desired therapeutic effect.
- **Fever:** Febrile reaction may decrease with continued therapy. Fever and chills generally occur within 15 to 20 min of the start of infusion.
- **Muscle weakness:** May occur from drug-related loss of potassium.

- **Topical use:** Thoroughly rub in the cream or lotion. Inform patients that topical amphotericin B may stain the skin, nails, and clothing. Clothing stains may be removed by soap and water or dry cleaning. Separate personal items that have come in direct contact with the affected area. Do not use other topical preparations or occlusive coverings without consulting the physician. Keep affected areas clean and dry.

SERIOUS ADVERSE REACTIONS

- **Anaphylaxis:** If anaphylaxis or severe respiratory distress occurs, the patient should not receive further infusions.
- **Reversible reactions:** Many reactions are reversible when amphotericin B is discontinued.
- **Acute reactions:** Fever, chills, hypotension, nausea, vomiting, and headache usually decrease with subsequent doses.
- **Other reactions:** Altered vision and hearing, seizures, hepatic failure, coagulation defects may improve with reduced dose of amphotericin B.

OVERDOSE/TOXICITY

- **Nephrotoxicity:** Acute renal failure is a more common serious reaction.
- **Cardiovascular:** Hypotension, ventricular fibrillation, cardiac arrest, and anaphylaxis occurs rarely.
- **Pulmonary:** Severe respiratory distress, pulmonary edema.
- **Hepatotoxicity:** Acute liver failure with jaundice, hepatitis.
- **Hematologic:** Agranulocytosis, thrombocytopenia, coagulation defects, leukopenia or leukocytosis, eosinophilia.
- **Management:** Dantrolene 50 mg PO or IV has been effective in both preventing and managing severe, shaking chills. Meperidine is used to manage severe, shaking chills. Use of alkaline agents such as sodium bicarbonate infusions may help to reduce renal tubular acidosis, which helps to support the kidneys.
- **GI decontamination:** No specific recommendations.

ANTIDOTE/DIALYSIS

- **Antidote:** No specific recommendations.
- **Dialysis:** Amphotericin B is not removed by hemodialysis, peritoneal dialysis, or high-permeability hemodialysis.

ampicillin sodium

See Antibiotics (p. 892)

ampicillin/sulbactam sodium

am'-pi-sill-in/sul-bac'-tam

Classes

Chemical: penicillin derivative, aminopenicillin, penicillinate (sulbactam)
Therapeutic: antibiotic

Pregnancy Category: B

Trade Names

Prescription: Unasyn

CLINICAL PHARMACOLOGY

Mechanism of Action

Ampicillin inhibits bacterial cell wall synthesis, whereas sulbactam inhibits bacterial beta-lactamase. **Therapeutic Effect:** Ampicillin is bactericidal in susceptible microorganisms. Sulbactam protects ampicillin from enzymatic degradation.

PHARMACOKINETICS

Protein binding: 28%-38%. Widely distributed. Partially metabolized in the liver. Primarily excreted in urine. Removed by hemodialysis. **Half-life:** 1 hr (increased in impaired renal function).

AVAILABILITY

Powder for injection: 1.5 g (ampicillin 1 g/sulbactam 500 g), 3 g (ampicillin 2 g/sulbactam 1 g).

INDICATIONS AND DOSAGE

Skin and skin-structure, intraabdominal, and gynecologic infections

IV, IM

Adults, Elderly: 1.5 g (1 g ampicillin/500 mg sulbactam) to 3 g (2 g ampicillin/1 g sulbactam) every 6 hr.

Skin and skin-structure infections

IV

Children 12 yr and younger: 150-400 mg/kg/day in divided doses every 6 hr. Maximum: 12 g/day.

Dosage in renal impairment

Dosage and frequency are modified based on creatinine clearance and the severity of the infection.

Creatinine Clearance	Dosage
Greater than 30 mL/min	0.5-3 g every 6-8 hr
15-29 mL/min	1.5-3 g every 12 hr
5-14 mL/min	1.5-3 g every 24 hr
Less than 5 mL/min	Not recommended

CONTRAINDICATIONS

Hypersensitivity to any penicillin or sulbactam, infectious mononucleosis

INTERACTIONS

Drug: **Allopurinol:** May increase incidence of rash. **Oral contraceptives:** May decrease effectiveness of oral contraceptives. **Probenecid:** May increase ampicillin blood concentration and risk of ampicillin toxicity. **Herbal:** None known. **Food:** None known.

DIAGNOSTIC TEST EFFECTS

May increase serum LDH, alkaline phosphatase, creatinine, AST (SGOT), and ALT (SGPT) levels. May cause a positive Coombs' test.

IV INCOMPATIBILITIES

Diltiazem (Cardizem), idarubicin (Idamycin), ondansetron (Zofran), sargramostim (Leukine), total parenteral nutrition (TPN)

IV COMPATIBILITIES

Famotidine (Pepcid), heparin, insulin (regular), morphine

SIDE-EFFECTS

Frequent: Diarrhea and rash (most common), urticaria, pain at IM injection site, thrombophlebitis with IV administration, oral or vaginal candidiasis. **Occasional:** Nausea, vomiting, headache, malaise, urine retention

CRITICAL CARE CONSIDERATIONS

ADMINISTRATION/HANDLING

IV ALERT

- **Storage/stability:** When reconstituted with 0.9% NaCl, the IV solution is stable for 8 hr at room temperature or 48 hr if refrigerated. Stability may differ with other diluents.
- **Precipitate:** Discard IV solution if a precipitate forms.
- **IV injection:** Dilute with 10 to 20 mL sterile water for injection. Administer IV injection slowly, over 10 to 15 min.
- **Intermittent IV infusion (piggyback):** Further dilute with 50-100 mL 0.9% NaCl. Administer over 15 to 30 min.
- **Avoid reactions:** Because of the potential for hypersensitivity and anaphylaxis, start the initial dose at a few drops per minute, and then increase the dose slowly to the ordered rate. Stay with the patient for the first 10 to 15 min; check the patient every 10 min during the infusion for signs and symptoms of hypersensitivity or anaphylaxis.

IM ALERT

- **Reconstitution:** Reconstitute each 1.5-g vial with 3.2 mL or each 3-g vial with 6.4 mL of sterile water for injection to provide a concentration of 250 mg ampicillin/125 mg sulbactam per milliliter.
- **Stability:** The reconstituted solution is stable for 1 hr.
- **Administration:** Inject deep into a large muscle mass within 1 hr of preparation.

PRECAUTIONS

HEALTH-RELATED

- ***Do not use in patients who are allergic to penicillin to avoid anaphylaxis.***
- **Renal impairment:** Higher than usual doses may cause seizures, especially in patients with renal impairment.
- Use ampicillin and sulbactam very cautiously in patients with antibiotic-associated colitis or a history of allergies, particularly to cephalosporins and beta-lactamase sensitivity.

AGE-RELATED

- **Neonates:** Elimination rate is markedly reduced.
- **Infants:** Ampicillin may lead to allergic sensitization, candidiasis, diarrhea, and a rash in infants.
- **Children:** Safety and efficacy of ampicillin and sulbactam have not been established in children under 1 yr. For children over 1 yr, use has been proven safe and effective for skin and suture infections.
- **Elderly:** Age-related renal impairment may require a dosage adjustment in the elderly.

PREGNANCY/LACTATION-RELATED

- Pregnancy category B; animal studies at doses 10 times the human dose reveal no evidence of harm; low concentrations excreted in breast milk.

MONITORING

- **Baseline assessment:** Determine history of allergies, especially to cephalosporins or penicillins, before starting drug therapy.
- **Lab work:** Biochemical profile including renal function studies (BUN, creatinine).
- **Rash or diarrhea:** Withhold ampicillin and promptly notify the physician if patients experience a rash or diarrhea.

Although rash is a common side effect of ampicillin, it also may indicate hypersensitivity. Severe diarrhea with abdominal pain, blood or mucus in stools, and fever may indicate antibiotic-associated colitis.

- **Phlebitis:** Evaluate the IV site for signs of phlebitis, such as heat, pain, and red streaking over the vein.
- **IM injection:** Check the IM injection site for pain and swelling. Inform patients that IM injections may cause discomfort.
- **Renal function:** Monitor intake and output, renal function tests, and urinalysis results.
- **Superinfection:** Assess for signs and symptoms of superinfection, such as anal or genital pruritus, black hairy tongue, changes in oral mucosa, diarrhea, increased fever, sore throat, and vomiting.
- **Evenly spaced dosing:** Space doses evenly around the clock and complete the full course of treatment.
- **Patient education:** Instruct patients to promptly report diarrhea, rash, or other new symptoms to a health care provider.

SERIOUS ADVERSE REACTIONS

- **Seizures:** Seen when higher than usual doses are used.
- **Hypersensitivity:** Severe hypersensitivity reactions, including anaphylaxis, acute interstitial nephritis, and blood dyscrasias may occur.
- **Colitis:** Antibiotic-associated colitis and other superinfections may result from altered bacterial balance.

OVERDOSE/TOXICITY

- **Seizures:** Overdose may produce seizures.
- **Gastrointestinal:** Nausea, vomiting, diarrhea. Severe diarrhea with abdominal pain, blood or mucus in stool, and fever may indicate antibiotic-associated colitis.
- **Hepatic/liver:** Elevated liver enzymes (AST [SGOT], ALT [SGPT]), confusion, altered behavior.
- **Management:** For severe symptoms, discontinue ampicillin, treat the allergic reaction (antihistamines, corticosteroids, epinephrine) and resuscitate as necessary.
- **GI decontamination:** No specific recommendations.

ANTIDOTE/DIALYSIS

- **Antidote:** No specific recommendations.
- **Dialysis:** Ampicillin sulbactam is removed by hemodialysis and is likely to be removed by high-permeability hemodialysis. It is not removed by peritoneal dialysis.

amprenavir

See HIV Medications (p. 961)

anagrelide

an-ag'-re-lide

Classes

Chemical: quinazoline derivative
Therapeutic: antiplatelet agent

Pregnancy Category: C

Trade Names

Prescription: Agrylin

CLINICAL PHARMACOLOGY

Mechanism of Action

A hematologic agent that reduces platelet production and prevents platelet shape changes caused by platelet-aggregating agents. **Therapeutic Effect:** Decreases platelet production and reduces platelet aggregation.

PHARMACOKINETICS

After oral administration, plasma concentration peak within 1 hr. Extensively metabolized. Primarily excreted in urine. **Half-life:** About 3 days.

AVAILABILITY

Capsules: 0.5 mg, 1 mg.

INDICATIONS AND DOSAGE

Thrombocythemia

PO

Adults, Elderly: Initially, 0.5 mg 4 times per day or 1 mg twice per day. Adjust to lowest effective dosage, increasing by up to 0.5 mg/day or less in any 1 wk. Maximum: 10 mg/day or 2.5 mg/dose. **Children:** Initially, 0.5 mg/day. Range: 0.5 mg 1-4 times per day.

CONTRAINDICATIONS

Severe hepatic impairment

INTERACTIONS

Drug: None known. **Herbal:** **Ginkgo biloba:** May increase the risk of bleeding. **Food:** None known.

DIAGNOSTIC TEST EFFECTS

May increase hepatic enzymes levels (rare).

SIDE-EFFECTS

Frequent: Headache (44%), palpitations (27%), diarrhea (26%), weakness (23%), nausea (17%), abdominal pain (16%), flatulence (16%), bloating (16%), dizziness (15%). **Occasional (less than 5%):** Tachycardia, chest pain, vomiting, paresthesia, peripheral edema, anorexia, dyspepsia, rash. **Rare:** Confusion, insomnia

CRITICAL CARE CONSIDERATIONS

ADMINISTRATION/HANDLING

PO ALERT

- May give anagrelide without regard to food.

PRECAUTIONS

HEALTH-RELATED

- **Impaired cardiac, renal, or liver function:** Use anagrelide cautiously in patients with cardiac disease or hepatic or renal impairment.

AGE-RELATED

- **Children:** Safety and efficacy of anagrelide have not been established in children under 16 yr.
- **Elderly:** Use cautiously in the elderly, who may have age-related cardiac disease and/or decreased renal or hepatic function.

PREGNANCY/LACTATION-RELATED

- Pregnancy category C; not recommended in women who are or may become pregnant; excretion into breast milk unknown.

MONITORING

- **Baseline assessment:** Assess for bruising and ecchymosis.
- **Lab work:** Hemoglobin, hematocrit, platelet, and white blood cell counts before treatment, every 2 days during the first week of treatment, and weekly thereafter until therapeutic range is achieved. Monitor BUN, serum creatinine levels, and hepatic enzymes.
- **Pregnancy concern:** Determine whether patients are or plan to become pregnant or are breast-feeding, because anagrelide may cause fetal harm.
- **Heart failure/dysrhythmias:** Assess patients with suspected heart disease for tachycardia, palpitations, and signs and symptoms of heart failure, such as dypsnea.
- **Bleeding risk:** Assess skin for bruises or petechiae. Inspect catheter and needle insertion sites for bleeding. Assess stools and oral secretions for blood, which may indicate GI bleeding. Platelet count should be decreased within 7-14 days of beginning therapy.
- **Clotting:** Monitor for vascular clotting/impaired circulation while platelet count is elevated during the first 7 days of treatment until anagrelide takes effect.
- **Patient education:** Instruct patients to promptly report chest discomfort, shortness of breath, and pain that is new or unusual to a health care provider.

SERIOUS ADVERSE REACTIONS

- Angina, myocardial infarction, vasodilation, heart failure, stroke, and dysrhythmias including complete heart block and atrial fibrillation occur rarely during treatment and may be related to elevated platelet count, which predisposes the patient to clotting.

OVERDOSE/TOXICITY

- **Clotting:** Acute MI, stroke, lethal dysrhythmias.
- **Drug discontinuation:** When anagrelide is discontinued for clotting, if the patient was having a reaction to the drug rather than a problem with elevated platelets, the symptoms should resolve. If the patient has clotting problems related to platelets, stopping anagrelide will not improve the symptoms, and clotting will continue.
- **GI decontamination:** No specific recommendations.

ANTIDOTE/DIALYSIS

- **Antidote:** No specific recommendations.
- **Dialysis:** No data are available on removal of anagrelide by hemodialysis, high permeability hemodialysis, or peritoneal dialysis.

anakinra

See Immunologics (p. 968)

anidulafungin

See Antifungals (p. 922)

A

anistreplase, anisoylated psac

an-ih-strep'-layz

Classes
Chemical: anisoylated plasminogen streptokinase activator complex
Therapeutic: thrombolytic

Pregnancy Category: C

Trade Names
Prescription: Eminase

CLINICAL PHARMACOLOGY

Mechanism of Action
An enzyme that activates the fibrinolytic system by converting plasminogen to plasmin and degrades fibrin clots. Action occurs within the thrombus, on its surface, and in circulating blood. **Therapeutic Effect:** Destroys thrombi.

PHARMACOKINETICS

Metabolized to plasminogen-streptokinase complex. Route of elimination is unknown. **Half-life:** 70 to 120 min.

AVAILABILITY

Powder for injection: 30 units/vial (Eminase).

INDICATIONS AND DOSAGE

Myocardial infarction
IV
Adults, Elderly: 30 units of a single injection over 2 to 5 min.

OFF-LABEL USES

Pulmonary embolism

CONTRAINDICATIONS

Recent intracranial or intraspinal surgery or trauma, cerebrovascular accident, active internal bleeding, severe hypertension, thrombocytopenia, prior course of anistreplase or streptokinase therapy within the past 12 mo, hypersensitivity to anistreplase or streptokinase

INTERACTIONS

Drug: Anticoagulants: May increase risk of hemorrhage. **Platelet aggregation inhibitors such as aspirin, nonsteroidal antiinflammatory drugs, ticlopidine:** May increase risk of bleeding. **Herbal:** None known. **Food:** None known.

DIAGNOSTIC TEST EFFECTS

Decreases serum plasminogen and fibrinogen levels during infusion, decreasing clotting time and confirming presence of lysis.

IV INCOMPATIBILITIES

Do not mix with other medications.

SIDE-EFFECTS

Frequent: Fever, superficial bleeding at puncture sites, decreased BP. **Occasional:** Allergic reaction, including rash and wheezing, ecchymosis

CRITICAL CARE CONSIDERATIONS

ADMINISTRATION/HANDLING

IV ALERT

- **Acute MI:** Anistreplase should be administered as soon as possible after the onset of acute symptoms of myocardial infarction, preferably in less than 4-6 hr.
- **Storage:** Refrigerate unopened vials.
- **Dilution:** Reconstitute at room temperature with 5 mL of sterile water for injection. Add diluent slowly to side of vial; roll and tilt to avoid foaming. Do not shake vial.
- **IV bolus administration:** 30 units over 2-5 min. Discontinue immediately if uncontrolled hemorrhage occurs.
- **Stability:** Reconstituted solution should be administered within 30 min after reconstitution.

PRECAUTIONS

HEALTH-RELATED

- Use anistreplase cautiously in patients at increased risk for bleeding, including those with GI bleeding or recent trauma injury and in those who have had major surgery within the past 10 days. See contraindications for more information about patients at high risk for bleeding.
- Effectiveness may be diminished if administered 5 days to 6 mo following prior infusions of anistreplase, streptokinase therapy, or streptococcal infections because high levels of antistreptococcal antibodies are present.

AGE-RELATED

- **Children:** Safety and efficacy of anistreplase have not been established in children.
- **Elderly:** May have increased risk of intracranial hemorrhage. Anistreplase should be used cautiously in the elderly.

PREGNANCY/LACTATION-RELATED

- Pregnancy category C.

MONITORING

- **Baseline assessment:** Evaluate chest discomfort and confirm acute MI before initiating thrombolytic therapy. Discontinue heparin (if heparin is a component of treatment) before giving anistreplase. Prothrombin time or aPTT should be less than twice the normal value before therapy starts. Determine female patients' usual amount of menstrual flow during menses.
- **Baseline lab work:** Assess activated partial thromboplastin time (aPTT), hemoglobin and hematocrit, fibrinogen level, platelet count, and prothrombin time before therapy starts. Cardiac markers (CPK, troponins, CKMB isoenzymes) should be evaluated to help confirm presence of MI, especially if 12-lead ECG is not diagnostic (ST elevation not seen) for acute MI.
- **Therapeutic effect:** Evaluate for resolution of ECG changes and chest discomfort. Vital signs should begin stabilizing.
- **Bleeding precautions:** Handle patients carefully and as infrequently as possible to prevent bleeding and ecchymosis. Examine stool for occult blood. Assess for abdominal or back pain, decrease in BP, increase in pulse rate, and severe headache, which may indicate hemorrhage. Monitor menstruating female patients for increased menstrual flow. Watch for excessive bleeding from minor cuts and scratches.
- **Ongoing lab work:** Monitor hemoglobin and hematocrit values, BP, and platelet count, aPTT, fibrinogen level, prothrombin time, and thrombin level every 4 hr after therapy begins if heparin infusion is initiated.
- **Patient education:** Instruct patients to report immediately chest pain, headache, palpitations, shortness of breath, black or red stool, coffee-ground vomitus, dark or red urine, red-speckled mucus from cough, and other signs of bleeding.

SERIOUS ADVERSE REACTIONS

- **Reperfusion dysrhythmias:** Lysis of coronary thrombi may produce life-threatening dysrhythmias, which should not be treated aggressively unless the patient's vital signs are unstable. These dysrhythmias generally resolve.

OVERDOSE/TOXICITY

- **Hemorrhage:** Severe internal or external bleeding may occur.
- **Management:** Discontinue infusion immediately at any sign of internal or external bleeding. Intracranial hemorrhage is considered the most severe complication of thrombolytic therapy.
- **GI decontamination:** No specific recommendations.

ANTIDOTE/DIALYSIS

- **Antidote:** No specific recommendations.
- **Dialysis:** Anistreplase is unlikely to be removed by hemodialysis and peritoneal dialysis. No data are available on removal by high-permeability hemodialysis.

antithrombin III

See Anticoagulants (p. 900)

antithymocyte globulin

See Immunologics (p. 968)

aprepitant

ap-re'-pi-tant

Classes
Chemical: triazolone derivative
Therapeutic: antiemetic

Pregnancy Category: B

Trade Names
Prescription: Emend, Emend 3-Day

CLINICAL PHARMACOLOGY

Mechanism of Action

A selective human substance P and neurokinin-1 (NK_1) receptor antagonist that inhibits chemotherapy-induced nausea and vomiting centrally in the chemoreceptor trigger zone. **Therapeutic Effect:** Prevents the acute and delayed phases of chemotherapy-induced emesis, including vomiting caused by high-dose cisplatin.

PHARMACOKINETICS

Crosses the blood-brain barrier. Extensively metabolized in the liver. Eliminated primarily by liver metabolism (not excreted renally). **Half-life:** 9-13 hr.

AVAILABILITY

Capsules (Emend): 80 mg, 125 mg.
Kit (Emend 3-Day): 125 mg-80 mg.

INDICATIONS AND DOSAGE

Prevention of chemotherapy-induced nausea and vomiting

PO

Adults, Elderly: 125 mg 1 hr before chemotherapy on day 1 and 80 mg once per day in the morning on days 2 and 3.

CONTRAINDICATIONS

Breast-feeding, concurrent use of astemizole, cisapride, pimozide, or terfenadine

INTERACTIONS

Drug: Alprazolam, docetaxel, etoposide, ifosfamide, imatinib, irinotecan, midazolam, paclitaxel, triazolam, vinblastine, vincristine, vinorelbine: May increase the plasma concentrations of these drugs. **Antifungals, clarithromycin, diltiazem, nefazodone, nelfinavir, ritonavir:** Increase aprepitant plasma concentration. **Carbamazepine, phenytoin, rifampin:** Decrease aprepitant plasma concentration. **Contraceptives:** May decrease the effectiveness of contraceptives. **Paroxetine:** May decrease the effectiveness of either drug. **Steroids:** Increases the blood levels and effects of steroids. Decreases PO dexamethasone dose by 50%; decreases methylprednisolone by 25% (IV) and 50% (PO). **Warfarin:** May decrease the effectiveness of warfarin. **Herbal:** None known. **Food:** None known.

DIAGNOSTIC TEST EFFECTS

May increase BUN level and serum creatinine, AST (SGOT), and ALT (SGPT) levels. May produce proteinuria.

SIDE-EFFECTS

Frequent (22%-10%): Fatigue, nausea, hiccups, diarrhea, constipation, anorexia. **Occasional (8%-4%):** Headache, vomiting, dizziness, dehydration, heartburn. **Rare (3% or less):** Tinnitus, insomnia, throat pain

CRITICAL CARE CONSIDERATIONS

ADMINISTRATION/HANDLING

DOSING ALERT

- Give aprepitant with 12 mg dexamethasone PO and 32 mg ondansetron IV on day 1, and with 8 mg dexamethasone PO on days 2 to 4.
- If patients are also receiving a steroid, reduce the IV steroid dose by 25% and the oral dose by 50%.

PO ALERT

- Give aprepitant without regard to food.
- First dose of 125 mg should be taken 1 hr before chemotherapy.

PRECAUTIONS

HEALTH-RELATED

- Use with caution in patients receiving steroids (will require reduction in steroid dose), chemotherapy agents that are metabolized through CYPA34 (drug levels may increase) and warfarin (prothrombin time and INR may be decreased).
- **Contraindications:** Do not use aprepitant concurrently with pimozide, terfenadine, astemizole, or cisapride because aprepitant is a moderate cytochrome P450 isoenzyme 3A4 (CYP3A4) inhibitor.

AGE-RELATED

- **Children:** Safety and efficacy of aprepitant have not been established in children.
- **Elderly:** No age-related precautions have been noted.

PREGNANCY/LACTATION-RELATED

- Pregnancy category B; excretion into breast milk unknown, use caution in nursing mothers.

MONITORING

- **Baseline assessment:** Assess the patient who experiences severe vomiting for dehydration, including dry mucous membranes, longitudinal furrow in the tongue, and poor skin turgor. Inform the patient nausea and vomiting should be relieved shortly after drug administration.
- **Lab work:** Patients on warfarin therapy should have coagulation studies (prothrombin time, INR) monitored at 7-10 days after receiving a 3-day regimen of aprepitant with chemotherapy to help avoid deep vein thrombosis, pulmonary embolus, MI, or other disorder related to clotting.
- **Bowel habits:** Monitor for diarrhea, constipation, or abdominal pain, which may be side effects of aprepitant. Hydrate as needed.
- **Cytochrome P450 pathway:** Note whether patients are receiving medications metabolized by this enzyme. The medications will not be appropriately metabolized, causing elevation of plasma levels.

SERIOUS ADVERSE REACTIONS

- Neutropenia and mucous membrane disorders occur rarely.
- Hypersensitivity occurs rarely; Stevens-Johnson syndrome has been reported.

OVERDOSE/TOXICITY

- **Symptoms:** Neutropenia leading to sepsis/septic shock, moderate liver enzyme elevation, proteinuria, diaphoresis, flushing, myalgia.
- **Management:** Symptoms should be managed by current accepted guidelines for each problem.
- **GI decontamination:** No special recommendations.

ANTIDOTE/DIALYSIS

- **Antidote:** No specific recommendations.
- **Dialysis:** Aprepitant is not removed by hemodialysis and is unlikely to be removed by high-permeability hemodialysis or peritoneal dialysis.

aprotinin bovine

a-proe-tye'-nin boe'-vyne

Classes
Chemical: blood product derivative
Therapeutic: hemostatic agent

Pregnancy Category: B

Trade Names
Prescription: Trasylol

CLINICAL PHARMACOLOGY

Mechanism of Action

A broad-spectrum protease inhibitor that inhibits multiple mediators such as kallikrein and plasmin. Inhibits proinflammatory cytokine release. Maintains glycoprotein homeostasis. Reduces glycoprotein loss in platelets. **Therapeutic Effect:** Results in the attenuation of inflammatory responses, fibrinolysis, and thrombin generation. Decreases the need for allogenic blood transfusions and reduces bleeding.

PHARMACOKINETICS

Rapid distribution into the extracellular space. Slowly degraded by lysosomal activity in the kidney. Excreted in urine. **Half-life:** 2.5 hr.

AVAILABILITY

Solution for injection: 1.4 mg/mL (10,000 kallikrein inhibitory units [KIU]/mL) in 100- or 200-mL vials.

INDICATIONS AND DOSAGE

Prophylaxis for perioperative blood loss during coronary artery bypass graft

IV

Adults: Test dose: 10,000 KIU 10 min before loading dose. Loading dose: 1 million-2 million KIU over 20-30 min and before sternotomy. Pump prime: 1 million-2 million KIU added to the recirculating priming fluid of the coronary artery bypass circuit. Constant infusion: 250,000-500,000 KIU/hr for duration of surgery.

OFF-LABEL USES

Liver transplantation

CONTRAINDICATIONS

Hypersensitivity to aprotinin or any component of the formulation

INTERACTIONS

Drug: Heparin: May prolong activated clotting time (ACT). **Herbal:** None known. **Food:** None known.

DIAGNOSTIC TEST EFFECTS

May increase creatine kinase (CK), serum creatinine, serum transaminases, partial thromboplastin time (PTT), activated clotting time (ACT), bleeding times, hemoglobin, mehatocrit, BUN, and creatinine.

IV INCOMPATIBILITIES

Do not administer with other medications.

SIDE-EFFECTS

Frequent: Fever (15%), nausea (11%). **Occasional:** Mental confusion, phlebitis, difficulty breathing, atrial fibrillation, MI, heart failure, atrial flutter, ventricular tachycardia, hypotension, supraventricular tachycardia. **Rare:** Allergic reaction, anaphylaxis

CRITICAL CARE CONSIDERATIONS

ADMINISTRATION/HANDLING

IV ALERT

- **Central IV access:** Administer via central line when patients have been prepared for surgery in the operating room.
- **Dedicated infusion line:** Do not infuse with other drugs present in the same line.
- **Possible hypotension:** Do not administer test dose or loading dose until patients can be made ready for rapid vessel cannulation, should it become necessary.

Administer loading dose with patients flat in supine position to help avoid hypotension. Delay addition of the pump priming solution until after the loading dose has been administered.
- **During cardiac surgical pump priming in the operating room:** To avoid physical incompatibility with heparin when adding to pump priming solution during cardiac surgery, each drug must be added separately during recirculation of the pump prime to ensure adequate dilution before admixture with the other medication.
- **Storage:** Store unopened vials at room temperature.

PRECAUTIONS

HEALTH-RELATED

- **Risk of anaphylaxis:** Increased risk in patients who are reexposed to aprotinin within 6 mo of previous exposures.
- **Hypotension:** Rapid IV infusion may cause a transient fall in BP.
- **Caution:** Use cautiously in patients with thromboembolic disease on anticoagulant therapy, history of other drug allergies, and renal insufficiency.
- **Aortic arch surgery:** May cause increased incidence of acute renal failure and mortality in patients undergoing hypothermic circulatory arrest during aortic arch surgical procedures.

AGE-RELATED

- **Children:** Safety and efficacy of aprotinin have not been established in children.
- **Elderly:** No age-related precautions have been noted.

PREGNANCY/LACTATION-RELATED

- Pregnancy category B.

MONITORING

- **Anesthesiologist:** Primary monitoring should be under the direction of an anesthesiologist in the operating room.
- **Baseline lab work:** Bleeding time, platelet counts, prothrombin time, activated clotting time, red blood cell counts, leukocyte counts, hematocrit, hemoglobin, and fibrinogen degradation products.
- **Premedication:** Premedicate with histamine blocker if needed. If patients have a history of allergic reactions, it may increase the risk for developing a hypersensitivity or anaphylactic reaction.
- **Ongoing lab work:** Monitor bleeding time, platelet counts, prothrombin time, international normalized ratio (INR), activated clotting time (ACT), red blood cell counts, leukocyte counts, hematocrit, hemoglobin, and fibrinogen degradation products. ACT and prothrombin time may remain elevated for several hours following surgery.
- **Other lab work effects:** May cause increased ALT (SGPT) with repeated administration. Serum creatinine, creatine kinase, and glucose may be elevated.
- **Hypersensitivity reactions:** Monitor for tachypnea, tachycardia, and hypotension throughout infusion. Reactions including anaphylaxis can occur at any time during administration, including when patients do not react to the test dose.
- **Circulation:** Monitor pulses, color of extremities, and ECG for ischemic changes because the drug is prothrombotic. Acute MI and saphenous vein closure are possible. Many reported side effects when aprotinin is used are also effects seen with any cardiac surgical procedure.

SERIOUS ADVERSE REACTIONS

- Hypersensitivity/anaphylactic reactions, thrombosis, and shock may occur.

OVERDOSE/TOXICITY

- **Symptoms:** Hypotension, tachycardia, tachypnea indicative of hypersensitivity. If thrombosis occurs, symptoms would be specific to the location of the occluded blood vessel.
- **Management:** For hypersensitivity, discontinue aprotinin immediately and manage anaphylaxis according to current accepted guidelines, which may include administration of epinephrine, corticosteroids, *diphenhydrAMINE (Benadryl), or ranitidine (Zantac); maintaining a patent airway with endotracheal tube; and oxygen and mechanical ventilation, as necessary.
- **GI decontamination:** No specific recommendations.

ANTIDOTE/DIALYSIS

- **Antidote:** There is no antidote specific for aprotinin. To reverse heparin activity, administer protamine based on the amount of heparin given, rather than using the ACT to calculate dosage.
- **Dialysis:** Aprotinin is unlikely to be removed by hemodialysis or peritoneal dialysis. No data are available on removal by high-permeability hemodialysis.

argatroban

ar-gat'-ro-ban

Classes

Chemical: L-arginine derivative, thrombin inhibitor

Therapeutic: anticoagulant, direct thrombin inhibitor

Pregnancy Category: B

Trade Names

Prescription: Argatroban

Do not confuse argatroban with Aggrestat, Orgaran, or Aggrenox.

CLINICAL PHARMACOLOGY

Mechanism of Action

A direct thrombin inhibitor that reversibly binds to thrombin-active sites. Inhibits thrombin-catalyzed or thrombin-induced reactions, including fibrin formation and activation of coagulant factors V, VIII, and XIII; also inhibits protein C formation and platelet aggregation. **Therapeutic Effect:** Produces anticoagulation.

PHARMACOKINETICS

Following IV administration, distributed primarily in extracellular fluid. Protein binding: 54%. Metabolized in the liver. Primarily excreted in the feces, presumably through biliary secretion. **Half-life:** 39-51 min.

AVAILABILITY

Injection: 100 mg/mL.

INDICATIONS AND DOSAGE

To prevent and treat heparin-induced thrombocytopenia

IV Infusion

Adults, Elderly: Initially, 2 mcg/kg/min administered as a continuous infusion. After initial infusion, dose may be adjusted until steady state aPTT is 1.5-3 times initial baseline value, not to exceed 100 sec.

Percutaneous coronary intervention

IV Infusion

Adults, Elderly: Initially, 25 mcg/kg/min and administer bolus of 350 mcg/kg over 3-5 min. ACT (activated clotting time) check 5-10 min following bolus. If ACT is less than 300 sec, give additional bolus 150 mcg/kg, increase infusion to 30 mcg/kg/min. If ACT is greater than 450 sec, decrease infusion to 15 mcg/kg/min. Once ACT of 300-450 sec achieved, proceed with procedure.

Dosage in hepatic impairment

Adults, Elderly: Initially, 0.5 mcg/kg/min.

OFF-LABEL USES

Cerebral thrombosis, MI

CONTRAINDICATIONS

Overt major bleeding

INTERACTIONS

Drug: **Antiplatelet agents, thrombolytics, other anticoagulants:** May increase the risk of bleeding. **Herbal:** **Arnica, astragalus, bilberry, black currant, cat's claw, chaparral, dandelion, evening primrose, feverfew, garlic, ginger, ginkgo biloba, hawthorn, kava, licorice, tan-shen, vitamin A:** May increase the risk of bleeding. **Food:** None known.

DIAGNOSTIC TEST EFFECTS

Increases aPTT, International Normalized Ratio (INR), and prothrombin time.

IV INCOMPATIBILITIES

Do not mix with other medications or solutions.

SIDE-EFFECTS

Frequent (8%-3%): Dyspnea (8%), hypotension (7%), fever, diarrhea, nausea, pain, vomiting, infection, cough

CRITICAL CARE CONSIDERATIONS

ADMINISTRATION/HANDLING

IV ALERT

- **Dilution:** Before infusion, dilute each 250-mg vial in 250 mL of NaCl, D_5W or lactated Ringer's solution to provide a final concentration of 1 mg/mL.
- **Mixing:** Mix the solution by repeatedly inverting the diluent bag for 1 min.
- **Following reconstitution:** The solution may briefly appear hazy because of formation of microprecipitates. These rapidly dissolve when the solution is mixed.
- **Precipitate:** Discard the solution if it is cloudy or has an insoluble precipitate.
- **Stability:** Following reconstitution, avoid exposing solution to direct sunlight. Solution is stable for 24 hr at room temperature and for 48 hr refrigerated.
- **Patients undergoing percutaneous coronary interventions:** Patients may require additional bolus doses of 150 mcg/kg and/or infusion rate increased to 40 mcg/kg/min if there is impending abrupt closure, dissection, or thrombus formation in the coronary vessel or the ACT is

unable to be maintained greater than 300 seconds. *Additional boluses are not recommended for patients with liver enzyme elevation greater than 3 times normal (AST [SGOT], ALT [SGPT]).*

- **Administration:** Rate of administration is based on body weight at 2 mcg/kg/min; (for example, for a 50-kg patient, infuse at rate of 6 mL/hr).

Argatroban Infusion Rates for mcg/kd/min Dose (1 mg/mL Final Concentration)

Body Weight (kg)	Infusion Rate (mL/hr)
50	6
60	7
70	8
80	10
90	11
100	12
110	13
120	14
130	16
140	17

PRECAUTIONS

HEALTH-RELATED

- **Medical:** Use argatroban cautiously in patients with congenital or acquired bleeding disorders, hepatic impairment, severe hypertension, or ulcerations.
- **Heparin-induced thrombocytopenia (HIT/HITTS):** Argatroban is often used as an alternative to heparin in patients with HIT/HITTS. There is a fourfold decrease in argatroban clearance in these patients, so dose must be carefully titrated.
- **Surgical:** Use cautiously immediately following administration of spinal anesthesia, lumbar puncture, and major surgery (especially brain, spinal, and eye).

AGE-RELATED

- **Children:** Safety and efficacy of argatroban have not been established in children under 18 yr.
- **Elderly:** No age-related precautions have been noted in the elderly.

PREGNANCY/LACTATION-RELATED

- Pregnancy category B; excretion into human milk unknown; use caution in nursing mothers.

MONITORING

- **Baseline assessment:** Obtain vital signs before infusion. Assess for bleeding disorders.
- **Baseline lab work:** CBC, prothrombin time, INR, ACT, and/or aPTT, liver enzymes, urinalysis.
- **Ongoing lab work:** Monitor activated coagulation time, aPTT, prothrombin time, INR, thrombin time (TT), and platelet count. Prothrombin time and INR may be prolonged. Liver enzymes (AST [SGOT], ALT [SGPT]) should be monitored in patients with ensuing multiorgan dysfunction syndrome or those who have baseline liver dysfunction.
- **Use following discontinuation of heparin:** Allow sufficient time for heparin's effects on the aPTT to resolve before checking aPTT to assess response to argatroban.
- **Deep vein thrombosis:** Do not obtain BP in the lower extremities if a deep-vein thrombus may be present.
- **Monitor ECG:** Note baseline rhythm and monitor for dysrhythmias. Ventricular dysrhythmias and atrial fibrillation may occur.
- **Assess for bleeding/bruising:** Assess for bleeding from surgical sites, gums, injection sites, stool, and for hematuria, ecchymosis, hematomas, and/or petechiae.
- **Prevent bruising/bleeding:** Handle patients carefully and as infrequently as possible without overlooking the need to turn every 2 hr. Minimize procedures that involve puncturing the skin. Avoid numerous blood draws, catheter insertions, and injections. Gently remove dressings and tape.
- **Possible hemorrhage:** Monitor for abdominal or back pain, hypotension, tachycardia, decreased central venous pressure (CVP) or pulmonary capillary wedge pressure (PCWP), and severe headache indicative of internal bleeding. Observe for an increase in menstrual flow.
- **Hematuria:** Review urinalysis for increased RBCs in urine.
- **Patient education:** Instruct patients to report black or red stool; coffee-ground vomitus; pink, red, or dark urine; or blood-tinged mucous from cough. Advise patients to use an electric razor and soft toothbrush to prevent bleeding.
- **Retroperitoneal bleeding:** Monitor groin puncture site following percutaneous coronary intervention.

SERIOUS ADVERSE REACTIONS

- **Symptomatic dysrhythmias:** Ventricular tachycardia and atrial fibrillation occur occasionally and may lead to hypotension, heart failure, and arrest if untreated.

- **Major bleeding:** Occurs rarely but is more likely in patients taking drugs that promote bleeding: heparin, bivalirudin (Angiomax), lepirudin (Refludan), aspirin, warfarin (Coumadin), thrombolytics (streptokinase, activase [Alteplase, rTPA], tenecteplase [TNKase], retivase [Reteplase]), glycoprotein IIb/IIa inhibitors (abciximab [Reo-Pro], eptifibatide [Integrilin], tirofiban [Aggrastat]), and other platelet inhibitors (ticlodipine [Ticlid], clopidogrel [Plavix], dipyridamole [Persantine]).
- **Allergic reaction, sepsis, cardiac arrest:** Occur rarely.

OVERDOSE/TOXICITY

- **Major bleeding:** Stroke; other significant internal or external hemorrhage that could lead to hypovolemic shock.
- **Management:** Discontinue argatroban for severe bleeding and reduce infusion rate for lesser bleeding. Obtain aPTT, ACT, and/or other anticoagulation tests. Prepare for blood transfusion if significant anemia has occurred (decreased Hgb, Hct). Follow accepted guidelines for management of hypovolemic shock due to hemorrhage including volume resuscitation and vasopressors if volume resuscitation is ineffective.
- **Animal studies:** Revealed toxicity symptoms including clonic seizures, coma, tremors, limb paralysis, and loss of righting reflex.
- **GI decontamination:** No specific recommendations.

ANTIDOTE/DIALYSIS

- **Antidote:** No specific recommendations.
- **Dialysis:** No data are available on removal of argatroban by hemodialysis, high-permeability hemodialysis, or peritoneal dialysis.

aripiprazole

ay-ri-pip'-ray-zole

Classes

Chemical: quinolinone derivative
Therapeutic: antipsychotic

Pregnancy Category: C

Trade Names

Prescription: Abilify

CLINICAL PHARMACOLOGY

Mechanism of Action

An antipsychotic agent that provides partial agonist activity at dopamine and serotonin ($5\text{-}HT_{1A}$) receptors and antagonist activity at serotonin ($5\text{-}HT_{2A}$) receptors. **Therapeutic Effect:** Diminishes schizophrenic behavior.

PHARMACOKINETICS

Well absorbed through the GI tract. Protein binding: 99% (primarily albumin). Reaches steady levels in 2 wk. Metabolized in the liver. Eliminated primarily in feces and, to a lesser extent, in urine. Not removed by hemodialysis. **Half-life:** 75 hr.

AVAILABILITY

Tablets: 2 mg, 5 mg, 10 mg, 15 mg, 20 mg, 30 mg.
Oral solution: 1 mg/mL.

INDICATIONS AND DOSAGE

Schizophrenia

PO

Adults, Elderly: Initially, 10-15 mg once per day. May increase up to 30 mg/day.

Bipolar disorder

PO

Adults, Elderly: 30 mg once per day. May decrease to 15 mg/day based on patient tolerance.

OFF-LABEL USES

Schizoaffective disorder

CONTRAINDICATIONS

None known.

INTERACTIONS

Drug: Carbamazepine: May decrease the aripiprazole blood concentration. **Fluoxetine, ketoconazole, quinidine, paroxetine:** May increase the aripiprazole blood concentration. **Herbal:** None known. **Food:** None known.

DIAGNOSTIC TEST EFFECTS

None known.

SIDE-EFFECTS

Frequent: Weight gain (8%-30%), headache (31%), insomnia (20%), vomiting (11%), agitation (25%), anxiety (20%), nausea (16%). **Occasional (4%-3%):** Light-headedness, akathisia. **Rare (2% or less):** Blurred vision, asthenia, or loss of energy and strength, fever, rash, cough, rhinitis, orthostatic hypotension

CRITICAL CARE CONSIDERATIONS

ADMINISTRATION/HANDLING

DOSAGE ALERT

- At least 2 wk should elapse between dosage adjustments.

PO ALERT

- Give aripiprazole without regard to food.

PRECAUTIONS

HEALTH-RELATED

- **CNS depressants:** Use aripiprazole cautiously in patients concurrently using CNS depressants, including alcohol.
- **Diseases:** Use cautiously in patients with cardiovascular or cerebrovascular diseases (may induce hypotension), history of seizures or conditions that may lower the seizure threshold (Alzheimer's disease), hepatic or renal impairment, or Parkinson's disease (potential for exacerbation).

AGE-RELATED

- **Children:** Safety and efficacy of aripiprazole have not been established in children.
- **Elderly:** No age-related precautions have been noted in the elderly.

PREGNANCY/LACTATION-RELATED

- Pregnancy category C; excreted in milk of rats during lactation; no human information.

MONITORING

- **Baseline assessment:** Assess appearance, vital signs, behavior, emotional status, response to environment, speech pattern, and thought content. Assess vital signs.
- **Lab work:** Biochemical profile including renal (BUN, creatinine) and liver function (AST [SGOT], ALT [SGPT], alkaline phosphatase, bilirubin) tests.
- **Hydration:** Correct dehydration and hypovolemia before beginning therapy.
- **Extrapyramidal symptoms:** Monitor for involuntary movements (jerking, twitching) and tardive dyskinesia (chewing or puckering of the mouth, puffing of the cheeks, or tongue protrusion). Occurs more commonly in elderly female patients.
- **Vital signs:** Monitor BP and pulse rate, particularly in patients with preexisting cardiovascular disease. Fluctuations in heart rate, orthostatic hypotension, and temperature elevation are possible.
- **Respiratory assessment:** Monitor breathing pattern and work of breathing because dyspnea and pneumonia (possibly from aspiration) may occur, especially in elderly patients. Dysphagia is seen more often in elderly patients.
- **Neurologic assessment:** Monitor for seizures, somnolence, altered cognitive and motor function, which occasionally leads to discontinuation of the drug.
- **Daily weight:** Monitor weight to ensure adequate nutrition and hydration is received. May cause weight gain with prolonged use.
- **Suicide precautions:** If patients are extremely depressed and/or have expressed suicidal ideations, initiate close monitoring.
- **Therapeutic response:** Increased interest in surroundings and ability to concentrate, improvement in self-care, and relaxed facial expression.
- **Patient education:** When aripiprazole is used outside the hospital, instruct patients to avoid alcohol, heat exposure leading to dehydration, and tasks that require mental alertness or motor skills until the response to the drug is known.

SERIOUS ADVERSE REACTIONS

- **Neurologic:** Extrapyramidal symptoms, tardive dyskinesia, and neuroleptic malignant syndrome occur rarely.
- **Tardive dyskinesia:** Has infrequently occurred in several patients after a brief period of treatment at low doses. Seen more commonly after a prolonged course of therapy and/or when using higher doses.

OVERDOSE/TOXICITY

- **Neuroleptic malignant syndrome:** High fever, muscle rigidity, altered mental status, irregular pulse, labile blood pressure, tachycardia, diaphoresis, and cardiac dysrhythmias.
- **NMS management:** Discontinue aripiprazole immediately. Aggressive management of BP, heart rate, and dysrhythmias according to accepted Advanced Cardiac Life Support (ACLS) guidelines. Manage other associated medical problems per accepted guidelines. When reintroducing aripiprazole, monitor carefully, as repeat episodes of NMS have been reported.

- **GI decontamination:** No specific recommendations.

ANTIDOTE/DIALYSIS

- **Antidote:** No specific recommendations.
- **Dialysis:** Aripiprazole is unlikely to be removed by hemodialysis, high-permeability hemodialysis, or peritoneal dialysis.

aspirin/acetylsalicylic acid/ASA

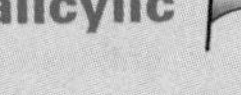

as'-pir-in

Classes

Chemical: salicylate derivative
Therapeutic: antiinflammatory, antiplatelet agent, antipyretic, nonnarcotic analgesic

Pregnancy Category: D (3rd trimester), C

Trade Names

Prescription: Entaprin, YSP Aspirin, Zero-Order Release, ZORprin
Over the Counter: Ascriptin, Asaphen E. C. ♣, Aspergum, Bayer, Bayer Children's Aspirin, Ecotrin, Ecotrin Maximum Strength, 8-Hour Bayer Extended Release, Empirin, Entrophen ♣, Maximum Bayer, Norwich, Novasen ♣

Combinations

Prescription: with butalbital (Fiorinal); with codeine (Empirin); with dihydrocodeine and caffeine (Synalgos DC); with dipyridamole (Aggrenox); with oxycodone (Percodan); with propoxyphene (Darvon)
Over the Counter: with antacids (Ascriptin, Bufferin, Magnaprin)

Do not confuse aspirin or Ascriptin with Aricept, Afrin, or Asendin, or Ecotrin with Edecrin.

CLINICAL PHARMACOLOGY

Mechanism of Action

A nonsteroidal salicylate that inhibits prostaglandin synthesis, acts on the hypothalamus heat-regulating center, and interferes with the production of thromboxane A, a substance that stimulates platelet aggregation. **Therapeutic Effect:** Reduces inflammatory response and intensity of pain; decreases fever; inhibits platelet aggregation.

PHARMACOKINETICS

Route	Onset	Peak	Duration
PO	1 hr	2 hr	4-6 hr

Rapidly and completely absorbed from GI tract; enteric-coated absorption delayed; rectal absorption delayed and incomplete. Protein binding: High. Widely distributed. Rapidly hydrolyzed to salicylate. **Half-life:** 15-20 min (aspirin); 2-3 hr (salicylate at low dose [300-600 mg]); more than 20 hr (salicylate at high dose).

AVAILABILITY

Tablets: 162 mg (Halfprin), 325 mg (Bayer), 500 mg (Bayer).
Tablets (chewable [Bayer, St. Joseph]): 81 mg.
Tablets (enteric coated [Bayer, Ecotrin, St. Joseph]): 81 mg, 325 mg, 500 mg, 650 mg.
Caplets (Bayer): 81 mg, 325 mg, 500 mg.
Gelcaps (Bayer): 325 mg, 500 mg.
Suppositories: 60 mg, 120 mg, 125 mg, 200 mg, 325 mg, 600 mg, 650 mg.

INDICATIONS AND DOSAGE

Analgesia, fever

PO, Rectal

Adults, Elderly: 325-1000 mg 4-6. Maximum: 4 g/day. **Children:** 10-15 mg/kg/dose 4-6. Maximum: 4 g/day.

Antiinflammatory

PO

Adults, Elderly: Initially, 2.4-3.6 g/day in divided doses; then 3.6-5.4 g/day. **Children:** Initially, 60-90 mg/kg/day in divided doses; then 80-100 mg/kg/day.

Platelet aggregation inhibitor

PO

Adults, Elderly: 75-325 mg/day.

Kawasaki disease

PO

Children: 80-100 mg/kg/day in divided doses. After fever resolves: 3-5 mg/kg once daily.

OFF-LABEL USES

Acute ischemic stroke, complications of pregnancy (prophylaxis), MI (prophylaxis), prevention of thromboembolism, rheumatic fever, treatment of Kawasaki disease

CONTRAINDICATIONS

Allergy to tartrazine dye, bleeding disorders, chicken pox or flu in children and teenagers, GI bleeding or ulceration, hepatic impairment, history of hypersensitivity to aspirin or NSAIDs

INTERACTIONS

Drug: **Alcohol, NSAIDs:** May increase the risk of adverse GI effects, including ulceration. **Antacids, urinary alkalinizers:**

Increase the excretion of aspirin. **Anticoagulants, heparin, thrombolytics:** Increase the risk of bleeding. **Insulin, oral antidiabetics:** May increase the effects of these drugs (with large doses of aspirin). **Methotrexate, zidovudine:** May increase the risk of toxicity of these drugs. **Ototoxic medications, vancomycin:** May increase the risk of ototoxicity. **Platelet aggregation inhibitors, valproic acid:** May increase the risk of bleeding. **Probenecid, sulfinpyrazone:** May decrease the effects of these drugs. Herbal: **Cat's claw, dong quai, evening primrose, feverfew, garlic, ginger, ginkgo biloba, red clover, green tea, ginseng:** All have additional antiplatelet activity and may increase the risk of bleeding. Food: None known.

DIAGNOSTIC TEST EFFECTS

May alter serum alkaline phosphatase, uric acid, AST (SGOT), and ALT (SGPT) levels. May prolong prothrombin time and bleeding time. May decrease serum cholesterol, serum potassium, and T_3 and T_4 levels.

SIDE-EFFECTS

Frequent: GI ulceration (6%-31%), bleeding, GI distress (including abdominal distention, cramping, heartburn, and mild nausea). Occasional: Severe bleeding, allergic reaction (including bronchospasm, pruritus, and urticaria), tinnitus

CRITICAL CARE CONSIDERATIONS

ADMINISTRATION/HANDLING

PO ALERT

- Give aspirin with water, milk, or meals if GI distress occurs.
- **Plain aspirin:** May chew (not enteric coated or extended release) if used as part of management of MI to speed up the effect on platelet inhibition.
- **Reye's syndrome:** Do not give aspirin to children or teenagers with chicken pox or the flu because this increases their risk of developing Reye's syndrome.
- **Stability:** Do not use aspirin that smells of vinegar; this odor indicates chemical breakdown of aspirin.
- **Enteric-coated/extended-release tablets:** Do not crush or break.

RECTAL ALERT

- **Storage:** Refrigerate suppositories.
- If the suppository is too soft, refrigerate it for 30 min or run cold water over the foil wrapper.
- **Administration:** Moisten the suppository with cold water before inserting it well into the rectum.

PRECAUTIONS

HEALTH-RELATED

- Use aspirin cautiously in patients with chronic renal insufficiency, vitamin K deficiency, or the "aspirin triad" of asthma, nasal polyps, and rhinitis.

AGE-RELATED

- **Children:** Use caution in giving aspirin to children with acute febrile illness. Do not give aspirin to children with chicken pox or the flu because this increases their risk of developing Reye's syndrome.
- **Elderly:** Lower aspirin dosages are recommended for elderly, who are more susceptible to salicylate toxicity. ***Elderly with altered mental status may have chronic salicylate toxicity that is overlooked.***

PREGNANCY/LACTATION-RELATED

- Pregnancy category C (category D if full doses used in third trimester); use in pregnancy should generally be avoided; in pregnancies at risk for the development of pregnancy-induced hypertension and preeclampsia, and in fetuses with intrauterine growth retardation, low-dose aspirin (40-150 mg/day) may be beneficial; excreted into breast milk in low concentrations.

MONITORING

- **Baseline assessment:** Assess the duration, location, and type of inflammation or pain including chest discomfort. Inspect the arthritic patient's affected joints for deformities, immobility, and skin condition.
- **Therapeutic serum aspirin level:** For antiarthritic effect, 20-30 mg/dL; peaks 2 hr after ingestion.
- **Toxic serum level:** Over 30 mg/dL.
- **Urine pH:** Monitor urine pH for signs of sudden acidification, indicated by a pH of 6.5 to 5.5. Sudden acidification may cause the serum salicylate level to increase greatly, leading to toxicity.
- **Bruising tendency:** Assess skin for evidence of ecchymosis.
- **Fever:** If aspirin is given as an antipyretic, take temperature just before and 1 hr after the drug is taken.

- **Response in arthritics:** Evaluate the arthritic patient for a therapeutic response to the drug, such as improved grip strength, increased joint mobility, reduced joint tenderness, and relief of pain, stiffness, and swelling.
- **Reye's syndrome:** Behavioral changes and vomiting may be early signs of Reye's syndrome. If these occur, contact the physician at once.
- **Patient education:** With ongoing use, inform patients that aspirin's antiinflammatory effect should occur within 1-3 wk, but antiplatelet effects that may create a bleeding tendency occur immediately. Because of the increased risk of GI bleeding, advise patients to avoid taking NSAIDs and drinking alcohol while taking aspirin. Do not crush or allow patients to chew enteric-coated or extended-release tablets. Caution patients to report ringing in the ears (tinnitus) or persistent abdominal or GI pain.

SERIOUS ADVERSE REACTIONS

- **GI bleeding:** High doses of aspirin may produce GI bleeding and gastric mucosal lesions.
- **Reye's syndrome:** Dehydrated, febrile children may experience aspirin toxicity quickly. Reye's syndrome may occur in children with chickenpox or flu.
- **Low-grade toxicity:** Characterized by tinnitus, generalized pruritus (possibly severe), headache, dizziness, flushing, tachycardia, hyperventilation, diaphoresis, and thirst.

OVERDOSE/TOXICITY

- **Rapid deterioration:** Patients who are awake and alert initially may expire within 6 hr while salicylate levels are declining because of distribution of salicylate coupled with acidemia.
- **Severe salicylate toxicity:** Characterized by hyperthermia, diaphoresis, restlessness, agitation, confusion, disorientation, hallucinations, hyperventilation, respiratory depression as condition progresses, seizures, and coma.
- **Metabolic derangements:** Respiratory alkalosis, metabolic acidosis, ketosis, hypokalemia, hyperglycemia, hypo- and hypercalcemia. If rhabdomyolysis ensues, DIC and acute tubular necrosis (renal failure) may follow. Renal failure is sometimes seen in the absence of rhabdomyolysis.
- **Hematologic:** Bleeding due to inhibition of platelet aggregation and prevention of activation of vitamin K-dependent coagulation factors; leukocytosis.
- **GI bleeding:** Hematemesis, abdominal pain, vomiting, and rare gastric perforation because of a corrosive effect on the GI tract.
- **Cardiopulmonary:** Sinus tachycardia, hypotension, ventricular dysrhythmias, shock, acute respiratory distress syndrome, asystole.
- **Severe neurotoxicity:** Confusion, agitation, seizures, coma, or deterioration in level of consciousness despite supportive care are ominous signs.
- **Lab work:** Arterial blood gases, complete metabolic panel, creatine kinase, prothrombin time, complete blood count, urine pH, salicylate level, and acetaminophen level (to ensure the patient/family is not confused about which medication the patient ingested).
- **Toxic salicylate levels:** Low-grade toxicity is generally greater than 20 mg/dL (greater than 1.46 mmol/L); severe toxicity is greater than 70 mg/dL (greater than 5.1 mmol/L).
- **Hypoglycemia:** Monitor closely for hypoglycemia.
- **Management:** Manage dehydration. Aspirin-toxic patients are often deficient by 5-6 L due to vomiting and may tolerate IV fluid at 500-600 mL/hr. Ringer's lactate is often used. Hematocrit may continue to rise despite aggressive hydration. Hydration should continue until crisis is under control. Following initial hydration, pH should be maintained greater than 7.4 with a goal of 7.5 to limit distribution of drug in the body. Aspirin-toxic patients have severe metabolic acidosis. Alkalinization of urine helps to maintain the desired pH. Alkaline urine enhances salicylate excretion. Continuous infusion of IV solution containing sodium bicarbonate is effective. Adequate urine output should be 2 to 3 mL/kg/hr in this setting. Hemodialysis effectively removes salicylates. Hemodialysis is indicated for patients with severe neurotoxicity, cardiovascular instability, and renal failure and for those whose salicylate levels are increasing despite other supportive measures.
- **GI decontamination:** Oral-activated charcoal is reported to be superior to using ipecac to induce vomiting. Repeat dosing of activated charcoal may be beneficial.

ANTIDOTE/DIALYSIS

- **Antidote:** No specific recommendations.
- **Dialysis:** Aspirin is removed by hemodialysis, peritoneal dialysis, and is likely removed by high-permeability hemodialysis.

atazanavir sulfate

See HIV Medications (p. 961)

atenolol

a-ten'-oh-lol

Classes

Chemical: β1-adrenergic blocker, cardioselective

Therapeutic: antianginal, antihypertensive

Pregnancy Category: D

Trade Names

Prescription: Tenormin

Combinations

Prescription: with chlorthalidone (Tenoretic)

Do not confuse atenolol with albuterol or timolol.

CLINICAL PHARMACOLOGY

Mechanism of Action

A $beta_1$-adrenergic blocker that acts as an antianginal, antidysrhythmic, and antihypertensive agent by blocking $beta_1$-adrenergic receptors in cardiac tissue. **Therapeutic Effect:** Slows sinus node heart rate, decreasing cardiac output and BP. Decreases myocardial oxygen demand.

PHARMACOKINETICS

Route	Onset	Peak	Duration
PO	1 hr	2-4 hr	12-24 hr

Incompletely absorbed from the GI tract. Protein binding: 6%-16%. Minimal liver metabolism. Primarily excreted unchanged in urine. Removed by hemodialysis. **Half-life:** 6-7 hr (increased in impaired renal function).

AVAILABILITY

Tablets: 25 mg, 50 mg, 100 mg.
Injection: 5 mg/10 mL.

INDICATIONS AND DOSAGE

Hypertension

PO

Adults: Initially, 25-50 mg once per day. May increase dose up to 100 mg once per day. **Elderly:** Usual initial dose, 25 mg per day. **Children:** Initially, 0.8-1 mg/kg/dose given once per day. Range: 0.8-1.5 mg/kg/day. Maximum: 2 mg/kg/day or 100 mg/day.

Angina pectoris

PO

Adults: Initially, 50 mg once per day. May increase dose up to 200 mg once per day. **Elderly:** Usual initial dose, 25 mg per day.

Acute MI

IV

Adults: Give 5 mg over 5 min; may repeat in 10 min. In those who tolerate full 10-mg IV dose, begin 50-mg tablets 10 min after last IV dose followed by another 50-mg oral dose 12 hr later. Thereafter, give 100 mg once per day or 50 mg twice per day for 6-9 days. For those who do not tolerate full IV dose, give 50 mg orally twice per day or 100 mg once per day for at least 7 days.

Dosage in Renal Impairment

Dosage interval is modified based on creatinine clearance.

Creatinine Clearance	Dosage interval
15-35 mL/min	50 mg per day
Less than 15 mL/min	50 mg every other day

OFF-LABEL USES

Acute alcohol withdrawal, dysrhythmia (especially supraventricular and ventricular tachycardia), improved survival in diabetics with heart disease, mild to moderately severe heart failure (adjunct); prevention of migraine, thyrotoxicosis, tremors; treatment of hypertrophic cardiomyopathy, pheochromocytoma, and syndrome of mitral valve prolapse

CONTRAINDICATIONS

Cardiogenic shock, overt heart failure, second- or third-degree heart block, severe bradycardia

INTERACTIONS

Drug: Cimetidine: May increase atenolol blood concentration. **Diuretics, other antihypertensives:** May increase hypotensive effect of atenolol. **Insulin, oral hypoglycemics:** May mask symptoms of hypoglycemia and prolong hypoglycemic effect of insulin and oral hypoglycemics. **NSAIDs:**

May decrease antihypertensive effect of atenolol. **Sympathomimetics, xanthines:** May mutually inhibit effects. Herbal: **Dong quai, ephedra, yohimbe, garlic, ginseng:** Should be avoided. Food: None known.

DIAGNOSTIC TEST EFFECTS

May increase serum antinuclear antibody titer and BUN, serum creatinine, potassium, lipoprotein, triglyceride, and uric acid levels.

IV INCOMPATIBILITIES

Amphotericin complex (Abelcet, Ambisome, Amphotec)

SIDE-EFFECTS

Frequent: Hypotension manifested as cold extremities, constipation or diarrhea, diaphoresis, dizziness, fatigue, headache, and nausea. Atenolol is generally well tolerated, with mild and transient side effects. Occasional: Insomnia, flatulence, urinary frequency, impotence or decreased libido, depression. Rare: Rash, arthralgia, myalgia, confusion (especially in the elderly), altered taste

CRITICAL CARE CONSIDERATIONS

ADMINISTRATION/HANDLING

PO ALERT

- May give atenolol without regard to meals.
- Crush tablets if necessary.

IV ALERT

- **Storage:** Store at room temperature. After reconstitution, store parenteral form for up to 48 hr at room temperature.
- **Dilution:** Give undiluted or dilute in 10 to 50 mL 0.9% NaCl or D_5W.
- **IV push/direct IV:** Give IV push over 5 min.
- **IV intermittent infusion:** Give IV infusion over 15 min.

PRECAUTIONS

HEALTH-RELATED

- Use atenolol cautiously in patients with bronchospastic disease, diabetes mellitus, thyroid disease, impaired renal or hepatic function, inadequate cardiac function, or peripheral vascular disease.

AGE-RELATED

- **Children:** No age-related precautions have been noted in children.
- **Elderly:** Are at increased risk for age-related peripheral vascular disease and impaired renal function.

PREGNANCY/LACTATION-RELATED

- Pregnancy category D; frequently used in the third trimester for treatment of hypertension (many studies of efficacy and safety of atenolol in pregnancy-induced hypertension); long-term use has been associated with intrauterine growth retardation; excreted into breast milk; observe for signs of beta-blockade.

MONITORING

- **Baseline assessment for heart rate or BP:** Assess heart rate and BP immediately before giving atenolol. If heart rate is less than 60 beats/min or systolic BP is less than 90 mmHg, withhold the medication.
- **Baseline assessment for angina:** If atenolol is being given as an antianginal, record the onset, quality (e.g., dull, sharp, or squeezing), radiation, location, intensity, and duration of anginal pain; document precipitating factors (e.g., emotional, stress, or exertion).
- **Baseline lab work:** Biochemical profile including blood glucose, renal and hepatic function test results, CBC to rule out anemia if patient is being managed for angina.
- **Heart failure:** Monitor for distended neck veins, night cough, peripheral edema, hypotension, bradycardia, activity intolerance, and difficulty breathing.
- **Cardiac:** Observe ECG for dysrhythmias including sinus bradycardia and heart block. If heart block progresses to second or third degree, atenolol should be withheld.
- **Fluid retention:** Monitor intake and output for oliguria and weight gain.
- **Hypoglycemia:** Assess blood glucose at least before meals and at bedtime in diabetics because atenolol may mask sympathetic nervous system effects (e.g., tachycardia and diaphoresis) associated with hypoglycemia.
- **Hyperglycemia:** Assess elderly carefully because they are at risk for developing hyperglycemia with long-term use.
- **Diarrhea:** Assess pattern of daily bowel activity and stool consistency.

A

- **Dizziness:** Assist with ambulation if dizziness occurs.
- **Patient education:** Warn patients not to discontinue atenolol abruptly. Advise that compliance with therapy is essential to control angina and hypertension. To reduce orthostatic effects, instruct patients to rise slowly from a lying to sitting position and pause momentarily before standing. Recommend avoidance of tasks requiring alertness or motor skills until the response to the drug is known. Instruct patients to report promptly to a health care provider confusion, depression, dizziness, rash, or unusual bruising or bleeding. Discharge teaching should include the correct technique for monitoring BP and pulse before taking atenolol. Urge patients to restrict alcohol and salt intake. Advise that therapeutic antihypertensive effects of atenolol are present within 1-2 wk.

SERIOUS ADVERSE REACTIONS

- **Abrupt withdrawal:** May result in diaphoresis, tachydysrhythmias, palpitations, tremors, headache, angina, or myocardial infarction in patients with heart disease; may result in thyroid storm in patients with hyperthyroidism.
- **Cardiovascular:** Atenolol administration may cause heart failure in patients with cardiac disease and peripheral ischemia in those with peripheral vascular disease.
- **Hypoglycemia:** May occur in patients with previously controlled diabetes.
- **Thrombocytopenia:** Unusual bruising or bleeding occurs rarely.
- **Hyperglycemia:** Long-term use may lead to hyperglycemia and development of diabetes mellitus.

OVERDOSE/TOXICITY

- **Symptoms:** Profound bradycardia, heart block, bronchospasm or wheezing with respiratory distress, heart failure, hypoglycemia, and hypotension.
- **Management:** Upon withdrawing atenolol following overdose, if acute angina, ST segment depression indicative of myocardial ischemia, or ST segment elevation indicative of MI are experienced, the patient must be provided with another therapy to promote myocardial perfusion immediately.
- **GI decontamination:** Activated charcoal is most effective versus whole bowel irrigation, which has not been thoroughly tested in humans.

ANTIDOTE/DIALYSIS

- **Antidote:** Beta agonist high-dose infusion such as DOPamine, epinephrine, *DOBUTamine, or isoproterenol (use cautiously to avoid extreme tachycardia) to counteract the effects of beta-blockade including bradycardia, hypotension, and bronchospasms. Glucagon is often successful in increasing heart rate in beta-blocker overdose. Phosphodiesterase inhibitors inamrinone and milrinone may be used to manage heart failure if other agents are ineffective. Other treatment options include glucose and insulin, cardiac pacing, crystalloid fluids, and vasopressors such as norepinephrine for hypotension. Aerosolized bronchodilators (e.g., albuterol) may be effective in counteracting bronchospastic effects.
- **Dialysis:** Atenolol is removed by hemodialysis and is likely removed by high-permeability hemodialysis. It is not removed by peritoneal dialysis.

atomoxetine hydrochloride

at′-oh-mox-e-teen hye-droe-klor′-ide

Classes

Chemical: propylamine derivative
Therapeutic: selective norepinephrine transporter inhibitor

Pregnancy Category: C

Trade Names

Prescription: Strattera

CLINICAL PHARMACOLOGY

Mechanism of Action

A norepinephrine reuptake inhibitor that enhances noradrenergic function by selective inhibition of the presynaptic norepinephrine transporter. **Therapeutic Effect:** Improves symptoms of attention-deficit/hyperactivity disorder (ADHD).

PHARMACOKINETICS

Rapidly absorbed after PO administration. Protein binding: 98% (primarily to albumin). Eliminated primarily in urine and, to a lesser extent, in feces. Not removed by hemodialysis. **Half-life:** 4-5 hr in general population, 22 hr in 7% of Caucasians, and 2% of African Americans (increased in moderate to severe hepatic insufficiency).

A

AVAILABILITY

Capsules: 10 mg, 18 mg, 25 mg, 40 mg, 60 mg, 80 mg, 100 mg.

INDICATIONS AND DOSAGE

ADHD

PO

Adults, Children weighing 70 kg and more: 40 mg once per day. May increase after at least 3 days to 80 mg as a single daily dose or in divided doses. Maximum: 100 mg.
Children weighing less than 70 kg: Initially, 0.5 mg/kg/day. May increase after at least 3 days to 1.2 mg/kg/day. Maximum: 1.4 mg/kg/day or 100 mg.

Dosage in hepatic impairment

Expect to administer 50% of normal atomoxetine dosage to patients with moderate hepatic impairment and 25% of normal dosage to those with severe hepatic impairment.

OFF-LABEL USES

Treatment of depression.

CONTRAINDICATIONS

Angle-closure glaucoma, use within 14 days of MAOIs

INTERACTIONS

Drug: **Fluoxetine, paroxetine, quinidine:** May increase atomoxetine blood concentration. **MAOIs:** May increase the risk of toxic effects. Herbal: None known. Food: None known.

DIAGNOSTIC TEST EFFECTS

None known.

SIDE-EFFECTS

Frequent: Headache (17%-27%); abdominal pain (20%); nausea (12%); vomiting (15%); fatigue, decreased appetite (14%); insomnia (16%); cough (11%). Occasional: Tachycardia (4%), hypertension (5%), weight loss, delayed growth in children. Rare: Irritability, jaundice, agitation

CRITICAL CARE CONSIDERATIONS

ADMINISTRATION/HANDLING

PO ALERT

- Give atomoxetine without regard to food.

PRECAUTIONS

HEALTH-RELATED

- Avoid concurrent use of medications that can increase heart rate or BP.
- Use atomoxetine cautiously in patients with cardiovascular disease, tachycardia, hypertension, moderate to severe hepatic impairment, or a risk of urine retention.

AGE-RELATED

- **Children:** Safety and efficacy of atomoxetine have not been established in children under 6 yr. Case reports indicate some children experience slowing of growth and lack of weight gain.
- **Elderly:** Age-related cardiovascular or cerebrovascular disease and hepatic or renal impairment may increase the risk of side effects.

PREGNANCY/LACTATION-RELATED

- Pregnancy category C; excretion into breast milk unknown; use caution in nursing mothers.

MONITORING

- **Baseline assessment:** Obtain vital signs before beginning atomoxetine therapy.
- **Lab work:** Biochemical profile including liver function tests (AST [SGOT], ALT [SGPT], alkaline phosphatase, bilirubin).
- **Ongoing vital signs:** Observe for tachycardia, hypertension, and orthostatic hypotension after dosage increases, and periodically during therapy.
- **Difficulty voiding:** Monitor urine output. Inability to urinate or urinary hesitancy may be an adverse reaction. Catheterization of the bladder may be necessary.
- **Dizziness:** Assist with ambulation if dizziness occurs. Orthostatic hypotension may be present.
- **Mood assessment:** Be alert for mood changes. Irritability may indicate adverse reaction.
- **Vomiting:** Monitor the fluid and electrolyte status of patients who experience significant vomiting. Patients may have decreased appetite.
- **Comprehensive program:** Patients receiving atomoxetine for ADHD should be enrolled in a comprehensive treatment program including psychologic, educational, and social measures.
- **Patient education:** When atomoxetine is used outside the hospital, instruct patients to take the last daily dose early in the evening to avoid insomnia, to avoid tasks that require mental alertness and motor skills until the response to the drug is known, and to report promptly fever, irritability, palpitations, or vomiting to a health care provider.

SERIOUS ADVERSE REACTIONS

- **Difficulty voiding:** Urine retention or urinary hesitance may occur.
- **MAOIs:** If patients receive atomoxetine while taking MAOIs, there have been reports of serious, sometimes fatal reactions including hyperthermia, rigidity, myoclonus, labile heart rate and BP, extreme agitation, delirium, coma, and occasionally symptoms similar to neuroleptic malignant syndrome (high fever, muscle rigidity, altered mental status, irregular pulse, labile BP, tachycardia, diaphoresis, and cardiac dysrhythmias).

OVERDOSE/TOXICITY

- **Symptoms:** Abdominal pain, weight loss, vomiting, dizziness, tachycardia, hypertension, headache, somnolence, irritability, mood swings, cough, dermatitis.
- **Management:** Atomoxetine should be discontinued and symptoms managed according to symptom-specific guidelines.
- **GI decontamination:** No specific recommendations. Repeated use of activated charcoal may be effective if the patient presents for treatment within 1 hr of overdose.

ANTIDOTE/DIALYSIS

- **Antidote:** No specific recommendations.
- **Dialysis:** Atomoxetine is generally not removed by hemodialysis, high-permeability hemodialysis, or peritoneal dialysis.

atorvastatin

a-tore'-va-sta-tin

Classes

Chemical: substituted hexahydronaphthalene

Therapeutic: HMG-CoA reductase inhibitor, antilipemic

Pregnancy Category: X

Trade Names

Prescription: Lipitor

Combinations

Prescription: with amlodipine (Caduet)

Do not confuse Lipitor with Levatol.

CLINICAL PHARMACOLOGY

Mechanism of Action

An antihyperlipidemic that inhibits hydroxamethylglutaryl-CoA (HMG-CoA) reductase, the enzyme that catalyzes the early step in cholesterol synthesis. **Therapeutic Effect:** Decreases LDL and VLDL cholesterol, and plasma triglyceride levels; increases HDL cholesterol concentration.

PHARMACOKINETICS

Poorly absorbed from the GI tract. Protein binding: greater than 98%. Metabolized in the liver. Minimally eliminated in urine. Plasma levels are markedly increased in chronic alcoholic hepatic disease but are unaffected by renal disease. **Half-life:** 14 hr.

AVAILABILITY

Tablets: 10 mg, 20 mg, 40 mg, 80 mg.

INDICATIONS AND DOSAGE

Prevention of cardiovascular disease (CVD)

PO

Adults, Elderly: 10 mg once daily.

Hyperlipidemias

PO

Adults, Elderly: Initially, 10-20 mg/day (40 mg in patients requiring greater than 45% reduction in LDL-C). Range: 10-80 mg/day.

Heterozygous hypercholesterolemia

PO

Children 10-17 yr: Initially, 10 mg/day. Maximum: 20 mg/day.

OFF-LABEL USES

Secondary prevention of ischemia in patients with heart failure

CONTRAINDICATIONS

Active hepatic disease, lactation, pregnancy, unexplained elevated liver function test results

INTERACTIONS

Drug: **Antacids, colestipol, propranolol:** Decreases atorvastatin activity. ***CycloSPORINE, erythromycin, gemfibrozil, nicotinic acid:** Increases the risk of acute renal failure and rhabdomyolysis with these drugs. **Digoxin, itraconazole, oral contraceptives, warfarin:** May increase atorvastatin blood concentration, producing severe muscle inflammation, pain, and weakness.
Herbal: **St. John's wort:** May decrease atorvastatin levels. **Food:** **Grapefruit juice:** May increase atorvastatin levels if more than 1 quart is consumed.

DIAGNOSTIC TEST EFFECTS

May increase serum creatine kinase (CK) and transaminase concentrations.

A

SIDE-EFFECTS

Atorvastatin is generally well tolerated. Side effects are usually mild and transient. **Frequent (3%-17%):** Headache. **Occasional (5%-2%):** Myalgia, rash or pruritus, allergy. **Rare (2%-1%):** Flatulence, dyspepsia

CRITICAL CARE CONSIDERATIONS

ADMINISTRATION/HANDLING

PO ALERT

- May give atorvastatin without regard to food.
- Do not break film-coated tablets.

PRECAUTIONS

HEALTH-RELATED

- Use atorvastatin cautiously in patients with a history of hepatic disease, hypotension, major surgery, severe acute infection, substantial alcohol consumption, uncontrolled seizures, severe endocrine, electrolyte, metabolic disorders, or trauma, and in those receiving anticoagulant therapy.
- **Serious illness:** Atorvastatin should be temporarily withheld or discontinued in acutely ill patients to avoid increased probability of development of a myopathy.
- **Increased probability of myopathy:** Increased when used concomitantly with *cycloSPORINE, erthyromycin, fibric acid derivatives, immunosuppressive drugs, niacin, and azole antifungal agents.

AGE-RELATED

- **Children:** Safety and efficacy of atorvastatin have not been established in children under 10 yr.
- **Elderly:** No age-related precautions are noted for the elderly.

PREGNANCY/LACTATION-RELATED

- Pregnancy category X; not recommended for nursing mothers.

MONITORING

- **Pregnancy concern:** Determine pregnancy before beginning atorvastatin therapy because it may cause fetal harm.
- **Lab work:** Assess baseline serum cholesterol and triglyceride levels and liver function test results. Monitor cholesterol and triglycerides for therapeutic response and liver enzymes every 12 wk after initial therapy and each time dosage is adjusted. Semiannual monitoring may be appropriate for patients on fixed doses with good response. Periodic laboratory tests are an essential part of ongoing therapy.
- **Side effects:** Constipation, abdominal pain, dyspepsia, flatulence. May require symptom-specific management to control.
- **Myalgias:** CPK level may be measured for patients with unexplained myalgias. Urine will appear brown if myoglobin is present.
- **Renal failure:** Monitor BUN, creatinine, and potassium levels if patients manifest myalgia or brown urine indicative of myoglobinuria. Urinalysis is used to diagnose myoglobinuria.
- **Diet instruction:** Patients must follow the prescribed diet because diet is an important part of lowering cholesterol and triglycerides.
- **Patient education:** When therapy is continued outside the hospital, warn patients not to take other medications without physician approval.

SERIOUS ADVERSE REACTIONS

- **Musculoskeletal pain:** Myopathy, arthralgia, myalgia, which may indicate impending rhabdomyolysis.
- **Renal failure:** Acute renal failure ensues when rhabdomyolysis is present.
- **Liver failure:** Liver enzyme elevation is indicative of impending liver failure.

OVERDOSE/TOXICITY

- **Rhabdomyolysis:** Rare cases; can lead to acute renal failure. Markedly elevated serum CK and possible myoglobinuria indicate the condition may be present. Should be managed according to accepted guidelines, which include aggressive volume replacement, hemodialysis, or continuous hemofiltration (CVVH) to support patient during acute renal failure. Use of bicarbonate to induce alkaline diuresis or mannitol for osmotic diuresis has not been well studied. Hyperkalemia and hyperphosphatemia are commonly seen with rhabdomyolysis and may require aggressive management.
- **Hypocalcemia:** Must be managed cautiously with rhabdomyolysis because calcium infusion may increase the deposition of calcium in the injured muscles.
- **Discontinue medication:** Atorvastatin should be discontinued if the patient develops myopathy and/or rhabdomyolysis.

A

- **GI decontamination:** No specific recommendations.

ANTIDOTE/DIALYSIS

- **Antidote:** No specific recommendations.
- **Dialysis:** Atorvastatin is not removed by hemodialysis and is unlikely to be removed by peritoneal dialysis. No data are available on removal by high-permeability hemodialysis.

atovaquone

a-toe'-va-kwone

Classes
Chemical: hydroxynapthoquinone derivative
Therapeutic: antiprotozoal

Pregnancy Category: C

Trade Names
Prescription: Mepron

Combinations
Prescription: with proguanil (Malarone)

CLINICAL PHARMACOLOGY

Mechanism of Action
A systemic antiinfective that inhibits the mitochondrial electron-transport system at the cytochrome bc1 complex (Complex III), which interrupts nucleic acid and adenosine triphosphate synthesis. **Therapeutic Effect:** Antiprotozoal and antipneumocystic activity.

PHARMACOKINETICS

Absorption increased with a high-fat meal. Protein binding: greater than 99%. Metabolized in liver. Primarily excreted in feces. **Half-life:** 2-3 days.

AVAILABILITY

Oral suspension: 750 mg/5 mL.

INDICATIONS AND DOSAGE

Pneumocystis carinii pneumonia (PCP)
PO
Adults, Children older than 12 yr: 750 mg twice per day with food for 21 days. **Children 12 yr and younger:** 40 mg/kg/day in two divided doses. Maximum: 1500 mg/day.
Prevention of PCP
PO
Adults: 1500 mg once per day with food. **Children 4-24 mo:** 45 mg/kg/day as single dose. Maximum: 1500 mg/day. **Children 1-3 mo and older than 24 mo:** 30 mg/kg/day as single dose. Maximum: 1500 mg/day.

CONTRAINDICATIONS

Development or history of potentially life-threatening allergic reaction to the drug

INTERACTIONS

Drug: Rifampin: May decrease atovaquone blood concentration and increase rifampin blood concentration. **Herbal:** None known. **Food: Fatty meals:** Increase absorption of atovaquone.

DIAGNOSTIC TEST EFFECTS

May increase serum alkaline phosphatase, amylase, AST (SGOT), and ALT (SGPT) levels. May decrease serum sodium levels.

SIDE-EFFECTS

Frequent (greater than 10%): Rash, nausea, diarrhea, headache, vomiting, fever, insomnia, cough. **Occasional (less than 10%):** Abdominal discomfort, thrush, asthenia, anemia, neutropenia

CRITICAL CARE CONSIDERATIONS

ADMINISTRATION/HANDLING

PO ALERT

- Atovaquone suspension should be administered with meals. Failure to administer with food may lower atovaquone concentrations and may limit response to therapy.

PRECAUTIONS

HEALTH-RELATED

- Use atovaquone cautiously in patients with chronic diarrhea, malabsorption syndromes, or severe PCP (*Pneumocystis carinii* pneumonia).
- **Renal impairment:** Atovaquone should not be used for malaria prophylaxis for patients with severe renal impairment (creatinine clearance less than 30 mL/min).

AGE-RELATED

- **Children:** Dosage for children under 13 yr is based on weight.
- **Elderly:** Monitor closely because of age-related cardiac, hepatic, and renal impairment. Use cautiously in elderly patients.

A

PREGNANCY/LACTATION-RELATED

- Pregnancy category C; human breast milk studies not available; in rats, concentrations in milk 30% of maternal serum.

MONITORING

- **Baseline assessment:** Determine history of allergies to atovaquone before beginning drug therapy. Evaluate history for medical problems that may interfere with drug absorption, such as GI disorders.
- **Lab work:** Hgb levels and renal function test results.
- **GI effects:** Assess for GI discomfort, anorexia, nausea, and vomiting. Assess the pattern of daily bowel activity for diarrhea.
- **Sensitivity:** Examine the skin for rash.
- **Fluid balance:** Monitor intake and output.
- **Do not discontinue:** Administer atovaquone for the full course of treatment.
- **Patient education:** Instruct patients not to take any other medications. Urge patients to report promptly diarrhea, rash, or other new symptoms to a health care provider. Explain that the full course of treatment must be completed.

SERIOUS ADVERSE REACTIONS

- Can develop life-threatening allergic reactions to any of the components of the formulations.

OVERDOSE/TOXICITY

- **Supportive treatment:** Atovaquone overdose information is limited. Treatment is symptomatic and supportive.
- **Hypotension:** Infuse isotonic fluid. If hypotension persists, administer dopamine or norepinephrine according to Advanced Cardiac Life Support (ACLS) guidelines titrated to desired response.
- **GI decontamination:** Administer oral activated charcoal treated within 1 hr of ingestion. Consider gastric lavage after ingestion of a potentially life-threatening amount if it can be performed soon after ingestion (generally within 1 hr). Protect airway by placing in Trendelenburg and left lateral decubitus position or by endotracheal intubation. Control any seizures first.

ANTIDOTE/DIALYSIS

- **Antidote:** No specific recommendations.
- **Dialysis:** Atovaquone is unlikely to be removed by hemodialysis or peritoneal dialysis. No data are available on removal by high-permeability hemodialysis.

atracurium besylate 

a-tra-kyoo'-ree-um bess'-il-ate

Classes

Chemical: nondepolarizing neuromuscular blocking agent

Therapeutic: skeletal muscle relaxant, paralytic agent

Pregnancy Category: C

Trade Names

Prescription: Tracrium

CLINICAL PHARMACOLOGY

Mechanism of Action

A nondepolarizing skeletal muscle relaxant that blocks the neurotransmitter action of acetylcholine by binding competitively with cholinergic receptor sites. **Therapeutic Effect:** Produces skeletal muscle relaxation.

PHARMACOKINETICS

Onset of action is dose-dependent and occurs within 2 to 3 min. Recovery begins in 20 to 35 min. Undergoes ester hydrolysis and Hofmann elimination. **Half-life:** 2 min (initial); 20 min (terminal).

AVAILABILITY

IV Solution: 10 mg/mL (Tracrium).

INDICATIONS AND DOSAGE

Adjunct to general anesthesia; administered to facilitate endotracheal intubation and/or to provide skeletal muscle relaxation during surgery or mechanical ventilation

IV

Adults, Elderly, Children 2 yr and older: Initially, 0.4-0.5 mg/kg as a bolus dose. The dose of 0.08-0.10 mg/kg is recommended for maintenance. After initial bolus dose is given, a diluted solution may be administered by continuous infusion. Infusion should be individualized for each patient. The rate of 5-9 mcg/kg/min should be adequate to maintain continuous neuromuscular blockade in most patients. **Infants, 1 mo to 2 yr:** Initially, 0.3-0.4 mg/kg. Maintenance doses may be required with slightly greater frequency in infants and children than in adults.

Long-term mechanical ventilation in intensive care unit

IV

Adults, Elderly, Children: Initially, 0.4-0.5 mg/kg as an IV bolus dose. Then 11-13 mcg/kg/min. Infusion rates may be higher for children than for adult patients.

A

CONTRAINDICATIONS

Hypersensitivity to atracurium, benzyl alcohol, or any component of the formulation

INTERACTIONS

Drug: **Isoflurane, halothane, aminoglycosides, corticosteroids, polymyxins, immunosuppressants, lithium, magnesium salts, procainamide, and quinidine:** May enhance neuromuscular blockade, which may lead to respiratory depression and paralysis. **Muscle relaxants:** May block the effects of atracurium. **Succinylcholine:** May accelerate the onset and/or increase the depth of neuromuscular blockade induced by atracurium. Herbal: **St. John's wort:** May increase the risk of cardiovascular collapse and/or delay emergence from anesthesia. Food: None known.

DIAGNOSTIC TEST EFFECTS

None known.

IV INCOMPATIBILITIES

Do not mix with alkaline solutions (e.g., barbiturate solutions).

SIDE-EFFECTS

Flushing, bradycardia, allergic reactions, rash, urticaria, reaction at injection site, inadequate or prolonged block, hypotension, tachycardia.

CRITICAL CARE CONSIDERATIONS

ADMINISTRATION/HANDLING

IM ALERT

- Do not give as IM injection due to tissue irritation.

IV ALERT

- **Skilled providers only:** Atracurium should be administered by adequately trained individuals familiar with its actions, characteristics, and hazards.
- **Unconsciousness:** Do not administer atracurium before unconsciousness has been induced.
- **Bolus injection:** May be given undiluted as a bolus injection. The first maintenance dose will generally be required 20 to 45 min after the initial injection.
- **IV infusion solutions:** Prepared by admixing atracurium besylate with an appropriate diluent such as D_5W, 0.9% NaCl, or D_5NS. Solutions containing 0.2 mg/mL or 0.5 mg/mL atracurium besylate in the suggested diluents may be stored either in the refrigerator or at room temperature for 24 hr without significant loss of potency. It is recommended that lactated Ringer's solution not be used as a diluent in the preparation of solutions of atracurium besylate for infusion. Unused solutions should be discarded.
- **Spontaneous degradation:** Has been demonstrated to occur more rapidly in lactated Ringer's solution than in 0.9% NaCl solution.
- **Additional maintenance doses:** Do not give additional doses of atracurium before there is a definite response to the first twitch. If no response is elicited, the infusion should be discontinued until response returns.
- **Cumulative effects:** Maintenance doses may be administered at relatively regular intervals for each patient, ranging from approximately 15 to 25 min once balanced anesthesia has been achieved and maintained. Higher doses of atracurium (up to 0.2 mg/kg) permit maintenance dosing at longer intervals.
- **Storage:** Vials of atracurium should be refrigerated. Use within 14 days on removal from refrigeration to room temperature.

PRECAUTIONS

HEALTH-RELATED

- Use cautiously in patients with cardiovascular disease, electrolyte disturbances, hypothermia, myasthenia gravis, Eaton-Lambert syndrome, amyotrophic lateral sclerosis, respiratory acidosis, or dystrophia myotonica.

AGE-RELATED

- **Neonates:** Atracurium 10-mL multiple-dose vials contain benzyl alcohol. In neonates, benzyl alcohol has been associated with an increased incidence of neurologic and other complications, which are sometimes fatal. Atracurium 5-mL single-use vials do not contain benzyl alcohol.
- **Children:** Safety and efficacy of atracurium have not been established in infants under 1 mo.
- **Elderly:** No age-related precautions noted in the elderly.

PREGNANCY/LACTATION-RELATED

- Pregnancy category C; unknown if excreted in breast milk; if used during labor and delivery, the potential need of forceps delivery increases for vaginal births.

A

MONITORING

- **Baseline assessment:** Assess vital signs, perform a complete physical assessment with focus on efficacy of breathing, neurologic status, level of pain or anticipated level of pain, and anxiety.
- **Lab work:** Biochemical profile including calcium, magnesium, and phosphates.
- **Sedation and analgesia:** Patients undergoing neuromuscular blockade with atracurium should be sedated and have appropriate pain management provided because patients are unable to express anxiety and discomfort during neuromuscular blockade. Atracurium produces apnea and paralysis.
- **Ongoing assessment:** Monitor heart rate, BP, and respiratory rate. Try to assess level of pain.
- **Sedation and neuromuscular blockade:** Monitor the degree of neuromuscular blockade using "train of four" technique with a peripheral nerve stimulator and sedation with a bispectral brain wave analysis device (BIS monitoring). Adjust atracurium and other medications to keep patients still, well ventilated, and as comfortable as possible. Because patients are totally dependent on health care providers to anticipate all needs and provide all care, most patients would rather not have awareness of the neuromuscular blockade experience.
- **Mechanical ventilation:** Assess ventilation status using lung assessment, vital signs, pulse oximetry, and end tidal CO_2 monitoring.
- **Weaning neuromuscular blockade:** Sedation with propofol (Diprivan), benzodiazepine infusion (lorazepam/Ativan), or morphine may provide enough relaxation to be able to wean atracurium without compromising the critically ill patient's ventilatory status.
- **Patient education:** Explain to patients they are unable to speak, open eyes, and move when full neuromuscular blockade is in place. When weaning atracurium, tell patients it will be difficult to talk because of head and neck muscle blockade.

SERIOUS ADVERSE REACTIONS

- Dysrhythmias, edema, and hypotension may occur.
- Anaphylaxis and hypersensitivity reactions have been reported.
- Malignant hyperthermia, a potentially fatal hypermetabolic state of skeletal muscle, occurs rarely.

OVERDOSE/TOXICITY

- **Symptoms:** Prolonged apnea; inability to maintain patent airway, move extremities, speak, or open eyes. May occur more often when agents that potentiate atracurium are given concomitantly. Seizures have been reported in critically ill patients but cause may be multifactorial.
- **Management:** Continue to keep the patient endotracheally intubated and mechanically ventilated until the patient is fully able to effectively maintain breathing and respiration. Antidote may be administered if needed.

ANTIDOTE/DIALYSIS

- **Antidote:** Pyridostigmine (Mestinon) or neostigmine (Prostigmin) given with atropine reverses muscle relaxation in most patients but may aggravate severe overdosage. Ensure the patient is endotracheally intubated and mechanical or manual ventilation is in place.
- **Dialysis:** Hemodialysis and peritoneal dialysis are unlikely to remove atracurium. No data are available on removal using high-permeability hemodialysis.

atropine sulfate

a'-troe-peen sul'-fate

Classes

Chemical: belladonna alkaloid

Therapeutic: antiasthmatic, anticholinergic, antispasmodic, bronchodilator, gastrointestinal, mydriatic, ophthalmic anticholinergic

Pregnancy Category: C

Trade Names

Prescription: Atropine Care, Atropen Autoinjector, Atropisol, Atrosulf-1, Isopto Atropine, Ocu-Tropine, Sal-Tropine

Do not confuse atropine sulfate with Akarpine or Aplisol.

CLINICAL PHARMACOLOGY

Mechanism of Action

An acetylcholine antagonist that inhibits the action of acetylcholine by competing with acetylcholine for common binding sites on muscarinic receptors, which are located on exocrine glands, cardiac and smooth-muscle ganglia, and intramural neurons. This action blocks all muscarinic effects. **Therapeutic Effect:** Decreases GI motility and secretory activity, and GU muscle tone (ureter, bladder); produces ophthalmic cycloplegia, and mydriasis.

PHARMACOKINETICS

AtroPen auto-injector: Rapidly and well absorbed after IM administration. Much of the drug is destroyed by enzymatic hydrolysis, particularly in the liver. Partially excreted unchanged in urine.

AVAILABILITY

Injection: 0.05 mg/mL, 0.1 mg/mL, 0.4 mg/0.5 mL, 0.4 mg/mL, 0.5 mg/mL, 1 mg/mL.
IM injection (AtroPen): 0.5 mg, 1 mg, 2 mg.
Ophthalmic ointment: 1%.
Ophthalmic solution: 0.5% (Isopto Atropine), 1% (Atropisol, Isopto Atropine), 2% (Atropisol).

INDICATIONS AND DOSAGE

Asystole, slow pulseless electrical activity

IV

Adults, Elderly: 1 mg; may repeat every 3-5 min up to total dose of 0.04 mg/kg.

Preanesthetic

IV, IM, Subcutaneous

Adults, Elderly: 0.4-0.6 mg 30-60 min preoperatively. **Children weighing 5 kg and more:** 0.01-0.02 mg/kg/dose to maximum of 0.4 mg/dose. **Children weighing less than 5 kg:** 0.02 mg/kg/dose 30-60 min preoperatively.

Bradycardia

IV

Adults, Elderly: 0.5-1 mg every 5 min not to exceed 2 mg or 0.04 mg/kg. **Children:** 0.02 mg/kg with a minimum of 0.1 mg to a maximum of 0.5 mg in children and 1 mg in adolescents. May repeat in 5 min. Maximum total dose: 1 mg in children, 2 mg in adolescents.

Cycloplegic refraction, postoperative mydriasis, uveitis

Ophthalmic Solution

Adults, Elderly: Instill 1 drop of 1% or 2% solution in affected eye(s) up to 4 times per day.

Ophthalmic Ointment

Adults, Elderly: Apply ointment in conjunctival sac up to 3 times per day. Apply ointment several hours before examination when used for refraction.

Poisoning by susceptible organophosphorous nerve agents having cholinesterase activity, organophosphorous or carbamate insecticides

IM

Adults, Children weighing more than 90 lb: AtroPen 2 mg (green). **Children weighing 40-90 lb:** AtroPen 1 mg (dark red). **Children weighing 15-39 lb:** AtroPen 0.5 mg (blue). **Infants weighing less than 15 lb:** AtroPen 0.25 mg (yellow) or 0.05 mg/kg.

OFF-LABEL USES

Malignant glaucoma.

CONTRAINDICATIONS

Bladder neck obstruction due to prostatic hypertrophy, cardiospasm, intestinal atony, myasthenia gravis in those not treated with neostigmine, narrow-angle glaucomaoma obstructive disease of the GI tract, paralytic ileus, severe ulcerative colitis, tachycardia secondary to cardiac insufficiency or thyrotoxicosis, toxic megacolon, unstable cardiovascular status in acute hemorrhage, asthma, adhesions between iris and lens.

INTERACTIONS

Drug: Anticholinergics: May increase effects of atropine. **Pralidoxime:** May increase the risk of atropinization (flushing, mydriasis, tachycardia, dryness of the mouth and nose) when used with the AtroPen auto-injector. **Herbal:** None known. **Food:** None known.

DIAGNOSTIC TEST EFFECTS

None known.

IV INCOMPATIBILITIES

Pentothal (Thiopental)

IV COMPATIBILITIES

*DiphenhydrAMINE (Benadryl), droperidol (Inapsine), fentanyl (Sublimaze), glycopyrrolate (Robinul), heparin, hydromorphone (Dilaudid), midazolam (Versed), morphine, potassium chloride, propofol (Diprivan), famotidine, nafcillin, inamrinone

SIDE-EFFECTS

Frequent: Dry mouth, nose, and throat that may be severe; decreased sweating, constipation, irritation at subcutaneous or IM injection site. **Occasional:** Swallowing difficulty, blurred vision, bloated feeling, impotence, urinary hesitancy. **Ophthalmic:** Mydriasis, blurred vision, photophobia, decreased visual

A

acuity, tearing, dry eyes or dry conjunctiva, eye irritation, crusting of eyelid. **Rare:** Allergic reaction, including rash and urticaria; mental confusion or excitement, particularly in children, fatigue

CRITICAL CARE CONSIDERATIONS

ADMINISTRATION/HANDLING

ADMINISTRATION ALERT

- Atropine may be discontinued if the patient experiences blurred vision, dizziness, or tachycardia.

IV ALERT

- For management of bradycardia, give atropine rapidly to prevent paradoxic slowing of the heart rate.

IM, SUBCUTANEOUS ALERT

- May give atropine by IM or subcutaneous injection.

PRECAUTIONS

HEALTH-RELATED

- Use atropine with extreme caution in patients with autonomic neuropathy, diarrhea, known or suspected GI infections, and mild to moderate ulcerative colitis.
- Use cautiously in patients with heart failure, chronic obstructive pulmonary disease, coronary artery disease, esophageal reflux or hiatal hernia associated with reflux esophagitis, gastric ulcer, hepatic or renal disease, hypertension, hyperthyroidism, and tachydysrhythmias.
- Patients with a transplanted heart will not respond to IV atropine for management of bradycardia. *DOPamine or epinephrine infusions may be used as an alternative.

AGE-RELATED

- **Infants and children:** Safety and efficacy of atropine have not been established in infants and children.
- **Elderly:** Use cautiously because it may induce agitation, confusion, memory impairment, or drowsiness; may precipitate undiagnosed glaucoma, constipation, or urinary retention.

PREGNANCY/LACTATION-RELATED

- Pregnancy category C; whether there is passage into breast milk still controversial; neonates are particularly sensitive to anticholinergic agents; compatible with breast-feeding.

MONITORING

- **Baseline assessment:** Instruct patients to urinate before giving atropine to reduce the risk of urine retention.
- **Lab work:** Biochemical profile including renal (BUN, creatinine) and liver function (AST [SGOT], ALT [SGPT], alkaline phosphatase, bilirubin) tests.
- **Vital signs:** Monitor for changes in BP, pulse, and temperature.
- **Tachycardia:** Monitor patients with heart disease for signs of tachycardia.
- **Dehydration:** Assess skin turgor and mucous membranes to evaluate hydration status. Encourage fluids unless the patient is to have nothing by mouth before surgery.
- **Constipation:** Assess bowel sounds for the presence of peristalsis; be alert for diminished bowel sounds. Assess pattern of daily bowel activity and stool consistency.
- **Hyperthermia:** Monitor for fever because patients receiving atropine are at an increased risk for hyperthermia.
- **Urinary retention:** Monitor intake and output and palpate the bladder to assess for urine retention.
- **Patient education:** Explain to patients that a warm, dry, flushing feeling may occur upon administration. Remind patients to remain in bed and not to eat or drink anything before surgery.

SERIOUS ADVERSE REACTIONS

- **Cardiac:** Tachycardia; palpitations; hot, dry, or flushed skin.
- **Gastrointestinal:** Absence of bowel sounds, nausea, vomiting.
- **Neurological:** Confusion, somnolence, slurred speech, dizziness, agitation, restlessness, excitement, rambling speech, visual hallucinations, paranoid behavior, and delusions, followed by depression.
- **Respiratory:** Tachypnea.
- **Visual:** Blurred vision.

OVERDOSE/TOXICITY

- **Physical assessment:** Tachycardia; palpitations; hot, dry, or flushed skin; absence of bowel sounds; increased respiratory rate; nausea; vomiting; confusion; somnolence; slurred speech; dizziness; and CNS stimulation.
- **Behavioral assessment:** Psychosis as evidenced by excitement, agitation, restlessness, rambling speech, visual hallucinations, paranoid behavior, and delusions, followed by depression.

- **Manage agitation:** Diazepam, phenobarbital, or chloral hydrate may be used to manage excitement.
- **GI decontamination:** No specific recommendations.

ANTIDOTE/DIALYSIS

- **Antidote:** Physostigmine reverses most cardiovascular and CNS effects but may cause bradycardia, seizures, or asystole. Neostigmine is the alternate antidote choice. Administer pilocarpine until the mouth is moist.
- **Dialysis:** Atropine is not removed by hemodialysis. No data are available on removal using peritoneal dialysis or high-permeability hemodialysis.

azatadine

See Antihistamines (p. 925)

azathioprine

ay-za-thye'-oh-preen

Classes

Chemical: 6-mercaptopurine derivative, purine analog
Therapeutic: immunosuppressant

Pregnancy Category: D

Trade Names

Prescription: Azasan, Azathioprine Sodium, Imuran

Do not confuse azathioprine with Azulfidine or azatadine, or Imuran with Elmiron or Imferon.

CLINICAL PHARMACOLOGY

Mechanism of Action

An immunologic agent that antagonizes purine metabolism and inhibits DNA, protein, and RNA synthesis. **Therapeutic Effect:** Suppresses cell-mediated hypersensitivities; alters antibody production and immune response in transplant recipients; reduces the severity of arthritis symptoms.

PHARMACOKINETICS

Well absorbed from the GI tract following PO administration. Protein binding: 30%. Metabolized in liver. Excreted in urine. **Half-life:** 5 hr.

AVAILABILITY

Tablets: 50 mg (Azasan, Imuran), 75 mg (Azasan), 100 mg (Azasan).
Injection (Imuran): 100-mg vial.

INDICATIONS AND DOSAGE

Adjunct in prevention of renal allograft rejection

PO, IV

Adults, Elderly, Children: 3-5 mg/kg/day on day of transplant, then 1-3 mg/kg/day as maintenance dose.

Rheumatoid arthritis

PO

Adults: Initially, 1 mg/kg/day as a single dose or in two divided doses. May increase by 0.5 mg/kg/day after 6-8 wk at 4-wk intervals up to maximum of 2.5 mg/kg/day. Maintenance: Lowest effective dosage. May decrease dose by 0.5 mg/kg or 25 mg/day every 4 wk (while other therapies, such as rest, physiotherapy, and salicylates, are maintained). **Elderly:** Initially, 1 mg/kg/day (50-100 mg); may increase by 25 mg/day until response or toxicity.

Dosage in renal impairment

Dosage is modified based on creatinine clearance.

Creatinine Clearance	Dose
10-50 mL/min	75% of usual dose
Less than 10 mL/min	50% of usual dose

OFF-LABEL USES

Treatment of biliary cirrhosis, chronic active hepatitis, glomerulonephritis, inflammatory bowel disease, inflammatory myopathy, multiple sclerosis, myasthenia gravis, nephrotic syndrome, pemphigoid, pemphigus, polymyositis, systemic lupus erythematosus

CONTRAINDICATIONS

Pregnant patients with rheumatoid arthritis

INTERACTIONS

Drug: Allopurinol: May increase activity and risk of toxicity of azathioprine. Decrease azathioprine dose to one third or one fourth of normal dose. **Bone marrow depressants:** May increase myelosuppression. **Live-virus vaccines:** May potentiate virus replication, increase the vaccine's side effects and decrease the patient's antibody response to the vaccine. **Other immunosuppressants:** May increase the risk of infection or neoplasms. **Amiosalicylates (olasalazine, mesalamine, sulfasalazine):** Increase toxicity to bone marrow (myelosuppression) caused by azathioprine. **Herbal: Cat's claw, echinacea:** Increase immunosuppressant effects. **Food:** None known.

A

DIAGNOSTIC TEST EFFECTS
May decrease serum albumin, Hgb, and serum uric acid levels. May increase serum alkaline phosphatase, amylase, bilirubin, AST (SGOT), and ALT (SGPT) levels.

IV INCOMPATIBILITIES
Methyl and propyl parabens, phenol

SIDE-EFFECTS
Frequent: Nausea, vomiting, anorexia (particularly during early treatment and with large doses). **Occasional:** Rash. **Rare:** Severe nausea and vomiting with diarrhea, abdominal pain, hypersensitivity reaction

CRITICAL CARE CONSIDERATIONS

ADMINISTRATION/HANDLING

PO ALERT
- Give azathioprine during or after meals to reduce the risk of GI disturbances.
- Store tablets at room temperature.

IV ALERT
- **Storage:** Store the parenteral form at room temperature.
- **Stability:** After reconstitution, the IV solution is stable for 24 hr at room temperature.
- **Reconstitution:** Reconstitute the 100-mg vial with 10 mL sterile water for injection to provide a concentration of 10 mg/mL. Swirl the vial gently to dissolve the solution.
- **Further dilution:** The solution may be further diluted in 50 mL D_5W or 0.9% NaCl.
- **IV infusion:** Infuse the solution over 30 to 60 min (range is 5 min to 8 hr).

PRECAUTIONS

HEALTH-RELATED
- Use azathioprine cautiously in immunosuppressed patients including patients previously treated for rheumatoid arthritis with alkylating agents (such as chlorambucil, cyclophosphamide, and melphalan) and patients with current or recent chicken pox.
- Azathioprine increases the possibility of neoplasia.
- Hematologic toxicities may be worse in renal transplant patients in rejection.

AGE-RELATED
- **Children:** Safety and efficacy of azathioprine have not been established in children.
- **Elderly:** May experience difficulty in tolerating azathioprine due to age-related organ dysfunction.

PREGNANCY/LACTATION-RELATED
- Pregnancy category D; appears in breast milk in small amounts; the World Health Organization does not recommend breastfeeding to mothers taking azathioprine.

MONITORING
- **Baseline assessment:** If azathioprine is being given for arthritis, assess the duration, location, onset, and type of fever, inflammation, and pain. Inspect affected joints for deformities, immobility, and skin condition.
- **Lab work:** Monitor CBC (especially platelet count), BUN, creatinine, and serum hepatic enzyme levels weekly during the first month of therapy, twice monthly during the second and third months of treatment, and monthly thereafter.
- **Infection:** Monitor vigilantly for signs of infection. Prophylactic antibiotics may be used for a febrile leukopenic patient.
- **Leukopenia and thrombocytopenia:** Expect to reduce the dosage or discontinue the drug if WBC or platelet count falls rapidly.
- **Delayed bone marrow suppression:** Assess laboratory test results, as well as signs and symptoms, for delayed myelosuppression.
- **Therapeutic response:** In patients receiving azathioprine for arthritis, evaluate for improved grip strength; increased joint mobility; reduced joint tenderness; and relief of pain, stiffness, and swelling.
- **Patient education:** Explain to patients with rheumatoid arthritis that azathioprine's therapeutic response may take up to 12 wk to appear. Instruct patients to promptly report abdominal pain, fever, mouth sores, sore throat, or unusual bleeding to a health care provider. Caution women of childbearing age to avoid pregnancy during treatment.

SERIOUS ADVERSE REACTIONS
- **Cancer/new tumors:** Azathioprine use increases the risk of developing neoplasia. Renal transplant patients are prone to develop malignant skin cancer and lymphomatous tumors.
- **Hematologic:** Significant leukopenia and thrombocytopenia may occur, particularly in those undergoing kidney transplant rejection.

- **Gastrointestinal:** Severe nausea and vomiting may indicate GI hypersensitivity.
- **Serious infections:** Fungal, viral, bacterial, and protozoal infections may be fatal.
- **Rejection of renal transplant:** If dose is too low, the patient may reject the kidney.

OVERDOSE/TOXICITY

- **Hematologic:** Extreme leukopenia, thrombocytopenia, and/or anemia indicative of bone marrow suppression may lead to bleeding.
- **Hepatotoxicity:** Elevated liver enzymes (AST [SGOT], ALT [SGPT], GGT, alkaline phosphatase, bilirubin) with jaundice occurs rarely.
- **GI hypersensitivity:** Nausea, vomiting, diarrhea, fever, malaise, with myalgias.
- **Management:** Most effects can be treated symptomatically and will resolve when either azathioprine is discontinued or dosage is reduced.
- **GI decontamination:** No specific recommendations.

ANTIDOTE/DIALYSIS

- **Antidote:** No specific recommendations.
- **Dialysis:** Azathioprine is removed by hemodialysis and is likely removed by high-permeability hemodialysis. No data are available on removal by peritoneal dialysis.

azelastine

a-zel'-as-teen

Classes

Chemical: phthalazinone derivative
Therapeutic: antihistamine

Pregnancy Category: C

Trade Names

Prescription: Astelin (nasal), Optivar (ophthalmic)

Do not confuse Optivar with Optiray.

CLINICAL PHARMACOLOGY

Mechanism of Action

An antihistamine that competes with histamine for histamine receptor sites on cells in the blood vessels, GI tract, and respiratory tract. **Therapeutic Effect:** Relieves symptoms associated with seasonal allergic rhinitis such as increased mucus production and sneezing and symptoms associated with allergic conjunctivitis, such as redness, itching, and excessive tearing.

PHARMACOKINETICS

Route	Onset	Peak	Duration
Nasal spray	0.5-1 hr	2-3 hr	12 hr
Ophthalmic	N/A	3 min	8 hr

Well absorbed through nasal mucosa. Primarily excreted in feces. **Half-life:** 22 hr.

AVAILABILITY

Nasal spray (Astelin): 137 mcg/spray.
Ophthalmic solution (Optivar): 0.05%.

INDICATIONS AND DOSAGE

Allergic rhinitis

Nasal

Adults, Elderly, Children 12 yr and older: 2 sprays in each nostril twice per day. **Children 5-11 yr:** 1 spray in each nostril twice per day.

Allergic conjunctivitis

Ophthalmic

Adults, Elderly, Children 3 yr or older: 1 drop into affected eye twice per day.

CONTRAINDICATIONS

History of hypersensitivity to antihistamines

INTERACTIONS

Drug: **Alcohol, other CNS depressants:** May increase CNS depression. **Cimetidine:** May increase azelastine blood concentration. **Herbal:** None known. **Food:** None known.

DIAGNOSTIC TEST EFFECTS

May increase ALT (SGPT) levels. May suppress flare and wheal reactions to antigen skin testing unless drug is discontinued 4 days before testing.

SIDE-EFFECTS

Frequent: Headache (15%), bitter taste (20%) **Ophthalmic:** Transient eye burning or stinging (30%). **Rare:** Nasal burning, paroxysmal sneezing, somnolence. **Ophthalmic:** Bitter taste, headache

CRITICAL CARE CONSIDERATIONS

ADMINISTRATION/HANDLING

NASAL ALERT

- Clear the nasal passages as much as possible before use.
- **Administration:** Tilt the head slightly forward. Insert the applicator tip into one nostril, pointing the tip toward the nasal passage and away from the nasal septum.

While holding the other nostril closed, spray into the nostril and inhale at the same time to deliver the drug as high into the nasal passages as possible. Repeat in the other nostril.
- Wipe the applicator tip with a clean, damp tissue and replace the cap immediately after use.

OPHTHALMIC ALERT
- **Administration:** Tilt the head back and instill the solution in the conjunctival sac of the affected eye. Close the eye, then press gently on the lacrimal sac for 1 min.
- Ensure the proper form is used in the eyes. Nasal preparation may not be sprayed into the eyes.

PRECAUTIONS
HEALTH-RELATED
- Use azelastine cautiously in patients with renal impairment.

AGE-RELATED
- **Children:** Safety and efficacy of ophthalmic azelastine have not been established in children under 3 yr; safety and efficacy of nasal azelastine have not been established in children under 5 yr.
- **Elderly:** No age-related precautions have been noted in the elderly.

PREGNANCY/LACTATION-RELATED
- Pregnancy category C; excretion into breast milk unknown.

MONITORING
- **Hypersensitivity:** Determine hypersensitivity to antihistamines before administration.
- **Therapeutic response:** Assess for clearing of the nasal passages after use.
- **Patient Education:** Teach patients to prime the pump with 4 sprays or until a fine mist appears before using the nasal spray the first time. After the first use and if the pump has not been used for 3 or more days, tell patients to prime the pump with 2 sprays or until a fine mist appears. Instruct patients to wipe the applicator tip with a clean, damp tissue and to replace the cap immediately after use. Azelastine should not be taken while using other antihistamines. Warn patients to avoid spraying the nasal drug into the eyes. Advise patients to avoid drinking alcoholic beverages during azelastine therapy.
- **Management:** Not likely to require extensive management with either nasal or oral routes of administration since systemic dosage is minimal.

SERIOUS ADVERSE REACTIONS
- Epistaxis occurs rarely.

OVERDOSE/TOXICITY
- May cause flushing, hypertension, tachycardia, severe headache, somnolence, extreme bitter taste, vertigo, anxiety, thought disorder, bronchospasm, hematuria, back pain, herpes/other viral infection, abdominal pain.
- **GI decontamination:** No specific recommendations.

ANTIDOTE/DIALYSIS
- **Antidote:** No specific recommendations.
- **Dialysis:** Azelastine is unlikely to be removed by hemodialysis, peritoneal dialysis, or high-permeability hemodialysis.

azithromycin

ay-zi-thro-mye'-sin

Classes
Chemical: macrolide derivative
Therapeutic: antibiotic

Pregnancy Category: B

Trade Names
Prescription: Zithromax, Zithromax TRI-PAK, Zithromax Z-PAK, Zmax

Do not confuse azithromycin with erythromycin.

CLINICAL PHARMACOLOGY
Mechanism of Action
A macrolide antibiotic that binds to ribosomal receptor sites of susceptible organisms, inhibiting RNA-dependent protein synthesis. **Therapeutic Effect:** Bacteriostatic or bactericidal, depending on the drug dosage.

PHARMACOKINETICS
Rapidly absorbed from the GI tract. Protein binding: 7%-50%. Widely distributed. Eliminated primarily unchanged by biliary excretion. **Half-life:** 68 hr.

AVAILABILITY
Oral suspension (Zithromax): 100 mg/5 mL, 200 mg/5 mL.

Oral suspension (extended release [Zmax]): 1 g single-dose packet, 2 g single-dose packet.
Tablets: 250 mg, 500 mg, 600 mg (Zithromax). Tri-Pak: 3 x 500 mg (Zithromax TRI-PAK). Z-Pak: 6 x 250 mg (Zithromax Z-PAK).
Powder for injection (Zithromax): 500 mg.
Powder for reconstitution (Zithromax): 1 g.

INDICATIONS AND DOSAGE

Acute exacerbations of chronic obstructive pulmonary disease (COPD)

PO

Adults, Elderly, Children 16 yr and older: 500 mg/day for 3 days or 500 mg on day 1, then 250 mg/day on days 2-5.

Acute bacterial sinusitis

PO (Zmax)

Adults, Elderly: 2 g as a single dose.

PO

Adults, Elderly: 500 mg/day for 3 days. **Children 6 mo and older:** 10 mg/kg for 3 days. Maximum: 500 mg/day.

Cervicitis

PO

Adults, Elderly: 1-2 g as single dose.

Chancroid

PO

Adults, Elderly: 1 g as single dose.

Mycobacterium avium complex (MAC) prevention

PO

Adults, Elderly: 1200 mg once weekly. **Children:** 20 mg/kg once weekly. Maximum: 1200 mg/dose.

MAC treatment

PO

Adults, Elderly: 600 mg/day with ethambutol 15 mg/kg/day. **Children:** 5 mg/kg/day (maximum 250 mg/day) in combination with ethambutol, with or without rifabutin.

Otitis media

PO

Children 6 mo and older: 30 mg/kg as single dose or 10 mg/kg/day for 3 days or 10 mg/kg on day 1 then 5 mg/kg on days 2-5.

Pharyngitis, tonsillitis

PO

Adults, Elderly, Children 16 yr and older: 500 mg on day 1, then 250 mg on days 2-5. **Children 2-15 yr:** 12 mg/kg daily for 5 days.

Pneumonia, community acquired

IV

Adults, Elderly, Children 16 yr and older: 500 mg on day 1, then 250 mg on days 2-5 or 500 mg/day IV for 2 days, then 500 mg/day PO to complete course of therapy (7-10 days). **Children 6 mo-15 yr:** 10 mg/kg on day 1, then 5 mg/kg on days 2-5. Maximum: 250 mg/day.

Skin/skin-structure infections

PO

Adults, Elderly, Children 16 yr and older: 500 mg on day 1, then 250 mg on days 2-5.

Pelvic inflammatory disease (PID)

IV

Adults, Elderly: 500 mg/day for at least 2 days, then 250 mg/day to complete a 7-day course of therapy.

OFF-LABEL USES

Chlamydial infections, gonococcal pharyngitis, uncomplicated gonococcal infections of the cervix, urethra, and rectum

CONTRAINDICATIONS

Hypersensitivity to other macrolide antibiotics

INTERACTIONS

Drug: **Aluminum- or magnesium-containing antacids:** May decrease azithromycin blood concentration. **Carbamazepine, *cycloSPORINE, theophylline, warfarin:** May increase the serum concentrations of these drugs. **Herbal:** None known. **Food:** None known.

DIAGNOSTIC TEST EFFECTS

May increase serum creatine kinase (CK), AST (SGOT), and ALT (SGPT) levels.

IV INCOMPATIBILITIES

Ceftriaxone (Rocephin), ciprofloxacin (Cipro), famotidine (Pepcid), furosemide (Lasix), ketorolac (Toradol), levofloxacin (Levaquin), morphine, piperacillin/tazobactam (Zosyn), potassium chloride

IV COMPATIBILITIES

*DiphenhydrAMINE (Benadryl)

SIDE-EFFECTS

Occasional: Nausea, vomiting, diarrhea, abdominal pain. **Rare:** Headache, dizziness, allergic reaction

CRITICAL CARE CONSIDERATIONS

ADMINISTRATION/HANDLING

PO ALERT

- **Antacids:** Give azithromycin 1 hr before or 2 hr after antacids.

- **Tablets:** Give tablets without regard to food.
- **Oral suspension:** Do not administer the oral suspension with food. Give it at least 1 hr before or 2 hr after a meal.
- **Storage/stability:** Store the oral suspension at room temperature. The suspension is stable for 10 days after reconstitution.

IV ALERT

- **Storage/stability:** Store vials at room temperature. After reconstitution, the solution is stable for 24 hr at room temperature or 7 days if refrigerated.
- **Initial dilution:** Reconstitute each 500-mg vial with 4.8 mL sterile water for injection to provide a concentration of 100 mg/mL. Shake well to ensure dissolution.
- **Final dilution:** Further dilute the solution with 250 or 500 mL 0.9% NaCl or D_5W to provide a final concentration of 2 mg/mL or 1 mg/mL, respectively.
- **Infusion:** Infuse the drug over 60 min.

PRECAUTIONS

HEALTH-RELATED

- **Hepatic/renal:** Use azithromycin cautiously in patients with hepatic or renal dysfunction.
- **Prolonged QT syndrome:** Use cautiously in patients with prolonged QT syndrome to avoid potentially lethal ventricular dysrhythmias.
- **Culture and sensitivity:** Specific sensitivity studies should be used to determine susceptibility of causative organism to azithromycin.
- **Resistant organisms:** Most strains of *Enterococcus faecalis* and methicillin-resistant staphylococcus are resistant to azithromycin.

AGE-RELATED

- **Children:** Safety and efficacy of aripiprazole have not been established in children under 16 yr for IV use and under 6 mo for oral use.
- **Elderly:** No age-related precautions have been noted in elderly patients with normal renal function.

PREGNANCY/LACTATION-RELATED

- Pregnancy category B; excretion into breast milk unknown.

MONITORING

- **Baseline assessment:** Assess for history of hepatitis or allergies to azithromycin or other macrolides before beginning therapy.
- **Lab work:** Monitor liver function test results.
- **GI system:** Assess for GI discomfort, nausea, or vomiting. Assess pattern of daily bowel activity and stool consistency for diarrhea.
- ***Clostridium difficile*–associated diarrhea:** Has been reported. Prolonged watery diarrhea with cramps warrants a stool culture.
- **Hepatotoxicity:** Assess for signs and symptoms of hepatotoxicity, such as abdominal pain, fever, GI disturbances, and malaise.
- **Superinfection:** Evaluate for signs and symptoms of superinfection, including genital or anal pruritus, sore mouth or tongue, and moderate to severe diarrhea.
- **Give suspension on empty stomach:** Administer oral suspension with 8 oz of water at least 1 hr before or 2 hr after consuming any food or beverages. If patients cannot tolerate the medication, food, milk, or antacids may be used to relieve symptoms using stated guidelines.
- **Evenly spaced doses:** Administer doses evenly around the clock and continue azithromycin for the full course of treatment.
- **Antacids:** If patients receive an antacid containing aluminum or magnesium, administer the drug 1 hr before or 2 hr after the antacid.

SERIOUS ADVERSE REACTIONS

- **Superinfection:** Antibiotic-associated colitis and other superinfections may result from altered bacterial balance, including pseudomembranous colitis.
- **Torsades de pointes:** Patients with prolonged QT syndrome are at risk for developing lethal dysrhythmias, including ventricular tachycardia, and torsades.
- **Other symptoms:** Palpitations, chest pain, melena, cholestatic jaundice, dizziness, angioedema. Acute interstitial nephritis and hepatotoxicity occur rarely.

OVERDOSE/TOXICITY

- Acute toxicity is uncommon with azithromycin.
- **Lab work:** Assess liver enzymes for liver failure because elimination is largely biliary. Assess pancreatic enzymes for pancreatitis.
- **Management:** Oral vancomycin (Vancocin) or metronidazole (Flagyl) are the treatments of choice for antibiotic-related pseudomembranous colitis. Mild cases of colitis may stop when the drug is

discontinued. Manage torsades de pointes according to Advanced Cardiac Life Support (ACLS) guidelines, including use of magnesium infusion, isoproterenol infusion, overdrive pacing, and possibly phenytoin.
- **GI decontamination:** Use gastric lavage if patients present within 1 hr of ingestion. Activated charcoal may be used following gastric lavage, or instead of gastric lavage.

ANTIDOTE/DIALYSIS
- **Antidote:** No specific recommendations.
- **Dialysis:** Azithromycin is not significantly removed by hemodialysis or peritoneal dialysis. No data are available on removal by high-permeability hemodialysis.

aztreonam

az'-tree-oh-nam

Classes
Chemical: monobactam
Therapeutic: antibiotic

Pregnancy Category: B

Trade Names
Prescription: Azactam

CLINICAL PHARMACOLOGY
Mechanism of Action
A monobactam antibiotic that inhibits bacterial cell wall synthesis. **Therapeutic Effect:** Bactericidal.

PHARMACOKINETICS
Completely absorbed after IM administration. Protein binding: 56%-60%. Partially metabolized by hydrolysis. Primarily excreted unchanged in urine. Removed by hemodialysis. **Half-life:** 1.4-2.2 hr (increased in impaired renal or hepatic function).

AVAILABILITY
Injection powder for reconstitution: 500 mg, 1 g, 2 g.

INDICATIONS AND DOSAGE
UTIs
IV, IM
Adults, Elderly: 500 mg-1 g every 8-12 hr.
Moderate to severe systemic infections
IV, IM
Adults, Elderly: 1-2 g every 8-12 hr.
Severe or life-threatening infections
IV
Adults, Elderly: 2 g every 6-8 hr.
Cystic fibrosis
IV
Children: 50 mg/kg/dose every 6-8 hr up to 200 mg/kg/day. Maximum: 8 g/day.
Mild to severe infections in children
IV
Children: 30 mg/kg every 6-8 hr. Maximum: 120 mg/kg/day. **Neonates:** 60-120 mg/kg/day every 6-12 hr.
Dosage in renal impairment
Dosage and frequency are modified based on creatinine clearance and the severity of the infection:

Creatinine Clearance	Dosage
10-30 mL/min	1-2 g initially, then half of usual dose at usual intervals
Less than 10 mL/min	1-2 g initially; then one quarter of usual dose at usual intervals

OFF-LABEL USES
Treatment of bone and joint infections

CONTRAINDICATIONS
Hypersensitivity to aztreonam

INTERACTIONS
Drug: None known. **Herbal:** None known. **Food:** None known.

DIAGNOSTIC TEST EFFECTS
May increase serum alkaline phosphatase, creatinine, LDH, AST (SGOT), and ALT (SGPT) levels. Produces a positive Coombs' test.

IV INCOMPATIBILITIES
Acyclovir (Zovirax), amphotericin (Fungizone), *DAUNOrubicin (Cerubidine), ganciclovir (Cytovene), lorazepam (Ativan), metronidazole (Flagyl), vancomycin (Vancocin).

IV COMPATIBILITIES
Aminophylline, bumetanide (Bumex), calcium gluconate, cimetidine (Tagamet), diltiazem (Cardizem), *DOBUTamine (Dobutrex), *DOPamine (Intropin), famotidine (Pepcid), furosemide (Lasix), heparin, hydromorphone (Dilaudid), insulin (regular), magnesium sulfate, morphine, potassium chloride, propofol (Diprivan), total parenteral nutrition (TPN).

SIDE-EFFECTS
Occasional (less than 3%): Discomfort and swelling at IM injection site, nausea, vomiting, diarrhea, rash. **Rare (less than 1%):** Phlebitis or thrombophlebitis at IV injection site, abdominal cramps, headache, hypotension

CRITICAL CARE CONSIDERATIONS

ADMINISTRATION/HANDLING

IM ALERT

- **Dilution:** Shake the vial immediately and vigorously after adding the diluent.
- **Administration:** Inject the drug deep into a large muscle mass.
- **Stability:** After reconstitution for IM injection, the solution is stable for 48 hr at room temperature and 7 days if refrigerated.

IV ALERT

- **Storage/stability:** Store vials at room temperature. After reconstitution, the solution is stable for 48 hr at room temperature and 7 days if refrigerated.
- **Solution:** Normally appears colorless to light yellow. Discard the solution if a precipitate forms. Discard unused portions of solution.
- **IV push:** Dilute each gram with 6 to 10 mL of sterile water for injection. Administer IV push over 3 to 5 min.
- **Intermittent IV infusion:** Further dilute with 50 to 100 mL of D_5W or 0.9% NaCl. Administer IV infusion over 20 to 60 min.

PRECAUTIONS

HEALTH-RELATED

- Use aztreonam cautiously in patients with hepatic or renal impairment or a history of allergies, especially to antibiotics.

AGE-RELATED

- **Children:** No age-related precautions have been noted in children. Side effects are similar to those in adults.
- **Elderly:** Age-related renal or hepatic impairment may require a dosage adjustment in the elderly.

PREGNANCY/LACTATION-RELATED

- Pregnancy category B; excreted in breast milk in concentrations less than 1% of maternal serum concentrations.

MONITORING

- **Baseline assessment:** Determine history of allergies, especially to antibiotics, before giving aztreonam. Watch for early symptoms of allergic reaction.
- **Lab work:** Biochemical profile including renal (BUN, creatinine) and liver function (AST [SGOT], ALT [SGPT], bilirubin, alkaline phosphatase) tests.
- **Phlebitis:** Evaluate for signs and symptoms of phlebitis, such as heat, pain, and red streaking over the vein, and pain at the IM injection site.
- **Bacterial imbalance in GI tract:** Observe for GI discomfort, nausea, or vomiting. Assess pattern of daily bowel activity and stool consistency. May develop antibiotic-induced colitis.
- **Rash:** Examine the skin for rash.
- **Superinfection:** Symptoms may include anal or genital pruritus, black hairy tongue, vomiting, diarrhea, fever, sore throat, and ulceration or changes of oral mucosa.
- **Labwork:** Monitor BUN, creatinine, and liver enzymes, especially in the elderly.

SERIOUS ADVERSE REACTIONS

- **Colitis:** Antibiotic-associated pseudomembranous colitis (*Clostridium difficile*–associated diarrhea) and other superinfections may result from altered bacterial balance.
- **Allergy:** Severe hypersensitivity reactions, anaphylaxis, bronchospasms, wheezing, and dyspnea occur rarely.
- **Dermatologic:** Toxic epidermal necrolysis, purpura, erythema multiforme, exfoliative dermatitis, urticaria, petechiae, pruritis.
- **Renal:** Increased serum creatinine, decreased creatinine clearance.

OVERDOSE/TOXICITY

- **Hematologic:** Pancytopenia, neutropenia, thrombocytopenia, anemia, leukocytosis, thrombocytosis, eosinophilia.
- **Hepatobiliary:** Hepatitis, jaundice.
- **Neurological:** Seizures, confusion, vertigo, paresthesia, insomnia, dizziness.
- **Management:** Most effects can be treated symptomatically and will resolve when either aztreonam is discontinued or dosage is reduced.
- **GI decontamination:** No specific recommendations.

ANTIDOTE/DIALYSIS

- **Antidote:** No specific recommendations.
- **Dialysis:** Aztreonam is removed by hemodialysis and is likely removed by high-permeability hemodialysis. No data are available on removal by peritoneal dialysis.

bacitracin

bass-i-tray'-sin

Classes

Chemical: bacillus subtilis derivative
Therapeutic: antibacterial, ophthalmic antibiotic

Pregnancy Category: C

Trade Names

Prescription: Ak-Tracin, Baci-IM, Baci-Rx, Ocu-Tracin, Ziba-Rx

Combinations

Prescription: with neomycin, polymixin, and hydrocortisone (Cortisporin)
Over the Counter: with neomycin and polymixin (Neosporin); with polymixin (Polysporin)

Do not confuse bacitracin with Bactrim or Bactroban.

CLINICAL PHARMACOLOGY

Mechanism of Action

An antibiotic that interferes with plasma membrane permeability and inhibits bacterial cell wall synthesis in susceptible bacteria. **Therapeutic Effect:** Bacteriostatic.

PHARMACOKINETICS

Not significantly absorbed following topical or ophthalmic administration.

AVAILABILITY

Powder for irrigation: 50,000 units.
Powder for injection (Baci-IM): 50,000 units.
Ophthalmic ointment (AK-Tracin): 500 units/g.
Topical ointment (Ocu-Tracin): 500 units/g.

INDICATIONS AND DOSAGE

Superficial ocular infections
Ophthalmic
Adults: One-quarter-to one-half-inch ribbon in conjunctival sac every 3-4 hr.

Skin abrasions, superficial skin infections
Topical
Adults, Children: Apply to affected area 1-5 times per day.

Surgical treatment and prophylaxis
Irrigation
Adults, Elderly: 50,000-150,000 units, as needed.

Pneumonia and empyema caused by staphylococci
IM
Infants weighing 2500 g and less: 900 units/kg/24 hr in 2-3 divided doses. **Infants weighing more than 2500 g:** 1000 units/kg/24 hr in 2-3 divided doses. **Children:** 800-1200 units/kg/day in 3 divided doses every 8 hr.

CONTRAINDICATIONS

IM use is contraindicated in patients with renal impairment.

INTERACTIONS

Drug: Nephrotoxic medications: May increase the risk of nephrotoxicity with IM bacitracin therapy. **Herbal:** None known. **Food:** None known.

DIAGNOSTIC TEST EFFECTS

IM injection form may produce albuninuria, cylindruria

SIDE-EFFECTS

Rare: Ophthalmic: Burning, itching, redness, swelling, pain
IM injection: Nausea, vomiting, pain at injection site, rash, azotemia, rising blood levels without any increase in dosage
Topical: Hypersensitivity reaction (allergic contact dermatitis, burning, inflammation, pruritus)

CRITICAL CARE CONSIDERATIONS

ADMINISTRATION/HANDLING

OPHTHALMIC ALERT

- **Administration:** Place a gloved finger on the lower eyelid and pull it out until a pocket is formed between the eye and lower lid. Place .25 to .5 inch of the ointment in the pocket. Close the eye gently for 1 to 2 min and roll the eyeball to increase bacitracin's contact with the eye. Remove excess ointment around the eye with a tissue.

PRECAUTIONS

HEALTH-RELATED

- Use cautiously with patients who have a sensitivity to any drug contained in the product. When administering a fixed-combination product containing bacitracin, familiarize yourself with the side effects of each of the product's drug components.

AGE-RELATED

- **Children:** No age-related precautions have been noted in children.
- **Elderly:** Age-related renal impairment may prompt a dosage adjustment.

PREGNANCY/LACTATION-RELATED
- Pregnancy category C.

MONITORING
- **Baseline assessment:** Determine history of allergies to bacitracin before beginning drug therapy.
- **Ophthalmic ointment:** Assess the eye for a therapeutic response or a hypersensitivity reaction (increased burning, pruritus, redness, and swelling).
- **Topical ointment:** Monitor for signs and symptoms of hypersensitivity, such as burning, inflammation, and pruritus.
- **Corticosteroids:** When using preparations containing corticosteroids, closely monitor for any unusual signs or symptoms because corticosteroids may mask clinical signs.
- **Evenly spaced doses:** Space drug doses evenly around the clock and continue using bacitracin for the full course of treatment.
- **Patient education:** Urge patients to report burning, itching, increased irritation, or rash.

SERIOUS ADVERSE REACTIONS
- Severe hypersensitivity reactions, including apnea and hypotension, occur rarely.

OVERDOSE/TOXICITY
- Overdose and toxicity are unlikely with any topical medication.

ANTIDOTE/DIALYSIS
- **Antidote:** No specific recommendations. Manage symptoms using accepted guidelines for the problems.
- **Dialysis:** No specific recommendations.

baclofen

bak'-loe-fen

Classes
Chemical: GABA chlorophenyl derivative
Therapeutic: skeletal muscle relaxant

Pregnancy Category: C

Trade Names
Prescription: Lioresal, Lioresal Intrathecal

Do not confuse baclofen with Bactroban or Beclovent.

CLINICAL PHARMACOLOGY
Mechanism of Action
A direct-acting skeletal muscle relaxant that inhibits transmission of reflexes at the spinal cord level. **Therapeutic Effect:** Relieves muscle spasticity.

PHARMACOKINETICS
Well absorbed from the GI tract. Protein binding: 30%. Partially metabolized in the liver. Primarily excreted in urine. **Half-life:** 2.5-4 hr; intrathecal: 1.5 hr.

AVAILABILITY
Tablets: 10 mg, 20 mg.
Intrathecal Injection: 50 mcg/mL, 500 mcg/mL, 2000 mcg/mL.

INDICATIONS AND DOSAGE
Spasticity
PO

Adults: Initially, 5 mg 3 times per day. May increase by 15 mg/day at 3-day intervals. Range: 40-80 mg/day. Maximum: 80 mg/day. **Elderly:** Initially, 5 mg 2-3 times per day. May gradually increase dosage. **Children:** Initially, 10-15 mg/day in divided doses every 8 hr. May increase by 5-15 mg/day at 3-day intervals. Maximum: 40 mg/day (children 2-7 yr); 60 mg/day (children 8 yr and older).

Usual intrathecal dosage
Intrathecal

Adults, Elderly, Children older than 12 yr: 300-800 mcg/day. **Children 12 yr and younger:** 100-300 mcg/day.

OFF-LABEL USES
Treatment of bladder spasms, cerebral palsy, intractable hiccups or pain, Huntington's chorea, trigeminal neuralgia

CONTRAINDICATIONS
Hypersensitivity to baclofen

INTERACTIONS
Drug: **Alcohol, other CNS depressants:** May increase CNS depression. **Herbal:** Avoid valerian, St. John's wort, kava kava, gotu kola. **Food:** None known.

DIAGNOSTIC TEST EFFECTS
May increase blood glucose level and serum alkaline phosphatase, AST (SGOT), and ALT (SGPT) levels.

SIDE-EFFECTS
Frequent (greater than 10%): Transient somnolence, asthenia, dizziness, lightheadedness, nausea, vomiting, weakness. **Occasional (10%-2%):** Headache, paresthesia, constipation, anorexia, hypotension, confusion, nasal congestion. **Rare (less than 1%):** Paradoxic CNS excitement or restlessness, tremor, dry mouth, diarrhea, nocturia, impotence

CRITICAL CARE CONSIDERATIONS

ADMINISTRATION/HANDLING

PO ALERT

- Give baclofen without regard to food.
- Crush tablets as needed.

INTRATHECAL ALERT

- Refer to pump manufacturer's specific instructions for pump operation.
- Before implanting pump, patients should demonstrate a positive response to a trial of intrathecal baclofen (i.e., significant decrease in muscle tone and spasms).
- Patients who do not respond to 100 mcg intrathecal bolus are not appropriate implantable-pump candidates.
- Extreme caution should be used when refilling pump reservoir to avoid overdose.

PRECAUTIONS

HEALTH-RELATED

- Use baclofen cautiously in patients with diabetes mellitus, epilepsy, impaired renal function, preexisting psychiatric disorders, or a history of stroke; patients with epilepsy and muscle spasticity; muscle spasms resulting from cerebral palsy, Parkinson's disease, rheumatic disorders.

AGE-RELATED

- **Children:** Safety and efficacy of oral baclofen have not been established in children under 12 yr. Children should be large enough to accommodate the implantable intrathecal pump if used. Safety and efficacy of intrathecal baclofen have not been established in children under 4 yr.
- **Elderly:** May require decreased dosage because of age-related renal impairment and are at increased risk for CNS toxicity, manifested as confusion, hallucinations, depression, and sedation.

PREGNANCY/LACTATION-RELATED

- Pregnancy category C; present in breast milk, 0.1% of mother's dose; compatible with breast-feeding.

MONITORING

- **Baseline assessment:** Record the duration, location, onset, and type of muscle spasm, and evaluate for signs and symptoms of immobility, stiffness, or swelling.
- **Lab work:** Complete blood count, liver and renal function tests periodically for those on long-term therapy.
- **Paradoxic reactions:** Assess for paradoxic reactions.
- **Risk for injury:** Assist patients with ambulation at all times.
- **Pump management:** Refilling of implantable-pump reservoir should be done by trained personnel. Refill intervals should be planned to avoid depletion of the reservoir, causing return of severe spasticity and possible withdrawal.
- **Therapeutic response:** Evaluate for decreased intensity of skeletal muscle pain.
- **Patient education:** Inform patients that drowsiness usually diminishes with continued therapy. If used after hospitalization, caution against discontinuing baclofen abruptly after long-term therapy. Warn patients to avoid alcohol and CNS depressants during therapy and to avoid tasks that require mental alertness or motor skills until response to the drug is known.

SERIOUS ADVERSE REACTIONS

- **Abrupt discontinuation:** May produce high fever, altered mental status, hallucinations, seizures, rebound spasticity that may lead to rhabdomyolysis, multiple organ failure, and death. Dantrolene may help manage withdrawal.
- **Signs of withdrawal:** Early signs show return of baseline spasticity, pruritis, hypotension, and paresthesias. Later signs reflect a hypermetabolic state.
- **Intrathecal pump infections:** May be treated by removal of the pump and IV antibiotic administration, or antibiotics may be given through the pump.

OVERDOSE/TOXICITY

- **Acute or chronic:** Signs of overdose may appear suddenly (acute) or gradually (chronic) after either intrathecal or oral therapy.
- **Acute overdose:** Respiratory depression and failure, tachycardia and/or bradycardia, hypotension and/or hypertension, atrial and/or ventricular dysrhythmias, heart block, headache, dizziness, myoclonus, areflexia, flaccid extremities, encephalopathy, coma, seizures (including both kinetic and akinetic status epilepticus), blurred vision, hypothermia, hypersalivation.
- **Brain death:** Deep coma and brainstem dysfunction may mimic brain death in baclofen-toxic patients. All diagnostic measures should be implemented over several days' time in critical care before making the diagnosis.

- **Chronic overdose:** Impaired memory, acute mania or catatonia, muscle weakness, sedation, respiratory depression, nausea, vomiting, seizures, and coma.
- **Supportive care:** Respiratory failure and coma should be managed with endotracheal intubation and mechanical ventilation. Use of succinylcholine should be limited to avoid cardiac arrest. Nitroprusside is recommended for hypertension due to its short duration of action. Norepinephrine is short acting and effective for hypotension. Diazepam or lorazepam manage seizures.
- **GI decontamination:** Ipecac is not recommended because of patients' altered level of consciousness. Oral activated charcoal can be used within several hours of ingestion if the patient's airway is secured. Gastric lavage is not necessary.

ANTIDOTE/DIALYSIS

- **Antidote:** Physostigmine, flumazenil, and ondansetron have been used as antidotes but are not consistently effective.
- **Dialysis:** No data are available on removal of baclofen using high-permeability hemodialysis and peritoneal dialysis. One source states that duration of toxicity is reduced by hemodialysis.

balsalazide disodium

bal-sal'-a-zide dye-soe'-dee-um

Classes

Chemical: 5-amino derivative of salicylic acid

Therapeutic: gastrointestinal antiinflammatory

Pregnancy Category: B

Trade Names

Prescription: Colazal

CLINICAL PHARMACOLOGY

Mechanism of Action

A 5-aminosalicylic acid derivative that changes intestinal microflora, altering prostaglandin production and inhibiting function of natural killer cells, mast cells, neutrophils, and macrophages. **Therapeutic Effect:** Diminishes inflammatory effect in colon.

PHARMACOKINETICS

Low and variable absorption following PO administration. Protein binding: greater than 99%. Extensively metabolized in colon. Minimal elimination in urine and feces. **Half-life:** Unknown.

AVAILABILITY

Capsules: 750 mg.

INDICATIONS AND DOSAGE

Ulcerative colitis

PO

Adults, Elderly: Three 750-mg capsules 3 times per day for 8-12 wk.

CONTRAINDICATIONS

Hypersensitivity to salicylates

SIDE-EFFECTS

Frequent (8%-5%): Headache, abdominal pain, nausea, diarrhea. **Occasional (4%-2%):** Vomiting, arthralgia, rhinitis, insomnia, fatigue, flatulence, coughing, dyspepsia

CRITICAL CARE CONSIDERATIONS

ADMINISTRATION/HANDLING

PO ALERT

- Administer capsules whole; do not open or crush.

PRECAUTIONS

HEALTH-RELATED

- Use balsalazide cautiously in patients with hepatic or renal impairment.

AGE-RELATED

- **Children:** Safety and efficacy of balsalazide have not been established in children.
- **Elderly:** No information available for the geriatric population.

PREGNANCY/LACTATION-RELATED

- Pregnancy category B; excretion into breast milk unknown; mesalamine has produced adverse effects in a nursing infant and should be used with caution during breast-feeding; observe nursing infant closely for changes in stool consistency.

MONITORING

- **Baseline assessment:** Assess symptoms of ulcerative colitis. Evaluate for dehydration and malnutrition.
- **Baseline lab work:** Serum chemistry values including BUN, alkaline phosphatase, bilirubin, creatinine, AST (SGOT), and ALT (SGPT) levels.

- **Ongoing lab work:** Monitor liver and kidney function test results for abnormalities.
- **Therapeutic response:** Reduction of abdominal discomfort and diarrhea.
- **Bowel activity:** Monitor bowel sounds for peristalsis. Assess stools for frequency and consistency. Evaluate for abdominal discomfort.
- **Patient education:** Instruct patients to take balsalazide as directed and not to chew or open balsalazide capsules. Instruct patients to report promptly abdominal pain, severe headache, chest pain, or unresolved diarrhea.

SERIOUS ADVERSE REACTIONS

- **Hepatotoxicity:** Jaundice, elevated liver enzymes, cirrhosis, hepatocellular damage, and liver failure occurs rarely. Some postmarketing data have included fatalities that were not seen during clinical trials.
- **Renal insufficiency:** Occurs only when the patient is also receiving other mesalamine products.

OVERDOSE/TOXICITY

- Liver and renal toxicity are discussed above.
- **Salicylate toxicity:** Vomiting, abdominal pain, diaphoresis, tachypnea, tachycardia, dehydration, leukocytosis, tinnitus, ketonuria in early stages. Progressive neurologic deterioration as severity of poisoning worsens. Rhabdomyolysis and acute respiratory distress syndrome are possible. Can progress to refractory shock with academia, acidosis, and lethal ventricular dysrhythmias. Clinical deterioration can be rapid. Death can occur within 6 hr of ingestion despite that salicylate levels may be declining.
- **Management:** *Managing dehydration*—salicylate-toxic patients are often deficient by 5-6 L because of vomiting and may tolerate IV fluid at 500-600 mL/hr. Ringer's lactate is often used. Hematocrit may continue to rise despite aggressive hydration. Hydration should continue until crisis is under control. *Managing acidosis*—following initial hydration, pH should be maintained greater than 7.4 with a goal of 7.5 to limit distribution of balsalazide in the body. Alkalinization of urine helps to maintain the desired pH. *Alkalinize urine:* Alkaline urine enhances salicylate excretion. Continuous infusion of IV solution containing sodium bicarbonate is effective. Adequate urine output should be 2-3 mL/kg/hr in this setting.
- **GI decontamination:** Oral activated charcoal is reported to be superior to using ipecac to induce vomiting. Repeat dosing of activated charcoal may be beneficial.

ANTIDOTE/DIALYSIS

- **Antidote:** No specific recommendations.
- **Dialysis:** Balsalazide may or may not be removed by hemodialysis but is unlikely to be removed by high-permeability hemodialysis or peritoneal dialysis.

basiliximab

See Immunologics (p. 968)

beclomethasone dipropionate

be-kloe-meth'-a-sone dye-pro'-pree-on-ate

Classes

Chemical: glucocorticoid, synthetic
Therapeutic: corticoseroid, antiinflammatory

Pregnancy Category: C

Trade Names

Prescription: Beconase AQ, Beconase, Beclovent, Qvar, Rivanase ♣, Vancenase, Vancenase AQ, Vancenase AQ DS, Vanceril, Vanceril DS

Do not confuse Becloforte or Beconase with baclofen.

CLINICAL PHARMACOLOGY

Mechanism of Action

An adrenocorticosteroid that prevents or controls inflammation by controlling the rate of protein synthesis, decreasing migration of polymorphonuclear leukocytes and fibroblasts, and reversing capillary permeability. **Therapeutic Effect:** Inhalation—Inhibits bronchoconstriction, produces smooth muscle relaxation, decreases mucus secretion. Intranasal—Decreases response to seasonal and perennial rhinitis.

PHARMACOKINETICS

Rapidly absorbed from pulmonary, nasal, and GI tissue. Undergoes extensive first-pass metabolism in the liver. Protein binding: 87%. Primarily eliminated in feces. **Half-life:** 3 hr.

AVAILABILITY

Oral inhalation (QVAR): 40 mcg per inhalation, 80 mcg/inhalation.
Nasal spray (Beconase AQ): 42 mcg/inhalation.

INDICATIONS AND DOSAGE

Long-term control of bronchial asthma, reduces need for oral corticosteriod therapy for asthma

Oral Inhalation

Adults, Elderly, Children 12 yr and older: 40-160 mcg twice per day. Maximum: 320 mcg twice per day.

Rhinitis, prevention of recurrence of nasal polyps

Nasal Inhalation

Adults, Elderly, Children 12 yr and older: 1-2 sprays in nostril 2-4 times daily. **Children 6-12 yr:** 1 spray 3 times per day.

OFF-LABEL USES

Prevention of seasonal rhinitis (nasal form)

CONTRAINDICATIONS

Hypersensitivity to beclomethasone, acute exacerbation of asthma, status asthmaticus

INTERACTIONS

Drug: None known. **Herbal:** None known. **Food:** None known.

DIAGNOSTIC TEST EFFECTS

None known.

SIDE-EFFECTS

Frequent: **Inhalation (14%-4%):** Throat irritation, dry mouth, hoarseness, cough, agitation, headache
Intranasal: Nasal burning, mucosal dryness
Occasional: **Inhalation (3%-2%):** Localized fungal infection (thrush)
Intranasal: Nasal-crusting epistaxis, sore throat, ulceration of nasal mucosa. **Rare:** **Inhalation:** Transient bronchospasm, esophageal candidiasis
Intranasal: Nasal and pharyngeal candidiasis, eye pain

CRITICAL CARE CONSIDERATIONS

ADMINISTRATION/HANDLING

INHALATION ALERT

- **Administration:** Shake the container well. Exhale completely and place the mouthpiece between the lips. Inhale and hold the breath for as long as possible before exhaling. Allow at least 1 min between inhalations. Rinse the mouth after each use to decrease dry mouth and hoarseness.

INTRANASAL ALERT

- **Administration:** Clear the nasal passages as much as possible. Insert the spray tip into the nostril, pointing toward the nasal passages, away from the nasal septum. Spray beclomethasone into the nostril while holding the other nostril closed and at the same time, inhale through the nose to deliver the medication as high into the nasal passages as possible.

PRECAUTIONS

HEALTH-RELATED

- Use beclomethasone cautiously in patients with cirrhosis, glaucoma, hypothyroidism, osteoporosis, tuberculosis, or untreated systemic infections.

AGE-RELATED

- **Children:** Safety and efficacy of beclomethasone have not been established in children under 6 yr. Prolonged treatment and high doses may decrease cortisol secretion and the short-term growth rate.
- **Elderly:** No age-related precautions have been noted.

PREGNANCY/LACTATION-RELATED

- Pregnancy category C; breast milk excretion unknown; other corticosteroids excreted in low concentrations with systemic administration; compatible with breast-feeding.

MONITORING

- **Baseline assessment:** Determine hypersensitivity to corticosteroids.
- **Response to treatment:** Evaluate for relief of wheezing, congestion, and dyspnea.
- **Dosing schedule:** Do not change the beclomethasone dosage schedule or stop the drug abruptly. Dosage must be tapered gradually.
- **Concomitant use of bronchodilator:** If using a bronchodilator inhaler concomitantly with a steroid inhaler, use the bronchodilator several minutes before using the corticosteroid to help the steroid penetrate into the bronchial tree.
- **Patient education:** Inform patients that symptoms should improve in several days. When using beclomethasone by inhalation, maintain fastidious oral care. Instruct patients to rinse the mouth with water immediately after inhalation to prevent dryness and fungal infection of the mouth. Instruct patients to notify the physician or

nurse of a sore throat or mouth (possible infection). When using beclomethasone intranasally, instruct patients to clear nasal passages before using beclomethasone and report nasal irritation, or if symptoms such as sneezing fail to improve.

SERIOUS ADVERSE REACTIONS

- **Hypersensitivity:** An acute hypersensitivity reaction including urticaria, angioedema, and severe bronchospasm, occurs rarely.
- **Masked bronchial asthma:** A transfer from systemic to local steroid therapy may unmask a previously suppressed bronchial asthma condition. Beclomethasone is not intended for treatment of acute asthma.

OVERDOSE/TOXICITY

- **Systemic corticosteroid effects:** A small number of patients may experience systemic steroid side effects including adrenal suppression. Dosage should be gradually tapered in these patients to help resolve symptoms.
- **Management:** Supportive care for significant symptoms should be implemented.

ANTIDOTE/DIALYSIS

- **Antidote:** No specific recommendations.
- **Dialysis:** Beclomethasone is not removed by hemodialysis, peritoneal dialysis, or high-permeability hemodialysis.

belladonna and opium

bell-a-don'-a oh'-pee-um

DEA Schedule: II

Classes

Chemical: belladonna alkaloid, opiate
Therapeutic: antispasmodic, narcotic analgesic

Pregnancy Category: C

Trade Names

Prescription: B&O Supprettes 15-A, B&O Supprettes 16-A

CLINICAL PHARMACOLOGY

Mechanism of Action

Anticholinergic alkaloid that inhibits the action of acetylcholine at postganglionic (muscarinic) receptor sites. Morphine (10% of opium) depresses cerebral cortex, hypothalamus, and medullary centers. Therapeutic Effect: Decreases digestive secretions, increases GI muscle tone, reduces GI force, alters pain perception and emotional response to pain.

PHARMACOKINETICS

Onset of action occurs within 30 min. Absorption is dependent on body hydration. Metabolized in liver to form glucuronide metabolites.

AVAILABILITY

Suppository: 16.2 mg belladonna extract/30 mg opium (B&O Supprettes 15-A), 16.2 mg belladonna extract/60 mg opium (B&O Supprettes 16-A).

INDICATIONS AND DOSAGE

Analgesic, antispasmodic

Rectal

Adults, Elderly. 1 suppository 1-2 times per day. Maximum: 4 doses per day.

OFF-LABEL USES

Glaucoma, severe renal or hepatic disease, bronchial asthma, respiratory depression, convulsive disorders, acute alcoholism, premature labor, hypersensitivity to belladonna or opium or its components

CONTRAINDICATIONS

Glaucoma, obstructive GI disease, myasthenia gravis, obstructive uropathy, intestinal atony, reflux esophagitis, toxic megacolon, ulcerative colitis

INTERACTIONS

Drug: **Alcohol, CNS depressants:** May increase CNS or respiratory depression, hypotension. **Anticholinergics:** May increase the effects of belladonna and opium. **Phenothiazines:** May decrease the antipsychotic effects of these drugs. Herbal: None known. Food: None known.

DIAGNOSTIC TEST EFFECTS

May increase serum AST (SGOT) and ALT (SGPT) levels.

SIDE-EFFECTS

Frequent: Dry mouth, nose, skin and throat, decreased sweating, constipation, irritation at site of administration, drowsiness, urinary retention, dizziness. Occasional: Blurred vision, decreased flow of breast milk, bloated feeling, drowsiness, headache, intolerance to light, nervousness, flushing. Rare: Dizziness, faintness, pruritis, urticaria

CRITICAL CARE CONSIDERATIONS

ADMINISTRATION/HANDLING

RECTAL ALERT

- **Administration:** Moisten finger and suppository before insertion.
- **Storage:** Store at room temperature.

PRECAUTIONS

HEALTH-RELATED

- Use extreme caution in patients with acute alcoholism, anoxia, CNS depression, hypercapnia, respiratory depression or dysfunction, seizures, shock, and untreated myxedema.
- Use cautiously in patients with acute abdominal conditions, Addison's disease, chronic obstructive pulmonary disease, hypothyroidism, impaired liver function, increased intracranial pressure, prostatic hypertrophy, and urethral stricture.

AGE-RELATED

- **Children:** May be more susceptible to respiratory depression.
- **Elderly:** May be more susceptible to respiratory depression and paradoxic excitement. Age-related prostatic hypertrophy or obstruction and renal impairment may increase risk of urinary retention; reduced dosage is recommended.

PREGNANCY/LACTATION-RELATED

- Pregnancy category C; excretion of belladonna into breast milk is controversial; neonates may be particularly sensitive to anticholinergic agents, therefore use caution in nursing mothers.

MONITORING

- **Baseline assessment:** Monitor vital signs and other signs of narcosis.
- **Lab work:** Biochemical profile including liver function tests (AST [SGOT], ALT [SGPT], alkaline phosphatase, bilirubin).
- **Hypotension:** Assess for paradoxic reactions.
- **Urinary retention:** Evaluate for difficulty voiding.
- **Constipation:** Assess daily pattern of bowel activity and stool consistency.
- **Therapeutic effect:** Assess for relief of bladder spasms, other pain; record onset of pain relief.
- **Patient education:** If belladonna and opium is to be used outside the hospital, instruct patients how to moisten the suppository before insertion. Urge avoidance of alcohol during therapy and avoidance of tasks that require mental alertness and motor skills until response to the drug is known. Instruct to change positions slowly to avoid orthostatic hypotension. Belladonna and opium use may cause dry mouth. Tell patients not to get overheated during hot weather because this may result in heat stroke and to avoid hot baths and saunas.

SERIOUS ADVERSE REACTIONS

- **Symptoms:** Increased intraocular pain, loss of memory, orthostatic hypotension, tachycardia.
- **Tolerance:** Develops to analgesic effect and physical dependence may occur with repeated use.

OVERDOSE/TOXICITY

- **Symptoms:** Respiratory failure and ventricular fibrillation rarely occur.
- **Management:** Supportive care to maintain airway and ventilation. Manage dysrhythmias according to Advanced Cardiac Life Support (ACLS) guidelines. Some patients may require sedation. Patient may have anticholinergic syndrome including anxiety, delirium, hallucinations, agitation, hyperactivity, hyperthermia, aphasia, myoclonus, seizures, urinary retention, paralytic ileus, intense dry mouth, and thirst.
- **GI decontamination:** No specific recommendations.

ANTIDOTE/DIALYSIS

- **Antidote:** Naloxone may help to reverse opium. Neostigmine may help to reverse effects of anticholinergic syndrome.
- **Dialysis:** No data are available on removal of belladonna and opium using hemodialysis, high-permeability hemodialysis, or peritoneal dialysis.

benazepril

See ACE Inhibitors (p. 883)

bendroflumethiazide

See Diuretics (p. 956)

benztropine mesylate

benz'-troe-peen mes'-sil-ate

Classes
Chemical: tertiary amine
Therapeutic: antiparkinson agent, anticholinergic

Pregnancy Category: C

Trade Names
Prescription: Apo-Benztropine ♣, Cogentin

Do not confuse benztropine with bromocriptine.

CLINICAL PHARMACOLOGY

Mechanism of Action
An antiparkinson agent that selectively blocks central cholinergic receptors, helping to balance cholinergic and dopaminergic activity. **Therapeutic Effect:** Reduces the incidence and severity of akinesia, rigidity, and tremor.

PHARMACOKINETICS

Well absorbed following oral and IM administration. Oral onset of action: 1-2 hr, IM onset of action: 30 min. The pharmacologic effects may not be apparent until 2-3 days after initiation of therapy and may persist for up to 48 hr after discontinuation of the drug. **Half-life:** Extended.

AVAILABILITY

Tablets: 0.5 mg, 1 mg, 2 mg.
Injection: 1 mg/mL.

INDICATIONS AND DOSAGE

Parkinsonism

PO

Adults: 0.5-6 mg/day as a single dose or in 2 divided doses. Titrate by 0.5 mg at 5-6 day intervals. **Elderly:** Initially, 0.5 mg once or twice per day. Titrate by 0.5 mg at 5-6 day intervals. Maximum: 4 mg/day.

Drug-induced extrapyramidal symptoms

PO, IM

Adults: 1-4 mg once or twice per day. **Children older than 3 yr:** 0.02-0.05 mg/kg/dose once or twice per day.

Acute dystonic reactions

IV, IM

Adults: Initially 1-2 mg, then 1-2 mg PO twice per day to prevent recurrence.

CONTRAINDICATIONS

Angle-closure glaucoma, benign prostatic hyperplasia, children younger than 3 yr, GI obstruction, intestinal atony, megacolon, myasthenia gravis, paralytic ileus, severe ulcerative colitis, bladder neck obstructions

INTERACTIONS

Drug: **Alcohol, other CNS depressants:** May increase sedation. **Amantadine, anticholinergics, MAOIs:** May increase the effects of benztropine. **Antacids, antidiarrheals:** May decrease the absorption and effects of benztropine. **Tricyclic antidepressants:** May cause excessive anticholinergic effects (dry mouth, constipation, sedation). **Herbal:** None known. **Food:** None known.

DIAGNOSTIC TEST EFFECTS

None known.

SIDE-EFFECTS

Frequent: Somnolence, dry mouth, blurred vision, constipation, decreased sweating or urination, GI upset, photosensitivity. **Occasional:** Headache, memory loss, muscle cramps, anxiety, peripheral paresthesia, orthostatic hypotension, abdominal cramps. **Rare:** Rash, confusion, eye pain

CRITICAL CARE CONSIDERATIONS

ADMINISTRATION/HANDLING

PO ALERT

- May give benztropine without regard to food.

IM AND IV ALERT

- For quick action, IV and IM routes of administration are equally effective.

PRECAUTIONS

HEALTH-RELATED

- Use benztropine cautiously in patients with dysrhythmias, heart disease, hypertension, hepatic or renal impairment, obstructive diseases of the GI or GU tracts, urine retention, benign prostatic hyperplasia, tachycardia, or treated open-angle glaucoma.
- For patients receiving phenothiazines, haloperidol, or other drugs with anticholinergic or antidopaminergic effects, the onset of GI symptoms, fever, or heat intolerance may lead to paralytic ileus, heat stroke, and hyperthermia which have been fatal in some patients.
- **Tardive dyskinesia:** Not recommended for treatment of tardive dyskinesia.
- **Anhidrosis:** May be a side effect. Administer with caution during hot weather.

B

AGE-RELATED

- **Children:** Should not be used in children under 3 yr; use with extreme caution in older children.
- **Elderly:** Patients over 60 yr are more likely to develop agitation, disorientation, confusion, and psychoticlike symptoms.

PREGNANCY/LACTATION-RELATED

- Pregnancy category C; an inhibitory effect on lactation may occur; infants may be particularly sensitive to anticholinergic effects

MONITORING

- **Baseline assessment:** Assess mental status for agitation, confusion, disorientation, and psychoticlike symptoms because benztropine frequently produces such side effects in patients over 60 yr.
- **Neurologic effects:** Monitor for agitation, headache, somnolence, and confusion which may indicate onset of toxic psychosis.
- **Therapeutic effect:** Assess for improvement of masklike facial expression, muscular rigidity, shuffling gait, and resting tremors.
- **Patient education:** Inform patients that dizziness, drowsiness, and dry mouth are expected responses to benztropine. Drowsiness may diminish or disappear with continued therapy. If benztropine is to be used outside of the hospital, warn patients to avoid tasks that require mental alertness or motor skills until response to the drug is known. Urge patients to avoid alcoholic beverages during benztropine therapy.

SERIOUS ADVERSE REACTIONS

- **Anticholinergic effects:** Tachycardia, paralytic ileus, severe dry mouth effecting swallowing and speech, urinary retention, dysuria, rash, heat stroke, fever, hyperthermia, toxic psychosis, and anhidrosis (absence of sweating).
- **Toxic psychosis:** Confusion, disorientation, hallucinations, memory impairment, and exacerbation of preexisting mental disorders.
- **Rhabdomyolysis:** May ensue in response to agitation combined with impaired thermoregulation.

OVERDOSE/TOXICITY

- **Intentional overdose:** Fairly common; associated with depression.
- **Drug abuse:** Benztropine is abused for its hallucinogenic and euphoric effects.
- **Anticholinergic syndrome:** Syndrome created by benztropine blocking acetylcholine from binding to acetylcholine receptor sites. Manifested by anticholinergic effects.
- **Symptoms:** Confusion, hallucination, incoherent speech and agitation with hyperthermia, tachycardia, dry axillae, decreased bowel sounds, and urinary retention.
- **Supportive care:** Maintenance of airway, supplemental oxygen, IV fluid replacement to correct intravascular volume deficit, cardiac monitoring and bladder catheterization, lab work to detect rhabdomyolysis.
- **GI decontamination:** Use of oral activated charcoal is effective if implemented within several hours of ingestion.

ANTIDOTE/DIALYSIS

- **Antidote:** Physostigmine is used in diagnosing anticholinergic syndrome and to help manage neuropsychiatric symptoms, but it may induce bronchospasm, seizures, and severe cardiac conduction abnormalities.
- **Dialysis:** No data are available on removal using hemodialysis, high-permeability hemodialysis, or peritoneal dialysis.

bepridil

See Antidysrhythmics (p. 919) and Calcium Channel Blockers (p. 950)

beractant

ber-akt'-ant

Classes

Chemical: phospholipid
Therapeutic: lung surfactant, natural bovine

Pregnancy Category: C

Trade Names

Prescription: Survanta

Do not confuse Survanta with Sufenta.

CLINICAL PHARMACOLOGY

Mechanism of Action

A natural bovine lung extract that reduces alveolar surface tension, stabilizing alveoli. Therapeutic Effect: Improves lung compliance and respiratory gas exchange.

PHARMACOKINETICS

Not absorbed systemically.

AVAILABILITY

Intratracheal suspension for inhalation: 25-mg/mL vials.

INDICATIONS AND DOSAGE

Prevention and rescue treatment of respiratory distress syndrome (RDS) or hyaline membrane disease in premature infants

Intratracheal

Infants: 100 mg of phospholipids/kg birth weight (4 mL/kg). Give within 15 min of birth if infant weighs less than 1250 g and has evidence of surfactant deficiency; give within 8 hr when RDS is confirmed by x-ray and requires mechanical ventilation. May repeat 6 hr or longer after preceding dose. Maximum: 4 doses in the first 48 hr of life.

CONTRAINDICATIONS

None known.

INTERACTIONS

Drug: None known. **Herbal:** None known. **Food:** None known.

DIAGNOSTIC TEST EFFECTS

None known.

SIDE-EFFECTS

Frequent: Transient bradycardia, oxygen (O_2) desaturation, increased carbon dioxide (CO_2) retention. **Occasional:** Endotracheal tube reflux. **Rare:** Apnea, endotracheal tube blockage, hypotension or hypertension, pallor, vasoconstriction

CRITICAL CARE CONSIDERATIONS

ADMINISTRATION/HANDLING

INTRATRACHEAL ALERT

- **Storage:** Refrigerate vials. Unopened, unused vials may be returned to the refrigerator only once and within 8 hr after having been warmed to room temperature.
- **Preparation:** Warm the vial by letting it stand at room temperature for 20 min or warming in your hand for 8 min. Gently swirl the vial, if needed, to redisperse contents. Do not shake. The solution normally appears off-white to light brown.
- **Single use only:** Enter each single-use vial only once; discard unused suspension.
- **Tracheal instillation:** Instill beractant through a catheter inserted into the infant's endotracheal tube. Do not instill into the main-stem bronchus. Monitor for bradycardia and hypoxemia during instillation.

PRECAUTIONS

HEALTH-RELATED

- Use cautiously in neonates at risk for circulatory overload.
- A higher incidence of patent ductus arteriosus has been evident is some studies following treatment.
- Beractant and all pulmonary surfactants have had disappointing results in studies of adults with acute respiratory distress syndrome.

AGE-RELATED

- **Neonates:** Beractant is for use only in neonates but has been studied for use in adults with acute respiratory distress syndrome with disappointing results.
- No age-related precautions have been noted because beractant is used for neonates only.

PREGNANCY/LACTATION-RELATED

- Pregnancy category C. This drug is not indicated for use in pregnant women.

MONITORING

- **Baseline assessment:** Assess for circulatory overload.
- **Bradycardia and hypoxemia:** Monitor for bradycardia and decreased arterial O_2 saturation during administration. *Stop the procedure if the infant experiences these effects and adjust support as needed before reinstituting therapy.*
- **Administration:** Administer beractant in a highly skilled setting; clinicians caring for the neonate must be experienced with intubation and ventilator management.
- **Ventilation and oxygenation:** Monitor with arterial or transcutaneous measurement of systemic O_2 and CO_2. Peak pressures and FiO_2 must be reduced when beractant is effective to avoid pneumothorax and oxygen toxicity. Effects may occur rapidly; close monitoring is essential.
- **Pulmonary assessment:** Auscultate breath sounds for crackles and rhonchi.
- **Therapeutic effect:** Observe for rapid chest expansion and improvement of oxygen saturation and measures of oxygenation.
- **Nosocomial infection:** Limit visitors during treatment, practice meticulous hand washing and other infection control measures to minimize the risk for infection.

B

- **Family education:** Offer emotional support to parents. Tell parents the purpose of the treatment and the expected outcome.

SERIOUS ADVERSE REACTIONS

- **Sepsis:** Life-threatening nosocomial sepsis possibly resulting from improper administration of beractant.
- **Other reactions:** Pulmonary hemorrhage, intracranial hemorrhage.
- **Complications:** Pneumothorax, oxygen toxicity, plugged endotracheal tube.

OVERDOSE/TOXICITY

- Highly unlikely because beractant is metabolized almost exclusively by the lungs.
- No cases have been reported of overdose or sensitivity.

ANTIDOTE/DIALYSIS

- **Antidote:** No specific recommendations.
- **Dialysis:** Beractant is not likely to be removed using hemodialysis, high-permeability hemodialysis, or peritoneal dialysis.

betamethasone

See Corticosteroids (p. 953)

betaxolol hydrochloride

See Beta-Adrenergic Blockers (p. 943)

bisacodyl

bis-a-koe'-dill

Classes

Chemical: diphenylmethane derivative
Therapeutic: laxative, stimulant

Pregnancy Category: C

Trade Names

Over the Counter: Alophen, Dulcolax, Fleet, Gentlax, Modane, Veracolate

Do not confuse Veracorate with Accorate or Modane with Mudrane.

CLINICAL PHARMACOLOGY

Mechanism of Action

A GI stimulant that has a direct effect on colonic smooth musculature by stimulating the intramural nerve plexi. **Therapeutic Effect:** Promotes fluid and ion accumulation in the colon, increasing peristalsis and producing a laxative effect.

PHARMACOKINETICS

Route	Onset	Peak	Duration
PO	6-10 hr	N/A	N/A
Rectal	15-60 min	N/A	N/A

Minimal absorption following oral and rectal administration. Absorbed drug is excreted in urine; remainder is eliminated in feces.

AVAILABILITY

Tablets (enteric-coated [Dulcolax, Fleet]): 5 mg.
Rectal enema (Fleet): 10 mg/30 mL.
Suppositories (Dulcolax, Fleet): 10 mg.

INDICATIONS AND DOSAGE

Treatment of constipation

PO

Adults, Children older than 12 yr: 5-15 mg as needed. Maximum: 30 mg. **Children 3-12 yr:** 5-10 mg or 0.3 mg/kg at bedtime or after breakfast. **Elderly:** Initially 5 mg/day.

Rectal, enema

Adults, Children 12 yr and older: One 1.25-oz bottle in a single daily dose.

Rectal, suppository

Adults, Children 12 yr and older: 10 mg to induce bowel movement. **Children 2-11 yr:** 5-10 mg as a single dose. **Children younger than 2 yr:** 5 mg. **Elderly:** 5-10 mg/day.

CONTRAINDICATIONS

Abdominal pain, intestinal obstruction, nausea, undiagnosed rectal bleeding, vomiting

INTERACTIONS

Drug: **Antacids, cimetidine, famotidine, ranitidine:** May cause rapid dissolution of bisacodyl, producing abdominal cramping and vomiting. **Oral medications:** May decrease transit time of concurrently administered oral medications, decreasing absorption of bisacodyl. **Herbal:** None known. **Food:** **Milk:** May cause rapid dissolution of bisacodyl (decreased effect).

DIAGNOSTIC TEST EFFECTS

None known.

SIDE-EFFECTS

Frequent: Some degree of abdominal discomfort, nausea, mild cramps, faintness. **Occasional:** **Rectal administration:** Burning of rectal mucosa, mild proctitis

CRITICAL CARE CONSIDERATIONS

ADMINISTRATION/HANDLING

PO ALERT

- Give bisacodyl on an empty stomach for faster action.
- Offer 6 to 8 glasses of water per day to aid in stool softening.
- Administer tablets whole; make sure the patient does not chew or crush them.
- Avoid giving within 1 hr of antacids, milk, or other oral medications.

RECTAL ALERT

- If the suppository is too soft, chill for 30 min in the refrigerator or run cold water over foil wrapper.
- **Administration:** Moisten the suppository with cold water before inserting deep into the rectum.

PRECAUTIONS

HEALTH-RELATED

- Excessive use of bisacodyl may lead to fluid and electrolyte imbalance.
- Bisacodyl should not be used when abdominal pain, nausea, and vomiting are present and should not be used for more than 7 days unless deemed necessary.

AGE-RELATED

- **Children:** Approved for use in children following evaluation of reason for constipation.
- **Elderly:** Repeated use of bisacodyl in the elderly may cause orthostatic hypotension and weakness due to electrolyte loss.

PREGNANCY/LACTATION-RELATED

- Pregnancy category C; excreted in breast milk.

MONITORING

- **Baseline assessment:** Before bisacodyl administration, assess abdomen for signs of tenderness, rigidity, and the presence of bowel sounds.
- **Baseline lab work:** Biochemical profile.
- **Ongoing lab work:** Monitor serum electrolyte levels in patients with excessive, frequent, or prolonged use of bisacodyl.
- **Medication history:** Determine whether other medications cause constipation.
- **Last bowel movement:** Try to determine the time of the last bowel movement and its amount and consistency.
- **Hydration:** Encourage maintenance of adequate fluid intake to help resolve constipation while in the hospital and at home.
- **Bowel assessment:** Assess for peristalsis and for pattern of daily bowel activity, stool consistency. Record time of evacuation. Monitor for abdominal distention and pain.
- **Patient education:** Instruct about measures to promote defecation, such as increasing fluid intake, exercising, and eating a high-fiber diet. Teach patients not to take antacids, milk, or other medications within 1 hr of taking bisacodyl because these substances may decrease the effectiveness of bisacodyl. Instruct patients to promptly report unrelieved constipation, dizziness, muscle cramps or pain, rectal bleeding, or weakness to a health care provider.

SERIOUS ADVERSE REACTIONS

- Long-term use may result in laxative dependence, chronic constipation, and loss of normal bowel function.

OVERDOSE/TOXICITY

- Prolonged use or overdose may result in electrolyte or metabolic disturbances (such as hypokalemia, hypocalcemia, and metabolic acidosis or alkalosis), as well as persistent diarrhea, vomiting, muscle weakness, malabsorption, and weight loss.
- **GI decontamination:** No specific recommendations, but if constipated, whole bowel irrigation may be beneficial in addition to oral activated charcoal.

ANTIDOTE/DIALYSIS

- **Antidote:** No specific recommendations.
- **Dialysis:** No data are available on removal of bisacodyl by hemodialysis, high-permeability hemodialysis, or peritoneal dialysis.

bismuth subsalicylate

See Antidiarrheals (p. 917)

bisoprolol fumarate ⚑

See Beta-Adrenergic Blockers (p. 943)

bitolterol

See Bronchodilators (p. 947)

B

bivalirudin

See Anticoagulants (p. 900)

bosentan

bo'-sen-tan or *boe-sen'-tan*

Classes
Chemical: pyrimidine derivative
Therapeutic: endothelin receptor antagonist

Pregnancy Category: X

Trade Names
Prescription: Tracleer

Do not confuse with Tricor.

CLINICAL PHARMACOLOGY

Mechanism of Action
An endothelin receptor antagonist that blocks endothelin-1, the neurohormone that constricts pulmonary arteries. **Therapeutic Effect:** Improves exercise ability and slows clinical worsening of pulmonary arterial hypertension (PAH).

PHARMACOKINETICS

Highly bound to plasma proteins, mainly albumin. Metabolized in the liver. Eliminated by biliary excretion. **Half-life:** Approximately 5 hr.

AVAILABILITY

Tablets: 62.5 mg, 125 mg.

INDICATIONS AND DOSAGE

Pulmonary arterial hypertension (PAH) in those with World Health Organization Class III or IV symptoms
PO
Adults, Elderly: 62.5 mg twice per day for 4 wk; then increase to maintenance dosage of 125 mg twice per day. **Alert:** When discontinuing, reduce dosage to 62.5 mg twice per day for 3-7 days to avoid clinical deterioration.

Dosage based on transaminase elevations
With any elevation accompanied by symptoms of liver injury or serum bilirubin 2 or more times upper limit of normal, stop treatment.
If AST (SGOT)/ALT (SGPT) is greater than 3 or less than 5 times upper limit of normal, reduce dose or interrupt treatment. If AST (SGOT)/ALT (SGPT) return to normal or pretreatment values, then either continue or reintroduce treatment. Monitor every 2 wk.
If AST (SGOT)/ALT (SGPT) is greater than 5 or less than 9 times upper limit of normal, stop treatment. If AST (SGOT)/ALT (SGPT) return to pretreatment values, reintroduce treatment. Monitor every 2 wk. If AST (SGOT)/ALT (SGPT) is greater than 8 times upper limit of normal, stop treatment.

OFF-LABEL USES

Heart failure, pulmonary hypertension secondary to scleroderma

CONTRAINDICATIONS

Administration with *cycloSPORINE or *glyBURIDE, pregnancy, hypersensitivity to bosentan

INTERACTIONS

Drug: Atorvastatin, *glyBURIDE, hormonal contraceptives (including oral, injectable, and implantable), lovastatin, simvastatin, warfarin: May decrease the plasma concentrations of these drugs. ***CycloSPORINE, ketoconazole:** May increase plasma concentration of bosentan. **Herbal: St. John's wort:** Decreases concentration of bosentan. **Food:** None known.

DIAGNOSTIC TEST EFFECTS

May increase serum bilirubin, AST (SGOT), and ALT (SGPT) levels. May decrease blood Hgb and Hct levels.

SIDE-EFFECTS

Frequent: Headache (16%-22%), nasopharyngitis (11%). **Occasional:** Flushing (7%-9%). **Rare:** Dyspepsia (heartburn, epigastric distress), fatigue, pruritus, hypotension

CRITICAL CARE CONSIDERATIONS

ADMINISTRATION/HANDLING

PO ALERT
- Give bosentan in the morning and evening, with or without food.
- Do not break or crush film-coated tablets. Have the patient swallow film-coated tablets whole and avoid chewing them.

PRECAUTIONS

HEALTH-RELATED
- Use bosentan extremely cautiously in patients with moderate to severe hepatic function impairment, and use cautiously in patients with mild hepatic impairment.

AGE-RELATED
- **Children:** Safety and efficacy of bosentan have not been established in children.
- **Elderly:** Use cautiously because the frequency of decreased cardiac, hepatic, and renal function is higher in older adults.

PREGNANCY/LACTATION-RELATED
- Pregnancy category X; expected to cause fetal harm if administered to pregnant women; excretion into human breast milk unknown.

MONITORING
- **Pretreatment pregnancy evaluation:** Because pregnancy must be avoided during bosentan therapy, determine pregnancy before the start of therapy. A negative result from a urine or serum pregnancy test performed during the first 5 days of a normal menstrual period and at least 11 days after the last act of sexual intercourse must be obtained before drug therapy begins.
- **Pregnancy evaluation:** Patients should have monthly pregnancy tests during bosentan therapy so medication may be discontinued to avoid fetal harm.
- **Lab work for liver function:** Assess baseline hepatic enzyme levels (serum aminotransferase, serum alkaline phosphatase, bilirubin, AST [SGOT], and ALT [SGPT]) before bosentan therapy begins and monthly thereafter. Increase frequency of monitoring and reduce the dose if a severe elevation in hepatic enzyme levels occurs. At least a threefold increase in hepatic enzymes (to upper level of normal) is expected. Stop treatment if symptoms of hepatic injury, including abdominal pain, fatigue, jaundice, nausea, and vomiting occur, or if the bilirubin level increases.
- **Lab work for anemia:** Monitor blood Hgb level at 1 and 3 mo after treatment begins and every 3 mo thereafter. A decrease in blood Hct and Hgb levels signifies anemia.
- ***GlyBURIDE:** Combined use of bosentan and *glyBURIDE is contraindicated because the combination causes further increases in liver enzymes, indicative of liver injury.
- **Cyclosporine-A:** Combined use of bosentan with *cycloSPORINE is contraindicated because it results in markedly increased plasma concentration of bosentan.
- **Use of contraceptives:** When bosentan is used outside the hospital, inform patients about the various methods of effective contraception.

SERIOUS ADVERSE REACTIONS
- Abnormal hepatic function indicative of liver injury, lower extremity edema, and palpitations occur rarely.

OVERDOSE/TOXICITY
- **Symptoms:** Liver failure, headache, nasopharyngitis, flushing, fatigue, hypotension, lower limb edema, possible anemia.
- **Drug discontinuation:** To manage liver failure, the drug must be discontinued. No evidence of acute rebound of pulmonary hypertension has been observed.
- **Management:** Supportive care based on accepted standards for treatment of liver failure, anemia, and other symptoms should be initiated.
- **GI decontamination:** No specific recommendations.

ANTIDOTE/DIALYSIS
- **Antidote:** No specific recommendations.
- **Dialysis:** Bosentan is unlikely to be removed using hemodialysis, peritoneal dialysis, or high-permeability hemodialysis.

botulinum toxin type a

bot′-yoo-lye-num

Classes
Chemical: clostridium botulinum derivative, neurotoxin
Therapeutic: muscle relaxation, paralysis

Pregnancy Category: C

Trade Names
Prescription: Botox

CLINICAL PHARMACOLOGY
Mechanism of Action
A neurotoxin that blocks neuromuscular conduction by binding to receptor sites on motor nerve endings and inhibiting the release of acetylcholine, resulting in muscle denervation. **Therapeutic Effect:** Reduces muscle activity.

PHARMACOKINETICS
In the treatment of blepharospasm, each treatment lasts approximately 3 mo. In the treatment of strabismus, the paralysis lasts for 2-6 wk and gradually resolves over an additional 2-6 wk. In the treatment of hemifacial spasm, treatment may last 6 mo.

AVAILABILITY
Injection: 100 units/vial.

B

INDICATIONS AND DOSAGE

Cervical dystonia in patients who have previously tolerated botulinum toxin type A

IM

Adults, Elderly: Mean dose of 236 units (range: 198-300 units) divided among the affected muscles, based on patient's head and neck position, localization of pain, muscle hypertrophy, patient response, and adverse reaction history.

Cervical dystonia in patients who have not previously been treated with botulinum toxin type A

IM

Adults, Elderly: Administer at lower dosage than for patients who have previously tolerated the drug.

Strabismus

IM

Adults, Children older then 12 yr: 1.25-2.5 units into any one muscle. **Children 2 mo-12 yr:** 1-2.5 units into any one muscle.

Blepharospasm

IM

Adults, Children 12 yr and older: Initially, 1.25-2.5 units. May increase up to 2.5-5.0 units at repeat treatments. Maximum: 5 units per injection or cumulative dose of 200 units over a 30-day period.

Cerebral palsy spasticity

IM

Children older than 18 mo: 1-6 units/kg (small muscle: 1-2 units/kg; large muscle: 3-6 units/kg). Maximum: 50 units per injection site. No more than 400 units per visit or during a 3-mo period.

Improvement of brow furrow

IM

Adults 65 yr and younger: Individualized.

OFF-LABEL USES

Treatment of dynamic muscle contracture in children with cerebral palsy, focal task-specific dystonia, head and neck tremor unresponsive to drug therapy, hemifacial spasms, laryngeal dystonia, oromandibular dystonia, spasmoditic torticollis, writer's cramp

CONTRAINDICATIONS

Infection at proposed injection sites, pregnancy

INTERACTIONS

Drug: **Aminoglycoside antibiotics, other drugs that interfere with neuromuscular transmission (such as curare-like compounds):** May potentiate the effects of botulinum toxin type A. **Herbal:** None known. **Food:** None known.

DIAGNOSTIC TEST EFFECTS

None known.

SIDE-EFFECTS

Alert: Side effects usually occur within the first week after injection. **Frequent (19%-11%):** Dysphagia (19%), localized pain, tenderness, or bruising at injection site; localized weakness in injected muscle; neck pain; headache. **Occasional (10%-2%):** Increased cough, flulike symptoms, upper respiratory tract infection, back pain, rhinitis, dizziness, hypertonia, soreness at injection site, asthenia, dry mouth, nausea, somnolence. **Rare:** Stiffness, numbness, diplopia, ptosis

CRITICAL CARE CONSIDERATIONS

ADMINISTRATION/HANDLING

DOSAGE ALERT

- Administer the drug at the lowest effective dosage and at the longest effective dosing interval to avoid formation of neutralizing antibodies.
- Botulinum toxins have been used as biological weapons.

IM ALERT

- ***Contraindication:*** *Do not give in any injection site that appears infected.*
- **Storage:** Store drug vials in the freezer. The reconstituted solution may be refrigerated for up to 4 hr.
- **Stability:** Administer the drug within 4 hr after reconstitution.
- **Appearance:** The solution normally appears as clear and colorless. Discard the solution if particulate matter is present.
- **Dilution:** Dilute with 0.9% NaCl. For a resulting dose of units/0.1 mL, draw up 1 mL of diluent to provide 10 units, 2 mL to provide 5 units, 4 mL to provide 2.5 units, or 8 mL to provide 1.25 units. Slowly and gently inject the diluent into the vial to avoid producing bubbles. Then rotate the vial gently to mix the drug. If a vacuum does not pull the diluent into the vial, discard it.
- **Injection:** Inject the drug into the affected muscles using a 25-, 27-, or 30-gauge

needle for superficial muscles, and a 22-gauge needle for deeper muscles.

PRECAUTIONS

HEALTH-RELATED

- Use botulinum toxin type A cautiously in patients with neuromuscular junctional disorders, such as amyotrophic lateral sclerosis, Lambert-Eaton syndrome, motor neuropathy, and myasthenia gravis because they may experience significant systemic effects, including respiratory compromise and severe dysphagia.

AGE-RELATED

- **Children:** Botulinum toxin type A has been used successfully in children over 2 mo.
- **Elderly:** May require lower doses for certain treatable conditions.

PREGNANCY/LACTATION-RELATED

- Pregnancy category C.

MONITORING

- **Baseline assessment:** Assess specific neuromuscular dysfunction before treatment.
- **Therapeutic effect:** Assess the onset, location, duration, and type of dystonia experienced. Assess for improvement.
- **Local reactions:** Examine the proposed injection site for signs of infection, such as erythema or swelling.
- **Systemic reactions:** Assess for signs of dysphagia and aspiration pneumonia, including fever, sputum production, and adventitious breath sounds. Urge patients to report respiratory, speech, or swallowing difficulties immediately.
- **Patient education:** Inform patients that clinical improvement should begin within 2 wk of the injection, but that the drug's maximum benefit will appear approximately 6 wk after the injection. Advise to resuming normal activity slowly and carefully.

SERIOUS ADVERSE REACTIONS

- Mild to moderate dysphagia occurs in approximately 20% of patients.
- Dysrhythmias and severe dysphagia (manifested as aspiration, pneumonia, and dyspnea) occur rarely.

OVERDOSE/TOXICITY

- **Symptoms:** Systemic weakness and descending, flaccid muscle paralysis beginning in the bulbar musculature. Gastrointestinal, cranial nerve (includes impaired, speech, swallowing, cough, and gag reflexes), and autonomic nervous system dysfunction are often the presenting symptoms. May progress to respiratory failure and arrest. Aspiration may occur, which can lead to pneumonia and acute respiratory distress syndrome in severe cases.
- **Management:** Patients with symptoms of botulism may require mechanical ventilation for 2-8 wk. Severe cases have required tracheostomy with ventilation up to 7 mo. Early recognition of botulinum poisoning is key to preventing severe complications and/or death.
- **GI decontamination:** No specific recommendations.

ANTIDOTE/DIALYSIS

- **Antidote:** The antitoxin used in North America is trivalent ABE and is produced by Aventis Pharmaceuticals (Bridgewater, NJ). One vial is administered using the revised Centers for Disease Control guidelines, which have reduced the dose from two vials and is effective in halting progression of the disease if given early. Steroids, guanidine, 4-aminopyridine have been tried, but placebo-controlled studies have shown no benefit. Antibiotics are not effective because the toxin is preformed.
- **Dialysis:** Plasmapheresis has been tried but has not proved beneficial.

botulinum toxin type b

bot'-yoo-lye-num

Classes

Chemical: clostridium botulinum derivative, neurotoxin

Therapeutic: muscle relaxation, paralysis

Pregnancy Category: C

Trade Names

Prescription: Myobloc

CLINICAL PHARMACOLOGY

Mechanism of Action

A neurotoxin that inhibits acetylcholine release at the neuromuscular junction. **Therapeutic Effect:** Produces flaccid paralysis.

PHARMACOKINETICS

The duration of effect is 12-16 wk at doses of 5000 or 10,000 units.

AVAILABILITY

Injection: 2500 units, 5000 units, 10,000 units.

B

INDICATIONS AND DOSAGE

To reduce the severity of symptoms in patients with cervical dystonia who have previously tolerated botulinum toxin type B

IM

Adults, Elderly: 2500-5000 units divided among the affected muscles.

To reduce the severity of symptoms in patients with cervical dystonia who have not previously been treated with botulinum toxin type B

IM

Adults, Elderly: Administer at lower dosage than for patients who have previously tolerated the drug.

CONTRAINDICATIONS

Infection at injection site, pregnancy

INTERACTIONS

Drug: Aminoglycoside antibiotics, other drugs that interfere with neuromuscular transmission (such as curare-like compounds): May potentiate the effects of botulinum toxin type B. **Herbal:** None known. **Food:** None known.

DIAGNOSTIC TEST EFFECTS

None known.

SIDE-EFFECTS

Alert: Side effects usually occur within the first week after the injection. **Frequent:** Headache (10%-16%), injection site pain (6%-13%), dry mouth. **Occasional (10%-4%):** Flulike symptoms, generalized pain, increased cough, back pain, myasthenia, dysphagia. **Rare:** Dizziness, nausea, rhinitis, vomiting, edema, allergic reaction

CRITICAL CARE CONSIDERATIONS

ADMINISTRATION/HANDLING

DOSAGE ALERT

- Botulinum toxins have been used as biological weapons.

IM ALERT

- **Storage:** Unreconstituted vials may be refrigerated for up to 21 mo. Do not freeze. The reconstituted solution may be stored in the refrigerator for up to 4 hr.
- **Stability:** Administer within 4 hr after reconstitution.
- **Appearance:** The solution normally appears clear and colorless. Discard the solution if particulate matter is present.
- **Dilution:** Dilute with 0.9% NaCl. Slowly and gently inject the diluent into the vial to avoid producing bubbles. Then rotate the vial gently to mix the drug. If a vacuum does not pull the diluent into the vial, discard it.
- **Injection:** Inject into the affected muscles using a 25-, 27-, or 30-gauge needle for superficial muscles and a 22-gauge needle for deeper muscles.

PRECAUTIONS

HEALTH-RELATED

- Use botulinum toxin type B cautiously in patients with neuromuscular junctional disorders, such as amyotrophic lateral sclerosis, Lambert-Eaton syndrome, motor neuropathy, and myasthenia gravis because they may experience significant systemic effects, including respiratory compromise and severe dysphagia.

AGE-RELATED

- **Children:** Botulinum toxin type B may be used in children.
- **Elderly:** May require lower doses for certain treatable conditions.

PREGNANCY/LACTATION-RELATED

- Pregnancy category C.

MONITORING

- **Baseline assessment:** Assess the onset, location, duration, and type of dystonia experienced. Assess for improvement. The drug's effect lasts for 12-16 wk at doses of 5000 or 10,000 units.
- **Local reactions:** Examine the proposed injection site for signs of infection, such as erythema or swelling.
- **Systemic reactions:** Assess for signs of dysphagia and aspiration pneumonia, including fever, sputum production, and adventitious breath sounds. Urge patients to immediately report respiratory, speech, or swallowing difficulties.
- **Patient education:** Advise resuming normal activity slowly and carefully.

SERIOUS ADVERSE REACTIONS

- Mild to moderate dysphagia occurs in approximately 10% of patients.
- Dysrhythmias and severe dysphagia (manifested as aspiration, pneumonia, and dyspnea) occur rarely.

OVERDOSE/TOXICITY

- **Symptoms:** Systemic weakness and descending, flaccid muscle paralysis beginning in the bulbar musculature. Gastrointestinal, cranial nerve (includes impaired speech, swallowing, cough, and gag reflexes) and autonomic nervous system dysfunction are often the presenting symptoms. May progress to respiratory failure and arrest. Aspiration may occur, which can lead to pneumonia and acute respiratory distress syndrome in severe cases.

- **Management:** Patients with symptoms of botulism may require mechanical ventilation for 2-8 wk. Severe cases have required tracheostomy with ventilation up to 7 mo. Early recognition of botulinum poisoning is key to preventing severe complications and/or death.
- **GI decontamination:** No specific recommendations.

ANTIDOTE/DIALYSIS

- **Antidote:** The antitoxin used in North America is trivalent ABE and is produced by Aventis Pharmaceuticals (Bridgewater, NJ). One vial is administered using the revised Centers for Disease Control and Prevention guidelines, which have reduced the dose from two vials and is effective in halting progression of the disease if given early. Steroids, guanidine, and 4-aminopyridine have been tried, but placebo-controlled studies have shown no benefit. Antibiotics are not effective because the toxin is preformed.
- **Dialysis:** Plasmapheresis has been tried but has not been proven beneficial.

bromocriptine mesylate

broe-moe-krip'-teen mes'-il-ate

Classes

Chemical: ergot alkaloid derivative
Therapeutic: anti-Parkinson's agent, dopaminergic, ovulation stimulant

Pregnancy Category: B

Trade Names

Prescription: Parlodel

Do not confuse bromocriptine with benztropine or Parlodel with pindolol.

CLINICAL PHARMACOLOGY

Mechanism of Action

A dopamine agonist that directly stimulates dopamine receptors in the corpus striatum and inhibits prolactin secretion. Also suppresses secretion of growth hormone. **Therapeutic Effect:** Improves symptoms of parkinsonism, suppresses galactorrhea, and reduces serum growth hormone concentrations in acromegaly.

PHARMACOKINETICS

Indication	Onset	Peak	Duration
Prolactin lowering	2 hr	8 hr	24 hr
Antiparkinson	0.5-1.5 hr	2 hr	N/A
Growth hormone suppressant	1-2 hr	4-8 wk	4-8 hr

Minimally absorbed from the GI tract. Protein binding: 90%-96%. Metabolized in the liver. Excreted in feces by biliary secretion. **Half-life:** 6-8 hr.

AVAILABILITY

Capsules: 5 mg.
Tablets: 2.5 mg.

INDICATIONS AND DOSAGE

Hyperprolactinemia

PO

Adults, Elderly: Initially, 1.25-2.5 mg at bedtime. May increase by 2.5 mg every 2-7 days. Range is 2.5-15 mg daily.

Pituitary prolactinomas

PO

Adults, Elderly: Initially, 1.25 mg 2-3 times per day. May gradually increase over several wk to 10-20 mg/day in divided doses. Maintenance: 2.5-20 mg/day in divided doses.

Parkinsonism

PO

Adults, Elderly: Initially, 1.25 mg 1-2 times per day. May take single doses at bedtime. May increase by 2.5 mg/day at 14- to 28-day intervals. Maintenance: 30-90 mg/day in 3 divided doses.

Acromegaly

PO

Adults, Elderly: Initially, 1.25-2.5 mg at bedtime. May increase by 1.25-2.5 mg every 3-7 days up to 30 mg/day in divided doses. Maintenance: 10-30 mg/day in divided doses. Maximum: 100 mg/day.

OFF-LABEL USES

Treatment of cocaine addiction, hyperprolactinemia associated with pituitary adenomas, neuroleptic malignant syndrome

CONTRAINDICATIONS

Hypersensitivity to ergot alkaloids, peripheral vascular disease, pregnancy, severe ischemic heart disease, uncontrolled hypertension, concurrent use with protease inhibitors, azole antifungals, some macrolide antibiotics, sibutramine

B

INTERACTIONS

Drug: Alcohol: May produce a disulfiram-like reaction (chest pain, confusion, flushed face, nausea, vomiting). **Erythromycin, ritonavir:** Use is contraindicated. May increase bromocriptine blood concentration and risk of toxicity. **Estrogens, progestins:** May decrease the effects of bromocriptine. **Haloperidol, MAOIs, phenothiazines, risperidone:** May decrease bromocriptine's prolactin-lowering effect. **Hypotension-producing medications:** May increase hypotension. **Levodopa:** May increase the effects of bromocriptine. **Metoclopramide:** Decreases the effects of bromocriptine. **Herbal:** None known. **Food:** None known.

DIAGNOSTIC TEST EFFECTS

May increase plasma growth hormone concentration.

SIDE-EFFECTS

Frequent: Nausea (49%), headache (19%), dizziness (17%). **Occasional (7%-3%):** Fatigue, lightheadedness, vomiting, abdominal cramps, diarrhea, constipation, nasal congestion, somnolence, dry mouth. **Rare:** Muscle cramps, urinary hesitancy

CRITICAL CARE CONSIDERATIONS

ADMINISTRATION/HANDLING

PO ALERT

- Administer the first dose with the patient lying down to avoid lightheadedness.
- Give bromocriptine after food to decrease the incidence of nausea.

PRECAUTIONS

HEALTH-RELATED

- Use bromocriptine cautiously in patients with impaired hepatic function.
- Use with caution in patients taking antihypertensive agents because additive hypotensive effects may occur.
- Use with caution in patients with dementia or psychosis; symptoms may worsen.
- Not recommended for women with pregnancy-induced hypertension, patients with severe ischemic heart disease or peripheral vascular disease, or patients taking other ergot alkaloids concomitantly.

AGE-RELATED

- **Children:** Safety and efficacy of bromocriptine have not been established in neonates and children under 15 yr.
- **Elderly:** More prone to CNS adverse effects, postural hypotension, neuropsychiatric disorders, nausea, vomiting, and dizziness.

PREGNANCY/LACTATION-RELATED

- Pregnancy category C; because it prevents lactation, should not be administered to mothers who elect to breast-feed infants.

MONITORING

- **Baseline assessment:** Pituitary gland tumor should be ruled out before beginning treatment of symptoms of hyperprolactinemia including amenorrhea with or without galactorrhea, infertility, or hypogonadism.
- **Lab work:** Biochemical profile with liver function tests (AST [SGOT], ALT [SGPT], bilirubin, alkaline phosphatase).
- **Therapeutic response:** Assess for improvement of condition being managed: decreased breast engorgement, decreased parkinsonian symptoms, or reduction of growth hormone levels with acromegaly.
- **Peak plasma concentration range:** 1.3-24.6 ng/mL (1-8.4 mmol/L).
- **Side effects:** Incidence of side effects including nausea, headache, dizziness, fatigue, lightheadedness, vomiting, abdominal cramps, nasal congestion, constipation, diarrhea, and drowsiness is high, especially at the beginning of therapy and with high dosages.
- **Patient education:** Instruct patients to change positions slowly and to sit before standing to avoid postural hypotension, which causes lightheadedness, dizziness, and fainting. Patients should avoid tasks that require mental alertness or motor skills until response to the drug is known. Urge use of nonhormonal contraceptives during treatment.

SERIOUS ADVERSE REACTIONS

- **Parkinson's disease:** Visual or auditory hallucinations.
- **Long-term, high-dose therapy:** May produce continuing rhinorrhea, syncope, GI hemorrhage, peptic ulcer, severe abdominal pain, confusion, and psychosis.
- **Cardiovascular:** Hypotension; stroke and MI are rare.
- **Seizures:** Rarely occur following development of visual disturbances, headache, and hypertension.

OVERDOSE/TOXICITY

- Only a few cases have been reported; symptoms may occur when therapy is initiated. No fatal dose has been determined.

- **Symptoms:** Symptoms reflect dopamine-receptor overstimulation: nausea, vomiting, dizziness, lethargy, sweating, hypotension, agitation, hallucinations, and dyskinesias. Seizures are possible.
- **Management:** If patients experience visual disturbances, headache, and hypertension, discontinue bromocriptine to avoid seizures.
- **GI decontamination:** No specific recommendations.

ANTIDOTE/DIALYSIS

- **Antidote:** No specific recommendations.
- **Dialysis:** Bromocriptine is unlikely to be removed by hemodialysis or peritoneal dialysis. No data are available on removal by high-permeability hemodialysis. Drug is 90%-96% protein bound and is excreted principally into bile and feces. Less than 5% of the parent drug is excreted in urine.

brompheneramine

See Antihistamines (p. 925)

budesonide

byoo-des'-oh-nide

Classes

Chemical: glucocorticoid, synthetic
Therapeutic: antiasthmatic, corticosteroid, antiinflammatory

Pregnancy Category: B (Inhaler), C (Oral)

Trade Names

Prescription: Entocort ♣, Entocort EC, Pulmicort ♣, Pulmicort Respules, Pulmicort Turbuhaler, Rhinocort, Rhinocort Aqua

CLINICAL PHARMACOLOGY

Mechanism of Action

A glucocorticoid that inhibits the accumulation of inflammatory cells and decreases and prevents tissues from responding to the inflammatory process. **Therapeutic Effect:** Relieves symptoms of allergic rhinitis or Crohn's disease.

PHARMACOKINETICS

Minimally absorbed from nasal tissue; moderately absorbed from inhalation. Protein binding: 88%. Primarily metabolized in the liver. **Half-life:** 2-3 hr.

AVAILABILITY

Capsules (Entocort EC): 3 mg.
Powder for oral inhalation (Pulmicort Turbuhaler): 200 mcg per inhalation.
Suspension for oral inhalation (Pulmicort Respules): 0.25 mg/2 mL; 0.5 mg/2 mg.
Nasal spray (Rhinocort Aqua): 32 mcg/spray.

INDICATIONS AND DOSAGE

Rhinitis

Intranasal (Rhinocort Aqua)

Adults, Elderly, Children 6 yr and older: 1 spray in each nostril once per day. Maximum: 8 sprays/day for adults and children 12 yr and older; 4 sprays/day for children younger than 12 yr.

Bronchial asthma

Nebulization

Children 6 mo-8 yr: 0.25-1 mg/day titrated to lowest effective dosage.

Inhalation

Adults, Elderly, Children 6 yr and older: Initially, 200-400 mcg twice per day. Maximum: Adults; 800 mcg twice per day; children; 400 mcg twice per day.

Crohn's disease

PO

Adults, Elderly: 9 mg once per day for up to 8 wk.

OFF-LABEL USES

Treatment of vasomotor rhinitis

CONTRAINDICATIONS

Hypersensitivity to any corticosteroid or its components, persistently positive sputum cultures for *Candida albicans*, primary treatment of status asthmaticus, systemic fungal infections, untreated localized infection involving nasal mucosa

INTERACTIONS

Drug: Bupropion: May lower the seizure threshold. **Itraconazole, ketoconazole, protease inhibitors, amiodarone:** May increase the plasma concentration of budesonide. **Herbal: St. John's wort:** Decreases budesonide levels. **Food: Grapefruit, grapefruit juice:** May increase the systemic exposure of budesonide.

DIAGNOSTIC TEST EFFECTS

None known.

SIDE-EFFECTS

Frequent (greater than 3%): Nasal: Mild nasopharyngeal irritation, burning, stinging, or dryness; headache; cough. **Inhalation:** Flulike symptoms, headache, pharyngitis. **Occasional (3%-1%): Nasal:** Dry mouth, dyspepsia, rebound congestion, rhinorrhea, loss of taste. **Inhalation:** Back pain, vomiting, altered taste, voice changes, abdominal pain, nausea, dyspepsia

B

CRITICAL CARE CONSIDERATIONS

ADMINISTRATION/HANDLING

PO ALERT

- Capsules should be swallowed whole and not chewed or broken.
- Patients should avoid drinking grapefruit juice for the duration of therapy.

INHALATION ALERT

- **Administration:** Shake the container well. Exhale completely and place the mouthpiece between the lips. Inhale and hold the breath for as long as possible before exhaling. Allow at least 1 min between inhalations. Rinse the mouth after each use to decrease dry mouth and hoarseness.

INTRANASAL ALERT

- **Administration:** Clear the nasal passages before using budesonide. Tilt the head slightly forward. Insert the spray tip into the nostril, pointing toward the nasal passages, away from the nasal septum. Spray the drug into the nostril while holding the other nostril closed, and at the same time inhale through the nose to deliver the drug as high into nasal passages as possible.

PRECAUTIONS

HEALTH-RELATED

- Use budesonide cautiously in patients with adrenal insufficiency, diabetes mellitus, cirrhosis, glaucoma, hypothyroidism, osteoporosis, tuberculosis, or untreated infection.

AGE-RELATED

- **Children:** Prolonged treatment and high doses may decrease cortisol secretion and short-term growth rate.
- **Elderly:** No age-related precautions have been noted in the elderly.

PREGNANCY/LACTATION-RELATED

- Pregnancy category C (oral), B (inhaled); unknown if excreted in breast milk.

MONITORING

- **Baseline assessment:** Determine hypersensitivity to corticosteroids or their components and whether the patient has been taking other forms of steroids. Patients can develop adrenal insufficiency if the amount of systemically available corticosteroids is markedly reduced.
- **Lab work:** Biochemical profile including blood glucose level. Monitor for hyperglycemia.
- **Therapeutic respiratory effects:** Monitor for relief of nasal congestion, sneezing, wheezing, or other symptoms. Advise patients taking budesonide intranasally to report if nasal irritation occurs or if symptoms, such as sneezing, fail to improve.
- **Therapeutic effects for Crohn's:** Observe for relief of diarrhea and abdominal cramping associated with mild to moderate Crohn's disease.
- **Hypercorticism:** Monitor for Cushing's syndrome if amiodarone, protease inhibitors, ketoconazole, itraconazole, ritonavir, or erythromycin are being taken. Plasma levels of budesonide can be increased sevenfold if given with medications that inhibit CYP3A4 (cytochrome P450 pathway).
- **Side effects:** For patients on oral budesonide, assess and manage more common complaints including headache, respiratory infection, nausea, indigestion, abdominal pain, dizziness, back pain, and fatigue.
- **Patient education:** Inform patients that symptoms may improve in 24 hr but budesonide's full effect may take 3-7 days to appear. Tell patients not to consume grapefruit juice while taking budesonide to avoid doubling the systemic drug level.

SERIOUS ADVERSE REACTIONS

- **Hypersensitivity:** Urticaria, angioedema, and severe bronchospasm occurs rarely.
- **Allergic reactions:** If moderate, use antihistamines with or without inhaled beta-agonists, corticosteroids, or epinephrine. If severe, use oxygen, aggressive airway management, antihistamines, epinephrine solution subcutaneously, corticosteroids, ECG monitoring, and IV fluids.
- **Hypercorticism:** Cushingoid appearance, osteoporosis, and muscle weakness are most common. Other effects include cataracts, glaucoma, peptic ulcer disease, hypertension, aseptic necrosis of the femur/femoral head, and pancreatitis.
- **Adrenal insufficiency:** Patients transferred from systemic to inhaled corticosteroids can develop adrenal insufficiency because a reduced amount of steroids are available from the inhaled form. This condition has been fatal.

B

OVERDOSE/TOXICITY

- **Symptoms:** Behavioral changes, psychosis, cardiac dysrhythmias, seizures rarely with some forms of corticosteroids.
- **Low toxicity:** Acute ingestion, even in massive doses, is rarely problematic. One case of suspected acute adrenal insufficiency has been reported after acute overdose.
- **Supportive therapy:** Manage symptoms as needed for overdose. Tapering of steroids is not necessary for acute ingestion.
- **GI decontamination:** No specific recommendations.

ANTIDOTE/DIALYSIS

- **Antidote:** No specific recommendations.
- **Dialysis:** Budesonide is unlikely to be removed by hemodialysis, peritoneal dialysis, or high-permeability hemodialysis.

bumetanide

byoo-met'-a-nide

Classes

Chemical: sulfonamide derivative
Therapeutic: diuretic, loop

Pregnancy Category: C

Trade Names

Prescription: Bumex, Burinex ♣

CLINICAL PHARMACOLOGY

Mechanism of Action

A loop diuretic that enhances excretion of sodium, chloride, and, to lesser degree, potassium, by direct action at the ascending limb of the loop of Henle and in the proximal tubule. **Therapeutic Effect:** Produces diuresis.

PHARMACOKINETICS

Route	Onset	Peak	Duration
PO	30-60 min	60-120 min	4-6 hr
IV	Rapid	15-30 min	2-3 hr
IM	40 min	60-120 min	4-6 hr

Completely absorbed from the GI tract (absorption decreased in heart failure and nephrotic syndrome). Protein binding: 94%-96%. Partially metabolized in the liver. Primarily excreted in urine. Not removed by hemodialysis. **Half-life:** 1-1.5 hr.

AVAILABILITY

Tablets: 0.5 mg, 1 mg, 2 mg.
Injection: 0.25 mg/mL.

INDICATIONS AND DOSAGE

Edema

PO

Adults, Children older than 18 yr: 0.5-2 mg 1-2 times daily. **Elderly:** 0.5 mg/day, increased as needed.

IV, IM

Adults, Elderly: 0.5-2 mg/dose; may repeat in 2-3 hr; or 0.5-2 mg/hr by continuous IV infusion. Maximum: 10 mg/day.

Hypertension

PO

Adults, Elderly: Initially, 0.5 mg/day. Range: 1-4 mg/day. Maximum: 5 mg/day. Larger doses may be given 2-3 doses/day.

Usual pediatric dosage

PO, IV, IM

Children: 0.015-0.1 mg/kg/dose every 6-24 hr. Maximum: 10 mg/day.

OFF-LABEL USES

Treatment of hypercalcemia, hypertension

CONTRAINDICATIONS

Anuria, hepatic coma, severe electrolyte depletion, hypersensitivity to sulfonylureas, pregnancy

INTERACTIONS

Drug: Amphotericin B, nephrotoxic and ototoxic medications: May increase the risk of nephrotoxicity and ototoxicity. **Anticoagulants, heparin:** May decrease the effects of these drugs. **Lithium:** May increase the risk of lithium toxicity. **Other hypokalemia-causing medications:** May increase the risk of hypokalemia. **Herbal:** Avoid ephedra, yohimbe, ginseng, dong quai, garlic. **Food:** None known.

DIAGNOSTIC TEST EFFECTS

May increase blood glucose, BUN, serum uric acid, and urinary phosphate levels. May decrease serum calcium, chloride, magnesium, potassium, and sodium levels.

IV INCOMPATIBILITIES

Midazolam (Versed)

IV COMPATIBILITIES

Aztreonam (Azactam), cefepime (Maxipime), diltiazem (Cardizem), *DOBUTamine (Dobutrex), furosemide (Lasix), lorazepam (Ativan), milrinone (Primacor), morphine, piperacillin and tazobactam (Zosyn), propofol (Diprivan)

SIDE-EFFECTS

Expected: Increased urinary frequency and urine volume. **Frequent:** Orthostatic hypotension, dizziness, hyperuricemia (18%), hypochloremia (15%), hypokalemia (15%).

Occasional: Blurred vision, diarrhea, headache, anorexia, premature ejaculation, impotence, dyspepsia, increased serum creatinine (7%). **Rare:** Rash, urticaria, pruritus, asthenia, muscle cramps, nipple tenderness

CRITICAL CARE CONSIDERATIONS

ADMINISTRATION/HANDLING

PO ALERT

- Give bumetanide with food to avoid GI upset, preferably with breakfast to help prevent nocturia.

IV ALERT

- **Storage/stability:** Store vials at room temperature. The solution remains stable for 24 hr if diluted.
- **Dilution:** Compatible with D_5W, 0.9% NaCl, and lactated Ringer's solution.
- **Undiluted:** May also be given undiluted. Administer the drug by IV push over 1 to 2 min.
- **Continuous IV infusion:** Bumetanide may be given as a continuous infusion.

PRECAUTIONS

HEALTH-RELATED

- Use bumetanide cautiously in debilitated patients and patients with diabetes mellitus, and hepatic or renal impairment.

AGE-RELATED

- **Children:** Safety and efficacy of bumetanide have not been established in children under 18 yr.
- **Elderly:** Older patients are at increased risk for circulatory collapse or thromboembolic episodes; they may be more sensitive to bumetanide's hypotensive and electrolyte effects. Age-related renal impairment may require reduced dosage or an extended dosage interval in the elderly. Renal function should be monitored.

PREGNANCY/LACTATION-RELATED

- Pregnancy category C (D if used in pregnancy-induced hypertension); cardiovascular disorders such as pulmonary edema, severe hypertension, or heart failure are probably the only valid indications for loop diuretics during pregnancy; excretion into breast milk unknown.

MONITORING

- **Baseline assessment:** Evaluate hydration status before giving bumetanide by checking vital signs for hypotension, poor skin turgor, and edema because bumetanide may lower BP following diuresis.
- **Lab work:** Assess baseline electrolyte levels for hypokalemia and renal and liver function tests for impairment.
- **Ongoing monitoring:** BP, electrolyte levels, fluid intake and output, vital signs, and daily weight.
- **Diuresis:** Note the extent of diuresis following administration of bumetanide. Instruct patients to rise slowly from a sitting or lying position.
- **Hypokalemia:** Monitor for electrolyte disturbances. Hypokalemia may cause dysrhythmias, altered mental status, muscle cramps, asthenia, and tremor.
- **Hyponatremia:** May result in cold and clammy skin, confusion, and thirst.
- **Patient education:** Advise about increased frequency and volume of urination. Explain that hearing abnormalities may occur: sense of fullness or ringing in ears. Encourage consumption of high-potassium foods: apricots, bananas, orange juice, raisins, potatoes, legumes, meat, and whole grains/cereals.

SERIOUS ADVERSE REACTIONS

- **Complications of vigorous diuresis:** Profound water and electrolyte depletion resulting in muscle cramps, hypokalemia, hyponatremia, dehydration, coma, acute hypotension, and circulatory collapse.
- **Ototoxicity:** Deafness, vertigo, or tinnitus may occur, especially in patients with severe renal impairment and those taking other ototoxic drugs.
- **Hematologic:** Blood dyscrasias have been reported.

OVERDOSE/TOXICITY

- **Symptoms:** Abdominal pain, arthritic pain, azotemia, dizziness, ECG changes, elevated BUN and creatinine, dehydration, encephalopathy, headache, hyperglycemia, hyperuricemia, hypochloremia, hyponatremia, hypokalemia, hypotension, metabolic acidosis, thrombocytopenia, vascular thrombosis, and embolism.
- **Management:** Rehydrate patients with IV fluids, replace electrolytes, support BP with vasopressors if hypotension is severe, resuscitate per Advanced Cardiac Life Support (ACLS) guidelines.
- **GI decontamination:** No specific recommendations.

ANTIDOTE/DIALYSIS

- **Antidote:** No specific recommendations.
- **Dialysis:** Bumetanide is not removed by hemodialysis and is unlikely to be removed by peritoneal dialysis. No data are available on removal by high-permeability hemodialysis.

bupivacaine hydrochloride

byoo-piv'-a-caine hye-droe-klor'-ide

Classes
Chemical: amide derivative
Therapeutic: anesthetic, local

Pregnancy Category: C

Trade Names
Prescription: Marcaine, Marcaine Spinal, Sensorcaine, Sensorcaine-MPF

Combinations
Prescription: with epinephrine (Marcaine with Epinephrine, Sensorcaine with Epinephrine, Sensorcaine-MPF with Epinephrine)

CLINICAL PHARMACOLOGY

Mechanism of Action
An amide-type anesthetic that stabilizes neuronal membranes and prevents initiation and transmission of nerve impulses thereby effecting local anesthetic actions. **Therapeutic Effect:** Produces local analgesia.

PHARMACOKINETICS

Onset of action occurs within 4-10 min depending on route of administration. Duration is 2-9 hr. Protein binding: 95%. Metabolized in liver. Excreted in urine. **Half life:** 1.5-5.5 hr (adults), 8.1 hr (neonates).

AVAILABILITY

Injection: 0.25% (Marcaine, Sensorcaine-MPF), 0.5% (Marcaine, Sensorcaine-MPF), 0.75% (Marcaine, Marcaine Spinal, Sensorcaine-MPF).

INDICATIONS AND DOSAGE

Dose varies with procedure, depth of anesthesia, vascularity of tissues, duration of anesthesia and condition of patient.

Analgesic, epidural (partial, moderate, complete motor blockade)
IV
Adults, Elderly: 10-20 mL (25-50 mg) of a 0.25% solution. Repeat once every 3 hr as needed. **Children more than 10 kg:** 1-2.5 mg/kg single dose as a 0.125% or 0.25% solution or 0.2-0.4 mg/kg/hr continuous infusion as a 0.1%, 0.125%, or 0.25% solution. Maximum: 0.4 mg/kg/hr. **Children less than 10 kg:** 1-1.25 mg/kg single dose as a 0.125% or 0.25% solution or 0.1-0.2 mg/kg/hr continuous infusion as a 0.1%, 0.125%, or 0.25% solution. Maximum: 0.2 mg/kg/hr.

Analgesic, intrapleural
IV
Adults, Elderly: 10-30 mL bolus of 0.25%, 0.375%, or 0.5% every 4-8 hr or 0.375% solution with epinephrine continuous infusion at 6 mL/hr after 20 mL loading dose.

Analgesic, dental
IV
Adults, Elderly: 1.8-3.6 mL of 0.5% solution (9-18 mg) with epinephrine. A second dose of 9 mg may be administered. Maximum: 90 mg total dose.

Analgesic, peripheral nerve block (moderate to complete motor blockade)
IV
Adults, Elderly: 5-37.5 mL (25-175 mg) of 0.5% solution or 5-70 mL (12.5-175 mg) of 0.25% solution. Repeat every 3 hr as needed. Maximum: up to 400 mg/day. **Children 12 yr and older:** 0.3-2.5 mg/kg as a 0.25% or 0.5% solution. Maximum: 1 mL/kg of 0.25% solution or 0.5 mL/kg of 0.5% solution.

Analgesic, retrobulbar (complete motor blockade)
IV
Adults, Elderly: 2-4 mL (15-30 mg) of 0.75% solution.

Analgesic, sympathetic blockade
IV
Adults, Elderly: 20-50 mL (50-125 mg) of 0.25% (no epinephrine) solution. Repeat once every 3 hr as needed.

Analgesic, hyperbaric spinal (obstetrical, normal vaginal delivery)
IV
Adults, Elderly: 0.8 mL (6 mg) bupivacaine in dextrose as 0.75% solution

Analgesic, hyperbaric spinal (obstetrical, cesarean section)
IV
Adults, Elderly: 1-1.4 mL (7.5-10.5 mg) bupivacaine in dextrose as 0.75% solution.

Anesthesia, hyperbaric spinal (surgical, lower extremity and perineal procedures)
IV
Adults, Elderly: 1 mL (7.5 mg) bupivacaine in dextrose as 0.75% solution **Children 12 yr and older:** 0.3-0.6 mg/kg bupivacaine in dextrose as a 0.75% solution

Anesthesia, spinal (surgical, lower abdominal procedures)
IV
Adults, Elderly: 1.6 mL (12 mg) bupivacaine in dextrose as 0.75% solution. **Children 12 yr and older:** 0.3-0.6 mg/kg bupivacaine in dextrose as a 0.75% solution
Anesthesia, spinal (surgical, hyperbaric, upper abdominal procedures)
IV
Adults, Elderly: 2 mL (15 mg) bupivacaine in dextrose as a 0.75% solution administered in horizontal position. **Children 12 yr and older:** 0.3-0.6 mg/kg bupivacaine in dextrose as a 0.75% solution
Analgesic, local infiltration
IV
Adults, Elderly: 0.25% solution. Maximum: 225 mg with epinephrine or 175 mg without epinephrine. **Children 12 yr and older:** 0.5-2.5 mg/kg as a 0.25% or 0.5% solution. Maximum: 1 mL/kg of 0.25% solution or 0.5 mL/kg of 0.5% solution.

CONTRAINDICATIONS

Local infection at the site of proposed lumbar puncture (spinal anesthesia), obstetrical paracervical block anesthesia, septicemia (spinal anesthesia), severe hemorrhage, severe hypotension or shock, dysrhythmias such as complete heart block that severely restrict cardiac output (spinal anesthesia), sulfite allergy (epinephrine containing solutions only), hypersensitivity to bupivacaine products or to other amide-type anesthetics

INTERACTIONS

Drug: **Angiotensin converting enzyme inhibitors:** May increase risk of bradycardia and hypotension as well as loss of consciousness. **Beta-blockers, ergot-type oxytocics, MAOIs, TCAs, phenothiazines, vasopressors:** May increase the risk of bupivacaine toxicity. **Cisatracurium, rapacuronium:** May increase neuromuscular blocking action. **Hyaluronidase:** May increase incidence of systemic reaction to bupivacaine. **Propofol:** May increase hypnotic effect of propofol. **Ropivacaine:** May prolong effect of intrathecal bupivacaine. **Verapamil:** May increase risk of heart block. Herbal: **St. John's wort:** May increase risk of cardiovascular collapse and/or delay emergence from anesthesia. Food: None known.

DIAGNOSTIC TEST EFFECTS

None known.

IV INCOMPATIBILITIES

None known.

IV COMPATIBILITIES

Fentanyl, hydromorphone (Dilaudid), morphine

SIDE-EFFECTS

Occasional: Hypotension, bradycardia, palpitations, respiratory depression, dizziness, headache, vomiting, nausea, restlessness, weakness, blurred vision, tinnitus, apnea

CRITICAL CARE CONSIDERATIONS

ADMINISTRATION/HANDLING

DOSAGE ALERT

- *Contraindication:* Solutions containing preservatives should *not* be used for epidural or caudal blocks. Local anesthetic preparations of bupivacaine contain preservatives.
- **Variable dosage:** Dose varies with anesthetic procedure, area to be anesthetized, vascularity of the tissues, number of neuronal segments to be blocked, depth of anesthesia and degree of muscle relaxation required, duration of anesthesia desired, individual tolerance, and physical condition of the patient.
- **Highly concentrated solutions:** *0.75% solutions should not used for obstetrical epidural anesthesia; reports of cardiac arrest and death have occurred with this concentration.*
- **Epidural anesthesia:** Concentrated solutions (0.5%-0.75%) should be given in incremental doses of 3-5 mL with sufficient time between doses to detect toxic manifestations of unintentional intravascular or intrathecal injection during epidural administration. Aspirate epidural needle or catheter before injecting bupivacaine to avoid accidental intravascular injection.
- **Repeated doses:** May cause significant increases in blood levels with repeated doses due to accumulation of bupivacaine/its metabolites or slow metabolization.
- **Spinal analgesia:** Use bupivacaine in dextrose only for spinal analgesia.
- **Lowest effective dosage:** Lowest effective anesthesia dose should be used to avoid high plasma levels and serious systemic side effects.
- **Storage:** Store at room temperature. Protect from light.
- **Stability:** Bupivacaine 1.25 mg/mL in 0.9% NaCl injection is stable for up to 32 days when refrigerated.

B

PRECAUTIONS

HEALTH-RELATED

- **Local preparations:** Local anesthetic preparations of bupivacaine contain antimicrobial preservatives and should not be used for caudal or epidural anesthesia.
- **Obstetric epidural anesthesia:** Use epidural bupivacaine cautiously and only at concentrations less than 0.75% to avoid cardiac arrest. The 0.75% concentration should be reserved for surgical procedures where high degree muscle relaxation is available.
- **Regional IV anesthesia (Bier block):** Use cautiously with hyperthyroidism, hepatic disease, impaired cardiovascular function, hypertension, and heart block. Patients are at higher risk for bupivacaine toxicity.
- **Retrobulbar blocks:** Use cautiously; bupivacaine has caused respiratory arrest.
- **Spinal anesthesia:** Spinal bupivacaine should not be injected during uterine contractions.
- **Cardiac dysrhythmias:** Bupivacaine may cause severe disturbances of cardiac rhythm, shock, or heart block after spinal anesthesia. Cardiac dysrhythmias may occur if preparations containing a vasoconstrictor such as epinephrine are used in patients during or following the administration of chloroform, cyclopropane, halothane, trichloroethylene, or other related agents.
- **Vasoconstrictors:** Use solutions containing vasoconstrictors cautiously in areas with limited blood supply in cardiac or peripheral vascular disease patients. Solutions containing epinephrine or other vasopressors should not be used concomitantly with ergot-type oxytocic drugs.
- **MAOIs and tricyclic antidepressants:** Use with extreme caution because severe hypertension can occur.
- **Reduced doses:** Should be given to debilitated, elderly, acutely ill, and young patients.
- **Malignant hyperthermia:** It is unknown if bupivacaine is a triggering agent.

AGE-RELATED

- **Children:** Bupivacaine spinal with dextrose is not recommended in children under 12 yr.
- **Elderly:** May require dosage reduction.

PREGNANCY/LACTATION-RELATED

- Pregnancy category C; excretion into breast milk unknown; regional use may prolong labor and delivery; use cautiously during pregnancy other than labor.

MONITORING

- **Before injection:** Where applicable, aspiration for blood or cerebrospinal fluid should be done before injecting bupivacaine for both original dose and all following doses to avoid intravascular or subarachnoid injection.
- **Test dose:** Administer a test dose containing epinephrine when possible to detect unintended intravenous or intrathecal injection. Monitor patients for onset and regression of anesthesia.
- **Therapeutic effect:** Assess for pain relief and record the onset of relief. Monitor the level of anesthesia, which is not always controllable in spinal techniques.
- **Hypotension:** Monitor for change in BP for detection of hypotension and signs of CNS toxicity. Monitor for change in rate and quality of pulse and respiration.
- **Therapeutic and toxic drug levels:** Monitor serum bupivacaine levels during continuous infusions. Levels above 4 mcg/mL in adult patients and above 5.4 mcg/mL in pediatric patients have been associated with toxic effects.
- **Paracervical anesthesia:** Monitor fetal heart rate during paracervical anesthesia.
- **Patient education:** Bupivacaine may cause ringing in ears, excitation, restlessness, or drowsiness. Warn patients to report skin rash or hives immediately. Instruct dental procedure patients not to chew gum or food while mouth is numb from injection because injury can occur without knowing it.

SERIOUS ADVERSE REACTIONS

- **Allergic reactions:** Solutions with epinephrine contain metabisulfite, a sulfite that may cause allergic-type reactions, including anaphylaxis. Severe reactions may require treatments including endotracheal intubation, mechanical ventilation, IV fluid infusion, vasopressors, epinephrine, steroids, and *diphenhydrAMINE.
- **Methemoglobinemia:** Generalized cyanosis, tachycardia, dyspnea, headache with a normal SpO_2. Arterial blood gas samples appear dark or chocolate colored. Pulse oximetry is inaccurate with methemoglobinemia (methemoglobin fractions greater than 10%). Managed with infusion of methylene blue.
- **Hemolysis:** Results from methemoglobinemia. When methemoglobinemia resolves, hemolysis may not be immediately apparent. Circulation may be compromised from hemolyzed blood cells. If extensive,

multiorgan dysfunction syndrome may ensue up to 3 days after methemoglobinemia resolves.

OVERDOSE/TOXICITY

- **Symptoms:** Arterial hypotension, bradycardia, ventricular dysrhythmias, CNS depression and excitation, convulsions, respiratory arrest, tinnitus have been reported.
- **Management:** Check position of infusion device to ensure bupivacaine has not been injected into the vasculature. Discontinue medication and resuscitate according to Advanced Cardiac Life Support (ACLS) guidelines.
- **GI decontamination:** No specific recommendations.

ANTIDOTE/DIALYSIS

- **Antidote:** No specific recommendations. IV methylene blue infusion is used for methemoglobinemia, if present, unless the patient has G6PD deficiency.
- **Dialysis:** Bupivacaine is unlikely to be removed by hemodialysis, high-permeability hemodialysis, or peritoneal dialysis.

*buPROPion hydrochloride

byoo-proe'-pee-on hye-droe-klor'-ide

Classes

Chemical: aminoketone derivative
Therapeutic: antidepressant

Pregnancy Category: B

Trade Names

Prescription: Wellbutrin, Wellbutrin SR, Zyban

Do not confuse *buPROPion with *busPIRone, Wellbutrin with Wellcovorin or Wellferon, or Zyban with Zagam.

CLINICAL PHARMACOLOGY

Mechanism of Action

An aminoketone that blocks the reuptake of neurotransmitters, including serotonin and norepinephrine at CNS presynaptic membranes, increasing their availability at postsynaptic receptor sites. Also reduces the firing rate of noradrenergic neurons. **Therapeutic Effect:** Relieves depression and nicotine withdrawal symptoms.

PHARMACOKINETICS

Rapidly absorbed from the GI tract. Protein binding: 84%. Crosses the blood-brain barrier. Undergoes extensive first-pass metabolism in the liver to active metabolite. Primarily excreted in urine. **Half-life:** 21 hr.

AVAILABILITY

Tablets (Wellbutrin): 75 mg, 100 mg.
Tablets (extended release [Wellbutrin XL]): 150 mg, 300 mg.
Tablets (sustained release [Wellbutrin SR]): 100 mg, 150 mg, 200 mg.
Tablets (sustained release [Zyban SR, Zyban SR refill]): 150 mg.

INDICATIONS AND DOSAGE

Depression

PO (Immediate Release)

Adults: Initially, 100 mg twice per day. May increase to 100 mg 3 times per day no sooner than 3 days after beginning therapy. Maximum: 450 mg/day. **Elderly:** 37.5 mg twice per day. May increase by 37.5 mg every 3-4 days. Maintenance: Lowest effective dosage.

PO (Sustained Release)

Adults: Initially, 150 mg/day as a single dose in the morning. May increase to 150 mg twice per day as early as day 4 after beginning therapy. Maximum: 400 mg/day. **Elderly:** Initially, 100 mg/day. May increase by 100 mg/day every 3-4 days. Maintenance: Lowest effective dosage. Maximum: 400 mg/day.

PO (Extended Release)

Adults: 150 mg once per day. May increase to 300 mg once per day. Maximum: 450 mg per day.

Smoking cessation

PO

Adults: Initially, 150 mg per day for 3 days; then 150 mg twice per day for 7-12 wk.

Dosage in liver impairment

Mild-moderate: Use caution, reduce dosage.
Severe: Use extreme caution, maximum dose:

- **Wellbutrin:** 75 mg/day.
- **Wellbutrin SR:** 100 mg/day or 150 mg every other day.
- **Wellbutrin XL:** 150 mg every other day.
- **Zyban:** 150 mg every other day.

OFF-LABEL USES

Treatment of attention-deficit/hyperactivity disorder in adults and children

CONTRAINDICATIONS

Current or prior diagnosis of anorexia nervosa or bulimia, seizure disorder, use within 14 days of MAOIs, concomitant use of other bupropion products.

INTERACTIONS

Drug: **Alcohol, lithium, ritonavir, steroids, trazodone, tricyclic antidepressants:** May increase the risk of seizures. **Fosphenytoin, phenytoin, phenobarbital:** May decrease the effectiveness of bupropion. **Haloperidol:** May increase plasma levels of haloperidol. **Levodopa:** May increase the risk of adverse effects including nausea, vomiting, excitation, restlessness, and postural tremor. **MAOIs:** May increase the risk of neuroleptic malignant syndrome and acute bupropion toxicity. **Theophylline:** May increase theophylline levels. Herbal: **Valerian, St. John's wort, SAMe, gotu kola, kava kava:** May cause increased CNS depression. Food: None known.

DIAGNOSTIC TEST EFFECTS

May decrease serum WBC count.

SIDE-EFFECTS

Frequent (25%-11%): Dizziness (11%), nausea (18%), dry mouth (24%), headache (25%), insomnia (16%). Occasional (9%-5%): Agitation (9%), diarrhea (7%), hostility, fatigue, anxiety (6%)

CRITICAL CARE CONSIDERATIONS

ADMINISTRATION/HANDLING

INTERACTION ALERT

- Make sure at least 14 days elapse between the use of MAOIs and *buPROPion.

PO ALERT

- Increase *buPROPion dosage gradually to minimize agitation, insomnia, and motor restlessness.
- Give *buPROPion with food to reduce GI irritation.
- Do not crush sustained-release tablets.
- Avoid bedtime administration to decrease risk of insomnia.
- **Evenly spaced doses:** Space doses 4 hr apart for immediate-onset tablets and 8 hr apart for sustained-release and extended-release tablets to avoid seizures.
- **Side effects:** Sustained-release *buPROPion causes fewer side effects than other forms of the drug.
- **Wellbutrin and Zyban:** To avoid overdose, patients undergoing smoking cessation should not use both medications because both contain *buPROPion.

PRECAUTIONS

HEALTH-RELATED

- Patients are at higher risk of increased seizures who have history of head trauma, prior seizures, CNS tumor, presence of severe hepatic cirrhosis, impaired renal function, and concomitant use of other medications which lower seizure threshold (antispsychotics, antidepressants, theophylline, systemic steroids).

AGE-RELATED

- **Children:** Safety and efficacy of *buPROPion have not been established in children.
- **Elderly:** More sensitive to the anticholinergic, cardiovascular, and sedative effects and may require a dosage adjustment for age-related renal impairment.

PREGNANCY/LACTATION-RELATED

- Pregnancy category B; excretion into breast milk unknown.

MONITORING

- **Baseline assessment:** Observe and record appearance, behavior, level of interest, mood, and sleep pattern. Assess for past history of seizures because patients on larger doses are at increased risk for seizures.
- **Baseline lab work:** Obtain blood chemistry studies before and periodically during long-term therapy to assess hepatic and renal function.
- **Suicide potential:** Closely supervise suicidal patients during early therapy. As depression lessens, energy level generally improves, increasing suicide potential.
- **Therapeutic effect:** Assess appearance, behavior, level of interest, mood, and sleep pattern to determine the drug's therapeutic effect. *BuPROPion's full therapeutic effect may take 4 wk to appear.
- **Dry mouth:** Suggest taking sips of tepid water or chewing sugarless gum to relieve dry mouth.
- **Patient education:** When using *buPROPion outside the hospital, warn patients to avoid tasks that require mental alertness or motor skills until response to the drug is known.

SERIOUS ADVERSE REACTIONS

- **Seizures:** The risk of seizures increases in patients taking more than 150 mg/dose of *buPROPion, in patients with a history of bulimia or seizure disorders, and in patients discontinuing drugs that may lower the seizure threshold.

OVERDOSE/TOXICITY

- **Low therapeutic index:** Toxicity can occur at or slightly below the maximal therapeutic dose of 450 mg per day.
- **Adult overdoses:** Overdoses of less than 450 mg are not associated with significant toxicity.
- **Symptoms:** Seizures, sinus tachycardia, possible QT prolongation, lethargy, tremors, confusion, vomiting, possible BP increases or decreases, possible fever. Seizures usually occur within the first 1-4 hr following ingestion of regular release *buPROPion.
- **Management:** Start IV for management of seizures, continuous cardiac monitoring for dysrhythmias. Supportive care alone is sufficient for most overdoses. Most seizures are short-lived and resolve without specific treatment. Phenytoin has effectively managed seizures.
- **Sustained release overdose:** Consult the poison control center or a medical toxicologist for treatment of overdose of sustained release preparations.
- **GI decontamination:** Oral activated charcoal is used for large overdoses and is generally effective if given within 1 hr of ingestion.

ANTIDOTE/DIALYSIS

- **Antidote:** No specific recommendations.
- **Dialysis:** *BuPROPrion is not removed by hemodialysis or peritoneal dialysis. No data are available on removal by high-permeability hemodialysis.

*busPIRone hydrochloride

byoo-spye'-rone hye-droe-klor'-ide

Classes

Chemical: azaspirodecanedione
Therapeutic: anxiolytic

Pregnancy Category: B

Trade Names

Prescription: BuSpar, BuSpar Dividose, Bustab ♣

Do not confuse busPIRone with *buPROPion.

CLINICAL PHARMACOLOGY

Mechanism of Action

Although its exact mechanism of action is unknown, this nonbarbiturate is thought to bind to serotonin and dopamine receptors in the CNS. The drug may also increase norepinephrine metabolism in the locus ceruleus. **Therapeutic Effect:** Produces anxiolytic effect.

PHARMACOKINETICS

Rapidly and completely absorbed from the GI tract. Protein binding: 95%. Undergoes extensive first-pass metabolism. Metabolized in the liver to active metabolite. Primarily excreted in urine. Not removed by hemodialysis. **Half-life:** 2-3 hr.

AVAILABILITY

Tablets: 5 mg (BuSpar), 7.5 mg, 10 mg (BuSpar), 15 mg (BuSpar, BuSpar Dividose), 30 mg (BuSpar Dividose).

INDICATIONS AND DOSAGE

Short-term management (up to 4 wk) of anxiety disorders

PO

Adults: 5 mg 2-3 times per day or 7.5 mg twice per day. May increase by 5 mg/day every 2-4 days. Maintenance: 15-30 mg/day in 2-3 divided doses. Maximum: 60 mg/day. **Elderly:** Initially 5 mg twice per day. May increase by 5 mg/day every 2-3 days. Maximum: 60 mg/day. **Children:** Initially 5 mg/day. May increase by 5 mg/day at weekly intervals. Maximum: 60 mg/day.

OFF-LABEL USES

Augmenting medication for antidepressants; management of aggression in mental retardation and secondary mental disorders, major depression, panic attack; premenstrual syndrome (aches, pain, fatigue, irritability).

CONTRAINDICATIONS

Concurrent use of MAOIs, severe hepatic or renal impairment

INTERACTIONS

Drug: Alcohol, other CNS depressants: Potentiates effects of *busPIRone and may increase sedation. **Diltiazem, verapamil, ketoconazole, ritonavir, nefazodone, erythromycin, itraconazole:** May increase *busPIRone blood concentration and risk of toxicity. **MAOIs:** May increase BP. **Rifampin:** May decrease blood level of *busPIRone. **Herbal: Ginkgo biloba, St. John's wort:** May cause changes in mental status. **Valerian, gotu kola, kava kava:** May increase sedation. **Food: Grapefruit, grapefruit juice:** May increase *busPIRone blood concentration and risk of toxicity.

DIAGNOSTIC TEST EFFECTS

None known.

SIDE-EFFECTS

Frequent (12%-6%): Dizziness, somnolence, nausea, headache. **Occasional (5%-2%):** Nervousness, fatigue, insomnia, dry mouth, lightheadedness, mood swings, blurred vision, poor concentration, diarrhea, paresthesia **Rare:** Muscle pain and stiffness, nightmares, chest pain, involuntary movements

CRITICAL CARE CONSIDERATIONS

ADMINISTRATION/HANDLING

PO ALERT

- Give *busPIRone without regard to food.
- ***Do not administer with grapefruit juice,*** which may increase risk of drug toxicity.
- Crush tablets as needed.

PRECAUTIONS

HEALTH-RELATED

- Use *busPIRone cautiously in patients with hepatic or renal impairment.
- **Withdrawal:** Withdraw patients gradually from other sedative, hypnotic, anxiolytic drugs before initiating *busPIRone to avoid withdrawal. *BusPIRone will not block the withdrawal syndrome.
- **Cytochrome P4503A4 metabolism:** Health care providers should be aware *busPIRone is metabolized through the cytochrome P4503A4 pathway; effect of *busPIRone can be altered significantly if patients are receiving another medication which increases or decreases metabolism via this pathway.

AGE-RELATED

- **Children:** Safety and efficacy of *busPIRone have not been established in children.
- **Elderly:** No age-related precautions have been noted in the elderly.

PREGNANCY/LACTATION-RELATED

- Pregnancy category B; excretion into breast milk unknown; use caution in nursing mothers.

MONITORING

- **Baseline assessment:** Assess for autonomic responses, such as cold, clammy hands and diaphoresis; and motor responses such as agitation, trembling, and tension.
- **Lab work:** Perform blood tests periodically to assess hepatic and renal function in patients on long-term therapy.
- **Inhibitors and inducers of cytochrome P450 3A4:** Use of *busPIRone with the following medications may increase the blood level of *busPIRone: diltiazem, verapamil, erythromycin, itraconazole, ketoconazole, ritonavir, nefazodone. May decrease the blood level of *busPIRone: rifampin.
- **Safety risk:** Assist patients with ambulation if drowsiness or lightheadedness occurs. Offer emotional support to anxious patients.
- **Therapeutic response:** Evaluate for a calm facial expression and decreased restlessness and insomnia. Improvement is seen within 7-10 days of starting therapy; optimum therapeutic effect generally takes 3-4 wk.
- **Patient education:** Drowsiness usually disappears with continued therapy. For dizziness, instruct patients to change positions slowly from recumbent to sitting before standing. When using *busPIRone outside the hospital, advise avoiding tasks that require mental alertness and motor skills until response to the drug is known. Caution patients not to take *busPIRone with grapefruit juice as this may increase the risk of drug toxicity.

SERIOUS ADVERSE REACTIONS

- **Symptoms:** Syncope, hypotension, hypertension, epistaxis, stupor, psychosis, photophobia, muscle weakness, muscle spasms.
- **Tolerance/dependence:** *BusPIRone does not appear to cause drug tolerance, psychological or physical dependence, or withdrawal syndrome, nor does it prevent withdrawal syndrome from other CNS depressant drugs.

OVERDOSE/TOXICITY

- **Symptoms:** Severe nausea, vomiting, dizziness, drowsiness, abdominal distention, and excessive pupil contraction.
- **GI decontamination:** Activated charcoal may be effective if given within 1 hr of ingestion.

- **Supportive care:** Management of overdose should be based on symptoms.

ANTIDOTE/DIALYSIS
- **Antidote:** No specific recommendations.
- **Dialysis:** *BusPIRone is not removed by hemodialysis. No data are available on removal using peritoneal dialysis or high-permeability hemodialysis.

butorphanol tartrate 

byoo-tor'-fa-nole tar'-trate

DEA Schedule: IV

Classes
Chemical: opiate derivative
Therapeutic: narcotic agonist-antagonist analgesic

Pregnancy Category: C, D

Trade Names
Prescription: Apo-Butorphanol ♣, Stadol, Stadol NS

Do not confuse butorphanol with butabarbital or Stadol with Haldol.

CLINICAL PHARMACOLOGY
Mechanism of Action
An opioid that binds to opiate receptor sites in the CNS. Reduces intensity of pain stimuli incoming from sensory nerve endings. Therapeutic Effect: Alters pain perception and emotional response to pain.

PHARMACOKINETICS

Route	Onset	Peak	Duration
IM	5-10 min	30-60 min	3-4 hr
IV	Less than 1 min	4-5 min	3-4 hr
Nasal	15 min	1-2 hr	4-5 hr

Rapidly absorbed after IM injection. Protein binding: 80%. Extensively metabolized in the liver. Primarily excreted in urine. Half-life: 2.5-4 hr.

AVAILABILITY
Injection (Stadol): 1 mg/mL, 2 mg/mL.
Nasal spray (Stadol NS): 10 mg/mL.

INDICATIONS AND DOSAGE
Analgesia
IV
Adults: 2 mg every 3-4 hr as needed. **Elderly:** 1 mg every 6 hr as needed. Dose should be half of recommended dose for adults.
IM
Adults: 1-4 mg every 3-4 hr as needed. **Elderly:** 1 mg every 6 hr as needed. Dose should be half of recommended dose for adults.
Migraine
Nasal
Adults: 1 mg or 1 spray in one nostril. May repeat in 60-90 min. May repeat 2-dose sequence every 3-4 hr as needed. Alternatively, 2 mg or 1 spray each nostril if patient remains recumbent, may repeat in 3-4 hr.

CONTRAINDICATIONS
CNS disease that affects respirations, hypersensitivity to the preservative benzethonium chloride, physical dependence on other opioid analgesics, preexisting respiratory depression, pulmonary disease, pregnancy

INTERACTIONS
Drug: **Alcohol, CNS depressants:** May increase CNS or respiratory depression and hypotension. **Buprenorphine:** Effects may be decreased with buprenorphine. **MAOIs:** May produce severe, fatal reaction unless dose is reduced by one-fourth. Herbal: **Valerian, St. John's wort, kava kava, gotu kola:** May increase CNS depressant effects. Food: None known.

DIAGNOSTIC TEST EFFECTS
None known.

IV INCOMPATIBILITIES
Amphotericin B complex (Abelcet, AmBisome, Amphotec)

IV COMPATIBILITIES
Atropine, *diphenhydrAMINE (Benadryl), droperidol (Inapsine), *hydrOXYzine (Vistaril), morphine, promethazine (Phenergan), propofol (Diprivan)

SIDE-EFFECTS
Frequent: **Parenteral:** Somnolence (43%), dizziness (19%). **Nasal:** Nasal congestion (13%), insomnia (11%) Occasional: **Parenteral (3%-9%):** Confusion, diaphoresis, clammy skin, lethargy, headache, nausea, vomiting, dry mouth. **Nasal (3%-9%):** Vasodilation, constipation, unpleasant taste, dyspnea, epistaxis, nasal irritation, upper respiratory tract infection, tinnitus. Rare: **Parenteral:** Hypotension, pruritus, blurred vision, sensation of heat, CNS stimulation, insomnia. **Nasal:** Hypertension, tremor, ear pain, paresthesia, depression, sinusitis

CRITICAL CARE CONSIDERATIONS

ADMINISTRATION/HANDLING

IM AND IV ALERT

- Butorphanol may be given by IM or IV push.

INTRANASAL ALERT

- **Administration:** Blow nose to clear nasal passages as much as possible. Spray into the nostril while holding the other nostril closed, and concurrently inspire through nose to permit medication as high into nasal passages as possible.

IV ALERT

- Store butorphanol at room temperature.
- May be given undiluted.
- Give over 3 to 5 min.

PRECAUTIONS

HEALTH-RELATED

- Butorphanol should not be used in narcotic-dependent patients to avoid severe pain due to antagonist properties.
- Use cautiously in patients with head injury, hypertension, impaired liver or renal function, MI, ventricular dysfunction, ischemic heart disease (may increase cardiac workload), and before biliary tract surgery (produces spasm of sphincter of Oddi).

AGE-RELATED

- **Children:** Safety and efficacy of butorphanol have not been established in children under 18 yr.
- **Elderly:** May be more sensitive to effects. Adjust drug dose and interval in the elderly. Use cautiously in patients who are debilitated or elderly. Mean half-life may be extended by 25%.

PREGNANCY/LACTATION-RELATED

- Pregnancy category C, D if used for prolonged time, high dose at term; excreted in breast milk.

MONITORING

- **Baseline assessment:** Obtain vital signs before giving butorphanol.
- **Lab work:** Biochemical profile including renal (BUN, creatinine) and liver function (AST [SGOT], ALT [SGPT], alkaline phosphatase, bilirubin) tests.
- **Respirations:** Withhold butorphanol and notify the physician if respirations are 12/min in adults or less or 20/min or less in children.
- **Pain:** Assess duration, location, onset, and type of pain experienced. The effect of butorphanol is reduced if full pain is experienced before the next dose. Instruct patients to alert provider to the onset of pain and not to wait until the pain is unbearable. Butorphanol is more effective when given at the onset of pain.
- **Patient safety:** Protect from falls, fainting, and respiratory depression.
- **Vital signs:** Monitor for hypotension, pulse rate and quality, and respirations.
- **Therapeutic effect:** Assess for clinical improvement; record the onset of pain relief.
- **Patient education:** Instruct patients to change positions slowly to avoid dizziness. Teach proper use of nasal spray. If butorphanol is to be taken outside of the hospital, warn patients to avoid tasks that require mental alertness or motor skills until response to the drug is known. Urge avoiding alcohol or CNS depressants to avoid somnolence, dizziness, and fainting. Initiate deep-breathing and coughing exercises, particularly in patients with impaired pulmonary function. Help change positions slowly every 2 to 4 hr.

SERIOUS ADVERSE REACTIONS

- **Abrupt withdrawal:** Sudden withdrawal of butorphanol after prolonged use may produce symptoms of narcotic withdrawal, such as abdominal cramping, rhinorrhea, lacrimation, anxiety, increased temperature, and piloerection or goose bumps.
- **Tolerance/dependence:** Tolerance to analgesic effect and physical dependence may occur with chronic use of butorphanol.

OVERDOSE/TOXICITY

- **Symptoms:** Severe respiratory depression, skeletal muscle flaccidity, cyanosis, hypotension, and extreme somnolence progressing to seizures, stupor, and coma.
- **Discontinue drug:** For progressively worsening symptoms, discontinue the drug and discuss alternatives with other health care providers.
- **Manage respiratory distress:** Patients may require endotracheal intubation and mechanical ventilation for prolonged respiratory depression. Ensure airway protection if obtunded, but do not induce vomiting if oral or nasal airway is inserted. Bag-valve-mask ventilation is appropriate

while deciding if endotracheal intubation is necessary.

- **Manage seizures:** Conventional management with benzodiazepines (lorazepam, diazepam) and/or barbiturates (phenobarbital) is generally effective. If seizures are refractory to initial treatment, higher doses of barbiturates or use of midazolam and propofol may be effective. Phenytoin is not as effective as other agents in toxic-induced seizures.
- **Manage responses:** Hypotension and bradycardia are commonly seen when using barbiturates or propofol to manage seizures.
- **GI decontamination:** No specific recommendations.

ANTIDOTE/DIALYSIS

- **Antidote:** Naloxone (Narcan) 2 mg IV (0.01 mg/kg for children) will relieve respiratory depression. Patients may require several doses because action of butorphanol exceeds that of naloxone.
- **Dialysis:** Generally not used to manage butorphanol overdose.

calcitonin

kal-si-toe'-nin

Classes

Chemical: polypeptide hormone

Therapeutic: antidote, hypercalcemia, anti-osteoporotic

Pregnancy Category: C

Trade Names

Prescription: Calcimar, Caltine ♣, Cibacalcin, Fortical, Miacalcin, Miacalcin Nasal

Do not confuse calcitonin with calcitriol.

CLINICAL PHARMACOLOGY

Mechanism of Action

A synthetic hormone that decreases osteoclast activity in bones, decreases tubular reabsorption of sodium and calcium in the kidneys, and increases absorption of calcium in the GI tract. **Therapeutic Effect:** Regulates serum calcium concentrations.

PHARMACOKINETICS

Injection form rapidly metabolized (primarily in kidneys); primarily excreted in urine. Nasal form rapidly absorbed. **Half-life:** 70-90 min (injection); 43 min (nasal).

AVAILABILITY

Injection (Miacalcin): 200 units/mL (calcitonin-salmon), 500 mg (calcitonin-human).
Nasal spray (Fortical, Miacalcin Nasal): 200 units/activation (calcitonin-salmon).

INDICATIONS AND DOSAGE

Skin testing before treatment in patients with suspected sensitivity to calcitonin-salmon

Intracutaneous

Adults, Elderly: Prepare a 10 units/mL dilution; withdraw 0.05 mL from a 200 units/mL vial in a tuberculin syringe; fill up to 1 mL with 0.9% NaCl. Take 0.1 mL and inject intracutaneously on inner aspect of forearm. Observe after 15 min; a positive response is the appearance of more than mild erythema or wheal.

Paget's disease

IM, Subcutaneous

Adults, Elderly: Initially, 100 units/day. Maintenance: 50 units/day or 50-100 units every 1-3 days.

Intranasal

Adults, Elderly: 200 units/day.

Osteoporosis imperfecta

IM, Subcutaneous

Adults: 2 units/kg 3 times per wk; given with an oral calcium supplement (230-345 mg/day).

Postmenopausal osteoporosis

IM, Subcutaneous

Adults, Elderly: 100 units every other day with adequate calcium and vitamin D intake.

Intranasal

Adults, Elderly: 200 units/day as a single spray, alternating nostrils daily.

Hypercalcemia

IM, Subcutaneous

Adults, Elderly: Initially, 4 units/kg every 12 hr; may increase to 8 units/kg every 12 hr if no response in 2 days; may further increase to 8 units/kg every 6 hr if no response in another 2 days.

OFF-LABEL USES

Treatment of secondary osteoporosis due to drug therapy or hormone disturbance

CONTRAINDICATIONS

Hypersensitivity to gelatin desserts, salmon protein, or synthetic calcitonin

INTERACTIONS

Drug: None known. **Herbal:** None known.
Food: None known.

DIAGNOSTIC TEST EFFECTS

None known.

SIDE-EFFECTS

Frequent: **IM, subcutaneous (10%):** Nausea (may occur 30 min after injection, usually diminishes with continued therapy), inflammation at injection site. **Nasal (12%-10%):** Rhinitis, nasal irritation, redness, sores. **Occasional:** **IM, subcutaneous (5%-2%):** Flushing of face or hands. **Nasal (5%-3%):** Back pain, arthralgia, epistaxis, headache. **Rare:** **IM, subcutaneous:** Epigastric discomfort, dry mouth, diarrhea, flatulence. **Nasal:** Itching of earlobes, pedal edema, rash, diaphoresis

CRITICAL CARE CONSIDERATIONS

ADMINISTRATION/HANDLING

IM, SUBCUTANEOUS ALERT

- Calcitonin may be administered subcutaneously or IM.

- No more than 2 mL should be given IM at any one site.
- Bedtime administration may reduce flushing and nausea.

INTRANASAL ALERT

- **Storage:** Refrigerate nasal spray. It may be stored at room temperature once the pump has been activated.
- **Administration:** Clear nasal passages as much as possible. Tilt the head slightly forward and insert the spray tip into the nostril, pointing toward the nasal passages and away from the septum. Spray into the nostril while holding the other nostril closed, and at the same time inhale through the nose to deliver the drug as high into the nasal passage as possible.

PRECAUTIONS

HEALTH-RELATED

- Use calcitonin cautiously in patients with a history of allergy or renal dysfunction.

AGE-RELATED

- **Children:** Safety and efficacy of calcitonin have not been established in children.
- **Elderly:** No age-related precautions have been noted.

PREGNANCY/LACTATION-RELATED

- Pregnancy category C; inhibits lactation in animals.

MONITORING

- **Baseline assessment:** Assess for symptoms of hypercalcemia and possible causes of hypercalcemia. Ask about allergy to salmon.
- **Baseline lab work:** Calcium and magnesium levels, electrolyte levels; arterial blood gas analysis to check for acidosis. Perform a skin test before beginning calcitonin therapy if patients may have sensitivity to calcitonin.
- **Diagnostic tests:** Perform tests for diseases causing hypercalcemia such as malignancy, acromegaly, thyroid/parathyroid/adrenal disease, kidney and liver disease in patients without prolonged immobility.
- **Drugs that increase calcium:** If patients are hypercalcemic, medications that may have helped to increase calcium include anabolic steroids, androgens, antacids, calcium supplements, chlorthalidone, diuretics, estrogens, indomethacin, lithium carbonate, theophylline, thyroid hormones, vitamins A and D.
- **IM injection:** Rotate sites and check them for inflammation.
- **ECG monitoring:** Hypercalcemia may prolong PR interval leading to heart block, shortened ST segment and QT interval; ventricular dysrhythmias can occur with severe hypercalcemia, leading to cardiac arrest.
- **Hypercalemia:** Symptoms are usually absent until calcium greater than 11 mg/dL. Symptoms include lethargy, weakness, anorexia, nausea, vomiting, polyuria, itching, bone pain, renal calculi, constipation, depression, confusion, paresthesias, personality changes, stupor, coma.
- **Therapeutic effect:** Assess calcium, phosphate, and magnesium levels if used for acute management of hypercalcemia; calcium should decrease in 2 days. If patients are acidotic, pH may require correction with bicarbonate rather than using calcitonin to reduce calcium. Improvement in biochemical abnormalities and symptoms should coincide with resolution of hypercalcemia. Bone pain improves in the first few months of treatment; in patients with neurologic lesions, improvement may take more than 1 yr.
- **Allergic reaction:** Assess for allergic reaction such as rash, urticaria, dyspnea, swelling, hypotension, and tachycardia.
- **Side effects:** Monitor for nausea/vomiting; nausea usually decreases with continued therapy.
- **Patient education:** If using calcitonin outside the hospital, teach patients and families how to administer the drug. Stress the need to use aseptic technique and rotate injection sites. Warn patients to notify the physician immediately of itching, rash, shortness of breath, or significant nasal irritation.

SERIOUS ADVERSE REACTIONS

- Patients with protein allergy may develop a hypersensitivity reaction.

OVERDOSE/TOXICITY

- **Symptoms:** Patients will likely be hypocalcemic with symptoms such as numbness, tingling, tetany, anxiety, depression, psychosis, spasms, muscle contraction, positive Chvostek's and Trousseau's sign, prolonged QT interval, and ST segment elevation; can lead to cardiac arrest.
- **Management:** Correct hypocalcemia while monitoring magnesium levels. If patients

had hypomagnesemia, hypocalciumia may be refractory to calcium therapy unless magnesium replacement is also initiated.
- **GI decontamination:** No specific recommendations.

ANTIDOTE/DIALYSIS
- **Antidote:** Calcium supplementation to manage hypocalcemia with 10% calcium gluconate or 10% calcium chloride slow IV push or by infusion. Calcium chloride contains more calcium than does calcium gluconate and requires careful infusion into a central IV line. Serum calcium is protein bound. Ionized calcium should be used as a guide to manage calcium levels if patients have low albumin levels.
- **Dialysis:** Calcitonin is unlikely to be removed by hemodialysis, high-permeability hemodialysis, or peritoneal dialysis.

calcium salts

kal'-see-um

Classes
Chemical: divalent cation
Therapeutic: antacid, antiosteoporotic, phosphate adsorbent (acetate)

Pregnancy Category: C

Trade Names
Prescription: Calcium acetate: PhosLo
Over the Counter: Calcium carbonate: Amitone, Cal-Carb Forte, Calci-Chew, Calci-Mix, Caltrate, Caltrate 600, Chooz, Dicarbosil, Florical, Maalox, Mallamint, Mylanta, Nephro-Calci, Os-Cal 500, Oysco 500, Oyst-Cal 500, Oyster Calcium, Quick Dissolve, Rolaids, Titralac, Tums, Tums Ex
Over the Counter: Calcium citrate: Citracal, Citracal Prenatal Rx, Cal-Citrate
Prescription: Calcium glubionate: Calcione, Calciquid
Over the Counter: Tricalcium phosphate: Posture

Combinations
Prescription: with cholecalciferol (Os-Cal-D)
Over the Counter: with sodium fluoride (Caltrate, Florical)

Do not confuse OsCal with Asacol, Citracal with Citrucel, or PhosLo with PhosChol.

CLINICAL PHARMACOLOGY
Mechanism of Action
An electrolyte that is essential for the function and integrity of the nervous, muscular, and skeletal systems. Calcium plays an important role in normal cardiac and renal function, respiration, blood coagulation, and cell membrane and capillary permeability. It helps regulate the release and storage of neurotransmitters and hormones, and it neutralizes or reduces gastric acid (increase pH). Calcium acetate combines with dietary phosphate to form insoluble calcium phosphate. **Therapeutic Effect:** Replaces calcium in deficiency states; controls hyperphosphatemia in end-stage renal disease.

PHARMACOKINETICS
Moderately absorbed from the small intestine (absorption depends on presence of vitamin D metabolites and pH). Primarily eliminated in feces.

AVAILABILITY
Calcium Acetate
Gelcap (Phoslo): 667 mg (equivalent to 169 mg elemental calcium).
Tablet (Phoslo): 667 mg (equivalent to 169 mg elemental calcium).
Calcium Carbonate
Tablets: equivalent to 500 mg elemental calcium (Os-Cal 500), equivalent to 600 mg elemental calcium (Caltrate 600).
Tablets (chewable): equivalent to 200 mg elemental calcium (Tums), equivalent to 500 mg elemental calcium (Os-Cal 500), 600 mg (Maalox Quick Dissolve), 750 mg (Smoothles).
Calcium Chloride
Injection: 10% (100 mg/mL) equivalent to 27.2 mg elemental calcium per mL.
Calcium Citrate
Tablets: 125 mg (Citracal Prenatal Rx), 250 mg (equivalent to 53 mg elemental calcium) (Cal-Citrate), 950 mg (equivalent to 200 mg elemental calcium) (Citracal).
Calcium Glubionate
Syrup: 1.8 g/5 mL (equivalent to 115 mg of elemental calcium per 5 mL).
Calcium Gluconate
Injection: 10% (equivalent to 9 mg elemental calcium per mL).

INDICATIONS AND DOSAGE
Hyperphosphatemia
PO (calcium acetate)
Adults, Elderly: 2-4 tablets 3 times per day with meals. May increase gradually to bring serum phosphate level to less than

6 mg/dL as long as hypercalcemia does not develop.

Hypocalcemia

PO (calcium carbonate)

Adults, Elderly: 1-2 g/day in 3-4 divided doses. **Children:** 45-65 mg/kg/day in 3-4 divided doses.

PO (calcium glubionate)

Adults, Elderly: 6-18 g/day in 4-6 divided doses. **Children, Infants:** 0.6-2 g/kg/day in 4 divided doses. **Neonates:** 1.2 g/kg/day in 4-6 divided doses.

IV (calcium chloride)

Adults, Elderly: 0.5-1 g repeated every 4-6 hr as needed. **Children:** 2.5-5 mg/kg/dose every 4-6 hr.

IV (calcium gluconate)

Adults, Elderly: 2-15 g/24 hr. **Children:** 200-500 mg/kg/day.

Antacid

PO (calcium carbonate)

Adults, Elderly: 1-2 tabs (5-10 mL) every 2 hr as needed.

Osteoporosis

PO (calcium carbonate)

Adults, Elderly: 1200 mg/day.

Cardiac arrest

IV (calcium chloride)

Adults, Elderly: 2-4 mg/kg. May repeat every 10 min. **Children:** 20 mg/kg. May repeat in 10 min.

Hypocalcemia tetany

IV (calcium chloride)

Adults, Elderly: 1 g may repeat in 6 hr. **Children:** 10 mg/kg over 5-10 min. May repeat in 6-8 hr.

IV (calcium gluconate)

Adults, Elderly: 1-3 g until therapeutic response achieved. **Children:** 100-200 mg/kg/dose every 6-8 hr.

Supplement

PO (calcium citrate)

Adults, Elderly: 0.5-2 g 2-4 times per day.

OFF-LABEL USES

Treatment of hyperphosphatemia (calcium carbonate)

CONTRAINDICATIONS

Calcium carbonate: Renal calculi, digoxin toxicity, hypercalcemia, hypercalciuria, sarcoidosis, ventricular fibrillation

Calcium acetate: Hypercalcemia, hypoparathyroidism

INTERACTIONS

Drug: Digoxin: May increase the risk of dysrhythmias. **Etidronate, gallium:** May antagonize the effects of these drugs. **Ketoconazole, phenytoin, tetracyclines:** May decrease the absorption of these drugs. **Magnesium (parenteral), methenamine:** May decrease the effects of these drugs. **Herbal:** None known. **Food:** None known.

DIAGNOSTIC TEST EFFECTS

May increase blood pH and serum gastrin and calcium levels. May decrease serum phosphate and potassium levels.

IV INCOMPATIBILITIES

Calcium chloride: amphotericin B complex (Abelcet, Ambisome, Amphotec), propofol (Diprivan), sodium bicarbonate **Calcium gluconate:** amphotericin B complex (Abelcet, Ambisome, Amphotec), fluconazole (Diflucan)

IV COMPATIBILITIES

Calcium chloride: Amikacin (Amikin), *DOBUTamine (Dobutrex), lidocaine, milrinone (Primacor), morphine, norepinephrine (Levophed) **Calcium gluconate:** Ampicillin, aztreonam (Azactam), cefazolin (Ancef), cefepime (Maxipime), ciprofloxacin (Cipro), *DOBUTamine (Dobutrex), enalapril (Vasotec), famotidine (Pepcid), furosemide (Lasix), heparin, lidocaine, magnesium sulfate, meropenem (Merrem IV), midazolam (Versed), milrinone (Primacor), norepinephrine (Levophed), piperacillin and tazobactam (Zosyn), potassium chloride, propofol (Diprivan)

SIDE-EFFECTS

Frequent: PO: Chalky taste. **Parenteral:** Hypotension; flushing; feeling of warmth; nausea; vomiting; pain, rash, redness, or burning at injection site; diaphoresis. **Occasional: PO:** Mild constipation, fecal impaction, peripheral edema, metabolic alkalosis (muscle pain, restlessness, slow breathing, altered taste). **Calcium carbonate:** Milk-alkali syndrome (headache, decreased appetite, nausea, vomiting, unusual tiredness). **Rare:** Difficult or painful urination

CRITICAL CARE CONSIDERATIONS

ADMINISTRATION/HANDLING

PO ALERT

- Give tablets with a full glass of water 30 min to 1 hr after meals.
- Chew chewable tablets well before swallowing.

- Dilute syrup in juice or water and administer before meals to increase absorption.
- Patients with end-stage renal disease may develop hypercalcemia when given with meals.

IV ALERT

- **Storage:** Store vials at room temperature.
- **Calcium chloride:** Calcium chloride may be given undiluted or may be diluted with an equal amount 0.9% NaCl or sterile water for injection into a central IV line. Give calcium chloride by slow IV push (0.5 to 1 mL/min). Rapid administration may produce bradycardia, hypotension, peripheral vasodilation, a chalky or metallic taste, and a feeling of warmth.
- **Calcium gluconate:** Calcium gluconate may be given undiluted or may be diluted in up to 1000 mL 0.9% NaCl. Give calcium gluconate by IV push at a rate of 0.5 to 1 mL/min; the maximum rate is 200 mg/min. Rapid administration may produce dysrhythmias, hypotension, MI, and vasodilation.

PRECAUTIONS

HEALTH-RELATED

- Use calcium cautiously in patients with chronic renal impairment, decreased cardiac function, dehydration, history of renal calculi, or ventricular fibrillation during cardiac resuscitation.
- Patients with progressive hypercalcemia due to overdose of calcium acetate may have severe symptoms requiring emergency management.

AGE-RELATED

- **Children:** Restrict IV use in children; small vasculature increases the risk of developing extreme vein irritation and possible tissue necrosis or sloughing.
- **Elderly:** Oral absorption may be decreased. Elderly with vascular disease are at risk of developing irritation of veins with possible tissue necrosis or sloughing.

PREGNANCY/LACTATION-RELATED

- Pregnancy category C; some oral supplemental calcium may be excreted in breast milk (chloride, gluconate, unknown); concentrations not sufficient to produce an adverse effect in neonates.

MONITORING

- **Baseline assessment:** Assess for hypocalcemia, monitor vital signs with attention to BP, which may increase with calcium administration.
- **Baseline lab work:** Biochemical profile including serum magnesium, potassium, phosphate levels; and renal function test results. Ionized calcium should be used as a guide to manage calcium levels if patients have low albumin levels. Serum calcium level should be monitored twice weekly during early therapy with calcium acetate.
- **Baseline diagnostic tests:** 12-lead ECG to evaluate for myocardial ischemia.
- **Hypocalcemia:** Symptoms include numbness, tingling, tetany, anxiety, depression, psychosis, spasms, muscle contraction, positive Chvostek's and Trousseau's sign, prolonged QT interval, and ST segment elevation; can lead to cardiac arrest.
- **ECG:** Monitor for changes in QT interval and ST segment. Hypocalcemia causes prolonged QT interval because ST segment is elevated and prolonged. ***Digitalis toxicity is potentiated by hypercalcemia.***
- **Renal failure patients:** Should provide phosphorous binding antacids before reducing elevated phosphorous before treating hypocalcemia.
- **Ongoing assessment:** Monitor BP, ECG, and serum magnesium, phosphate, and potassium levels, urine calcium concentrations, as well as renal function test results. Monitor resolution of hypocalcemia and for development of hypercalcemia. If patients had hypomagnesemia, hypocalcemia may be refractory to calcium therapy unless magnesium replacement is also initiated.
- **Hypercalemia:** Usually absent until calcium is greater than 11 mg/dL. Symptoms include lethargy, weakness, anorexia, nausea, vomiting, polyuria, itching, bone pain, renal calculi, constipation, depression, confusion, paresthesias, personality changes, stupor, coma.
- **Patient education:** Instruct patients to take tablets with a full glass of water 30 min to 1 hr after meals, not to take calcium within 2 hr of consuming other oral drugs or fiber-containing foods, and to drink liquids before meals. Emphasize the importance of diet if receiving calcium as an antacid or a supplement. Patients should be aware of the need for adequate amounts of vitamin D and be made aware of food sources of calcium. Urge patients to avoid consuming excessive amounts of alcohol, caffeine, and tobacco.

SERIOUS ADVERSE REACTIONS

- **Hypercalcemia:** A serious adverse effect of all calcium salts, particularly calcium acetate use. Symptoms are not usually apparent until calcium level greater than 11 mg/dL. Early signs include constipation, headache, dry mouth, increased thirst, irritability, decreased appetite, metallic taste, fatigue, weakness, and depression. Chronic hypercalcemia may result in vascular calcification. The serum calcium times phosphate (CaXP) product should not be allowed to exceed 66.

OVERDOSE/TOXICITY

- **Hypercalcemia symptoms:** Later signs include confusion, somnolence, hypertension, photosensitivity, dysrhythmias, nausea, vomiting, and increased painful urination. Hypercalcemia may prolong PR interval leading to heart block, shortened ST segment and QT interval; ventricular dysrhythmias can occur with severe hypercalcemia, leading to cardiac arrest. Radiographic evaluation is used to evaluate areas of possible soft tissue calcification.
- **GI decontamination:** No specific recommendations.

ANTIDOTE/DIALYSIS

- **Antidote:** Acute hypercalcemia is managed with rapid administration of IV normal saline to increase urinary calcium excretion. Concomitant administration of furosemide prevents development of fluid volume excess. Administration of sodium bicarbonate may help lower calcium level by creating mild alkalosis, but administration must be done carefully. IV calcitonin may be used but generally takes 1-2 days for action.
- **Dialysis:** Renal failure patients are at higher risk of hypercalcemia because of altered elimination of body chemicals including phosphates, calcium, and magnesium. Calcium may be lowered by using dialysate low in calcium during hemodialysis.

calfactant

cal-fac'-tant

Classes

Chemical: phospholipid
Therapeutic: lung surfactant, natural bovine

Pregnancy Category: X

Trade Names

Prescription: Infasurf

CLINICAL PHARMACOLOGY

Mechanism of Action

A natural lung extract that reduces alveolar surface tension, stabilizing the alveoli. **Therapeutic Effect:** Restores surface activity to infant lungs, improves lung compliance and respiratory gas exchange.

PHARMACOKINETICS

No studies have been performed.

AVAILABILITY

Intratracheal suspension: 35-mg/mL vials.

INDICATIONS AND DOSAGE

Respiratory distress syndrome (RDS)

Intratracheal

Neonates: 3 mL/kg of birth weight administered as soon as possible after birth in 2 doses of 1.5 mL/kg. Repeat 3-mL/kg doses, up to a total of 3 doses given 12 hr apart.

CONTRAINDICATIONS

Known hypersensitivity to calfactant.

INTERACTIONS

Drug: None known. **Herbal:** None known. **Food:** None known.

DIAGNOSTIC TEST EFFECTS

None known.

SIDE-EFFECTS

Frequent: Cyanosis (65%), airway obstruction (39%), bradycardia (34%), reflux of surfactant into endotracheal tube (21%), need for manual ventilation (16%). **Occasional:** Need for reintubation (3%)

CRITICAL CARE CONSIDERATIONS

ADMINISTRATION/HANDLING

INTRATRACHEAL ALERT

- **Storage:** Refrigerate vials. Unopened, unused vials may be returned to the refrigerator only once after having been warmed to room temperature.
- **Preparation:** Gently swirl the vial to redisperse contents. Do not shake. Enter

each single-use vial only once; discard unused suspension.

- **Instillation:** Instill the drug intratracheally through a side port adapter into the infant's endotracheal tube. Give each aliquot over 20-30 ventilatory breaths. Administer only during the inspiratory cycle.
- **Positioning:** Between aliquot dosages, turn infants so that the opposite lung is in the dependent position.

PRECAUTIONS

HEALTH-RELATED

- Use calfactant cautiously in patients who are not endotracheally intubated.

AGE-RELATED

- Calfactant is for use only in neonates. No age-related precautions have been noted.

PREGNANCY/LACTATION-RELATED

- Pregnancy category X; this drug is not indicated for use in pregnant women but poses minimal risk in pregnant women.

MONITORING

- **Skilled clinicians:** Calfactant should be administered by critical care clinicians experienced with intubation and ventilator management for the neonate.
- **Transcutaneous:** Monitor oxygenation and ventilation using arterial or transcutaneous measurement of systemic oxygen (O_2) and carbon dioxide (CO_2). Oxygen level should increase and carbon dioxide level should decrease as respiratory failure resolves.
- **Respiratory:** Auscultate breath sounds for crackles and rhonchi. Breath sounds should improve as medication is administered over time.
- **Family education:** Tell parents the purpose of the treatment and the expected outcome. Explain why visitors are limited during treatment. Teach hand washing and other infection control measures to minimize the risk of nosocomial infections.

SERIOUS ADVERSE REACTIONS

- **Respiratory:** Cyanosis, airway obstruction, respiratory distress or failure.
- **Cardiac:** Bradycardia.

OVERDOSE/TOXICITY

- No specific recommendations.

ANTIDOTE/DIALYSIS

- **Antidote:** No specific recommendations.
- **Dialysis:** No data are available on removal of calfactant by hemodialysis, high-permeability hemodialysis, or peritoneal dialysis.

candesartan cilexetil

See Angiotensin II Receptor Antagonists (p. 889)

captopril

cap'-toe-pril

Classes

Chemical: angiotensin-converting enzyme (ACE) inhibitor, sulfhydryl

Therapeutic: antihypertensive

Pregnancy Category: C (1st trimester) D (2nd, 3rd trimesters)

Trade Names

Prescription: Capoten

Combinations

Prescription: with hydrochlorothiazide (Capozide)

Do not confuse captopril with Capitrol.

CLINICAL PHARMACOLOGY

Mechanism of Action

An angiotensin-converting enzyme (ACE) inhibitor that suppresses the renin-angiotensin-aldosterone system and prevents conversion of angiotensin I to angiotensin II, a potent vasoconstrictor; may also inhibit angiotensin II at local vascular and renal sites. Decreases plasma angiotensin II, increases plasma renin activity, and decreases aldosterone secretion. **Therapeutic Effect:** Reduces peripheral arterial resistance, pulmonary capillary wedge pressure; improves cardiac output and exercise tolerance.

PHARMACOKINETICS

Route	Onset	Peak	Duration
PO	0.25 hr	1-1.5 hr	Dose-related

Rapidly well absorbed from the GI tract (absorption is decreased in the presence of food). Protein binding: 25%-30%. Metabolized in the liver. Primarily excreted in urine. Removed by hemodialysis. **Half-life:** less than 3 hr (increased in those with impaired renal function).

AVAILABILITY

Tablets: 12.5 mg, 25 mg, 50 mg, 100 mg.

C

INDICATIONS AND DOSAGE

Hypertension

PO

Adults, Elderly: Initially, 12.5-25 mg 2-3 times per day. After 1-2 wk, may increase to 50 mg 2-3 times per day. Diuretic may be added if no response in additional 1-2 wk. If taken in combination with diuretic, may increase to 100-150 mg 2-3 times per day after 1-2 wk. Maintenance: 25-150 mg 2-3 times per day. Maximum: 450 mg/day.

Heart failure

PO

Adults, Elderly: Initially, 6.25-25 mg 3 times per day. Maintenance: increase to 12.5-25 mg 3 times per day. After at least 2 wk, may increase to 50-100 mg 3 times per day. Maximum: 450 mg/day.

Post–myocardial infarction, impaired liver function

PO

Adults, Elderly: 6.25 mg per day, then 12.5 mg 3 times per day. Increase to 25 mg 3 times per day for several weeks. Maintenance: goal is 50 mg given 3 times per day.

Diabetic nephropathy prevention of kidney failure

PO

Adults, Elderly: 25 mg 3 times per day. **Children:** Initially 0.3-0.5 mg/kg/dose titrated up to a maximum of 6 mg/kg/day in 2-4 divided doses. **Neonates:** Initially, 0.05-0.1 mg/kg/dose every 8-24 hr titrated up to 0.5 mg/kg/dose given every 6-24 hr.

Dosage in renal impairment

Creatinine clearance 10-50 mL/min: 75% of normal dosage.

Creatinine clearance less than 10 mL/min: 50% of normal dosage.

OFF-LABEL USES

Diagnosis of anatomic renal artery stenosis, hypertensive crisis, rheumatoid arthritis

CONTRAINDICATIONS

History of angioedema from previous treatment with ACE inhibitors, hypersensitivity to captopril, bilateral renal artery stenosis.

INTERACTIONS

Drug: Alcohol, antihypertensives, diuretics: May increase the effects of captopril. **Lithium:** May increase lithium blood concentration and risk of lithium toxicity. **NSAIDs:** May decrease the effects of captopril. **Potassium-sparing diuretics, potassium supplements:** May cause hyperkalemia. **Herbal: Ephedra, yohimbe, ginseng:** May decrease effects of captopril. **Garlic:** May cause hypotension. **Food: All food:** Food significantly reduces drug absorption by 30%-40%.

DIAGNOSTIC TEST EFFECTS

May increase BUN, serum alkaline phosphatase, serum bilirubin, serum creatinine, serum potassium, AST (SGOT), and ALT (SGPT) levels. May decrease serum sodium levels. May cause positive antinuclear antibody titer.

SIDE-EFFECTS

Frequent (7%-4%): Rash. **Occasional (4%-2%):** Pruritus, dysgeusia (altered taste). **Rare (less than 2%-0.5%):** Headache, cough, insomnia, dizziness, fatigue, paraesthesia, malaise, nausea, diarrhea or constipation, dry mouth, tachycardia, angioedema, anaphylactoid reactions

CRITICAL CARE CONSIDERATIONS

ADMINISTRATION/HANDLING

PO ALERT

- Give captopril 1 hr before meals for maximum absorption because food significantly decreases drug absorption.
- May crush tablets if necessary.

PRECAUTIONS

HEALTH-RELATED

- Use captopril cautiously in patients with cerebrovascular or coronary insufficiency, hypovolemia, renal impairment, and sodium depletion, as this increases probability of hypotension.
- Use cautiously in patients on dialysis and in those receiving diuretics because hypovolemia increases the probability of hypotension.

AGE-RELATED

- **Children:** Safety and efficacy of captopril have not been established in children.
- **Elderly:** May be more sensitive to the hypotensive effects of captopril. Use cautiously in elderly patients.

PREGNANCY/LACTATION-RELATED

- Pregnancy category C (first trimester) and D (second and third trimesters—fetal and neonatal hypotension, neonatal skull hypoplasia, anuria, reversible or irreversible renal failure, death, oligohydramnios); excreted into breast milk in small amounts; compatible with breast-feeding.

MONITORING

- **Baseline assessment:** Assess baseline heart rate and BP immediately before each captopril dose. Determine whether diuretics or medications for heart failure or angina (e.g., nitrates, other vasodilators) were being taken or if patient is pregnant or has liver or kidney disease. All are at higher risk of developing hypotension.
- **Baseline lab work:** CBC and blood chemistry including liver enzymes. Test the first urine of the day for protein by dipstick method before beginning captopril therapy.
- **Proteinuria:** Monitor for proteinuria periodically thereafter in patients with prior renal disease and in those receiving captopril dosages greater than 150 mg/day.
- **Infection:** Monitor CBC and blood chemistry every 2 wk for the next 3 mo and periodically thereafter in patients with autoimmune disease or renal impairment, and in those who are taking drugs that affect immune response or leukocyte count.
- **Renal insufficiency:** Monitor CBC, BUN, serum creatinine, and serum potassium levels in patients receiving a diuretic.
- **Liver failure:** Monitor liver enzymes (AST [SGOT], ALT [SGPT], alkaline phosphotase, bilirubin) periodically. If enzymes are elevated, discontinue captopril.
- **Hypotension and tachycardia:** Monitor for increased heart rate and decreased BP regularly throughout therapy. If an excessive reduction in BP occurs, place patients in the supine position with feet slightly elevated and administer IV normal saline rapid infusion to increase BP. Patients undergoing general anesthesia are at higher risk of hypotension.
- **Hydration:** Offer fluids frequently or administer IV fluids to maintain hydration. Hypotension is common in volume depleted patients.
- **Cough:** Many develop a cough while taking ACE inhibitors, which resolves when the medication is discontinued. If cough is severe, consider discontinuation of captopril.
- **Angioedema or allergic reaction:** Examine the skin for swelling of the face, lips, tongue, pruritus, rash, respiratory distress, or any sign of adverse reaction to medication; patients receiving ACE inhibitors are more likely to have these reactions because of the drug's impact inflammatory mediators.
- **Patient education:** For patients using captopril outside the hospital, explain that the full therapeutic effect of captopril may not occur for several weeks, that noncompliance with drug therapy or skipping captopril doses may cause severe, rebound hypertension and not to consume alcohol while taking captopril.

SERIOUS ADVERSE REACTIONS

- **Excessive hypotension (first-dose syncope):** May occur in patients with heart failure and in those who are severely sodium and volume depleted.
- **Angioedema:** Rarely occurs but is more common with all ACE inhibitors. Discontinue captopril and consider other medications to manage hypertension.
- **Hyperkalemia:** Rare occurrence seen more commonly with renal-insufficient patients, those with diabetes mellitus, those using potassium-sparing diuretics, potassium supplements, or salt substitutes.
- **Hyponatremia:** Seen in patients on a low sodium diet or receiving diuretics.
- **Agranulocytosis and neutropenia:** Sometimes seen in those with collagen vascular disease, including scleroderma and systemic lupus erythematosus, and impaired renal function.
- **Anaphylaxis:** ACE inhibitors affect the metabolism of eicosanoids and polypeptides which may prompt serious allergic reactions.

OVERDOSE/TOXICITY

- **Hypotension:** Should be managed with rapid IV infusion of normal saline solution to correct volume depletion created by vasodilation. Tachycardia is compensatory for hypotension and will resolve when BP is increased. Other measures for management of hypotension include vasopressors (e.g., *DOPamine, norepinephrine) if BP does not respond to volume infusion.
- **Nephrotic syndrome:** May be noted in those with history of renal disease.
- **Liver failure:** Rare complication that starts with cholestatic jaundice and progresses to fulminant hepatic necrosis and sometimes death.
- **Other complications:** Should be managed according to current accepted

standards, including Advanced Cardiac Life Support (ACLS) guidelines.
- **GI decontamination:** No specific recommendations.

C

ANTIDOTE/DIALYSIS
- **Antidote:** No specific recommendations.
- **Dialysis:** Captopril is removed by hemodialyis and is likely to be removed by high-permeability (high-flux) hemodialysis. No data are available on removal by peritoneal dialysis. Hypersensitivity type reactions have been noted in patients undergoing hemodialysis using high-flux dialysis membranes (e.g., AN69) when receiving captopril and other ACE inhibitors. Consideration should be given to using another type dialysis membrane for patients on ACE inhibitors.

carbamazepine

kar-ba-maz'-e-peen

Classes
Chemical: iminostilbene derivative
Therapeutic: anticonvulsant, antimanic, antineuralgic, antipsychotic

Pregnancy Category: D

Trade Names
Prescription: Apo-Carbamazepine ♣, Atretol, Carbatrol, Epitol, Tegretol, Tegretol-XR

Do not confuse Tegretol with Cartrol, Topamax, Toprol XL, Toradol, or Trental.

CLINICAL PHARMACOLOGY
Mechanism of Action
An iminostilbene derivative that decreases sodium and calcium ion influx into neuronal membranes, reducing posttetanic potentiation at synapses. **Therapeutic Effect:** Reduces seizure activity.

PHARMACOKINETICS
Slowly and completely absorbed from the GI tract. Protein binding: 75%. Metabolized in the liver to active metabolite. Primarily excreted in urine. Not removed by hemodialysis. **Half-life:** 25-65 hr (decreased with chronic use).

AVAILABILITY
Capsules (extended release): 100 mg (Carbatrol, Equetro), 200 mg (Carbatrol, Equetro), 300 mg (Carbatrol, Equetro), 400 mg (Carbatrol).
Suspension (Tegretol): 100 mg/5 mL.
Tablets (Epitol, Tegretol): 200 mg.
Tablets (chewable [Tegretol]): 100 mg.
Tablets (extended release [Tegretol XR]): 100 mg, 200 mg, 400 mg.

INDICATIONS AND DOSAGE
Seizure control
PO
Adults, Children older than 12 yr: Oral suspension: 100 mg given 4 times per day. **Adults, Children older than 12 yr:** Initially, 200 mg twice per day. May increase dosage by 200 mg/day at weekly intervals. Range: 400-1200 mg/day in 2-4 divided doses. Maximum: 1.6-2.4 g/day. **Children 6-12 yr:** Initially, 100 mg twice per day. May increase by 100 mg/day at weekly intervals. Range: 400-800 mg/day. Maximum: 1000 mg/day. Oral suspension: 50 mg given 4 times/day. **Children younger than 6 yr:** Initially 5 mg/kg/day. May increase at weekly intervals to 10-20 mg/kg/day. Maximum: 35 mg/kg/day. Oral suspension given 4 times/day. **Elderly:** Initially 100 mg 1-2 times per day. May increase by 100 mg/day at weekly intervals. Usual dose 400-1000 mg/day.

Trigeminal neuralgia, diabetic neuropathy
PO
Adults: Initially, 100 mg twice per day. May increase by 100 mg twice per day up to 400-800 mg/day. Maximum: 1200 mg/day. **Elderly:** Initially 100 mg 1-2 times per day. May increase by 100 mg/day at weekly intervals. Usual dose 400-1000 mg/day.

Bipolar disorder
PO (Equetro)
Adults, Elderly: Initially, 400 mg/day in 2 divided doses. May adjust dose in 200 mg increments. Maximum: 1600 mg/day in divided doses.

OFF-LABEL USES
Treatment of alcohol withdrawal, diabetes insipidus, neurogenic pain, psychotic disorders

CONTRAINDICATIONS
Concomitant use of MAOIs, history of myelosuppression, hypersensitivity to carbemazepine or tricyclic antidepressants, MAOIs should be discontinued for a minimum of 14 days before administration of carbamazepine, pregnancy

INTERACTIONS
Drug: Anticoagulants, clarithromycin, diltiazem, erythromycin, estrogens, propoxyphene, quinidine, steroids: May decrease the effects of these drugs.

Antipsychotics, haloperidol, tricyclic antidepressants: May increase CNS depressant effects. **Cimetidine:** May increase carbamazepine blood concentration and risk of toxicity. **Isoniazid:** May increase metabolism of isoniazid; may increase carbamazepine blood concentration and risk of toxicity. **MAOIs:** May cause seizures and hypertensive crisis. **Other anticonvulsants, barbiturates, benzodiazepines, valproic acid:** May increase the metabolism of these drugs. **Verapamil:** May increase the toxicity of carbamazepine. **Herbal: Evening primrose:** Decreases seizure threshold. **Valerian, St. John's wort, kava kava, gotu kola:** Increase CNS depression. **Food: Grapefruit, grapefruit juice:** May increase the absorption and blood concentration of carbamazepine.

DIAGNOSTIC TEST EFFECTS

May increase BUN and blood glucose levels and serum alkaline phosphatase, bilirubin, AST (SGOT), ALT (SGPT), protein, cholesterol, HDL, and triglyceride levels. May decrease serum calcium and thyroid hormone (T_3, T_4, T_4 index) levels. Therapeutic serum level is 4-12 mcg/mL; toxic serum level is greater than 12 mcg/mL.

SIDE-EFFECTS

Frequent: Drowsiness, dizziness, nausea, vomiting, somnolence, headache. **Occasional:** Visual abnormalities (spots before eyes, difficulty focusing, blurred vision), dry mouth or pharynx, tongue irritation, headache, fluid retention, diaphoresis, constipation or diarrhea, behavioral changes in children

CRITICAL CARE CONSIDERATIONS

ADMINISTRATION/HANDLING

DOSAGE ALERT

- **Changing anticonvulsants:** If patients must change to another anticonvulsant, plan to decrease the carbamazepine dose gradually as therapy begins with a low dose of the replacement drug.
- **Changing drug forms:** When transferring from tablets to suspension, divide the total daily tablet dose into smaller, more frequent doses of suspension (4 times per day). Administer extended-release tablets in 2 divided doses.
- **Altered levels:** Carbamazepine effects the enzymes involved in the cytochrome P450 (CYP3A4) pathway which help to metabolize numerous medications. Numerous medications may either increase or decrease carbamazepine levels.

PO ALERT

- Give carbamazepine with meals to reduce the risk of GI distress.
- Do not administer carbamazepine with grapefruit juice because it may increase the drug's concentration in the blood.
- Shake the oral suspension well. Do not administer simultaneously with any other liquid medicine.
- Do not crush extended-release tablets.
- **Storage:** Store tablets, capsules, and oral suspension at room temperature.

PRECAUTIONS

HEALTH-RELATED

- Use cautiously in patients with impaired cardiac, hepatic, or renal function.

AGE-RELATED

- **Children:** Children are more likely than adults to develop behavioral changes.
- **Elderly:** Are more susceptible to agitation, AV block, bradycardia, confusion, and syndrome of inappropriate antidiuretic hormone secretion.

PREGNANCY/LACTATION-RELATED

- Pregnancy category D; concentration in milk approximately 60% of maternal plasma concentration; compatible with breast-feeding.

MONITORING

- **Baseline assessment:** Before starting therapy, assess the LOC and review the history of the seizure disorder, including the duration, frequency, and intensity of seizures. Screen for use of MAOIs and cyclic antidepressants. Screen for prior bone marrow disease or bone marrow depression.
- **Baseline lab work:** BUN, creatinine, CBC, serum iron determination, and urinalysis before therapy.
- **Ongoing lab work:** Monitor for therapeutic serum levels of carbamazepine. BUN, creatinine, CBC, serum iron determination, and urinalysis periodically during therapy. Inform patients that blood tests will be repeated frequently during the first 3 mo of therapy and monthly thereafter for 2 to 3 yr.
- **Blood levels:** Therapeutic level: 4-12 mcg/mL; toxic level: greater than 12 mcg/mL.
- **Seizure precautions:** Have airway management equipment at the bedside. Do

not force anything into the mouth when patients are seizing. Provide a quiet, dark environment and institute safety precautions. Observe seizure patients frequently for recurrence of seizure activity.

- **Therapeutic effect:** Assess seizure patients for evidence of clinical improvement, such as a decrease in the frequency and intensity of seizures.
- **Toxicity:** Assess for early signs of toxicity, such as ecchymosis, fever, joint pain, mouth ulcerations, sore throat, and unusual bleeding from any site.
- **Neuralgia patients:** Avoid anything that could trigger tic douloureux, such as cold or hot foods or liquids and jarring the bed.
- **Patient education:** When carbamazepine will be used outside the hospital, instruct patients not to take the oral suspension of carbamazepine simultaneously with other liquid medicines or with grapefruit juice. Caution against abruptly discontinuing carbamazepine after long-term use because this may precipitate seizures. Strict maintenance of drug therapy is essential for seizure control.
- **Side effects:** Dizziness and unsteadiness are common. Drowsiness usually disappears with continued therapy. Caution patients to avoid tasks that require mental alertness or motor skills until response to the drug is known. Instruct patients to notify the health care provider of visual disturbances.
- **Medic alert bracelet:** Advise patients to always carry an identification card or wear an identification bracelet that displays their seizure disorder and anticonvulsant therapy.

SERIOUS ADVERSE REACTIONS

- **Status epilepticus:** Abrupt withdrawal may precipitate status epilepticus.
- **Blood dyscrasias:** Aplastic anemia, agranulocytosis, thrombocytopenia, leukopenia, leukocytosis, and eosinophilia.
- **Cardiovascular:** Heart failure, hypotension or hypertension, thrombophlebitis, and dysrhythmias.
- **Dermatologic:** Rash, urticaria, pruritus, Stevens–Johnson syndrome, toxic epidermal necrolysis, and photosensitivity.
- **Anticonvulsant hypersensitivity syndrome:** Potentially fatal hypersensitivity reaction that occurs rarely with carbamazepine, phenytoin, and phenobarbital

OVERDOSE/TOXICITY

- **Hepatotoxicity:** Elevated liver enzymes, hepatitis, cholestatic and hepatocellular jaundice, rarely liver failure.
- **Overdose:** Encephalopathy, coma, respiratory failure, seizures, tachycardia, cardiac conduction disturbance (prolonged QRS complex), and hypotension.
- **GI decontamination:** No specific recommendations, but if patients are seen within the first 3 hr of overdose, activated charcoal and gastric lavage are both recommended as part of treatment.
- **Supportive care:** Endotracheal intubation, mechanical ventilation, fluid volume resuscitation done carefully to avoid development of pulmonary edema, possible use of hypertonic sodium bicarbonate therapy, intravenous vasopressor infusions, and seizure control with benzodiazepines and barbiturates.

ANTIDOTE/DIALYSIS

- **Antidote:** No specific recommendations.
- **Dialysis:** Carbamazepine is not removed by hemodialysis or peritoneal dialysis. No data are available on removal by high-permeability hemodialysis. Charcoal hemoperfusion may be attempted to help improve drug clearance.

carbenicillin

See Antibiotics (p. 892)

carbidopa; levodopa

kar-bi-doe'-pa; lee-voe-doe'-pa

Classes

Chemical: catecholamine precursor
Therapeutic: anti-Parkinson's agent, antidyskinetic

Pregnancy Category: C

Trade Names

Prescription: Apo-Levotard ♣, Atamet, Parcopa, Sinemet, Sinemet CR

Do not confuse Atamet with Aldomet or Sinemet with Sinequan.

CLINICAL PHARMACOLOGY

Mechanism of Action

Levodopa is converted to dopamine in the basal ganglia thus increasing dopamine concentration in the brain and inhibiting hyperactive cholinergic activity. Carbidopa prevents peripheral breakdown of levodopa, allowing more levodopa to be available for transport into the brain. **Therapeutic Effect:** Reduces tremor.

PHARMACOKINETICS

Carbidopa is rapidly and completely absorbed from the GI tract. Widely distributed. Excreted primarily in urine. Levodopa is converted to dopamine. Excreted primarily in urine. **Half-life:** 1-2 hr (carbidopa); 1-3 hr (levodopa).

AVAILABILITY

Tablets (Atamet, Sinemet): 10 mg carbidopa/100 mg levodopa, 25 mg carbidopa/100 mg levodopa, 25 mg carbidopa/250 mg levodopa.
Tablets (oral disintegrating [Parcopa]): 10 mg carbidopa/100 mg levodopa, 25 mg carbidopa/100 mg levodopa, 25 mg carbidopa/250 mg levodopa.
Tablets (extended release [Sinemet CR]): 25 mg carbidopa/100 mg levodopa, 50 mg carbidopa/200 mg levodopa.

INDICATIONS AND DOSAGE

Parkinsonism

PO

Adults: Initially, 25/100 mg 3 times per day. May increase by 1 tablet every other day to a maximum of 200/2000 mg daily.
Elderly: Initially 25/100 mg twice per day. May increase as necessary.
When converting a patient from Sinemet to Sinemet CR (50 mg/200 mg), dosage is based on the total daily dose of levodopa, as follows:

Sinemet	Sinemet CR
300-400 mg	1 tablet twice per day
500-600 mg	1.5 tablet twice per day or 1 tablet 3 times per day
700-800 mg	4 tablets in 3 or more divided doses
900-1000 mg	5 tablets in 3 or more divided doses

Intervals between doses of Sinemet CR should be 4-8 hr while awake.

CONTRAINDICATIONS

Angle-closure or narrow angle glaucoma, use within 14 days of MAOIs (MAO type B may be used), skin lesions (Sinemet CR), history of melanoma (Sinemet CR), known hypersensitivity to any component of the drug

INTERACTIONS

Drug: Anticonvulsants, benzodiazepines, haloperidol, phenothiazines: May decrease the effects of carbidopa and levodopa. **MAOIs:** May increase the risk of hypertensive crisis. **Selegiline:** May increase levodopa-induced dyskinesias, nausea, orthostatic hypotension, confusion, and hallucinations.
Herbal: Kava kava: May decrease effects of carbidopa and levodopa. **Food:** Avoid high protein diets and high intake of vitamin B_6.

DIAGNOSTIC TEST EFFECTS

May increase BUN level and serum LDH, alkaline phosphatase, bilirubin, AST (SGOT), and ALT (SGPT) levels.

SIDE-EFFECTS

Frequent (90%-10%): Uncontrolled movements of face, tongue, arms, or upper body; nausea and vomiting (80%); anorexia (50%).
Occasional: Depression, anxiety, confusion, nervousness, urine retention, palpitations, dizziness, lightheadedness, decreased appetite, blurred vision, constipation, dry mouth, flushed skin, headache, insomnia, diarrhea, unusual fatigue, darkening of urine and sweat. **Rare:** Hypertension, ulcer, hemolytic anemia (marked by fatigue)

CRITICAL CARE CONSIDERATIONS

ADMINISTRATION/HANDLING

DOSAGE ALERT

- Plan to discontinue levodopa at least 12 hr before giving carbidopa and levodopa. Expect the initial dose to provide at least 25% of the previous levodopa dose.
- Instruct patients to void before giving carbidopa and levodopa to reduce the risk of urine retention.

PO ALERT

- Carbidopa and levodopa may be given without regard to food, but if nausea occurs, take drug with food.
- Scored tablets may be crushed as needed. Extended-release tablets may be cut in half but not crushed.

PRECAUTIONS

HEALTH-RELATED

- Use carbidopa and levodopa cautiously in patients with active peptic ulcer; severe cardiac, endocrine, hepatic, pulmonary, or renal impairment; treated open-angle glaucoma; or a history of MI, bronchial asthma (because of tartrazine sensitivity), or emphysema.

AGE-RELATED

- **Children:** Safety and efficacy of carbidopa and levodopa have not been established in children under 18 yr.

C

- **Elderly:** More sensitive to the effects of levodopa. Elderly patients receiving anticholinergics are at increased risk for adverse CNS effects, such as anxiety, confusion, and nervousness.

PREGNANCY/LACTATION-RELATED

- Pregnancy category C; should not be given to nursing mothers.

MONITORING

- **Baseline assessment:** Assess mental status including affect, mood, and evidence of CNS depression, before and at regular intervals throughout drug therapy.
- **Baseline lab work:** Biochemical profile including renal (BUN, creatinine) and liver (AST [SGOT], ALT [SGPT], alkaline phosphatase, bilirubin) function tests; CBC with differential.
- **Side effects:** Note dyskinesia and neurologic effects, including agitation, headache, lethargy, confusion, dry mouth, difficulty urinating, irregular heartbeats, mental changes, severe nausea or vomiting, or uncontrolled movement of the hands, arms, legs, eyelids, face, mouth, or tongue.
- **Therapeutic effects:** Assess for relief of symptoms such as improvement of mask-like facial expression, muscular rigidity, shuffling gait, and resting tremors of the hands and head. The drug's therapeutic effects may be delayed from several weeks to months.
- **Colored secretions/excretions:** Carbidopa and levodopa may darken sweat and urine. This is not harmful.
- **Patient education:** Patients should avoid tasks that require mental alertness or motor skills until response to the drug is known. Caution patients to avoid alcoholic beverages during therapy. May take sips of tepid water and chew sugarless gum to relieve dry mouth.

SERIOUS ADVERSE REACTIONS

- **Long-term therapy:** There is a high incidence of involuntary choreiform, dystonic, and dyskinetic movements for patients on long-term therapy.
- **Neuroleptic malignant syndrome:** Seen occasionally when dose of carbidopa and levodopa is reduced or drug is discontinued, especially if patients are receiving neuroleptic medications. Symptoms include fever, muscular rigidity, altered mental status, and autonomic dysfunction.
- **Mild to severe CNS and psychiatric disturbances:** Reduced attention span, anxiety, nightmares, daytime somnolence, euphoria, fatigue, paranoia, psychotic episodes, depression, and hallucinations.
- **Cardiovascular:** Irregular heart rhythm, syncope, hypotension, hypertension, tachycardia, tachypnea, chest pain.
- **Reactivation of melanoma:** Sinemet CR may prompt recurrence of melanoma in patients with previously diagnosed disease.

OVERDOSE/TOXICITY

- **Symptoms:** Agitation, confusion, dyskinesia, dystonia, tachycardia, tachypnea, hypertension, nausea, hallucinations, dizziness, irregular heart beat, nausea, vomiting, hypotension, respiratory distress.
- **Potential for abuse:** Parkinsonian patients who desire a particular psychologic effect or CNS stimulation from the drug may abuse it.
- **Acute psychosis:** May be managed by withholding anti-Parkinsonian drugs and using benzodiazepines to manage severe agitation. Standard neuroleptics should be avoided due to pro-Parkinsonian effects. A neurologist should be consulted.
- **Management:** Maintain airway with endotracheal intubation and mechanical ventilation if necessary. Maintain BP with IV fluids and vasoactive drugs. Hypertension should be managed with nitroprusside rather than beta-blockers. Hypotension is best managed with alpha-agonists (e.g., norepinephrine). *DOPamine should be avoided to reduce possibility of vasodilation. Agitation and dyskinesia are initially managed with IV benzodiazepines (e.g., lorazepam, diazepam). Neuromuscular blockade may be used to control extreme movement disorders or unmanageable behavior as a last resort.
- **GI decontamination:** Oral activated charcoal may be effective in reducing some adverse effects if given within several hours of ingestion. No published evidence supports gastric lavage.

ANTIDOTE/DIALYSIS

- **Antidote:** No specific recommendations.
- **Dialysis:** No data are available on removal of carbidopa; it is unlikely that levodopa is removed by hemodialysis, high-permeability hemodialysis, or peritoneal dialysis.

carbinoxamine

See Antibiotics (p. 892)

carisoprodol

kar-i-so-pro'-dol

Classes

Chemical: meprobamate congener
Therapeutic: skeletal muscle relaxant

Pregnancy Category: C

Trade Names

Prescription: Soma, Vanadom

Combinations

Prescription: with aspirin (Soma Compound); with aspirin and codeine (Soma Compound with Codeine)

Do not confuse carisoprodol with carvedilol or carteolol.

CLINICAL PHARMACOLOGY

Mechanism of Action

A centrally acting skeletal muscle relaxant whose exact mechanism is unknown. Effects may be due to its CNS depressant actions. **Therapeutic Effect:** Relieves muscle spasms and pain.

PHARMACOKINETICS

Metabolized in the liver to meprobamate. Excreted in urine. **Half-life:** 8 hr.

AVAILABILITY

Tablets (Soma, Vanadom): 350 mg.

INDICATIONS AND DOSAGE

Adjunct to rest, physical therapy, analgesics, and other measures for relief of discomfort from acute, painful musculoskeletal conditions

PO

Adults, Elderly: 350 mg 4 times per day. Use lower initial dose and increase gradually as needed and tolerated in patients with hepatic disease.

CONTRAINDICATIONS

Acute intermittent porphyria, sensitivity to meprobamate, mebutamate, or tybamate, known sensitivity to carisoprodol

INTERACTIONS

Drug: **Alcohol, other CNS depressants:** May increase CNS depression. **Herbal:** None known. **Food:** None known.

DIAGNOSTIC TEST EFFECTS

None known.

SIDE-EFFECTS

Frequent (greater than 10%): Somnolence.
Occasional (10%-1%): Tachycardia, facial flushing, dizziness, headache, lightheadedness, dermatitis, nausea, vomiting, abdominal cramps, dyspnea, hiccups

CRITICAL CARE CONSIDERATIONS

ADMINISTRATION/HANDLING

PO ALERT

- Give carisoprodol with food to decrease GI upset.
- Give the last dose at bedtime.

PRECAUTIONS

HEALTH-RELATED

- Use carisoprodol cautiously in patients with hepatic or renal impairment.
- The metabolite meprobamate has prompted seizures in epileptic patients.

AGE-RELATED

- **Children:** Safety and efficacy of carisoprodol have not been established in children under 6 yr for meprobamate, an active metabolite of carisoprodol.
- **Elderly:** The lowest effective dose should be used to prevent oversedation.

PREGNANCY/LACTATION-RELATED

- Pregnancy category C; crosses placenta; excreted in breast milk (2-4 times maternal plasma).

MONITORING

- **Baseline assessment:** Assess for other medications being taken, especially CNS depressants.
- **Baseline lab work:** Liver and renal function test results.
- **Therapeutic effect:** Assess for relief of muscle spasm and pain.
- **Patient education:** Inform patients carisoprodol may cause dizziness or drowsiness. Urge patients to avoid alcohol and other CNS depressants. Drug dependence has been reported with long-term use.

SERIOUS ADVERSE REACTIONS

- **Withdrawal:** When dose is reduced or discontinued, anxiety, insomnia, irritability, headache, and muscular pain may occur. If noted, carisoprodol should be resumed and withdrawn more gradually.

C

- **Idiosyncratic reactions:** Extreme weakness, transient quadriplegia, hallucinations, encephalopathy, slurred speech, bradycardia, areflexia, hypotonia, dizziness; seen within minutes to hours after receiving first dose.

OVERDOSE/TOXICITY
- **Overdose:** CNS and respiratory depression, shock, stupor, and coma.
- **Management:** Supportive care including ensuring patent airway and ventilation using endotracheal intubation and mechanical ventilation if needed. If in shock, support with IV hydration and use vasopressors if BP is not corrected with fluid infusions.
- **GI decontamination:** No specific recommendations.

ANTIDOTE/DIALYSIS
- **Antidote:** Some case reports suggest that flumazenil has the ability to reverse CNS depressant effects of carisoprodol.
- **Dialysis:** Carisoprodol is removed by hemodialysis and peritoneal dialysis and is likely to be removed by high-permeability hemodialysis. The metabolite meprobamate is moderately dialyzable. Charcoal hemoperfusion has been shown to reduce the half-life from 8.3 hr to 2.6 hr.

carteolol

See Beta-Adrenergic Blockers (p. 943)

carvedilol

kar'-ve-dil-ol

Classes

Chemical: α-adrenergic blocker, peripheral; β-adrenergic blocker, nonselective
Therapeutic: antihypertensive

Pregnancy Category: C, D (2nd, 3rd trimesters)

Trade Names

Prescription: Coreg

Do not confuse carvedilol with carteolol or carisoprodol.

CLINICAL PHARMACOLOGY

Mechanism of Action

An antihypertensive that possesses nonselective beta-blocking and alpha-adrenergic blocking activity. Causes vasodilation. **Therapeutic Effect:** Reduces cardiac output, exercise-induced tachycardia, and reflex orthostatic tachycardia; reduces peripheral vascular resistance.

PHARMACOKINETICS

Route	Onset	Peak	Duration
PO	30 min	1-2 hr	24 hr

Rapidly and extensively absorbed from the GI tract. Protein binding: 98%. Metabolized in the liver. Excreted primarily via bile into feces. Minimally removed by hemodialysis. **Half-life:** 7-10 hr. Food delays rate of absorption.

AVAILABILITY

Tablets: 3.125 mg, 6.25 mg, 12.5 mg, 25 mg.

INDICATIONS AND DOSAGE

Hypertension

PO

Adults, Elderly: Initially, 6.25 mg twice per day. May double at 7- to 14-day intervals to highest tolerated dosage. Maximum: 50 mg/day.

Heart failure

PO

Adults, Elderly: Initially, 3.125 mg twice per day. May double at 2-wk intervals to highest tolerated dosage. Maximum: for patients weighing more than 85 kg, give 50 mg twice per day, for those weighing 85 kg or less, give 25 mg twice per day.

Left ventricular dysfunction

PO

Adults, Elderly: Initially, 3.125-6.25 mg twice per day. May increase at intervals of 3-10 days up to 25 mg twice per day.

OFF-LABEL USES

Treatment of angina pectoris, idiopathic cardiomyopathy

CONTRAINDICATIONS

Bronchial asthma or related bronchospastic conditions, cardiogenic shock, pulmonary edema, second- or third-degree AV block, severe bradycardia (unless patient has a permanent implanted pacemaker), hypersensitivity to carvedilol, second and third trimesters of pregnancy, decompensated heart failure requiring IV inotropic therapy

INTERACTIONS

Drug: **Calcium blockers:** Increase risk of conduction disturbances. **Catapres:** May potentiate BP effects. **Cimetidine:** May increase carvedilol blood concentration. **Digoxin:** Increases concentrations of this drug. **Diuretics, other antihypertensives:** May increase hypotensive effect. **Insulin, oral hypoglycemics:** May mask symptoms of hypoglycemia and prolong hypoglycemic effect of these drugs. **Rifampin:** Decreases carvedilol blood concentration. Herbal: **Ephedra, yohimbe, ginseng:** Decrease effects of carvedilol. **Garlic:** Increase antihypertensive effects. Food: None known.

DIAGNOSTIC TEST EFFECTS

None known.

SIDE-EFFECTS

Frequent (over 10%): Carvedilol is generally well tolerated, with mild and transient side effects. Hypotension (9%-20%), fatigue (4%-24%), dizziness (6%-32%). Occasional (3%-10%): Diarrhea, bradycardia, rhinitis, back pain. Rare (2% or less): Orthostatic hypotension (2%), somnolence (2%), urinary tract infection, viral infection

CRITICAL CARE CONSIDERATIONS

ADMINISTRATION/HANDLING

PO ALERT

- Give carvedilol with food to slow the rate of absorption and reduce the risk of orthostatic hypotension.
- To assess tolerance for carvedilol, assess a standing systolic BP 1 hr following drug administration.

PRECAUTIONS

HEALTH-RELATED

- Use carvedilol cautiously in patients undergoing anesthesia; with heart failure managed with ACE inhibitors, digoxin, or diuretics; diabetes mellitus; hypoglycemia; impaired hepatic function; peripheral vascular disease; and thyrotoxicosis. Patients with renal insufficiency may have 40%-50% higher plasma levels than patients without kidney disease.
- **Cytochrome P450 enzyme metabolism:** Level of carvedilol may be affected by drugs which induce or inhibit cytochrome P450 enzymes.

AGE-RELATED

- **Children:** Safety and efficacy of carvedilol have not been established in children.
- **Elderly:** Plasma levels may be 50% higher compared with younger patients. Incidence of dizziness may be increased.

PREGNANCY/LACTATION-RELATED

- Pregnancy category C (D if used in the second or third trimester).

MONITORING

- **Baseline assessment:** Assess heart rate and BP immediately before giving carvedilol. If heart rate is less than 60 beats/min or systolic BP is less than 90 mmHg, withhold the medication. Assess for history of diabetes and cardiovascular disease.
- **Baseline lab work:** Biochemical profile with renal (BUN, creatinine) and liver (AST [SGOT], ALT [SGPT]), alkaline phosphatase, bilirubin) function tests.
- **Dyspnea:** Monitor respiratory status for dyspnea.
- **Hypotension:** Monitor BP for hypotension.
- **Bradycardia:** Assess pulse for rate and quality; monitor ECG for heart block and/or bradycardia.
- **Heart failure:** Evaluate for signs of heart failure including distended neck veins, rales, increased weight, progressively positive fluid balance, dyspnea (particularly on exertion or lying down), night cough, and peripheral edema.
- **Drug discontinuation:** Do not abruptly discontinue carvedilol. Compliance with the therapy regimen is essential to control hypertension.
- **Hypoglycemia:** Monitor blood glucose carefully in diabetics as carvedilol may mask symptoms of hypoglycemia.
- **Patient education:** When using carvedilol outside the hospital, explain that the full antihypertensive effect will be noted in 1-2 wk. Advise patients who wear contact lenses they may experience decreased tearing. Advise patients not to take nasal decongestants and OTC cold preparations, especially those containing stimulants, without physician approval. To manage heart failure, instruct patients to check their pulse rate and BP before taking carvedilol and to limit alcohol and salt intake. Advise patients to avoid tasks that require mental alertness or motor skills until response to the drug is known and to report excessive fatigue or prolonged dizziness.

SERIOUS ADVERSE REACTIONS

- **Abrupt withdrawal:** Diaphoresis, palpitations, headache, and tremors.
- **Cardiovascular:** Heart failure, heart block, dyspnea, and MI in patients with

heart disease; peripheral ischemia in those with peripheral vascular disease.

- **Thyroid storm:** May occur in patients with thyrotoxicosis because carvedilol masks symptoms of hyperthyroidism.
- **Hypoglycemia:** May occur in patients with previously controlled diabetes.

OVERDOSE/TOXICITY

- **Hematologic:** Anemia, thrombocytopenia, purpura.
- **Overdose:** Profound bradycardia, hypotension, bronchospasm, cardiac insufficiency, heart failure, cardiogenic shock, and cardiac arrest.
- **Management:** Manage airway with endotracheal intubation and mechanical ventilation if necessary. Support BP by working to increase cardiac output using antidotes. If antidotes are insufficient to increase BP, fluid status should be evaluated and managed appropriately to adjust intravascular volume to a level the heart can manage. Vasopressors such as norepinephrine or high-dose *DOPamine may help increase BP if beta-agonists fail. Cardiac pacing may be attempted if medications fail. If bronchospasms occur, both IV and aerosolized $beta_2$-agonists should help relieve spasms.
- **GI decontamination:** Activated charcoal may reduce blood concentration; ipecac and gastric lavage are unlikely to have any significant effect.

ANTIDOTE/DIALYSIS

- **Antidote:** Glucagon or insulin may have positive inotropic action to increase cardiac output. Beta-agonists such as isoproterenol, epinephrine, *DOBUTamine, and prenalterol (not available in the United States) may help increase heart rate to correct bradydysrhythmias. Inamrinone or milrinone may also help increase cardiac output. Atropine may prompt transient increases in heart rate.
- **Dialysis:** Carvediolol is not removed by hemodialysis. No data are available on removal by peritoneal dialysis and high-permeability hemodialysis. Plasma concentrations of carvedilol may be 40%-50% higher when used by hypertensive patients with moderate to severe renal impairment.

cascara sagrada

cass-care'-ah sah-graud'-ah

Classes
Chemical: anthraquinone derivative
Therapeutic: laxative, stimulant

Pregnancy Category: C

Trade Names
Over the Counter: Aromatic Cascara Fluid extract, Cascara Sagrada, Cascara Aromatic

CLINICAL PHARMACOLOGY

Mechanism of Action
A GI stimulant that has a direct effect on colonic smooth musculature by stimulating intramural nerve plexi. **Therapeutic Effect:** Promotes fluid and ion accumulation in the colon, increasing peristalsis and promoting a laxative effect.

PHARMACOKINETICS

Poorly absorbed following PO administration. Metabolized in the liver. Excreted in urine and bile. **Half-life:** Unknown.

AVAILABILITY

Liquid: (18% alcohol) 1 g/mL.
Tablets: 150 mg, 325 mg.

INDICATIONS AND DOSAGE

Treatment of constipation
PO
Adults, Elderly: 5 mL or 1-2 tablets at bedtime. **Children 2-11 yr:** 2.5 mL, 1-3 mL as a single dose. **Infants:** 1.25 mL, 0.5-2 mL as a single dose.

CONTRAINDICATIONS

Abdominal pain, appendicitis, intestinal obstruction, nausea, vomiting, hypersensitivity to cascara sagrada

INTERACTIONS

Drug: **Oral medications:** May decrease transit time of concurrently administered oral medications, decreasing the absorption of cascara sagrada. **Herbal:** None known. **Food:** None known.

DIAGNOSTIC TEST EFFECTS

May increase blood glucose level. May decrease serum calcium and potassium levels.

SIDE-EFFECTS

Frequent: Pink-red, red-violet, red-brown, or yellow-brown discoloration of urine. **Occasional:** Some degree of abdominal discomfort, nausea, mild cramps, faintness

CRITICAL CARE CONSIDERATIONS

ADMINISTRATION/HANDLING

PO ALERT

- Give cascara sagrada on an empty stomach for faster action.
- Avoid giving within 1 hr of antacids, milk, or other oral medications to ensure maximal effectiveness of the drug.

PRECAUTIONS

HEALTH-RELATED

- Excessive use of cascara sagrada may lead to fluid and electrolyte imbalance.

AGE-RELATED

- **Children:** No specific precautions.
- **Elderly:** No specific precautions.

PREGNANCY/LACTATION-RELATED

- Pregnancy category C; excreted in breast milk.

MONITORING

- **Baseline assessment:** Before administration, assess the abdomen for tenderness, rigidity, and bowel sounds. Try to determine when the last bowel movement occurred and its the amount and consistency.
- **Lab work:** Monitor serum electrolyte levels, especially potassium and calcium in patients with excessive, frequent, or prolonged use of cascara sagrada.
- **Hydration:** Maintain adequate fluid intake.
- **Bowel activity:** Assess bowel sounds for peristalsis and pattern of daily bowel activity and stool consistency.
- **Urine color:** Urine may temporarily turn pink-red, red-violet, red-brown, or yellow-brown.
- **Drug interactions:** Do not administer other oral medications within 1 hr of taking cascara sagrada because other drugs may decrease effectiveness of cascara sagrada.
- **Patient education:** When using cascara sagrada outside the hospital, tell patients to institute other measures to promote defecation such as increasing fluid intake, exercising, and eating a high-fiber diet. Warn patients not to use cascara sagrada if abdominal pain, nausea, or vomiting lasting longer than 1 wk occurs because this may indicate bowel obstruction is present. Inform patients the liquid form contains alcohol.

SERIOUS ADVERSE REACTIONS

- Long-term use may result in laxative dependence, chronic constipation, and loss of normal bowel function.
- Prolonged use may produce profuse diarrhea leading to dehydration and severe electrolyte and acid-base imbalance.

OVERDOSE/TOXICITY

- **Symptoms:** May result in electrolyte or metabolic disturbances (such as hypokalemia, hypocalcemia, and metabolic acidosis or alkalosis), as well as persistent diarrhea, vomiting, muscle weakness, malabsorption, and weight loss.
- **Management:** Provide rehydration, correct electrolyte and acid-base imbalance.
- **GI decontamination:** No specific recommendations.

ANTIDOTE/DIALYSIS

- **Antidote:** May use current accepted standard medications to manage diarrhea if symptoms persist.
- **Dialysis:** No data are available on removal using hemodialysis, high-permeability hemodialysis, or peritoneal dialysis.

caspofungin acetate

cas-poe-fun′-gin ass′-eh-tayte

Classes

Chemical: glucan synthesis inhibitor
Therapeutic: fungistatic, antifungal

Pregnancy Category: C

Trade Names

Prescription: Cancidas

CLINICAL PHARMACOLOGY

Mechanism of Action

An antifungal that inhibits the synthesis of glucan, a vital component of fungal cell formation, thereby damaging the fungal cell membrane. **Therapeutic Effect:** Fungi-static.

PHARMACOKINETICS

Distributed in tissue. Extensively bound to albumin. Protein binding: 97%. Slowly metabolized in liver to active metabolite. Excreted primarily in urine and to a lesser extent in feces. Not removed by hemodialysis. **Half-life:** 40-50 hr.

AVAILABILITY

Powder for injection: 50-mg and 70-mg vials.

C

INDICATIONS AND DOSAGE

Aspergillosis

IV

Adults, Elderly, Children older than 12 yr: Give single 70-mg loading dose on day 1, followed by 50 mg/day thereafter. For patients with moderate hepatic insufficiency (Child-Pugh score 7-9), daily dose reduced to 35 mg.

Invasive candidiasis

IV

Adults, Elderly: Initially, 70 mg followed by 50 mg daily.

Esophageal candidiasis

IV

Adult, Elderly: 50 mg per day.

Empiric therapy

IV

Adults, Elderly: Initially, 70 mg then 50 mg/day. May increase to 70 mg/day.

CONTRAINDICATIONS

Hypersensitivity to caspofungin or any components of the product.

INTERACTIONS

Drug: Carbamazepine, *cycloSPORINE, dexamethasone, efavirenz, nelfinavir, nevirapine, phenytoin, rifampin: May increase blood concentration of caspofungin. **Tacrolimus:** May decrease the effect of tacrolimus. **Herbal:** None known. **Food:** None known.

DIAGNOSTIC TEST EFFECTS

May increase prothrombin time as well as serum alkaline phosphatase, serum bilirubin, serum creatinine, LDH, AST (SGOT), ALT (SGPT), serum uric acid, urine pH, urine protein, urine RBC, and urine WBC levels. May decrease Hgb, Hct, platelet count, and serum albumin, serum bicarbonate, serum protein, and serum potassium levels.

IV INCOMPATIBILITIES

Do not mix caspofungin with any other medication or use dextrose as a diluent.

SIDE-EFFECTS

Frequent (26%): Fever. **Occasional (16%-4%):** Headache, nausea, phlebitis (16%), chills (14%), increased transaminases (AST [SGOT], ALT [SGPT]) (13%), increased alkaline phosphatase (11%). **Rare (3% or less):** Paresthesia, vomiting, diarrhea, abdominal pain, myalgia, tremor, insomnia

CRITICAL CARE CONSIDERATIONS

ADMINISTRATION/HANDLING

IV ALERT

- **Storage:** Refrigerate caspofungin but warm to room temperature before reconstituting. Reconstituted solution may be stored at room temperature for 1 hr before infusion. Final infusion solution may be stored at room temperature for 24 hr; discard the solution if it contains particles or is discolored.
- **70-mg dose:** Add 10.5 mL 0.9% NaCl to the 70-mg vial. Transfer 10 mL of the reconstituted solution to 250 mL 0.9% NaCl.
- **50-mg dose:** Add 10.5 mL 0.9% NaCl to the 50-mg vial. Transfer 10 mL of the reconstituted solution to 100 mL or 250 mL 0.9% NaCl.
- **35-mg dose:** Add 10.5 mL 0.9% NaCl to the 50-mg vial. Transfer 7 mL of the reconstituted solution to 100 mL or 250 mL 0.9% NaCl. Moderate liver insufficiency, transfer 7 mL to 100 or 250 mL 0.9% NaCl.
- **Infusion:** Infuse over 60 min. Do not mix or coinfuse with any other medications.

PRECAUTIONS

HEALTH-RELATED

- Use caspofungin cautiously in patients with impaired hepatic function.
- Caspofungin is not recommended for concomitant use in patients receiving *cycloSPORINE unless the potential benefits outweigh the probable risk of liver impairment.

AGE-RELATED

- **Children:** Safety and efficacy of caspofungin have not been established in children.
- **Elderly:** Age-related renal or hepatic impairment may require a dosage adjustment.

PREGNANCY/LACTATION-RELATED

- Pregnancy category C; excreted in breast milk of laboratory rats; use only with caution in lactating women or discontinue breast-feeding.

MONITORING

- **Baseline assessment:** Obtain temperature, history of allergies, and history of hepatic dysfunction.
- **Baseline lab work:** Liver function tests.
- **Ongoing lab work:** Liver function tests, especially in patients with preexisting hepatic dysfunction.
- **Patient education:** Urge patients to report pain, burning, or swelling at the IV infusion site and to report increased shortness of breath, itching, facial swelling, or rash, which may indicate an allergic reaction.

SERIOUS ADVERSE REACTIONS

- Hypersensitivity reactions (characterized by rash, facial swelling, pruritus, and a sensation of warmth) may occur.

OVERDOSE/TOXICITY

- **Symptoms:** May produce hepatotoxicity or allergic reaction leading to anaphylaxis.
- **Management:** Caspofungin should be discontinued if patients show signs of anaphylaxis or liver failure. Patients should be managed according to accepted standards for liver failure. Maintenance of patent airway and treatment of hypotension are priorities with anaphylaxis. Endotracheal intubation with mechanical ventilation may be used for airway management, along with vasopressors and fluid infusion to manage hypotension.
- **GI decontamination:** No specific recommendations.

ANTIDOTE/DIALYSIS

- **Antidote:** No specific recommendations.
- **Dialysis:** Caspofungin is not removed by hemodialysis and is unlikely to be removed by peritoneal dialysis or high-permeability hemodialysis.

cefaclor

See Antibiotics (p. 892)

cefadroxil

sef-ah-drox'-il

Classes

Chemical: cephalosporin (first generation)
Therapeutic: antibiotic

Pregnancy Category: B

Trade Names

Prescription: Duricef

Do not confuse Duricef with Duramorph.

CLINICAL PHARMACOLOGY

Mechanism of Action

A first-generation cephalosporin that binds to bacterial cell membranes and inhibits cell wall synthesis. **Therapeutic Effect:** Bactericidal.

PHARMACOKINETICS

Well absorbed from the GI tract. Protein binding: 15%-20%. Widely distributed. Primarily excreted unchanged in urine. Removed by hemodialysis. **Half-life:** 1-2 hr (increased in impaired renal function to 20-24 hr).

AVAILABILITY

Capsules: 500 mg.
Oral Suspension: 125 mg/5 mL, 250 mg/5 mL, 500 mg/5 mL.
Tablets: 1 g.

INDICATIONS AND DOSAGE

UTIs
PO

Adults, Elderly: 1-2 g/day as a single dose or in 2 divided doses. **Children:** 30 mg/kg/day in 2 divided doses. Maximum: 2 g/day.

Skin and skin-structure infections, group A beta-hemolytic streptococcal pharyngitis, tonsillitis
PO

Adults, Elderly: 1-2 g in 2 divided doses. **Children:** 30 mg/kg/day in 2 divided doses. Maximum: 2 g/day.

Impetigo
PO

Children: 30 mg/kg/day as a single or in 2 divided doses. Maximum: 2 g/day.

Dosage in renal impairment

After an initial 1-g dose, dosage and frequency are modified based on creatinine clearance and the severity of the infection.

Creatinine Clearance	Dosage Interval
25-50 mL/min	500 mg every 12 hr
10-25 mL/min	500 mg every 24 hr
0-10 mL/min	500 mg every 36 hr

C

CONTRAINDICATIONS

History of anaphylactic reaction to penicillins or hypersensitivity to cefadroxil or other cephalosporins

INTERACTIONS

Drug: Probenecid: Increases cefadroxil blood concentration. **Herbal:** None known. **Food:** None known.

DIAGNOSTIC TEST EFFECTS

May increase BUN level and serum alkaline phosphatase, bilirubin, creatinine, LDH, AST (SGOT), and ALT (SGPT) levels. May cause a positive direct or indirect Coombs' test.

SIDE-EFFECTS

Frequent: Oral candidiasis, mild diarrhea, mild abdominal cramping, vaginal candidiasis. **Occasional:** Nausea, unusual bruising or bleeding, serum sickness–like reaction (marked by fever and joint pain; usually occurs after the second course of therapy and resolves after the drug is discontinued). **Rare:** Allergic reaction (rash, pruritus, urticaria), thrombophlebitis (pain, redness, swelling at injection site)

CRITICAL CARE CONSIDERATIONS

ADMINISTRATION/HANDLING

PO ALERT

- After reconstitution, oral solution is stable for 14 days if refrigerated.
- Shake the oral suspension well before using.
- Give cefadroxil without regard to food; however, if GI upset occurs, give with food or milk.

PRECAUTIONS

HEALTH-RELATED

- **Penicillin allergy:** Use very cautiously in patients with history of antibiotic allergies (especially penicillin). Cross-sensitivity of beta-lactam antibiotics may occur in up to 10% of penicillin allergic patients.
- **Colitis:** Use cefadroxil cautiously in patients with colitis (antibiotic-associated or ulcerative colitis).
- **Renal impairment:** Use cefadroxil cautiously in patients with renal impairment and those using nephrotoxic drugs concurrently.

AGE-RELATED

- **Children:** No age-related precautions have been noted in children.
- **Elderly:** Age-related renal impairment may require a dosage adjustment.

PREGNANCY/LACTATION-RELATED

- Pregnancy category B; low concentrations in milk.

MONITORING

- **Baseline assessment:** Determine history of allergies, particularly to cefadroxil, other cephalosporins, or penicillins, before beginning drug therapy.
- **Lab work:** Culture and sensitivity tests of the site of infection. Renal function tests to assess baseline renal status and then ongoing for increased BUN/creatinine to monitor for nephrotoxicity.
- **Superinfections:** Assess the mouth for white patches on the mucous membranes and tongue; assess for abdominal pain or cramping, anal or genital pruritus or discharge, moderate to severe diarrhea, and severe mouth or tongue soreness.
- ***Clostridium difficile* colitis:** Assess the pattern of daily bowel activity and stool consistency. Although mild GI effects may be tolerable, severe effects may indicate the onset of antibiotic-associated colitis.
- **Hand washing:** If *C. difficile* colitis develops, wash hands with antibacterial soap; alcohol-based foam is ineffective against *C. difficile* spores.
- **Nephrotoxicity:** Monitor intake and output. Oliguria may indicate onset of renal insufficiency or inadequate hydration. Renal excretion of cefadroxil is inhibited by probenecid.
- **Patient education:** Space doses evenly around the clock and continue administration of cefadroxil for the full course of treatment. Patients should be advised to continue the dosage regime if treatment will continue outside the hospital.

SERIOUS ADVERSE REACTIONS

- **Hypersensitivity:** Patients with a history of allergies, especially to penicillin, are at increased risk for developing a severe hypersensitivity reaction marked by severe pruritus, angioedema, bronchospasm, and anaphylaxis.

- **Manage hypersensitivity:** May require treatment with epinephrine and other emergency measures including oxygen, endotracheal intubation, mechanical ventilation, IV fluids, IV antihistamines, corticosteroids, and vasopressors.
- **Hepatic dysfunction:** Cholestasis and elevation of serum transaminase.
- **Seizures:** Have occurred, especially in renal impaired patients.
- **Serum sickness–like reaction:** Erythema multiforme, rashes, other skin lesions, accompanied by arthralgia/arthritis with or without fever.

OVERDOSE/TOXICITY

- **Nephrotoxicity:** May occur, especially in patients with preexisting renal disease.
- **Superinfections:** Antibiotic-associated colitis (pseudomembranous colitis) and other superinfections may result from altered bacterial balance.
- **Management of *C. difficile* (antibiotic-associated) colitis:** Discontinue cefadroxil. Oral vancomycin (Vancocin) or metronidazole (Flagyl) are the most effective treatments for antibiotic-associated (pseudomembranous) colitis.
- **GI decontamination:** No specific recommendations.

ANTIDOTE/DIALYSIS

- **Antidote:** No specific recommendations.
- **Dialysis:** Cefadroxil is removed by hemodialysis and is likely to be removed by high-permeability hemodialysis. It is not removed by peritoneal dialysis.

cefazolin sodium

sef-a'-zoe-lin soe'-dee-um

Classes

Chemical: cephalosporin (first generation)
Therapeutic: antibiotic

Pregnancy Category: B

Trade Names

Prescription: Ancef, Kefzol

Do not confuse cefazolin with cefprozil or Cefzil or cefditoren.

CLINICAL PHARMACOLOGY

Mechanism of Action

A first-generation cephalosporin that binds to bacterial cell membranes and inhibits cell wall synthesis. **Therapeutic Effect:** Bactericidal.

PHARMACOKINETICS

Widely distributed. Protein binding: 85%. Primarily excreted unchanged in urine. Moderately removed by hemodialysis. **Half-life:** 0.5-2 hr (increased in impaired renal function).

AVAILABILITY

Powder for injection (Ancef, Kefzol): 500 mg, 1 g, 5 g, 10 g.
Ready-to-hang infusion (Ancef): 500 mg/50 mL, 1 g/50 mL.

INDICATIONS AND DOSAGE

Uncomplicated urinary tract infections
IV, IM
Adults, Elderly: 1 g every 12 hr.

Mild to moderate infections
IV, IM
Adults, Elderly: 250-500 mg every 8-12 hr.

Severe infections
IV, IM
Adults, Elderly: 0.5-1 g every 6-8 hr.

Life-threatening infections
IV, IM
Adults, Elderly: 1-1.5 g every 6 hr. Maximum: 12 g/day.

Perioperative prophylaxis
IV, IM
Adults, Elderly: 1 g 30-60 min before surgery, 0.5-1 g during surgery, and every 6-8 hr for up to 24 hr postoperatively.

Usual pediatric dosage
Children: 50-100 mg/kg/day in divided doses every 8 hr. Maximum: 6 g/day. **Neonates older than 7 days:** 40-60 mg/kg/day in divided doses every 8-12 hr. **Neonates 7 days and younger:** 40 mg/kg/day in divided doses every 12 hr.

Dosage in renal impairment
Dosing frequency is modified based on creatinine clearance.

Creatinine Clearance	Dosage Interval
10-30 mL/min	Usual dose every 12 hr
Less than 10 mL/min	Usual dose every 24 hr

CONTRAINDICATIONS

History of anaphylactic reaction to penicillins or hypersensitivity to cefazolin or other cephalosporins

INTERACTIONS

Drug: Probenecid: Increases cefazolin blood concentration. **Herbal:** None known. **Food:** None known.

DIAGNOSTIC TEST EFFECTS

May increase BUN level and serum alkaline phosphatase, bilirubin, creatinine, LDH, AST

(SGOT), and ALT (SGPT) levels. May cause a positive direct or indirect Coombs' test

IV INCOMPATIBILITIES

Amikacin (Amikin), amiodarone (Cordarone), hydromorphone (Dilaudid)

IV COMPATIBILITIES

Calcium gluconate, diltiazem (Cardizem), famotidine (Pepcid), heparin, insulin (regular), lidocaine, magnesium sulfate, midazolam (Versed), morphine, multivitamins, potassium chloride, propofol (Diprivan), some formulas of total parenteral nutrition (TPN), vecuronium (Norcuron)

SIDE-EFFECTS

Frequent: Discomfort with IM administration, oral candidiasis, mild diarrhea, mild abdominal cramping, vaginal candidiasis. **Occasional:** Nausea, serum sickness–like reaction (marked by fever and joint pain; usually occurs after the second course of therapy and resolves after the drug is discontinued). **Rare:** Allergic reaction (rash, pruritus, urticaria), thrombophlebitis (pain, redness, swelling at injection site)

CRITICAL CARE CONSIDERATIONS

ADMINISTRATION/HANDLING

IV ALERT

- **IV push dilution:** Reconstitute each 1-g vial with at least 10 mL of sterile water for injection.
- **Solution:** Normally appears light yellow to yellow. Discard the solution if a precipitate forms.
- **IV push:** Administer the IV push over 3 to 5 min.
- **IV infusion (piggyback) dilution:** The solution may be further diluted in 50-100 mL D_5W or 0.9% NaCl to decrease the incidence of thrombophlebitis.
- **IV infusion (piggyback):** Infuse over 20 to 30 min.
- **Stability:** IV infusion (piggyback) is stable for 24 hr at room temperature and 96 hr if refrigerated.

IM ALERT

- Reconstitute each 500-mg vial with 2 mL of sterile water for injection and each 1-g vial with 2.5 mL of sterile water for injection.
- To minimize discomfort, slowly inject the drug deep into the gluteus maximus rather than the lateral aspect of the thigh.

PRECAUTIONS

HEALTH-RELATED

- **Penicillin allergy:** Use very cautiously in patients with history of antibiotic allergies (especially penicillin). Cross sensitivity of beta-lactam antibiotics may occur in up to 10% of penicillin-allergic patients.
- **Colitis:** Use cefazolin cautiously in patients with colitis (antibiotic-associated or ulcerative colitis).
- **Renal impairment:** Use cefazolin cautiously in patients with renal impairment and those using nephrotoxic drugs concurrently.

AGE-RELATED

- **Children:** No age-related precautions have been noted in children.
- **Elderly:** Age-related renal impairment may require a dosage adjustment.

PREGNANCY/LACTATION-RELATED

- Pregnancy category B; low milk concentrations.

MONITORING

- **Baseline assessment:** Determine history of allergies, particularly to cefazolin, other cephalosporins, or penicillins, before beginning drug therapy to help avoid possible allergic reaction to cefazolin.
- **Baseline lab work:** Basic chemical profile including liver function tests (AST [SGOT], ALT [SGPT], bilirubin, alkaline phosphatase), K+, BUN, and creatinine levels to evaluate renal function. Obtain culture of infected area before drug administration (wound, blood, sputum, urine).
- **IM injection site:** Evaluate the IM injection site for induration and tenderness.
- **Superinfections:** Assess the mouth for white patches on the mucous membranes or tongue and for severe mouth or tongue soreness; assess for severe anal or genital pruritus or discharge.
- ***Clostridium difficile* colitis:** Assess the pattern of daily bowel activity and stool consistency. Although mild GI effects may be tolerable, severe symptoms including abdominal pain or cramping, and moderate to severe diarrhea may indicate the onset of antibiotic-associated colitis.
- **Hand washing:** If *C. difficile* colitis develops, wash hands with antibacterial soap; alcohol-based foam is ineffective against *C. difficile* spores.

- **Nephrotoxicity:** Monitor intake and output and renal function test results to assess for nephrotoxicity. Renal excretion may be inhibited by probenicid.
- **Patient education:** Space doses evenly around the clock and continue administration of cefazolin for the full course of treatment. Advise patients to continue the dosage regime if treatment will continue outside the hospital.

SERIOUS ADVERSE REACTIONS

- **Hypersensitivity:** Patients with a history of allergies, especially to penicillin, are at increased risk for developing a severe hypersensitivity reaction marked by severe pruritus, angioedema, bronchospasm, and anaphylaxis.
- **Manage hypersensitivity:** May require treatment with epinephrine and other emergency measures including oxygen, endotracheal intubation, mechanical ventilation, IV fluids, IV antihistamines, corticosteroids, and vasopressors.

OVERDOSE/TOXICITY

- **Nephrotoxicity:** May occur, especially in patients with preexisting renal disease.
- **Superinfections:** Antibiotic-associated colitis (pseudomembranous colitis) and other superinfections may result from altered bacterial balance.
- **Management of *C. difficile* (antibiotic-associated) colitis:** Discontinue cefazolin. Oral vancomycin (Vancocin) or metronidazole (Flagyl) are the most effective treatments for antibiotic-associated (pseudomembranous) colitis.
- **GI decontamination:** No specific recommendations.

ANTIDOTE/DIALYSIS

- **Antidote:** No specific recommendations.
- **Dialysis:** Cefazolin is removed by hemodialysis and high-permeability hemodialysis. It is not removed by peritoneal dialysis. Patients with creatinine clearance of less than 10 mL/min should be given half the usual dose every 18-24 hr.

cefdinir

See Antibiotics (p. 893)

cefditoren pivoxil

See Antibiotics (p. 893)

cefepime hydrochloride

sef′-e-pim hye-droe-klor′-ide

Classes

Chemical: cephalosporin (fourth generation)
Therapeutic: antibiotic

Pregnancy Category: B

Trade Names

Prescription: Maxipime

Do not confuse cefepime with ceftidine.

CLINICAL PHARMACOLOGY

Mechanism of Action

A fourth-generation cephalosporin that binds to bacterial cell membranes and inhibits cell wall synthesis. **Therapeutic Effect:** Bactericidal.

PHARMACOKINETICS

Well absorbed after IM administration. Protein binding: 20%. Widely distributed. Primarily excreted unchanged in urine. Removed by hemodialysis. **Half-life:** 2 hr (increased in impaired renal function, and in the elderly).

AVAILABILITY

Powder for Injection: 500 mg, 1 g, 2 g.

INDICATIONS AND DOSAGE

Pneumonia

IV

Adults, Elderly: 1-2 g every 8-12 hr for 7-10 days. **Children 2 mo and older:** 50 mg/kg every 12 hr. Maximum: 2 g/dose.

Intraabdominal infections

IV

Adults, Elderly: 2 g every 12 hr for 10 days.

Skin and skin-structure infections

IV

Adults, Elderly: 2 g every 12 hr for 10 days. **Children 2 mo and older:** 50 mg/kg every 12 hr. Maximum: 2 g/dose.

UTIs

IV

Adults, Elderly: 0.5-2 g every 12 hr for 7-10 days. **Children 2 mo and older:** 50 mg/kg every 12 hr. Maximum: 2 g/dose.

Febrile neutropenia

IV

Adults, Elderly: 2 g every 8 hr. **Children 2 mo and older:** 50 mg/kg every 8 hr. Maximum: 2 g/dose.

Dosage in renal impairment

Dosage and frequency are modified based on creatinine clearance and the severity of the infection.

Normal Dose	Creatinine Clearance		
	30-60 mL/min	11-29 mL/min	Less than 11 mL/min
500 mg every 12 hr	500 mg every 24 hr	500 mg every 24 hr	250 mg every 24 hr
1 g every 12 hr	1 g every 24 hr	500 mg every 24 hr	250 mg every 24 hr
2 g every 12 hr	2 g every 24 hr	1 g every 24 hr	500 mg every 24 hr
2 g every 8 hr	2 g every 12 hr	2 g every 24 hr	1 g every 24 hr

CONTRAINDICATIONS

History of anaphylactic reaction to penicillins or hypersensitivity to cefipime or other cephalosporins

INTERACTIONS

Drug: Aminoglycosides: May increase the risk of nephrotoxicity and ototoxicity. **Probenecid:** May increase cefepime blood concentration. **Herbal:** None known. **Food:** None known.

DIAGNOSTIC TEST EFFECTS

May increase serum alkaline phosphatase, bilirubin, LDH, AST (SGOT), and ALT (SGPT) levels. May cause a positive direct or indirect Coombs' test.

IV INCOMPATIBILITIES

Acyclovir (Zovirax), amphotericin (Fungizone), cimetidine (Tagamet), ciprofloxacin (Cipro), cisplatin (Platinol), dacarbazine (DTIC), *DAUNOrubicin (Cerubidine), diazepam (Valium), *diphenhydrAMINE (Benadryl), *DOBUTamine (Dobutrex), *DOPamine (Intropin), *DOXOrubicin (Adriamycin), droperidol (Inapsine), famotidine (Pepcid), ganciclovir (Cytovene), haloperidol (Haldol), magnesium, magnesium sulfate, mannitol, meperidine (Demerol), metoclopramide (Reglan), morphine, ofloxacin (Floxin), ondansetron (Zofran), vancomycin (Vancocin)

IV COMPATIBILITIES

Bumetanide (Bumex), calcium gluconate, furosemide (Lasix), hydromorphone (Dilaudid), lorazepam (Ativan), propofol (Diprivan)

SIDE-EFFECTS

Frequent: Discomfort with IM administration, oral candidiasis, mild diarrhea, mild abdominal cramping, vaginal candidiasis. **Occasional:** Nausea, serum sickness–like reaction (marked by fever and joint pain; usually occurs after the second course of therapy and resolves after the drug is discontinued). **Rare:** Allergic reaction (rash, pruritus, urticaria), thrombophlebitis (pain, redness, swelling at injection site), seizures (if renal impaired)

CRITICAL CARE CONSIDERATIONS

ADMINISTRATION/HANDLING

IV ALERT

- **IV push dilution:** Add 5 mL of diluent recommended by the manufacturer to each 500-mg vial (10 mL to each 1-g or 2-g vial).
- **IV infusion (piggyback) dilution:** Further dilute the resulting solution with 50-100 mL 0.9% NaCl, or D_5W.
- **IV infusion:** Administer intermittent IV infusion (piggyback) over 30 min.
- **IV push:** Administer the IV push over 3-5 min.
- **Stability:** Solution is stable for 24 hr at room temperature, 7 days refrigerated.

IM ALERT

- To dilute, add 1.3 mL of sterile water for injection, 0.9% NaCl, or D_5W to 500-mg vial (or 2.4 mL to each 1-g and 2-g vial).
- To minimize discomfort, slowly inject the drug deep into the gluteus maximus rather than the lateral aspect of the thigh.

PRECAUTIONS

HEALTH-RELATED

- **Penicillin allergy:** Use very cautiously in patients with history of antibiotic allergies (especially penicillin). Cross-sensitivity of beta-lactam antibiotics may occur in up to 10% of penicillin allergic patients.
- **Colitis:** Use cefepime cautiously in patients with colitis (antibiotic-associated or ulcerative colitis).
- **Renal impairment:** Use cefepime cautiously in patients with renal impairment and those using nephrotoxic drugs concurrently; may cause seizures.

AGE-RELATED

- **Children:** No age-related precautions have been noted in children over 2 mo.
- **Elderly:** Age-related renal impairment may require decreased dosage or increased dosing interval.

PREGNANCY/LACTATION-RELATED

- Pregnancy category B; excreted into breast milk in very low concentrations (0.5 mcg/mL).

MONITORING

- **Baseline assessment:** Determine history of allergies, particularly to cefepime, other cephalosporins, or penicillins before beginning drug therapy to help avoid possible allergic reaction to cefepime.
- **Baseline lab work:** Basic chemical profile including liver function tests (AST [SGPT], ALT [SGOT], alkaline phosphatase, bilirubin), K+, BUN, and creatinine levels to evaluate renal function. Obtain culture of infected area before drug administration (wound, blood, sputum, urine).
- **Superinfections:** Assess the mouth for white patches on the mucous membranes or tongue and for severe mouth or tongue soreness; assess for severe anal or genital pruritus or discharge.
- ***Clostridium difficile* colitis:** Assess the pattern of daily bowel activity and stool consistency. Although mild GI effects may be tolerable, severe symptoms including abdominal pain or cramping, and moderate to severe diarrhea may indicate the onset of antibiotic-associated colitis.
- **Hand washing:** If *C. difficile* colitis develops, wash hands with antibacterial soap; alcohol-based foam is ineffective against *C. difficile* spores.
- **Nephrotoxicity:** Monitor intake and output and renal function test results to assess for nephrotoxicity. Renal excretion may be inhibited by probenicid and may require reduction in dosage of cefepime.
- **IM injection:** Check the injection site for redness and induration.
- **Patient education:** Space doses evenly around the clock and continue administration of cefepime for the full course of treatment. Patients should be advised to continue the dosage regime if treatment will continue outside the hospital.

SERIOUS ADVERSE REACTIONS

- **Hypersensitivity:** Patients with a history of allergies, especially to penicillin, are at increased risk for developing a severe hypersensitivity reaction marked by severe pruritus, angioedema, bronchospasm, and anaphylaxis.
- **Manage hypersensitivity:** May require treatment with epinephrine and other emergency measures including oxygen, endotracheal intubation, mechanical ventilation, IV fluids, IV antihistamines, corticosteroids, and vasopressors.
- **Serum sickness–like reaction:** Erythema multiforme, rashes, other skin lesions, accompanied by arthralgia/arthritis with or without fever.

OVERDOSE/TOXICITY

- **Nephrotoxicity:** May occur, especially in patients with preexisting renal disease.
- **Superinfections:** Antibiotic-associated colitis (pseudomembranous colitis) and other superinfections may result from altered bacterial balance. Severity of colitis ranges from mild to life threatening.
- **Management of *C. difficile* (antibiotic-associated) colitis:** Discontinue cefepime. Oral vancomycin (Vancocin) or metronidazole (Flagyl) are the most effective treatments for antibiotic-associated (pseudomembranous) colitis.
- **GI decontamination:** No specific recommendations.

ANTIDOTE/DIALYSIS

- **Antidote:** No specific recommendations.
- **Dialysis:** Cefepime is removed by hemodialysis, high-permeability hemodialysis, and peritoneal dialysis. On hemodialysis days, the drug should be administered following hemodialysis, dosing 1 g on the first day and 500 mg daily thereafter.

cefixime

See Antibiotics (p. 892)

cefmandole

See Antibiotics (p. 892)

cefmetazole

See Antibiotics (p. 892)

cefoperazone

See Antibiotics (p. 892)

cefotaxime sodium

See Antibiotics (p. 892)

cefoxitin sodium

se-fox'-i-tin soe'-dee-um

Classes
Chemical: cephamycin
Therapeutic: antibiotic

Pregnancy Category: B

Trade Names
Prescription: Mefoxin

Do not confuse cefoxitin with cefotaxime, cefotetan, or Cytoxan.

CLINICAL PHARMACOLOGY

Mechanism of Action

A second-generation cephalosporin that binds to bacterial cell membranes and inhibits cell wall synthesis. **Therapeutic Effect:** Bactericidal.

PHARMACOKINETICS

Well distributed. Protein binding: 65%-80%. Primarily excreted in urine. Removed by hemodialysis. **Half-life:** 0.8-1 hr.

AVAILABILITY

Powder for injection: 1 g, 2 g, 10 g.
Intravenous solution: 1 g/50 mL, 2 g/50 mL.

INDICATIONS AND DOSAGE

Mild to moderate infections

IV, IM

Adults, Elderly: 1-2 g every 6-8 hr.

Severe infections

IV, IM

Adults, Elderly: 1 g every 4 hr or 2 g every 6-8 hr up to 2 g every 4 hr.

Perioperative prophylaxis

IV, IM

Adults, Elderly: 1-2 g 30-60 min before surgery, then 1-2 g every 6-8 hr for up to 24 hr after surgery. **Children older than 3 mo:** 30-40 mg/kg 30-60 min before surgery, then every 6 hr for up to 24 hr after surgery.

Cesarean section

IV

Adults: 2 g as soon as umbilical cord is clamped, then 2 g 4 and 8 hr after first dose, then every 6 hr for up to 24 hr.

Usual pediatric dosage

IV, IM

Children older than 3 mo: 80-160 mg/kg/day in 4-6 divided doses. Maximum: 12 g/day. **Neonates:** 90-100 mg/kg/day in divided doses every 8 hr.

Dosage in renal impairment

After a loading dose of 1-2 g, dosage and frequency are modified based on creatinine clearance and the severity of the infection.

Creatinine Clearance	Dosage
30-50 mL/min	1-2 g every 8-12 hr
10-29 mL/min	1-2 g every 12-24 hr
5-9 mL/min	500 mg-1 g every 12-24 hr
Less than 5 mL/min	500 mg-1 g every 24-48 hr

CONTRAINDICATIONS

History of anaphylactic reaction to penicillins or hypersensitivity to cefoxitin or other cephalosporins

INTERACTIONS

Drug: Probenecid: Increases serum concentration of cefoxitin. **Herbal:** None known. **Food:** None known.

DIAGNOSTIC TEST EFFECTS

May increase BUN level and serum alkaline phosphatase, creatinine, AST (SGOT), and ALT (SGPT) levels. May produce a positive direct or indirect Coombs' test. Interferes with cross-matching procedures and hematologic tests.

IV INCOMPATIBILITIES

Filgrastim (Neupogen), pentamidine (Pentam IV), vancomycin (Vancocin)

IV COMPATIBILITIES

Diltiazem (Cardizem), famotidine (Pepcid), heparin, hydromorphone (Dilaudid), magnesium sulfate, morphine, multivitamins, propofol (Diprivan)

SIDE-EFFECTS

Frequent: Discomfort with IM administration, oral candidiasis, mild diarrhea, mild abdominal cramping, vaginal candidiasis. **Occasional:** Nausea, serum sickness–like reaction (marked by fever and joint pain; usually occurs after the second course of therapy and resolves after the drug is discontinued). **Rare:** Allergic reaction (pruritus, rash, urticaria), thrombophlebitis (pain, redness, swelling at injection site)

CRITICAL CARE CONSIDERATIONS

ADMINISTRATION/HANDLING

IV ALERT

- **IV push dilution:** Reconstitute each 1-g vial with 10 mL of sterile water for injection to provide a concentration of 95 mg/mL. The solution normally appears colorless to light amber. A darker color does not indicate loss of potency. Discard the solution if a precipitate forms.

- **IV infusion (piggyback) dilution:** The resulting solution may be further diluted with 50 to 100 mL of sterile water for injection, 0.9% NaCl, or D_5W. Discard the solution if a precipitate forms.
- **IV push:** Administer over 3-5 min.
- **IV infusion:** Administer the intermittent IV infusion over 15-30 min.
- **Stability:** IV infusion (piggyback) is stable for 24 hr at room temperature and 48 hr if refrigerated.

IM ALERT

- **Dilution:** Reconstitute each 1-g vial with 2 mL of sterile water for injection or lidocaine to provide a concentration of 400 mg/mL.
- **Injection:** To minimize discomfort, slowly inject the drug deep into the gluteus maximus rather than the lateral aspect of the thigh.

PRECAUTIONS

HEALTH-RELATED

- **Penicillin allergy:** Use very cautiously in patients with history of antibiotic allergies (especially penicillin). Incidence of cross sensitivity may range from 3% to 16%.
- **Colitis:** Use cefoxitin cautiously in patients with colitis (antibiotic-associated or ulcerative colitis).
- **Renal impairment:** Use cefoxitin cautiously in patients with renal impairment and those using nephrotoxic drugs concurrently.

AGE-RELATED

- **Children:** Safety and efficacy of cefoxitin have not been established in children under 3 mo. Higher doses of cefoxitin have prompted increased incidence of eosinophilia and elevated AST (SGOT) in patients over 3 mo.
- **Elderly:** Age-related renal impairment may require a dosage adjustment.

PREGNANCY/LACTATION-RELATED

- Pregnancy category B; low milk concentrations.

MONITORING

- **Baseline assessment:** Determine history of allergies, particularly to cefoxitin, other cephalosporins, or penicillins, before beginning drug therapy to help avoid possible allergic reaction to cefoxitin.
- **Baseline lab work:** Basic chemical profile including liver function tests (AST [SGOT], ALT [SGPT], alkaline phosphatase, bilirubin), K+, BUN, and creatinine levels to evaluate renal function. Obtain culture of infected area prior to drug administration (wound, blood, sputum, urine).
- **Altered lab values:** Drug administration may prompt positive direct Coombs' test, eosinophilia, and thrombocytosis. May create false positive urine glucose test results by standard methods. High cefoxitin levels may cause false elevation of serum and urine creatinine levels.
- **Superinfections:** Assess the mouth for white patches on the mucous membranes or tongue and for severe mouth or tongue soreness; assess for severe anal or genital pruritus or discharge.
- ***Clostridium difficile* colitis:** Assess the pattern of daily bowel activity and stool consistency. Although mild GI effects may be tolerable, severe symptoms including abdominal pain or cramping, and moderate to severe diarrhea may indicate the onset of antibiotic-associated colitis.
- **Hand washing:** If *C. difficile* colitis develops, wash hands with antibacterial soap; alcohol-based foam is ineffective against *C. difficile* spores.
- **Nephrotoxicity:** Monitor intake and output and renal function test results to assess for nephrotoxicity.
- **IM injection:** Check the injection site for redness and induration.
- **Patient education:** Space doses evenly around the clock and continue administration of cefoxitin for the full course of treatment. Advise patients to continue the dosage regime if treatment will continue outside the hospital.

SERIOUS ADVERSE REACTIONS

- **Hypersensitivity:** Patients with a history of allergies, especially to penicillin, are at increased risk for developing a severe hypersensitivity reaction marked by severe pruritus, angioedema, bronchospasm, and anaphylaxis.
- **Manage hypersensitivity:** May require treatment with epinephrine and other emergency measures including oxygen, endotracheal intubation, mechanical ventilation, IV fluids, IV antihistamines, corticosteroids, and vasopressors.
- **Serum sickness–like reaction:** Erythema multiforme, rashes, other skin lesions, accompanied by arthralgia/arthritis with or without fever.

C

OVERDOSE/TOXICITY

- **Hepatic dysfunction:** Elevation of AST (SGOT), ALT (SGPT), LDH, and alkaline phosphatase.
- **Nephrotoxicity:** May occur, especially in patients with preexisting renal disease.
- **Superinfections:** Antibiotic-associated colitis (pseudomembranous colitis) and other superinfections may result from altered bacterial balance.
- **Management of *C. difficile* (antibiotic-associated) colitis:** Discontinue cefoxitin. Oral vancomycin (Vancocin) or metronidazole (Flagyl) are the most effective treatments for antibiotic-associated (pseudomembranous) colitis.
- **GI decontamination:** No specific recommendations.

ANTIDOTE/DIALYSIS

- **Antidote:** No specific recommendations.
- **Dialysis:** Cefoxitin is removed by hemodialysis and is likely to be removed by high-permeability hemodialysis. It is not removed by peritoneal dialysis.

cefpodoxime proxetil

sef-pode-ox'-eem proks'-eh-till

Classes

Chemical: cephalosporin (3rd generation)
Therapeutic: antibiotic

Pregnancy Category: B

Trade Names

Prescription: Vantin

Do not confuse Vantin with Ventolin or Vancocin or cefpodoxime with cefepime.

CLINICAL PHARMACOLOGY

Mechanism of Action

A third-generation cephalosporin that binds to bacterial cell membranes and inhibits cell wall synthesis. **Therapeutic Effect:** Bactericidal.

PHARMACOKINETICS

Well absorbed from the GI tract (food increases absorption). Protein binding: 18%-20%. Widely distributed. Primarily excreted unchanged in urine. Partially removed by hemodialysis. **Half-life:** 2.3 hr (increased in impaired renal function and elderly patients).

AVAILABILITY

Oral Suspension: 50 mg/5 mL, 100 mg/5 mL.
Tablets: 100 mg, 200 mg.

INDICATIONS AND DOSAGE

Chronic bronchitis, pneumonia

PO

Adults, Elderly, Children older than 13 yr: 200 mg every 12 hr for 10-14 days.

Gonorrhea, rectal gonococcal infection (female patients only)

PO

Adults, Children older than 13 yr: 200 mg as a single dose.

Skin and skin-structure infections

PO

Adults, Elderly, Children older than 13 yr: 400 mg every 12 hr for 7-14 days.

Pharyngitis, tonsillitis

PO

Adults, Elderly, Children older than 13 yr: 100 mg every 12 hr for 5-10 days. **Children 2 mo-12 yr:** 5 mg/kg every 12 hr for 5-10 days. Maximum: 100 mg/dose.

Acute maxillary sinusitis

PO

Adults, Children older than 13 yr: 200 mg twice per day for 10 days. **Children 2 mo-12 yr:** 5 mg/kg every 12 hr for 10 days. Maximum: 200 mg/dose.

Urinary tract infections

PO

Adults, Elderly, Children older than 13 yr: 100 mg every 12 hr for 7 days.

Acute otitis media

PO

Children 2 mo-12 yr: 5 mg/kg every 12 hr for 5 days. Maximum: 200 mg/dose.

Dosage in renal impairment

For patients with creatinine clearance less than 30 mL/min, usual dose is given every 24 hr. For patients on hemodialysis, usual dose is given 3 times/wk after dialysis.

CONTRAINDICATIONS

History of anaphylactic reaction to penicillins or hypersensitivity to cefpodoxime or cephalosporins

INTERACTIONS

Drug: Antacids, H_2 antagonists: May decrease cefpodoxime absorption. **Probenecid:** May increase cefpodoxime blood concentration. **Herbal:** None known. **Food:** None known.

DIAGNOSTIC TEST EFFECTS

May increase BUN level and serum alkaline phosphatase, bilirubin, creatinine, LDH, AST (SGOT), and ALT (SGPT) levels. May produce a positive direct or indirect Coombs' test.

SIDE-EFFECTS

Frequent: Oral candidiasis, mild diarrhea (15% in infants and toddlers), mild abdominal cramping, vaginal candidiasis, diaper rash (12%). **Occasional:** Nausea, serum sickness–like reaction (marked by fever and joint pain; usually occurs after the second course of therapy and resolves after the drug is discontinued). **Rare:** Allergic reaction (pruritus, rash, urticaria)

CRITICAL CARE CONSIDERATIONS

ADMINISTRATION/HANDLING

PO ALERT

- Administer cefpodoxime with food to enhance drug absorption.
- After reconstitution, refrigerated oral suspension is stable for 14 days.

PRECAUTIONS

HEALTH-RELATED

- **Penicillin allergy:** Use very cautiously in patients with history of antibiotic allergies (especially penicillin). Cross-sensitivity of beta-lactam antibiotics may occur in up to 10% of penicillin allergic patients.
- **Colitis:** Use cefpodoxime cautiously in patients with colitis (antibiotic-associated or ulcerative colitis).
- **Renal impairment:** Use cefpodoxime cautiously in patients with renal impairment and those using nephrotoxic drugs concurrently.

AGE-RELATED

- **Children:** Safety and efficacy of cefpodoxime have not been established in children under 2 mo.
- **Elderly:** Age-related renal impairment may require a dosage adjustment.

PREGNANCY/LACTATION-RELATED

- Pregnancy category B; excreted into breast milk; average 2% of serum levels at 4 hr following 200-mg dose

MONITORING

- **Baseline assessment:** Determine history of allergies, particularly to cefpodoxime, other cephalosporins, or penicillins, before beginning drug therapy to help avoid possible allergic reaction to cefpodoxime.
- **Baseline lab work:** Basic chemical profile including liver enzymes (AST [SGOT], ALT [SGPT], alkaline phosphatase, LDH, bilirubin), K+, BUN, and creatinine levels to evaluate renal function. Obtain culture of infected area before drug administration (wound, blood, sputum, urine).
- **Superinfections:** Assess the mouth for white patches on the mucous membranes or tongue and for severe mouth or tongue soreness; assess for severe anal or genital pruritus or discharge.
- ***Clostridium difficile* colitis:** Assess the pattern of daily bowel activity and stool consistency. Although mild GI effects may be tolerable, severe symptoms including abdominal pain or cramping, and moderate to severe diarrhea may indicate the onset of antibiotic-associated colitis.
- **Hand washing:** If *C. difficile* colitis develops, wash hands with antibacterial soap; alcohol-based foam is ineffective against *C. difficile* spores.
- **Nephrotoxicity:** Monitor intake and output and renal function test results to assess for nephrotoxicity.
- **Patient education:** Space doses evenly around the clock and continue administration of cefpodoxime for the full course of treatment. Advise patients to continue the dosage regime if treatment will continue outside the hospital. Instruct patients using oral suspension outside the hospital to refrigerate it, shake well before using, and take with food.

SERIOUS ADVERSE REACTIONS

- **Hypersensitivity:** Patients with a history of allergies, especially to penicillin, are at increased risk for developing a severe hypersensitivity reaction marked by severe pruritus, angioedema, bronchospasm, and anaphylaxis.
- **Manage hypersensitivity:** May require treatment with epinephrine and other emergency measures including oxygen, endotracheal intubation, mechanical ventilation, IV fluids, IV antihistamines, corticosteroids, and vasopressors.
- **Serum sickness–like reaction:** Erythema multiforme, rashes, other skin lesions, accompanied by arthralgia/arthritis with or without fever.

OVERDOSE/TOXICITY

- **Hepatic dysfunction:** Elevation of AST (SGOT), ALT (SGPT), LDH, and alkaline phosphatase.
- **Nephrotoxicity:** May occur, especially in patients with preexisting renal disease.
- **Superinfections:** Antibiotic-associated colitis (pseudomembranous colitis) and other

superinfections may result from altered bacterial balance.

- **Management of *C. difficile* (antibiotic-associated) colitis:** Discontinue cefpodoxime. Oral vancomycin (Vancocin) or metronidazole (Flagyl) are the most effective treatments for antibiotic-associated (pseudomembranous) colitis.
- **GI decontamination:** No specific recommendations.

ANTIDOTE/DIALYSIS

- **Antidote:** No specific recommendations.
- **Dialysis:** Cefpodoxime is removed by hemodialysis and is likely to be removed by high-permeability hemodialysis. It is not removed by peritoneal dialysis. In patients on hemodialysis, cefpodoxime should be given 3 times weekly following dialysis.

cefprozil

See Antibiotics (p. 892)

ceftazidime

sef-tay'-zi-deem

Classes

Chemical: cephalosporin (third generation)
Therapeutic: antibiotic

Pregnancy Category: B

Trade Names

Prescription: Ceptaz, Fortaz, Tazicef, Tazidime

Do not confuse ceftazidime with ceftizoxime.

CLINICAL PHARMACOLOGY

Mechanism of Action

A third-generation cephalosporin that binds to bacterial cell membranes and inhibits cell wall synthesis. **Therapeutic Effect:** Bactericidal.

PHARMACOKINETICS

Widely distributed (including to cerebrospinal fluid [CSF]). Protein binding: 17%. Primarily excreted unchanged in urine. Removed by hemodialysis. **Half-life:** 2 hr (increased in impaired renal function).

AVAILABILITY

Powder for injection (Fortaz, Tazicef, Tazidime): 500 mg, 1 g, 2 g.

INDICATIONS AND DOSAGE

Urinary tract infections

IV, IM

Adults: 250-500 mg every 8-12 hr.

Mild to moderate infections

IV, IM

Adults: 1 g every 8-12 hr.

Uncomplicated pneumonia, skin and skin-structure infections

IV, IM

Adults: 0.5-1 g every 8 hr.

Bone and joint infections

IV, IM

Adults: 2 g every 12 hr.

Meningitis, serious gynecologic and intraabdominal infections

IV, IM

Adults: 2 g every 8 hr.

Pseudomonal pulmonary infections in patients with cystic fibrosis

IV

Adults: 30-50 mg/kg every 8 hr. Maximum: 6 g/day.

Usual elderly dosage

IV

Elderly (normal renal function): 500 mg-1 g every 12 hr.

Usual pediatric dosage

IV

Children 1 mo-12 yr: 100-150 mg/kg/day in divided doses every 8 hr. Maximum: 6 g/day. **Neonates 0-4 wk:** 100 mg/kg/day in divided doses every 8-12 hr. **Neonates 0-4 wk (less than 1200 g):** 100 mg/kg/day divided every 12 hr. **Neonates under 7 days (1200-2000 g):** 100 mg/kg/day divided every 12 hr. **Neonates under 7 days (more than 2000 g):** 100-150 mg/kg/day divided every 8 hr.

Dosage in renal impairment

After an initial 1-g dose, dosage and frequency are modified based on creatinine clearance and the severity of the infection.

Creatinine Clearance	Dosage
31-50 mL/min	1 g every 12 hr
10-30 mL/min	1 g every 24 hr
Less than 10 mL/min	500 mg every 48-72 hr

CONTRAINDICATIONS

History of anaphylactic reaction to penicillins or hypersensitivity to ceftazidime or other cephalosporins

INTERACTIONS

Drug: **Aminoglycosides, diuretics (e.g., furosemide):** May increase the risk of nephrotoxicity. **Herbal:** None known. **Food:** None known.

DIAGNOSTIC TEST EFFECTS

May increase BUN level and serum alkaline phosphatase, creatinine, LDH, AST (SGOT), and ALT (SGPT) levels. May produce a positive direct or indirect Coombs' test. Interferes with crossmatching procedures and hematologic tests.

IV INCOMPATIBILITIES

Amphotericin B complex (Ambisome, Amphotec, Abelcet), *DOXOrubicin liposomal (Doxil), fluconazole (Diflucan), idarubicin (Idamycin), midazolam (Versed), pentamidine (Pentam IV), vancomycin (Vancocin), total parenteral nutrition (TPN)

IV COMPATIBILITIES

Diltiazem (Cardizem), famotidine (Pepcid), heparin, hydromorphone (Dilaudid), morphine, propofol (Diprivan), acyclovir, aminophylline, ciprofloxacin (Cipro)

SIDE-EFFECTS

Frequent: Discomfort with IM administration, oral candidiasis, mild diarrhea, mild abdominal cramping, vaginal candidiasis. **Occasional:** Nausea, serum sickness–like reaction (marked by fever and joint pain; usually occurs after the second course of therapy and resolves after the drug is discontinued). **Rare:** Allergic reaction (pruritus, rash, urticaria), thrombophlebitis (pain, redness, swelling at injection site)

CRITICAL CARE CONSIDERATIONS

ADMINISTRATION/HANDLING

IV ALERT

- **IV push dilution:** Add 10 mL of sterile water for injection to each 1-g vial to provide a concentration of 90 mg/mL. The solution normally appears light yellow to amber, but tends to darken; color change does not indicate loss of potency. Discard the solution if a precipitate forms.
- **IV infusion (piggyback) dilution:** Resulting solution may be further diluted with 50 to 100 mL of 0.9% NaCl, D_5W, or another compatible diluent. Discard the solution if a precipitate forms.
- **IV infusion:** Administer intermittent infusion (piggyback) over 15 to 30 min.
- **IV push:** Administer the IV push over 3-5 min.
- **Stability:** IV infusion (piggyback) is stable for 18 hr at room temperature and 7 days if refrigerated.

IM ALERT

- **Dilution:** Add 1.5 mL of sterile water for injection or lidocaine 1% to 500-mg vial, (if prescribed) or 3 mL to 1-g vial to provide a concentration of 280 mg/mL.
- **Injection:** To minimize discomfort, slowly inject the drug deep into the gluteus maximus rather than the lateral aspect of the thigh.

PRECAUTIONS

HEALTH-RELATED

- **Penicillin allergy:** Use very cautiously in patients with history of antibiotic allergies (especially penicillin). Cross-sensitivity of beta-lactam antibiotics may occur in up to 10% of penicillin allergic patients.
- **Colitis:** Use ceftazidime cautiously in patients with colitis (antibiotic-associated or ulcerative colitis).
- **Renal impairment:** Use ceftazidime cautiously in patients with renal impairment and those using nephrotoxic drugs concurrently.

AGE-RELATED

- **Children:** Safety and efficacy of ceftazidime have not been established in children under 12 yr. If treatment is needed for children under 12 yr, a sodium carbonate formulation should be used.
- **Elderly:** Age-related renal impairment may require a dosage adjustment.

PREGNANCY/LACTATION-RELATED

- Pregnancy category B; excreted in human milk in low concentrations.

MONITORING

- **Baseline assessment:** Determine history of allergies, particularly to ceftazidime, other cephalosporins, or penicillins, before beginning drug therapy to avoid possible allergic reaction to ceftazidime.
- **Baseline lab work:** Basic chemical profile including liver enzymes (AST [SGOT], ALT [SGPT], LDH, alkaline phosphatase, bilirubin), K+, BUN, and creatinine levels to evaluate renal function. Obtain culture of infected area before drug administration (wound, blood, sputum, urine).
- **Superinfections:** Assess the mouth for white patches on the mucous membranes or tongue and for severe mouth or tongue soreness; assess for severe anal or genital pruritus or discharge.
- ***Clostridium difficile* colitis:** Assess the pattern of daily bowel activity and stool consistency. Although mild GI effects

may be tolerable, severe symptoms including abdominal pain or cramping, and moderate to severe diarrhea may indicate the onset of antibiotic-associated colitis.

- **Hand washing:** If *C. difficile* colitis develops, wash hands with antibacterial soap; alcohol-based foam is ineffective against *C. difficile* spores.
- **Nephrotoxicity:** Monitor intake and output and renal function test results to assess for nephrotoxicity.
- **IM injection:** Check the injection site for redness and induration.
- **Patient education:** Space doses evenly around the clock and continue administration of ceftazidime for the full course of treatment. Advise patients to continue the dosage regime if treatment will continue outside the hospital.

SERIOUS ADVERSE REACTIONS

- **Hypersensitivity:** Patients with a history of allergies, especially to penicillin, are at increased risk for developing a severe hypersensitivity reaction marked by severe pruritus, angioedema, bronchospasm, and anaphylaxis.
- **Manage hypersensitivity:** May require treatment with epinephrine and other emergency measures including oxygen, endotracheal intubation, mechanical ventilation, IV fluids, IV antihistamines, corticosteroids, and vasopressors.
- **Serum sickness–like reaction:** Erythema multiforme, rashes, other skin lesions, accompanied by arthralgia/arthritis with or without fever.

OVERDOSE/TOXICITY

- **Hepatic dysfunction:** Elevation of AST (SGOT), ALT (SGPT), LDH and alkaline phosphatase.
- **Nephrotoxicity:** May occur, especially in patients with preexisting renal disease.
- **Superinfections:** Antibiotic-associated colitis (pseudomembranous colitis) and other superinfections may result from altered bacterial balance.
- **Management of *C. difficile* (antibiotic-associated) colitis:** Discontinue ceftazidime. Oral vancomycin (Vancocin) or metronidazole (Flagyl) are the most effective treatments for antibiotic-associated (pseudomembranous) colitis.
- **GI decontamination:** No specific recommendations.

ANTIDOTE/DIALYSIS

- **Antidote:** No specific recommendations.
- **Dialysis:** Ceftazidime is removed by hemodialysis and peritoneal dialysis and is likely removed by high-permeability hemodialysis. Ceftazidime should be given following completion of the dialysis treatment. Both hemodialysis and peritoneal dialysis patients should receive a loading dose of 1 g.

ceftibuten

See Antibiotics (p. 892)

ceftizoxime sodium

sef-ti-zox'-eem soe'-dee-um

Classes

Chemical: cephalosporin (third generation)
Therapeutic: antibiotic

Pregnancy Category: B

Trade Names

Prescription: Cefizox

Do not confuse ceftizoxime with cefotaxime or ceftazidime.

CLINICAL PHARMACOLOGY

Mechanism of Action

A third-generation cephalosporin that binds to bacterial cell membranes and inhibits cell wall synthesis. **Therapeutic Effect:** Bactericidal.

PHARMACOKINETICS

Widely distributed (including to CSF). Protein binding: 30%. Primarily excreted unchanged in urine. Moderately removed by hemodialysis. **Half-life:** 1.7 hr (increased in impaired renal function).

AVAILABILITY

Intravenous Solution: 1 g/50 mL, 2 g/50 mL.
Powder for Injection: 500 mg, 1 g, 2 g, 10 g.

INDICATIONS AND DOSAGE

Uncomplicated urinary tract infections

IV, IM

Adults, Elderly: 500 mg every 12 hr.

Mild, moderate, or severe infections of the biliary, respiratory, and GU tracts; skin, bone, and intraabdominal infections; meningitis; and septicemia

IV, IM

Adults, Elderly: 1-2 g every 8-12 hr.

Life-threatening infections of the biliary, respiratory, and GU tracts; skin, bone, and intraabdominal infections; meningitis; and septicemia

IV

Adults, Elderly: 3-4 g every 8 hr, up to 2 g every 4 hr.

Pelvic inflammatory disease

IV

Adults: 2 g every 4-8 hr.

Uncomplicated gonorrhea

IM

Adults: 1 g one time. Disseminated: 1 g every 8 hr.

Usual pediatric dosage

IM

Children older than 6 mo: 50 mg/kg every 6-8 hr. Maximum: 12 g/day.

Dosage in renal impairment

After a loading dose of 0.5-1 g, dosage and frequency are modified based creatinine clearance and the severity of the infection. For dialysis patients with less severe infections, give 500 mg every 48 hr or 250 mg every 24 hr. For life-threatening infections, give 0.5-1 g every 48 hr or 0.5 g every 24 hr. Patients should receive medication after hemodialysis on dialysis days.

Creatinine Clearance	Dosage
50-79 mL/min	0.5 g-1.5 g every 8 hr
5-49 mL/min	0.25 g-1 g every 12 hr
Less than 5 mL/min	0.25-0.5 g every 24 hr or 0.5 g-1 g every 48 hr (dialysis patients)

CONTRAINDICATIONS

History of anaphylactic reaction to penicillins or hypersensitivity to ceftizoxime or other cephalosporins

INTERACTIONS

Drug: Probenecid: Increases serum concentration of ceftizoxime. **Herbal:** None known. **Food:** None known.

DIAGNOSTIC TEST EFFECTS

May increase BUN level and serum alkaline serum phosphatase, creatinine, AST (SGOT), and ALT (SGPT) levels. May produce a positive direct or indirect Coombs' test.

IV INCOMPATIBILITIES

Filgrastim (Neupogen)

IV COMPATIBILITIES

Hydromorphone (Dilaudid), morphine, propofol (Diprivan), acyclovir, allopurinol, aztreonam, esmolol, famotidine, gatifloxacin

SIDE-EFFECTS

Frequent: Discomfort with IM administration, oral candidiasis, mild diarrhea, mild abdominal cramping, vaginal candidiasis. **Occasional:** Nausea, serum sickness–like reaction (fever, joint pain; usually occurs after the second course of therapy and resolves after the drug is discontinued). **Rare:** Allergic reaction (rash, pruritus, urticaria), thrombophlebitis (pain, redness, swelling at injection site)

CRITICAL CARE CONSIDERATIONS

ADMINISTRATION/HANDLING

IV ALERT

- **IV push dilution:** To reconstitute, add 5 mL of sterile water for injection to each 0.5-g vial to provide a concentration of 95 mg/mL. The solution normally appears clear to pale yellow. A change from yellow to amber does not indicate loss of potency. Discard the solution if a precipitate forms.
- **IV infusion (piggyback) dilution:** Resulting solution may be further diluted with 50 to 100 mL of 0.9% NaCl, D_5W, or another compatible fluid. Discard the solution if a precipitate forms.
- **IV infusion:** Infuse intermittent IV infusion (piggyback) over 15-30 min.
- **IV push:** Administer the IV push over 3-5 min.
- **Stability:** IV infusion (piggyback) is stable for 24 hr at room temperature and 96 hr if refrigerated.

IM ALERT

- **Dilution:** Add 1.5 mL of sterile water for injection to each 0.5-g vial to provide a concentration of 270 mg/mL.
- **Injection:** Give deep IM injections slowly to minimize patient discomfort.
- **2-g injection:** When giving a 2 g dose, divide the dose and give in different large muscle masses.

PRECAUTIONS

HEALTH-RELATED

- **Penicillin allergy:** Use very cautiously in patients with history of antibiotic allergies (especially penicillin). Cross-sensitivity of beta-lactam antibiotics may occur in up to 10% of penicillin allergic patients.
- **Colitis:** Use ceftizoxime cautiously in patients with colitis (antibiotic-associated or ulcerative colitis).

- **Renal impairment:** Use ceftizoxime cautiously in patients with renal impairment and those using nephrotoxic drugs concurrently.

AGE-RELATED

- **Children:** Safety and efficacy of ceftizoxime have not been established in children under 6 mo. Ceftizoxime use in children is associated with transient elevations of blood eosinophil count and serum CPK, AST (SGOT), and ALT (SGPT) levels. CPK elevation may be related to IM injection.
- **Elderly:** Age-related renal impairment may require a dosage adjustment.

PREGNANCY/LACTATION-RELATED

- Pregnancy category B; excreted in human milk in low concentrations.

MONITORING

- **Baseline assessment:** Determine history of allergies, particularly to ceftizoxime, other cephalosporins, or penicillins, before beginning drug therapy to help avoid possible allergic reaction to ceftizoxime.
- **Baseline lab work:** Basic chemical profile including liver enzymes (AST [SGOT], ALT [SGPT], LDH, alkaline phosphatase, bilirubin), K+, BUN, and creatinine levels to evaluate renal function. Obtain culture of infected area before drug administration (wound, blood, sputum, urine). CBC with WBC differential to evaluate infection.
- **Superinfections:** Assess the mouth for white patches on the mucous membranes or tongue and for severe mouth or tongue soreness; assess for severe anal or genital pruritus or discharge.
- ***Clostridium difficile* colitis:** Assess the pattern of daily bowel activity and stool consistency. Although mild GI effects may be tolerable, severe symptoms including abdominal pain or cramping, and moderate to severe diarrhea may indicate the onset of antibiotic-associated colitis.
- **Hand washing:** If *C. difficile* colitis develops, wash hands with antibacterial soap; alcohol-based foam is ineffective against *C. difficile* spores.
- **Nephrotoxicity:** Monitor intake and output and renal function test results to assess for nephrotoxicity.
- **IM injection:** Monitor the injection site for redness, pain, and induration.
- **Patient education:** Space doses evenly around the clock and continue administration of ceftizoxime for the full course of treatment. Patients should be advised to continue the dosage regime if treatment will continue outside the hospital.

SERIOUS ADVERSE REACTIONS

- **Hypersensitivity:** Patients with a history of allergies, especially to penicillin, are at increased risk for developing a severe hypersensitivity reaction marked by severe pruritus, angioedema, bronchospasm, and anaphylaxis.
- **Manage hypersensitivity:** May require treatment with epinephrine and other emergency measures including oxygen, endotracheal intubation, mechanical ventilation, IV fluids, IV antihistamines, corticosteroids, and vasopressors.
- **Serum sickness-like reaction:** Erythema multiforme, rashes, other skin lesions, accompanied by arthralgia/arthritis with or without fever.

OVERDOSE/TOXICITY

- **Hepatic dysfunction:** Elevation of AST (SGOT), ALT (SGPT), LDH, and alkaline phosphatase.
- **Hemolytic anemia:** Severe muscle pain, aching, respiratory distress, possible cardiac arrest occur very rarely.
- **Nephrotoxicity:** May occur, especially in patients with preexisting renal disease.
- **Superinfections:** Antibiotic-associated colitis (pseudomembranous colitis) and other superinfections may result from altered bacterial balance.
- **Management of *C. difficile* (antibiotic-associated) colitis:** Discontinue ceftizoxime. Oral vancomycin (Vancocin) or metronidazole (Flagyl) are the most effective treatments for antibiotic-associated (pseudomembranous) colitis.
- **GI decontamination:** No specific recommendations.

ANTIDOTE/DIALYSIS

- **Antidote:** No specific recommendations.
- **Dialysis:** Ceftizoxime is removed by hemodialysis and is likely removed by high-permeability hemodialysis. It is not removed by peritoneal dialysis. For dialysis patients (creatinine clearance less than 5 mL/min) with less severe infections, dose should be 500 mg every 48 hr or 250 mg every 24 hr. For life-threatening

infections, dose should be 0.5 to 1 g every 48 hr or 0.5 g every 24 hr. Patients should receive medication following hemodialysis on dialysis days.

ceftriaxone sodium

sef-try-ax'-one soe'-dee-um

Classes
Chemical: cephalosporin (third generation)
Therapeutic: antibiotic

Pregnancy Category: B

Trade Names
Prescription: Rocephin, Rocephin IM Convenience Kit

CLINICAL PHARMACOLOGY

Mechanism of Action

A third-generation cephalosporin that binds to bacterial cell membranes and inhibits cell wall synthesis. **Therapeutic Effect:** Bactericidal.

PHARMACOKINETICS

Widely distributed (including to cerebrospinal fluid). Protein binding: 83%-96%. Primarily excreted unchanged in urine. Not removed by hemodialysis. **Half-life:** 4.3-4.6 hr IV; 5.8-8.7 hr IM (increased in impaired renal function).

AVAILABILITY

Kit (intramuscular [Rocephin IM Convenience Kit]): 500 mg, 1 g.
Intravenous solution (Rocephin): 1 g/50 mL, 2 g/50 mL.
Powder for injection (Rocephin): 250 mg, 500 mg, 1 g, 2 g, 10 g.

INDICATIONS AND DOSAGE

Mild to moderate infections
IV, IM
Adults, Elderly: 1-2 g as a single dose or in 2 divided doses. **Children:** 50-75 mg/kg/day in divided doses every 12 hr. Maximum: 2 g/day.

Serious infections
IV, IM
Adults, Elderly: Up to 4 g/day in 2 divided doses. **Children:** 80-100 mg/kg/day in 1-2 divided doses every 12 hr. Maximum: 4 g/day.

Skin and skin-structure infections
IV, IM
Children: 50-75 mg/kg/day as a single dose or in 2 divided doses. Maximum: 2 g/day.

Meningitis
IV
Children: Initially, 75 mg/kg, then 100 mg/kg/day as a single dose or in divided doses every 12 hr. Maximum: 4 g/day.

Lyme disease
IV
Adults, Elderly: 2 g per day for 10-14 days.

Acute bacterial otitis media
IM
Children: 50 mg/kg as a single dose.

Perioperative prophylaxis
IV, IM
Adults, Elderly: 1 g 0.5-2 hr before surgery.

Uncomplicated gonorrhea
IM
Adults: 250 mg plus doxycycline one time.

Dosage in renal impairment
Dosage modification is usually unnecessary, but liver and renal function test results should be monitored in those with both renal and liver impairment or severe renal impairment.

CONTRAINDICATIONS

History of anaphylactic reaction to penicillins or hypersensitivity to ceftriaxone or other cephalosporins

INTERACTIONS

Drug: None known. **Herbal:** None known. **Food:** None known.

DIAGNOSTIC TEST EFFECTS

May increase BUN level and serum alkaline phosphatase, bilirubin, creatinine, AST (SGOT), and ALT (SGPT) levels. May produce a positive direct or indirect Coombs' test. Interferes with cross-matching procedures and hematologic tests.

IV INCOMPATIBILITIES

Aminophylline, amphotericin B complex (AmBisome, Amphotec, Abelcet), filgrastim (Neupogen), fluconazole (Diflucan), labetalol (Normodyne), pentamidine (Pentam IV), vancomycin (Vancocin)

IV COMPATIBILITIES

Diltiazem (Cardizem), heparin, lidocaine, morphine, propofol (Diprivan), total parenteral nutrition (TPN)

SIDE-EFFECTS

Frequent: Discomfort with IM administration, oral candidiasis, mild diarrhea, mild abdominal cramping, vaginal candidiasis, local induration at injection site (5%-17%).

Occasional: Nausea, serum sickness–like reaction (marked by fever and joint pain; usually occurs after the second course of therapy and resolves after the drug is discontinued). **Rare:** Allergic reaction (rash, pruritus, urticaria), thrombophlebitis (pain, redness, swelling at injection site)

C

CRITICAL CARE CONSIDERATIONS

ADMINISTRATION/HANDLING

IV ALERT

- **First IV infusion dilution:** Add 2.4 mL of sterile water for injection to each 250-mg vial, 4.8 mL to each 500-mg vial, 9.6 mL to each 1-g vial, and 19.2 mL to each 2-g vial to provide a concentration of 100 mg/mL. The solution normally appears light yellow to amber.
- **Second dilution for IV infusion (piggyback):** Resulting solution may be further diluted with 50-100 mL of 0.9% NaCl or D_5W. Discard the solution if a precipitate forms.
- **IV infusion:** Infuse the intermittent IV infusion (piggyback) over 15-30 min for adults and over 10 to 30 min for children or neonates.
- **Reduce risk of phlebitis:** Alternate IV sites and use large veins.
- **Stability:** IV infusion (piggyback) is stable for up to 3 days at room temperature and 10 days if refrigerated. Must be protected from light while stored.

IM ALERT

- **Dilution:** Add 0.9 mL of sterile water for injection, 0.9% NaCl, D_5W, bacteriostatic water and 0.9% benzyl alcohol, or lidocaine to each 250-mg vial, 1.8 mL to each 500-mg vial, 3.6 mL to each 1-g vial, and 7.2 mL to each 2-g vial to provide a concentration of 250 mg/mL.
- **Injection:** To minimize discomfort, slowly inject the drug deep into the gluteus maximus rather than the lateral aspect of the thigh.

PRECAUTIONS

HEALTH-RELATED

- **Penicillin allergy:** Use very cautiously in patients with history of antibiotic allergies (especially penicillin).
- **Colitis:** Use ceftriaxone cautiously in patients with colitis (antibiotic-associated or ulcerative colitis).
- **Renal impairment:** Use ceftriaxone cautiously in patients with renal or hepatic impairment, particularly if both organs are impaired. Ceftriaxone is excreted by both renal and biliary excretion.

AGE-RELATED

- **Children:** Ceftriaxone use in children may displace serum bilirubin from serum albumin. Use ceftriaxone cautiously in neonates, who may become hyperbilirubinemic.
- **Elderly:** No dosage adjustment required.

PREGNANCY/LACTATION-RELATED

- Pregnancy category B; excreted in breast milk.

MONITORING

- **Baseline assessment:** Determine history of allergies, particularly to ceftriaxone, other cephalosporins, or penicillins, before beginning drug therapy to help avoid possible allergic reaction to ceftriaxone.
- **Baseline lab work:** Basic chemical profile including liver enzymes (AST [SGOT], ALT [SGPT], LDH, bilirubin, alkaline phosphatase), K+, BUN, and creatinine levels to evaluate renal function. Obtain culture of infected area before drug administration (wound, blood, sputum, urine, CSF) as appropriate. CBC with differential to evaluate infection.
- **Superinfections:** Assess the mouth for white patches on the mucous membranes or tongue and for severe mouth or tongue soreness; assess for severe anal or genital pruritus or discharge.
- ***Clostridium difficile* colitis:** Assess the pattern of daily bowel activity and stool consistency. Although mild GI effects may be tolerable, severe symptoms including abdominal pain or cramping, and moderate to severe diarrhea may indicate the onset of antibiotic-associated colitis.
- **Hand washing:** If *C. difficile* (antibiotic-associated) colitis develops, wash hands with antibacterial soap; alcohol-based foam is ineffective against *C. difficile* spores.
- **Nephrotoxicity:** Monitor intake and output and renal function test results to assess for nephrotoxicity.
- **IM injection:** Monitor the injection site for redness, pain, and induration.
- **Patient education:** Space doses evenly around the clock and continue administration of ceftriaxone for the full course of

treatment. Advise patients to continue the dosage regime if treatment will continue outside the hospital.

SERIOUS ADVERSE REACTIONS

- **Hypersensitivity:** Patients with a history of allergies, especially to penicillin, are at increased risk for developing a severe hypersensitivity reaction marked by severe pruritus, angioedema, bronchospasm, and anaphylaxis.
- **Manage hypersensitivity:** May require treatment with epinephrine and other emergency measures including oxygen, endotracheal intubation, mechanical ventilation, IV fluids, IV antihistamines, corticosteroids, and vasopressors.
- **Gallbladder disease:** May cause symptoms of cholecystitis. Gallbladder appears abnormal (sludge present) on ultrasound. Symptoms resolve upon discontinuing the medication. May be due to precipitated calcium salt from ceftriaxone.
- **Serum sickness–like reaction:** Erythema multiforme, rashes, other skin lesions, accompanied by arthralgia/arthritis with or without fever.

OVERDOSE/TOXICITY

- **Hepatic dysfunction:** Elevation of AST (SGOT), ALT (SGPT), LDH, and alkaline phosphatase.
- **Nephrotoxicity:** May occur, especially in patients with preexisting renal disease.
- **Superinfections:** Antibiotic-associated colitis (pseudomembranous colitis) and other superinfections may result from altered bacterial balance.
- **Management of *C. difficile* (antibiotic-associated) colitis:** Discontinue ceftriaxone. Oral vancomycin (Vancocin) or metronidazole (Flagyl) are the most effective treatments for antibiotic-associated (pseudomembranous) colitis.
- **GI decontamination:** No specific recommendations.

ANTIDOTE/DIALYSIS

- **Antidote:** No specific recommendations.
- **Dialysis:** Ceftriaxone is not removed by hemodialysis or peritoneal dialysis. No data are available on removal using high-permeability hemodialysis. Patients with both liver and kidney disease should receive no more than 2 g daily, with close monitoring of serum ceftriaxone levels. May be given following hemodialysis on dialysis days.

cefuroxime

See Antibiotics (p. 892)

celecoxib

sel-eh-cox'-ib

Classes

Chemical: cyclooxygenase-2 (COX-2) inhibitor

Therapeutic: COX-2 specific inhibitor, NSAID, nonnarcotic analgesic

Pregnancy Category: C, D (3rd trimester or near delivery)

Trade Names

Prescription: Celebrex

Do not confuse Celebrex with Cerebyx or Celexa.

CLINICAL PHARMACOLOGY

Mechanism of Action

An NSAID that inhibits cyclooxygenase-2, the enzyme responsible for prostaglandin synthesis. Mechanism of action in treating familial adenomatous polyposis is unknown. **Therapeutic Effect:** Reduces inflammation and relieves pain.

PHARMACOKINETICS

Widely distributed. Protein binding: 97%. Metabolized in the liver. Primarily eliminated in feces. **Half-life:** 11.2 hr.

AVAILABILITY

Capsules: 100 mg, 200 mg, 400 mg.

INDICATIONS AND DOSAGE

Osteoarthritis

PO

Adults, Elderly: 200 mg/day as a single dose or 100 mg twice per day.

Rheumatoid arthritis

PO

Adults, Elderly: 100-200 mg twice per day.

Acute pain

PO

Adults, Elderly: Initially, 400 mg with additional 200 mg on day 1, if needed. Maintenance: 200 mg twice per day as needed.

Familial adenomatous polyposis

PO

Adults, Elderly: 400 mg twice daily (with food).

Primary dysmenorrhea

PO

Adults: Initial dose is 400 mg followed by 200 mg on day 1 if needed. Maintenance dose is 200 mg twice per day as needed (with food).

Ankylosing spondylitis

PO

Adults, Elderly: 200 mg/day as a single dose or in 2 divided doses. May increase to 400 mg/day if no effect is seen after 6 wk.

CONTRAINDICATIONS

Hypersensitivity to celecoxib, aspirin, NSAIDs, or sulfonamides

INTERACTIONS

Drug: Fluconazole: May increase celecoxib blood level twofold. **Lithium:** May increase lithium blood levels. **Warfarin:** May increase the risk of bleeding. **Herbal:** None known. **Food:** None known.

DIAGNOSTIC TEST EFFECTS

May increase AST (SGOT) and ALT (SGPT) levels.

SIDE-EFFECTS

Frequent (greater than 5%): Diarrhea, dyspepsia, headache, upper respiratory tract infection. **Occasional (5%-1%):** Abdominal pain, flatulence, nausea, back pain, peripheral edema, dizziness, rash

CRITICAL CARE CONSIDERATIONS

ADMINISTRATION/HANDLING

PO ALERT

- Give celecoxib without regard to food.
- Capsules should not be broken or crushed.

PRECAUTIONS

HEALTH-RELATED

- Celecoxib is used cautiously in patients more than 60 yr, smokers, renal or liver impaired patients, asthmatics, those with active alcoholism, or history of peptic ulcer disease, and those receiving anticoagulant or steroid therapy.
- Celecoxib has been associated with the development of life-threatening cardiovascular disease and gastrointestinal bleeding.
- When high doses of celecoxib are given to prevent colon cancer, risk of cardiovascular events increases.

AGE-RELATED

- **Children:** Safety and efficacy of celecoxib have not been established in children under 18 yr.
- **Elderly:** No age-related precautions have been noted.

PREGNANCY/LACTATION-RELATED

- Pregnancy category C (D if used in third trimester or near delivery); breast milk secretion unknown.

MONITORING

- **Baseline assessment:** Assess for history of cardiovascular disease including chest discomfort, carotid artery disease, transient ischemic attack (TIA), heart attack, stroke, or GI bleeding because celecoxib may prompt worsening of cardiovascular and GI symptoms. Assess for location, severity, and type of pain being managed.
- **Baseline lab work:** Biochemical profile including renal and liver function studies.
- **Baseline diagnostic tests:** 12-lead ECG to evaluate for myocardial ischemia. X-ray affected joints to evaluate deformities.
- **Therapeutic effect:** Assess for relief of pain and improvement in mobility, decreased stiffness and joint swelling, improved grip strength.
- **Patient education:** Advise patients to take celecoxib with food if GI upset occurs. Inform patients that alcohol and aspirin with celecoxib increases risk of GI bleeding. Celecoxib may decrease the cardiovascular protective effects of aspirin.

SERIOUS ADVERSE REACTIONS

- Risk of developing significant cardiovascular disease; GI ulceration, bleeding, and perforation; elevated liver enzymes rarely progressing to hepatic necrosis; elevated BUN and creatinine, sometimes progressing to acute renal failure; anemia; fluid retention; edema; hypertension; and bronchospasms in asthma patients.

OVERDOSE/TOXICITY

- **Symptoms:** Seizures, coma or encephalopathy, respiratory failure or potential for obstructive airway angioedema, hypotension, shock, cardiac dysrhythmias, GI hemorrhage.

- **GI decontamination:** No specific recommendations.

ANTIDOTE/DIALYSIS

- **Antidote:** No specific recommendations.
- **Dialysis:** Celecoxib is unlikely to be removed by hemodialysis or peritoneal dialysis. No data are available on removal by high-permeability hemodialysis.

cephalexin

sef-a-lex'-in

Classes

Chemical: cephalosporin (1st generation)
Therapeutic: antibiotic

Pregnancy Category: B

Trade Names

Prescription: Biocef, Keflex, Keftab

CLINICAL PHARMACOLOGY

Mechanism of Action

A first-generation cephalosporin that binds to bacterial cell membranes and inhibits cell wall synthesis. **Therapeutic Effect:** Bactericidal.

PHARMACOKINETICS

Rapidly absorbed from the GI tract. Protein binding: 10%-15%. Widely distributed. Primarily excreted unchanged in urine. Moderately removed by hemodialysis (20%-50%). **Half-life:** 0.9-1.2 hr (increased in impaired renal function).

AVAILABILITY

Capsules: 250 mg (Keflex), 500 mg (Biocef, Keflex).
Powder for oral suspension (Biocef, Keflex): 125 mg/5 mL, 250 mg/5 mL.
Tablets: 250 mg, 500 mg.

INDICATIONS AND DOSAGE

Bone infections, prophylaxis of rheumatic fever, follow-up to parenteral therapy

PO

Adults, Elderly: 250-500 mg every 6 hr up to 4 g/day.

Streptococcal pharyngitis, skin and skin-structure infections, uncomplicated cystitis

PO

Adults, Elderly: 500 mg every 12 hr.

Usual pediatric dosage

Children: 25-100 mg/kg/day in 2-4 divided doses.

Otitis media

PO

Children: 75-100 mg/kg/day in 4 divided doses.

Dosage in renal impairment

After usual initial dose, dosing frequency is modified based on creatinine clearance and the severity of the infection.

Creatinine Clearance	Dosage Interval
Less than 10 mL/min	250-500 mg every 12 hr

CONTRAINDICATIONS

History of anaphylactic reaction to penicillins or hypersensitivity to cephalexin or other cephalosporins

INTERACTIONS

Drug: Probenecid: Increases serum concentration of cephalexin. **Herbal:** None known. **Food:** None known.

DIAGNOSTIC TEST EFFECTS

May increase serum alkaline phosphatase, AST (SGOT), and ALT (SGPT) levels. May produce a positive direct or indirect Coombs' test. Interferes with crossmatching procedures and hematologic tests.

SIDE-EFFECTS

Frequent: Oral candidiasis, mild diarrhea, mild abdominal cramping, vaginal candidiasis. **Occasional:** Nausea, serum sickness–like reaction (marked by fever and joint pain; usually occurs after the second course of therapy and resolves after the drug is discontinued). **Rare:** Allergic reaction (rash, pruritus, urticaria)

CRITICAL CARE CONSIDERATIONS

ADMINISTRATION/HANDLING

PO ALERT

- After reconstitution, refrigerated oral suspension is stable for 14 days.
- Shake oral suspension well before using.
- Give oral cephalexin without regard to meals; however, if GI upset occurs, give with food or milk.

PRECAUTIONS

HEALTH-RELATED

- **Penicillin allergy:** Use very cautiously in patients with history of antibiotic allergies (especially penicillin).

C

- **Colitis:** Use cephalexin cautiously in patients with colitis (antibiotic-associated or ulcerative colitis).
- **Renal impairment:** Use cephalexin cautiously in patients with renal impairment and those using nephrotoxic drugs concurrently.

AGE-RELATED

- **Children:** No age-related precautions have been noted in children.
- **Elderly:** Age-related renal impairment may require a dosage adjustment.

PREGNANCY/LACTATION-RELATED

- Pregnancy category B; excreted in breast milk.

MONITORING

- **Baseline assessment:** Determine history of allergies, particularly to cephalexin, other cephalosporins, or penicillins, before beginning drug therapy to help avoid possible allergic reaction to cephalexin.
- **Baseline lab work:** Basic chemical profile including liver enzymes (AST [SGOT], ALT [SGPT], alkaline phosphatase, LDH, bilirubin), K+, BUN, and creatinine levels to evaluate renal function. Obtain culture of infected area before drug administration (wound, blood, sputum, urine, CSF) as appropriate. CBC with differential to evaluate infection.
- **Superinfections:** Assess the mouth for white patches on the mucous membranes or tongue and for severe mouth or tongue soreness; assess for severe anal or genital pruritus or discharge.
- ***Clostridium difficile* colitis:** Assess the pattern of daily bowel activity and stool consistency. Although mild GI effects may be tolerable, severe symptoms including abdominal pain or cramping, and moderate to severe diarrhea may indicate the onset of antibiotic-associated colitis.
- **Hand washing:** If *C. difficile* colitis develops, wash hands with antibacterial soap; alcohol-based foam is ineffective against *C. difficile* spores.
- **Nephrotoxicity:** Monitor intake and output and renal function test results to assess for nephrotoxicity.
- **Patient education:** Space doses evenly around the clock and continue administration of cephalexin for the full course of treatment. Advise patients to continue the dosage regimen if treatment will continue outside the hospital.

SERIOUS ADVERSE REACTIONS

- **Hypersensitivity:** Patients with a history of allergies, especially to penicillin, are at increased risk for developing a severe hypersensitivity reaction marked by severe pruritus, angioedema, bronchospasm, and anaphylaxis.
- **Manage hypersensitivity:** May require treatment with epinephrine and other emergency measures including oxygen, endotracheal intubation, mechanical ventilation, IV fluids, IV antihistamines, corticosteroids, and vasopressors.
- **Serum sickness–like reaction:** Erythema multiforme, rashes, other skin lesions, accompanied by arthralgia/arthritis with or without fever.
- **Seizures:** Rare but reported primarily in renal failure patients not treated with reduced doses.

OVERDOSE/TOXICITY

- **Hepatic dysfunction:** Elevation of liver enzymes.
- **Nephrotoxicity:** May occur, especially in patients with preexisting renal disease.
- **Superinfections:** Antibiotic-associated colitis (pseudomembranous colitis) and other superinfections may result from altered bacterial balance.
- **Management of *C. difficile* (antibiotic-associated) colitis:** Discontinue cephalexin. Oral vancomycin (Vancocin) or metronidazole (Flagyl) are the most effective treatments for antibiotic-associated (pseudomembranous) colitis.
- **GI decontamination:** No specific recommendations.

ANTIDOTE/DIALYSIS

- **Antidote:** No specific recommendations.
- **Dialysis:** Cephalexin is removed by hemodialysis and is likely removed by high-permeability hemodialysis. It is not removed by peritoneal dialysis.

cephradine

See Antibiotics (p. 892)

cetirizine hydrochloride

se-ti'-ra-zeen hye-droe-klor'-ide

Classes
Chemical: piperazine derivative
Therapeutic: antihistamine

Pregnancy Category: B

Trade Names
Prescription: Reactine ♣, Zyrtec

Combinations
Prescription: with pseudoephedrine (Zyrtec-D 12-hour tablets)

Do not confuse Zyrtec with Zantac or Zyprexa.

CLINICAL PHARMACOLOGY

Mechanism of Action

A second-generation piperazine that competes with histamine for H_1-receptor sites on effector cells in the GI tract, blood vessels, and respiratory tract. **Therapeutic Effect:** Prevents allergic response, produces mild bronchodilation, blocks histamine-induced bronchitis.

PHARMACOKINETICS

Route	Onset	Peak	Duration
PO	15-30 min	4-8 hr	Less than 24 hr

Rapidly and almost completely absorbed from the GI tract (absorption not affected by food). Protein binding: 93%. Undergoes low first-pass metabolism; not extensively metabolized. Primarily excreted in urine (more than 80% as unchanged drug). **Half-life:** 6.5-10 hr.

AVAILABILITY

Syrup: 5 mg/5 mL.
Tablets: 5 mg, 10 mg.
Tablets (chewable): 5 mg, 10 mg.

INDICATIONS AND DOSAGE

Allergic rhinitis, urticaria

PO

Adults, Elderly, Children older than 5 yr: Initially, 5-10 mg/day as a single dose. **Children 2-5 yr:** 2.5 mg/day. May increase up to 5 mg/day as a single or in 2 divided doses. **Children 12-23 mo:** Initially, 2.5 mg/day. May increase up to 5 mg/day in 2 divided doses. **Children 6-11 mo:** 2.5 mg once per day.

Dosage in renal or hepatic impairment

For adult and elderly patients with renal impairment (creatinine clearance of 11-31 mL/min), those receiving hemodialysis (creatinine clearance of less than 7 mL/min), and those with hepatic impairment, dosage is decreased to 5 mg once per day.

OFF-LABEL USES

Treatment of bronchial asthma

CONTRAINDICATIONS

Hypersensitivity to cetirizine or *hydrOXYzine

INTERACTIONS

Drug: Alcohol, other CNS depressants: May increase CNS depression. **Herbal:** None known. **Food:** None known.

DIAGNOSTIC TEST EFFECTS

May suppress wheal and flare reactions to antigen skin testing unless drug is discontinued 4 days before testing.

SIDE-EFFECTS

Occasional (14%-2%): Pharyngitis; dry mucous membranes, nose, or throat; nausea and vomiting; abdominal pain; headache (children: 11%-14%); dizziness; fatigue; thickening of mucus; somnolence (adults: 14%); photosensitivity; urine retention

CRITICAL CARE CONSIDERATIONS

ADMINISTRATION/HANDLING

PO ALERT

- Give cetirizine without regard to food.

PRECAUTIONS

HEALTH-RELATED

- Use cetirizine cautiously in patients with renal or hepatic impairment; clearance of the drug is reduced in these cases.
- May cause drowsiness at dosages greater than 10 mg/day.

AGE-RELATED

- **Children:** Cetirizine is less likely to cause anticholinergic effects in children.
- **Elderly:** Elderly patients are more likely to experience anticholinergic effects, such as dry mouth and urine retention, as well as dizziness, sedation, and confusion. Decreased cetirizine clearance may be due to age-related renal impairment.

PREGNANCY/LACTATION-RELATED

- Pregnancy category B; excreted into breast milk.

C

MONITORING

- **Baseline assessment:** Auscultate breath sounds. Assess severity of rhinitis, urticaria, or other symptoms.
- **Baseline lab work:** Biochemical profile including renal (BUN, creatinine) and liver (AST [SGOT], ALT [SGPT], alkaline phosphatase, bilirubin) tests. CBC to evaluate for eosinophilia.
- **Hydration:** Increase fluids in patients with upper respiratory allergies to maintain thin secretions and offset thirst.
- **Therapeutic response:** Reduced sneezing, resolution of nasal congestion and coughing, resolution of urticaria.
- **Patient education:** If taking cetirizine outside the hospital, instruct patients to avoid performing tasks requiring alertness or motor skills until response to the drug is known. Cetirizine may cause drowsiness. Urge patients to avoid alcohol during cetirizine therapy and to avoid prolonged exposure to sunlight.

SERIOUS ADVERSE REACTIONS

- **Children:** May experience paradoxical reactions, including restlessness, insomnia, euphoria, nervousness, and tremor.
- **Elderly:** Dizziness, sedation, and confusion are more likely to occur.

OVERDOSE/TOXICITY

- **Symptoms:** Extreme somnolence, coma, seizures, confusion, cardiac dysrhythmias (widened QRS, ventricular tachycardia), fatigue, dizziness, abdominal pain, sore throat, coughing, bronchospasms, diarrhea.
- **Management:** Symptom directed supportive treatment is recommended. Endotracheal intubation may be needed to maintain patent airway. Cardiac monitoring should be initiated for identification of dysrhythmias.
- **GI decontamination:** No specific recommendations.

ANTIDOTE/DIALYSIS

- **Antidote:** No specific recommendations.
- **Dialysis:** Cetirizine is not removed by hemodialysis or peritoneal dialysis. No data are available on removal by high-permeability hemodialysis. Patients with creatinine clearance of less than 32 mL/min, including hemodialysis patients, should receive a reduced dose of 5 mg once daily.

chloral hydrate ⚑

klor'-al hye'-drate

DEA Schedule: IV

Classes

Chemical: halogenated alcohol
Therapeutic: sedative/hypnotic

Pregnancy Category: C

Trade Names

Prescription: Aquachloral Supprettes, Somnote

CLINICAL PHARMACOLOGY

Mechanism of Action

A nonbarbiturate chloral derivative that produces CNS depression. **Therapeutic Effect:** Induces quiet, deep sleep, with only a slight decrease in respiratory rate and BP.

PHARMACOKINETICS

Readily absorbed from the GI tract following PO administration. Well absorbed following rectal administration. Protein binding: 70%-80%. Metabolized in liver and erythrocytes to the active metabolite, trichloroethanol, which may be further metabolized to inactive metabolites. Excreted in urine. **Half-life:** 7-10 hr (trichloroethanol).

AVAILABILITY

Capsules (Somnote): 500 mg.
Syrup: 500 mg/5 mL.
Suppositories (Aquachloral supprettes): 324 mg, 648 mg.

INDICATIONS AND DOSAGE

Premedication for dental or medical procedures

PO, Rectal

Adults: 0.5-1 g, 30 min before procedure.
Children: 75 mg/kg up to 1 g total.

Premedication for EEG

PO, Rectal

Adults: 0.5-1.5 g. **Children:** 25-50 mg/kg/dose 30-60 min before EEG. May repeat in 30 min. Maximum: 1 g for infants, 2 g for children.

CONTRAINDICATIONS

Gastritis, marked hepatic or renal impairment, severe cardiac disease

INTERACTIONS

Drug: Alcohol, other CNS depressants: May increase the effects of chloral hydrate. **Furosemide (IV):** May alter BP and cause diaphoresis if given within 24 hr after chloral hydrate. **Warfarin:** May increase the effect of warfarin. **Herbal:** **Valerian, St. John's wort, kava kava, gotu kola:** May increase effects of chloral hydrate. **Food:** None known.

DIAGNOSTIC TEST EFFECTS

May interfere with copper sulfate test for glycosuria, fluorometric tests for urine catecholamines, urinary 17-hydroxycorticosteroid determinations.

SIDE-EFFECTS

Occasional: Gastric irritation (nausea, vomiting, flatulence, diarrhea), rash, sleepwalking. **Rare:** Headache, paradoxic CNS hyperactivity or nervousness in children, excitement or restlessness in the elderly (particularly in patients with pain).

CRITICAL CARE CONSIDERATIONS

ADMINISTRATION/HANDLING

PO ALERT

- Administer chloral hydrate capsules with a full glass of water or juice.
- Capsules should be swallowed whole; capsules should not be chewed.
- Dilute dose of syrup in water to minimize gastric irritation.

RECTAL ALERT

- Store suppositories at room temperature; do not refrigerate.

PRECAUTIONS

HEALTH-RELATED

- Use chloral hydrate cautiously in patients with clinical depression or a history of drug abuse because the drug is highly addictive and dangerous if overdose is taken.
- Chloral hydrate has been known to cause acute intermittent porphyria and should be used with caution in susceptible patients.

AGE-RELATED

- **Children:** No age-related precautions have been noted. Children are more prone to paradoxical reactions (CNS hyperactivity, nervousness).
- **Elderly:** No age-related precautions have been noted. Elderly are more prone to paradoxical reactions (excitement, restlessness).

PREGNANCY/LACTATION-RELATED

- Pregnancy category C; excreted into breast milk; may cause mild drowsiness in infant, otherwise compatible with breast-feeding.

MONITORING

- **Baseline assessment:** Assess BP, pulse rate, and respiratory rate, rhythm, and depth immediately before administering chloral hydrate.
- **Baseline lab work:** Blood chemistry studies to assess renal and hepatic function.
- **Safety:** Institute safety measures including raising bed rails and putting call bell within easy reach.
- **Sleep:** Provide an environment conducive to sleep. Offer back rub, quiet environment, and low lighting.
- **Large doses:** Assess the breath for a "pear-like" odor often noted when patients have consumed a large dose of chloral hydrate.
- **Ongiong assessment:** Monitor mental status and vital signs.
- **Pediatric and elderly patients:** Assess for paradoxic reactions such as excitability, nervousness, restlessness.

SERIOUS ADVERSE REACTIONS

- **Symptoms:** Somnolence, confusion, slurred speech, severe incoordination, respiratory depression.
- **"Mickey Finn" effect:** When combined with alcohol, sedative action occurs very rapidly and has been used to induce prolonged, profound sedation in recreational settings.

OVERDOSE/TOXICITY

- **Symptoms:** Respiratory failure, coma, seizures, premature ventricular beats, ventricular tachycardia, ventricular fibrillation, accelerated junctional rhythm, torsades de pointes, asystole, upper GI hemorrhage, gastric necrosis and perforation, esophagitis.
- **Management:** Symptom-directed supportive treatment including cardiac monitoring, oxygen, endotracheal intubation, mechanical ventilation, IV fluid volume replacement. Manage tachydysrhythmias with beta-adrenergic blocking agents (propranolol, metoprolol) which seem superior to other types of agents used for ventricular dysrhythmias. Cardioversion and defibrillation may be successful. Repeat doses of beta-blockers may be needed to control prolonged dysrhythmias. Use of *DOPamine

C

and norepinephrine may exacerbate dysrhythmias. Alpha-selective agonists such as phenylephrine may be superior for management of hypotension. Monitor for at least 3 hr following overdose ingestion.
- **GI decontamination:** No specific recommendations.

ANTIDOTE/DIALYSIS
- **Antidote:** No specific recommendations.
- **Dialysis:** Chloral hydrate is removed by hemodialysis and is likely to be removed by high-permeability hemodialysis. It is not removed by peritoneal dialysis.

chloramphenicol

klor-am-fen'-i-kole

Classes
Chemical: dichloroacetic acid derivative
Therapeutic: antibiotic

Pregnancy Category: C

Trade Names
Prescription: Systemic: AK-Chlor, Chloromycetin, Chloromycetin Ophthalmic, Chloromycetin Sodium Succinate, Chloroptic, Chloroptic S.O.P., Diochloram ♣, Ophtho-Chloram ♣, Pentamycetin ♣

Combinations
Prescription: Ophthalmic: Hydrocortisone acetate and polymixin B sulfate (Opthocort); hydrocortisone acetate (Chloromycetin Hydrocortisone)

Do not confuse chloramphenicol with chlorambucil.

CLINICAL PHARMACOLOGY
Mechanism of Action
A dichloroacetic acid derivative that inhibits bacterial protein synthesis by binding to bacterial ribosomal receptor sites. **Therapeutic Effect:** Bacteriostatic (may be bactericidal in high concentrations).

PHARMACOKINETICS
Rapidly and completely absorbed from the GI tract following PO administration. Well absorbed after IM administration. Some systemic absorption following ophthalmic and otic administration. Protein binding: 60%. Metabolized in liver. Excreted in urine. **Half-life:** 1.5-3.5 hr with normal renal function; 3-7 hr with end-stage renal disease; 10-12 hr with cirrhosis (hepatic).

AVAILABILITY
Powder for injection (Chloromycetin Sodium Succinate): 1 g.
Powder for reconstitution (ophthalmic [Chloromycetin Ophthalmic]): 25 mg.
Ophthalmic ointment (AK-Chlor, Chloroptic S.O.P., Ocu-Chlor): 1%.
Ophthalmic solution (Chloroptic, AK-Chlor, Ocu-Chlor): 0.5%.

INDICATIONS AND DOSAGE
Mild to moderate infections caused by organisms resistant to other less toxic antibiotics
IV
Adults, Elderly: 50-100 mg/kg/day in divided doses every 6 hr. Maximum: 4 g/day.
Children older than 1 mo: 50-75 mg/kg/day in divided doses every 6 hr. Maximum: 4 g/day

Meningitis
IV
Children older than 1 mo: 50-100 mg/kg/day in divided doses every 6 hr.

Usual ophthalmic dosage
Adults, Elderly, Children: 1-2 drops 4-6 times/day.

CONTRAINDICATIONS
Hypersensitivity to chloramphenicol; must not be used to treat trivial infections or as a prophylactic agent to prevent bacterial infections

INTERACTIONS
Drug: Anticonvulsants, bone marrow depressants: May increase myelosuppression. **Clindamycin, erythromycin:** May antagonize the effects of these drugs. **Fosphenytoin, phenobarbital, phenytoin, warfarin:** May increase blood concentrations of these drugs. **Oral antidiabetics:** May increase the effects of these drugs. **Vitamin B_{12}:** May decrease the effects of vitamin B_{12} in patients with pernicious anemia. **Herbal:** None known. **Food: Vitamin B_{12}:** May decrease intestinal absorption of vitamin B_{12}.

DIAGNOSTIC TEST EFFECTS
Therapeutic blood level: 10-20 mcg/mL; toxic blood level: greater than 25 mcg/mL. When administered with iron salts, may increase serum iron levels.

SIDE-EFFECTS
Occasional: Systemic: Nausea, vomiting, diarrhea
Ophthalmic: Blurred vision, burning, stinging, hypersensitivity reaction

Otic: Hypersensitivity reaction. **Rare:** Peripheral neuritis (numbness and weakness in feet and hands), rash, shortness of breath, confusion, headache, optic neuritis (blurred vision, eye pain), aplastic anemia

CRITICAL CARE CONSIDERATIONS

ADMINISTRATION/HANDLING

IV ALERT

- **IV push dilution:** Reconstitute each 1-g vial with at least 10 mL of sterile water for injection or D_5W to prepare a 10% solution (100 mg/mL).
- **IV push:** Administer IV push over 1-5 min.
- **IV infusion (piggyback) dilution:** Solution may be further diluted in 50-100 mL D_5W to decrease the incidence of thrombophlebitis.
- **IV infusion (piggyback):** Infuse over 10-30 min.
- **Stability:** IV infusion (piggyback) is stable for 24 hr at room temperature.

PRECAUTIONS

HEALTH-RELATED

- **Potentially lethal:** Chloramphenicol is potentially lethal and should not be used to treat trivial infections. If sensitivity studies indicate another antibiotic is effective, chloramphenicol should be discontinued and the other drug should be used.
- **Bone marrow suppression:** Use chloramphenicol cautiously in patients with bone marrow suppression, and in those who have previously undergone cytotoxic drug therapy or radiation therapy. Bone marrow suppression and blood dyscrasias have occurred with both short-term and longer-term therapy.
- **Renal and/or liver impairment:** Use chloramphenicol cautiously in patients with renal impairment and in those using nephrotoxic drugs concurrently.

AGE-RELATED

- **Children:** Use chloramphenicol cautiously in children under 2 yr. Sources vary on dosing in neonates under 2 kg, but a loading dose of 20 mg/kg is recommended followed by a total dose of at least 25 mg/kg daily. Blood concentration in all premature and full-term neonates differs from that of all other neonates. Use caution, lower doses, and/or extended dosing intervals.
- **Elderly:** Age-related renal impairment may require a dosage adjustment.

PREGNANCY/LACTATION-RELATED

- Pregnancy category C; use caution at term due to potential for "gray baby syndrome" toxicity; excreted into breast milk; milk levels are too low to precipitate the gray baby syndrome, but a theoretical risk does exist for bone marrow depression.

MONITORING

- **Baseline assessment:** Determine if other myelosuppressive drugs are being taken; chloramphenicol should not be given concurrently with these drugs.
- **Baseline lab work:** Complete blood count with WBC differential, complete biochemical profile. Obtain culture of infected area before drug administration (wound, blood, sputum, urine, cerebrospinal fluid) as appropriate.
- **Blood levels:** Monitor drug blood levels. Therapeutic blood level is 10 to 20 mcg/mL; toxic blood level is greater than 25 mcg/mL.
- **Infants/gray syndrome:** Monitor for gray syndrome: abdominal distension with or without emesis, progressive cyanosis, hypotension, shock, irregular respirations, and death within a few hours of onset of symptoms.
- **Superinfections:** Assess the mouth for white patches on the mucous membranes or tongue and for severe mouth or tongue soreness; assess for severe anal or genital pruritus or discharge.
- ***Clostridium difficile* colitis:** Assess the pattern of daily bowel activity and stool consistency. Although mild GI effects may be tolerable, severe symptoms including abdominal pain or cramping, and moderate to severe diarrhea may indicate the onset of antibiotic-associated colitis.
- **Hand washing:** If *C. difficile* (antibiotic-associated) colitis develops, wash hands with antibacterial soap; alcohol-based foam is ineffective against *C. difficile* spores.
- **Nephrotoxicity:** Monitor intake and output and renal function test results to assess for nephrotoxicity.
- **Patient education:** Space doses evenly around the clock and continue administration of chloramphenicol for the full course of treatment. Advise patients to continue the dosage regimen if treatment will continue outside the hospital.

- **Nausea/vomiting/diarrhea:** Treat side effects with current standard agents.
- **Visual disturbances:** Determine whether visual disturbances are being experienced. Differentiate between optic neuritis and bacterial/fungal overgrowth on the eyes. Drug should be discontinued for optic neuritis.
- **Eyedrops/ointment:** Use the ophthalmic form for at least 48 hr after the eye returns to normal appearance.

SERIOUS ADVERSE REACTIONS

- **Manage hypersensitivity/allergic reaction:** May require treatment with epinephrine and other emergency measures including oxygen, endotracheal intubation, mechanical ventilation, IV fluids, IV antihistamines, corticosteroids, and vasopressors.
- **Blood dyscrasias/bone marrow suppression:** There is a narrow margin between effective therapy and toxic levels producing blood dyscrasias. Myelosuppression, with resulting aplastic anemia, hypoplastic anemia, and pancytopenia, may occur weeks or months later. Aplastic anemia may occur 3 wk to 12 mo after beginning therapy.

OVERDOSE/TOXICITY

- **Bone marrow suppression:** Anemia, leukopenia, reticulcytopenia, thrombocytopenia. Drug should be discontinued. Drug may cause fatality if toxic effects are not recognized and managed appropriately.
- **Optic and peripheral neuritis:** Visual disturbances, paresthesias, motor disturbances can occur. Drug should be discontinued.

ANTIDOTE/DIALYSIS

- **Antidote:** No specific recommendations.
- **Dialysis:** Chloramphenicol is removed by hemodialysis and is likely to be removed by high-permeability hemodialysis. It is not removed by peritoneal dialysis.

chlordiazepoxide hydrochloride

See Antianxiety Agents (p. 890)

*chlorproMAZINE

See Antipsychotics (p. 934)

*chlorproPAMIDE

See Antidiabetics (p. 911)

chlorthalidone

klor-thal'-i-doan

Classes

Chemical: phthalimidine derivative
Therapeutic: antihypertensive, diuretic, thiazide

Pregnancy Category: B, D (if used in pregnancy-induced hypertension)

Trade Names

Prescription: Apo-Chlorthalidone ♣, Hygroton, Thalitone

Do not confuse Hygroton with Hycodan.

Combinations

Prescription: with atenolol (Tenoretic); with clonidine (Combipres, Chlorpres); with reserpine (Demi-Regroton, Regroton)

CLINICAL PHARMACOLOGY

Mechanism of Action

A thiazide diuretic that blocks reabsorption of sodium, potassium, and water at the distal convoluted tubule; also decreases plasma and extracellular fluid volume and peripheral vascular resistance. **Therapeutic Effect:** Produces diuresis; lowers BP.

PHARMACOKINETICS

Route	Onset	Peak	Duration
PO (diuretic)	2 hr	2-6 hr	Up to 72 hr

Rapidly absorbed from the GI tract. Excreted unchanged in urine. **Half-life:** 35-50 hr. Onset of antihypertensive effect: 3-4 days; optimal therapeutic effect: 3-4 wk.

AVAILABILITY

Tablets (Hygroton, Thalitone): 15 mg, 25 mg, 50 mg, 100 mg.

INDICATIONS AND DOSAGE

Hypertension, edema

PO

Adults: 25-100 mg/day or 100 mg 3 times per wk. **Elderly:** Initially, 12.5-25 mg/day or every other day.

CONTRAINDICATIONS

Anuria, history of hypersensitivity to sulfonamides, chlorthalidone, or other thiazide diuretics, renal decompensation

INTERACTIONS

Drug: **Cholestyramine, colestipol:** May decrease the absorption and effects of chlorthalidone. **Digoxin:** May increase the risk of digoxin toxicity associated with chlorthalidone-induced hyperkalemia. **Lithium:** May increase the risk of lithium toxicity. **Herbal:** **Licorice:** May increase the risk of hypokalemia, reduce the effectiveness of chlorthalidone, or both. **Food:** None known.

DIAGNOSTIC TEST EFFECTS

May increase blood glucose and serum cholesterol, LDL, bilirubin, calcium, creatinine, uric acid, and triglyceride levels. May decrease urinary calcium and serum magnesium, potassium, and sodium levels.

SIDE-EFFECTS

Expected: Increase in urinary frequency and urine volume. **Frequent:** Potassium depletion (rarely produces symptoms), photosensitivity. **Occasional:** Anorexia, impotence, diarrhea, orthostatic hypotension, GI disturbances. **Rare:** Rash

CRITICAL CARE CONSIDERATIONS

ADMINISTRATION/HANDLING

PO ALERT

- Give chlorthalidone with food or milk if GI upset occurs.
- Administer with breakfast to help prevent nocturia.
- Crush scored tablets if needed.

PRECAUTIONS

HEALTH-RELATED

- Use chlorthalidone cautiously in debilitated patients and in patients with diabetes mellitus, gout, hypercholesterolemia, hepatic impairment, or severe renal disease.
- **Renal disease:** Chlorthalidone may prompt azotemia; do not use with anuria.
- **Progressive liver disease:** May prompt hepatic coma by minor alterations in fluid and electrolyte balance.
- **Systemic lupus erythematosus:** Exacerbation is reported with thiazide diuretics, which are structurally similar, but has not been seen with chlorthalidone.

AGE-RELATED

- **Children:** Safety and efficacy of chlorthalidone have not been established in children.
- **Elderly:** Use with caution; elderly patients may be more sensitive to hypotensive and electrolyte effects.

PREGNANCY/LACTATION-RELATED

- Pregnancy category B (D if used in pregnancy-induced hypertension); therapy for preexisting hypertension can be continued throughout pregnancy with minimal risk; initiating for simple edema not recommended; few unequivocal indications for diuretic therapy in pregnancy except for pulmonary edema or congestive heart failure; compatible with breast-feeding.

MONITORING

- **Baseline assessment:** Assess for hypotension before administering chlorthalidone. Examine for edema and assess mucous membranes and skin turgor to determine hydration status. Evaluate mental status and muscle strength.
- **Baseline lab work:** Assess electrolyte levels, particularly serum sodium, potassium, and chloride levels.
- **Fluid and electrolyte imbalance:** Monitor for electrolyte disturbances. *Hypokalemia:* altered mental status, muscle cramps, nausea and vomiting, tachycardia, asthenia, and tremor. *Hyponatremia:* cold and clammy skin, confusion, and thirst.
- **Hyperglycemia:** For patients receiving prolonged therapy, periodically check the blood glucose level for hyperglycemia. Insulin and/or oral hypoglycemic agent dose may need to be increased.
- **Patient education:** When using chlorthalidone outside the hospital, teach patients to eat foods high in potassium such as apricots, bananas, raisins, orange juice, potatoes, legumes, meat, and whole grains (including cereals). Urge patients to avoid prolonged exposure to sunlight to avoid sunburn. Instruct patients to change positions slowly to reduce the drug's hypotensive effect.

SERIOUS ADVERSE REACTIONS

- **Dehydration/electrolyte imbalance:** Vigorous diuresis may lead to profound water and electrolyte depletion resulting in hypokalemia, hyponatremia, mild hypochloremia, and dehydration.
- **Hypotension:** Acute hypotensive episodes may occur.
- **Hyperglycemia:** May occur during prolonged therapy.

C

OVERDOSE/TOXICITY

- **Symptoms:** Lethargy and coma without changes in electrolytes or hydration. Hepatic coma may be seen in patients with underlying liver disease.
- **GI decontamination:** No specific recommendations.

ANTIDOTE/DIALYSIS

- **Antidote:** No specific recommendations.
- **Dialysis:** Chlorthalidone is not removed by hemodialysis and is unlikely to be removed by peritoneal dialysis. No data are available on removal by high-permeability hemodialysis.

cholestyramine resin

koe-less-tir'-a-meen reh'-zin

Classes
Chemical: bile acid sequestrant
Therapeutic: antilipemic, bile acid sequestrant

Pregnancy Category: C

Trade Names
Prescription: Questran, Questran Light, LoCHOLEST, LoCHOLEST Light, Prevalite

Do not confuse Questran with Quarzan.

CLINICAL PHARMACOLOGY

Mechanism of Action

An antihyperlipoproteinemic that binds with bile acids in the intestine, forming an insoluble complex. Binding results in partial removal of bile acid from enterohepatic circulation. **Therapeutic Effect:** Removes LDL cholesterol from plasma.

PHARMACOKINETICS

Not absorbed from the GI tract. Decreases in serum LDL apparent in 5-7 days and in serum cholesterol in 1 mo. Serum cholesterol returns to baseline levels about 1 mo after drug is discontinued.

AVAILABILITY

Powder for oral suspension: 4 g/5 g (Questran Light), 4 g/9 g (Prevalite, Questran).

INDICATIONS AND DOSAGE

Hypercholesterolemia

PO

Adults, Elderly: Initially, 4 g 1-2 times per day. Maintenance: 8-16 g/day in divided doses. Maximum: 24 g/day. **Children:** 80 mg/kg 3 times per day.

Pruritis

PO

Adults, Elderly. Initially, 4 g 1-2 times per day. Maintenance: 8-16 g/day in divided doses. Maximum: 24 g/day.

OFF-LABEL USES

Treatment of diarrhea (due to bile acids), hyperoxaluria

CONTRAINDICATIONS

Complete biliary obstruction, hypersensitivity to cholestyramine or tartrazine (frequently seen in aspirin hypersensitivity)

INTERACTIONS

Drug: Anticoagulants: May increase effects of these drugs by decreasing level of vitamin K. **Digoxin, folic acid, penicillins, propranolol, tetracyclines, thiazides, thyroid hormones, other medications:** May bind and decrease absorption of these drugs. **Mycophenolate mofetil:** May reduce mycophenolic acid exposure. **Oral vancomycin:** Binds and decreases the effects of oral vancomycin. **Warfarin:** May decrease warfarin absorption. **Herbal:** None known. **Food: Folic acid, calcium, iron:** Cholestyramine may decrease absorption of these items.

DIAGNOSTIC TEST EFFECTS

May increase serum alkaline phosphatase, serum magnesium, AST (SGOT), and ALT (SGPT) levels. May decrease serum calcium, potassium, and sodium levels. May prolong prothrombin time.

SIDE-EFFECTS

Frequent: Constipation (may lead to fecal impaction), nausea, vomiting, abdominal pain, indigestion. **Occasional:** Diarrhea, belching, bloating, headache, dizziness. **Rare:** Gallstones, peptic ulcer disease, malabsorption syndrome

CRITICAL CARE CONSIDERATIONS

ADMINISTRATION/HANDLING

PO ALERT

- **Other medications:** Give other drugs at least 1 hr before or 4-6 hr after cholestyramine because this drug is capable of binding drugs in the GI tract.
- **Dry form:** Highly irritating to the GI tract. Mix with 3-6 ounces of fruit juice, milk, soup, or water. Allow powder to sit on the surface of liquid for 1-2 min to prevent lumping; then mix thoroughly. When

mixing powder with carbonated beverages, stir liquid slowly in an extra large glass to avoid excessive foaming.
- Administer cholestyramine before meals to promote binding with bile acids.

PRECAUTIONS

HEALTH-RELATED
- Use cholestyramine cautiously in patients with bleeding disorders, GI dysfunction (especially constipation), hemorrhoids, or osteoporosis.
- May cause hyperchloremic acidosis in children, smaller patients, those with renal insufficiency, volume depletion, and those receiving spironolactone.

AGE-RELATED
- **Children:** No age-related precautions have been noted, but cholestyramine use is limited in children under 10 yr.
- **Elderly:** Are at increased risk for experiencing adverse nutritional effects and GI side effects.

PREGNANCY/LACTATION-RELATED
- Pregnancy category C; should be used cautiously in nursing mothers; lack of vitamin absorption may affect nursing infants.

MONITORING
- **Baseline assessment:** Determine history of hypersensitivity to aspirin, cholestyramine, and tartrazine before beginning cholestyramine therapy.
- **Baseline lab work:** Blood chemistry, serum cholesterol, and triglyceride levels.
- **Constipation:** Assess pattern of daily bowel activity and stool consistency. Encourage several glasses of water between meals.
- **Abdominal symptoms:** Evaluate for pain, flatulence, and food tolerance.
- **Therapeutic effect:** Monitor for lower cholesterol levels.
- **Administration:** Give other drugs at least 1 hr before or 4-6 hr after cholestyramine.
- **Patient education:** When using cholestyramine outside the hospital, advise patients to complete a full course of therapy. Caution against omitting or changing drug doses. Warn to never take cholestyramine in its dry form. Teach proper mixing with liquids. Instruct patients to take cholestyramine before meals. Explain prevention of constipation: drink several glasses of water between meals, eat high-fiber foods such as fruits, whole-grain cereals, and vegetables.

SERIOUS ADVERSE REACTIONS
- High dosage may interfere with fat absorption, resulting in steatorrhea.

OVERDOSE/TOXICITY
- Bowel obstruction, hyperchloremic acidosis, and osteoporosis secondary to calcium excretion may occur.
- **Vitamin deficiencies:** Bleeding due to hypoprothrombinemia (vitamin K deficiency), night blindness due to vitamin A deficiency, vitamin D deficiency (causes symptoms of hypocalcemia). Two deaths have been reported in pediatric patients.
- **GI decontamination:** Whole bowel irrigation may be of additional use to help clear bound bile acid complexes. Drug is not absorbed systemically.

ANTIDOTE/DIALYSIS
- **Antidote:** No specific recommendations.
- **Dialysis:** Cholestyramine is unlikely to be removed by hemodialysis, high-permeability hemodialysis, or peritoneal dialysis.

choline salicylate

See Salicylates (p. 982)

cidofovir

See Antivirals (p. 937)

cilostazol

sil-oh'-sta-zol

Classes
Chemical: quinolinone derivative
Therapeutic: hemorrheologic agent

Pregnancy Category: C

Trade Names
Prescription: Pletal

Do not confuse Pletal with Plendil.

CLINICAL PHARMACOLOGY

Mechanism of Action
A phosphodiesterase III inhibitor that inhibits platelet aggregation. Dilates vascular beds with greatest dilation in femoral beds. **Therapeutic Effect:** Improves walking distance in patients with intermittent claudication.

C

PHARMACOKINETICS

Moderately absorbed from the GI tract. Protein binding: 95%-98%. Extensively metabolized in the liver. Excreted primarily in the urine and, to a lesser extent, in the feces. Not removed by hemodialysis. **Half-life:** 11-13 hr. Therapeutic effect is usually noted in 2-4 wk but may take as long as 12 wk.

AVAILABILITY

Tablets: 50 mg, 100 mg.

INDICATIONS AND DOSAGE

Intermittent claudication

PO

Adults, Elderly: 100 mg twice per day at least 30 min before or 2 hr after meals. 50 mg twice per day during concurrent therapy with clarithromycin, diltiazem, erythromycin, fluconazole, fluoxetine, omeprazole, or sertraline.

CONTRAINDICATIONS

Heart failure of any severity; hemostatic disorders or active pathologic bleeding, such as bleeding peptic ulcer and intracranial bleeding; hypersensitivity to cilostazol

INTERACTIONS

Drug: Clarithromycin, diltiazem, erythromycin, fluconazole, fluoxetine, omeprazole, sertraline: May increase concentration of cilostazol. Decrease dose of cilostazol by 50%. **Aspirin:** May potentiate inhibition of platelet aggregation. **Herbal:** None known. **Food: Grapefruit, grapefruit juice:** May increase blood concentration and risk of toxicity of cilostazol.

DIAGNOSTIC TEST EFFECTS

May increase BUN and serum creatinine levels. May decrease Hgb and Hct.

SIDE-EFFECTS

Frequent (34%-10%): Headache, diarrhea, palpitations, dizziness, pharyngitis. **Occasional (7%-3%):** Nausea, rhinitis, back pain, peripheral edema, dyspepsia, abdominal pain, tachycardia, cough, flatulence, myalgia. **Rare (2%-1%):** Leg cramps, paresthesia, rash, vomiting

CRITICAL CARE CONSIDERATIONS

ADMINISTRATION/HANDLING

PO ALERT

- Give at least 30 min before or 2 hr after meals.
- Do not give cilostazol with grapefruit juice.

PRECAUTIONS

HEALTH-RELATED

- Cilostazol is contraindicated in patients with any degree of heart failure.

AGE-RELATED

- **Children:** Safety and efficacy of cilostazol have not been established in children.
- **Elderly:** No age-related precautions have been noted in the elderly.

PREGNANCY/LACTATION-RELATED

- Pregnancy category C; excreted in breast milk.

MONITORING

- **Baseline assessment:** Assess Hgb, Hct, and platelet count before and periodically during cilostazol treatment.
- **Therapeutic effect:** Assess for relief of cramping in the feet, calf muscles, thighs, and buttocks during exercise. Assess for improved walking endurance.
- **Cardiac monitoring:** Assess for tachycardia, ventricular premature beats.

SERIOUS ADVERSE REACTIONS

- Asthenia, hypertension, hematuria, angina pectoris, arthritis, bronchitis.
- Heart failure leading to death when given to patients with underlying heart failure.
- Interaction with other medications metabolized by the cytochrome P450 pathway (erythromycin, ketoconazole, omerprazole, diltiazem).

OVERDOSE/TOXICITY

- Headache, diarrhea, hypotension, and cardiac dysrhythmias including ventricular tachycardia.
- **GI decontamination:** No specific recommendations.

ANTIDOTE/DIALYSIS

- **Antidote:** No specific recommendations.
- **Dialysis:** Cilostazol is not removed by hemodialysis or peritoneal dialysis. No data are available on removal by high-permeability hemodialysis.

cimetidine

See Acid Secretion Inhibitors (p. 884)

cinoxacin

See Antibiotics (p. 892)

ciprofloxacin hydrochloride

sip-ro-floks'-a-sin hye-droe-klor'-ide

Classes
Chemical: fluoroquinolone derivative
Therapeutic: antibiotic

Pregnancy Category: C

Trade Names
Prescription: Ciloxan (ophthalmic), Cipro, Cipro I.V., Cipro XR, Proquin XR

Do not confuse ciprofloxacin or Ciproxin with Ciloxan, cinoxacin, or Cytoxan.

CLINICAL PHARMACOLOGY

Mechanism of Action
A fluoroquinolone that inhibits the enzyme DNA gyrase in susceptible bacteria, interfering with bacterial cell replication. **Therapeutic Effect:** Bactericidal.

PHARMACOKINETICS

Well absorbed from the GI tract (food delays absorption). Protein binding: 20%-40%. Widely distributed (including to cerebrospinal fluid). Metabolized in the liver to active metabolite. Primarily excreted in urine. Minimal removal by hemodialysis. **Half-life:** 4-6 hr (increased in impaired renal function and the elderly).

AVAILABILITY

Tablets (Cipro): 100 mg, 250 mg, 500 mg, 750 mg.
Tablets (Extended Release): 500 mg (Cipro XR, Proquin XR), 1000 mg (Cipro XR).
Infusion (Cipro I.V.): 200 mg/100 mL, 400 mg/200 mL.
Intravenous Solution (Cipro I.V.): 10 mg/mL.
Ophthalmic Ointment (Ciloxan): 0.3%.
Ophthalmic Suspension (Ciloxan): 0.3%.
Oral Suspension, Powder for Reconstitution (Cipro): 250 mg/5 mL, 500 mg/5 mL.

INDICATIONS AND DOSAGE

Bone and joint infections
IV
Adults, Elderly: 400 mg every 12 hr for 4-6 wk.
PO
Adults, Elderly: 500 mg every 12 hr for 4-6 wk.

Conjunctivitis
Ophthalmic
Adults, Elderly: 1-2 drops every 2 hr for 2 days, then 2 drops every 4 hr for next 5 days.

Corneal ulcer
Ophthalmic
Adults, Elderly: 2 drops every 15 min for 6 hr, then 2 drops every 30 min for the remainder of first day, 2 drops every 1 hr on second day, and 2 drops every 4 hr on days 3-14.

Cystic fibrosis
IV
Children 5-17 yr: 30 mg/kg/day in 3 divided doses for 1 wk followed by oral therapy. Maximum: 1.2 g/day.
PO
Children: 40 mg/kg/day in divided doses every 12 hr following 1 wk of IV therapy. Maximum: 2 g/day.

Febrile neutropenia
IV
Adults, Elderly: 400 mg every 8 hr for 7-14 days (in combination).

Gonorrhea
PO
Adults, Elderly: 250-500 mg as a single dose.

Infectious diarrhea
PO
Adults, Elderly: 500 mg every 12 hr for 5-7 days.

Intraabdominal infections (with metronidazole)
IV
Adults, Elderly: 400 mg every 12 hr for 7-14 days.
PO
Adults, Elderly: 500 mg every 12 hr for 7-14 days.

Lower respiratory tract infections
IV
Adults, Elderly: 400 mg every 12 hr for 7-14 days.
PO
Adults, Elderly: 500 mg every 12 hr for 7-14 days (750 mg every 12 hr for 7-14 days for severe or complicated infections).

Nosocomial pneumonia
IV
Adults, Elderly: 400 mg every 8 hr for 10-14 days.

Prostatitis
IV
Adults, Elderly: 400 mg every 12 hr for 28 days.
PO
Adults, Elderly: 500 mg every 12 hr for 28 days.

Sinusitis
IV
Adults, Elderly: 400 mg every 12 hr for 10 days.

PO
Adults, Elderly: 500 mg every 12 hr for 10 days.
Skin and skin structure infections
IV
Adults, Elderly: 400 mg every 12 hr for 7-14 days.
PO
Adults, Elderly: 500 mg every 12 hr for 7-14 days (750 mg every 12 hr for severe or complicated infections).
Susceptible infections
IV
Adults, Elderly: 400 mg every 8-12 hr.
PO
Adults, Elderly: 500-750 mg every 12 hr.
Typhoid fever
PO
Adults, Elderly: 500 mg every 12 hr for 10 days.
UTIs
IV
Adults, Elderly: 200 mg every 12 hr for 7-14 days (400 mg every 12 hr for severe or complicated infections).
PO
Adults, Elderly: 100-250 mg every 12 hr for 3 days for acute uncomplicated infections; 250 mg every 12 hr for 7-14 days for mild to moderate infections; 500 mg every 12 hr for 7-14 days for severe or complicated infections.
Dosage in renal impairment
Dosage and frequency are modified based on creatinine clearance and the severity of the infection.

Creatinine Clearance	Dosage
Less than 30 mL/min	PO: 250-500 mg every 18 hr; IV: 200-400 mg every 18-24 hr

Hemodialysis
Adults, Elderly: 250-500 mg every 24 hr (after dialysis).
Peritoneal Dialysis
Adults, Elderly: 250-500 mg every 24 hr (after dialysis).

OFF-LABEL USES
Treatment of chancroid

CONTRAINDICATIONS
Hypersensitivity to ciprofloxacin or other quinolones; for ophthalmic administration: vaccinia, varicella, epithelial herpes simplex, keratitis, mycobacterial infection, fungal disease of ocular structure, use after uncomplicated removal of a foreign body

INTERACTIONS
Drug: Antacids, iron preparations, sucralfate: May decrease ciprofloxacin absorption. **Antidiabetic agents:** May produce changes in blood glucose and increase the risk of hypoglycemia or hyperglycemia. **Caffeine, oral anticoagulants:** May increase the effects of these drugs. **Corticosteroids:** May increase the risk for tendon rupture. **Fosphenytoin, phenytoin:** May increase or decrease fosphenytoin or phenytoin levels. **Probenecid:** May increase the serum levels of ciprofloxacin. **Theophylline:** Decreases clearance and may increase blood concentration and risk of toxicity of theophylline. **Herbal: Dong quai, St. John's wort:** Increased photosensitivity. **Fennel:** May decrease the bioavailability of ciprofloxacin and cause possible treatment failure. **Guar gum:** May cause changes in blood glucose and increase the risk of hypoglycemia or hyperglycemia. **Food: Dairy food or calcium-fortified juices:** May decrease ciprofloxacin concentrations.

DIAGNOSTIC TEST EFFECTS
May increase BUN and serum alkaline phosphatase, bilirubin, creatinine, LDH, AST (SGOT), and ALT (SGPT) levels.

IV INCOMPATIBILITIES
Aminophylline, ampicillin and sulbactam (Unasyn), cefepime (Maxipime), dexamethasone (Decadron), furosemide (Lasix), heparin, hydrocortisone (Solu-Cortef), *methylPREDNISolone (Solu-Medrol), phenytoin (Dilantin), sodium bicarbonate, total parenteral nutrition (TPN)

IV COMPATIBILITIES
Calcium gluconate, diltiazem (Cardizem), *DOBUTamine (Dobutrex), *DOPamine (Intropin), lidocaine, lorazepam (Ativan), magnesium, midazolam (Versed), potassium chloride

SIDE-EFFECTS
Frequent (5%-2%): Nausea, diarrhea, dyspepsia, vomiting, constipation, flatulence, confusion, crystalluria
Ophthalmic: Burning, crusting in corner of eye. **Occasional (less than 2%):** Abdominal pain or discomfort, headache, rash, dizziness, bad taste, sensation of something in eye, eyelid redness or itching. **Rare (less than 1%):** Dizziness, confusion, tremors, hallucinations, hypersensitivity reaction, insomnia, dry mouth, paresthesia

C

CRITICAL CARE CONSIDERATIONS

ADMINISTRATION/HANDLING

PO ALERT

- Preferred administration time is 2 hr after a meal, but ciprofloxacin may be given without regard to food.
- Do not administer oral suspension by nasogastric tube.
- Oral suspension may be stored for 14 days at room temperature.
- Do not administer antacids containing aluminum or magnesium within 2 hr of ciprofloxacin.
- Provide patients with sufficient amounts of citrus fruits and cranberry juice to acidify urine to prevent crystalluria.

IV ALERT

- **Storage:** Store the injection form at room temperature protected from light and heat. IV ciprofloxacin is available prediluted in ready-to-use infusion containers.
- **Dilution:** After withdrawing the drug from a 200-mg or 400-mg vial, further dilute it with D_5W or 0.9% NaCl for injection to a final concentration of 1 to 2 mg/mL. The solution normally appears clear and colorless or slightly yellow. Stable for 14 days if refrigerated.
- **Infusion:** Infuse the drug over 60 min.

OPHTHALMIC ALERT

- **Administration:** Tilt the head back and place the solution in the conjunctival sac of the affected eye. Close the eye and then press gently on the lacrimal sac for 1 min.
- Do not use ophthalmic solutions for injection.
- Unless the eye infection is very superficial, systemic administration is generally used along with ophthalmic treatment.

PRECAUTIONS

HEALTH-RELATED

- Use ciprofloxacin cautiously in patients with CNS disorders, renal impairment, cardiomyopathy, hypokalemia, seizures, and those taking caffeine or theophylline. May cause serious and fatal reactions when given with theophylline including cardiac arrest, seizures, respiratory failure, and dysrhythmias.

AGE-RELATED

- **Children:** Safety and efficacy of ciprofloxacin have not been established in children under 18 yr. May erode cartilage of weight bearing joints in infants and children.
- **Elderly:** Age-related renal impairment may require a dosage adjustment.

PREGNANCY/LACTATION-RELATED

- Pregnancy category C; appears in breast milk at levels similar to serum; allow 48 hr to elapse after last dose before resuming breast-feeding.

MONITORING

- **Baseline assessment:** Determine history of hypersensitivity to ciprofloxacin or other quinolones before beginning drug therapy.
- **Baseline lab work:** Basic chemical profile including K+, BUN, and creatinine levels to evaluate renal function. Obtain culture of infected area before drug administration (wound, blood, sputum, urine).
- **Superinfections:** Assess the mouth for white patches on the mucous membranes or tongue and for severe mouth or tongue soreness; assess for severe anal or genital pruritus or discharge.
- ***Clostridium difficile*** **colitis:** Assess the pattern of daily bowel activity and stool consistency. Although mild GI effects may be tolerable, severe symptoms including abdominal pain or cramping, and moderate to severe diarrhea may indicate the onset of antibiotic-associated colitis.
- **Hand washing:** If *C. difficile* colitis develops, wash hands with antibacterial soap; alcohol-based foam is ineffective against *C. difficile* spores.
- **Nephrotoxicity:** Monitor intake and output and renal function test results to assess for nephrotoxicity.
- **Therapeutic response:** Observe patients receiving the ophthalmic form for a therapeutic response.
- **Side effects:** Evaluate for dizziness, headache, tremors, and visual problems. Assess for chest and joint pain.
- **Patient education:** When using ciprofloxacin outside the hospital, advise patients not to skip drug doses and to take ciprofloxacin for the full course of therapy. Ciprofloxacin should be taken during meals with 8 oz of water. Patients should drink several glasses of water between meals. Shake the oral suspension well before taking it and instruct patients not to chew the microcapsules in the suspension.

Sugarless gum or hard candy may relieve ciprofloxacin's bad taste. Explain to patients receiving the ophthalmic form that a crystal precipitate may form but usually resolves in 1-7 days.

SERIOUS ADVERSE REACTIONS

- Superinfection (especially enterococcal or fungal), nephropathy, cardiopulmonary arrest, chest pain, and cerebral thrombosis may occur.
- **Arthropathy:** May occur if ciprofloxacin is given to children under 18 yr.
- **Sensitization to ophthalmic drug form:** May contraindicate later systemic use of ciprofloxacin.
- **Hypersensitivity:** Patients with a history of allergies, especially to penicillin, are at increased risk for developing a severe hypersensitivity reaction marked by severe pruritus, angioedema, bronchospasm, and anaphylaxis.
- **Manage hypersensitivity:** May require treatment with epinephrine and other emergency measures including oxygen, endotracheal intubation, mechanical ventilation, IV fluids, IV antihistamines, corticosteroids, and vasopressors.

OVERDOSE/TOXICITY

- **Neurologic:** Seizures, increased intracranial pressure, confusion, depression, hallucinations, tremors, and toxic psychosis.
- **Ophthalmic:** Cataracts and other eye abnormalities.
- **Cardiac:** Prolonged QT syndrome, ventricular dysrhythmias, torsades de pointes; more common when patients are receiving other antidysrhythmic drugs that prolong the QT interval (procainamide, quinidine, amiodarone, sotalol).
- **Nephrotoxicity:** May occur, especially in patients with preexisting renal disease.
- **Superinfections:** Antibiotic-associated colitis (pseudomembranous colitis) and other superinfections may result from altered bacterial balance.
- **GI decontamination:** No specific recommendations.

ANTIDOTE/DIALYSIS

- **Antidote:** No specific recommendations.
- **Dialysis:** Ciprofloxacin is partially removed by both hemodialysis and peritoneal dialysis. No data are available on removal by high-permeability hemodialysis. Ciprofloxacin should be given following hemodialysis on dialysis days and following last exchange if peritoneal dialysis is used.

cisatracurium besylate 

sis-a-tra-kyoo'-ree-um bess'-il-ate

Classes

Chemical: nondepolarizing neuromuscular blocking agent

Therapeutic: skeletal muscle relaxation, paralysis

Pregnancy Category: B

Trade Names

Prescription: Nimbex

CLINICAL PHARMACOLOGY

Mechanism of Action

A nondepolarizing skeletal muscle relaxant that blocks the neurotransmitter action of acetylcholine by binding competitively with cholinergic receptor sites. **Therapeutic Effect:** Produces skeletal muscle relaxation.

PHARMACOKINETICS

Onset of action is dose-dependent and occurs within 2-3 min. Recovery begins in 20-35 min. Protein binding: Unknown. Undergoes ester hydrolysis and Hofmann elimination. Primarily excreted in urine. **Half-life:** 22 min.

AVAILABILITY

IV solution: 2 mg/mL, 10 mg/mL (Nimbex).

INDICATIONS AND DOSAGE

Adjunct to general anesthesia; to facilitate endotracheal intubation and to provide skeletal muscle relaxation during surgery or mechanical ventilation

IV

Adults, Elderly, Children 12 yr and older: 0.15-0.2 mg/kg as bolus injection. A dose of 0.03 mg/kg cisatracurium besylate is recommended for maintenance of neuromuscular blockade during prolonged surgical procedures. Maintenance dosing is generally required 40-50 min following an initial dose of 0.15 mg/kg cisatracurium besylate and 50-60 min following an initial dose of 0.20 mg/kg cisatracurium besylate, but the need for maintenance doses should be determined by clinical criteria. **Children 2-12 yr:** 0.1 mg/kg administered over 5-10 sec during either halothane or opioid anesthesia.

Long-term mechanical ventilation in the intensive care unit (ICU)

IV

Adults, Elderly: 3 mcg/kg/min (range: 0.5-10.2 mcg/kg/min) continuous infusion. **Children:** Infusion rates may be higher in pediatric patients than in adult patients.

CONTRAINDICATIONS

Hypersensitivity to cisatracurium or any component of the formulation

INTERACTIONS

Drug: **Isoflurane, enflurane, aminoglycosides, polymyxins, lithium, magnesium salts, procainamide, and quinidine:** May enhance neuromuscular blockade, which may lead to respiratory depression and paralysis. **Muscle relaxants:** May block the effects of cisatracurium. Herbal: **St. John's wort:** May increase the risk of cardiovascular collapse and/or delay emergence from anesthesia. Food: None known.

DIAGNOSTIC TEST EFFECTS

None known.

IV INCOMPATIBILITIES

Alkaline solutions (e.g., barbiturate solutions), propofol (Diprivan), ketorolac (Toradol)

IV COMPATIBILITIES

Alfentanil (Alfenta), droperidol (Inapsine), fentanyl (Sublimaze), midazolam (Versed), sufentanil (Sufenta)

SIDE-EFFECTS

Rare: Bradycardia, hypotension, flushing, bronchospasm, rash

CRITICAL CARE CONSIDERATIONS

ADMINISTRATION/HANDLING

IM ALERT

- Do not give as IM injection because tissue irritation may result.

IV ALERT

- **High potency:** Neuromuscular blocking potency is 3-5 times that of atracurium.
- **Skilled providers only:** Cisatracurium should be used only by those skilled in airway management and respiratory support. Nimbex injection, 20-mL vial containing 10 mg of cisatracurium per milliliter, is intended only for use in the ICU.
- **IV bolus:** May be administered undiluted as bolus injection.
- **IV infusion:** Infusions should be initiated only after early evidence of spontaneous recovery from the initial bolus dose has been observed.
- **Dilution:** Cisatracurium besylate injection diluted in D_5W, 0.9% NaCl, or D_5NS solution to 0.1 mg/mL may be stored either in the refrigerator or at room temperature for 24 hr without significant loss of potency. Dilutions to 0.1 or 0.2 mg/mL in D_5W may be stored under refrigeration for 24 hr. Cisatracurium besylate injection should not be diluted in lactated Ringer's solution because of chemical instability.
- **Storage:** Refrigerate intact vials. Use vials within 21 days on removal from refrigerator at room temperature.

CISATRACURIUM (CONCENTRATION 0.1 MG/ML) INFUSION RATE TABLE

WEIGHT	DRUG DOSE (MCG/KG/MIN)				
	1	1.5	2	3	5
5 kg	3	4.5	6	9	15
10 kg	6	9	12	18	30
45 kg	27	41	54	81	135
50 kg	30	45	60	90	150
70 kg	42	63	84	126	210
100 kg	60	90	120	180	300

CISATRACURIUM (CONCENTRATION 0.4 MG/ML) INFUSION RATE TABLE

WEIGHT	DRUG DOSE (MCG/KG/MIN)				
	1	1.5	2	3	5
5 kg	0.8	1.2	1.5	2.3	3.8
10 kg	1.5	2.3	3	4.5	7.5
45 kg	6.8	10.1	13.5	20.3	33.8
50 kg	7.5	11.3	15	22.5	37.5
70 kg	10.5	15.8	21	31.5	52.5
100 kg	15	22.5	30	45	75

PRECAUTIONS

HEALTH-RELATED

- Use cautiously in patients with electrolyte disturbances, hypothermia, myasthenia gravis, Eaton-Lambert syndrome, amyotrophic lateral sclerosis, respiratory acidosis, severe obesity, dystrophia myotonica, or impaired renal or liver function.
- Not recommended for use in rapid sequence intubation; succinylcholine is the drug of choice.

AGE-RELATED

- **Children:** Safety and efficacy of cisatracurium have not been established in children under 2 yr.
- **Elderly:** No age-related precautions have been noted.

PREGNANCY/LACTATION-RELATED

- Pregnancy category B; breast-feeding should be deferred until patients are fully recovered.

MONITORING

- **Baseline assessment:** Assess vital signs, perform a complete physical assessment with focus on efficacy of breathing, neurologic status, level of pain or anticipated level of pain, and anxiety.

- **Sedation and analgesia:** Patients undergoing neuromuscular blockade with cisatracurium should be sedated and have appropriate pain management provided because patients are unable to express anxiety and discomfort during neuromuscular blockade. Cisatracurium besylate produces apnea and paralysis.
- **Ongoing assessment:** Monitor heart rate, continuous ECG, BP, pulse oximetry, and respiratory rate. Try to assess level of pain. Assess renal and liver function if the patient is in the intensive care unit.
- **Sedation and neuromuscular blockade:** Monitor the degree of neuromuscular blockade using "train of four" technique with a peripheral nerve stimulator and sedation with a bispectral brain wave analysis device (BIS monitoring). Adjust cisatracurium and other medications to keep patients still, well ventilated, and as comfortable as possible. Because patients are totally dependent on health care providers to anticipate all needs and provide all care, most patients would rather not be aware of the neuromuscular blockade experience.
- **Provide mechanical ventilation:** Assess ventilation status using lung assessment, vital signs, pulse oximetry, and end tidal CO_2 monitoring. Tachycardia and dysrhythmias may indicate hypoxemia is present.
- **Weaning neuromusclar blockade:** Sedation with propofol (Diprivan), benzodiazepine infusion (lorazepam/Ativan), or morphine may provide enough relaxation to be able to wean cisatracurium without compromising the critically ill patients' ventilatory status. Confirm recovery with 5-second head lift and grip strength once cisatracurium is weaned.
- **Patient education:** Explain to patients they are unable to speak, open eyes, and move when full neuromuscular blockade is in place. When weaning cisatracurium, explain it will be difficult to talk due to head and neck muscle blockade.

SERIOUS ADVERSE REACTIONS

- Dysrhythmias, edema, and hypotension may occur.
- Anaphylaxis and hypersensitivity reactions have been reported.

OVERDOSE/TOXICITY

- **Symptoms:** Prolonged apnea, respiratory depression, inability to maintain patent airway, to move extremities, speak, or open eyes. May occur more often when agents that potentiate cisatracurium besylate are given concomitantly. Seizures have been reported in critically ill patients, but the cause may be multifactorial. Cardiovascular collapse occurs rarely.
- **Management:** Continue to keep patients endotracheally intubated and mechanically ventilated until they are fully able to effectively maintain breathing and respiration. Antidote may be administered if needed. Resuscitate per Advanced Cardiac Life Support (ACLS) guidelines for cardiac arrest.
- **GI decontamination:** No specific recommendations.

ANTIDOTE/DIALYSIS

- **Antidote:** Edrophonium (Enlon) or neostigmine (Prostigmin) 1-3 mg IV push (0.5 mg IV push for children) given with atropine reverses muscle relaxation in most patients but may aggravate severe overdosage. Ensure that patients are endotracheally intubated and that mechanical or manual ventilation is in place.
- **Dialysis:** Hemodialysis or peritoneal dialysis is unlikely to remove cisatracurium. No data are available on removal by high-permeability hemodialayis.

citalopram hydrobromide

sye-tal'-oh-pram hye-droe-broe'-mide

Classes

Chemical: bicyclic phthalane derivative
Therapeutic: antidepressant, selective serotonin reuptake inhibitor (SSRI)

Pregnancy Category: C

Trade Names

Prescription: Celexa

Do not confuse Celexa with Celebrex, Zyprexa, or Cerebyx.

CLINICAL PHARMACOLOGY

Mechanism of Action

A selective serotonin reuptake inhibitor that blocks the uptake of the neurotransmitter serotonin at CNS presynaptic neuronal membranes, increasing its availability at postsynaptic receptor sites. **Therapeutic Effect:** Relieves depression.

PHARMACOKINETICS
Well absorbed after PO administration. Protein binding: 80%. Primarily metabolized in the liver. Primarily excreted in feces with a lesser amount eliminated in urine. **Half-life:** 35 hr.

AVAILABILITY
Oral solution: 10 mg/5 mL.
Tablets: 10 mg, 20 mg, 40 mg.
Tablets (orally disintegrating): 10 mg, 20 mg, 40 mg.

INDICATIONS AND DOSAGE
Depression
PO
Adults: Initially, 20 mg once per day in the morning or evening. May increase in 20-mg increments at intervals of no less than 1 wk. Maximum: 60 mg/day. **Elderly, Patients with hepatic impairment:** 10-20 mg/day. May titrate to 40 mg/day only for nonresponding patients.

OFF-LABEL USES
Treatment of alcohol abuse, dementia, diabetic neuropathy, obsessive–compulsive disorder, panic disorder, smoking cessation

CONTRAINDICATIONS
Sensitivity to citalopram, use within 14 days of MAOIs

INTERACTIONS
Drug: Antifungals, cimetidine, macrolide antibiotics: May increase the citalopram plasma level. **Carbamazepine:** May decrease the citalopram plasma level. **Lithium:** May increase lithium concentration and/or increase the risk of serotonin syndrome. **MAOIs:** May cause serotonin syndrome, marked by autonomic hyperactivity, coma, diaphoresis, excitement, hyperthermia, and rigidity, and neuroleptic malignant syndrome. **Metoprolol:** Increases the metoprolol plasma level. **Herbal: Ginkgo biloba, St. John's wort:** May increase the risk of serotonin syndrome. **Food:** None known.

DIAGNOSTIC TEST EFFECTS
May reduce serum sodium level.

SIDE-EFFECTS
Frequent (21%-11%): Nausea, dry mouth, somnolence, insomnia, diaphoresis. **Occasional (8%-4%):** Tremor, diarrhea, abnormal ejaculation, dyspepsia, fatigue, anxiety, vomiting, anorexia. **Rare (3%-2%):** Sinusitis, sexual dysfunction, menstrual disorder, abdominal pain, agitation, decreased libido

CRITICAL CARE CONSIDERATIONS

ADMINISTRATION/HANDLING
PO ALERT
- Give citalopram without regard to food.
- Crush scored tablets if necessary.
- Allow 14 days to elapse between the use of MAOIs and citalopram to avoid serious, possibly fatal reactions.

PRECAUTIONS
HEALTH-RELATED
- Use citalopram cautiously in patients with hepatic or renal impairment and in those with a history of hypomania, mania, or seizures.

AGE-RELATED
- **Children:** Use in children may increase anticholinergic effects and hyperexcitability.
- **Elderly:** Are more sensitive to the drug's anticholinergic effects, such as dry mouth, and are more likely to experience confusion, dizziness, hyperexcitability, and sedation.

PREGNANCY/LACTATION-RELATED
- Pregnancy category C; breast-feeding: unknown, two cases of infants experiencing excessive somnolence, decreased feeding, and weight loss have been reported.

MONITORING
- **Baseline assessment:** Observe and record appearance, behavior, interest in the environment, mood, sleep pattern, and thought content.
- **Baseline lab work:** CBC and blood chemistry tests before and periodically during therapy for patients on long-term therapy.
- **Suicidal patients:** Closely supervise during early therapy; also when depression lessens, energy level improves, thus increasing risk of suicide.
- **Therapeutic effect:** Assess appearance, behavior, level of interest, mood, and sleep pattern to determine the drug's therapeutic effect.
- **Gradual dosage change:** Do not abruptly discontinue citalopram or increase the dosage.
- **Patient education:** When using citalopram outside of the hospital, urge patients to avoid alcohol and to avoid tasks that

require mental alertness or motor skills until response to the drug is known. Sipping tepid water and chewing sugarless gum may help relieve dry mouth.

C

SERIOUS ADVERSE REACTIONS

- **Serotonin syndrome:** Altered cognition, abnormal behavior, and possibly neuromuscular dysfunction (myoclonus, hyperreflexia, muscle rigidity, extreme tremor), which can lead to seizures, hyperthermia, coma, disseminated intravascular coagulation (DIC), hypotension, ventricular tachycardia, and metabolic acidosis. Occurs when citalopram is given within 14 days of an MAOI (phenelzine [Nardil], tranylcypromine [Parnate]).

OVERDOSE/TOXICITY

- **Symptoms:** Dizziness, hypotension, paresthesia, headache, coughing, sweating, tremors, polyuria, altered taste sensation, drowsiness, tachycardia, somnolence, confusion, and seizures.
- **GI decontamination:** No specific recommendations.

ANTIDOTE/DIALYSIS

- **Antidote:** No specific recommendations.
- **Dialysis:** Citalopram is not removed by hemodialysis or high-permeability hemodialysis and is unlikely to be removed by peritoneal dialysis.

clarithromycin

clare-i-thro-mye'-sin

Classes

Chemical: macrolide derivative
Therapeutic: antibiotic

Pregnancy Category: C

Trade Names

Prescription: Biaxin, Biaxin BID ♣, Biaxin XL, Biaxin XL-Pak

CLINICAL PHARMACOLOGY

Mechanism of Action

A macrolide that binds to ribosomal receptor sites of susceptible organisms, inhibiting protein synthesis of the bacterial cell wall. Therapeutic Effect: Bacteriostatic; may be bactericidal with high dosages or very susceptible microorganisms.

PHARMACOKINETICS

Well absorbed from the GI tract. Protein binding: 65%-75%. Widely distributed. Metabolized in the liver to active metabolite. Primarily excreted in urine. Not removed by hemodialysis. Half-life: 3-7 hr; metabolite 5-7 hr (increased in impaired renal function).

AVAILABILITY

Oral suspension (Biaxin): 125 mg/5 mL, 250 mg/5 mL.
Tablets (Biaxin): 250 mg, 500 mg.
Tablets (extended release [Biaxin XL, Biaxin XL Pak]): 500 mg.

INDICATIONS AND DOSAGE

Bronchitis

PO

Adults, Elderly: 250-500 mg every 12 hr for 7-14 days.

PO (Extended Release)

Adults, Elderly: 1 g once daily for 7 days.

Skin, soft tissue infections

PO

Adults, Elderly: 250 mg every 12 hr for 7-14 days. **Children:** 7.5 mg/kg every 12 hr for 10 days. Maximum: 1 g/day.

Myobacterium avium complex (MAC) prophylaxis

PO

Adults, Elderly: 500 mg twice per day. **Children:** 7.5 mg/kg every 12 hr. Maximum: 500 mg twice per day.

MAC treatment

PO

Adults, Elderly: 500 mg twice per day in combination. **Children:** 7.5 mg/kg every 12 hr in combination. Maximum: 500 mg twice per day.

Pharyngitis, tonsillitis

PO

Adults, Elderly: 250 mg every 12 hr for 10 days. **Children:** 7.5 mg/kg every 12 hr for 10 days. Maximum: 1 g/day.

Pneumonia

PO

Adults, Elderly: 250 mg every 12 hr for 7-14 days. **Children:** 7.5 mg/kg every 12 hr.

PO (Extended Release)

Adults, Elderly: 1 g/day.

Maxillary sinusitis

PO

Adults, Elderly: 500 mg every 12 hr or 1000 mg (two 500 mg extended release) once daily for 14 days. **Children:** 7.5 mg/kg every 12 hr. Maximum: 500 mg twice per day.

Heliobacter pylori

PO

Adults, Elderly: 500 mg every 8-12 hr for 10-14 days in combination.

Acute otitis media

PO

Children: 7.5 mg/kg every 12 hr for 10 days.

Dosage in renal impairment

For patients with creatinine clearance less than 30 mL/min, reduce dose by 50% or double dosing interval.

CONTRAINDICATIONS

Hypersensitivity to clarithromycin or other macrolide antibiotics

INTERACTIONS

Drug: Carbamazepine, digoxin, theophylline: May increase blood concentration and toxicity of these drugs. **Rifampin:** May decrease clarithromycin blood concentration. **Warfarin:** May increase warfarin effects. **Zidovudine:** May decrease blood concentration of zidovudine. **Herbal: St. John's wort:** Decreases clarithromycin levels. **Food:** None known.

DIAGNOSTIC TEST EFFECTS

May (rarely) increase BUN, AST (SGOT), and ALT (SGPT) levels.

SIDE-EFFECTS

Occasional (6%-3%): Diarrhea, nausea, altered taste, abdominal pain. **Rare (2%-1%):** Headache, dyspepsia

CRITICAL CARE CONSIDERATIONS

ADMINISTRATION/HANDLING

PO ALERT

- Give clarithromycin without regard to food.
- Do not crush or break tablets.
- Clarithromycin should be administered with a full 8-oz glass of water.

PRECAUTIONS

HEALTH-RELATED

- Use clarithromycin cautiously in patients with known sensitivity to erythromycin or other macrolides, hepatic or renal dysfunction, and in elderly patients with severe renal impairment.

AGE-RELATED

- **Children:** Safety and efficacy of clarithromycin have not been established in children under 6 mo.
- **Elderly:** Age-related renal impairment may require a dosage adjustment. Elderly with severe renal impairment may require reduced dosage.

PREGNANCY/LACTATION-RELATED

- Pregnancy category C; excretion into breast milk unknown; use caution in nursing mothers.

MONITORING

- **Baseline assessment:** Determine history of allergies, particularly to clarithromycin or other macrolides before beginning drug therapy to help avoid possible allergic reaction to clarithromycin.
- **Baseline lab work:** Chemical profile including K+, BUN, and creatinine levels to evaluate renal function, and serum transaminases (AST [SGOT], ALT [SGPT], GGT), LDH, bilirubin to evaluate liver function. Obtain culture of infected area before drug administration (wound, blood, sputum, urine).
- **Superinfections:** Assess the mouth for white patches on the mucous membranes or tongue and for severe mouth or tongue soreness; assess for severe anal or genital pruritus or discharge.
- ***Clostridium difficile* colitis:** Assess the pattern of daily bowel activity and stool consistency. Although mild GI effects may be tolerable, severe symptoms including abdominal pain or cramping, and moderate to severe diarrhea may indicate the onset of antibiotic-associated colitis.
- **Hand washing:** If *C. difficile* colitis develops, wash hands with antibacterial soap; alcohol-based foam is ineffective against *C. difficile* spores.
- **Nephrotoxicity and hepatotoxicity:** Monitor for fluid retention (edema, positive fluid balance), liver and renal function test results to assess for toxicity.
- **Patient education:** Space doses evenly around the clock. If clarithromycin is used outside the hospital, instruct patients to continue taking clarithromycin for the full course of treatment.

SERIOUS ADVERSE REACTIONS

- **Hypersensitivity:** Patients with a history of allergies, especially to erythromycin and other macrolides, are at increased risk for developing a severe hypersensitivity reaction marked by severe pruritus, angioedema, bronchospasm, and anaphylaxis.
- **Manage hypersensitivity:** May require treatment with epinephrine and other emergency measures including oxygen, endotracheal intubation, mechanical ventilation, IV fluids, IV antihistamines, corticosteroids, and vasopressors.

OVERDOSE/TOXICITY

- **Nephrotoxicity:** Increased BUN and creatinine, decreased urine output, anuria, possible hyperkalemia, fluid overload indicative of acute renal failure.
- **Superinfections:** Antibiotic-associated colitis (pseudomembranous colitis) and other superinfections may result from altered bacterial balance. Discontinue clarithromycin. Oral vancomycin (Vancocin) or metronidazole (Flagyl) are the most effective treatments for pseudomembranous colitis.
- **Hepatotoxicity and thrombocytopenia:** Occur rarely.
- **GI decontamination:** No specific recommendations.

ANTIDOTE/DIALYSIS

- **Antidote:** No specific recommendations.
- **Dialysis:** No data are available on removal of clarithromycin by hemodialysis, peritoneal dialysis, or high-permeability hemodialysis.

clemastine fumarate

klem'-as-teen foo'-mah-rate

Classes

Chemical: ethanolamine derivative
Therapeutic: antihistamine

Pregnancy Category: B

Trade Names

Prescription: Contac 12 Hour Allergy, Dayhistol Allergy, Tavist Allergy

Combinations

Over the Counter: with pseudoephedrine and acetaminophen (Tavist Allergy/Sinus/Headache Tablets)

CLINICAL PHARMACOLOGY

Mechanism of Action

An ethanolamine that competes with histamine on effector cells in the GI tract, blood vessels, and respiratory tract. **Therapeutic Effect:** Relieves allergy symptoms, including urticaria, rhinitis, and pruritus.

PHARMACOKINETICS

Route	Onset	Peak	Duration
PO	15-60 min	5-7 hr	10-12 hr

Well absorbed from the GI tract. Metabolized in the liver. Excreted primarily in urine. **Half-life:** 21 hr.

AVAILABILITY

Syrup (Tavist): 0.67 mg/5 mL.
Tablets: 1.34 mg (1 mg base [Contac 12 Hour Allergy]), 2.68 mg (2 mg base [Tavist]).

INDICATIONS AND DOSAGE

Allergic rhinitis, urticaria

PO

Adults, Children older than 11 yr: 1.34 mg twice per day up to 2.68 mg three times per day. Maximum: 8.04 mg/day. **Children 6-11 yr:** 0.67-1.34 mg (clemastine fumarate 0.5-1 mg base) twice per day. Maximum: 4.02 mg/day (3 mg base). **Children younger than 6 yr:** 0.05 mg/kg/day as clemastine base divided into 2-3 doses per day. Maximum: 1.34 mg/day (1 mg base). **Elderly:** 1.34 mg 1-2 times per day.

CONTRAINDICATIONS

Angle-closure glaucoma, hypersensitivity to clemastine, use within 14 days of MAOIs

INTERACTIONS

Drug: **Alcohol, other CNS depressants:** May increase CNS depression. **MAOIs:** May increase the anticholinergic and CNS depressant effects of clemastine. **Herbal:** None known. **Food:** None known.

DIAGNOSTIC TEST EFFECTS

May suppress wheal and flare reactions to antigen skin testing unless drug is discontinued 4 days before testing.

SIDE-EFFECTS

Frequent: Somnolence, dizziness, urine retention, thickening of bronchial secretions, dry mouth, nose, or throat; in elderly, sedation, dizziness, hypotension. **Occasional:** Epigastric distress, flushing, blurred vision, tinnitus, paresthesia, diaphoresis, chills

CRITICAL CARE CONSIDERATIONS

ADMINISTRATION/HANDLING

PO ALERT

- Give clemastine without regard to food.
- Crush scored tablets as needed.
- Fixed-combination form Tavist-D may produce mild CNS stimulation.

PRECAUTIONS

HEALTH-RELATED

- Use clemastine cautiously in patients with bronchial asthma, increased intraocular pressure, narrow angle glaucoma, pyloroduodenal obstruction, peptic ulcer disease, bladder neck obstruction, or benign prostatic hyperplasia.

AGE-RELATED

- **Children:** Safety and efficacy of clemastine have not been established in children under 12 yr.
- **Elderly:** More likely to cause dizziness, sedation, and hypotension in the elderly.

PREGNANCY/LACTATION-RELATED

- Pregnancy category B; excreted into breast milk; may cause drowsiness and irritability in nursing infant; use with caution during breast-feeding.

MONITORING

- **Baseline history:** For patients undergoing an allergic reaction, obtain history of recently ingested drugs and foods, environmental exposure, and emotional stress.
- **Baseline assessment:** Monitor pulse rate, pulse quality respiratory rate, rhythm, and depth. Auscultate breath sounds for crackles, rhonchi, and wheezing.
- **Hypotension:** Monitor BP, especially in elderly patients who are at increased risk for developing hypotension.
- **Paradoxic reaction:** Monitor children closely for paradoxical reaction.
- **Patient education:** When clemastine will be used outside the hospital, inform patients that dizziness, drowsiness, and dry mouth may occur. Tolerance to sedative effects may ensue. Coffee and tea may help reduce drowsiness. Warn patients to avoid performing tasks that require mental alertness or motor skills until response to the drug is known. Patients should avoid alcohol during clemastine therapy.

SERIOUS ADVERSE REACTIONS

- **Hypersensitivity:** Eczema, pruritus, rash, cardiac disturbances, angioedema, and photosensitivity.
- **Paradoxical reactions:** Children may experience restlessness, insomnia, euphoria, nervousness, and tremors.
- **Addictive effects:** Clemastine has addictive effects with alcohol and other CNS depressants (hypnotics, sedatives, tranquilizers, "sleeping pills," etc.).
- **Anticholinergic syndrome:** Dry skin, flushing, hyperthermia, urinary retention, diminished bowel sounds, mydriasis, myoclonus, tachycardia, hypertension, peripheral vasodilation, dysrhythmias, cardiogenic shock, agitation, altered mental status, anxiety, ataxia, cardiopulmonary arrest, coma, delirium, disorientation, extrapyramidal reactions, hallucinations, incoherent speech, lethargy, paranoia, psychosis, seizures. Management is symptom specific.

OVERDOSE/TOXICITY

- **Adults:** Symptoms may vary from CNS depression, including sedation, apnea, cardiovascular collapse, and death to severe paradoxical reaction, such as hallucinations, tremor, and seizures.
- **Children:** May result in hallucinations, seizures, and death.
- **GI decontamination:** No specific recommendations.

ANTIDOTE/DIALYSIS

- **Antidote:** No specific recommendations.
- **Dialysis:** No data are available on removal of clemastine by hemodialysis, peritoneal dialysis, or high-permeability hemodialysis.

clindamycin

klin-da-mye'-sin

Classes

Chemical: lincomycin derivative
Therapeutic: antibiotic

Pregnancy Category: B

Trade Names

Prescription: Cleocin HCl, Cleocin Ovules, Cleocin Pediatric, Cleocin Phosphate, Cleocin T, Cleocin Vaginal, Clinda-Derm, Clindagel, Clindamax, Clindesse, Clindets Pledget, Dalacin C ♣

CLINICAL PHARMACOLOGY

Mechanism of Action

A lincosamide antibiotic that inhibits protein synthesis of the bacterial cell wall by binding to bacterial ribosomal receptor sites. Topically, it decreases fatty acid concentration on the skin. **Therapeutic Effect:** Bacteriostatic. Prevents outbreaks of acne vulgaris.

PHARMACOKINETICS

Rapidly absorbed from the GI tract. Protein binding: 92%-94%. Widely distributed. Metabolized in the liver to some active metabolites. Primarily excreted in urine. Not removed by hemodialysis. **Half-life:** 2.4-3 hr (increased in impaired renal function and premature infants).

C

AVAILABILITY

Capsules (Cleocin HCl): 75 mg, 150 mg, 300 mg.
Powder for reconstitution (Cleocin Pediatric): 75 mg/5 mL.
Intravenous solution (Cleocin Phosphate): 150 mg/mL, 300 mg-5%/50 mL, 600 mg-5%/50 mL, 900 mg-5%/50 mL.
Topical gel (Cleocin T, Clindagel, Clindamax): 1%.
Topical lotion (Cleocin T): 1%.
Topical solution (Cleocin T, Clinda-Derm): 1%.
Topical swab (Cleocin T, Clindets Pledget): 1%.
Vaginal cream (Cleocin Vaginal): 2%.
Vaginal suppository (Cleocin Ovules): 100 mg.

INDICATIONS AND DOSAGE

Susceptible infections

IV, IM

Adults, Elderly: 600-2700 mg/day in 2-4 divided doses. **Children 1 mo-16 yr:** 20-40 mg/kg/day in 2-4 divided doses. Maximum: 4.8 g/day. **Children younger than 1 mo:** 15-20 mg/kg/day in 2-3 divided doses.

PO

Adults, Elderly: 150-450 mg every 6 hr. **Children:** 8-20 mg/kg/day in 3-4 divided doses.

Bacterial vaginosis

PO

Adults, Elderly: 300 mg twice per day for 7 days.

Intravaginal

Adults: One applicatorful at bedtime for 3-7 days or one suppository at bedtime for 3 days.

Intravaginal (Clindesse cream)

Adults: One applicatorful once at any time of the day.

Acne vulgaris

Topical

Adults: Apply thin layer to affected area twice per day.

OFF-LABEL USES

Treatment of actinomycosis, babesiosis, erysipelas, malaria, otitis media, *Pneumocystis carinii* pneumonia, sinusitis, toxoplasmosis

CONTRAINDICATIONS

History of antibiotic-associated colitis, regional enteritis, or ulcerative colitis; hypersensitivity to clindamycin or lincomycin; known allergy to tartrazine dye

INTERACTIONS

Drug: **Adsorbent antidiarrheals:** May delay absorption of clindamycin. **Chloramphenicol, erythromycin:** May antagonize the effects of clindamycin. **Neuromuscular blockers:** May increase the effects of these drugs. Herbal: None known. Food: None known.

DIAGNOSTIC TEST EFFECTS

May increase serum alkaline phosphatase, AST (SGOT), and ALT (SGPT) levels.

IV INCOMPATIBILITIES

Allopurinol (Aloprim), filgrastim (Neupogen), fluconazole (Diflucan), idarubicin (Idamycin)

IV COMPATIBILITIES

Amiodarone (Cordarone), diltiazem (Cardizem), heparin, hydromorphone (Dilaudid), magnesium sulfate, midazolam (Versed), morphine, multivitamins, propofol (Diprivan), total parenteral nutrition (TPN)

SIDE-EFFECTS

Frequent: **Systemic:** Abdominal pain, nausea, vomiting, diarrhea
Topical: Dry scaly skin
Vaginal: Vaginitis, pruritus. Occasional: **Systemic:** Phlebitis or thrombophlebitis with IV administration, pain and induration at IM injection site, allergic reaction, urticaria, pruritus
Topical: Contact dermatitis, abdominal pain, mild diarrhea, burning or stinging
Vaginal: Headache, dizziness, nausea, vomiting, abdominal pain. Rare: **Vaginal:** Hypersensitivity reaction

CRITICAL CARE CONSIDERATIONS

ADMINISTRATION/HANDLING

PO ALERT

- **Storage:** Store capsules at room temperature.
- **Food:** Capsules may be taken without regard to food; give capsules with 8 oz of water.
- **Oral solution:** After reconstitution, oral solution is stable for 2 wk at room temperature. Do not refrigerate oral solution to avoid thickening.

IV ALERT

- **Stability:** IV infusion (piggyback) is stable at room temperature for up to 16 days.
- **Dilution:** Dilute 300-600 mg with 50 mL D_5W or 0.9% NaCl (900-1200 mg with 100 mL). Never exceed a concentration of 18 mg/mL.

- **Infusion:** Infuse 50-mL (300- to 600-mg) piggyback solution over 10-20 min; infuse 100-mL (900-mg to 1.2-g) piggyback solution over 30-40 min. Severe hypotension or cardiac arrest can occur with rapid administration.
- **Maximum infusion dose:** Do not administer more than 1.2 g (1200 mg) in a single infusion.

IM ALERT

- **Maximum IM dose:** Do not exceed 600 mg/dose.
- Give by deep IM injection.

TOPICAL ALERT

- **Avoid eyes:** Do not apply topical preparations to abraded areas or near the eyes.

PRECAUTIONS

HEALTH-RELATED

- Use clindamycin cautiously in patients with severe renal or hepatic dysfunction
- **Neuromuscular blocking agents:** Use cautiously in patients receiving neuromuscular blocking agents concurrently.
- **Colitis:** Use clindamycin cautiously in patients with colitis or history of colitis (antibiotic-associated or ulcerative colitis).
- **Lincosamide allergy:** Use very cautiously in patients with history of antibiotic allergies (especially preparations containing clindamycian or lincomycin).
- **Transplant patients:** May decrease *cycloSPORINE (Sandimmune) levels.

AGE-RELATED

- **Children:** Use clindamycin cautiously in children under 1 mo. For topical preparations, safety and efficacy have not been established in children under 12 yr.
- **Elderly:** No age-related precautions have been noted.

PREGNANCY/LACTATION-RELATED

- Pregnancy category B; excreted into breast milk; compatible with breast-feeding.

MONITORING

- **Baseline assessment:** Determine history of allergies, particularly to clindamycin or lincomycin, before beginning drug therapy.
- **Neuromuscular blockade:** Avoid concurrent use, if possible, to avoid potentiating neuromuscular blockade causing severe respiratory depression.
- **Baseline lab work:** Chemical profile including K+, BUN, and creatinine levels to evaluate renal function, and serum transaminases (AST [SGOT], ALT [SGPT], GGT), LDH, bilirubin to evaluate liver function. Obtain culture of infected area before drug administration (wound, blood, sputum, urine).
- **Superinfections:** Assess the mouth for white patches on the mucous membranes or tongue and for severe mouth or tongue soreness; assess for severe anal or genital pruritus or discharge.
- ***C. difficile* colitis:** Assess the pattern of daily bowel activity and stool consistency. Although mild GI effects may be tolerable, severe symptoms including abdominal pain or cramping, and moderate to severe diarrhea may indicate the onset of antibiotic-associated colitis.
- **Hand washing:** If *C. difficile* colitis develops, wash hands with antibacterial soap; alcohol-based foam is ineffective against *C. difficile* spores.
- **Skin:** Assess skin for dryness, irritation, and rash with topical application.
- **Eye irritation:** If topical/vaginal clindamycin accidentally comes in contact with the eyes, rinse eyes with copious amounts of cool tap water.
- **Nephrotoxicity and hepatotoxicity:** Monitor for fluid retention (edema, positive fluid balance), liver and renal function test results to assess for toxicity.
- **IM injection site:** Evaluate the injection site for induration and tenderness.
- **Patient education:** Space doses evenly around the clock. If clindamycin is used outside the hospital, instruct patients to continue taking clindamycin for the full course of treatment. Instruct patients to take oral doses with 8 oz water. Use caution when applying topical clindamycin concurrently with abrasive, peeling acne agents, soaps, or alcohol-containing cosmetics to avoid irritation. Instruct patients not to apply topical preparations near the eyes or on abraded areas. Advise patients not to engage in sexual intercourse during treatment with the vaginal form of clindamycin.

SERIOUS ADVERSE REACTIONS

- **Hypersensitivity:** Patients with a history of allergies, especially to lincomycin and other lincosamides, are at increased risk for developing a severe hypersensitivity reaction marked by severe pruritus, angioedema, bronchospasm, and anaphylaxis.
- **Manage hypersensitivity:** May require treatment with epinephrine and other emergency measures including oxygen,

endotracheal intubation, mechanical ventilation, IV fluids, IV antihistamines, corticosteroids, and vasopressors.
- **Respiratory depression:** May potentiate neuromuscular blocking agents (tubocurarine, mivacurium), including drugs not primarily used for neuromuscular blockade (streptomycin, kanamycin), to cause severe respiratory depression.

OVERDOSE/TOXICITY
- **Nephrotoxicity:** Increased BUN and creatinine, decreased urine output, anuria, possible hyperkalemia, fluid overload indicative of acute renal failure.
- **Superinfections:** Antibiotic-associated colitis (pseudomembranous colitis) and other superinfections may result from altered bacterial balance.
- **Manage pseudomembranous colitis:** Fluids, electrolytes, protein supplements, oral vancomycin (Vancocin), or IV metronidazole (Flagyl).
- **Hepatotoxicity and thrombocytopenia:** Occur rarely.
- **GI decontamination:** No specific recommendations.

ANTIDOTE/DIALYSIS
- **Antidote:** No specific recommendations.
- **Dialysis:** Clindamycin is not removed by hemodialysis or peritoneal dialysis. No data are available on removal by high-permeability hemodialysis.

clofazimine

kloe-faz'-i-meen

Classes
Chemical: iminophenazine dye
Therapeutic: leprostatic, mycobacterium avium complex

Pregnancy Category: C

Trade Names
Prescription: Lamprene

CLINICAL PHARMACOLOGY
Mechanism of Action
An antibiotic that binds to mycobacterial DNA. Therapeutic Effect: Inhibits mycobacterial growth and produces antiinflammatory action.

PHARMACOKINETICS
Variable absorption following PO administration. Because of its high lipophilicity, clofazimine is deposited primarily in fatty tissue. Metabolized in liver. Primarily excreted in feces and minimal elimination in urine. Half-life: 70 days (following long-term therapy).

AVAILABILITY
Capsules: 50 mg.

INDICATIONS AND DOSAGE
Leprosy
PO

Adults, Elderly: 100 mg/day in combination with dapsone and rifampin for 3 yr then 100 mg/day as monotherapy. **Children:** 1 mg/kg/day in combination with dapsone and rifampin.

Erythema nodosum
PO

Adults, Elderly: 100-200 mg/day for up to 3 mo, then 100 mg/day.

CONTRAINDICATIONS
Hypersensitivity to clofazimine

INTERACTIONS
Drug: **Aluminum- and magnesium-containing antacids:** May decrease plasma concentrations of clofazimine. **Dapsone:** May decrease the effects of clofazimine. Herbal: None significant. Food: **All foods:** May increase the absorption of clofazimine.

DIAGNOSTIC TEST EFFECTS
May increase blood glucose levels.

SIDE-EFFECTS
Frequent (greater than 10%): Dry skin, abdominal pain, nausea, vomiting, diarrhea, skin discoloration (pink to brownish-black). Occasional (10%-1%): Rash; pruritus; eye irritation; discoloration of sputum; sweat and urine

CRITICAL CARE CONSIDERATIONS

ADMINISTRATION/HANDLING
PO ALERT
- Clofazimine may be given with food to reduce GI discomfort.

PRECAUTIONS
HEALTH-RELATED
- Use clofazimine cautiously in patients with GI problems, including abdominal pain and diarrhea.

AGE-RELATED
- **Children:** No age-related precautions have been noted.

- **Elderly:** No age-related precautions have been noted.

PREGNANCY/LACTATION-RELATED

- Pregnancy category C; excreted into breast milk; do not administer to nursing mothers unless clearly indicated.

MONITORING

- **Baseline assessment:** Assess for sensitivity to clofazimine.
- **Mild GI discomfort:** Monitor for colicky abdominal pain, nausea, vomiting, diarrhea, and reduce dose if symptoms occur to avoid severe pain.
- **Severe abdominal pain:** Clofazimine has prompted severe pain that required exploratory laparotomy.
- **Skin discoloration:** Clofazimine may cause skin discoloration.
- **Concomitant use of corticosteroids:** Clofazimine administered in dosages of 100-200 mg daily for up to 3 mo may be useful in eliminating or reducing steroid requirements when treating severe erythema nodosum leprosum reactions.

SERIOUS ADVERSE REACTIONS

- **Severe abdominal symptoms:** GI bleeding, severe abdominal pain due to splenic infarction or bowel obstruction. Fatalities have been reported following onset of these symptoms.

OVERDOSE/TOXICITY

- **Dapsone resistant leprosy:** If dosage of clofazimine is 200 mg day or greater and patients do not respond, risk of abdominal symptoms may increase. Patients should be managed with a combination of one or more antileprosy drugs for 3 yr. For advice about combination drug regimens, contact the U.S. Public Health Service, Gillis W. Long Hansen's Disease Center, Carville, LA (504) 642-7771.
- **GI decontamination:** No specific recommendations.

ANTIDOTE/DIALYSIS

- **Antidote:** No specific recommendations.
- **Dialysis:** Clofazimine is not removed by hemodialysis or peritoneal dialysis. No data are available on removal by high-permeability hemodialysis.

clomipramine hydrochloride

See Antidepressants (p. 906)

clonazepam

See Anticonvulsants (p. 903)

clonidine

kloe'-ni-deen

Classes

Chemical: imidazoline derivative

Therapeutic: antihypertensive, centrally acting sympathoplegic

Pregnancy Category: C

Trade Names

Prescription: Catapres, Catapres-TTS-1, Catapres-TTS-2, Catapres-TTS-3, Clonidine TTS-1, Clonidine TTS-2, Clonidine TTS-3, Duraclon

Combinations

Prescription: with chlorthalidone (Chlorpres, Combipress)

Do not confuse clonidine with clomiphene, Klonopin, or quinidine or Catapres with with Cetapred.

CLINICAL PHARMACOLOGY

Mechanism of Action

An antiadrenergic, sympatholytic agent that prevents pain signal transmission to the brain and produces analgesia at pre- and post-alpha-adrenergic receptors in the spinal cord. **Therapeutic Effect:** Reduces peripheral resistance; decreases BP and heart rate.

PHARMACOKINETICS

Route	Onset	Peak	Duration
PO	0.5-1 hr	2-4 hr	Up to 8 hr

Well absorbed from the GI tract. Transdermal best absorbed from the chest and upper arm; least absorbed from the thigh. Protein binding: 20%-40%. Metabolized in the liver. Primarily excreted in urine. Not removed by hemodialysis. **Half-life:** 12-16 hr (increased with impaired renal function).

AVAILABILITY

Tablets (Catapres): 0.1 mg, 0.2 mg, 0.3 mg.
Transdermal patch: 2.5 mg (release at 0.1 mg/24 hr) (Catapres-TTS-1, Clonidine TTS-1), 5 mg (release at 0.2 mg/24 hr) (Catapres-TTS-2, Clonidine TTS-2), 7.5 mg (release at 0.3 mg/24 hr) (Catapres-TTS-3, Clonidine TTS-3).
Injection (Duraclon): 100 mcg/mL, 500 mcg/mL.

INDICATIONS AND DOSAGE

Hypertension

PO

Adults: Initially, 0.1 mg twice per day. Increase by 0.1-0.2 mg every 2-4 days. Maintenance: 0.2-1.2 mg/day in 2-4 divided doses up to maximum of 2.4 mg/day. **Elderly:** Initially, 0.1 mg at bedtime. May increase gradually. **Children:** Initially, 5-10 mcg/kg/day in divided doses every 8-12 hr. Increase at 5- to 7-day intervals up to 25 mcg/kg/day in divided doses every 6 hr. Maximum: 0.9 mg/day.

Transdermal

Adults, Elderly: System delivering 0.1 mg/24 hr up to 0.6 mg/24 hr every 7 days.

Attention-deficit/hyperactivity disorder (ADHD)

PO

Children: Initially 0.05 mg/day. May increase by 0.05 mg/day every 3-7 days up to 3-5 mcg/kg/day in divided doses 3-4 times per day. Maximum: 0.3-0.4 mg/day.

Severe pain

Epidural

Adults, Elderly: 30-40 mcg/hr. **Children:** Initially, 0.5 mcg/kg/hr, not to exceed adult dose.

OFF-LABEL USES

ADHD, diagnosis of pheochromocytoma, opioid withdrawal, prevention of migraine headaches, treatment of diarrhea in diabetes mellitus, treatment of dysmenorrhea, menopausal flushing

CONTRAINDICATIONS

Hypersensitivity to clonidine; epidural clonidine is contraindicated in those patients with bleeding diathesis, infection at the injection site, and those receiving anticoagulation therapy; administration of epidural clonidine is contraindicated above the C4 dermatome

INTERACTIONS

Drug: **Beta-blockers:** Discontinuing these drugs may increase risk of clonidine withdrawal hypertensive crisis. **Tricyclic antidepressants:** May decrease effect of clonidine. **Herbal:** **Yohimbe:** May decrease the effectiveness of clonidine. **Food:** None known.

DIAGNOSTIC TEST EFFECTS

None known.

IV INCOMPATIBILITIES

None known.

IV COMPATIBILITIES

Bupivacaine (Marcaine, Sensorcaine), fentanyl (Sublimaze), heparin, ketamine (Ketalar), lidocaine, lorazepam (Ativan)

SIDE-EFFECTS

Frequent: Dry mouth (40%), somnolence (33%), dizziness (16%), sedation, constipation (10%). **Occasional (5%-1%):** **Tablets, injection:** Depression, swelling of feet, loss of appetite, decreased sexual ability, itching eyes, dizziness, nausea, vomiting, nervousness. **Transdermal:** Itching, reddening or darkening of skin. **Rare (less than 1%):** Nightmares, vivid dreams, cold feeling in fingers and toes

CRITICAL CARE CONSIDERATIONS

ADMINISTRATION/HANDLING

PO ALERT

- Give clonidine without regard to food.
- Tablets may be crushed.
- Give last oral dose just before bedtime.

TRANSDERMAL ALERT

- Apply transdermal system to dry, hairless area of intact skin on upper arm or chest.
- Rotate sites to prevent skin irritation.
- Do not trim patch to adjust dose.

EPIDURAL ALERT

- Dilute 500 mcg/mL strength product before use in 0.9% sodium chloride for injection to a final concentration of 100 mcg/mL.
- Clonidine should be administered using an appropriate infusion pump to facilitate accurate dosing.

PRECAUTIONS

HEALTH-RELATED

- Use clonidine cautiously in patients with cardiovascular disease, recent MI, renal insufficiency, hemodynamic instability, Raynaud's disease, severe coronary insufficiency, cerebrovascular disease, or thromboangiitis obliterans.
- Epidural clonidine is not recommended for obstetrical, postpartum, or perioperative pain management due to risk of hemodynamic instability related to bradycardia and hypotension.

AGE-RELATED

- **Children:** Are more sensitive to hypotensive effects. Use epidural clonidine with caution in children. Safety and efficacy have not been established for PO clonidine in children and for transdermal clonidine in children under 12 yr.
- **Elderly:** May be more sensitive to the hypotensive effect of clonidine. Age-

related renal impairment may require dosage adjustment.

PREGNANCY/LACTATION-RELATED

- Pregnancy category C; secreted into breast milk; hypotension has not been observed in nursing infants, although clonidine was found in the serum of the infants.

MONITORING

- **Baseline assessment:** Obtain BP immediately before giving each dose.
- **Lab work:** Biochemical profile including renal (BUN, creatinine) and liver (AST [SGOT], ALT [SGPT], alkaline phosphatase, bilirubin) function tests.
- **Ongoing assessment:** Monitor for hypertension, hypotension, and BP fluctuations. Hypertension should be controlled without fluctuations in BP.
- **Diagnostic tests:** 12-lead ECG to evaluate for myocardial ischemia.
- **Epidural infusion:** Monitor pain control in cancer patients resistant to opioid analgesics alone. Clonidine is more effective with neuropathic pain than with visceral or somatic pain. Monitor catheter insertion site for redness, tenderness, and leakage. When discontinuing epidural infusion, dose should be gradually reduced over 2-4 days to avoid withdrawal symptoms.
- **Implantable epidural catheter:** Monitor site for catheter-related infection including epidural abscess and meningitis, which occur in 5%-20% of patients.
- **Dry mouth:** Offer sips of water and sugarless gum to help relieve dry mouth.
- **Timely dose administration:** Skipping doses or voluntarily discontinuing clonidine may produce severe, rebound hypertension.
- **Patient education:** Advise patients that clonidine's side effects tend to diminish during therapy. Clonidine may have a sedative effect. Patients should not operate machinery or drive until response to the drug is known. Instruct patients to sit up slowly from lying to a sitting position and to dangle legs before standing to avoid dizziness and fainting.

SERIOUS ADVERSE REACTIONS

- **Abrupt withdrawal:** May result in rebound hypertension associated with nervousness, agitation, anxiety, insomnia, hand tingling, tremor, flushing, and diaphoresis.
- **Concurrent beta-blocker use:** Discontinue beta-blocker therapy several days before discontinuing clonidine to prevent clonidine-withdrawal hypertensive crisis. Reduce clonidine dosage over 2-4 days.
- **Manage withdrawal:** May be treated by administration of clonidine or IV phentolamine (Regitine).

OVERDOSE/TOXICITY

- **Symptoms:** Hypotension, coma, respiratory depression, bradycardia, transient hypertension, apnea, hypoglycemia, miosis (constricted pupils), periods of agitation alternating with coma, hypothermia.
- **Management:** Endotracheal intubation, mechanical ventilation, high-dose naloxone may relieve respiratory depression, IV fluids for hypotension, *DOPamine for bradycardia rather than atropine (atropine can prolong hypertensive crisis in some patients), atropine only for significant bradycardia with hypotension.
- **GI decontamination:** Single dose of activated charcoal may be more effective when patients present early in tablet rather than solution overdoses. Solutions are more rapidly absorbed. In clonidine patch ingestion, whole bowel irrigation with polyethylene glycol/balanced solution has been reported to be effective in enhancing GI tract clearance.

ANTIDOTE/DIALYSIS

- **Antidote:** No antidote has been proven consistently safe and effective. Ephedrine, along with IV fluids, may be used to manage hypotension.
- **Dialysis:** Clonidine is not removed by hemodialysis or peritoneal dialysis, and no data are available on removal by high-permeability hemodialysis.

clopidogrel bisulfate

kloh-pid'-oh-grel bye-sul'-fate

Classes

Chemical: thienopyridine derivative
Therapeutic: antiplatelet agent

Pregnancy Category: B

Trade Names

Prescription: Plavix

Do not confuse Plavix with Paxil.

CLINICAL PHARMACOLOGY

Mechanism of Action

A thienopyridine derivative that inhibits binding of the enzyme adenosine phosphate (ADP) to its platelet receptor and subsequent ADP-mediated activation of a glycoprotein complex. **Therapeutic Effect:** Inhibits platelet aggregation.

C

PHARMACOKINETICS

Route	Onset	Peak	Duration
PO	1 hr	2 hr	N/A

Rapidly absorbed. Protein binding: 98%. Extensively metabolized by the liver. Eliminated equally in the urine and feces. **Half-life:** 8 hr.

AVAILABILITY

Tablets: 75 mg.

INDICATIONS AND DOSAGE

MI, stroke reduction

PO

Adults, Elderly: 75 mg once per day.

Acute coronary syndrome

PO

Adults, Elderly: Initially, 300 mg loading dose, then 75 mg once per day (in combination with aspirin).

OFF-LABEL USES

Graft patency (saphenous vein), mitral regurgitation, mitral stenosis, noncardioembolic stroke, percutaneous coronary intervention

CONTRAINDICATIONS

Active bleeding, coagulation disorders, severe hepatic disease, hypersensitivity to clopidogrel

INTERACTIONS

Drug: **Atorvastatin, fluvastatin, other NSAIDs, phenytoin, tamoxifen, tolbutamide, torsemide, warfarin:** May interfere with metabolism of these drugs. **Herbal:** **Ginger, ginkgo biloba:** May increase the risk of bleeding. **Food:** None known.

DIAGNOSTIC TEST EFFECTS

Prolongs bleeding time.

SIDE-EFFECTS

Frequent (15%): Abdominal pain, vomiting, gastritis, constipation. **Occasional (8%-6%):** Upper respiratory tract infection, chest pain, flulike symptoms, headache, dizziness, arthralgia. **Rare (5%-3%):** Fatigue, edema, hypertension, abdominal pain, dyspepsia, diarrhea, nausea, epistaxis, dyspnea, rhinitis

CRITICAL CARE CONSIDERATIONS

ADMINISTRATION/HANDLING

PO ALERT

- Give clopidogrel without regard to food.
- Do not crush coated tablets.

PRECAUTIONS

HEALTH-RELATED

- Use clopidrogel cautiously in preoperative patients, patients with history of hematologic disorders or bleeding, peptic ulcer disease, other lesions at risk for bleeding, hypertension, hepatic or renal impairment.

AGE-RELATED

- **Children:** Safety and efficacy of clopidogrel have not been established in children.
- **Elderly:** No age-related precautions have been noted.

PREGNANCY/LACTATION-RELATED

- Pregnancy category B; excreted into breast milk in rats.

MONITORING

- **Baseline lab work:** Platelet count before clopidogrel therapy; Hgb, WBC count, and BUN, serum bilirubin, creatinine, AST (SGOT), and ALT (SGPT) levels.
- **Ongoing lab work:** Platelet count every 2 days during the first week of treatment and weekly thereafter until therapeutic maintenance dose is reached. Monitor for thrombocytopenia.
- **Abrupt discontinuation:** Produces an elevated platelet count within 5 days.
- **Hepatic insufficiency:** Monitor for jaundice and elevated serum transaminases.
- **Bleeding:** Monitor for bleeding from invasive/puncture sites. Inform patients it may take longer to stop bleeding during drug therapy. Instruct patients to report unusual bleeding.
- **Cardiac:** Monitor for dysrhythmias in patients with acute coronary syndrome.
- **Neurologic:** Monitor for changes in level of consciousness, motor function, and sensation if patients are at risk for stroke.
- **Neurovascular:** Assess peripheral pulses, temperature, sensation, and movement of extremities if patients have peripheral vascular disease.
- **Patient education:** Tell patients to notify all health care/dental health providers of clopidogrel therapy before procedures are

scheduled or new drugs prescribed so they are prepared to manage for increased risk of bleeding.

SERIOUS ADVERSE REACTIONS

- **TTP:** Thrombotic thrombocytopenic purpura (TTP) manifested by thrombocytopenia, microangiopathic hemolytic anemia, altered level of consciousness, hepatic and/or renal insufficiency and fever. Generally occurs within the first 2 wk of therapy.
- **Management:** May respond to discontinuation of clopidogrel and plasma exchange (TPE).

OVERDOSE/TOXICITY

- **Symptoms:** Bleeding from wounds, puncture sites and/or GI bleeding, intracranial bleeding, rash or other skin disorders, elevated liver enzymes. May require platelet transfusion to help control severe bleeding.
- **GI decontamination:** No specific recommendations.

ANTIDOTE/DIALYSIS

- **Antidote:** No specific recommendations. Plasma exchange and platelet transfusions may help control bleeding.
- **Dialysis:** Clopidogrel is unlikely to be removed by hemodialysis or peritoneal dialysis. No data are available on removal by high-permeability hemodialysis.

clorazepate dipotassium

See Antianxiety Agents (p. 890)

clozapine

klo'-za-peen

Classes

Chemical: dibenzodiazepine derivative
Therapeutic: antipsychotic

Pregnancy Category: B

Trade Names

Prescription: Clozaril, FazaClo

Do not confuse clozapine with Cloxapen or clofazimine or Clozaril with Clinoril or Colazal.

CLINICAL PHARMACOLOGY

Mechanism of Action

A dibenzodiazepine derivative that interferes with the binding of dopamine at dopamine receptor sites; binds primarily at non dopamine receptor sites. **Therapeutic Effect:** Diminishes schizophrenic behavior.

PHARMACOKINETICS

Absorbed rapidly and almost completely. Distributed rapidly and extensively. Crosses the blood–brain barrier. Protein binding: 95%. Metabolized in the liver. Excreted in urine and feces. **Half-life:** 8 hr.

AVAILABILITY

Tablets (Clozaril): 12.5 mg, 25 mg, 100 mg, 200 mg.
Tablets (oral-disintegrating [FazaClo]): 25 mg, 100 mg.

INDICATIONS AND DOSAGE

Alert: For initiation of therapy, the patient must have a WBC count equal to or greater than 3500/mm^3 and an ANC count equal to or greater than 2000/mm^3.

Schizophrenic disorders, reduce suicidal behavior

PO

Adults: Initially, 12.5 mg once or twice per day. May increase by 25-50 mg/day over 2 wk until dosage of 300-450 mg/day is achieved. May further increase by 50-100 mg/day no more than once or twice per wk. Range: 200-600 mg/day. Maximum: 900 mg/day. **Elderly:** Initially, 25 mg/day. May increase by 25 mg/day. Maximum: 450 mg/day.

CONTRAINDICATIONS

Coma, concurrent use of other drugs that may suppress bone marrow function, history of clozapine-induced agranulocytosis or severe granulocytopenia, myeloproliferative disorders, paralytic ileus, severe CNS depression, hypersensitivity to clozapine

INTERACTIONS

Drug: Alcohol, other CNS depressants: May increase CNS depressant effects. **Bone marrow depressants:** May increase myelosuppression. **Citalopram:** May increase clozapine blood concentration. **Lithium:** May increase the risk of confusion, dyskinesia, and seizures. **Phenobarbital:** Decreases clozapine blood concentration. **Herbal: St. John's wort:** Decreases clozapine levels **Food:** None known.

DIAGNOSTIC TEST EFFECTS

May increase serum glucose, cholesterol, and triglycerides.

SIDE-EFFECTS

Frequent: Somnolence (39%), salivation (31%), tachycardia (25%), dizziness (19%), constipation (14%). **Occasional:** Hypotension (9%); headache (7%); tremor, syncope, diaphoresis, dry mouth (6%); nausea, visual disturbances (5%); nightmares, restlessness, akinesia, agitation, hypertension, abdominal discomfort or heartburn, weight gain (4%). **Rare:** Rigidity, confusion, fatigue, insomnia, diarrhea, rash

CRITICAL CARE CONSIDERATIONS

ADMINISTRATION/HANDLING

PO ALERT

- Give clozapine without regard to food.

PRECAUTIONS

HEALTH-RELATED

- Use of clozapine should be reserved for severely ill schizophrenia patients who have not responded to standard antipsychotic drug treatment because of risk for potentially life-threatening agranulocytosis, seizures, fatal myocarditis, and respiratory and cardiac arrest.
- Clozapine is available only through a distribution system that ensures WBC monitoring according to the mandated schedule.
- Clozapine is a substrate for many CYP450 enzymes, so numerous drug reactions may occur while taking this medication.
- Use clozapine cautiously in patients with history of seizures; myocarditis; cardiovascular disease; glaucoma; benign prostatic hyperplasia; urine retention; impaired hepatic, renal, or respiratory function; and those undergoing alcohol withdrawal.

AGE-RELATED

- **Children:** Safety and efficacy of clozapine have not been established in children.
- **Elderly:** May be more susceptible to orthostatic hypotension, urinary retention, and constipation.

PREGNANCY/LACTATION-RELATED

- Pregnancy category B; breast-feeding should be discontinued.

MONITORING

- **Baseline assessment:** Assess vital signs, appearance, behavior, emotional status, response to environment, speech pattern, and thought content.
- **Baseline lab work:** WBC count with differential, liver enzymes, and biochemical profile before beginning treatment.
- **Ongoing lab work:** Monitor CBC for agranulocytosis and leukopenia every week for the first 6 mo of continuous therapy, then biweekly for patients with acceptable WBC counts throughout treatment and for 4 wk after treatment is discontinued. Monitor for elevation of serum transaminases (AST [SGOT], ALT [SGPT]) and hyperglycemia.
- **ECG:** Observe for sinus tachycardia, prolongation of the PR, QRS, and QT intervals; ST depression; T wave and U wave notching or inversion; and heart block.
- **BP:** Monitor for hypertension or hypotension, which may indicate the onset of an adverse drug reaction.
- **Neurologic:** Observe for involuntary movements, tremors, drowsiness, restlessness, agitation, confusion, fatigue, visual disturbances, sweating, and excessive salivation.
- **Suicidal patients:** Closely supervise during early therapy. As depression lessens, energy level improves, which increases the suicide potential.
- **Therapeutic response:** Assess for increased interest in surroundings and ability to concentrate, improvement in self-care, and relaxed facial expression.
- **Abrupt discontinuation:** Do not abruptly discontinue clozapine to avoid recurrence of psychotic symptoms.
- **Anticholinergic effects:** Monitor for urinary retention, constipation, and dry mouth.
- **Patient education:** Inform patients that drowsiness generally subsides with continued therapy and to avoid alcohol during clozapine therapy. Avoid tasks that require mental alertness or motor skills until response to the drug is known.

SERIOUS ADVERSE REACTIONS

- **Seizures:** Occur in about 3% of patients.
- **Neurologic:** Extrapyramidal symptoms, akathisia, tardive dyskinesia, and neuroleptic malignant syndrome occur rarely.
- **Tardive dyskinesia:** Has infrequently occurred in several patients after a brief period of treatment at low doses. Seen more commonly after a prolonged course of therapy and/or when using higher doses.

- **Pulmonary embolism:** Sudden onset chest pain with dyspnea seen more frequently in patients with deep vein thrombosis.
- **Cardiomyopathy:** Exertional dyspnea, orthopnea, paroxysmal noctural dyspnea, and peripheral edema.

OVERDOSE/TOXICITY

- **Symptoms:** CNS depression (sedation, coma, delirium), hypersalivation, seizures, aganulocytosis, respiratory depression, respiratory arrest, fatal myocarditis, dysrhythmias, orthostatic hypotension, and cardiac arrest. Diazepam 5-10 mg every 15 min to total 30 mg for seizures.
- **Neuroleptic malignant syndrome (NMS):** High fever, muscle rigidity, altered mental status, irregular pulse, labile BP, tachycardia, diaphoresis, and cardiac dysrhythmias.
- **Management of NMS:** Discontinue clozapine immediately, aggressive management of BP, heart rate, and dysrhythmias according to accepted Advanced Cardiac Life Support (ACLS) guidelines, manage other associated medical problems per accepted guidelines. When reintroducing clozapine, monitor carefully because repeat episodes of NMS have been reported.
- **GI decontamination:** No specific recommendations.

ANTIDOTE/DIALYSIS

- **Antidote:** Cautiously use flumazenil (Romazicon) 0.2 mg (2 mL) over 30 sec; may repeat after 30 sec with 0.3 mL (3 mL) over 30 sec. Further doses may be given up to 0.5 mg (5 mL) up to a total of 3 mg (30 mL). Flumazenil reverses CNS depressive effects. Naloxone (Narcan) should be considered in addition to flumazenil if patients have significant respiratory depression.
- **Dialysis:** Clozapine is not removed by hemodialysis and is unlikely to be removed by peritoneal dialysis. No data are available on removal by high-permeability hemodialysis.

cocaine hydrochloride ⚑

koe-kane' hye-droe-klor'-ide

Classes

Chemical: natural tropane alkaloid
Therapeutic: local anesthetic

DEA Schedule: II

Pregnancy Category: D

Trade Names

Prescription: Cocaine

CLINICAL PHARMACOLOGY

Mechanism of Action

A topical anesthetic that decreases membrane permeability and increases norepinephrine at postsynaptic receptor sites, producing intense vasoconstriction. **Therapeutic Effect:** Blocks conduction of nerve impulses.

PHARMACOKINETICS

Readily absorbed from all mucous membranes. Cocaine penetrates the CNS but is rapidly metabolized. Rapidly hydrolyzed in blood by serum cholinesterases. Metabolized in liver. Excreted in urine. **Half-life:** 1 hr.

AVAILABILITY

Powder, as hydrochloride: 1 g, 5 g, 25 g (Cocaine HCl).
Topical solution, as hydrochloride: 40 mg/mL (40%), 100 mg/mL (10% [Cocaine HCl]).

INDICATIONS AND DOSAGE

Anesthesia

Topical

Adults, Elderly, Children: 1%-4% to mucous membranes. Maximum: 1-3 mg/kg (four 400 mg). Dosage varies depending on the area to be anesthetized, vascularity of the tissues, individual tolerance, and anesthetic technique. Administer lowest effective dose.

OFF-LABEL USES

Horner's syndrome (diagnosis)

CONTRAINDICATIONS

Hypersensitivity to cocaine or any component of the formulation

INTERACTIONS

Drug: **Alcohol:** May increase heart rate and BP. **Beta-blockers:** May decrease effects of beta-blockers. **Cholinesterase inhibitors:** May increase effects and risk of toxicity. **Sympathomimetics:** May increase CNS stimulation and risk of cardiovascular effects. **Tricyclic antidepressants, digoxin, methyldopa:** May increase risk of dysrhythmias. **Herbal:** **Hemp:** May increase toxic effects of cocaine. **St. John's wort:**

May increase risk of cardiovascular collapse and/or delayed emergence from anesthesia.
Food: None known.

DIAGNOSTIC TEST EFFECTS

C

May give false-negative results of scintigraphy.

SIDE-EFFECTS

Frequent: Loss of sense of smell and taste.
Occasional: Anxiety, central nervous system stimulation or depression.

CRITICAL CARE CONSIDERATIONS

ADMINISTRATION/HANDLING

DOSAGE ALERT

- The lowest effective dose should be used to avoid complications.
- Concentrations greater than 4% are not recommended because of difficulty in controlling dosage and increased risk of toxic reactions.
- Solutions are incompatible with alkali and with alkaloidal precipitants.
- Direct instillation of cocaine into the eye is not recommended.
- Apply with cotton applicators or packs, instilled into cavity, or as a spray.
- Store powder and solution at room temperature in a well-closed, light-resistant container. Ethylene oxide is recommended for sterilization of the external surface of glass bottles containing the solution. Do not steam autoclave.

PRECAUTIONS

HEALTH-RELATED

- Use cocaine hydrochloride cautiously in critically ill patients, children, and debilitated or elderly patients.
- Topical cocaine should be used with caution on severely traumatized mucosa or when sepsis is present in the area of intended application.
- Use cocaine hydrochloride cautiously in patients with a history of drug sensitivities or drug abuse; drug can cause strong psychologic dependence and some tolerance.
- Cocaine hydrochloride has been abused for cortical stimulant effect. When abused, cocaine may be orally ingested, smoked (freebasing "crack" [alkaline cocaine]), sniffed intranasally, or injected intravenously.

AGE-RELATED

- **Children:** Safety and efficacy of cocaine hydrochloride have not been established in children.
- **Elderly:** Risk of cocaine-induced adverse effects may be increased.

PREGNANCY/LACTATION-RELATED

- Pregnancy category D; breast-feeding is not recommended.

MONITORING

- **Baseline assessment:** Assess duration, intensity, location, and type of pain.
- **Therapeutic effect:** Monitor for anesthetic response or pain relief.
- **CNS stimulation:** Assess for euphoria, restlessness, increased BP, pulse, and respirations. Be prepared to provide ventilatory support and emergency medications in the event of progression of CNS response.
- **Overdose:** Monitor ECG continuously for myocardial ischemia or infarction, BP for hypertension, temperature for hyperthermia, for signs of other organ failure or bleeding/clotting abnormality. Both hemorrhage and thrombus formation are associated with cocaine abuse.
- **Patient education:** Inform patients that nothing may be ingested by mouth until sensation returns when drug is used for throat anesthesia. Isolated use of cocaine for procedures will not cause dependence. Warn patients to report feelings of euphoria, restlessness, or rapid heartbeat if these develop during the procedure.

SERIOUS ADVERSE REACTIONS

- **Repeated nasal application:** May produce stuffy nose, chronic rhinitis, and may eventually damage intranasal structures.
- **Hyperthermia:** Results from psychomotor agitation, reduced heat dissipation due to vasoconstriction, altered temperature control in the hypothalamus. Degree of hyperthermia correlates with survival rate in overdose patients.
- **Chest discomfort:** Pain, diaphoresis, palpitations, and shortness of breath. Myocardial ischemia may lead to acute MI.
- **Hypertension:** CNS stimulation may cause BP elevation.

OVERDOSE/TOXICITY

- **Early signs:** Increased BP, increased pulse, chest pain, irregular heartbeat, chills/fever, agitation, nervousness, confusion, inability to remain still, nausea, vomiting, abdominal pain, hemoptysis, increased sweating, rapid breathing, respiratory distress, and large pupils.
- **Advanced signs:** Dysrhythmias, CNS hemorrhage, ischemic or hemorrhagic stroke, heart failure, seizures, delirium, hyperreflexia, acute dystonia, pulmonary hemorrhage, pulmonary thrombus, rare renal infarction, and rhabdomyolysis.
- **Late signs:** Loss of reflexes, muscle paralysis, dilated pupils, loss of consciousness, cyanosis, pulmonary edema, cardiac and respiratory failure.
- **Management:** Hyperthermia may resolve with control of agitation with benzodiazepines (lorazepam/Ativan or diazepam/Valium), IV hydration with fluids and electrolyte replacement, hypertension with nitroprusside or phentolamine (Regitine); manage seizures with benzodiazepines; use nitroglycerin for chest discomfort (avoid beta-blockers); ventricular tachycardia may be treated with lidocaine and defibrillation.
- **GI decontamination:** Charcoal and whole bowel irrigation if packets were ingested.

ANTIDOTE/DIALYSIS

- **Antidote:** No specific recommendations.
- **Dialysis:** Cocaine is not removed effectively by hemodialysis or peritoneal dialysis. No data are available on removal by high-permeability hemodialysis.

codeine phosphate/ codeine sulfate

koe'-deen foss'-fate/koe'-deen sul'-fate

DEA Schedule: II (analgesic), III (fixed-combination form)

Classes

Chemical: natural opium alkaloid, phenanthrene derivative

Therapeutic: antitussive, narcotic analgesic

Pregnancy Category: C, D

Trade Names

Prescription: Codeine Phosphate, Codeine Sulfate

Combinations

Prescription: with acetaminophen (Tylenol no. 2, Tylenol no. 3, Tylenol no. 4); with aspirin (Empirin no. 3, Empirin no. 4); with chlorpheniramine (Codeprex); with guaifenesin (Robitussin AC); with APAP (Capital, Aceta); with APAP butalbital, caffeine (Fioricet, Phenaphen); with aspirin (Fiorinal)

Do not confuse codeine with Cardene or Lodine or colchicine.

CLINICAL PHARMACOLOGY

Mechanism of Action

An opioid agonist that binds to opioid receptors at many sites in the CNS, particularly in the medulla. This action inhibits the ascending pain pathways. **Therapeutic Effect:** Alters the perception of and emotional response to pain, suppresses cough reflex.

PHARMACOKINETICS

Well absorbed following PO administration. Protein binding: 7%. Metabolized in liver. Excreted in urine. **Half-life:** 2.5-3.5 hr.

AVAILABILITY

Tablets (phosphate): 30 mg, 60 mg.
Tablets (sulfate): 15 mg, 30 mg, 60 mg.
Oral solution: 15 mg/5 mL.
Injection: 15 mg/mL, 30 mg/mL, 60 mg/mL.

INDICATIONS AND DOSAGE

Analgesia

PO, IM, Subcutaneous

Adults, Elderly: 30 mg every 4-6 hr. Range: 15-60 mg. **Children:** 0.5-1 mg/kg every 4-6 hr. Maximum: 60 mg/dose.

Cough

PO

Adults, Elderly, Children 12 yr and older: 10-20 mg every 4-6 hr. **Children 6-11 yr:** 5-10 mg every 4-6 hr. Maximum: 60 mg/day. **Children 2–5 yr:** 2.5-5 mg every 4-6 hr. Maximum: 30 mg/day.

Dosage in renal impairment

Dosage is modified based on creatinine clearance.

Creatinine Clearance	Dosage
10–50 mL/min	75% of usual dose
Less than 10 mL/min	50% of usual dose

OFF-LABEL USES

Treatment of diarrhea

CONTRAINDICATIONS

Hypersensitivity to codeine

INTERACTIONS

Drug: **Alcohol, other CNS depressants:** May increase CNS or respiratory depression, and hypotension. **MAOIs:** May produce a severe, sometimes fatal reaction; plan to administer a test dose, which is one quarter of usual codeine dose. **Herbal:** None known. **Food:** None known.

C

DIAGNOSTIC TEST EFFECTS

May increase serum amylase and lipase levels.

SIDE-EFFECTS

Frequent: Constipation, somnolence, nausea, vomiting. **Occasional:** Paradoxic excitement, confusion, palpitations, facial flushing, decreased urination, blurred vision, dizziness, dry mouth, headache, hypotension (including orthostatic hypotension), decreased appetite, injection site redness, burning, or pain. **Rare:** Hallucinations, depression, abdominal pain, insomnia

CRITICAL CARE CONSIDERATIONS

ADMINISTRATION/HANDLING

PO ALERT

- Ambulatory patients and those with mild/moderate pain are more likely to have dizziness, hypotension, nausea, and vomiting than recumbent or supine positioned patients or patients in severe pain.
- Reduce initial dosage in elderly and debilitated patients; those with renal insufficiency, hypothyroidism, Addison's disease, or using other CNS depressants concurrently.
- Give codeine with food or milk to minimize adverse GI effects.

IM, SUBCUTANEOUS ALERT

- Discard drug if cloudiness or precipitates are present.

PRECAUTIONS

HEALTH-RELATED

- Use codeine extremely cautiously in patients with acute alcoholism, anoxia, CNS depression, hypercapnia, respiratory depression or dysfunction, seizures, shock, or untreated myxedema.
- Use codeine cautiously in patients with acute abdominal conditions, Addison's disease, chronic obstructive pulmonary disease, hypothyroidism, hepatic impairment, increased intracranial pressure, benign prostatic hyperplasia, or urethral stricture.

AGE-RELATED

- **Children:** More prone to experience paradoxical excitement. Children under 2 yr are more susceptible to the drug's respiratory depressant effects.
- **Elderly:** More prone to experience respiratory depression and paradoxic reactions. Age-related renal impairment may increase the risk of codeine-induced urinary retention.

PREGNANCY/LACTATION-RELATED

- Pregnancy category C (category D if used for prolonged periods or in high doses at term); use during labor produces neonatal respiratory depression; passes into breast milk in very small amounts; compatible with breast-feeding.

MONITORING

- **Baseline assessment:** Assess the duration, location, onset, and type of pain. If cough is being treated, assess the frequency, severity, and type of cough, as well as sputum production.
- **Lab work:** Biochemical profile including liver function studies (AST [SGOT], ALT [SGPT], alkaline phosphatase, bilirubin).
- **Therapeutic effect:** Assess for clinical improvement and record the onset of pain or cough relief. Drug's effect is reduced if the full pain response recurs before the next dose. Find the dosage regimen most effective to provide steady control of pain without inducing constant somnolence or sleep.
- **Constipation:** Assess daily pattern of bowel activity and stool consistency. Manage constipation with additional fluids, adding fiber to diet, and laxatives or stool softeners if needed.
- **Congestion:** Increase fluid intake and environmental humidity to help improve the viscosity of lung secretions. Encourage deep-breathing and coughing exercises.
- **Orthostatic hypotension:** Instruct patients to change positions slowly to avoid orthostatic hypotension.
- **Patient education:** Caution patients that drug dependence or tolerance may occur with prolonged use of high doses and to avoid alcohol during codeine therapy. Warn patients to avoid tasks that require

mental alertness or motor skills until response to the drug is known.

SERIOUS ADVERSE REACTIONS

- **Paralytic ileus/bowel obstruction:** Too-frequent use may result in ileus or obstruction.
- **Tolerance/dependence:** Patients who use codeine repeatedly may develop a tolerance to the drug's analgesic effect as well as physical dependence.
- **Chest discomfort:** Pain, diaphoresis, palpitations, shortness of breath. Myocardial ischemia may lead to acute myocardial infarction.
- **Hypertension:** CNS stimulation may cause BP elevation.

OVERDOSE/TOXICITY

- **Symptoms:** Cold or clammy skin, confusion, seizures, decreased BP, restlessness, pinpoint pupils, bradycardia, respiratory depression, decreased LOC, and severe weakness.
- **Management:** Administer antidote naloxone and provide supportive care, which may include endotracheal intubation, mechanical ventilation, management of hypotension with fluids and vasopressors, unless bradycardic. Manage bradycardia according to Advanced Cardiac Life Support (ACLS) guidelines (atropine IV, *DOPamine infusion).
- **GI decontamination:** Patients suspected of concealing large amounts of drugs by ingesting packages (called "body packers") can be detected using a contrast-enhanced upper GI series with small bowel follow-through if initial GI radiograph is negative. "Body packers" may benefit from whole bowel irrigation. Simple ingestions may benefit from a single dose of activated charcoal.

ANTIDOTE/DIALYSIS

- **Antidote:** Naloxone 2 mg IV for adults and 0.01 mg/kg for children, up to a total of 10 mg, with dose calculation based on the likelihood of drug dependence. If patients initially respond but then experience resedation, rebolus with naloxone or begin continuous naloxone infusion starting at two thirds of the initial reversal dose hourly titrated to effect.
- **Dialysis:** Codeine is not removed by hemodialysis and is unlikely to be removed by peritoneal dialysis. No data are available on removal by high-permeability hemodialysis.

colchicine 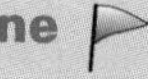

kol'-chi-seen

Classes

Chemical: colchicum autumnale alkaloid
Therapeutic: antigout agent

Pregnancy Category: D (parenteral), C (oral)

Trade Names

Prescription: Colchicine

Combinations

Prescription: with probenicid (Proben-C, Colbenemid)

Do not confuse colchicine with codeine.

CLINICAL PHARMACOLOGY

Mechanism of Action

An alkaloid that decreases leukocyte motility, phagocytosis, and lactic acid production. Therapeutic Effect: Decreases urate crystal deposits and reduces inflammatory process.

PHARMACOKINETICS

Rapidly absorbed from the GI tract. Highest concentration is in the liver, spleen, and kidney. Protein binding: 30%-50%. Reenters the intestinal tract by biliary secretion and is reabsorbed from the intestines. Partially metabolized in the liver. Eliminated primarily in feces.

AVAILABILITY

Tablets: 0.5 mg, 0.6 mg.
Injection: 0.5 mg/mL.

INDICATIONS AND DOSAGE

Acute gouty arthritis

PO

Adults, Elderly: Initially, 0.6-1.2 mg; then 0.6 mg every 1-2 hr until pain is relieved or nausea, vomiting, or diarrhea occurs. Total dose: 6 mg. Wait at least 3 days before initiating another course of therapy.

IV

Adults, Elderly: Initially, 1-2 mg; then 0.5 mg every 6 hr until satisfactory response. Maximum: 4 mg/wk or 4 mg/one course of treatment. If pain recurs, may give 1-2 mg/day for several days but no sooner than 7 days after a full course of IV therapy (total of 4 mg).

Chronic gouty arthritis

PO

Adults, Elderly: 0.6 mg every other day up to 3 times per day.

C

OFF-LABEL USES

To reduce frequency of recurrence of familial Mediterranean fever; treatment of acute calcium pyrophosphate deposition, amyloidosis, biliary cirrhosis, recurrent pericarditis, sarcoid arthritis

CONTRAINDICATIONS

Blood dyscrasias; severe cardiac, GI, hepatic, or renal disorders, hypersensitivity to colchicine

INTERACTIONS

Drug: **Bone marrow depressants:** May increase the risk of blood dyscrasias. **Clarithromycin, erythromycin:** May increase plasma levels of colchicine and increase the risk of toxicity. **NSAIDs:** May increase the risk of bone marrow depression, neutropenia, and thrombocytopenia. Herbal: None known. Food: **Vitamin B_{12}:** Absorption may be decreased.

DIAGNOSTIC TEST EFFECTS

May increase serum alkaline phosphatase and AST (SGOT) levels. May decrease platelet count.

IV INCOMPATIBILITIES

No information available via Y-site administration.

SIDE-EFFECTS

Frequent: **PO:** Nausea, vomiting, abdominal discomfort. Occasional: **PO:** Anorexia. Rare: Hypersensitivity reaction, including angio-edema. **Parenteral:** Nausea, vomiting, diarrhea, abdominal discomfort, pain or redness at injection site, neuritis in injected arm

CRITICAL CARE CONSIDERATIONS

ADMINISTRATION/HANDLING

PO ALERT

- Give colchicine without regard to meals.

IM, SUBCUTANEOUS ALERT

- Subcutaneous or IM administration produces severe local reaction. Administer via IV route only.

IV ALERT

- **Storage:** Store at room temperature.
- **Dilution:** May dilute with 0.9% NaCl or sterile water for injection; do not dilute with D_5W.
- **Administration:** Administer over 2-5 min.

PRECAUTIONS

HEALTH-RELATED

- Use colchicine cautiously in debilitated or elderly patients and in patients with impaired hepatic function. Patients with impaired renal function may experience myopathy and neuropathy manifested as generalized weakness.

AGE-RELATED

- **Children:** Safety and efficacy of colchicine have not been established in children.
- **Elderly:** May be more susceptible to cumulative toxicity, and age-related renal impairment may increase risk of myopathy. IV colchine is relatively contraindicated in elderly.

PREGNANCY/LACTATION-RELATED

- Pregnancy category D for IV (known teratogen); unknown if excreted in breast milk.
- Pregnancy category C for PO.

MONITORING

- **Baseline assessment:** Assess feet and toes for severity of gouty arthritis and pain level. Neurologic exam to establish baseline sensation, muscle strength, and movement. Ensure no significant GI dysfunction or cardiac history: both contraindicate use of colchicine.
- **Baseline lab work:** Uric acid level, complete chemical profile to assess renal and hepatic function.
- **Ongoing lab work:** Serum uric acid level.
- **Diet:** Limit intake of high purine foods to avoid additional uric acid generation.
- **Hydration:** Provide a high fluid intake (3000 mL/day) while taking colchicine to aid renal excretion of uric acid.
- **Intake and output:** Monitor fluid intake and output; output should be at least 2000 mL/day.
- **Onset of adverse effects:** Discontinue colchicine immediately if GI, cardiac, renal symptoms, or liver problems occur.
- **Therapeutic effect:** Assess for improved joint range of motion and reduced joint tenderness, redness, and swelling.
- **Patient education:** When using colchicine outside the hospital, limit intake of high-purine foods (fish and organ meats) and drink 8-10 eight-ounce glasses of fluid daily. Warn patients to report if fever, numbness, skin rash, sore throat, fatigue, unusual bleeding or bruising, or weakness occurs. Colchicine should be discontinued

as soon as gout pain is relieved, or at the first appearance of diarrhea, nausea, or vomiting.

SERIOUS ADVERSE REACTIONS

- **GI symptoms:** If patients have GI symptoms shortly following ingestion, colchicine should be discontinued immediately. Onset of GI symptoms at any point in therapy indicates therapy should be discontinued.
- **Hematologic effects:** Bone marrow depression, including aplastic anemia, agranulocytosis, and thrombocytopenia may occur with long-term therapy.
- **Electrolyte imbalance:** Hypokalemia, hyponatremia, hypocalcemia, hypophosphatemia.

OVERDOSE/TOXICITY

- **Progression of symptoms:** Initially causes burning sensation of skin or throat, severe nausea, vomiting, diarrhea, and abdominal pain. Multiple organ failure (fever, seizures, ascending paralysis, delirium, hepatic and renal failure, acute respiratory distress syndrome, possible rhabdomyolysis and hemorrhage) may ensue. The third stage is marked by hair loss, leukocytosis, and stomatitis.
- **Death:** Cumulative IV doses of colchicine above 4 mg (or 0.8 mg/kg) have resulted in irreversible organ failure and death.
- **Management:** Supportive care, including IV volume replacement, blood products, intubation and mechanical ventilation, hemodynamic monitoring with vasopressor support if needed. Manage seizures with benzodiazepines or barbiturates. Manage underlying acidosis aggressively. Hemodialysis or continuous renal replacement therapy are used for renal failure. Monitor closely for infection if neutropenia ensues.
- **GI decontamination:** Activated charcoal administered in multiple doses, unless patients have a paralytic ileus. Gastric lavage is helpful only if the patient presents within 1 hr of overdose.

ANTIDOTE/DIALYSIS

- **Antidote:** No specific recommendations.
- **Dialysis:** Colchicine is not removed by hemodialysis or peritoneal dialysis. No data are available on removal by high-permeability hemodialysis.

colesevelam

koh-le-sev′-e-lam

Classes

Chemical: hydrophilic nonabsorbed polymer

Therapeutic: antilipemic, bile acid sequestrant

Pregnancy Category: B

Trade Names

Prescription: Welchol

Do not confuse Welchol with Wellbutrin.

C

CLINICAL PHARMACOLOGY

Mechanism of Action

A bile acid sequestrant and nonsystemic polymer that binds with bile acids in the intestines, preventing their reabsorption and removing them from the body. Therapeutic Effect: Decreases LDL cholesterol.

PHARMACOKINETICS

Not absorbed. Primarily eliminated in feces.

AVAILABILITY

Tablets: 625 mg.

INDICATIONS AND DOSAGE

To decrease LDL cholesterol level in primary hypercholesterolemia (Fredrickson type IIa)

PO

Adults, Elderly: 3 tablets with meals twice per day or 6 tablets once per day with a meal. May increase daily dose to 7 tablets per day.

CONTRAINDICATIONS

Complete biliary obstruction, hypersensitivity to colsevelam

INTERACTIONS

Drug: **Aspirin, clindamycin, digoxin, furosemide, *glipiZIDE, hydrocortisone, imipramine, NSAIDs, phenytoin, propranolol, tetracyclines, thiazide diuretics, and vitamins A, D, E, K:** May decrease the absorption of these drugs. Herbal: None known. Food: None known.

DIAGNOSTIC TEST EFFECTS

None known.

SIDE-EFFECTS

Frequent (12%-8%): Flatulence, constipation, infection, dyspepsia (heartburn, epigastric distress)

C

CRITICAL CARE CONSIDERATIONS

ADMINISTRATION/HANDLING

PO ALERT

- Administer colesevelam with meals.
- Give colesevelam with a liquid.

PRECAUTIONS

HEALTH-RELATED

- Use colesevelam cautiously in patients with dysphagia, severe GI motility disorders, liver disease, and those with history of major GI tract surgery. Colesevelam facilitates depletion of bile acids which prompts increased conversion of cholesterol into bile acids.
- Colesevelam has not been tested in patients with triglyceride levels greater than 300 mg/dL and should be used cautiously in these patients.
- **Fat-soluble vitamin deficiency:** Animal studies revealed large drug doses caused vitamin K deficiency resulting in bleeding and hemorrhage. Colesevelam did not significantly reduce absorption of vitamins A, D, E, or K in normal doses.

AGE-RELATED

- **Children:** Safety and efficacy of colesevelam have not been established in children.
- **Elderly:** No age-related precautions have been noted.

PREGNANCY/LACTATION-RELATED

- Pregnancy category B (no harm in animal studies, but no adequate and well-controlled studies in pregnant women; no expected excretion into breast milk.

MONITORING

- **Baseline assessment:** Assess for cardiovascular disease risk factors including history of diabetes, hyperglycemia, chest discomfort, intermittent claudication, headaches, dizziness, confusion, activity intolerance, and poor peripheral circulation.
- **Baseline lab work:** Assess lipid profile (total cholesterol, LDL-C, and triglyceride levels), blood glucose, and serum transaminases (AST [SGOT], ALT [SGPT]).
- **Therapeutic effect:** Monitor for reduction in lipid profile values including cholesterol and triglyceride levels.
- **Bowel obstruction:** Assess for constipation, bloating, abdominal pain, hyperactive or slow to absent bowel sounds, and hard stool consistency. Encourage PO fluid intake or provide adequate hydration.
- **GI side effects:** Assess for and manage dyspepsia, heartburn, and steatorrhea.
- **Patient education:** Advise following the prescribed diet, exercise, monitor lab values as prescribed (cholesterol, triglycerides, blood glucose) because all are an important part of treatment. Explain not to take any medications, including OTC drugs, without physician approval.

SERIOUS ADVERSE REACTIONS

- **Bowel obstruction:** GI tract obstruction may occur.
- **Other reactions:** Other bile acid sequestrants (cholestyramine) have caused reduced absorption of warfarin resulting in bleeding.

OVERDOSE/TOXICITY

- **GI decontamination:** No specific recommendations, but since colesevelam binds to bile acids secreted into the intestine, bowel irrigation may be effective following use of activated charcoal as appropriate.

ANTIDOTE/DIALYSIS

- **Antidote:** No specific recommendations.
- **Dialysis:** Colesevelam is unlikely to be removed by hemodialysis, peritoneal dialysis, or high-permeability hemodialysis.

corticotropin (ACTH)

kor-ti-koe-troe'-pin

Classes

Chemical: adrenocorticotropic hormone
Therapeutic: corticosteroid, adrenal

Pregnancy Category: C

Trade Names

Prescription: ACTH-80, ACTH Gel, Acthar, Acthar Gel, Acthar Gel H.P.

Do not confuse corticotropin with cortisone.

CLINICAL PHARMACOLOGY

Mechanism of Action

An adrenocortical steroid that stimulates the adrenal cortex to secrete cortisol, corticosterone, aldosterone, and androgenic substances. Acts to stimulate synthesis of adrenocortical hormones. Therapeutic Effect: Suppresses immune response and inflammation.

PHARMACOKINETICS

Half-life: 15 min.

AVAILABILITY

Powder for injection: 25 units (Acthar).
Injection: 40 units/mL (Acthar Gel, Acthar Gel H.P.), 80 units/mL (ACTH-80, Acthar Gel H.P.).

INDICATIONS AND DOSAGE

Diagnostic testing

IV

Adults: 10-25 units in 500 mL D_5W infused over 8 hr.

Acute exacerbation of multiple sclerosis

IM, Subcutaneous

Adults: 80-120 units/day for 2-3 wk.

Infantile spasms

IM

Infants: 20-40 units/day or 80 units every other day for 3 mo (or 1 mo after cessation of seizures).

Usual repository injection

IM, Subcutaneous

Adults: 40-80 units every 24-72 hr.

CONTRAINDICATIONS

Hypersensitivity to any corticosteroid, corticotropin, or porcine proteins; systemic fungal infection; peptic ulcers (except in life-threatening situations); scleroderma; primary adrenocortical insufficiency; live virus vaccine; long-term therapy in children; ocular herpes simplex

INTERACTIONS

Drug: **Amphotericin:** May increase hypokalemia. **Digoxin:** May increase the toxicity of digoxin caused by hypokalemia. **Diuretics, insulin, oral hypoglycemics, potassium supplements:** May decrease the effects of diuretics, insulin, oral hypoglycemics, and potassium supplements. **Hepatic enzyme inducers:** May decrease the effects of corticotropin. **Live virus vaccines:** May decrease antibody response to vaccine, increase vaccine side effects, and potentiate virus replication. Herbal: None known. Food: None known.

DIAGNOSTIC TEST EFFECTS

May decrease serum calcium, potassium, and thyroxine levels. May increase cholesterol, lipids, glucose, sodium, and amylase.

SIDE-EFFECTS

Frequent: Insomnia, heartburn, nervousness, abdominal distention, increased sweating, acne, mood swings, increased appetite, facial flushing, delayed wound healing, increased susceptibility to infection, diarrhea or constipation. Occasional: Headache, edema, change in skin color, frequent urination. Rare: Tachycardia, allergic reaction (rash, hives), pain, erythema, swelling at injection site, psychic changes, hallucinations, depression

C

CRITICAL CARE CONSIDERATIONS

ADMINISTRATION/HANDLING

IM/SUBCUTANEOUS ALERT

- Give corticotropin zinc hydroxide preparation IM only.
- **Acthar:** Must be reconstituted at the time of use by dissolving in a volume of sterile water for injection or sodium chloride injection to create an individual dose contained in 1-2 mL of solution. The reconstituted solution should be refrigerated and used within 24 hr.

IV ALERT

- **Cosyntropin (Cortrosyn):** Use IV only (corticotropin injection). May be given by direct IV injection.
- **Reconstitution:** Dilute with at least 1.1 mL normal saline (NS). May dilute with up to 2-5 mL. Discard unused reconstituted solution. Administer single dose over 2 min.
- **Further dilution:** Dilute with 250 mL normal saline (250 mcg in 250 mL NS) for a concentration of 1 mcg/mL. Administer over 4-8 hr.
- **Storage:** Store corticotropin for injection at room temperature.

PRECAUTIONS

HEALTH-RELATED

- Use corticotropin cautiously in patients with thromboembolic disorders, history of tuberculosis (may reactivate disease), hypothyroidism, cirrhosis, nonspecific ulcerative colitis, heart failure, hypertension, psychosis, renal insufficiency, and seizures.
- Discontinue prolonged therapy slowly.
- Corticotropin will not increase cortisol secretion in patients with primary adrenal insufficiency.

AGE-RELATED

- **Children:** Prolonged use of corticotropin in children will inhibit skeletal growth.
- **Elderly:** No studies of corticotropin use in the elderly have been performed.

PREGNANCY/LACTATION-RELATED

- Pregnancy category C; use cautiously in breast-feeding women.

MONITORING

- **Baseline assessment:** Determine hypersensitivity to any of the corticosteroids. Assess vital signs, height, and weight.
- **Lab work:** Plasma cortisol level to diagnose deficiency and response to corticotropin. CBC including WBC differential; baseline biochemical profile including blood glucose levels, calcium, magnesium, phosphorous, renal (BUN, creatinine), and liver (AST [SGOT], ALT [SGPT], bilirubin, alkaline phosphatase) function studies.
- **Diagnostic tests:** Corticotropin stimulation test is used to diagnose adrenal insufficiency; adrenal function is considered abnormal if plasma cortisol level is less the 18 mcg/dL after an injection of ACTH (cosyntropin).
- **Immunosuppression:** Assess for signs of infection caused by reduced immune response, including fever, sore throat, or vague symptoms.
- **Pulmonary artery catheter:** Swan Ganz catheter may be needed to help assess volume and overall hemodynamic status when managing adrenal insufficiency. Hypovolemia may be present. With primary adrenal insufficiency, IV glucocorticoids (hydrocortisone), and mineralcorticoids, (fludrocortisone) must be replaced as adrenal glands are unable to respond to corticotropin.
- **Long-term therapy:** Monitor for signs of either hypercortisolism (dose is too high) and adrenal insufficency (dose is too low). High dosage may prompt hypocalcemia (muscle twitching, cramps, positive Chvostek's or Trousseau's signs), hypokalemia (weakness and muscle cramps, numbness or tingling, especially in the lower extremities, nausea and vomiting, irritability, ventricular dysrhythmias), and hyperglycemia (polyuria, polydipsia, polyphagia leading to dehydration). Low dosage may prompt hyponatremia (confusion, irritability, dizziness, seizures, coma, possible muscle spasms), hyperkalemia (irritability, abdominal cramping, diarrhea, ascending weakness, paresthesias, irregular pulse, metabolic acidosis, widening QRS, loss of P wave), and hypoglycemia (confusion, tremors, tachycardia, diaphoresis, dysrhythmias).
- **Taper dosage gradually:** Assess for signs of adrenal insufficiency (hypotension, tachycardia, confusion, weakness, nausea, abdominal pain, possible fever, hyperkalemia, hypoglycemia, hyponatremia, hypocalcemia) when tapering the drug because cortisol levels may decrease quickly.
- **Insomnia and mood swings:** Assess ability to sleep and emotional status.
- **Weight gain/BP elevation:** Monitor for salt and retention-induced weight gain, edema, and increase in BP.
- **Patient education:** Instruct patients not to change the dose or schedule of corticotropin. Caution against discontinuing the drug. Taper corticotropin dosage gradually under supervision of a health care provider with appropriate educational preparation to manage adrenal insufficiency and pituitary dysfunction. Instruct patients to report fever, muscle aches, sore throat, sudden weight gain, or swelling, and inform dentists and other health care providers of corticotropin therapy now or within the past 12 mo.

SERIOUS ADVERSE REACTIONS

- **Long-term therapy:** Electrolyte imbalances (hypocalcemia, hypokalemia, hyponatremia), muscle wasting in arms and legs, osteoporosis, spontaneous fractures, amenorrhea, cataracts, glaucoma, peptic ulcer, and fluid retention.
- **Abrupt discontinuation after long-term therapy:** May prompt adrenal insufficiency (anorexia, nausea, fever, headache, joint pain, rebound inflammation, fatigue, weakness, lethargy, dizziness, and orthostatic hypertension).

OVERDOSE/TOXICITY

- **Hypercortisolism:** Generally seen with long-term therapy rather than isolated dosage error. Symptoms include severe behavioral changes including extreme euphoria, personality changes, severe depression, frank psychosis (more likely in patients with mental health history), significant weight gain (greater than 15 lb), pitting edema, heart failure, difficulty breathing, GI bleeding (hematemesis, bloody stools, expectoration of blood). Patients with underlying infection or who acquire a significant infection may develop fatal septic shock. Electrolyte imbalances include hyperglycemia, hypernatremia, and hypokalemia.
- **Management:** Corticotropin must be tapered rather than discontinued to avoid adrenal insufficiency. Symptom specific supportive care should be provided.

Hyperglycemia should be managed with insulin infusion until the patient's blood glucose stabilizes.

- **GI decontamination:** No specific recommendations.

ANTIDOTE/DIALYSIS

- **Antidote:** No specific recommendations.
- **Dialysis:** No data are available on removal of corticotropin by hemodialysis, high-permeability hemodialysis, or peritoneal dialysis.

cortisone acetate

kor'-ti-sone ass'-eh-tayte

Classes
Chemical: glucocorticoid
Therapeutic: corticosteroid, systemic

Pregnancy Category: D

Trade Names
Prescription: Cortone

Do not confuse cortisone with Cort-Dome or corticotropin.

CLINICAL PHARMACOLOGY

Mechanism of Action

An adrenocortical steroid that inhibits the accumulation of inflammatory cells at inflammation sites, phagocytosis, lysosomal enzyme release and synthesis, and release of mediators of inflammation. Therapeutic Effect: Prevents or suppresses cell-mediated immune reactions. Decreases or prevents tissue response to inflammatory process.

PHARMACOKINETICS

Slowly absorbed after PO administration. Protein binding: 90%. Metabolized in liver. Excreted in urine and feces. Half-life: 0.5-2 hr.

AVAILABILITY

Tablets: 5 mg, 10 mg, 25 mg.
Injectable suspension: 25 mg/mL, 50 mg/mL.

INDICATIONS AND DOSAGE

Adrenocortical insufficiency

PO

Adults, Elderly: 12-15 mg/m^2 divided as two thirds in the morning and one third in the afternoon. **Children:** 0.5-0.75 mg/kg/day in 3 divided doses.

IM

Children: 0.25-0.35 mg/kg/day.

Dosage is dependent on the condition being treated and patient response.

Inflammatory conditions

PO

Adults, Elderly: 25-300 mg/day. **Children.** 2.5-10 mg/kg/day in 3-4 divided doses.

IM

Adults, Elderly: 25-300 mg/day. **Children:** 1-5 mg/kg/day in 1-2 doses/day.

CONTRAINDICATIONS

Hypersensitivity to cortisone or other corticosteroids, administration of live virus vaccine, peptic ulcers (except in life-threatening situations), systemic fungal infection

INTERACTIONS

Drug: **Amphotericin:** May increase hypokalemia. **Bupropion:** May lower the seizure threshold. **Digoxin:** May increase digoxin toxicity caused by hypokalemia. **Diuretics, insulin, oral hypoglycemics, potassium supplements:** May decrease the effects of these drugs. **Fluoroquinolones:** May increase the risk for tendon rupture. **Hepatic enzyme inducers:** May decrease the effects of cortisone. **Live-virus vaccines:** May decrease antibody response to vaccine, increase vaccine side effects, and potentiate virus replication. Herbal: **Echinacea, Ma huang:** May decrease corticosteroid effectiveness. Food: None known.

DIAGNOSTIC TEST EFFECTS

May increase blood glucose and serum lipid, amylase, and sodium levels. May decrease serum calcium, potassium, and thyroxine levels.

SIDE-EFFECTS

Frequent: Insomnia, heartburn, anxiety, abdominal distention, increased diaphoresis, acne, mood swings, increased appetite, facial flushing, delayed wound healing, increased susceptibility to infection, diarrhea or constipation, nervousness. Occasional: Headache, edema, change in skin color, frequent urination. Rare: Tachycardia, allergic reaction (such as rash and hives), psychological changes, hallucinations, depression

CRITICAL CARE CONSIDERATIONS

ADMINISTRATION/HANDLING

PO ALERT

- May administer cortisone without regard to meals; food may help to reduce heartburn or other GI discomfort.

C

IM ALERT

- Cortone acetate sterile suspension contains 50 mg/mL of cortisone acetate, which is sensitive to heat. Do not alter suspension. Dilution may change rate of absorption and reduce effectiveness.
- If PO dosage cannot be tolerated, one daily injection is generally sufficient to provide dosage because the IM route has a long duration of action.

PRECAUTIONS

HEALTH-RELATED

- Use cortisone cautiously in patients with cirrhosis or other liver disease, heart failure, history of tuberculosis (it may reactivate disease), ocular herpes simplex, history of GI bleeding, hypertension, hypothyroidism, nonspecific ulcerative colitis, possible infection, possible psychosis, seizure disorders, or thromboembolic disorders.
- **Cytochrome P450 enzyme metabolism:** Patients receiving phenytoin, phenobarbital, rifampin (increase clearance of cortisone) may require an increased dose of cortisone. Troleandomycin and ketoconazole decrease clearance of cortisone; patients receiving these drugs may require decreased doses of cortisone.
- Cortisone increases clearance of high-dose aspirin; patients receiving chronic therapy may require higher doses of aspirin. Aspirin should be used cautiously with cortisone in patients with hypoprothrombinemia to avoid bleeding.
- **Anticoagulants:** Effects on blood coagulation may increase or decrease when cortisone is administered with anticoagulants.

AGE-RELATED

- **Children:** Monitor growth and development of children receiving long-term steroid therapy.
- **Elderly:** No special dosage precautions; all patients on prolonged therapy may develop subcapsular cataracts and glaucoma and are at higher risk for ocular infections.

PREGNANCY/LACTATION-RELATED

- Pregnancy category D; excreted in breast milk.

MONITORING

- **Baseline assessment:** Determine hypersensitivity to corticosteroids; measure height, weight, and vital signs. If diabetes mellitus is present, increase antidiabetic drug regimen or consider IV insulin infusion to manage steroid-induced hyperglycemia initially. Assess drugs being taken that are affected by cortisone and adjust dosage.
- **Baseline lab work:** Serum electrolyte levels; if digoxin is being taken, measure serum digoxin level or levels of any other medication affected by cortisone.
- **Adjusted drug doses:** If drug dosages had been increased or decreased in relation to cortisone administration, when the drug is withdrawn, ensure that other medication doses are readjusted to avoid toxicity or ineffective levels of the other medications.
- **Infection:** Be alert for infection caused by reduced immune response, including fever, sore throat, and vague symptoms.
- **Weight gain/elevated BP:** Monitor for salt and retention-induced weight gain, edema, and increases in BP.
- **Hypokalemia:** Monitor ECG for dysrhythmias induced by increased potassium excretion such as premature ventricular beats and ventricular and supraventricular tachycardias.
- **Electrolyte imbalance:** Monitor for hypocalcemia (muscle twitching, cramps, and positive Chvostek's or Trousseau's signs), or hypokalemia (ECG changes, nausea and vomiting, irritability, weakness and muscle cramps, numbness and tingling, especially in lower extremities).
- **Avoid adrenal insufficiency:** Wean cortisone slowly to discontinue both aggressive short term and prolonged therapy.
- **Sleep disturbance and emotional lability:** Assess sleep pattern and emotional status; cortisone may cause sleeplessness, euphoria, high energy, or labile emotional state. Inform patients that cortisone often causes mood swings.
- **Patient education:** When using cortisone outside the hospital, instruct patients to take cortisone exactly as prescribed (not to change the dosage or schedule). Caution against abruptly discontinuing the drug; cortisone must be withdrawn gradually under medical supervision. Tell patients to report fever, muscle aches, sore throat, and sudden weight gain or swelling and to inform dentists and other physicians about taking/having taken cortisone within the past 12 mo.

SERIOUS ADVERSE REACTIONS

- **Long-term therapy:** May cause hypocalcemia, hypokalemia, muscle wasting in arms and legs, osteoporosis, spontaneous fractures, amenorrhea, cataracts, glaucoma, peptic ulcer disease, Cushing's syndrome (moon face, fat pads), and heart failure.

- **Abrupt discontinuation after long-term therapy:** May cause anorexia, nausea, fever, headache, joint pain, rebound inflammation, fatigue, weakness, lethargy, dizziness, and orthostatic hypotension.

OVERDOSE/TOXICITY

- **Severe behavioral changes:** Extreme euphoria, personality changes, severe depression, frank psychosis (more likely in patients with mental health history).
- **Edema/weight gain:** Significant weight gain (greater than 15 lb), pitting edema, heart failure, difficulty breathing.
- **GI bleeding:** Hematemesis, bloody stools, expectoration of blood.
- **Severe infection:** Patients who have underlying infection or acquire a significant infection may develop fatal septic shock.
- **GI decontamination:** No specific recommendations.

ANTIDOTE/DIALYSIS

- **Antidote:** No specific recommendations.
- **Dialysis:** Cortisone is not removed by hemodialysis or peritoneal dialysis. No data are available on removal by high-permeability hemodialysis.

cromolyn sodium

See Bronchodilators (p. 947)

cyclobenzaprine hydrochloride

sye-kloe-ben'-za-preen hye-droe-klor'-ide

Classes

Chemical: tricyclic amine
Therapeutic: skeletal muscle relaxant

Pregnancy Category: B

Trade Names

Prescription: Flexeril, Riva-Cycloprine ♣

Do not confuse cyclobenzaprine with *cycloSERINE or cyproheptadine or Flexeril with Floxin.

CLINICAL PHARMACOLOGY

Mechanism of Action

A centrally acting skeletal muscle relaxant that reduces tonic somatic muscle activity at the level of the brainstem. **Therapeutic Effect:** Relieves local skeletal muscle spasm.

PHARMACOKINETICS

Route	Onset	Peak	Duration
PO	1 hr	3-8 hr	12-24 hr

Well but slowly absorbed from the GI tract. Protein binding: 93%. Metabolized in the GI tract and the liver. Primarily excreted in urine. **Half-life:** 18 hr.

AVAILABILITY

Tablets: 5 mg, 10 mg.

INDICATIONS AND DOSAGE

Acute, painful musculoskeletal conditions
PO
Adults: Initially, 5 mg 3 times per day. May increase to 10 mg 3 times per day. **Elderly:** 5 mg 3 times per day.
Dosage in hepatic impairment
Mild: 5 mg 3 times per day.
Moderate and severe: Not recommended.

OFF-LABEL USES

Treatment of fibromyalgia

CONTRAINDICATIONS

Acute recovery phase of MI, dysrhythmias, heart failure, heart block, conduction disturbances, hyperthyroidism, use within 14 days of MAOIs, hypersensitivity to cyclobenzaprine

INTERACTIONS

Drug: **Alcohol, other CNS depression-producing medications (such as tricyclic antidepressants):** May increase CNS depression. **MAOIs:** May increase the risk of hypertensive crisis and severe seizures. **Tramadol:** May increase the risk of seizures. **Herbal:** None known. **Food:** None known.

DIAGNOSTIC TEST EFFECTS

None known.

SIDE-EFFECTS

Frequent: Somnolence (39%), dry mouth (27%), dizziness (11%). **Rare (3%-1%):** Fatigue, asthenia, blurred vision, headache, nervousness, confusion, nausea, constipation, dyspepsia, unpleasant taste

CRITICAL CARE CONSIDERATIONS

ADMINISTRATION/HANDLING

PO ALERT

- Give cyclobenzaprine without regard to food.

C

- Do not administer cyclobenzaprine for longer than 2-3 wk.

PRECAUTIONS

HEALTH-RELATED

- Use cyclobenzaprine cautiously in patients with angle-closure glaucoma, impaired hepatic or renal function, increased intraocular pressure, or a history of urinary retention.

AGE-RELATED

- **Children:** Safety and efficacy of cyclobenzaprine have not been established in children.
- **Elderly:** Have an increased sensitivity to the drug's anticholinergic effects, such as confusion and urine retention.

PREGNANCY/LACTATION-RELATED

- Pregnancy category B; no data are available, but closely related tricyclic antidepressants are excreted into breast milk.

MONITORING

- **Baseline assessment:** Assess duration, location, onset, and type of muscle spasm. Examine for immobility, stiffness, and swelling.
- **Lab work:** Biochemical profile including renal (BUN, creatinine) and liver (AST [SGOT], ALT [SGPT], bilirubin, alkaline phosphatase) function tests.
- **Prevent falls:** Assist patients with ambulation to avoid falls related to ataxia. Instruct patients to change positions slowly to help avoid cyclobenzaprine's hypotensive effects.
- **Therapeutic response:** Assess for decreased skeletal muscle pain, stiffness, tenderness, and improved mobility.
- **Drowsiness:** Usually diminishes with continued therapy.
- **Dry mouth:** Have patients sip water or chew sugarless gum to relieve dry mouth.
- **Patient education:** When cyclobenzaprine will be used outside the hospital, tell patients to avoid tasks that require mental alertness or motor skills until response to the drug is known. Urge patients to avoid alcohol and other CNS depressants while taking cyclobenzaprine.

SERIOUS ADVERSE REACTIONS

- Cyclobenzaprine is related to tricyclic antidepressants and when used in higher doses for conditions other than muscle spasm associated with musculoskeletal conditions, it has rarely produced syncope, tachycardia, other cardiac dysrhythmias, general malaise, ataxia, vertigo, anxiety, tremors, and liver dysfunction.

OVERDOSE/TOXICITY

- **Symptoms:** Visual hallucinations, hyperactive reflexes, muscle rigidity, vomiting and hyperpyrexia, respiratory depression, sinus and/or ventricular tachycardia, widening of QRS complex on ECG, right axis deviation, seizures, hypotension.
- **Management:** Supportive therapy to alleviate symptoms including maintenance of patent airway, intubation and mechanical ventilation if needed, IV fluids initially to correct hypotension, vasopressors to correct refractory hypotension, benzodiazepines (lorazepam, diazepam) to manage seizures. Ventilator driven serum alkalization and/or IV administration of sodium bicarbonate to help increase serum pH may help correct cardiac conduction defects since many common antidysrhythmic agents are ineffective or may worsen dysrhythmias. Flumazenil should not be given, as it may prompt seizures.
- **GI decontamination:** Activated charcoal followed by gastric lavage for patients who present within 1-3 hr following ingestion.

ANTIDOTE/DIALYSIS

- **Antidote:** No specific recommendations.
- **Dialysis:** Cyclobenzaprine is unlikely to be removed by hemodialysis, peritoneal dialysis, or high-permeability hemodialysis.

cyclophosphamide 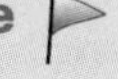

sye-kloe-fos'-fa-mide

Classes

Chemical: nitrogen mustard, synthetic
Therapeutic: antineoplastic

Pregnancy Category: D

Trade Names

Prescription: Cytoxan, Cytoxan Lyophilized, Neosar, Procytox ♣

Do not confuse Cytoxan with cefoxitin, Ciloxan, cyclosporine, or Cytotec.

CLINICAL PHARMACOLOGY

Mechanism of Action

An alkylating agent that inhibits DNA and RNA protein synthesis by cross-linking with DNA and RNA strands, preventing cell growth. Cell cycle-phase nonspecific. **Therapeutic Effect:** Potent immunosuppressant.

C

PHARMACOKINETICS

Well absorbed from the GI tract. Protein binding: Low. Crosses the blood–brain barrier. Metabolized in the liver to active metabolites. Primarily excreted in urine. Removed by hemodialysis. **Half-life:** 3-12 hr.

AVAILABILITY

Tablets (Cytoxan): 25 mg, 50 mg.
Powder for injection (Neosar): 100 mg, 200 mg, 500 mg, 1 g, 2 g.
Powder for injection (Lyophilized [Cytoxan Lyophilized]): 100 mg, 200 mg, 500 mg, 1 g, 2 g.

INDICATIONS AND DOSAGE

Ovarian adenocarcinoma, breast carcinoma, Hodgkin's disease, non-Hodgkin's lymphoma, multiple myeloma, leukemia (acute lymphoblastic, acute myelogenous, acute monocytic, chronic granulocytic, chronic lymphocytic), mycosis fungoides, disseminated neuroblastoma, retinoblastoma

PO

Adults: 1-5 mg/kg/day. **Children:** Initially, 2-8 mg/kg/day. Maintenance: 2-5 mg/kg twice per wk.

IV

Adults: 40-50 mg/kg in divided doses over 2-5 days or 10-15 mg/kg every 7-10 days or 3-5 mg/kg twice per wk. **Children:** 2-8 mg/kg/day for 6 days or total dose for 7 days once per wk.

Biopsy-proven minimal-change nephrotic syndrome

PO

Adults, Children: 2.5-3 mg/kg/day for 60-90 days.

OFF-LABEL USES

Adrenocortical, bladder, cervical, endometrial, prostatic, testicular carcinomas; Ewing's sarcoma; multiple sclerosis: non–small cell, small cell lung cancer; organ transplant rejection; osteosarcoma; ovarian germ cell, primary brain, trophoblastic tumors; rheumatoid arthritis; soft-tissue sarcomas, systemic dermatomyositis, systemic lupus erythematosus, Wilms's tumor

CONTRAINDICATIONS

Severe bone marrow suppression

INTERACTIONS

Drug: Allopurinol, bone marrow depressants: May increase myelosuppression. **Antigout medications:** May decrease the effects of these drugs. **Cytarabine:** May increase the risk of cardiomyopathy. **Immunosuppressants:** May increase the risk of infection and development of neoplasms. **Live-virus vaccines:** May potentiate virus replication, increase vaccine side effects, and decrease antibody response to the vaccine. **Herbal:** None known. **Food:** None known.

DIAGNOSTIC TEST EFFECTS

May increase serum uric acid levels.

IV INCOMPATIBILITIES

Amphotericin B complex (Abelcet, AmBisome, Amphotec)

IV COMPATIBILITIES

Granisetron (Kytril), heparin, hydromorphone (Dilaudid), lorazepam (Ativan), morphine, ondansetron (Zofran), propofol (Diprivan)

SIDE-EFFECTS

Expected: Marked leukopenia 8-15 days after initial therapy. **Frequent:** Nausea, vomiting (beginning about 6 hr after administration and lasting about 4 hr); alopecia (33%). **Occasional:** Diarrhea, darkening of skin and fingernails, stomatitis, headache, diaphoresis. **Rare:** Pain or redness at injection site

CRITICAL CARE CONSIDERATIONS

ADMINISTRATION/HANDLING

DOSAGE ALERT

- Cyclophosphamide dosage is individualized based on the patient's clinical response.
- **Combination therapy:** When used in specific protocols, follow optimum dosage and drug sequencing guidelines.
- **Carcinogenic:** Cyclophosphamide should be handled with extreme care during preparation to avoid undue exposure to the carcinogenic, mutagenic, and teratogenic effects.

PO ALERT

- Give cyclophosphamide on an empty stomach. If GI upset occurs, may give with food.

IV ALERT

- **IV push reconstitution:** Reconstitute each 100 mg to 5 mL sterile water for injection or bacteriostatic water for injection for a concentration of 20 mg/mL. Shake to dissolve; allow solution to stand until clear.
- **Further dilution:** Dilute with 250 mL D_5W, 0.9% NaCl, 0.45% NaCl, lactated Ringer's solution (LR), or D_5W/LR.

- **IV infusion:** Give each 100 mg or fraction thereof over at least 15 min. The IV route may cause facial flushing, faintness, and oropharygeal odd sensations.

C

PRECAUTIONS

HEALTH-RELATED

- Use cyclophosphamide cautiously in patients with severe leukopenia, thrombocytopenia, tumor infiltration of bone marrow, or previous therapy with other antineoplastic agents or radiation.

AGE-RELATED

- **Children:** No age-related precautions have been noted; children are more prone to developing hemorrhagic cystitis than are adults.
- **Elderly:** Age-related renal impairment may prompt a dosage reduction.

PREGNANCY/LACTATION-RELATED

- Pregnancy category D; excreted in breast milk; contraindicated because of potential for adverse effects relating to immune suppression, growth, and carcinogenesis.

MONITORING

- **Baseline assessment:** Assess for history of cancer or nephrotic syndrome in children. If used off label, assess for history and management of disease state.
- **Lab work:** CBC with WBC differential; biochemical profile including renal (BUN, creatinine) function tests and uric acid levels.
- **Hydration:** Keep patients well hydrated to avoid cystitis.
- **Anemia:** Assess for weakness, activity intolerance, excessive fatigue.
- **Leukopenia:** Recovery from severe leukopenia due to bone marrow depression occurs in 17-28 days.
- **Thrombocytopenia:** Assess for easy bruising, ecchymoses, bleeding from gums or from invasive sites, hematuria or coffee ground emesis or nasogastric tube output.
- **Patient education:** Encourage patients to consume large amounts of fluid before, during, and after cyclophosphamide therapy to create enough urine to require frequent voiding to help avoid cystitis. Discuss the need to review all other medications and for patients not to receive vaccinations while on therapy because resistance is very low. Patients should avoid contact with anyone who has recently received a vaccination. Instruct on importance of promptly reporting any unusual bruising or bleeding to a health care provider. Explain that alopecia is reversible, but new hair growth may be a different color or texture than original hair.

SERIOUS ADVERSE REACTIONS

- **Cystitis:** Hemorrhagic cystitis is a common occurrence in long-term therapy, especially in pediatric patients.
- **Hyperkalemia:** Seen with prolonged use or large doses.
- **Infertility:** Amenorrhea and azoospermia may occur.

OVERDOSE/TOXICITY

- **Hematologic:** Bone marrow depression resulting in anemia, leucopenia, thrombocytopenia, and hypoprothrombinemia. Thrombocytopenia may occur 10-15 days after drug is initiated. Anemia generally occurs after large doses or prolonged therapy.
- **Pulmonary fibrosis:** Shortness of breath, cough, activity intolerance; diagnosis is made initially by chest x-ray, then lung biopsy.
- **Cardiotoxicity:** Heart failure, dysrhythmias.
- **GI decontamination:** No specific recommendations.

ANTIDOTE/DIALYSIS

- **Antidote:** No specific recommendations.
- **Dialysis:** Cyclophosphamide is removed by hemodialysis and is likely removed by high-permeability hemodialysis. No data are available on removal by peritoneal dialysis.

*cycloSPORINE

sye-kloe-spor'-in

Classes

Chemical: cyclic peptide
Therapeutic: immunosuppressant

Pregnancy Category: C

Trade Names

Prescription: Gengraf, Neoral, Restasis, Sandimmune

Do not confuse cyclosporine with *cycloSERINE, cyclophosphamide, or Cyklokapron.

CLINICAL PHARMACOLOGY

Mechanism of Action

A cyclic polypeptide that inhibits both cellular and humoral immune responses by inhibiting interleukin-2, a proliferative factor needed for T-cell activity. **Therapeutic Effect:** Prevents organ rejection and relieves symptoms of psoriasis and arthritis.

PHARMACOKINETICS

Variably absorbed from the GI tract. Protein binding: 90%. Widely distributed. Metabolized in the liver. Eliminated primarily by biliary or fecal excretion. Not removed by hemodialysis. **Half-life:** Adults, 10-27 hr; children, 7-19 hr.

AVAILABILITY

Capsules (Softgel [Gengraf, Neoral, Sandimmune]): 25 mg, 100 mg.
Oral solution (Sandimmune): 50-mL bottle with calibrated liquid measuring device.
Injection (Sandimmune): 50 mg/mL.
Ophthalmic emulsion (Restasis): 0.05%.

INDICATIONS AND DOSAGE

Transplantation, prevention of organ rejection

PO

Adults, Elderly, Children: 14-18 mg/kg/dose given 4-12 hr before organ transplantation; 10-14 mg/kg/day used for kidney transplant; continued for 1-2 wk. Maintenance: Pretransplant dose is decreased by 5% weekly to 5-15 mg/kg/day in divided doses, then tapered to 3-10 mg/kg/day.

IV

Adults, Elderly, Children: Initially, 5-6 mg/kg/dose given 4-12 hr before organ transplantation. Maintenance: 3-8 mg/kg/day in divided doses.

Rheumatoid arthritis

PO

Adults, Elderly: Initially, 2.5 mg/kg per day in 2 divided doses. May increase by 0.5-0.75 mg/kg/day after 8 wk of treatment if insufficient response is seen. Maximum: 4 mg/kg/day.

Psoriasis

PO

Adults, Elderly: Initially, 2.5 mg/kg/day in 2 divided doses. May increase by 0.5 mg/kg/day after 4 wk of treatment if insufficient response is seen. Maximum: 4 mg/kg/day.

Dry eye

Ophthalmic

Adults, Elderly: Instill 1 drop in each affected eye every 12 hr.

OFF-LABEL USES

Treatment of alopecia areata, aplastic anemia, atopic dermatitis, Behet's disease, biliary cirrhosis, prevention of corneal transplant rejection

CONTRAINDICATIONS

History of hypersensitivity to *cycloSPORINE or polyoxyethylated castor oil

INTERACTIONS

Drug: **ACE inhibitors, potassium-sparing diuretics, potassium supplements:** May cause hyperkalemia. **Cimetidine, danazol, diltiazem, erythromycin, itraconazole, ketoconazole, voraconazole:** May increase *cycloSPORINE concentration and risk of hepatotoxicity and nephrotoxicity. **Immunosuppressants:** May increase risk of infection and lymphoproliferative disorders. **Live-virus vaccines:** May increase vaccine side effects, potentiate virus replication, and decrease antibody response to the vaccine. **Lovastatin:** May increase the risk of acute renal failure and rhabdomyolysis. **Warfarin:** May decrease anticoagulant effects. **Herbal:** **St. John's wort:** May alter *cycloSPORINE absorption. **Food:** **Grapefruit, grapefruit juice:** May increase the absorption and risk of toxicity of *cycloSPORINE.

DIAGNOSTIC TEST EFFECTS

May increase BUN and serum alkaline phosphatase, amylase, bilirubin, creatinine, potassium, uric acid, AST (SGOT), and ALT (SGPT) levels. May decrease serum magnesium level. Therapeutic peak serum level is 50-300 ng/mL; toxic serum level is greater than 400 ng/mL.

IV INCOMPATIBILITIES

Amphotericin B complex (Abelcet, AmBisome, Amphotec), magnesium

IV COMPATIBILITIES

Propofol (Diprivan)

SIDE-EFFECTS

Frequent: Mild to moderate hypertension (26%), nausea (23%), hirsutism (21%), tremor (12%). **Occasional (4%-2%):** Acne, leg cramps, gingival hyperplasia (marked by red, bleeding, and tender gums), paresthesia, diarrhea, nausea, vomiting, headache. **Rare (less than 1%):** Hypersensitivity reaction, abdominal discomfort, gynecomastia, sinusitis

CRITICAL CARE CONSIDERATIONS

ADMINISTRATION/HANDLING

PO ALERT

- Oral solution available in 50-mL bottles with a calibrated liquid measuring device.

Begin therapy with the oral form as soon as possible. Patients should be managed in facilities equipped and staffed with adequate laboratory and supportive medical resources familiar with immunosuppressive therapy.

- Avoid grapefruit and grapefruit juice because they increase the drug's blood concentration and risk of side effects.
- **Preparation:** In a glass container, mix oral solution with room-temperature milk, chocolate milk, or orange juice.
- **Administration:** Stir the mixture well and drink it immediately. Avoid using Styrofoam containers because the liquid form of the drug may adhere to the wall of the container. Add more diluent to the glass container and mix it with the remaining solution to ensure that the total amount of *cycloSPORINE is swallowed.
- **Following administration:** Dry the outside of the measuring device before replacing it in its cover. Do not rinse with water.
- **Stability:** Do not refrigerate the oral solution because it may separate. Discard the oral solution 2 mo after the bottle has been opened.
- **Steroids:** Give *cycloSPORINE with adrenal corticosteroids.

IV ALERT

- **Storage:** Store the parenteral form at room temperature and protect it from light.
- **Dilution:** Dilute each milliliter of concentrate with 20-100 mL 0.9% NaCl or D_5W.
- **Stability:** After dilution, solution is stable for 24 hr. Discard diluted solution after 24 hr.
- **Infusion:** Infuse the solution over 2-6 hr.
- **Hypersensitivity:** Monitor patients continuously for the first 30 min of the infusion and frequently thereafter for hypersensitivity reaction, marked by facial flushing and dyspnea.

OPHTHALMIC ALERT

- Before administration, invert the vial several times to obtain a uniform suspension. Instruct patients to remove any contact lenses. May use with artificial tears.
- Following administration, may reinsert lenses 15 min after drug administration.

PRECAUTIONS

HEALTH-RELATED

- Use *cycloSPORINE cautiously in patients with cardiac impairment, chicken pox, herpes zoster infection, hypokalemia, malabsorption syndrome, or renal or hepatic impairment.
- Use ophthalmic form cautiously in patients with eye infection.
- **Infection and lymphoma:** Administering other immunosuppressive agents with *cycloSPORINE increases susceptibility to infection and lymphoma.

AGE-RELATED

- **Children:** No age-related precautions have been noted in pediatric transplant patients.
- **Elderly:** Are at increased risk for hypertension and increased serum creatinine.

PREGNANCY/LACTATION-RELATED

- Pregnancy category C; excreted into breast milk; avoid nursing.

MONITORING

- **Baseline assessment:** Assess for pregnancy, history of cardiac problems, herpes zoster, malabsorption syndrome, and liver or kidney disease. Only physicians experienced in the management of systemic immunosuppressive therapy and management of organ transplantation should prescribe *cycloSPORINE.
- **Baseline lab work:** Monitor renal function studies, liver function tests, and drug blood levels before beginning *cycloSPORINE therapy and regularly during treatment.
- **Ongoing lab work:** Diligently monitor BUN and serum LDH, bilirubin, creatinine, AST (SGOT), and ALT (SGPT) levels for hepatotoxicity or nephrotoxicity. Mild toxicity is characterized by a slow rise in serum levels; more overt toxicity by a rapid rise in serum levels.
- **Hematuria:** May be indicative of nephrotoxicity.
- **Hyperkalemia:** Monitor serum potassium level for hyperkalemia.
- **Hypertension:** Monitor BP for hypertension.
- **Follow trough level:** Administer *cycloSPORINE after trough serum level has been drawn when levels are being aggressively followed.
- **Serum levels:** Therapeutic peak serum level is 50-300 ng/mL; toxic serum level is greater than 400 ng/mL.
- **Dosing:** Effective dosage in organ transplant patients balances suppressing organ rejection against developing severe infections. Immunosuppression is a delicate balance in order to avoid near-lethal

situations with either exacerbation of the primary problem or development of infection caused by immune dysfunction.

- **Evenly spaced doses:** Administer *cycloSPORINE at the same times each day to maintain maximal effects.
- **Side effects:** Headache, excessive hair growth, gum disease, and tremor. Provide good oral hygiene to prevent gingivitis.
- **Patient education:** When *cycloSPORINE is used outside the hospital, instruct patients to consult a health care provider for further instructions if they forget to take a dose. Inform patients that routine blood testing is essential during *cycloSPORINE therapy. Patients should not drink grapefruit juice to facilitate accurate dosing and to avoid side effects. Capsules should be kept in the original foil wrapping and stored in a dry, cool environment away from direct light. The liquid form should be kept in the amber-colored glass container.

SERIOUS ADVERSE REACTIONS

- **Mild nephrotoxicity:** Occurs in 25% of renal transplant patients, 38% of cardiac transplant patients, and 37% of liver transplant patients generally 2-3 mo after transplantation (more severe toxicity generally occurs soon after transplantation).
- **Hepatotoxicity:** Occurs in 4% of renal transplant patients, 7% of cardiac transplant patients, and 4% of liver transplant patients, generally within the first month after transplantation. Both toxicities usually respond to dosage reduction.
- **Severe hyperkalemia and hyperuricemia:** Occur occasionally.

OVERDOSE/TOXICITY

- **Symptoms:** Nephrotoxicity, hepatotoxicity, hyperkalemia, hyperuricemia, Stevens–Johnson syndrome, toxic epidermal necrolysis, leukopenia, lymphoma.
- **Management:** Supportive care for organ-specific or biochemical-specific problem. Dosage reduction may be required.
- **GI decontamination:** No specific recommendations.

ANTIDOTE/DIALYSIS

- **Antidote:** No specific recommendations.
- **Dialysis:** *CycloSPORINE is not removed by hemodialysis or peritoneal dialysis. No data are available on removal by high-permeability hemodialysis.

cyproheptadine

See Antihistamines (p. 925)

daclizumab

da-kliz'-yoo-mab

Classes
Chemical: monoclonal antibody
Therapeutic: immunosuppressive

Pregnancy Category: C

Trade Names
Prescription: Zenapax

Do not confuse Zenapax with Zovirax.

CLINICAL PHARMACOLOGY

Mechanism of Action
A monoclonal antibody that binds to the interleukin-2 (IL-2) receptor complex, inhibiting the IL-2-mediated activation of T lymphocytes, a critical pathway in the cellular immune response involved in allograft rejection. **Therapeutic Effect:** Prevents organ rejection.

PHARMACOKINETICS

Half-life: Adults: 20 days. Children: 13 days.

AVAILABILITY

Injection: 5 mg/mL.

INDICATIONS AND DOSAGE

Prevention of acute renal transplant rejection (in combination with an immunosuppressive)

IV

Adults, Children: 1 mg/kg over 15 min every 14 days for 5 doses, beginning no more than 24 hr before transplantation. Maximum: 100 mg.

OFF-LABEL USES

Treatment of aplastic anemia, graft versus host disease

CONTRAINDICATIONS

Hypersensitivity to daclizumab

INTERACTIONS

Drug: None known. **Herbal:** None known. **Food:** None known.

DIAGNOSTIC TEST EFFECTS

None known.

IV INCOMPATIBILITIES

Do not mix daclizumab with any other drugs.

SIDE-EFFECTS

Occasional (greater than 5%): Constipation, nausea, diarrhea, vomiting, abdominal pain, edema, headache, dizziness, fever, pain, fatigue, insomnia, weakness, arthralgia, myalgia, diaphoresis

CRITICAL CARE CONSIDERATIONS

ADMINISTRATION/HANDLING

IV ALERT

- **Storage:** Refrigerate vials and protect them from light. Do not freeze.
- **Dilution:** Dilute daclizumab in 50 mL 0.9% NaCl. Invert vial gently. Avoid shaking. Use within 4 hr of dilution.
- **Infusion:** Infuse daclizumab over 15 min.
- **Stability:** Reconstituted solution is stable for 4 hr at room temperature, 24 hr if refrigerated.

PRECAUTIONS

HEALTH-RELATED

- Use daclizumab cautiously in patients with diabetes, an infection, or a history of malignancy. Daclizumab is given in combination with an immunosuppresive regimen (*cycloSPORINE, corticosteroids) for prevention of organ rejection.

AGE-RELATED

- **Children:** Safety and efficacy of daclizumab have not been established in children.
- **Elderly:** Use with caution and observe closely.

PREGNANCY/LACTATION-RELATED

- Pregnancy category C; unknown if excreted in breast milk; breast-feeding should be discontinued.

MONITORING

- **Baseline assessment:** Temperature for fever, BP, and pulse rate. Ask about sensitivity to human, murine, or any antibodies in the past.
- **Baseline lab work:** CBC with differential, platelet count, and renal and liver function tests. Note blood glucose, as drug may cause hyperglycemia.
- **Ongoing lab work:** Monitor for renal (elevated BUN, creatinine) or liver dysfunction (elevated AST [SGOT], ALT [SGPT], alkaline phosphatase, LDH), thrombocytopenia, markedly decreased white blood cell count.
- **Allergic reaction:** Monitor vital signs. Early signs include hypertension, hypotension, and tachycardia, then respiratory distress.

- **GI/GU disturbances:** Monitor for GI disturbances or urinary changes.
- **Infection:** Monitor symptoms of systemic infection: neutropenia, fever or sore throat, unusual bleeding or bruising, and wound infection. Wound healing may be impaired.
- **Bleeding:** Assess for bleeding, especially in thrombocytopenic patients.
- **Patient education:** Tell patients to report difficulty breathing or swallowing, itching or swelling of the lower extremities, rash, rapid heartbeat, or weakness. When using daclizumab outside the hospital, caution women to avoid pregnancy during therapy. Urge patients to avoid crowded areas and other circumstances that place them at risk for infection.

SERIOUS ADVERSE REACTIONS

- **Rare hypersensitivity:** Dyspnea, tachycardia, dysphagia, peripheral edema, rash, and pruritus. Manage with oxygen, epinephrine, corticosteroids, and/or antihistamines (*diphenhydrAMINE/Benadryl). Resuscitate if needed.

OVERDOSE/TOXICITY

- **Symptoms:** Abdominal distention or pain, nausea, constipation, diarrhea, edema, headache, tremors, acute renal failure, thrombosis, bleeding, liver dysfunction, weakness, urinary retention, chest pain, pulmonary edema.
- **GI decontamination:** No specific recommendations.

ANTIDOTE/DIALYSIS

- **Antidote:** No specific recommendations.
- **Dialysis:** Daclizumab is unlikely to be removed by hemodialysis, peritoneal dialysis, or continuous renal replacement therapy. No data are available on removal by high-permeability hemodialysis.

dalteparin sodium

See Anticoagulants (p. 900)

dantrolene sodium

dan'-troe-leen soe'-dee-um

Classes

Chemical: hydantoin derivative
Therapeutic: antidote, malignant hyperthermia; skeletal muscle relaxant

Pregnancy Category: C

Trade Names

Prescription: Dantrium

Do not confuse Dantrium with Daraprim.

CLINICAL PHARMACOLOGY

Mechanism of Action

A skeletal muscle relaxant that reduces muscle contraction by interfering with release of calcium ion. Reduces calcium ion concentration. **Therapeutic Effect:** Dissociates excitation-contraction coupling. Interferes with catabolic process associated with malignant hyperthermic crisis.

PHARMACOKINETICS

Poorly absorbed from the GI tract. Protein binding: High. Metabolized in the liver. Primarily excreted in feces (45%-50%). **Half-life:** IV: 4-8 hr; PO: 8.7 hr.

AVAILABILITY

Capsules (Dantrium): 25 mg, 50 mg, 100 mg.
Powder for injection (Dantrium Intravenous): 20-mg vial.

INDICATIONS AND DOSAGE

Spasticity

PO

Adults, Elderly: Initially, 25 mg/day. Increase to 25 mg 2-4 times per day, then by 25-mg increments every 4-7 days up to 100 mg 2-4 times per day. **Children:** Initially, 0.5 mg/kg twice per day. Increase to 0.5 mg/kg 3-4 times per day every 4-7 days, then in increments of 0.5 mg/kg/day up to 3 mg/kg 2-4 times per day. Maximum: 400 mg/day.

Prevention of malignant hyperthermic crisis

PO

Adults, Elderly, Children: 4-8 mg/kg/day in 3-4 divided doses 1-2 days before surgery; give last dose 3-4 hr before surgery.

IV

Adults, Elderly, Children: 2.5 mg/kg about 1.25 hr before surgery.

Management of malignant hyperthermic crisis

IV

Adults, Elderly, Children: Initially a minimum of 1 mg/kg rapid IV; may repeat up to total cumulative dose of 10 mg/kg. May follow with 4-8 mg/kg/day PO in 4 divided doses up to 3 days after crisis.

OFF-LABEL USES

Relief of exercise-induced pain in patients with muscular dystrophy, treatment of flexor spasms and neuroleptic malignant syndrome

CONTRAINDICATIONS

Active hepatic disease, hypersensitivity to dantrolene

INTERACTIONS

Drug: Central nervous system (CNS) depressants: May increase CNS depression with short-term use. **Liver toxic medications:** May increase the risk of liver toxicity with chronic use. **Herbal: Valerian, kava kava, gotu kola:** May increase CNS depression. **Food:** None known.

DIAGNOSTIC TEST EFFECTS

May alter liver function test results.

IV INCOMPATIBILITIES

None known.

SIDE-EFFECTS

Frequent: Drowsiness, dizziness, weakness, general malaise, diarrhea (mild). **Occasional:** Confusion, diarrhea (may be severe), headache, insomnia, constipation, urinary frequency. **Rare:** Paradoxic CNS excitement or restlessness, paresthesia, tinnitus, slurred speech, tremor, blurred vision, dry mouth, nocturia, impotence, rash, pruritus

CRITICAL CARE CONSIDERATIONS

ADMINISTRATION/HANDLING

PO ALERT

- Give dantrolene without regard to meals.
- Begin with low-dose therapy, then increase gradually at 4- to 7-day intervals to reduce incidence of side effects.

IV ALERT

- **Storage:** Store at room temperature.
- **Stability:** Use within 6 hr after reconstitution.
- **Dilution:** Reconstitute 20-mg vial with 60 mL sterile water for injection to provide a concentration of 0.33 mg/mL. Solution appears clear, colorless. Discard if cloudy or precipitate is present.
- **IV infusion:** Administer over 1 hr.
- **Extravasation:** Diligently monitor for extravasation due to high pH of IV preparation. May produce severe complications.

PRECAUTIONS

HEALTH-RELATED

- Use dantrolene cautiously in patients with a history of liver disease, impaired cardiac or pulmonary function.

AGE-RELATED

- **Children:** No age-related precautions noted in children 5 yr and older.
- **Elderly:** No information available on dantrolene use in the elderly.

PREGNANCY/LACTATION-RELATED

- Pregnancy category C; breast-feeding should be discontinued.

MONITORING

- **Baseline assessment:** Record the duration, location, onset, and type of muscle spasm. Examine for immobility, stiffness, and swelling. Assess for prior symptoms of malignant hyperthermia in perioperative patients if used for prevention of malignant hyperthermia.
- **Baseline lab work:** Biochemical profile including renal (BUN, creatinine) and liver (alkaline phosphatase, AST [SGOT], ALT [SGPT], bilirubin) function tests.
- **Ongoing lab work:** Liver and renal function tests; especially for patients on long-term therapy or those at risk for malignant hyperthermia.
- **Dysrhythmias:** Monitor ECG continuously if used in perioperative patients at risk for malignant hyperthermia. Conduction may be altered due to dantrolene altering release of calcium ions.
- **Metabolic acidosis:** Monitor arterial blood gases to assess for metabolic acidosis associated with malignant hyperthermia.
- **Oliguria:** Monitor for decreasing urine output; patients should be well hydrated throughout the procedure and especially if malignant hyperthermia occurs.
- **Fever:** If malignant hyperthermia occurs, institute cooling measures immediately.
- **Therapeutic effect:** Evaluate for decreased intensity of skeletal muscle pain or spasm. If used for malignant hyperthermia prevention, monitor for occurrence of fever associated with anesthesia, tachycardia, hypoxemia (decreasing pulse oximetry reading), and hypercapnia.
- **Patient education:** Explain to patients that drowsiness usually diminishes with continued therapy. Caution avoidance of tasks that require mental alertness or motor skills until response to the drug is known. Urge patients to avoid alcohol or other depressants while taking dantrolene. Advise using sunscreen when outdoors because photosensitivity may occur. Warn patients to notify the physician if they experience bloody or tarry stools, continued weakness, diarrhea, fatigue, itching, and nausea.

SERIOUS ADVERSE REACTIONS

- **Hepatitis:** Noted most frequently between third and twelfth month of therapy.
- **Malignant hyperthermia:** May occur in susceptible patients who are not given an adequate dose of dantrolene. All anesthetics should be discontinued immediately when onset of malignant hyperthermia is recognized. Symptoms include tachycardia, fever, tachypnea, hypoxemia, hypercapnia, skeletal muscle rigidity, cyanosis with mottling of the extremities and trunk.

OVERDOSE/TOXICITY

- **Symptoms:** Vomiting, muscular hypotonia, muscle twitching, respiratory depression, and seizures.
- **Liver toxicity:** Noted most often in females, those 35 yr and older, and those taking other medications concurrently.
- **GI decontamination:** No specific recommendations.

ANTIDOTE/DIALYSIS

- **Antidote:** No specific recommendations.
- **Dialysis:** No data are available on removal of dantrolene using hemodialysis, peritoneal dialysis, continuous renal replacement therapy, or high-permeability hemodialysis.

dapsone

dap'-sone

Classes

Chemical: sulfone
Therapeutic: antiprotozoal, leprostatic

Pregnancy Category: C

Trade Names

Prescription: Dapsone

CLINICAL PHARMACOLOGY

Mechanism of Action

An antibiotic that is a competitive antagonist of para-aminobenzoic acid (PABA); it prevents normal bacterial utilization of PABA for synthesis of folic acid. **Therapeutic Effect:** Inhibits bacterial growth.

PHARMACOKINETICS

Slowly absorbed from the GI tract. Protein binding: 70%-90%. Metabolized in liver. Excreted in urine. **Half-life:** 10-50 hr.

AVAILABILITY

Tablets: 25 mg, 100 mg.

INDICATIONS AND DOSAGE

Leprosy

PO

Adults, Elderly: 50-100 mg/day for 3-10 yr. **Children:** 1-2 mg/kg/24 hr. Maximum: 100 mg/day.

Dermatitis herpetiformis

PO

Adults, Elderly: Initially, 50 mg/day. May increase up to 300 mg/day.

Pneumocystis carinii pneumonia (PCP)

PO

Adults, Elderly: 100 mg/day in combination with trimethoprim for 21 days.

Prevention of PCP

PO

Adults, Elderly: 100 mg/day. **Children older than 1 mo:** 2 mg/kg/day. Maximum: 100 mg/day.

OFF-LABEL USES

Treatment of inflammatory bowel disorders, malaria

CONTRAINDICATIONS

Hypersensitivity to dapsone and/or its derivatives

INTERACTIONS

Drug: Methotrexate: May increase hematologic reactions. **Probenecid:** May decrease the excretion of dapsone. **Protease inhibitors (including ritonavir):** May increase dapsone blood concentration. **Rifampin:** May decrease rifampin blood concentration. **Trimethoprim:** May increase the risk of toxic effects. **Herbal: St. John's wort:** May decrease dapsone blood concentration. **Food:** None known.

DIAGNOSTIC TEST EFFECTS

None known.

SIDE-EFFECTS

Frequent (greater than 10%): Hemolytic anemia, methemoglobinemia, rash. **Occasional (10%-1%):** Hemolysis, photosensitivity reaction

CRITICAL CARE CONSIDERATIONS

ADMINISTRATION/HANDLING

PO ALERT

- Give dapsone without regard to food.

PRECAUTIONS

HEALTH-RELATED

- Use dapsone cautiously in patients with agranulocytosis, severe anemia, aplastic anemia, glucose-6-phosphate dehydrogenase deficiency, or a hypersensitivity to dapsone or its derivatives (such as sulfoxone sodium).
- Drug resistance to dapsone is increasing when used to treat *Mycobacterium leprae* (for leprosy) and chloroquine-resistant malaria.
- **Brown recluse spider bites:** Although dapsone is touted as effective for treatment of resultant necrotic lesions, there are few data to support this practice.

AGE-RELATED

- **Children:** Children under 4 yr are more prone to developing severe methemoglobinemia. Doses of 100 mg (1 tablet) have been reported to cause hemolysis and methemoglobinemia.
- **Elderly:** No special precautions have been noted.

PREGNANCY/LACTATION-RELATED

- Pregnancy category C; extensive, but uncontrolled, experience and two published surveys in pregnant women have not shown increases in the risk for fetal abnormalities if administered during all trimesters; excreted in breast milk, hemolytic reactions can occur in neonates, discontinue nursing or discontinue drug; alternatively, some authors have suggested infants should be kept with mothers infected with leprosy, and breast-feeding during drug therapy encouraged

MONITORING

- **Baseline assessment:** Determine hypersensitivity to dapsone or its derivatives, such as sulfoxone sodium.
- **Lab work:** Complete blood count (CBC) at baseline and weekly, biochemical profile, culture and sensitivity results to determine whether organism is sensitive to dapsone, as appropriate. Explain to patients that frequent blood tests are necessary, especially during early dapsone therapy.
- **Hemolytic anemia:** Observe for tachycardia, jaundice, hypoxia, pallor, acidemia, and shock. Monitor for decreased hemoglobin and hematocrit.
- **Methemoglobinemia and sulfhemoglobinemia:** Monitor for cyanosis, respiratory distress, tachypnea with a decrease in pulse oximetry reading (low SpO_2) with a normal pO_2 noted on arterial blood gas analysis. ABG will reveal abnormal hemoglobins.
- **Skin lesions:** Assess the skin for a dermatologic reaction. Discontinue dapsone if rash occurs. Exfoliative dermatitis may occur.
- **Patient education:** When dapsone is used outside the hospital, advise patients to report persistent fatigue, fever, or sore throat. Encourage avoidance of overexposure to sun or ultraviolet light.

SERIOUS ADVERSE REACTIONS

- Agranulocytosis; hemolytic anemia; 'sulfone (hypersensitivity) syndrome,' which can develop as long as 2 mo after starting therapy; maculopathy (noted in eye ground exam); and acute renal failure may occur.

OVERDOSE/TOXICITY

- **Hemolysis, sulfhemoglobinemia, and methemoglobinemia:** Clinical presentation of dapsone-induced methemoglobinemia may be delayed up to 3 days owing to the delayed peak level of dapsone (up to 20 hr in overdose) and long half-life (30 hr when therapeutic, possibly 77 hr with overdose). Heinz bodies on peripheral blood smear may provide an early sign of hemolysis.
- **Other effects:** Nausea, vomiting, rash including exfoliative dermatitis, fulminant hepatic necrosis with jaundice, and psychosis. Any immunocompromised patient who presents with cyanosis or hemodynamic instability should be suspected of dapsone poisoning.
- **Exchange transfusion:** If patients fail to respond to other treatments for methemoglobinemia or sulfhemoglobinemia, exchange transfusion may be used.
- **GI decontamination:** Single or multiple dose activated charcoal is recommended if patients present within 1-2 hr of ingestion.

ANTIDOTE/DIALYSIS

- **Antidote:** Methylene blue 1-2 mg/kg IV over 5-10 min for methemoglobinemia; may repeat in 1 hr if cyanosis persists.
- **Dialysis:** Dapsone is removed by conventional hemodialysis, but is likely better removed by high-permeability dialysis and charcoal hemoperfusion. No data are available regarding removal by peritoneal dialysis.

daptomycin

dap'-toe-mye-sin

Classes

Chemical: lipopeptide, cyclic
Therapeutic: antibiotic

Pregnancy Category: B

Trade Names

Prescription: Cubicin

CLINICAL PHARMACOLOGY

Mechanism of Action

A lipopeptide antibacterial agent that binds to bacterial membranes and causes a rapid depolarization of the membrane potential. The loss of membrane potential leads to inhibition of protein, DNA, and RNA synthesis. Therapeutic Effect: Bactericidal.

PHARMACOKINETICS

Widely distributed. Protein binding: 90%. Primarily excreted unchanged in urine. Moderately removed by hemodialysis. Half-life: 7-8 hr (increased in impaired renal function in up to 28% of patients).

AVAILABILITY

Powder for injection: 250 mg/vial, 500 mg/vial.

INDICATIONS AND DOSAGE

Complicated skin and skin structure infections

IV

Adults, Elderly: 4 mg/kg every 24 hr for 7-14 days.

Dosage in renal impairment

For patients with creatinine clearance of less than 30 mL/min, dosage is 4 mg/kg every 48 hr for 7-14 days. For hemodialysis and continuous ambulatory peritoneal disease (CAPD) patients, administer same dose as in less than 30 mL/min after hemodialysis or CAPD.

CONTRAINDICATIONS

Hypersensitivity to daptomycin

INTERACTIONS

Drug: **Hydroxamethylglutaryl-CoA (HMG-CoA) reductase inhibitors:** May cause myopathy. **Tobramycin:** Increases the serum concentration of daptomycin. Herbal: None known. Food: None known.

DIAGNOSTIC TEST EFFECTS

May increase serum CPK levels. May alter liver function test results.

IV INCOMPATIBILITIES

Diluents containing dextrose. If the same IV line is used to administer different drugs, the line should be flushed with 0.9% NaCl.

SIDE-EFFECTS

Frequent (6%-5%): Constipation, nausea, peripheral injection site reactions, headache, diarrhea. Occasional (4%-3%): Insomnia, rash, vomiting. Rare (less than 3%): Pruritus, dizziness, hypotension

CRITICAL CARE CONSIDERATIONS

ADMINISTRATION/HANDLING

IV ALERT

- **Storage:** Store daptomycin in the refrigerator.
- **Appearance:** Normally appears as a pale yellow to light brown lyophilized cake.
- **Dilution:** Reconstitute the 250-mg vial with 5 mL 0.9% NaCl and the 500-mg vial with 10 mL 0.9% NaCl. Further dilute in 50 mL 0.9% NaCl. Discard the solution if it contains particulate matter.
- **Stability:** Reconstituted solution is stable for 12 hr at room temperature and up to 48 hr if refrigerated.
- **Infusion:** Infuse the intermittent IV (piggyback) infusion over 30 min.

PRECAUTIONS

HEALTH-RELATED

- Use daptomycin cautiously in patients with a history of or current musculoskeletal disorders or liver or renal impairment.
- Avoid concurrent use of HMG-CoA reductase inhibitors because they may cause rhabdomyolysis.

AGE-RELATED

- **Children:** Safety and efficacy of daptomycin have not been established in children under 18 yr.
- **Elderly:** No age-related precautions have been noted, but elderly may be more prone to experience side effects.

PREGNANCY/LACTATION-RELATED

- Pregnancy category B; breast milk excretion unknown.

MONITORING

- **Baseline lab work:** Obtain culture and sensitivity of target organism before giving the first dose. Therapy may begin before the test results are known. Biochemical profile to assess both kidney and liver function and to note baseline CPK level.

- **Ongoing lab work:** Monitor CPK if muscle weakness is experienced. Discontinue daptomycin if CPK is 5 times upper limit of normal in symptomatic patients or 10 times upper limit of normal in asymptomatic patients.
- **Colitis:** Severe diarrhea with abdominal pain, blood or mucus in stools, and fever may indicate antibiotic-associated colitis.
- **Nausea/vomiting:** Manage with standard measures. Provide IV hydration if severe symptoms occur. Consider use of another antibiotic.
- **Superinfection:** Be alert for signs and symptoms of superinfection, including anal or genital pruritus, black hairy tongue, diarrhea, increased fever, sore throat, ulceration or changes of oral mucosa, and vomiting.
- **Hand washing:** If *Clostridium difficile* colitis develops, wash hands with antibacterial soap; alcohol-based foam is ineffective against *C. difficile* spores.
- **IV site:** Monitor for redness, tenderness, or swelling.
- **Evenly spaced dosing:** Administer doses evenly around the clock.
- **Dizziness:** Institute appropriate safety measures if dizziness occurs.
- **Patient education:** If daptomycin is used outside the hospital, instruct patients to report headache, nausea, rash, severe diarrhea, new muscle weakness, or any other new symptoms to a health care provider. Over-the-counter medications, especially those for pain and relief of cold or sinus symptoms, should be discussed with the health care provider before taking the medication.

SERIOUS ADVERSE REACTIONS

- **Superinfections:** Antibiotic-associated colitis and other superinfections may result from altered bacterial balance. Management includes oral vancomycin (Vancocin) and metronidazole (Flagyl).

OVERDOSE/TOXICITY

- **Rhabdomyolysis/skeletal muscle myopathy:** Symptoms including muscle pain and weakness, particularly of the distal extremities, occur rarely.
- **GI decontamination:** No specific recommendations.

ANTIDOTE/DIALYSIS

- **Antidote:** No specific recommendations.
- **Dialysis:** Daptomycin is not significantly removed by hemodialysis or peritoneal dialysis. No data are available on removal by high-permeability hemodialysis. Administer following dialysis on hemodialysis days.

darbepoetin alfa

dar-be-poe'-e-tin al'-fa

Classes

Chemical: amino acid glycoprotein
Therapeutic: hematopoietic agent

Pregnancy Category: C

Trade Names

Prescription: Aranesp

Do not confuse Aranesp with Aricept.

CLINICAL PHARMACOLOGY

Mechanism of Action

A glycoprotein that stimulates formation of RBCs in bone marrow; increases serum half-life of epoetin. **Therapeutic Effect:** Induces erythropoiesis and release of reticulocytes from bone marrow.

PHARMACOKINETICS

Well absorbed after subcutaneous administration. **Half-life:** 48.5 hr.

AVAILABILITY

Injection: 25 mcg/mL, 40 mcg/mL, 60 mcg/mL, 100 mcg/mL, 150 mcg/mL, 200 mcg/mL, 300 mcg/mL.
Prefilled syringe: 25 mcg/0.42 mL, 40 mcg/0.4 mL, 60 mcg/0.3 mL, 100 mcg/0.5 mL, 200 mcg/0.4 mL, 300 mcg/0.6 mL, 500 mcg/mL.

INDICATIONS AND DOSAGE

Anemia in chronic renal failure

IV Bolus, Subcutaneous

Adults, Elderly: Initially, 0.45 mcg/kg once weekly. Adjust dosage to achieve and maintain a target Hgb not to exceed 12 g/dL. Do not increase dosage more frequently than once monthly. Limit increases in Hgb by less than 1 g/dL over any 2-wk period.

Anemia associated with chemotherapy

IV, Subcutaneous

Adults, Elderly: 2.25 mcg/kg/dose once per wk or 500 mcg every 3 wk. May increase up to 4.5 mcg/kg/dose once per wk.

CONTRAINDICATIONS

History of sensitivity to darbepoeitin, other mammalian cell-derived products, or human albumin; uncontrolled hypertension

INTERACTIONS

Drug: None known. **Herbal:** None known. **Food:** None known.

DIAGNOSTIC TEST EFFECTS

May increase BUN, serum phosphorus, potassium, serum creatinine, serum uric acid, and sodium levels. May decrease bleeding time, serum iron concentration, and serum ferritin.

IV INCOMPATIBILITIES

Do not mix with other medications.

SIDE-EFFECTS

Frequent: Myalgia, hypertension or hypotension, headache, diarrhea. **Occasional:** Fatigue, edema, vomiting, reaction at administration site, asthenia, dizziness

CRITICAL CARE CONSIDERATIONS

ADMINISTRATION/HANDLING

IV ALERT

- **Storage:** Refrigerate vials.
- **Dilution:** Do not shake vials vigorously because it may denature medication, rendering it inactive. Reconstitution is not necessary.
- **IV bolus:** May be given as an IV bolus.

SUBCUTANEOUS ALERT

- **One dose per vial:** Do not reenter vial. Discard unused portion.
- **Dilution:** May be mixed in a syringe with bacteriostatic 0.9% NaCl with benzyl alcohol 0.9% or bacteriostatic saline at a 1:1 ratio. Benzyl alcohol acts as a local anesthetic and may reduce injection site discomfort.

PRECAUTIONS

HEALTH-RELATED

- Use darbepoetin alfa cautiously in patients with hemolytic anemia, history of seizures, known porphyria (impairment of erythrocyte formation in bone marrow), sickle cell anemia, or thalassemia.
- Iron studies should be done before and throughout darbepoeitin therapy because the drug will not effectively increase hematocrit if iron stores are insufficient.

AGE-RELATED

- **Children:** Safety and efficacy of darbepoetin alfa have not been established in children.
- **Elderly:** Age-related renal impairment may require dosage adjustment.

PREGNANCY/LACTATION-RELATED

- Pregnancy category C; unknown if excreted in human milk.

MONITORING

- **Baseline assessment:** Assess BP before administering darbepoetin. BP may rise during early therapy in patients with history of hypertension.
- **Baseline lab work:** Assess CBC; note Hct. Assess serum iron level: transferrin saturation should be greater than 20%, and serum ferritin level should be greater than 100 ng/mL before and during therapy.
- **Supplemental iron:** All patients will eventually need supplemental iron therapy.
- **Ongoing lab work:** Monitor Hct level weekly. Reduce dosage if Hct level increases more than 4 points in 2 wk. Monitor CBC with differential, Hgb, reticulocyte count, BUN, phosphorus, potassium, serum creatinine, and serum ferritin levels.
- **Hypertension:** Monitor for increased BP; 25% of patients taking darbepoetin alfa require antihypertensive therapy and sodium restriction.
- **Vascular access:** Monitor patency of dialysis access as clotting may occur.
- **Patient education:** Inform patients that frequent blood tests will be needed to determine correct dosage. Tell patients to report severe headache. Warn patients to avoid tasks that require mental alertness or motor skills until response to the drug is known. Risk of seizures is higher in first months of therapy.

SERIOUS ADVERSE REACTIONS

- Vascular access thrombosis, seizures, heart failure, sepsis, dysrhythmias, and anaphylactic reaction occur rarely.
- Resuscitate as needed for anaphylaxis using IV fluids, vasopressors, medications to reduce allergic reaction, and to control other shock-related symptoms.

OVERDOSE/TOXICITY

- **Excessive hypertension:** May require discontinuation of darbepoetin until BP is controlled.

- **Excessive increase in hemoglobin:** Dose of darbepoetin should be reduced if hemoglobin increases more than 1 g/dL in 2 wk or in patients with hemoglobin over 12 g/dL.
- **Phlebotomy:** May be considered to treat overdose or polycythemia.
- **GI decontamination:** No specific recommendations.

ANTIDOTE/DIALYSIS

- **Antidote:** No specific recommendations.
- **Dialysis:** Darbepoetin alfa is unlikely to be removed by hemodialysis, peritoneal dialysis, or high-permeability hemodialysis. Dialysis prescription may require adjustment to avoid clotting of vascular access.

deferoxamine mesylate

de-fer-ox'-a-meen mes'-sil-ate

Classes
Chemical: siderochrome
Therapeutic: antidote, heavy metal

Pregnancy Category: C

Trade Names
Prescription: Desferal

CLINICAL PHARMACOLOGY

Mechanism of Action
An antidote that binds with iron to form complex. **Therapeutic Effect:** Promotes urine excretion of acute iron poisoning.

PHARMACOKINETICS

Well absorbed after IM, subcutaneous administration. Widely distributed. Rapidly metabolized in tissues, plasma. Excreted in urine. Removed by hemodialysis. **Half-life:** 6 hr.

AVAILABILITY

Injection: 500 mg (Desferal Mesylate), 2 g.

INDICATIONS AND DOSAGE

Acute iron intoxication

IM
Adults: Initially 1 g, then 500 mg every 4 hr up to 2 doses. Maximum: 6 g/day. Subsequent doses of 500 mg have been given every 4-12 hr. **Children:** 90 mg/kg every 8 hr. Maximum: 6 g/24 hr.

IV
Adults: 1 g, then 500 mg every 4 hr up to 2 doses, then 500 mg every 4-12 hr. **Children:** 15 mg/kg/hr. Maximum: 6 g/24 hr.

Chronic iron overload

Subcutaneous
Adults: 1-2 g/day (20-40 mg/kg) over 8-24 hr. **Children:** 1-2 g/day (20-40 mg/kg) over 8-12 hr.

IM
Adults: 0.5-1 g/day. In addition to IM, 2 g infused at rate not to exceed 15 mg/kg/hr.

Renal impairment

IM, IV, Subcutaneous
Adults: Creatinine clearance less than 10 mL/min, give 50% of normal dose.

CONTRAINDICATIONS

Severe renal disease, anuria, primary hemochromatosis, hypersensitivity to deferoxamine mesylate or any component of the formulation

INTERACTIONS

Drug: **Vitamin C:** May increase effect of deferoxamine. **Herbal:** None known. **Food:** None known.

DIAGNOSTIC TEST EFFECTS

May cause a falsely high total iron-binding capacity (TIBC).

IV INCOMPATIBILITIES

Do not mix with any other intravenous medications.

SIDE-EFFECTS

Frequent: Pain, induration at injection site, urine color change (to orange-rose). **Occasional:** Abdominal discomfort, diarrhea, leg cramps, impaired vision

CRITICAL CARE CONSIDERATIONS

ADMINISTRATION/HANDLING

SUBCUTANEOUS ALERT

- **Reconstitution:** Mix 500-mg vial with 2 mL sterile water for injection to provide a concentration of 250 mg/mL.
- **Injection:** Administer very slowly; may give undiluted.

IM/IV ALERT

- **Reconstitution:** Mix 500-mg vial with 2 mL sterile water for injection to provide a concentration of 250 mg/mL.
- **Injection:** Inject deeply into upper outer quadrant of buttock; may give undiluted.

IV ALERT

- **Reconstitution:** Mix 500-mg vial with 2 mL sterile water for injection to provide a concentration of 250 mg/mL.

- **Further dilution:** Dilute with 0.9% NaCl or D_5W, and administer at maximum rate of 15 mg/kg/hr. Too-rapid IV administration may produce skin flushing, urticaria, hypotension, or shock.

PRECAUTIONS

HEALTH-RELATED

- Use deferoxamine cautiously in patients with aluminum overload or aluminum-related encephalopathy.

AGE-RELATED

- **Children:** Safety and efficacy of deferoxamine have not been established in children.
- **Elderly:** Age-related renal impairment may require dosage reduction.

PREGNANCY/LACTATION-RELATED

- Pregnancy category C; excretion into breast milk unknown; use caution in nursing mothers.

MONITORING

- **Baseline assessment:** Determine history of allergies and amount of iron ingested or infused.
- **Baseline lab work:** Serum iron levels, iron binding capacity before and during therapy to assess severity of iron poisoning and effectiveness of chelation. CBC and coagulation profile to assess for bleeding/bleeding potential, biochemical panel to assess for liver and/or renal failure, and for high anion gap metabolic acidosis with elevated lactate level which indicates multiple organ dysfunction resulting from serious iron toxicity; requires chelation therapy.
- **Iron toxicity:** Monitor for dehydration, respiratory distress, metabolic acidosis, dysrhythmias, hypotension, and shock.
- **Therapeutic effect:** Deferoxamine should help resolve metabolic acidosis and systemic toxicity (multiple organ dysfunction) associated with iron toxicity.
- **Renal failure:** Provide adequate IV hydration to help reduce incidence of acute renal failure during deferoxamine infusion.
- **Deafness:** Assess for hearing loss (neurotoxicity).
- **Eye damage:** Obtain periodic slit-lamp ophthalmic exams in those treated for chronic iron overload.
- **Subcutaneous skin irritation:** Monitor for pruritus, erythema, skin irritation, and swelling if using subcutaneous technique.
- **Patient education:** Inform patients that urine will appear reddish. Discomfort may occur at site of injection.

SERIOUS ADVERSE REACTIONS

- Altered mental status, acidosis, high-frequency hearing loss, visual changes, which may be due to iron toxicity rather than deferoxamine infusion.

OVERDOSE/TOXICITY

- **Nephrotoxicity:** Acute renal failure.
- **Respiratory:** Acute respiratory distress syndrome.
- **Sepsis:** Deferoxamine-iron complex may promote *Yersinia enterocolitica* sepsis following chelation therapy. Prophylactic antibiotics should be considered.
- **GI decontamination:** Whole bowel irrigation is sometimes effective for iron toxicity due to ingestion of multiple iron tablets.

ANTIDOTE/DIALYSIS

- **Antidote:** No specific recommendations.
- **Dialysis:** Deferoxamine is removed by hemodialysis and is likely removed using high-permeability hemodialysis. No data are available regarding removal using peritoneal dialysis.

delavirdine mesylate

de-la-vir′-deen mes′-il-ate

Classes

Chemical: arylpiperazine derivative, nonnucleoside reverse transcriptase inhibitor
Therapeutic: antiretroviral

Pregnancy Category: C

Trade Names

Prescription: Rescriptor

Do not confuse Rescriptor with Retrovin or Ritonavir.

CLINICAL PHARMACOLOGY

Mechanism of Action

A nonnucleoside reverse transcriptase inhibitor that binds directly to HIV-1 reverse transcriptase and blocks RNA- and DNA-dependent DNA polymerase activities. **Therapeutic Effect:** Interrupts HIV replication, slowing the progression of HIV infection.

PHARMACOKINETICS

Rapidly absorbed after PO administration. Protein binding: 98%. Primarily distributed in plasma. Metabolized in the liver. Eliminated in feces and urine. **Half-life:** 2-11 hr.

AVAILABILITY

Tablets: 100 mg, 200 mg.

INDICATIONS AND DOSAGE

HIV infection (in combination with other antiretrovirals)

PO

Adults: 400 mg 3 times per day.

CONTRAINDICATIONS

Hypersensitivity to delavirdine. Delavirdine should not be administered with the following medications: astemizole and terfenadine (antihistamines), dihydroergotamine, ergonovine, ergotamine, methylergonovine (ergot derivatives), cisapride (motility agent), pimozide (neuroleptic), alprazolam, midazolam, triazolam

INTERACTIONS

Drug: **Atorvastatin, simvastatin:** May decrease delavirdine blood concentration. **Benzodiazepines, calcium channel blockers:** May cause life-threatening adverse reactions. **Carbamazepine, phenobarbital, phenytoin:** May decrease delavirdine blood concentration. **Didanosine:** May decrease concentrations of delavirdine; separate administration by 1 hr. **H_2 blockers:** May decrease delavirdine absorption. **Lovastatin, simvastatin:** May decrease delavirdine blood concentration. **Rifampin:** May decrease delavirdine blood concentrations. **Sildenafil:** May increase sildenafil concentrations, leading to hypotension, visual changes, and priapism. Herbal: **St. John's wort:** May decrease delavirdine blood concentration. Food: None known.

DIAGNOSTIC TEST EFFECTS

May increase AST (SGOT) and ALT (SGPT) levels. May decrease neutrophil count.

SIDE-EFFECTS

Frequent (18%): Rash, pruritus. Occasional (greater than 2%): Headache, nausea, diarrhea, fatigue, anorexia. Rare (less than 2%): Erythema multiforme, Stevens–Johnson syndrome

CRITICAL CARE CONSIDERATIONS

ADMINISTRATION/HANDLING

PO ALERT

- Give delavirdine without regard to food.
- Tablets may be dissolved in water before consumption.
- Give delavirdine with orange juice or cranberry juice if achlorhydria (absence of hydrochloric acid in the stomach) is present.

PRECAUTIONS

HEALTH-RELATED

- Use delavirdine cautiously in patients with hepatic impairment.
- CYP3A4 pathway and HMG-CoA reductase inhibitor pathway interactions may occur when delavirdine is administered with other medications metabolized by these pathways.

AGE-RELATED

- **Children:** Safety and efficacy of delavirdine have not been established in children under 16 yr.
- **Elderly:** Safety and efficacy have not been established in patients over 65 yr.

PREGNANCY/LACTATION-RELATED

- Pregnancy category C; teratogenic in rats; excreted in breast milk at high concentrations.

MONITORING

- **Baseline assessment:** Assess history of HIV infection and medications used for management.
- **Baseline lab work:** Liver function tests before and periodically during delavirdine therapy.
- **Ongoing lab work:** Liver function tests and biochemical profile.
- **Severe rash:** Assess skin for rash.
- **Medication interactions:** Delavirdine may inhibit the metabolism of many drugs used in critical care including antidysrythmics, calcium channel blockers, sedative hypnotics, to create altered drug effects or reduced delavirdine concentrations.
- **Antacids:** Administer at least 1 hr apart from delavirdine.
- **Possible *Clostridium difficile* colitis:** Severe diarrhea with abdominal pain, blood or mucus in stools, and fever may indicate antibiotic-associated colitis.
- **Hand washing:** If *C. difficile* colitis develops, wash hands with antibacterial soap; alcohol-based foam is ineffective against *C. difficile* spores.
- **Nausea/vomiting:** Manage with standard measures. Provide IV hydration if severe symptoms occur. Consider use of another medication. Assess eating pattern and monitor for nausea and weight loss. Small, frequent meals may offset nausea and anorexia.

- **Superinfection:** Be alert for signs and symptoms of superinfection, including anal or genital pruritus, black hairy tongue, diarrhea, increased fever, sore throat, ulceration or changes of oral mucosa, and vomiting.
- **Patient education:** When using delavirdine outside the hospital, advise patients to ask the health care provider before taking any other medications, including OTC drugs. Explain that delavirdine is not a cure for HIV infection nor does it reduce the risk of transmitting HIV to others.

SERIOUS ADVERSE REACTIONS

- **Severe rash:** With fever, blistering, oral lesions, conjunctivitis, swelling, muscle and joint aches.
- Erythema multiforme and Stevens–Johnson syndrome.

OVERDOSE/TOXICITY

- **Liver failure:** Elevated liver enzymes, jaundice, ascites, fluid retention, bleeding.
- **GI decontamination:** No specific recommendations.

ANTIDOTE/DIALYSIS

- **Antidote:** No specific recommendations.
- **Dialysis:** It is unknown if delavirdine is removed by hemodialysis, high-permeability dialysis, or peritoneal dialysis.

demeclocycline hydrochloride

dem-e-kloe-sye'-kleen hye-droe-klor'-ide

Classes

Chemical: tetracycline derivative
Therapeutic: antibiotic

Pregnancy Category: D

Trade Names

Prescription: Declomycin

CLINICAL PHARMACOLOGY

Mechanism of Action

A tetracycline antibiotic that inhibits bacterial protein synthesis by binding to ribosomal receptor sites; also inhibits antidiuretic hormone (ADH)-induced water reabsorption. **Therapeutic Effect:** Bacteriostatic; also produces water diuresis.

PHARMACOKINETICS

Food and dairy products interfere with absorption. Protein binding: 41%-50%. Metabolized in liver. Excreted in urine. Removed by hemodialysis. **Half-life:** 10-15 hr.

AVAILABILITY

Tablets: 150 mg, 300 mg.

INDICATIONS AND DOSAGE

Mild to moderate infections, including acne, pertussis, chronic bronchitis, and urinary tract infections

PO

Adults, Elderly: 150 mg 4 times per day or 300 mg 2 times per day. **Children older than 8 yr:** 8-12 mg/kg/day in 2-4 divided doses.

Uncomplicated gonorrhea

PO

Adults: Initially, 600 mg, then 300 mg every 12 hr for 4 days for total of 3 g.

Syndrome of inappropriate ADH secretion (SIADH)

PO

Adults, Elderly: Initially 900-1200 mg/day in 3-4 divided doses, then decrease dose to 600-900 mg/day in divided doses.

CONTRAINDICATIONS

Children 8 yr and younger, pregnancy, concurrent use with methoxyflurane, hypersensitivity to demeclocycline

INTERACTIONS

Drug: Antacids containing aluminum, calcium, or magnesium; laxatives containing magnesium; oral iron preparations: Impair the absorption of demeclocycline. **Cholestyramine, colestipol:** May decrease demeclocycline absorption. **Oral contraceptives:** May decrease the effects of oral contraceptives. **Herbal:** None known. **Food: Dairy products:** May decrease demeclocycline absorption.

DIAGNOSTIC TEST EFFECTS

May increase BUN and serum alkaline phosphatase, amylase, bilirubin, AST (SGOT), and ALT (SGPT) levels.

SIDE-EFFECTS

Frequent: Anorexia, nausea, vomiting, diarrhea, dysphagia, possibly severe photosensitivity (with moderate to high demeclocycline dosage). **Occasional:** Urticaria, rash; diabetes insipidus syndrome, marked by polydipsia, polyuria, and weakness (with long-term therapy)

CRITICAL CARE CONSIDERATIONS

ADMINISTRATION/HANDLING

PO ALERT

- Give antacids containing aluminum, calcium, or magnesium; laxatives containing magnesium; or oral iron preparations 1-2 hr before or after demeclocycline to avoid impaired drug absorption.

- Administer demeclocycline with a full glass of water.
- Demeclocycline should be taken on an empty stomach.

PRECAUTIONS

HEALTH-RELATED

- Use demeclocycline cautiously in patients with renal impairment and in those who cannot avoid sun or ultraviolet exposure, which may produce a severe photosensitivity reaction.

AGE-RELATED

- **Children:** Not recommended for use in children under 8 yr; demeclocycline may cause permanent yellow, gray, or brown discoloration of teeth.
- **Elderly:** Age-related changes of renal and liver function may prompt poorer clearance of the drug and may exacerbate renal or liver dysfunction.

PREGNANCY/LACTATION-RELATED

- Pregnancy category D; problems associated with use of the tetracyclines during or around pregnancy include adverse effects on fetal teeth and bones, maternal liver toxicity, and congenital defects; excreted into breast milk in low concentrations; use caution in nursing mothers.

MONITORING

- **Baseline assessment:** Determine history of allergies, especially to tetracyclines, and renal insufficiency before beginning drug therapy.
- **Baseline lab work:** Biochemical profile reflective of renal and liver function.
- **Possible *Clostridium difficile* colitis:** Severe diarrhea with abdominal pain, blood or mucus in stools, and fever may indicate antibiotic-associated colitis.
- **Hand washing:** If *C. difficile* colitis develops, wash hands with antibacterial soap; alcohol-based foam is ineffective against *C. difficile* spores.
- **Nausea/vomiting:** Manage with standard measures. Provide IV hydration if severe symptoms occur. Consider use of another medication. Assess eating pattern and monitor for nausea and weight loss. Small, frequent meals may offset nausea and anorexia.
- **Superinfection:** Be alert for signs and symptoms of superinfection, including anal or genital pruritus, black hairy tongue, diarrhea, increased fever, sore throat, ulceration or changes of oral mucosa, and vomiting.
- **Renal impairment:** Monitor intake and output and renal function tests. Nephrogenic diabetes insipidus has been reported.
- **Increased intracranial pressure:** Monitor for headache and visual changes, which may indicate benign increased intracranial pressure (ICP) (pseudotumor cerebri).
- **Evenly spaced doses:** Space doses evenly around the clock and administer demeclocycline for the full course of treatment.
- **Patient education:** When using demeclocycline outside the hospital, instruct patients to take doses on an empty stomach with a full glass of water; to space doses evenly around the clock, and to continue taking demeclocycline for the full course of treatment. Encourage patients to avoid overexposure to sun or ultraviolet light to prevent photosensitivity reactions. Advise patients to avoid dosage directly before lying down to sleep at night to help prevent esophageal inflammation and ulceration. Instruct patients to report diarrhea, rash, or if other new symptoms occur.

SERIOUS ADVERSE REACTIONS

- Superinfection (especially fungal) and anaphylaxis. Manage *C. difficile*–associated colitis with oral vancomycin (Vancocin) or metromidazole (Flagyl).
- **Bulging fontanelles:** Occurs rarely in infants.
- **Increased intracranial pressure:** Usually benign but can have permanent sequelae even after medication is discontinued.
- **Diabetes insipidus:** Polyuria, polydipsia, and weakness, which resolves after medication is discontinued.

OVERDOSE/TOXICITY

- **Nephrotoxicity:** Acute renal failure reflected by oliguria, increased BUN and creatinine, hyperkalemia.
- **Pseudotumor cerebri:** Increased intracranial pressure, which generally resolves following discontinuation of the drug.
- **GI decontamination:** No specific recommendations.

ANTIDOTE/DIALYSIS

- **Antidote:** No specific recommendations.
- **Dialysis:** No data are available regarding removal of demeclocycline using hemodialysis, high-permeability dialysis, or peritoneal dialysis.

desipramine hydrochloride

dess-ip′-ra-meen hye-droe-klor′-ide

Classes

Chemical: dibenzazepine derivative, secondary amine

Therapeutic: antidepressant, tricyclic

Pregnancy Category: C

Trade Names

Prescription: Norpramin

Do not confuse desipramine with clomipramine, disopyramide, imipramine, or nortriptyline.

CLINICAL PHARMACOLOGY

Mechanism of Action

A tricyclic antidepressant that blocks the reuptake of neurotransmitters, such as norepinephrine and serotonin, at presynaptic membranes, increasing their availability at postsynaptic receptor sites. Also has strong anticholinergic activity. **Therapeutic Effect:** Relieves depression.

PHARMACOKINETICS

Rapidly, and well absorbed from the GI tract. Protein binding: 90%. Metabolized in the liver. Primarily excreted in urine. Not removed by hemodialysis. **Half-life:** 12-27 hr.

AVAILABILITY

Tablets: 10 mg, 25 mg, 50 mg, 75 mg, 100 mg, 150 mg.

INDICATIONS AND DOSAGE

Depression

PO

Adults: 75 mg/day. May gradually increase to 150-200 mg/day. Maximum: 300 mg/day. **Elderly:** Initially 10-25 mg/day. May gradually increase by 10-25 mg every 7 days to 75-100 mg/day. Maximum: 300 mg/day. **Children older than 12 yr:** Initially, 25-50 mg/day. May gradually increase to 100 mg/day. Maximum: 150 mg/day. **Children 6-12 yr:** 1-3 mg/kg/day. Maximum: 5 mg/kg/day.

OFF-LABEL USES

Treatment of attention-deficit/hyperactivity disorder, bulimia nervosa, cataplexy associated with narcolepsy, cocaine withdrawal, neurogenic pain, panic disorder

CONTRAINDICATIONS

Angle-closure (narrow angle) glaucoma, use within 14 days of MAOIs, hypersensitivity to desipramine or other dibenzapine tricyclic antidepressants; desipramine should not be used in the acute recovery period following myocardial infarction

INTERACTIONS

Drug: Alcohol, other CNS depressants: May increase CNS and respiratory depression and the hypotensive effects of desipramine. **Antithyroid agents:** May increase the risk of agranulocytosis. **Cimetidine:** May increase desipramine blood concentration and risk of toxicity. **Clonidine, guanadrel:** May decrease the effects of these drugs. **MAOIs:** May increase the risk of neuroleptic malignant syndrome, hyperpyrexia, hypertensive crisis, and seizures. **Phenothiazines:** May increase the anticholinergic and sedative effects of desipramine. **Phenytoin:** May decrease the desipramine blood concentration. **Sympathomimetics:** May increase the risk of cardiac effects. **Herbal: St. John's wort:** May increase desipramine's pharmacologic effects and risk of toxicity. **Food:** None known.

DIAGNOSTIC TEST EFFECTS

May alter blood glucose level and ECG readings.

SIDE-EFFECTS

Frequent: Somnolence, fatigue, dry mouth, blurred vision, constipation, delayed micturition, orthostatic hypotension, diaphoresis, impaired concentration, increased appetite, urine retention. **Occasional:** GI disturbances (such as nausea, GI distress, metallic taste). **Rare:** Paradoxic reactions (agitation, restlessness, nightmares, insomnia), extrapyramidal symptoms (particularly fine hand tremor)

CRITICAL CARE CONSIDERATIONS

ADMINISTRATION/HANDLING

PO ALERT

- Give desipramine with food or milk if GI distress occurs.
- Make sure at least 14 days elapse between the use of MAOIs and desipramine.

PRECAUTIONS

HEALTH-RELATED

- Use desipramine cautiously in patients with cardiac conduction disturbances,

D

cardiovascular disease, hyperthyroidism, seizure disorders, urinary retention, and those taking thyroid replacement therapy.

- **Cytochrome P450 2D6 pathway:** Patients who have a deficiency in this pathway may experience elevated plasma levels of desipramine.

D

AGE-RELATED

- **Children:** Desipramine use is not recommended for children under 6 yr.
- **Elderly:** Administer lower dosages to elderly patients because of increased risk for drug toxicity.

PREGNANCY/LACTATION-RELATED

- Pregnancy category C; excreted into breast milk; effect on the nursing infant unknown but may be of concern.

MONITORING

- **Baseline lab work:** CBC and blood chemistry tests before and periodically during long-term therapy to assess hepatic and renal function.
- **Baseline diagnostic tests:** Baseline ECG if risk for dysrhythmias is present.
- **Suicide precautions:** Closely monitor suicidal patients during early therapy. As depression lessens, energy level improves, increasing the likelihood of suicide attempts.
- **Therapeutic effect:** Assess for improved appearance, behavior, level of interest, mood, and sleep pattern.
- **Drug levels:** Therapeutic serum level for desipramine is 115-300 ng/mL; toxic serum level is greater than 400 ng/mL.
- **Dysrhythmias:** Continuously monitor ECG for dysrhythmias including heart block, ventricular tachycardia, and ventricular fibrillation, especially if history of abnormal heart rhythms is present.
- **Abrupt withdrawal:** Do not abruptly discontinue desipramine to avoid withdrawal.
- **Patient education:** Inform patients that desipramine's full therapeutic effect may be noted in 2-4 wk. Instruct patients to change positions slowly to help prevent dizziness. Explain a tolerance will be developed to desipramine's anticholinergic, sedative, and hypotensive effects during early therapy.

SERIOUS ADVERSE REACTIONS

- Abrupt discontinuation after prolonged therapy may produce severe headache, malaise, nausea, vomiting, and vivid dreams.

OVERDOSE/TOXICITY

- **Cardiovascular toxicity:** Sudden death, myocardial infarction, stroke, hypotension, and hypertension.
- **Neuroleptic malignant syndrome:** Fever, muscular rigidity, tremors or other extrapyramidal movements, altered mental status (includes coma and unresponsive catatonia) and autonomic dysfunction, which contributes to cardiovascular changes. Rhabdomyolysis leading to other complications may be seen if muscle rigidity is severe.
- **Overdose:** Confusion, seizures, somnolence, dysrhythmias, fever, hallucinations, dyspnea, vomiting, and unusual fatigue or weakness.
- **GI decontamination:** No specific recommendations.

ANTIDOTE/DIALYSIS

- **Antidote:** For neuroleptic malignant syndrome, dantrolene, bromocryptine, amantadine, and carbidopa-levodopa may be given.
- **Dialysis:** Desipramine is not removed by hemodialysis or peritoneal dialysis. No data are available for removal by high-permeability dialysis.

desirudin

See Anticoagulants (p. 900)

desloratadine

des-lor-at'-a-deen

Classes

Chemical: piperidine derivative
Therapeutic: antihistamine

Pregnancy Category: C

Trade Names

Prescription: Aerius ♣, Clarinex, Clarinex RediTabs

Combinations

Prescription: with pseudoephedrine (Clarinex-D 12 Hour)

Do not confuse Clarinex with Claritin.

CLINICAL PHARMACOLOGY

Mechanism of Action

A nonsedating antihistamine that exhibits selective peripheral histamine H_1 receptor blocking action. Competes with histamine at receptor sites. **Therapeutic Effect:** Prevents allergic responses mediated by histamine, such as rhinitis and urticaria.

PHARMACOKINETICS

Rapidly and almost completely absorbed from the GI tract. Distributed mainly in liver, lungs, GI tract, and bile. Metabolized in the liver to active metabolite and undergoes extensive first-pass metabolism. Eliminated in urine and feces. **Half-life:** 27 hr (increased in the elderly and in renal or hepatic impairment).

AVAILABILITY

Tablets (Clarinex): 5 mg.
Tablets (orally disintegrating [Clarinex Reditabs]): 2.5 mg, 5 mg.
Syrup (Clarinex): 2.5 mg/5 mL.

INDICATIONS AND DOSAGE

Allergic rhinitis, urticaria

PO

Adults, Elderly, Children older than 12 yr: 5 mg once per day. **Children 6-11 yr:** 2.5 mg once per day. **Children 1-5 yr:** 1.25 mg once per day. **Children 6-11 mo:** 1 mg once per day.

Dosage in hepatic or renal impairment

Dosage is decreased to 5 mg every other day.

CONTRAINDICATIONS

Hypersensitivity to desloratadine, loratidine, or any components of the product

INTERACTIONS

Drug: **Erythromycin, ketoconazole:** May increase desloratadine blood concentration. **Herbal:** None known. **Food:** None known.

DIAGNOSTIC TEST EFFECTS

May suppress wheal and flare reactions to antigen skin testing unless the drug is discontinued 4 days before testing.

SIDE-EFFECTS

Frequent (14%): Headache. **Occasional (3%):** Dry mouth, somnolence. **Rare (less than 3%):** Fatigue, dizziness, diarrhea, nausea

CRITICAL CARE CONSIDERATIONS

ADMINISTRATION/HANDLING

PO ALERT

- Do not crush or break film-coated tablets.
- Desloratadine is 2.5-4 times more potent than its parent compound, loratadine.

PRECAUTIONS

HEALTH-RELATED

- Use desloratadine cautiously in patients with hepatic impairment.

AGE-RELATED

- **Children:** Safety and efficacy of desloratadine have not been established in children under 12 yr. Children are more sensitive to the drug's anticholinergic effects.
- **Elderly:** Are more sensitive to the drug's anticholinergic effects, such as dry mouth, nose, and throat.

PREGNANCY/LACTATION-RELATED

- Pregnancy category C; passes into breast milk, use caution in nursing mothers.

MONITORING

- **Baseline assessment:** Auscultate breath sounds for wheezing.
- **Lab work:** CBC with differential to evaluate for infection and eosinophil count.
- **Chronic urticaria:** Examine patients being treated for urticaria.
- **Skin testing:** Discontinue desloratadine 4 days before antigen skin testing.
- **PO fluids:** Increase the fluid intake in patients with upper respiratory allergies to decrease the viscosity of secretions, offset thirst, and replace fluids lost from diaphoresis.
- **Therapeutic effects:** Monitor for resolution of allergic rhinitis or urticaria.
- **Patient education:** Inform patients that desloratadine should not cause drowsiness but to avoid performing tasks that require mental alertness or motor skills until response to the drug is known. Urge patients to avoid consuming alcohol during desloratadine therapy.

SERIOUS ADVERSE REACTIONS

- Tachycardia.
- **Hypsensitivity reaction:** Rash, pruritis, urticaria, dyspnea, edema, and anaphylaxis.

OVERDOSE/TOXICITY

- **Liver dysfunction:** Rare elevated liver enzymes including bilirubin.
- **GI decontamination:** No specific recommendations.

ANTIDOTE/DIALYSIS

- **Antidote:** No specific recommendations.
- **Dialysis:** Desloratadine is not removed by hemodialysis or peritoneal dialysis. No data are available on removal by high-permeability dialysis.

desmopressin

des-moe-press'-in

Classes

Chemical: arginine vasopressin analog
Therapeutic: antidiuretic, antihemophilic, hemostatic

Pregnancy Category: B

Trade Names

Prescription: DDAVP, DDAVP Nasal, DDAVP Rhinal Tube, Minirin, Stimate

CLINICAL PHARMACOLOGY

Mechanism of Action

A synthetic pituitary hormone that increases reabsorption of water by increasing permeability of collecting ducts of the kidneys. Also serves as a plasminogen activator. Therapeutic Effect: Increases plasma factor VIII (antihemophilic factor). Decreases urinary output.

PHARMACOKINETICS

Route	Onset	Peak	Duration
PO	1 hr	2-7 hr	6-8 hr
IV	15-30 min	1.5-3 hr	N/A
Intranasal	15 min-1 hr	1-5 hr	5-21 hr

Poorly absorbed after oral or nasal administration. Metabolism: Unknown. Half-life: Oral: 1.5-2.5 hr. Intranasal: 3.3-3.5 hr. IV: 0.4-4 hr.

AVAILABILITY

Tablets (DDAVP): 0.1 mg, 0.2 mg.
Injection (DDAVP): 4 mcg/mL.
Nasal solution (DDAVP): 0.01%.
Nasal spray: 0.01 mg/inhalation (DDAVP Nasal), 0.15 mg/inhalation (Stimate).

INDICATIONS AND DOSAGE

Primary nocturnal enuresis

PO

Children 12 yr and older: 0.2-0.6 mg once before bedtime.

Intranasal

Children 6 yr and older: Initially, 20 mcg (0.2 mL) at bedtime; use one-half dose in each nostril. Adjust to maximum of 40 mcg/day. Range: 10-40 mcg.

Central cranial diabetes insipidus

PO

Adults, Elderly, Children 12 yr and older: Initially, 0.05 mg twice per day. Range: 0.1-1.2 mg/day in 2-3 divided doses. **Children younger than 12 yr:** Initially, 0.05 mg; then twice per day. Range: 0.1-0.8 mg daily.

IV, Subcutaneous

Adults, Elderly, Children 12 yr and older: 2-4 mcg/day in 2 divided doses or one tenth of maintenance intranasal dose.

Intranasal (use 100 mcg/mL concentration)

Adults, Elderly, Children older than 12 yr: 5-40 mcg (0.05-0.4 mL) in 1-3 doses/day. **Children 3 mo-12 yr:** Initially, 5 mcg (0.05 mL)/day. Range: 5-30 mcg (0.05-0.3 mL)/day.

Hemophilia A, von Willebrand's disease (type I)

IV Infusion

Adults, Elderly, Children weighing more than 10 kg: 0.3 mcg/kg diluted in 50 mL 0.9% NaCl. **Children weighing 10 kg and less:** 0.3 mcg/kg diluted in 10 mL 0.9% NaCl.

Intranasal (use 1.5 mg/mL concentration providing 150 mcg/spray)

Adults, Elderly, Children 12 yr and older weighing more than 50 kg: 300 mcg; use 1 spray in each nostril. **Adults, Elderly, Children 12 yr and older weighing 50 kg or less:** 150 mcg as a single spray.

OFF-LABEL USES

Prophylaxis and treatment of central diabetes insipidus, treatment of hemophilia A, primary nocturnal enuresis, von Willebrand's disease

CONTRAINDICATIONS

Hemophilia A with factor VIII levels less than 5%; hemophilia B; severe type I, type IIB, or platelet-type von Willebrand's disease

INTERACTIONS

Drug: **Carbamazepine, *chlorproPAMIDE, clofibrate:** May increase the effects of desmopressin. **Demeclocycline, lithium, norepinephrine:** May decrease effects of desmopressin. Herbal: None known. Food: None known.

DIAGNOSTIC TEST EFFECTS

None known.

SIDE-EFFECTS

Occasional: **IV:** Pain, redness, or swelling at injection site; headache; abdominal cramps; vulval pain; flushed skin; mild BP elevation; nausea with high dosages
Nasal: Rhinorrhea, nasal congestion, slight BP elevation

CRITICAL CARE CONSIDERATIONS

ADMINISTRATION/HANDLING

PO ALERT

- Store away from light and excessive heat.

IV ALERT

- **Storage:** Refrigerate, although desmopressin is stable for 2 wk at room temperature.
- **IV infusion:** Dilute in 10-50 mL 0.9% NaCl and prepare to infuse over 15-30 min.
- **Preoperative use:** Administer 30 min before procedure, as prescribed.
- Remember that the IV dose is one tenth the intranasal dose.

INTRANASAL ALERT

- **Storage:** Refrigerate DDAVP nasal solution and Stimate nasal spray. DDAVP nasal spray is stable at room temperature.
- **Stability:** Nasal solution and Stimate nasal spray are stable for 3 wk at room temperature if unopened.
- **Administration:** Draw up a measured quantity of desmopressin with a calibrated catheter (rhinyle). Insert one end in the nose and have patients blow on the other end to deposit the solution deep in the nasal cavity. For infants, young children, and obtunded patients, an air-filled syringe may be attached to the catheter to deposit the solution.

SUBCUTANEOUS ALERT

- **Therapeutic response:** Estimate by adequacy of sleep duration when used for noctural enuresis.
- **Timing:** Expect to adjust morning and evening dosages separately.

PRECAUTIONS

HEALTH-RELATED

- Use desmopressin cautiously in patients with fluid or electrolyte imbalances, coronary artery disease, hypertensive cardiovascular disease, or predisposition to thrombus formation.

AGE-RELATED

- **Children:** Use cautiously in neonates under 3 mo because this age group is at high risk for fluid balance problems. Careful fluid restrictions are recommended in infants. Safety for use in children under 12 yr with diabetes insipidus has not been established.
- **Elderly:** Are at increased risk for hyponatremia and water intoxication.

PREGNANCY/LACTATION-RELATED

- Pregnancy category B (no uterotonic action at antidiuretic doses); compatible with breast-feeding.

MONITORING

- **Baseline assessment:** BP, pulse rate, and weight.
- **Baseline lab work:** Factor VIII coagulant concentration (in hemophilia A and von Willebrand's disease), bleeding times, serum electrolyte levels, urine specific gravity.
- **Hypertension and tachycardia:** Monitor BP and pulse during infusion.
- **Therapeutic effect for resolution of diabetes insipidus:** Monitor for polyuria, polydipsia, and weakness. Assess fluid intake, serum osmolality, urine volume, urine specific gravity, and weight.
- **Ongoing labwork:** Assess serum electrolyte levels, factor VIII antigen level, aPTT, and factor VIII activity level for hemophilia.
- **Patient education:** When using desmopressin outside the hospital, caution patients to avoid overhydration. Teach the proper technique for intranasal administration. Warn patients to report abdominal cramps, headache, heartburn, nausea, or shortness of breath. Tell parents of children treated for nocturnal enuresis to monitor sleep pattern carefully.

SERIOUS ADVERSE REACTIONS

- Water intoxication or hyponatremia, marked by headache, somnolence, confusion, decreased urination, rapid weight gain, seizures, and coma may occur in overhydration. Children, elderly, and infants are especially at risk.

OVERDOSE/TOXICITY

- Water intoxication and hyponatremia leading to seizures and coma.
- **GI decontamination:** No specific recommendations.

ANTIDOTE/DIALYSIS

- **Antidote:** No specific recommendations.
- **Dialysis:** No data are available regarding removal of desmopressin using hemodialysis, peritoneal dialysis, or high-permeability dialysis.

dexamethasone

dex-a-meth'-a-sone

Classes

Chemical: glucocorticoid, synthetic
Therapeutic: corticosteroid, ophthalmic, corticosteroid, systemic

D

Pregnancy Category: C

Trade Names

Prescription: Adrenocot, Cortastat, Cortastat 10, Cortastat LA, Dalalone, Dalalone D.P., Dalalone L.A., Decadron, Decadron 5-12 Pak, Decadron Phosphate Injectable, Decaject, De-Sone LA, Dexacen-4, Dexamethasone Intensol, Dexasone, Dexasone LA, Dexpak Taperpak, Hexadrol, Hexadrol Phosphate, Maxidex, Solurex, Solurex LA

Combinations

Prescription: with neomycin, (NeoDecadron, Ak-Neo-Dex); with neomycin and polymixin B (Dexacidin, Maxitrol, Dexasporin); with tobramycin (Tobradex); with lidocaine (Decadron with Xylocaine)

Do not confuse dexamethasone with desoximetasone or dextromethorphan or Maxidex with Maxzide.

CLINICAL PHARMACOLOGY

Mechanism of Action

A long-acting glucocorticoid that inhibits accumulation of inflammatory cells at inflammation sites, phagocytosis, lysosomal enzyme release and synthesis, and release of mediators of inflammation. **Therapeutic Effect:** Prevents and suppresses cell and tissue immune reactions and inflammatory process.

PHARMACOKINETICS

Rapidly, completely absorbed from the GI tract after oral administration. Widely distributed. Protein binding: High. Metabolized in the liver. Primarily excreted in urine. Minimally removed by hemodialysis. **Half-life:** 3-4.5 hr (biologic half-life: 36-54 hr).

AVAILABILITY

Nasal aerosol: 100 mcg.
Ophthalmic ointment (Decadron, Maxidex): 0.05% .
Ophthalmic solution (Decadron): 0.1%.
Ophthalmic suspension (Maxidex): 0.1%.
Oral concentrate (Dexamethasone Intensol): 1 mg/mL.
Oral solution: 0.5 mg/5 mL, 1 mg/mL.
Tablets: 0.25 mg, 0.5 mg (Decadron), 0.75 mg (Decadron, Decadron 5-12 Pak), 1 mg, 1.5 mg (Dexpak Taperpak), 2 mg, 4 mg (Decadron, Hexadrol), 6 mg.
Topical aerosol: 0.01%, 0.04%.
Topical cream (Decadron): 0.1%,
Topical gel: 0.1%.
Injectable solution: 4 mg/mL (Adrenocot, Cortastat, Dalalone, Decadron Phosphate Injectable, Decaject, Dexacen-4, Dexasone, Hexadrol Phosphate, Solurex), 10 mg/mL (Cortastat 10, Dexasone, Hexadrol Phosphate).
Injectable Suspension: 8 mg/mL (Cortastat LA, Dalalone LA, De-Sone LA, Dexasone LA, Solurex LA), 16 mg/mL (Dalalone D.P.).

INDICATIONS AND DOSAGE

Antiinflammatory

PO, IV, IM

Adults, Elderly: 0.75-9 mg/day in divided doses every 6-12 hr. **Children:** 0.08-0.3 mg/kg/day in divided doses every 6-12 hr.

Cerebral edema

IV

Adults, Elderly: Initially, 10 mg, then 4 mg (IV or IM) every 6 hr.

PO, IV, IM

Children: Loading dose of 1-2 mg/kg, then 1-1.5 mg/kg/day in divided doses every 4-6 hr for 5 days, then taper over 5 days, then discontinue.

Nausea and vomiting in chemotherapy patients

IV

Adults, Elderly: 8-20 mg once, then 4 mg (PO) every 4-6 hr or 8 mg every 8 hr. **Children:** 10 mg/m^2/dose (Maximum: 20 mg), then 5 mg/m^2/dose every 6 hr.

Usual topical dosage

Topical

Adults, Elderly, Children: Apply to affected area 3-4 times per day.

Physiologic replacement

PO, IV, IM

Children: 0.03-0.15 mg/kg/day in divided doses every 6-12 hr.

Usual ophthalmic dosage, ocular inflammatory conditions

Ointment

Adults, Elderly, Children: Thin coating 3-4 times/day.

Suspension

Adults, Elderly, Children: Initially, 2 drops every 1 hr while awake and every 2 hr at night for 1 day, then reduce to 3-4 times/day.

OFF-LABEL USES

Antiemetic, croup

CONTRAINDICATIONS

Active untreated infections, fungal, tuberculosis, viral diseases of the eye, hypersensitivity to dexamethasone, (for topical) sensitivity to any component of the product

INTERACTIONS

Drug: Amphotericin: May increase hypokalemia. **Digoxin:** May increase digoxin toxicity caused by hypokalemia. **Diuretics, insulin, oral hypoglycemics, potassium supplements:** May decrease the effects of these drugs. **Hepatic enzyme inducers:** May decrease the effects of dexamethasone. **Live-virus vaccines:** May decrease antibody response to vaccine, increase vaccine side effects, and potentiate virus replication. **Herbal:** None known. **Food:** None known.

DIAGNOSTIC TEST EFFECTS

May increase blood glucose and serum lipid, amylase, and sodium levels. May decrease serum calcium, potassium, and thyroxine levels.

IV INCOMPATIBILITIES

Ciprofloxacin (Cipro), *DAUNOrubicin (Cerubidine), idarubicin (Idamycin), midazolam (Versed)

IV COMPATIBILITIES

Aminophylline, cimetidine (Tagamet), cisplatin (Platinol), cyclophosphamide (Cytoxan), cytarabine (Cytosar), docetaxel (Taxotere), *DOXOrubicin (Adriamycin), etoposide (VePesid), granisetron (Kytril), heparin, hydromorphone (Dilaudid), lorazepam (Ativan), morphine, ondansetron (Zofran), paclitaxel (Taxol), potassium chloride, propofol (Diprivan), total parenteral nutrition (TPN)

SIDE-EFFECTS

Frequent: **Inhalation:** Cough, dry mouth, hoarseness, throat irritation. **Intranasal:** Burning, mucosal dryness. **Ophthalmic:** Blurred vision. **Systemic:** Insomnia, facial swelling or cushingoid appearance, moderate abdominal distention, indigestion, increased appetite, nervousness, facial flushing, diaphoresis. **Occasional:** **Inhalation:** Localized fungal infection, such as thrush. **Intranasal:** Crusting inside nose, nosebleed, sore throat, ulceration of nasal mucosa. **Ophthalmic:** Decreased vision, watering of eyes, eye pain, burning, stinging, redness of eyes, nausea, vomiting. **Systemic:** Dizziness, decreased or blurred vision. **Topical:** Allergic contact dermatitis, purpura or blood-containing blisters, thinning of skin with easy bruising, telangiectasis or raised dark red spots on skin. **Rare:** **Inhalation:** Increased bronchospasm, esophageal candidiasis. **Intranasal:** Nasal and pharyngeal candidiasis, eye pain. **Systemic:** General allergic reaction (such as rash and hives); pain, redness, or swelling at injection site; psychologic changes; false sense of well-being; hallucinations; depression

CRITICAL CARE CONSIDERATIONS

ADMINISTRATION/HANDLING

PO ALERT

- Give dexamethasone with milk or food.

IV ALERT

- Dexamethasone sodium phosphate may be given by IV push or IV infusion.
- **IV push:** Give over 1-4 min.
- **IV infusion:** Mix with 0.9% NaCl or D_5W and infuse over 15-30 min.
- **Neonates:** If administering to a neonate, solution must be preservative-free.
- **Stability:** IV solution must be used within 24 hr.

IM ALERT

- Give deep IM, preferably in the gluteus maximus.

OPHTHALMIC ALERT

- **Solution or ointment:** Place a gloved finger on the lower eyelid and pull it out until a pocket is formed between the eye and lower lid. Hold the dropper above the pocket and place the correct number of drops (or .25 to .5 inches of ointment) into the pocket. Close the eye gently. Remove excess solution or ointment around the eye with a tissue.
- **Ophthalmic solution:** Apply digital pressure to the lacrimal sac for 1-2 min to minimize drainage to the nose and throat and reduce risk of systemic effects.
- **Ophthalmic ointment:** Close the eye for 1-2 min. Roll the eyeball to increase the contact area of dexamethasone to the eye. Use ointment at night to reduce the frequency of solution administration.
- **Taper dose:** Taper the dosage slowly when discontinuing dexamethasone.

TOPICAL ALERT

- Gently cleanse the area before applying dexamethasone. Apply sparingly and rub into area thoroughly. Use occlusive dressings only as ordered.

PRECAUTIONS

HEALTH-RELATED

- Use dexamethasone cautiously in patients with cirrhosis, heart failure, diabetes mellitus, high thromboembolic risk, hypertension, hyperthyroidism, ocular herpes simplex, osteoporosis, peptic ulcer disease, respiratory tuberculosis, seizure disorders, ulcerative colitis, or untreated systemic infections.

D

- Use the ophthalmic form cautiously in patients on long-term therapy because prolonged use may result in cataracts or glaucoma.

AGE-RELATED

- **Children:** Prolonged treatment with high dosages may decrease the short-term growth rate and cortisol secretion in children.
- **Elderly:** Are at higher risk for developing hypertension or osteoporosis. May require reduced dose due to reduced muscle mass. Elderly patients should avoid use of aluminum-based antacids to reduce risk of developing Alzheimer's disease.

PREGNANCY/LACTATION-RELATED

- Pregnancy category C; used in patients with premature labor at about 24-36 wk gestation to stimulate fetal lung maturation; excreted in breast milk; could suppress infant growth and interfere with endogenous corticosteroid production.

MONITORING

- **Baseline assessment:** Determine hypersensitivity to corticosteroids. Obtain BP, height, and weight.
- **Baseline lab work:** Obtain blood glucose levels, hemoglobin A1C, serum electrolyte levels including calcium and magnesium levels.
- **Hyperglycemia:** Determine presence of diabetes mellitus. Increase antidiabetic drug regimen if blood glucose becomes elevated.
- **Digoxin:** When giving digoxin, draw a serum digoxin level.
- **Fluid retention:** Monitor intake and output; record weight daily.
- **GI distress:** Evaluate food tolerance. Assess pattern of daily bowel activity. Instruct patients to report hyperacidity promptly.
- **Masked infection:** Monitor for fever, sore throat, and vague symptoms.
- **Fluid/electrolyte imbalance:** Monitor electrolyte levels. Monitor for hypercalcemia (cramps and muscle twitching) or hypokalemia (irritability, nausea and vomiting, muscle cramps and weakness, and numbness or tingling, especially of the lower extremities).
- **Mood swings:** Assess sleep ability and emotional status; moods vary from euphoria to depression.
- **Abrupt discontinuation:** Dexamethasone must be withdrawn gradually to avoid adrenal insufficiency.
- **Topical application:** Apply dexamethasone after a bath or shower for best absorption.
- **Patient education:** Caution patients against abruptly discontinuing dexamethasone or changing the dosage or schedule. Tell patients to report fever, muscle aches, sore throat, and sudden weight gain or swelling. Explain that severe stress, including serious infection, surgery, or trauma, may require an increase in dexamethasone dosage. Tell patients to inform dentists and other physicians they are taking dexamethasone or have taken it within the past 12 mo. Explain that steroids often cause mood swings.

SERIOUS ADVERSE REACTIONS

- **Long-term therapy:** May cause muscle wasting (especially in arms and legs), osteoporosis, spontaneous fractures, amenorrhea, cataracts, glaucoma, peptic ulcer disease, and heart failure.
- **Abrupt withdrawal after long-term therapy:** May cause severe joint pain, severe headache, anorexia, nausea, fever, rebound inflammation, fatigue, weakness, lethargy, dizziness, and orthostatic hypotension.
- **Ophthalmic form:** May cause glaucoma, ocular hypertension, and cataracts.

OVERDOSE/TOXICITY

- **Cushing's syndrome:** May be unavoidable and should resolve if medication dose can be reduced or discontinued. Syndrome reflects fluid retention, muscle wasting, possible hyperglycemia, vascular fragility which leads to bleeding and easy bruising, abnormal fat distribution, and the classic "moon face."
- **Severe hyperglycemia:** May occur if blood glucose is not monitored and managed appropriately. Thick blood viscosity secondary to associated dehydration may lead to thrombus formation and embolism.
- **GI decontamination:** No specific recommendations.

ANTIDOTE/DIALYSIS

- **Antidote:** No specific recommendations.
- **Dialysis:** Dexamethasone is not removed by hemodialysis or peritoneal dialysis. No data are available on removal by high-permeability dialysis.

dexchlorpheniramine

See Antihistamines (p. 925)

dexmedetomidine hydrochloride

decks-meh-deh-tome'-ih-deen hye-droe-klor'-ide

Classes

Chemical: selective $alpha_2$-adrenergic agonist

Therapeutic: sedative hypnotic, analgesic

Pregnancy Category: C

Trade Names

Prescription: Precedex

Do not confuse Precedex with Peridex or Percocet.

CLINICAL PHARMACOLOGY

Mechanism of Action

A selective $alpha_2$-adrenergic agonist. Therapeutic Effect: Produces analgesic, hypnotic, and sedative effects.

PHARMACOKINETICS

Rapidly distributed throughout body. Protein binding: 94%. Extensively metabolized in liver. Primarily excreted in urine; minimal elimination in feces. Half-life: 2 hr (terminal).

AVAILABILITY

Injection: 100 mcg/mL.

INDICATIONS AND DOSAGE

Sedation before, during, and after intubation and mechanical ventilation while in intensive care unit

IV

Adults: Loading dose of 1 mcg/kg over 10 min followed by maintenance infusion of 0.2-0.7 mcg/kg/hr. **Elderly:** May require decreased dosage. No guidelines available.

OFF-LABEL USES

Pain relief, treatment of shivering

CONTRAINDICATIONS

Hypersensitivity to dexmedetomidine; drug should not be used outside of critical care

INTERACTIONS

Drug: **Anesthetics, opioids, other sedative-hypnotics:** May enhance the effects of dexmedetomidine. Herbal: None known. Food: None known.

DIAGNOSTIC TEST EFFECTS

May increase serum potassium, alkaline phosphatase, AST (SGOT), and ALT (SGPT) levels.

IV INCOMPATIBILITIES

Do not mix dexmedetomidine with any other medications

SIDE-EFFECTS

Frequent: Hypotension (30%), nausea (11%). Occasional (3%-2%): Pain, fever, oliguria, thirst

CRITICAL CARE CONSIDERATIONS

ADMINISTRATION/HANDLING

IV ALERT

- **Storage:** Store vials at room temperature.
- **Dilution:** Dilute dexmedetomidine with 48 mL 0.9% NaCl before use.
- **Infusion:** Administer as a maintenance infusion for no longer than 24 hr.

PRECAUTIONS

HEALTH-RELATED

- Use dexmedetomidine cautiously in patients with heart failure, advanced heart block, hypovolemia, or hepatic or renal impairment.
- **Cytochrome P450 pathway metabolism:** Dexmedetomidine is almost completely metabolized by the liver via direct glucurondidation and cytochrome P450-mediated metabolism but has few clinically significant drug interactions.
- Make sure that patients are on a continuous cardiac monitor and pulse oximeter to assess for dysrhythmias and hypoxemia before and during drug administration.

AGE-RELATED

- **Children:** Safety and efficacy of dexmedetomidine for children under 18 yr have not been established.
- **Elderly:** Have a higher incidence of bradycardia and hypotension, possibly due to age-related organ impairment.

PREGNANCY/LACTATION-RELATED

- Pregnancy category C; unknown if excreted in breast milk.

MONITORING

- **Baseline assessment:** Obtain vital signs, including BP and heart rate.
- **Baseline lab work:** Liver function tests and serum electrolyte levels.
- **Baseline diagnostic tests:** Perform a baseline ECG to help rule out underlying cardiac disease.

- **Continuous ECG:** Monitor for heart block. Rapid bolus administration may cause bradycardia, atrial fibrillation, and sinus arrest.
- **Continuous pulse oximetry:** Assess for hypoxemia. Increase FiO_2 and adjust ventilator settings and dexmedetomidine dose. Assess respiratory rate, rhythm, and work of breathing.
- **Hypotension/transient hypertension:** Monitor BP for hypotension and pulse rate for bradycardia. Dexmedetomidine is a vasodilator and may also cause heart block. Transient hypertension may be seen during loading and is managed by slowing the rate of infusion.
- **Ventilator settings:** Monitor and adjust ventilator settings as needed if hypoxemia occurs or if patients require varying doses of dexmedetomidine for effective sedation.
- **Comfort measures:** Perform mouth care and repositioning while patients are sedated. Patients may be arousable and alert when stimulated but then will resume sedated state without an increase in drug dosage.
- **Patient education:** Explain that dexmedetomidine will provide relaxation and sedation before, during, and after insertion of the endotracheal tube and during mechanical ventilation. Inform patients that hands and arms may be restrained (if warranted) during mechanical ventilation to avoid accidental self extubation.

SERIOUS ADVERSE REACTIONS

- Bradycardia, atrial fibrillation, hypoxia, anemia, pain, and pleural effusion may occur with too-rapid IV infusion.

OVERDOSE/TOXICITY

- **Vasodilated shock with respiratory distress:** Resuscitate to increase BP, increase heart rate, and administer oxygen and mechanical ventilation to maintain oxygenation.
- **GI decontamination:** No specific recommendations.

ANTIDOTE/DIALYSIS

- **Antidote:** No specific antidote. Use of anticholinergic agents (atropine, glycopyrrolate) may be considered to modify vagal tone if hypotension ensues, along with increasing IV fluids, elevating legs, and using vasopressors (*DOPamine, norepinephrine [Levophed]).
- **Dialysis:** No data are available on removal of dexmedetomidine using hemodialysis, high-permeability dialysis, or peritoneal dialysis.

dexmethylphenidate hydrochloride

dex-meth-ill-fen'-i-date hye-droe-klor'-ide

DEA Schedule: II

Classes

Chemical: piperidine derivative of amphetamine

Therapeutic: central nervous system stimulant

Pregnancy Category: C

Trade Names

Prescription: Focalin, Focalin XR

CLINICAL PHARMACOLOGY

Mechanism of Action

A CNS stimulant that blocks the reuptake of norepinephrine and *DOPamine into presynaptic neurons, increasing the release of these neurotransmitters into the synaptic cleft. **Therapeutic Effect:** Decreases motor restlessness and fatigue; increases motor activity, mental alertness, and attention span; elevates mood.

PHARMACOKINETICS

Route	Onset	Peak	Duration
PO	30 min	1-1.5 hr	4-5 hr

Readily absorbed from the GI tract. Plasma concentrations increase rapidly. Metabolized in the liver. Excreted unchanged in urine. **Half-life:** 2.2 hr.

AVAILABILITY

Tablets (Focalin): 2.5 mg, 5 mg, 10 mg.
Capsules (extended release [Focalin XR]): 5 mg, 10 mg, 20 mg.

INDICATIONS AND DOSAGE

Attention-deficit/hyperactivity disorder (ADHD)

PO (Patients new to dexmethylphenidate or methylphenidate)

Adults, Elderly: 2.5 mg twice per day (5 mg/day). May adjust dosage in 2.5- to 5-mg increments every 7 days. Maximum: 20 mg/day.

PO (Patients currently taking methylphenidate)

Adults, Elderly: Half the methylphenidate dosage. Maximum: 20 mg/day.

PO (Extended release [Patients new to dexmethylphenidate or methylphenidate])

Adults, Elderly: Initially, 10 mg/day; adjust dose every 7 days. Maximum: 20 mg/day.

Children: Initially, 5 mg/day. May increase dosage at weekly intervals. Maximum: 20 mg/day.

PO (Extended release [Patients currently taking methylphenidate])

Adults, Elderly: Half the methylphenidate dosage. Maximum: 20 mg/day. Patients using Focalin may be switched to the same daily dose for Focalin XR.

CONTRAINDICATIONS

Hypersensitivity to dexmethylphenidate or methylphenidate, diagnosis or family history of Tourette syndrome; glaucoma; history of marked agitation, anxiety, or tension; motor tics; use within 14 days of MAOIs

INTERACTIONS

Drug: **Amitriptyline, phenobarbital, phenytoin, primidone:** Dosage of these drugs may need to be decreased. **MAOIs:** May increase the effects of dexmethylphenidate. **Other CNS stimulants:** May have an additive effect. **Warfarin:** May inhibit the metabolism of warfarin. **Herbal:** None known. **Food:** None known.

DIAGNOSTIC TEST EFFECTS

None known.

SIDE-EFFECTS

Frequent: Abdominal pain (15%), nausea (19%), anorexia (30%), headache (25%), jitteriness (12%). **Occasional:** Tachycardia, dysrhythmias, palpitations, insomnia, twitching, anxiety. **Rare:** Blurred vision, rash, arthralgia

CRITICAL CARE CONSIDERATIONS

ADMINISTRATION/HANDLING

PO ALERT

- Give dexmethylphenidate without regard to food.
- Crush tablets as needed.
- Administer the last dose of the day several hours before bedtime to prevent insomnia. Tablets should be administered at least 4 hr apart.

PRECAUTIONS

HEALTH-RELATED

- Use dexmethylphenidate cautiously in patients with cardiovascular disease, psychosis, or seizure disorders.
- Avoid dexmethylphenidate use in patients with a history of substance abuse. Chronic abusive use leads to marked tolerance and psychologic dependence may occur along with varying degrees of abnormal behavior. When withdrawing drug from abusive use, severe depression has been reported as well as unmasking of other mental health disorders.
- Use of dexmethylphenidate is not recommended when patients are taking antihypertensive or vasopressors.

AGE-RELATED

- **Children:** Safety and efficacy of dexmethylphenidate have not been established in children under 6 yr. Children are more prone to abdominal pain, insomnia, anorexia, and weight loss. Long-term dexmethylphenidate use may inhibit growth in children.
- **Elderly:** No age-related precautions have been noted.

PREGNANCY/LACTATION-RELATED

- Pregnancy category C; excretion into breast milk unknown; use caution in nursing mothers.

MONITORING

- **Baseline assessment:** Obtain baseline height and weight.
- **Baseline lab work:** CBC with WBC differential and platelet count.
- **Ongoing lab work:** Monitor CBC with WBC differential and platelet count routinely during therapy.
- **Growth delay:** Weigh patients regularly to detect delayed growth in children when used long term.
- **Therapeutic effect:** Discontinue dexmethylphenidate or reduce the dose if symptoms of ADHD return.
- **Insomnia:** Administer last daily dose several hours before bedtime to prevent insomnia.
- **Patient education:** When dexmethylphenidate is used outside the hospital, instruct patients to take the last dose of the day several hours before bedtime to prevent insomnia. Warn patients to avoid tasks that require mental alertness or motor skills until response to the drug is known.

SERIOUS ADVERSE REACTIONS

- **Withdrawal after prolonged therapy:** May unmask symptoms of the underlying disorder.

- **Seizures:** Dexmethylphenidate may lower the seizure threshold in patients with a history of seizures.
- **Growth delay:** Prolonged administration to children may delay growth.

OVERDOSE/TOXICITY
- **Excessive sympathomimetic effects:** Vomiting, tremor, hyperreflexia, seizures, confusion, hallucinations, and diaphoresis.
- **GI decontamination:** No specific recommendations.

ANTIDOTE/DIALYSIS
- **Antidote:** No specific recommendations.
- **Dialysis:** No data are available on removal of dexmethylphenidate using dialysis, high-permeability dialysis, or peritoneal dialysis.

dextran 40

See Anticoagulants (p. 900)

dextroamphetamine sulfate

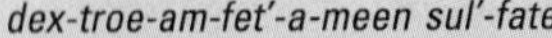

dex-troe-am-fet'-a-meen sul'-fate

DEA Schedule: II

Classes
Chemical: D-β-phenyl-isopropylamine
Therapeutic: central nervous system stimulant

Pregnancy Category: C

Trade Names
Prescription: Dexedrine, Dexedrine Spansule, Dextrostat

Do not confuse dextroamphetamine with dextromethorphan or Dexedrine with Dextran or Excedrin.

CLINICAL PHARMACOLOGY
Mechanism of Action
An amphetamine that enhances the action of dopamine and norepinephrine by blocking their reuptake from synapses; also inhibits monoamine oxidase and facilitates the release of catecholamines. **Therapeutic Effect:** Increases motor activity and mental alertness; decreases motor restlessness, drowsiness, and fatigue; suppresses appetite.

PHARMACOKINETICS
Well absorbed following PO administration. Metabolized in liver. Excreted in urine. Removed by hemodialysis. **Half-life:** 10-13 hr.

AVAILABILITY
Capsules (sustained release [Dexedrine Spansule]): 5 mg, 10 mg, 15 mg.
Tablets: 5 mg (Dexedrine), 10 mg (Dexedrine, Dextrostat).

INDICATIONS AND DOSAGE
Narcolepsy
PO
Adults, Children older than 12 yr: Initially, 10 mg/day. Increase by 10 mg/day at weekly intervals until therapeutic response is achieved. **Children 6-12 yr:** Initially, 5 mg/day. Increase by 5 mg/day at weekly intervals until therapeutic response is achieved. Maximum: 60 mg/day.
Attention-deficit/hyperactivity disorder (ADHD)
PO
Children 6 yr and older: Initially, 5 mg once or twice per day. Increase by 5 mg/day at weekly intervals until therapeutic response is achieved. **Children 3-5 yr:** Initially, 2.5 mg/day. Increase by 2.5 mg/day at weekly intervals until therapeutic response is achieved. Range: 0.1-0.5 mg/kg/dose. Maximum: 40 mg/day.
Appetite suppressant
PO
Adults: 5-30 mg daily in divided doses of 5-10 mg each, given 30-60 min before meals; or 1 extended-release capsule in the morning.

CONTRAINDICATIONS
Hypersensitivity to dextroamphetamine, advanced arteriosclerosis, agitated states, glaucoma, history of drug abuse, hypersensitivity to sympathomimetic amines, hyperthyroidism, moderate to severe hypertension, symptomatic cardiovascular disease, use within 14 days of MAOIs

INTERACTIONS
Drug: Beta-blockers: May increase the risk of bradycardia, heart block, and hypertension. **Digoxin:** May increase the risk of dysrhythmias. **MAOIs:** May prolong and intensify the effects of dextroamphetamine. **Meperidine:** May increase the risk of hypotension, respiratory depression, seizures, and vascular collapse. **Other CNS stimulants:** May increase the effects of dextroamphetamine. **Thyroid hormones:** May

increase the effects of either drug. **Tricyclic antidepressants:** May increase cardiovascular effects. **Herbal:** **Ephedra:** May increase stimulant effects of dextroamphetamine. **Food:** **Acidic foods and vitamin C:** May increase serum levels.

DIAGNOSTIC TEST EFFECTS

May increase plasma corticosteroid concentration.

SIDE-EFFECTS

Frequent: Irregular pulse, increased motor activity, talkativeness, nervousness, mild euphoria, insomnia. **Occasional:** Headache, chills, dry mouth, GI distress, worsening depression in patients who are clinically depressed, tachycardia, palpitations, chest pain, dizziness, decreased appetite

CRITICAL CARE CONSIDERATIONS

ADMINISTRATION/HANDLING

PO ALERT

- Take before meals to use as appetite suppressant.
- May administer with or without food unless used to suppress appetite.
- Administer medication early in the day to avoid insomnia.

PRECAUTIONS

HEALTH-RELATED

- Use dextroamphetamine cautiously in debilitated or tartrazine-sensitive patients.

AGE-RELATED

- **Children:** Use cautiously in children under 3 yr.
- **Elderly:** Use cautiously in elderly to avoid adverse cardiovascular effects.

PREGNANCY/LACTATION-RELATED

- Pregnancy category C; excreted in breast milk.

MONITORING

- **Baseline assessment:** Assess vital signs, including heart rate and BP.
- **CNS overstimulation:** Monitor for agitation, hypertension, cardiac dysrhythmias, and weight loss.
- **Patient education:** When using dextroamphetamine outside the hospital, instruct patients to take the drug early in the day. Inform patients that they may develop a tolerance to the drug's appetite-suppressant and mood-elevating effects within a few weeks. Warn to avoid performing tasks that require mental alertness or motor skills until response to the drug is known. Dextroamphetamine may mask signs and symptoms of extreme fatigue. Patients should report decreased appetite, dizziness, dry mouth, or pronounced nervousness. Suggest taking sips of tepid water and chewing sugarless gum to relieve dry mouth.

SERIOUS ADVERSE REACTIONS

- Abrupt withdrawal after prolonged use of high doses may produce lethargy lasting for weeks.
- Prolonged administration to children with ADHD may inhibit growth.

OVERDOSE/TOXICITY

- **Symptoms:** May produce agitation, dysrhythmias, and psychosis.
- **Severe cases of amphetamine/amphetamine derivative overdose:** May manifest cardiac ischemia, hyperthermia, severe hypertension, coma, intractable seizures, stroke, fever, and multisystem organ failure often secondary to rhabdomyolysis.
- **GI decontamination:** No specific recommendations.

ANTIDOTE/DIALYSIS

- **Antidote:** Depending on severity of overdose, various agents may be used to control agitation including lorazepam, diazepam, midazolam, phenobarbial, propofol, and haloperidol. Fever may be controlled with sedation, physical cooling measures, and paralysis.
- **Dialysis:** Dextroamphetamine is removed by hemodialysis and peritoneal dialysis. No data are available on removal using high-permeability hemodialysis.

diazepam ⚑

dye-az'-e-pam

DEA Schedule: IV

Classes

Chemical: benzodiazepine

Therapeutic: anesthesia adjunct, anticonvulsant, anxiolytic, sedative/hypnotic, skeletal muscle relaxant

Pregnancy Category: D

Trade Names

Prescription: Apo-Diazepam ♣, Diastat, Diastat Pediatric, Dizac, Valium

Do not confuse diazepam with diazoxide or Ditropan or Valium with Valcyte.

D

CLINICAL PHARMACOLOGY

Mechanism of Action

A benzodiazepine that depresses all levels of the CNS by enhancing the action of gamma-aminobutyric acid, a major inhibitory neurotransmitter in the brain. Therapeutic Effect: Produces anxiolytic effect, elevates the seizure threshold, produces skeletal muscle relaxation.

PHARMACOKINETICS

Route	Onset	Peak	Duration
PO	30 min	1-2 hr	2-3 hr
IV	1-5 min	15 min	15-30 min
IM	15 min	30-90 min	30-90 min

Well absorbed from the GI tract. Widely distributed. Protein binding: 98%. Metabolized in the liver to active metabolite. Excreted in urine. Not removed by hemodialysis. Half-life: 20-70 hr (increased in hepatic dysfunction and the elderly).

AVAILABILITY

Oral concentrate (Diazepam Intensol): 5 mg/mL.
Oral solution: 5 mg/5 mL.
Tablets (Valium): 2 mg, 5 mg, 10 mg.
Injection: 5 mg/mL.
Rectal gel (Diastat): 5 mg/mL.

INDICATIONS AND DOSAGE

Anxiety, skeletal muscle relaxation

PO

Adults: 2-10 mg 2-4 times per day. **Elderly:** 2-5 mg 2-4 times per day. **Children:** 0.12-0.8 mg/kg/day in divided doses every 6-8 hr.

IV, IM

Adults: 2-10 mg repeated in 3-4 hr. **Children:** 0.04-0.3 mg/kg/dose every 2-4 hr. Maximum: 0.6 mg/kg in an 8-hr period. **Children 1 mo to 5 yr:** 1-2 mg every 3-4 hr. **Children older than 5 yr:** 5-10 mg every 3-4 hr.

Preanesthesia

IV

Adults, Elderly: 5-15 mg 5-10 min before procedure. **Children:** 0.2-0.3 mg/kg. Maximum: 10 mg.

Alcohol withdrawal

PO

Adults, Elderly: 10 mg 3-4 times during first 24 hr then reduced to 5-10 mg 3-4 times per day as needed

IV, IM

Adults, Elderly: Initially 10 mg, followed by 5-10 mg every 3-4 hr.

Status epilepticus

IV

Adults, Elderly: 5-10 mg every 10-15 min up to 30 mg/8 hr. **Children 5 yr and older:** 1 mg IV/IM every 2-5 min. May repeat every 2-4 hr. Maximum: 10 mg/dose. **Children 1 mo to younger than 5 yr:** 0.1-0.3 mg/kg/dose every 2 min. Maximum: 5 mg/dose.

Control of increased seizure activity in patients with refractory epilepsy who are on stable regimens of anticonvulsants

Rectal Gel

Adults, Children 12 yr and older: 0.2 mg/kg; may be repeated in 4-12 hr. **Children 6-11 yr:** 0.3 mg/kg; may be repeated in 4-12 hr. **Children 2-5 yr:** 0.5 mg/kg; may be repeated in 4-12 hr.

OFF-LABEL USES

Treatment of panic disorder, tension headache, tremors

CONTRAINDICATIONS

Angle-closure (narrow angle) glaucoma, coma, preexisting CNS depression, respiratory depression, severe, uncontrolled pain, hypersensitivity to diazepam

INTERACTIONS

Drug: **Alcohol, other CNS depressants:** May increase CNS depression. Herbal: **Kava kava, valerian:** May increase CNS depression. Food: None known.

DIAGNOSTIC TEST EFFECTS

May elevate serum LDH, alkaline phosphatase, bilirubin, AST (SGOT), and ALT (SGPT) levels. May produce abnormal renal function test results. Therapeutic serum drug level is 0.5-2 mcg/mL; toxic serum drug level is greater than 3 mcg/mL.

IV INCOMPATIBILITIES

Amphotericin B complex (Abelcet, AmBisome, Amphotec), cefepime (Maxipime), diltiazem (Cardizem), fluconazole (Diflucan), foscarnet (Foscavir), heparin, hydrocortisone (Solu-Cortef), hydromorphone (Dilaudid), meropenem (Merrem IV), potassium chloride, propofol (Diprivan), vitamins

IV COMPATIBILITIES

*DOBUtamine (Dobutrex), fentanyl, morphine

SIDE-EFFECTS

Frequent: Pain with IM injection, somnolence, fatigue, ataxia, hypotension. **Occasional:** Slurred speech, orthostatic hypotension, headache, hypoactivity, constipation, nausea, blurred vision. **Rare:** Paradoxic CNS reactions, such as hyperactivity or nervousness in children and excitement or restlessness in the elderly or debilitated (generally noted during first 2 wk of therapy, particularly in presence of uncontrolled pain)

CRITICAL CARE CONSIDERATIONS

ADMINISTRATION/HANDLING

PO ALERT

- Give diazepam without regard to food. Dilute with juice, water, or a carbonated beverage or mix with a semisolid food such as applesauce or pudding to improve flavor.
- Crush tablets as needed.
- Do not crush or break capsules.

IV ALERT

- **Storage:** Store unopened vials at room temperature.
- **Administration site:** Administer into free flowing IV solution close to the IV insertion site into a large vein to reduce the risk of phlebitis and thrombosis. Avoid small veins, such as those of the wrist or dorsum of hand.
- **Adult rate:** Administer IV at a rate not exceeding 5 mg/min.
- **Child rate:** Give over a 3-min period for children, because a too-rapid IV may result in hypotension and respiratory depression.

IM ALERT

- Inject the IM dose deep into the deltoid muscle. IM injection may be painful.

RECTAL ALERT

- Do not administer the rectal gel more often than once every 5 days or 5 times per mo.

PRECAUTIONS

HEALTH-RELATED

- Use diazepam cautiously in patients with hypoalbuminemia, hepatic or renal impairment, and in those who are taking other CNS depressants.

AGE-RELATED

- **Children:** Chronic diazepam use during pregnancy may produce withdrawal symptoms, CNS depression in the neonate. Administer a reduced dose initially to prevent oversedation.
- **Elderly:** Administer a reduced dose initially and increase dosage gradually to prevent ataxia and excessive sedation.

PREGNANCY/LACTATION-RELATED

- Pregnancy category D; drug and metabolite enter breast milk; lethargy and loss of weight in nursing infant have been reported.

MONITORING

- **Baseline assessment:** Assess BP, pulse rate, and respiratory rate, rhythm, and depth immediately before giving diazepam.
- **Lab work:** Biochemical profile including renal (BUN, creatinine) and liver (AST [SGOT], ALT [SGPT], bilirubin, alkaline phosphatase) function tests.
- **Autonomic responses:** Monitor for cold, clammy hands and diaphoresis, and motor responses such as agitation, trembling, and tension.
- **Respiratory depression:** Monitor respirations every 5-15 min for 2 hr.
- **Hypotension:** Keep patients recumbent for up to 3 hr after parenteral administration to reduce the drug's hypotensive effect.
- **Treatment of musculoskeletal spasms:** Record the duration, location, onset, and type of pain, and check for immobility, stiffness, and swelling.
- **Treatment of seizures:** Assess LOC and review the history of the seizure disorder, including the duration, frequency, and intensity of seizures. Initiate seizure precautions and observe patients frequently for a recurrence of seizure activity.
- **Ongoing vital signs:** Monitor BP, heart rate, and respiratory rate.
- **Paradoxic CNS reactions:** Assess for paradoxic CNS reactions, particularly early in therapy for children and elderly.
- **Therapeutic response:** For patients with seizure disorder, assess for a decrease in the frequency or intensity of seizures; in patients with anxiety, assess for a calm facial expression and decreased restlessness; in patients with musculoskeletal spasm, assess for decreased intensity of skeletal muscle pain.

D

- **Drug levels:** Monitor therapeutic serum drug levels. Therapeutic serum level for diazepam is 0.5 to 2 mcg/mL. Toxic serum level is greater than 3 mcg/mL.
- **Abrupt discontinuation:** Abrupt discontinuation of the drug may prompt withdrawal symptoms.
- **Patient education:** Caution patients not to discontinue diazepam abruptly after prolonged use. Explain that diazepam may be habit forming. Urge patients to avoid consuming alcohol and to limit caffeine intake during diazepam therapy. Warn patients to avoid tasks that require mental alertness and motor skills until response to the drug is known. Urge female patients on long-term therapy to use effective contraception during therapy and to report pregnancy. Instruct patients not to take the rectal form of the drug more than once every 5 days or more than 5 times per mo.

SERIOUS ADVERSE REACTIONS

- **IV administration:** May produce pain, swelling, thrombophlebitis, and carpal tunnel syndrome.
- **Withdrawal symptoms:** Abrupt discontinuation or too-rapid withdrawal may result in pronounced restlessness, irritability, insomnia, hand tremor, abdominal or muscle cramps, diaphoresis, vomiting, and seizures.
- **Patients with epilepsy:** Abrupt withdrawal in epileptic patients may produce an increase in the frequency or severity of seizures.

OVERDOSE/TOXICITY

- **Symptoms:** Somnolence, ataxia, dysarthria, confusion, diminished reflexes, non-life-threatening respiratory depression and coma.
- **Severe symptoms:** Severe overdose may result in respiratory failure (signals another drug may be "on board" in patients), prolonged or profound level of obtundation.
- **GI decontamination:** No specific recommendations.

ANTIDOTE/DIALYSIS

- **Antidote:** Flumazenil (Romazicon) if only diazepam is likely present in the body. If other agents have been given or ingested, flumazenil may not be effective. Naloxone (Narcan) should be considered if severe hypoventilation or respiratory failure ensues. Treatment of overdose should be supportive. Vomiting is common, so airway must be protected to avoid aspiration.
- **Dialysis:** Diazepam is not removed by hemodialysis and is not likely to be removed by peritoneal dialysis. There are no data on removal by high-permeability dialysis.

diclofenac

dye-kloe'-fen-ak

Classes

Chemical: phenylacetic acid derivative
Therapeutic: NSAID, antipyretic, nonnarcotic analgesic

Pregnancy Category: C

Trade Names

Prescription: Cataflam, Solaraze, Voltaren, Voltaren Ophthalmic, Voltaren Ophta ♣, Voltaren XR

Combinations

Prescription: with misoprostol (Arthotec)

Do not confuse diclofenac with Diflucan or Duphalac or Voltaren with Verelan.

CLINICAL PHARMACOLOGY

Mechanism of Action

An NSAID that inhibits prostaglandin synthesis, reducing the intensity of pain. Also constricts the iris sphincter. May inhibit angiogenesis (the formation of blood vessels) by inhibiting substance P or blocking the angiogenic effects of prostaglandin E. **Therapeutic Effect:** Produces analgesic and antiinflammatory effects. Prevents miosis during cataract surgery. May reduce angiogenesis in inflamed tissue.

PHARMACOKINETICS

Route	Onset	Peak	Duration
PO	30 min	2-3 hr	Up to 8 hr

Completely absorbed from the GI tract; penetrates cornea after ophthalmic administration (may be systemically absorbed). Protein binding: greater than 99%. Widely distributed. Metabolized in the liver. Primarily excreted in urine. Minimally removed by hemodialysis. **Half-life:** 1.2-2 hr.

AVAILABILITY

Topical gel (Solaraze): 3%.

Tablets (immediate release [Cataflam]): 50 mg.
Tablets (delayed release [Voltaren]): 25 mg, 50 mg, 75 mg.
Tablets (extended release [Voltaren XR]): 100 mg.
Ophthalmic solution (Voltaren Ophthalmic): 0.1%.

INDICATIONS AND DOSAGE

Osteoarthritis

PO (Cataflam, Voltaren)

Adults, Elderly: 50 mg 2-3 times per day.

PO (Voltaren XR)

Adults, Elderly: 100-200 mg/day as a single dose.

Rheumatoid arthritis

PO (Cataflam, Voltaren)

Adults, Elderly: 50 mg 2-4 times per day. Maximum: 225 mg/day.

PO (Voltaren XR)

Adults, Elderly: 75 mg twice per day or 100 mg once or twice per day. Maximum: 225 mg/day.

Ankylosing spondylitis

PO (Voltaren)

Adults, Elderly: 100-125 mg/day in 4-5 divided doses.

Analgesia, primary dysmenorrhea

PO (Cataflam)

Adults, Elderly: 50 mg 3 times per day.

Usual pediatric dosage

Children: 2-3 mg/kg/day in 2-4 divided doses.

Actinic keratoses

Topical

Adults, Adolescents: Apply twice per day to lesion for 60-90 days.

Cataract surgery

Ophthalmic

Adults, Elderly: Apply 1 drop to eye 4 times per day commencing 24 hr after cataract surgery. Continue for 2 wk afterward.

Pain, relief of photophobia in patients undergoing corneal refractive surgery

Ophthalmic

Adults, Elderly: Apply 1-2 drops to affected eye 1 hr before surgery, within 15 min after surgery, then 4 times per day for up to 3 days.

OFF-LABEL USES

Treatment of vascular headaches (oral); to reduce the occurrence and severity of cystoid macular edema after cataract surgery (ophthalmic form)

CONTRAINDICATIONS

Hypersensitivity to aspirin, diclofenac, and other NSAIDs; porphyria

INTERACTIONS

Drug: Acetylcholine, carbachol: May decrease the effects of these drugs (with ophthalmic diclofenac). **Antihypertensives, diuretics:** May decrease the effects of these drugs. **Aspirin, other salicylates:** May increase the risk of GI side effects such as bleeding. **Bone marrow depressants:** May increase the risk of hematologic reactions. **Epinephrine, other antiglaucoma medications:** May decrease the antiglaucoma effect of these drugs. **Heparin, oral anticoagulants, thrombolytics:** May increase the effects of these drugs. **Lithium:** May increase the blood concentration and risk of toxicity of lithium. **Methotrexate:** May increase the risk of methotrexate toxicity. **Probenecid:** May increase diclofenac blood concentration. **Herbal: Ginkgo biloba:** May increase the risk of bleeding. **Food:** None known.

DIAGNOSTIC TEST EFFECTS

May increase BUN level; urine protein level; and serum LDH, potassium, alkaline phosphatase, creatinine, AST (SGOT), and ALT (SGPT) levels. May decrease serum uric acid level.

SIDE-EFFECTS

Frequent (15%-4%): PO: Headache, abdominal cramps, constipation, diarrhea, nausea, rash, dyspepsia, elevated liver enzymes (up to 15%). **Ophthalmic:** Burning or stinging on instillation, ocular discomfort.
Occasional (3%-1%): PO: Flatulence, dizziness, epigastric pain, ulcer of GI tract, edema. **Ophthalmic:** Ocular itching or tearing.
Rare (less than 1%): PO: Rash, peripheral edema or fluid retention, visual disturbances, vomiting, drowsiness

CRITICAL CARE CONSIDERATIONS

ADMINISTRATION/HANDLING

PO ALERT

- Do not crush or break enteric-coated tablets.
- Give diclofenac with food, milk, or antacids if GI distress occurs.

OPHTHALMIC ALERT

- **Administration:** Place a gloved finger on the lower eyelid, pull it out until a pocket is formed between the eye and lower lid, hold the dropper above the pocket, and place the prescribed number of drops in the pocket. Gently close the eye and apply digital pressure to the lacrimal sac for 1 to 2 min to minimize drainage into the nose and throat to reduce the risk of systemic effects. Remove excess solution with a tissue.

PRECAUTIONS

HEALTH-RELATED

- Use diclofenac cautiously in patients with heart failure, hypertension, hepatic or renal impairment, or a history of GI disease.
- Avoid applying the gel around eyes or on open skin wounds, infected areas, or areas affected by exfoliative dermatitis.

AGE-RELATED

- **Children:** Safety and efficacy of diclofenac have not been established in children. Do not use diclofenac topical gel on children, infants, or neonates.
- **Elderly:** GI bleeding or ulceration is more likely to cause serious complications, and age-related renal impairment may increase the risk of hepatotoxicity or renal toxicity; a decreased drug dosage is recommended.

PREGNANCY/LACTATION-RELATED

- Pregnancy category C.

MONITORING

- **Baseline assessment:** Assess duration, location, onset, and type of inflammation or pain. Inspect affected joints in arthritic patients for deformity, immobility, and skin condition.
- **Baseline lab work:** Obtain a biochemical profile including BUN, creatinine, serum potassium, LDH, alkaline phosphatase, creatinine, AST (SGOT), and ALT (SGPT) levels. Obtain urine sample for urinary protein levels.
- **Side effects:** Monitor for dyspepsia, headache and changes in daily bowel activity and stool consistency.
- **Therapeutic response:** Evaluate for improved grip strength, increased joint mobility, and decreased joint pain, tenderness, stiffness, and swelling.
- **Patient education:** Instruct patients to swallow diclofenac tablets whole and not to crush or chew. Advise taking diclofenac with food or milk if experiencing GI upset. Warn patients to avoid alcohol and aspirin during diclofenac therapy because these substances increase the risk of GI bleeding. Tell patients to report a persistent headache, black stools, changes in vision, pruritus, rash, or weight gain. Instruct not to use hydrogel soft contact lenses during ophthalmic diclofenac therapy. Instruct females to report pregnancy or planned pregnancy.

SERIOUS ADVERSE REACTIONS

- Rare reactions with long-term use include peptic ulcer disease, GI bleeding, gastritis, a severe hepatic reaction (jaundice), and a severe hypersensitivity reaction (bronchospasm or angioedema).

OVERDOSE/TOXICITY

- **Nephrotoxicity:** Hematuria, dysuria, proteinuria leading to acute renal failure.
- **Overdose symptoms:** Hypotonia, muscle fasciculations, twitching, bone marrow suppression, metabolic acidosis, nausea, vomiting, diarrhea, GI bleeding, abdominal pain, volume depletion with secondary hypotension, tachycardia, pulmonary edema and acute respiratory distress syndrome, acute psychosis, sezures, CNS depression following agitation.
- **GI decontamination:** No specific recommendations.

ANTIDOTE/DIALYSIS

- **Antidote:** No specific antidote. Treatment should be supportive and directed at symptoms.
- **Dialysis:** Diclofenac is not likely to be removed by hemodialysis or peritoneal dialysis. No data are available regarding removal with high-permeability dialysis.

dicloxacillin

See Antibiotics (p. 892)

dicyclomine hydrochloride

dye-sye'-kloe-meen hye-droe-klor'-ide

Classes

Chemical: tertiary amine
Therapeutic: anticholinergic, antispasmodic, gastrointestinal

Pregnancy Category: B

Trade Names

Prescription: Bentyl, Bentylol ♣, Dicyclocot, Formulex ♣, Lomine ♣

Do not confuse dicyclomine with doxycycline or dyclonine or Bentyl with Aventyl or Benadryl.

CLINICAL PHARMACOLOGY

Mechanism of Action

A GI antispasmodic and anticholinergic agent that directly acts as a relaxant on smooth muscle. **Therapeutic Effect:** Reduces tone and motility of GI tract.

PHARMACOKINETICS

Route	Onset	Peak	Duration
PO	30 min	1-1.5 hr	4 hr

Readily absorbed from the GI tract. Widely distributed. Metabolized in the liver. Eliminated by the kidneys. **Half-life:** 2 hr.

AVAILABILITY

Capsules (Bentyl): 10 mg.
Tablets (Bentyl): 20 mg.
Syrup (Bentyl): 10 mg/5 mL.
Injection (Bentyl, Dicyclocot): 10 mg/mL.

INDICATIONS AND DOSAGE

Functional disturbances of GI motility

PO

Adults: 10-20 mg 3-4 times per day up to 40 mg 4 times/day. **Children older than 2 yr:** 10 mg 3 times per day. **Children 6 mo-2 yr:** 5-10 mg 3-4 times per day. Maximum: 40 mg/day. **Elderly:** 10-20 mg 4 times per day. May increase up to 160 mg/day.

IM

Adults: 20 mg every 4-6 hr.

CONTRAINDICATIONS

Hypersensitivity to dicyclomine, bladder neck obstruction due to prostatic hyperplasia, coronary vasospasm, intestinal atony, myasthenia gravis in patients not treated with neostigmine, narrow-angle glaucoma, obstructive disease of the GI tract, paralytic ileus, severe ulcerative colitis, tachycardia secondary to cardiac insufficiency or thyrotoxicosis, toxic megacolon, unstable cardiovascular status in acute hemorrhage

INTERACTIONS

Drug: **Antacids, antidiarrheals:** May decrease the absorption of dicyclomine. **Ketoconazole:** May decrease the absorption of ketoconazole. **Other anticholinergics:** May increase the effects of dicyclomine. **Potassium chloride:** May increase the severity of GI lesions with the wax matrix formulation of potassium chloride. **Herbal:** **Betel nut:** May decrease effectiveness of dicyclomine. **Food:** None known.

DIAGNOSTIC TEST EFFECTS

None known.

SIDE-EFFECTS

Frequent: Dry mouth (sometimes severe), constipation, diminished sweating ability, urinary retention. **Occasional:** Blurred vision; photophobia; urinary hesitancy; somnolence (with high dosage); agitation, excitement, confusion, or severe somnolence noted in elderly (even with low dosages); transient lightheadedness (with IM route), irritation at injection site (with IM route). **Rare:** Confusion, hypersensitivity reaction, increased intraocular pressure, nausea, vomiting, unusual fatigue

CRITICAL CARE CONSIDERATIONS

ADMINISTRATION/HANDLING

PO ALERT

- Store capsules, tablets, syrup, and parenteral form at room temperature.
- Dilute syrup with an equal volume of water just before administration.
- Give dicyclomine without regard to meals. Food may slightly decrease absorption.

IM ALERT

- **IM only:** Do not administer IV or subcutaneously.
- **IM injection:** Inject deep in large muscle mass.
- **Treatment:** Do not give for longer than 2 days.

PRECAUTIONS

HEALTH-RELATED

- Use dicyclomine extremely cautiously in patients with autonomic neuropathy, diarrhea, known or suspected GI infections, or mild to moderate ulcerative colitis.
- Use cautiously in patients with heart failure, chronic obstructive pulmonary disease, coronary artery disease, esophageal reflux or hiatal hernia associated with reflux esophagitis, gastric ulcer, hyperthyroidism, hypertension, hepatic or renal disease, or tachydysrhythmias.

AGE-RELATED

- **Children:** Dicyclomine is contraindicated in infants under 6 mo. Infants and young children are more susceptible to toxic effects.
- **Elderly:** Dicyclomine may cause agitation, confusion, somnolence, or excitement.

PREGNANCY/LACTATION-RELATED

- Pregnancy category B; single case report of apnea in nursing infant; contraindicated in nursing women

MONITORING

- **Baseline assessment:** Assess bowel symptoms necessitating use of the drug and determine history of tachycardia; dicyclomine may increase heart rate.
- **Lab work:** Biochemical profile with renal (BUN, creatinine) and liver (AST [SGOT], ALT [SGPT], bilirubin, alkaline phosphatase) function tests.
- **Before administration:** Instruct patients to void before giving dicyclomine to reduce the risk of urine retention.
- **Urinary retention:** Evaluate for urine retention. May require insertion of a urinary catheter to manage in some patients.
- **Therapeutic effect:** Decreased muscle spasms in the small intestine, resulting in less abdominal discomfort and more normal bowel habits. Assess pattern of daily bowel activity and stool consistency.
- **Decreased perspiration:** Monitor changes in heart rate, BP, and body temperature. Patients will be less able to lower body temperature with reduced sweating.
- **Paralytic ileus:** Assess bowel sounds for peristalsis.
- **Dehydration:** Assess mucous membranes and skin turgor. Encourage adequate fluid intake.
- **Patient education:** Tell patients not to become overheated while exercising in hot weather (may cause heat stroke) and to avoid hot baths and saunas. Avoid tasks that require mental alertness or motor skills until response to the drug is known. Instruct not to take antacids or antidiarrheals within 1 hr of taking dicyclomine because these drugs decrease dicyclomine's effectiveness.

SERIOUS ADVERSE REACTIONS

- Heat stroke, paralytic ileus, dehydration, high fever, urinary tract infection from urinary retention.

OVERDOSE/TOXICITY

- **Anticholinergic syndrome:** Pupillary dilation; tachycardia; palpitations; hot, dry, or flushed skin; absence of bowel sounds; hyperthermia; increased respiratory rate; ECG abnormalities; nausea; vomiting; rash over face or upper trunk; CNS stimulation; and psychosis (marked by agitation, restlessness, rambling speech, visual hallucinations, paranoid behavior, and delusions) followed by depression.
- **Rhabdomyolysis:** May be seen in severe cases of anticholinergic syndrome.
- **GI decontamination:** No specific recommendations.

ANTIDOTE/DIALYSIS

- **Antidote:** No specific antidote, but significantly agitated patients may be treated with an anticholinesterase (physostigmine) or sedative. Restraints should be used as a last resort because patient fighting increases the chance of rhabdomyolysis. Supportive care should be directed at symptoms.
- **Dialysis:** No data are available on removal of dicyclomine with hemodialysis, high-permeability hemodialysis, or peritoneal dialysis.

didanosine

dye-dan'-o-seen

Classes

Chemical: nucleoside analog
Therapeutic: antiretroviral

Pregnancy Category: B

Trade Names

Prescription: Videx, Videx-EC

CLINICAL PHARMACOLOGY

Mechanism of Action

A purine nucleoside analogue that is intracellularly converted into a triphosphate, which interferes with RNA-directed DNA polymerase (reverse transcriptase). **Therapeutic Effect:** Inhibits replication of retroviruses, including HIV.

PHARMACOKINETICS

Variably absorbed from the GI tract. Protein binding: less than 5%. Rapidly metabolized intracellularly to active form. Primarily excreted in urine. Partially (20%) removed by hemodialysis. **Half-life:** 1.5 hr; metabolite: 8-24 hr.

AVAILABILITY

Capsules (delayed release): 125 mg (Videx), 200 mg (Videx-EC), 250 mg (Videx-EC), 400 mg (Videx-EC).
Pediatric powder for oral solution (Videx): 10 mg/mL.
Powder for oral solution (Videx): 100 mg, 167 mg, 250 mg.
Tablets (chewable [Videx]): 25 mg, 50 mg, 100 mg, 150 mg, 200 mg.

INDICATIONS AND DOSAGE

HIV infection (in combination with other antiretrovirals)

PO (Delayed-Release Capsules)

Adults, Children 13 yr and older, weighing 60 kg and more: 400 mg once per day. **Adults, Children 13 yr and older, weighing less than 60 kg:** 250 mg once per day.

PO (Oral Solution)

Adults, Children 13 yr and older weighing 60 kg and more: 250 mg every 12 hr. **Adults, Children 13 yr and older weighing less than 60 kg:** 167 mg every 12 hr.

PO (Pediatric Powder for Oral Solution)

Children younger than 2 wk: 50 mg/m^2 every 12 hr. **Children 2 wk-8 mo:** 100 mg/m^2/day in divided doses every 12 hr. **Children 8 mo and older:** 120 mg/m^2 every 12 hr.

Dosage in renal impairment

Patients weighing less than 60 kg:

Creatinine Clearance	Oral Solution	Delayed-Release Capsules
30-59 mL/min	100 mg twice per day	125 mg once per day
10-29 mL/min	100 mg once per day	125 mg once per day
Less than 10 mL/min	100 mg once per day	N/A

Patients weighing 60 kg or more:

Creatinine Clearance	Oral Solution	Delayed-Release Capsules
30-59 mL/min	100 mg twice per day	200 mg once per day
10-29 mL/min	167 mg once per day	125 mg once per day
Less than 10 mL/min	100 mg once per day	125 mg once per day

CONTRAINDICATIONS

Hypersensitivity to didanosine or any of its components

INTERACTIONS

Drug: Dapsone, fluoroquinolones, itraconazole, ketoconazole, tetracyclines: May decrease absorption of these drugs. **Medications producing pancreatitis or peripheral neuropathy:** May increase the risk of pancreatitis or peripheral neuropathy. **Stavudine:** May increase the risk of fatal lactic acidosis in pregnancy. **Herbal:** None known. **Food: All foods:** Decreases absorption of didanosine.

DIAGNOSTIC TEST EFFECTS

May increase serum alkaline phosphatase, amylase, bilirubin, lipase, triglyceride, AST (SGOT), ALT (SGPT), and uric acid levels. May decrease serum potassium levels.

SIDE-EFFECTS

Frequent: Adults (greater than 10%): Diarrhea, neuropathy, chills, fever, nausea, vomiting, abdominal pain

Children (greater than 25%): Chills, fever, decreased appetite, pain, malaise, nausea, vomiting, diarrhea, abdominal pain, headache, nervousness, cough, rhinitis, dyspnea, asthenia, rash, pruritus. **Occasional: Adults (9%-2%):** Rash, pruritus, headache, abdominal pain, nausea, vomiting, pneumonia, myopathy, decreased appetite, dry mouth, dyspnea. **Children (25%-10%):** Failure to thrive, weight loss, stomatitis, oral thrush, ecchymosis, arthritis, myalgia, insomnia, epistaxis, pharyngitis

CRITICAL CARE CONSIDERATIONS

ADMINISTRATION/HANDLING

PO ALERT

- Swallow enteric-coated capsules whole on an empty stomach.
- Thoroughly crush and disperse chewable tablets in at least 30 mL of water. Stir the mixture well (2 to 3 min) and swallow immediately.
- **Storage:** Store at room temperature.
- **Stability:** Tablets dispersed in water are stable for 1 hr at room temperature; after reconstitution of buffered powder, oral solution is stable for 4 hr at room temperature.
- **Pediatric stability:** Pediatric powder for oral solution is stable for 30 days if refrigerated after reconstitution as directed.
- **Oral solution reconstitution:** Reconstitute buffered powder for oral solution by pouring contents of the packet into 4 oz of water; stir the mixture until completely dissolved (2-3 min). Do not mix powder with fruit juice or any other acidic liquid since didanosine is unstable in acidic pH.
- **Pediatric oral solution:** Add 100-200 mL of water to 2 g or 4 g of the unbuffered pediatric powder, respectively, to provide a concentration of 20 mg/mL. Immediately mix with an equal amount of an antacid to provide a concentration of 10 mg/mL. Shake thoroughly before administering each dose.

PRECAUTIONS

HEALTH-RELATED

- Use didanosine cautiously in patients with alcoholism, elevated serum triglyceride levels, renal or hepatic dysfunction, or T-cell counts less than 100 cells/mm^3.
- Use cautiously in patients with phenylketonuria and those on sodium-restricted diets since didanosine contains phenylalanine and sodium.
- **Pancreatitis:** Use with extreme caution in patients with a history of pancreatitis.

AGE-RELATED

- **Children:** Didanosine is well tolerated in children over 2 wk.
- **Elderly:** Age-related renal impairment may require a dosage adjustment.

PREGNANCY/LACTATION-RELATED

- Pregnancy category B; unknown if excreted in breast milk; discontinuation of breast-feeding recommended.

MONITORING

- **Baseline assessment:** Monitor vital signs and weight.
- **Baseline lab work:** Obtain baseline CBC and serum renal and liver function tests.
- **Ongoing lab work:** Monitor blood chemistry values and CBC.
- **Pancreatitis:** Monitor for abdominal pain, elevated serum amylase or triglyceride levels, nausea, and vomiting, which may indicate pancreatitis.
- **Peripheral neuropathy:** Assess for burning feet, restless leg syndrome (inability to find a comfortable position for legs and feet), and lack of coordination.
- **Diarrhea:** Monitor pattern of daily bowel activity and stool consistency.
- **Rash:** Check the skin for eruptions and rash.
- **Opportunistic infections:** Assess for cough or other respiratory symptoms, fever, and oral mucosa changes.
- **Nausea, vomiting, food intolerance:** Check weight at least twice per wk.
- **Sensory deficits:** Assess for visual or auditory difficulty and provide protection from light if photophobia occurs.
- **Patient education:** Teach patients to shake the oral suspension well before using, to keep it refrigerated, to discard the solution after 30 days and obtain a new supply. Advise against consuming alcohol and to report nausea or vomiting, numbness, or persistent, severe abdominal pain. Explain that didanosine is not a cure for HIV infection nor does it reduce the risk of transmitting HIV to others.

SERIOUS ADVERSE REACTIONS

- Pneumonia, hepatomegaly, hyperuricemia, and opportunistic infections occur occasionally.

OVERDOSE/TOXICITY

- Peripheral neuropathy, potentially fatal pancreatitis, potentially fatal lactic acidosis, retinal changes, and optic neuritis are the major toxic effects.
- **GI decontamination:** No specific recommendations.

ANTIDOTE/DIALYSIS

- **Antidote:** No specific recommendations.
- **Dialysis:** Didanosine is not removed by hemodialysis, high-permeability hemodialysis, or peritoneal dialysis. Drug dose should be reduced in renal impaired patients.

difenoxine with atropine

See Antidiarrheals (p. 917)

diflunisal

dye-floo'-ni-sal

Classes

Chemical: salicylate derivative
Therapeutic: NSAID, antipyretic, nonnarcotic analgesic

Pregnancy Category: C

Trade Names

Prescription: Dolobid

Do not confuse diflunisal with Dicarbosil or Dolobid with Slo-bid.

CLINICAL PHARMACOLOGY

Mechanism of Action

A nonsteroidal antiinflammatory that inhibits prostaglandin synthesis, reducing inflammatory response and intensity of pain stimulus reaching sensory nerve endings. **Therapeutic Effect:** Produces analgesic and antiinflammatory effect.

PHARMACOKINETICS

Route	Onset	Peak	Duration
PO	1 hr	2-3 hr	8-12 hr

Completely absorbed from the GI tract. Widely distributed. Protein binding: greater than 99%. Metabolized in liver. Primarily excreted in urine. Not removed by hemodialysis. **Half-life:** 8-12 hr.

AVAILABILITY

Tablets: 250 mg, 500 mg.

INDICATIONS AND DOSAGE

Mild to moderate pain

PO

Adults, Elderly: Initially 1 g, then 250-500 mg every 8-12 hr. Maximum: 1.5 g/day.

Osteoarthritis

PO

Adults, Elderly: 500-1000 mg/day in 2 divided doses. Maximum: 1500 mg/day.

Rheumatoid arthritis

PO

Adults, Elderly: 0.5-1 g/day in 2 divided doses. Maximum: 1.5 g/day.

OFF-LABEL USES

Treatment of psoriatic arthritis, vascular headache

CONTRAINDICATIONS

Active GI bleeding, factor VII or factor IX deficiencies, hypersensitivity to diflunisal, aspirin, or NSAIDs

INTERACTIONS

Drug: **Antihypertensives, diuretics:** May decrease the effects of these drugs. **Aspirin, salicylates:** May increase the risk of GI bleeding and side effects. **Bone marrow depressants:** May increase the risk of hematologic reactions. **Heparin, oral anticoagulants, thrombolytics:** May increase the effects of these drugs. **Lithium:** May increase the blood concentration and risk of toxicity of lithium. **Methotrexate:** May increase the risk of toxicity of methotrexate. **Probenecid:** May increase diflunisal blood concentration. **Herbal:** **Ginkgo biloba:** May increase the risk of bleeding. **Food:** None known.

DIAGNOSTIC TEST EFFECTS

May increase serum AST (SGOT) and ALT (SGPT) levels. May decrease serum uric acid levels.

SIDE-EFFECTS

Side effects are less common with short-term treatment. **Occasional (9%-3%):** Nausea, dyspepsia (heartburn, indigestion, constipation, epigastric pain), diarrhea, headache, rash. **Rare (3%-1%):** Vomiting, flatulence, dizziness, somnolence, insomnia, fatigue, tinnitus

CRITICAL CARE CONSIDERATIONS

ADMINISTRATION/HANDLING

PO ALERT

- May give diflunisal with meals, milk, or water.
- Do not crush or break enteric-coated tablets.

PRECAUTIONS

HEALTH-RELATED

- Use diflunisal cautiously in patients with edema, elevated liver function tests, erosive gastritis, impaired renal or liver function, peptic ulcer disease, platelet and bleeding disorders, and vitamin K deficiency.

AGE-RELATED

- **Children:** Safety and efficacy of diflunisal have not been established in children.
- **Elderly:** GI bleeding or ulceration is more likely to cause serious adverse effects. Age-related renal impairment may increase risk of liver or renal toxicity; a decreased drug dosage is recommended.

PREGNANCY/LACTATION-RELATED

- Pregnancy category C; excreted into breast milk; use caution in nursing mothers.

MONITORING

- **Baseline assessment:** Assess duration, location, onset, and type of inflammation or pain. Inspect the affected joints in arthritic patients for deformities, immobility, and skin condition. Determine history of adverse reactions to aspirin or other NSAIDs.
- **Baseline lab work:** Obtain baseline CBC, prothrombin time, aPTT, and renal and liver function studies.
- **GI side effects:** Monitor for dyspepsia and nausea, diarrhea, constipation, and flatulence.
- **Rash:** Assess the skin for rash.
- **Therapeutic response:** Improved grip strength, increased joint mobility, reduced joint tenderness, and relief of pain, stiffness, and swelling.
- **Patient education:** Instruct patients to swallow tablets whole; do not chew or crush. If GI upset occurs, take diflunisal with food or milk. Warn patients to report GI distress, headache, or rash. Have female patients report if pregnancy is suspected or planned.

SERIOUS ADVERSE REACTIONS

- **GI system:** Peptic ulcer, GI bleeding, gastritis, and severe hepatic reaction,

D

including cholestasis, and jaundice occur rarely.
- **Severe hypersensitivity:** Bronchospasm and angioedema occur rarely.

OVERDOSE/TOXICITY

- **Nephrotoxicity:** Dysuria, hematuria, proteinuria, and nephrotic syndrome.
- **Overdose symptoms:** Hypotonia, muscle fasciculations, twitching, bone marrow suppression, metabolic acidosis, nausea, vomiting, diarrhea, GI bleeding, abdominal pain, volume depletion with secondary hypotension, tachycardia, pulmonary edema and acute respiratory distress syndrome, acute psychosis, seizures, CNS depression following agitation.
- **GI decontamination:** No specific recommendations.

ANTIDOTE/DIALYSIS

- **Antidote:** No specific recommendations. Treatment should be supportive and directed at symptoms.
- **Dialysis:** Diflunisal is not removed by hemodialysis and is not likely removed by peritoneal dialysis. There are no data on removal by high-permeability dialysis.

digoxin

di-jox'-in

Classes

Chemical: digitalis glycoside
Therapeutic: antidysrhythmic, cardiac glycoside

Pregnancy Category: C

Trade Names

Prescription: Digitek, Lanoxicaps, Lanoxin

Do not confuse digoxin with Desoxyn or doxepin, or Lanoxin with Levsinex or Lonox.

CLINICAL PHARMACOLOGY

Mechanism of Action

A cardiac glycoside that increases the influx of calcium from extracellular to intracellular cytoplasm. Therapeutic Effect: Potentiates the activity of the contractile cardiac muscle fibers and increases the force of myocardial contraction. Slows the heart rate by decreasing conduction through the SA and AV nodes.

PHARMACOKINETICS

Route	Onset	Peak	Duration
PO	0.5-2 hr	2-6 hr	3-4 days
IV	5-30 min	1-4 hr	3-4 days

Readily absorbed from the GI tract. Widely distributed. Protein binding: 30%. Partially metabolized in the liver. Primarily excreted in urine. Removed by hemodialysis. Half-life: 36-48 hr (increased with impaired renal function and in the elderly).

AVAILABILITY

Capsules (Lanoxicaps): 50 mcg, 100 mcg, 200 mcg.
Elixir (Lanoxin): 50 mcg/mL.
Tablets (Digitek, Lanoxin): 125 mcg, 250 mcg, 500 mcg.
Injection (Lanoxin): 100 mcg/mL, 250 mcg/mL.

INDICATIONS AND DOSAGE

Rapid loading dose for the management and treatment of heart failure; control of ventricular rate in patients with atrial fibrillation; treatment and prevention of recurrent paroxysmal atrial tachycardia

PO

Adults, Elderly: Initially, 0.5-0.75 mg, additional doses of 0.125-0.375 mg at 6- to 8-hr intervals. Range: 0.75-1.25 mg. **Children 10 yr and older:** 10-15 mcg/kg. **Children 5-9 yr:** 20-35 mcg/kg. **Children 2-4 yr:** 30-40 mcg/kg. **Children 1-23 mo:** 35-60 mcg/kg. **Neonate, full-term:** 25-35 mcg/kg. **Neonate, premature:** 20-30 mcg/kg.

IV

Adults, Elderly: 0.6-1 mg. **Children 10 yr and older:** 8-12 mcg/kg. **Children 5-9 yr:** 15-30 mcg/kg. **Children 2-4 yr:** 25-35 mcg/kg. **Children 1-23 mo:** 30-50 mcg/kg **Neonates, full-term:** 20-30 mcg/kg. **Neonates, premature:** 15-25 mcg/kg.

Maintenance dosage for heart failure; control of ventricular rate in patients with atrial fibrillation; treatment and prevention of recurrent paroxysmal atrial tachycardia

PO, IV

Adults, Elderly: 0.125-0.375 mg/day. **Children:** 25%-35% loading dose (20%-30% for premature neonates).

Dosage in renal impairment

Dosage adjustment is based on creatinine clearance. Total digitalizing dose: decrease by 50% in end-stage renal disease.

Creatinine Clearance	Dosage
10-50 mL/min	25%-75% usual
Less than 10 mL/min	10%-25% usual

CONTRAINDICATIONS

Ventricular fibrillation, ventricular tachycardia unrelated to heart failure, hypersensitivity to digoxin

INTERACTIONS

Alert: Digoxin and regular human insulin are physically compatible for 3 hr in 0.9% NaCl. In D_5W, a slight haze develops in 1 hr. Do not allow digoxin and insulin to come in contact with each other in an IV for more than 15 min. Drug: **Amiodarone:** May increase digoxin blood concentration and risk of toxicity; may have an additive effect on the SA and AV nodes. **Amphotericin, glucocorticoids, potassium-depleting diuretics:** May increase risk of toxicity caused by hypokalemia. **Antidysrhythmics, parenteral calcium, sympathomimetics:** May increase risk of dysrhythmias. **Antidiarrheals, cholestyramine, colestipol, sucralfate:** May decrease absorption of digoxin. **Diltiazem, fluoxetine, quinidine, verapamil:** May increase digoxin blood concentration. **Parenteral magnesium:** May cause cardiac conduction changes and heart block. Herbal: **Siberian ginseng:** May increase serum digoxin levels. **St. John's wort:** May reduce digoxin efficacy. Food: **All food:** May decrease peak digoxin concentrations.

DIAGNOSTIC TEST EFFECTS

None known.

IV INCOMPATIBILITIES

Amphotericin B complex (Abelcet, Amphotec, AmBisome), fluconazole (Diflucan), foscarnet (Foscavir), propofol (Diprivan)

IV COMPATIBILITIES

Cimetidine (Tagamet), diltiazem (Cardizem), furosemide (Lasix), heparin, insulin ([regular] in 0.9% NaCl, physically compatible for 3 hr; in D_5W, a slight haze develops within 1 hr), lidocaine, midazolam (Versed), milrinone (Primacor), morphine, potassium chloride, propofol (Diprivan)

SIDE-EFFECTS

Occasional: diarrhea, anorexia, nausea, vomiting, headache, visual disturbances. There is a very narrow margin of safety between a therapeutic and toxic result. Long-term therapy may produce mammary gland enlargement in women but is reversible when drug is withdrawn.

CRITICAL CARE CONSIDERATIONS

ADMINISTRATION/HANDLING

PO ALERT

- May give digoxin without regard to meals.
- Crush tablets if necessary.

IV ALERT

- **Dilution:** Give undiluted or dilute with at least a fourfold volume of sterile water for injection or normal saline; using less than this amount may cause a precipitate to form. Use immediately following dilution or preparation.
- **IV injection:** Give IV slowly over at least 5 min.
- **Loading dose:** Administer digoxin loading dose in several doses at 4- to 8-hr intervals, as prescribed.
- **Atrial fibrillation or flutter:** Larger digoxin doses are often required for adequate control of ventricular rate in patients with atrial fibrillation or flutter.

IM ALERT

- Avoid giving digoxin IM because it may cause severe local irritation and is erratically absorbed. If no other route is possible, give deep into the muscle followed by massage. Give no more than 2 mL at any one site.

PRECAUTIONS

HEALTH-RELATED

- Use digoxin cautiously in patients with acute MI, advanced cardiac disease, cor pulmonale, hypokalemia, hypothyroidism, impaired hepatic or renal function, incomplete AV block, or pulmonary disease.

AGE-RELATED

- **Children:** Neonates vary in tolerance to digoxin. Premature and immature infants are more sensitive to drug effects. Dose should be reduced and individualized to level of maturity.
- **Elderly:** Age-related hepatic or renal function impairment may require dosage adjustment. There is an increased risk of loss of appetite in this age group.

PREGNANCY/LACTATION-RELATED

- Pregnancy category C; passes readily to fetus; excreted into breast milk; considered compatible with breast-feeding.

MONITORING

- **Baseline assessment:** Assess apical pulse for 60 sec or 30 sec if the patient is receiving maintenance therapy. If heart rate is 60 beats/min or lower in adults or 70 beats/min or less in children, withhold digoxin. Note heart rhythm on continuous ECG monitor. The prescriber should be aware of all instances of symptomatic bradycardia.
- **Baseline and ongoing lab work:** Obtain biochemical panel including potassium, calcium, and magnesium levels. Obtain blood samples for digoxin level 6-8 hr after digoxin administration or just before administration of next digoxin dose.
- **Cardiac:** Monitor ECG for dysrhythmias and pulse for bradycardia for 1-2 hr after digoxin administration. Excessive slowing of the pulse may be the first sign of toxicity. Development and progression of heart block may follow, along with ventricular dysrhythmias.
- **Toxicity:** Assess for GI disturbances and neurologic abnormalities every 2-4 hr during loading dose and daily during maintenance therapy.
- **Hypokalemia, hypomagnesemia, hypercalcemia:** Monitor serum potassium, magnesium, and calcium levels. Hypokalemia, hypomagnesemia, and hypercalcemia can potentiate digoxin's effects and promote toxicity.
- **Drug levels:** Monitor serum drug levels. Therapeutic serum level is 0.8-2 ng/mL. Toxic serum level is greater than 2 ng/mL. Some patients remain free of symptoms of toxicity despite digoxin levels of greater than 2 ng/mL. Asymptomatic patients with high drug levels may not be toxic but rather have a higher tolerance for the drug.
- **Patient education:** Stress the importance of follow-up visits and blood tests. Teach how to take the apical pulse correctly and to report a pulse rate of 60 beats/min or less, as directed by the health care provider. Advise patients carrying or wearing identification that they are taking digoxin. Inform dentists and other physicians about digoxin therapy. Caution patients not to increase or skip digoxin doses. Explain not to take OTC medications without physician approval. Teach patients how to recognize digoxin toxicity and to report decreased appetite, diarrhea, nausea, visual changes, or vomiting.

SERIOUS ADVERSE REACTIONS

- Facial pain, personality change, and ocular disturbances (photophobia, light flashes, halos around bright objects, yellow or green color perception) may be noted.

OVERDOSE/TOXICITY

- **Early manifestations of adult digoxin toxicity:** GI disturbances (anorexia, nausea, vomiting) and neurologic abnormalities (fatigue, headache, depression, weakness, drowsiness, confusion, nightmares).
- **Overdose in children:** Infants and children experience signs of overdose differently than adults. The first sign of overdose in children is usually a dysrhythmia, such as bradycardia, followed by nausea, vomiting, diarrhea, anorexia, and CNS disturbances.
- **Life-threatening overdose:** Severe ventricular dysrhythmias (ventricular tachycardia or ventricular fibrillation), progressive bradycardia, progressive heart block, and third-degree heart block not responsive to atropine.
- **GI decontamination:** No specific recommendations.

ANTIDOTE/DIALYSIS

- **Antidote:** Digoxin immune FAB is the antidote for digitalis (digoxin) intoxication; indicated for ingestion of 10 mg or more of digoxin in previously healthy adults or ingestion of 4 mg or more in previously healthy children. Other medications may be required to support the patient including atropine, phenytoin, procainamide, disodium edetate, replacement of potassium, magnesium, or control of hypercalcemia.
- **Dialysis:** Digoxin is not removed by hemodialysis or peritoneal dialysis. There are no data regarding removal of digoxin by high-permeability dialysis.

digoxin immune FAB

di-jox'-in

Classes

Chemical: antibody fragment
Therapeutic: antidote, digitalis

Pregnancy Category: C

Trade Names

Prescription: Digibind, DigiFab

Do not confuse digoxin immune FAB with Desoxyn or doxepin.

CLINICAL PHARMACOLOGY

Mechanism of Action

An antidote that binds molecularly to digoxin in the extracellular space. Therapeutic Effect: Makes digoxin unavailable for binding at its site of action on cells in the body.

PHARMACOKINETICS

Route	Onset	Peak	Duration
IV	30 min	3-4 hr	3-4 days

Widely distributed into extracellular space. Excreted in urine. Half-life: 15-20 hr.

AVAILABILITY

Powder for injection: 38-mg vial (Digibind), 40-mg vial (DigiFab).

INDICATIONS AND DOSAGE

Potentially life-threatening digoxin overdose

IV

Adults, Elderly, Children: Dosage varies according to amount of digoxin to be neutralized. Refer to manufacturer's dosing guidelines.

CONTRAINDICATIONS

Hypersensitivity to digoxin immune FAB

INTERACTIONS

Drug: None known. Herbal: None known. Food: None known.

DIAGNOSTIC TEST EFFECTS

May decrease serum potassium level. Serum digoxin concentration may increase precipitously and persist for up to 1 wk until FAB/digoxin complex is eliminated from the body.

IV INCOMPATIBILITIES

None known.

SIDE-EFFECTS

Rare: Allergic reaction, hypokalemia

CRITICAL CARE CONSIDERATIONS

ADMINISTRATION/HANDLING

IV ALERT

- **Storage:** Refrigerate vials.
- **First dilution:** Reconstitute each 38-mg vial with 4 mL sterile water for injection to provide a concentration of 9.5 mg/mL. Reconstitute each 40-mg vial with 4 mL of sterile water for injection to provide a concentration of 10 mg/mL.
- **Further dilution:** Further dilute with 50 mL 0.9% NaCl.
- **Stability:** After reconstitution, use the solution immediately. If it is not used immediately, store the solution in the refrigerator for up to 4 hr.
- **Infusion:** Infuse over 30 min. It is recommended that the solution be infused through a 0.22-micron filter.
- **Imminent cardiac arrest:** If cardiac arrest is imminent, may give drug by IV push.

PRECAUTIONS

HEALTH-RELATED

- Use digoxin immune FAB cautiously in patients with impaired cardiac or renal function.
- **Sensitivity to ovine proteins:** Allergy testing is not practical when patients are experiencing life-threatening toxicity, but patients allergic to ovine proteins or those who have previously received antibodies or FAB fragments produced from sheep are at risk for hypersensitivity.

AGE-RELATED

- **Children:** No age-related precautions have been noted in children.
- **Elderly:** Age-related renal impairment may require cautious use.

PREGNANCY/LACTATION-RELATED

- Pregnancy category C; excretion into breast milk unknown; use caution in nursing mothers.

MONITORING

- **Baseline assessment:** Assess for cardiac history or other significant impairment including sensitivity to ovine proteins. Drug is intended for use in previously healthy people. Note baseline symptoms indicative of toxicity so they can be monitored for improvement. Assess mental status and muscle strength.
- **Baseline lab work:** Obtain serum digoxin level before administering the drug. If the serum digoxin level was drawn less than 6 hr before the last digoxin dose, the serum digoxin level may be unreliable. Patients with impaired renal function may require more than 1 wk before serum digoxin assay is reliable.
- **Vital signs:** Closely monitor BP, heart rate and rhythm, ECG, serum potassium level, and temperature during and after drug administration.
- **Therapeutic effect:** Observe for changes from the initial assessment. Hypokalemia

may result in cardiac dysrhythmias, changes in mental status, muscle cramps, muscle strength changes, or tremor. Hyperkalemia may result in cold and clammy skin, confusion, and diarrhea. Patients may require electrolyte and dysrhythmia management in addition to receiving digoxin immune FAB.
- **Continuous ECG:** Assess for dysrhythmias (heart block, ventricular dysrhythmias, bradycardia). May attempt managing with other appropriate antidysrhythmic agents.
- **Heart failure:** Monitor for dyspnea, lung crackles, and peripheral edema. Occasionally, aggressive management causes digoxin level to fall below the therapeutic level.
- **Patient education:** Before discharge, review digoxin dosages carefully with patients, making sure they understand how to take the drug as prescribed. Instruct about follow-up care, including monitoring serum digoxin level. Make sure patients know the signs and symptoms of digoxin toxicity, including anorexia, nausea, and vomiting, as well as visual changes.

SERIOUS ADVERSE REACTIONS
- **Hyperkalemia:** May occur as a result of digitalis toxicity. Symptoms of hyperkalemia include diarrhea, paresthesia of extremities, heaviness of legs, decreased BP, cold skin, grayish pallor, hypotension, mental confusion, irritability, flaccid paralysis, tented T waves, widening QRS interval, and ST depression.
- **Hypokalemia:** May develop rapidly when the effect of digitalis is reversed. Symptoms of hypokalemia include muscle cramping, nausea, vomiting, hypoactive bowel sounds, abdominal distention, difficulty breathing, and orthostatic hypotension.

OVERDOSE/TOXICITY
- **Heart failure:** Low cardiac output and heart failure occur rarely.
- **Hypersensitivity:** Patients may be sensitive to ovine proteins: urticaria, respiratory distress, and vascular collapse. Patients should be resuscitated per standards of managing anaphylaxis including epinephrine, corticosteroids, *diphenhydrAMINE, oxygen, IV fluids, and vasopressors.
- **GI decontamination:** No specific recommendations.

ANTIDOTE/DIALYSIS
- **Antidote:** No specific recommendations.
- **Dialysis:** Digoxin immune FAB is not removed by hemodialysis or peritoneal dialysis and is unlikely to be removed by high-permeability hemodialysis.

dihydroergotamine mesylate

dye-hye-droe-er-got'-a-meen mes'-sil-ate

Classes
Chemical: ergot alkaloid
Therapeutic: antimigraine agent

Pregnancy Category: X

Trade Names
Prescription: D.H.E.45, Dihydroergotamine-Sandoz ♣, Migranal

CLINICAL PHARMACOLOGY
Mechanism of Action
An ergotamine derivative, alpha-adrenergic blocker that directly stimulates vascular smooth muscle. May also have antagonist effects on serotonin. **Therapeutic Effect:** Peripheral and cerebral vasoconstriction.

PHARMACOKINETICS
Slow, incomplete absorption from the GI tract; rate of absorption of intranasal varies. Protein binding: greater than 90%. Undergoes extensive first-pass metabolism in liver. Metabolized to active metabolite. Eliminated in feces via biliary system. **Half-life:** 9-10 hr.

AVAILABILITY
Injection: 1 mg/mL (D.H.E.45).
Nasal spray: 4 mg/mL (0.5 mg/spray) (Migranal).

INDICATIONS AND DOSAGE
Migraine headaches, cluster headaches
IM/Subcutaneous

Adults, Elderly: 1 mg at onset of headache; repeat hourly. Maximum: 3 mg/day; 6 mg/wk.

IV

Adults, Elderly: 1 mg at onset of headache; repeat hourly. Maximum: 2 mg/day; 6 mg/wk.

Intranasal

Adults, Elderly: 1 spray (0.5 mg) into each nostril; repeat in 15 min. Maximum: 4 sprays/day; 8 sprays/wk.

CONTRAINDICATIONS

Coronary artery disease, hypertension, impaired liver or renal function, malnutrition, peripheral vascular diseases, such as thromboangiitis obliterans, syphilitic arteritis, severe arteriosclerosis, thrombophlebitis, Raynaud's disease, sepsis, severe pruritus, hypersensitivity to dihydroergotamine

INTERACTIONS

Drug: Beta-blockers, erythromycin: May increase the risk of vasospasm. **Ergot alkaloids, systemic vasoconstrictors:** May increase pressor effect. **Fluoxetine:** May increase risk of ergotism. **Nitroglycerin:** May decrease the effect of nitroglycerin. **Protease inhibitors:** May increase the risk of toxicity of dihydroergotamine. **Herbal:** None known. **Food:** None known.

DIAGNOSTIC TEST EFFECTS

None known.

SIDE-EFFECTS

Occasional: Cough, dizziness, rhinitis, altered taste, throat and nose irritation, nausea, vomiting, dizziness. **Rare:** Muscle pain, fatigue, diarrhea, upper respiratory infection, dyspepsia

CRITICAL CARE CONSIDERATIONS

ADMINISTRATION/HANDLING

INTRANASAL ALERT

- **Storage:** Do not refrigerate or freeze.
- **Early administration:** Administer at the first signs of acute migraine or cluster headache. Initiate treatment at the first sign of symptom of an attack.
- **Before administration:** Nasal spray must be primed (pumped 4 times).
- **Administration:** Patients should not tilt head back or inhale through the nose. Patients must inhale deeply through the nose while spraying or immediately after spraying to let the drug be absorbed through the skin in the nose.
- **Nasal spray:** May be administered at any time during a migraine attack.
- **Stability:** Once spray is prepared, use within 8 hr. Discard unused solution.

PRECAUTIONS

HEALTH-RELATED

- Dihydroergotamine should be used with caution in patients with peripheral vascular disease, coronary artery disease, cerebrovascular disease, or liver or renal impairment.
- **CYP 3A4 inhibitors:** Serious and/or life-threatening peripheral ischemia resulting from vasospasms has occurred when patients received dihydroergotamine while taking drugs such as macrolide antibiotics or protease inhibitors.

AGE-RELATED

- **Neonates:** Dihydroergotamine may cause diarrhea or vomiting in neonates.
- **Children:** Dihydroergotamine may be used safely in children over 6 yr, but only use when patients are unresponsive to other medication.
- **Elderly:** Age-related occlusive peripheral vascular disease increases risk of peripheral vasoconstriction; age-related renal impairment may require dosage reduction.

PREGNANCY/LACTATION-RELATED

- Pregnancy category X; likely excreted into breast milk; ergotamine has caused symptoms of ergotism (e.g., vomiting, diarrhea) in the infant; excessive dosage or prolonged administration may inhibit lactation.

MONITORING

- **Baseline assessment:** Determine history of peripheral vascular disease, liver or renal impairment. Assess peripheral circulation, including the temperature, color, and strength of pulses in the extremities. Determine pregnancy status.
- **Lab work:** Biochemical profile including renal (BUN, creatinine) and liver (AST [SGOT], ALT [SGPT], alkaline phosphatase, bilirubin) function tests.
- **Baseline migraine assessment:** Determine the duration, location, onset, and precipitating symptoms of the migraine.
- **Ergotamine dosage:** Monitor closely for ergotamine overdose as a result of prolonged administration or excessive dosage.
- **Patient education:** When using dihydroergotamine outside the hospital, instruct patients to take at the first sign of a migraine headache. Tell patients to report if the drug dosage does not relieve vascular headaches or if they experience irregular heartbeat, chest discomfort, nausea, numbness or tingling of the fingers and toes, pain or weakness of the extremities, and vomiting after taking the drug. Advise not to tilt head back or inhale through the nose while spraying. Warn women to avoid pregnancy and to report any

suspected pregnancy immediately to a health care provider. Explain that this drug is contraindicated in pregnancy. Advise about other methods of contraception.

SERIOUS ADVERSE REACTIONS

- **Peripheral vasoconstriction:** Localized edema and itching; feet or hands becoming cold, pale, and numb; muscle pain when walking and after, even at rest; gangrene may occur.
- **Cerebral vasoconstriction:** Occasionally confusion, depression, drowsiness, and seizures occur.
- **Cardiac ischemia/MI:** Chest discomfort, chest pain radiating to arms to jaw, diaphoresis, nausea, and possible vomiting.
- **Spontaneous abortion:** Has been reported in pregnant women.

OVERDOSE/TOXICITY

- **Fibrosis:** Pleural and retroperitoneal fibrosis, rarely cardiac valvular fibrosis.
- **Ergotamine toxicity:** Prolonged administration or excessive dosage may produce ergotamine poisoning manifested as seizures, stroke, nausea, vomiting, weakness of legs, flank pain, hematuria, azotemia, pain in limb muscles, numbness and tingling of fingers or toes, precordial pain, tachycardia or bradycardia, and hypertension or hypotension.
- **GI decontamination:** No specific recommendations.

ANTIDOTE/DIALYSIS

- **Antidote:** For neuroleptic malignant syndrome, dantrolene, bromocryptine, amantadine, carbidopa-levodopa may be given.
- **Dialysis:** No data are available regarding removal of dihydroergotamine using hemodialysis, high-permeability hemodialysis, or peritoneal dialysis.

diltiazem hydrochloride

dil-tye'-a-zem hye-droe-klor'-ide

Classes

Chemical: benzothiazepine

Therapeutic: antianginal; antidysrhythmic, class IV; antihypertensive; calcium channel blocker

Pregnancy Category: C

Trade Names

Prescription: Cardizem, Cardizem CD, Cardizem LA, Cardizem SR, Cartia, Dilacor XR, Diltia XT, Taztia XT, Tiazac

Combinations

Prescription: with enalapril (Teczem)

Do not confuse Cardizem with Cardene or Cardene SR or Tiazac with Ziac.

CLINICAL PHARMACOLOGY

Mechanism of Action

An antianginal, antihypertensive, and antidysrhythmic agent that inhibits calcium movement across cardiac and vascular smooth-muscle cell membranes. This action causes the dilation of coronary arteries, peripheral arteries, and arterioles. **Therapeutic Effect:** Decreases heart rate and myocardial contractility, slows SA and AV conduction and decreases total peripheral vascular resistance by vasodilation.

PHARMACOKINETICS

Route	Onset	Peak	Duration
PO	0.5-1 hr	1.5-4 hr	N/A
PO (extended release)	2-3 hr	3-6 hr	N/A
IV	3 min	2-7 min	1-3 hr

Well absorbed from the GI tract. Protein binding: 70%-80%. Undergoes first-pass metabolism in the liver to active metabolite. Primarily excreted in urine. Not removed by hemodialysis. **Half-life:** 3-6 hr.

AVAILABILITY

Capsules (sustained release [Cardizem SR]): 60 mg, 90 mg, 120 mg.

Capsules (extended release [Cardizem CD]): 120 mg (Cardizem CD, Cartia XT, Dilacor XR, Diltia XT, Taztia XT, Tiazac), 180 mg (Cardizem CD, Cartia XT, Dilacor XR, Diltia XT, Taztia XT, Tiazac), 240 mg (Cardizem CD, Cartia XT, Dilacor XR, Diltia XT, Taztia XT, Tiazac), 300 mg (Cardizem CD, Cartia XT, Taztia XT, Tiazac), 360 mg (Cardizem CD, Taztia XT, Tiazac), 420 mg (Tiazac).

Tablets (Cardizem): 30 mg, 60 mg, 90 mg, 120 mg.

Tablets (extended release [Cardizem LA]): 120 mg, 180 mg, 240 mg, 300 mg, 360 mg, 420 mg.

Injection (ready-to-hang infusion): 1 mg/mL.

INDICATIONS AND DOSAGE

Angina

PO (Cardizem)

Adults, Elderly: Initially 30 mg 4 times per day. Range: 180-360 mg/day.

PO (Cardizem CD, Cartia XT, Dilacor XR, Diltia XT, Tiazac)

Adults, Elderly: Initially 120-180 mg/day. Maximum: 480 mg/day.

PO (Cardizem LA)

Adults, Elderly: Initially 180 mg/day. May increase at intervals of 7-14 days. Maximum: 360 mg/day.

Hypertension

PO (Cardizem CD, Cartia XT, Dilacor XR, Diltia XT, Tiazac)

Adults, Elderly: Initially 180-240 mg/day. Range: 180-420 mg/day, Tiazac: 120-540 mg/day.

PO (Cardizem SR)

Adults, Elderly: Initially 60-120 mg twice per day. May increase at 14-day intervals. Maintenance: 240-360 mg/day.

PO (Cardizem LA)

Adults, Elderly: Initially 180-240 mg/day. May increase at 14-day intervals. Range: 120-540 mg/day.

Temporary control of rapid ventricular rate in atrial fibrillation or flutter, rapid conversion of paroxysmal supraventricular tachycardia to normal sinus rhythm

IV push

Adults, Elderly: Initially, 0.25 mg/kg actual body weight over 2 min. May repeat in 15 min at dose of 0.35 mg/kg actual body weight. Subsequent doses individualized.

IV Infusion

Adults, Elderly: After initial bolus injection, may begin infusion at 5-10 mg/hr; may increase by 5 mg/hr up to a maximum of 15 mg/hr. Infusion duration should not exceed 24 hr.

CONTRAINDICATIONS

Acute MI, pulmonary congestion, hypersensitivity to diltiazem or other calcium channel blockers, second- or third-degree AV block (except in the presence of a pacemaker), severe hypotension (less than 90 mmHg, systolic), sick sinus syndrome, or cardiogenic shock. IV diltiazem should not be given at the same time or within a few hours of IV beta-blockers, in patients with Wolfe-Parkinson-White syndrome or short PR syndrome (accessory pathway mediated tachycardias), for ventricular tachycardia, or to newborns (contains benzyl alcohol)

INTERACTIONS

Drug: **Beta-blockers:** May have additive effect. **Carbamazepine, quinidine, theophylline:** May increase diltiazem blood concentration and risk of toxicity. **Digoxin:** May increase serum digoxin concentration. **Procainamide, quinidine:** May increase risk of QT-interval prolongation. **Herbal:** None known. **Food:** None known.

DIAGNOSTIC TEST EFFECTS

PR interval may be increased.

IV INCOMPATIBILITIES

*AcetaZOLAMIDE (Diamox), acyclovir (Zovirax), aminophylline, ampicillin, ampicillin/sulbactam (Unasyn), cefoperazone (Cefobid), diazepam (Valium), furosemide (Lasix), heparin, insulin, nafcillin, phenytoin (Dilantin), rifampin (Rifadin), sodium bicarbonate

IV COMPATIBILITIES

Albumin, aztreonam (Azactam), bumetanide (Bumex), cefazolin (Ancef), cefotaxime (Claforan), ceftazidime (Fortaz), ceftriaxone (Rocephin), cefuroxime (Zinacef), cimetidine (Tagamet), ciprofloxacin (Cipro), clindamycin (Cleocin), digoxin (Lanoxin), *DOBUTamine (Dobutrex), *DOPamine (Intropin), gentamicin (Garamycin), hydromorphone (Dilaudid), lidocaine, lorazepam (Ativan), metoclopramide (Reglan), metronidazole (Flagyl), midazolam (Versed), morphine, multivitamins, nitroglycerin, norepinephrine (Levophed), potassium chloride, potassium phosphate, tobramycin (Nebcin), vancomycin (Vancocin)

SIDE-EFFECTS

Frequent (10%-5%): Peripheral edema, dizziness, lightheadedness, headache, bradycardia, asthenia (loss of strength, weakness). **Occasional (5%-2%):** Nausea, constipation, flushing, ECG changes. **Rare (less than 2%):** Rash, micturition disorder (polyuria, nocturia, dysuria, frequency of urination), abdominal discomfort, somnolence

CRITICAL CARE CONSIDERATIONS

ADMINISTRATION/HANDLING

PO ALERT

- Give diltiazem before meals and at bedtime.
- Crush tablets as needed.
- Do not crush or open sustained-release capsules.

IV ALERT

- **Storage:** Refrigerate vials.
- **Stability:** After dilution, solution is stable for 24 hr.
- **Dilution:** Depends on manufacturer. For Cardizem Lyo-ject syringe or Cardizem injectable, add 125 mg to 100 mL D_5W or

0.9% NaCl to provide a concentration of 1 mg/mL. Add 250 mg to 250 or 500 mL diluent to provide a concentration of 0.83 mg/mL or 0.45 mg/mL, respectively. The maximum concentration is 1.25 g/250 mL or 5 mg/mL.

- **Dilution of Monovial:** 100 mg Cardizem is added to 100 mL diluent for a final concentration of 1 mg/mL. Add 200 mg (2 monovials) to 250 mL for a final concentration of 0.8 mg/mL or 200 mg (2 monovials) to 500 mL for a final concentration of 0.4 mg/mL.

PRECAUTIONS

HEALTH-RELATED

- Use diltiazem cautiously in patients with heart failure, liver disease, or impaired renal function.
- Accurate pretreatment diagnosis differentiating wide complex supraventricular from ventricular tachycardia is imperative. Diltiazem is ineffective against ventricular tachycardia.

AGE-RELATED

- **Children:** Newborns should not receive diltiazem (contains benzyl alcohol). No age-related precautions have been noted in children.
- **Elderly:** Age-related renal impairment may require cautious use.

PREGNANCY/LACTATION-RELATED

- Pregnancy category C; excreted into breast milk in concentrations that may approximate those in maternal serum; use caution in nursing mothers.

MONITORING

- **Baseline assessment:** Assess heart rate, BP, LOC, and whether chest discomfort is present. Concurrent nitroglycerin therapy may be used for relief of anginal pain.
- **Baseline lab work:** Assess liver and renal function test results.
- **Chest discomfort:** Note onset, type (sharp, dull, or squeezing), radiation, location, intensity, and duration of anginal pain and its precipitating factors, such as exertion and emotional stress.
- **Cardiac:** Assess heart rate, BP, and ECG tracing immediately before diltiazem administration. Continuous ECG monitoring should be in place if diltiazem infusion is used. Monitor for normalization of heart rate and ECG rhythm to baseline rhythm or normal sinus rhythm.
- **Dizziness:** Assist patients with ambulation if dizziness occurs.
- **Peripheral edema:** Assess for peripheral edema behind the medial malleolus in ambulatory patients or in the sacral area in bedridden patients.
- **Bradycardia:** Monitor pulse for bradycardia during administration.
- **Side effects:** Assess for signs and symptoms of asthenia or headache.
- **Patient education:** Caution patients against abruptly discontinuing diltiazem. Instruct patients to rise slowly from a lying to a sitting position and wait momentarily before standing to avoid dizziness from the hypotensive effect. Warn patients to avoid tasks that require mental alertness or motor skills until response to the drug is known. Instruct to report constipation, irregular heartbeat, nausea, pronounced dizziness, or shortness of breath.

SERIOUS ADVERSE REACTIONS

- **Abrupt discontinuation:** May manifest accelerated heart rate, which may lead to chest discomfort. Some patients receive diltiazem for refractory angina (unlabelled use).
- **Cardiac disturbances:** Heart failure and second- or third-degree AV block occur rarely.

OVERDOSE/TOXICITY

- Nausea, somnolence, confusion, slurred speech; profound bradycardia, ventricular tachycardia, ventricular fibrillation, heart block, or asystole may ensue. Manage dysrhythmias per Advanced Cardiac Life Support (ACLS) guidelines.
- **GI decontamination:** No specific recommendations.

ANTIDOTE/DIALYSIS

- **Antidote:** Calcium chloride may be helpful in reversing undesirable effects of diltiazem. Depending on the situation, maintain IV fluids as appropriate. Rapid ventricular response may respond to cardioversion. Refer to ACLS guidelines for management of specific tachycardias.
- **Dialysis:** Diltiazem is not removed by hemodialysis or peritoneal dialysis. No data are available regarding removal using high-permeability dialysis.

*dimenhyDRINATE

See Antihistamines (p. 925)

*diphenhydrAMINE hydrochloride

See Antihistamines (p. 925)

atropine sulfate; diphenoxylate hydrochloride

a'-troe-peen sul'-fate; dye-fen-ox'-i-late hye-droe-klor'-ide

DEA Schedule: V

Classes
Chemical: meperidine analog
Therapeutic: antidiarrheal

Pregnancy Category: C

Trade Names
Prescription: Lomocot, Lomotil, Lonox, Vi-Atro

Do not confuse Lomotil with Lamictal or Lonox with Lanoxin, Loprox, or Lovenox.

CLINICAL PHARMACOLOGY

Mechanism of Action

A meperidine derivative that acts locally and centrally on gastric mucosa. **Therapeutic Effect:** Reduces intestinal motility.

PHARMACOKINETICS

Well absorbed from the GI tract. Metabolized in the liver to active metabolite. Primarily eliminated in feces. **Half-life:** 2.5 hr; onset of antidiarrheal effect, 45-60 min with peak at 2 hr and duration of action 3-4 hr; metabolite, 12-24 hr.

AVAILABILITY

Tablets (Lomotil, Lonox): 2.5 mg diphenoxylate/0.025 mg atropine.
Liquid (Lomotil): 2.5 mg/5 mL.

INDICATIONS AND DOSAGE

Diarrhea

PO

Adults, Elderly: Initially, 15-20 mg/day in 3-4 divided doses; then 5-15 mg/day in 2-3 divided doses. **Children 9-12 yr:** 2 mg 5 times per day. **Children 6-8 yr:** 2 mg 4 times per day. **Children 2-5 yr:** 2 mg 3 times per day.

CONTRAINDICATIONS

Children younger than 2 yr, dehydration, jaundice, narrow-angle glaucoma, severe hepatic disease

INTERACTIONS

Drug: Alcohol, other CNS depressants: May increase CNS depressant effects. **Anticholinergics:** May increase the effects of atropine. **Digoxin:** May increase serum digoxin levels. **MAOIs:** May precipitate hypertensive crisis. **Herbal:** None known. **Food:** None known.

DIAGNOSTIC TEST EFFECTS

May increase serum amylase level.

SIDE-EFFECTS

Frequent: Somnolence, lightheadedness, dizziness, nausea. **Occasional:** Headache, dry mouth. **Rare:** Flushing, tachycardia, urine retention, constipation, paradoxical reaction (marked by restlessness and agitation), blurred vision

CRITICAL CARE CONSIDERATIONS

ADMINISTRATION/HANDLING

PO ALERT

- Give without regard to meals. If GI irritation occurs, give with food.

PRECAUTIONS

HEALTH-RELATED

- Use diphenoxylate cautiously in patients with acute ulcerative colitis, cirrhosis, hepatic or renal disease, or renal impairment.

AGE-RELATED

- **Children:** Diphenoxylate is not recommended for use in children because of the increased risk of toxicity, which can lead to respiratory depression. Administer the liquid form to children 2-12 yr using a graduated dropper for accurate measurement.
- **Elderly:** Are more susceptible to the anticholinergic effects of diphenoxylate, and they may experience confusion and respiratory depression.

PREGNANCY/LACTATION-RELATED

- Pregnancy category C; excreted in breast milk.

MONITORING

- **Baseline assessment:** Assess for dehydration: dry mucous membranes, poor skin turgor, and low urine output. Check abdomen for tenderness, distention, and guarding, as well as the presence and activity of bowel sounds.

- **Lab work:** Biochemical profile including renal (BUN, creatinine) and liver (AST [SGOT], ALT [SGPT], bilirubin, alkaline phosphatase) function tests.
- **Dehydration:** Maintain adequate fluid intake. Monitor intake and output. Tachycardia and mild drop in BP may indicate hypovolemia and dehydration.
- **Urinary retention:** Palpate bladder to check for urinary retention.
- **Ileus:** Assess bowel sounds for peristalsis, pattern of daily bowel activity, and stool consistency. Discontinue medication if patients experience abdominal distention or markedly reduced to absent bowel sounds.
- **Patient education:** When using diphenoxylate outside the hospital, warn to avoid tasks requiring mental alertness or motor skills until response to the drug is known. Urge avoidance of alcohol and barbiturates during drug therapy. Instruct to report abdominal distention, fever, palpitations, or persistent diarrhea to the health care provider.

SERIOUS ADVERSE REACTIONS

- **Paralytic ileus and toxic megacolon:** Constipation, decreased appetite, and stomach pain with nausea or vomiting occur rarely.

OVERDOSE/TOXICITY

- **Toxicity:** Dehydration may predispose to diphenoxylate toxicity.
- **Anticholinergic syndrome:** CNS depression, including hypotonic reflexes, hallucinations, tremor, seizures, anxiety, agitation, sedation, hypotension, severe respiratory depression, coma, cardiovascular collapse, and death. Most cases are not life-threatening and require symptom directed, supportive care only.
- **Overdose in children:** May result in hallucinations, seizures, and death.
- **GI decontamination:** No specific recommendations.

ANTIDOTE/DIALYSIS

- **Antidote:** No specific recommendations.
- **Dialysis:** No data are available on removal of diphenoxylate and atropine using hemodialysis, high-permeability hemodialysis, or peritoneal dialysis.

dipyridamole

See Anticoagulants (p. 900)

dirithromycin

See Antibiotics (p. 892)

disopyramide phosphate

See Antidysrhythmics (p. 919)

*DOBUTamine hydrochloride

doe-byoo'-ta-meen hye-droe-klor'-ide

Classes

Chemical: catecholamine, synthetic
Therapeutic: sympathomimetic, ß-adrenergic agonist

Pregnancy Category: B

Do not confuse *DOBUTamine with *DOPamine.

CLINICAL PHARMACOLOGY

Mechanism of Action

A direct-acting inotropic agent acting primarily on beta$_1$-adrenergic receptors. Therapeutic Effect: Decreases preload and afterload, and enhances myocardial contractility, stroke volume, and cardiac output. Improves renal blood flow and urine output.

PHARMACOKINETICS

Route	Onset	Peak	Duration
IV	1-2 min	10 min	Length of infusion

Metabolized in the liver. Primarily excreted in urine. Not removed by hemodialysis. Half-life: 2 min.

AVAILABILITY

Infusion (ready-to-use): 1 mg/mL, 2 mg/mL, 4 mg/mL.
Injection: 12.5-mg/mL vial.

INDICATIONS AND DOSAGE

Short-term management of cardiac decompensation

IV Infusion

Adults, Elderly, Children: 2.5-20 mcg/kg/min. Rarely, drug can be infused at a rate of up to 40 mcg/kg/min to increase cardiac output. **Neonates:** 2-15 mcg/kg/min.

CONTRAINDICATIONS

Hypovolemia patients, idiopathic hypertrophic subaortic stenosis, sulfite sensitivity, hypersensitivity to *DOBUTamine

INTERACTIONS

Drug: Beta-blockers: May antagonize the effects of *DOBUTamine. **Digoxin:** May increase the risk of dysrhythmias and enhance the inotropic effect of both drugs. **Entacapone:** May increase the risk of dysrhythmias, hypertension, and tachycardias. **MAOIs, oxytocics, tricyclic antidepressants:** May increase the adverse effects of *DOBUTamine, such as dysrhythmias and hypertension. **Herbal:** None known. **Food:** None known.

DIAGNOSTIC TEST EFFECTS

Decreases serum potassium level

IV INCOMPATIBILITIES

Acyclovir (Zovirax), alteplase (Activase), amphotericin B complex (Abelcet, AmBisome, Amphotec), bumetanide (Bumex), cefepime (Maxipime), foscarnet (Foscavir), furosemide (Lasix), heparin, piperacillin/tazobactam (Zosyn)

IV COMPATIBILITIES

Amiodarone (Cordarone), calcium chloride, calcium gluconate, diltiazem (Cardizem), *DOPamine (Intropin), enalapril (Vasotec), famotidine (Pepcid), hydromorphone (Dilaudid), insulin (regular), lidocaine, lorazepam (Ativan), magnesium sulfate, midazolam (Versed), milrinone (Primacor), morphine, nitroglycerin, norepinephrine (Levophed), potassium chloride, propofol (Diprivan), total parenteral nutrition (TPN)

SIDE-EFFECTS

Frequent (greater than 5%): Increased heart rate, increased BP. **Occasional (5%-3%):** Pain at injection site. **Rare (3%-1%):** Nausea, headache, anginal pain, shortness of breath, fever

CRITICAL CARE CONSIDERATIONS

ADMINISTRATION/HANDLING

IV ALERT

- **Dosage:** *DOBUTamine dosage is determined by patient response to the drug. Titrate dosage to individual response.
- **Hypovolemia:** Correct hypovolemia with volume expanders before *DOBUTamine infusion.
- **Digitalization:** Administer digoxin to patients with atrial fibrillation before infusion. Digitalize by IV route only to ensure a more predictable response.
- **Storage:** Store at room temperature because freezing produces crystallization. Pink discoloration of the solution, caused by oxidation, does not indicate loss of potency if the solution is used within the recommended time period.
- **Dilution:** Dilute 250-mg ampule with 10 mL sterile water for injection or D_5W for injection; the resulting solution is 25 mg/mL. Add additional 10 mL of diluent if contents of ampule are not completely dissolved; the resulting solution is 12.5 mg/mL.
- **Further dilution:** Further dilute 250-mg vial with D_5W or 0.9% NaCl. Maximum concentration is 3.125 g/250 mL, or 12.5 mg/mL (12,500 mcg/mL). Further diluted solution for infusion must be used within 24 hr.
- **Pediatric dilution:** 6 mg/kg in 100 mL diluent; 1 mg/kg/min equals 1 mg/hr.
- **Infusion pump:** Use infusion pump to control flow rate.
- **Manufacturer recommendations:** Manufacturer recommends not adding other medications to *DOBUTamine, not using in conjunction with other agents, or using with diluents that contain both ethanol and sodium bisulfate. Do not add to any strong alkaline solution, including sodium bicarbonate.

***DOBUTAMINE 1000 mcg/mL (250 mg/250 mL) INFUSION RATES (mgtt/min OR mL/hr)**

Dosage mcg/kg/min	WEIGHT (kg) 5	10	20	30	40	50	60	70	80	90	100
0.5	0.15	0.3	0.6	0.9	1.2	1.5	1.8	2.1	2.4	2.7	3
1	0.3	0.6	1.2	1.8	2.4	3	3.6	4.2	4.8	5.4	6
2.5	0.75	1.5	3	4.5	6	7.5	9	10.5	12	13.5	15
5	1.5	3	6	9	12	15	18	21	24	27	30
7.5	2.25	4.5	9	13.5	18	22.5	27	31.5	36	40.5	45
10	3	6	12	18	24	30	36	42	48	54	60
12.5	3.75	7.5	15	22.5	30	37.5	45	52.5	60	67.5	75
15	4.5	9	18	27	36	45	54	63	72	81	90
17.5	5.25	10.5	21	31.5	42	52.5	63	73.5	84	94.5	105
20	6	12	24	36	48	60	72	84	96	108	120

PRECAUTIONS

HEALTH-RELATED

- Use *DOBUTamine cautiously in patients with atrial fibrillation or hypertension.

AGE-RELATED

- **Children:** No age-related precautions have been noted.

- **Elderly:** No age-related precautions, but lower dosages may be warranted in elderly with age-related organ dysfunction.

PREGNANCY/LACTATION-RELATED

- Pregnancy category B; excreted in breast milk.

D

MONITORING

- **Baseline assessment:** Assess history of heart failure, BP, respiratory rate, heart rate, and heart rhythm.
- **Baseline lab work:** Basic biochemical profile to assess for electrolyte imbalance. Hypokalemia should be corrected before use of *DOBUTamine to avoid induction of ventricular dysrhythmias.
- **Continuous ECG:** Monitor cardiac rhythm continuously for dysrhythmias or tachycardia.
- **Weight:** Determine body weight in kilograms for dosage calculation. Estimated weights are sometimes significantly inaccurate.
- **Hypovolemia:** Hydrate patients before beginning *DOBUTamine therapy to avoid lowering of BP caused by vasodilation.
- **Dosage parameters:** Establish heart rate and BP parameters for adjusting the drug rate or stopping infusion.
- **IV infiltration:** Watch for infiltration of IV solution, which can cause local inflammatory changes and rarely, dermal necrosis.
- **Maintain hydration:** Maintain accurate intake and output records. Measure the urine output at least every 4 hr; more often in unstable patients. Urine output may increase as cardiac output improves.
- **Ongoing lab work:** Assess serum potassium and *DOBUTamine plasma levels.
- **Therapeutic levels:** *DOBUTamine's therapeutic range is 40-190 ng/mL. Serum levels are not routinely used as part of monitoring therapy.
- **BP changes:** Monitor BP at least hourly and as needed for changes in the physical assessment. Hypertension sometimes ensues in patients with preexisting hypertension. Hypotension may be seen if patients are dehydrated.
- **Hemodynamic monitoring:** If pulmonary artery catheter is in place, check for improvement in cardiac output and decreasing pulmonary wedge pressures and/or central venous pressure in heart failure patients. Monitor mixed venous oxygen saturations if SVO_2 catheter is in place. SVO_2 should increase if *DOBUTamine is successfully improving cardiac output and perfusion.
- **Manage ECG or hemodynamic changes:** Consider dosage reduction or changing to a non-catecholamine-based positive inotropic agent if patients experience cardiac dysrhythmias, decreased urine output, or a significant increase or decrease in BP or heart rate. Phosphodiesterase inhibitors such as milrinone (Primacor) or inamrinone (Inocor) may also be effective in managing heart failure.
- **Patient education:** Instruct patients to report chest pain or palpitations during the infusion or pain or burning at the IV site.

SERIOUS ADVERSE REACTIONS

- Tachycardia (heart rate increase of more than 10% of baseline), hypotension, slight chest discomfort, tachypnea, IV insertion site redness due to infiltration.

OVERDOSE/TOXICITY

- **Significant tachycardia:** Increase in heart rate more than 30 beats/min.
- **Cardiac ischemia:** Severe chest discomfort, dyspnea, nausea, diaphoresis, and premature ventricular contractions (PVCs).
- **Hypertension:** Marked increase in BP (by 50 mmHg or higher).
- **Management:** Reduction in infusion rate or temporarily discontinuing the infusion until patients stabilize should correct ventricular dysrhythmias and BP changes. Restart at low dose and titrate upward slowly to effect. If ineffective, beta-blockers may be administered. Hypotension requires treatment with vasopressors (*DOPamine, norepinephrine [Levophed]) if volume infusion is not warranted or is ineffective.
- **GI decontamination:** No specific recommendations.

ANTIDOTE/DIALYSIS

- **Antidote:** Beta-blockers (e.g., metoprolol [Lopressor] or propranolol [Inderal]) may best manage tachycardia and ventricular dysrhythmias because these problems are likely catecholamine induced. If ineffective, lidocaine or amiodarone may be administered.
- **Dialysis:** *DOBUTamine is not removed by hemodialysis or peritoneal dialysis. No data are available on drug removal using high-permeability dialysis.

docusate

dok'-yoo-sate

Classes

Chemical: anionic surfactant
Therapeutic: laxative, stool softener

Pregnancy Category: C

Trade Names

Over the Counter: *Docusate Sodium:* Colace, Dioeze, Diocto, DOK, DOSS DSS, Modane Soft, Regulax SS; *Docusate Calcium:* Selax ♣, Soflax ♣, Sulfolax, Surfak Stool Softener

Combinations

Over the Counter: with senna concentrate (Senokot-S); with phenolphthalein (Doxidan); with casanthranol (Peri-Colace); with cascara sagrada (Nature's Remedy)

CLINICAL PHARMACOLOGY

Mechanism of Action

A bulk-producing laxative that decreases surface film tension by mixing liquid and bowel contents. **Therapeutic Effect:** Increases infiltration of liquid to form a softer stool.

PHARMACOKINETICS

Minimal absorption from the GI tract. Acts in small and large intestines. Results usually occur 1-2 days after first dose, but may take 3-5 days.

AVAILABILITY

Capsules: 50 mg (Colace), 100 mg (Colace, Ducosoft-S), 240 mg (Surfak).
Liquid (Colace): 50 mg/5 mL (sodium).
Syrup (Colace, Diocto): 60 mg/15 mL.

INDICATIONS AND DOSAGE

Stool softener

PO

Adults, Elderly: 50-300 mg/day in 2-4 divided doses. **Children 12 yr and older:** 50-200 mg/day in 2-4 divided doses. **Children 6-11 yr:** 40-150 mg/day in 1-4 divided doses. **Children 3-5 yr:** 20-60 mg/day in 1-4 divided doses. **Children younger than 3 yr:** 10-40 mg in 1-4 divided doses.

CONTRAINDICATIONS

Acute abdominal pain, concomitant use of mineral oil, intestinal obstruction, nausea, vomiting, hypersensitivity to docusate

INTERACTIONS

Drug: Danthron, mineral oil: May increase the absorption of danthron or mineral oil. **Herbal:** None known. **Food:** None known.

DIAGNOSTIC TEST EFFECTS

None known.

SIDE-EFFECTS

Occasional: Mild GI cramping, throat irritation (with liquid preparation). **Rare:** Rash

CRITICAL CARE CONSIDERATIONS

ADMINISTRATION/HANDLING

PO ALERT

- **Hydration:** Provide IV fluid hydration or have patients drink 6-8 glasses of water per day to aid in stool softening. Give each dose with full glass of water or fruit juice if possible.
- **Infants:** Administer docusate liquid with infant formula, fruit juice, or milk to mask the bitter taste.

PRECAUTIONS

HEALTH-RELATED

- Use docusate with caution in dehydrated patients because efficacy is reliant on having water available to mix with stool to provide softening effect.

AGE-RELATED

- **Children:** Not recommended in children under 6 yr.
- **Elderly:** No age-related precautions have been noted.

PREGNANCY/LACTATION-RELATED

- Pregnancy category C; no reports linking use of docusate with congenital defects have been located; diarrhea has been reported in one infant exposed to docusate while breast-feeding, but relationship between symptom and drug is unknown.

MONITORING

- **Baseline assessment:** Before docusate administration, assess abdomen for tenderness, rigidity, and the presence of bowel sounds. Determine when the last bowel movement occurred; find out the amount and consistency.
- **Lab work:** Biochemical profile to help assess fluid and electrolyte status.
- **Hydration:** Ensure patients receive adequate fluid intake.
- **Underlying ileus:** Assess bowel sounds for peristalsis, pattern of daily bowel activity, and stool consistency. If ileus

is suspected, evaluate with abdominal x-rays.

- **Patient education:** Advise patients to increase fluid intake, to exercise, and to eat a high-fiber diet to promote defecation. Tell patients to report unrelieved constipation, dizziness, muscle cramps or pain, rectal bleeding, or weakness to the health care provider.

D

SERIOUS ADVERSE REACTIONS

- None known.

OVERDOSE/TOXICITY

- Excessive dosing may result in diarrhea leading to dehydration.
- **GI decontamination:** No specific recommendations.

ANTIDOTE/DIALYSIS

- **Antidote:** No specific recommendations.
- **Dialysis:** Docusate is not systemically absorbed from the stomach and acts in the intestines. All modes of dialysis are ineffective for nonsystemic drugs.

dofetilide

doe-fet'-il-ide

Classes

Chemical: methanesulfonanilide derivative
Therapeutic: antidysrhythmic, class III

Pregnancy Category: C

Trade Names

Prescription: Tikosyn

CLINICAL PHARMACOLOGY

Mechanism of Action

A selective potassium channel blocker that prolongs repolarization without affecting conduction velocity by blocking one or more time-dependent potassium currents. Dofetilide has no effect on sodium channels or adrenergic alpha- or beta-receptors. Therapeutic Effect: Terminates reentrant tachydysrhythmias, preventing reinduction.

PHARMACOKINETICS

Well absorbed from the GI tract. Protein binding: 60%-70%. Metabolized in liver. Primarily excreted in urine; minimal elimination in feces. Half-life: 7.5-10 hr.

AVAILABILITY

Capsules: 125 mcg, 250 mcg, 500 mcg.

INDICATIONS AND DOSAGE

Maintain normal sinus rhythm after conversion from atrial fibrillation or flutter

PO

Adults, Elderly: Individualized using a seven-step dosing algorithm dependent on calculated creatinine clearance and QT interval measurements.

CONTRAINDICATIONS

Concurrent use of drugs that prolong the QT interval; concurrent use of amiodarone, megestrol, prochlorperazine, or verapamil; congenital or acquired prolonged QT syndrome; paroxysmal atrial fibrillation; severe renal impairment (GFR less than 20 mL/min), hypersensitivity to dofetilide

INTERACTIONS

Drug: **Amiloride, megestrol, metformin, prochlorperazine, triamterene:** May increase plasma levels of dofetilide. **Bepridil, phenothiazines, tricyclic antidepressants:** May prolong the QT interval. **Cimetidine, verapamil:** Increases levels of dofetilide. **Ketoconazole, trimethoprim:** Increases plasma concentration of dofetilide. Herbal: None known. Food: **Grapefruit, grapefruit juice:** Can increase dofetilide plasma levels.

DIAGNOSTIC TEST EFFECTS

None known.

SIDE-EFFECTS

Occasional (less than 11%): Headache (11%); chest pain (10%); dizziness (8%); dyspnea (6%); nausea (5%); insomnia, back and abdominal pain, diarrhea (3%); rash (less than 3%)

CRITICAL CARE CONSIDERATIONS

ADMINISTRATION/HANDLING

PO ALERT

- Administer dofetilde at the same time each day without regard to food.
- Dose should not be doubled if a dose is missed.
- Before dofetilide therapy begins, previous antidysrhythmic drugs should be discontinued for at least 3 plasma half-lives of the other medications. Amiodarone may have to be withdrawn for at least 3 mo before starting dofetilide.

PRECAUTIONS

HEALTH-RELATED

- Patients started or restarted on dofetilide should be hospitalized for a minimum of 3 days in a facility capable of performing a creatinine clearance and highly competent in dysrhythmia monitoring/management and resuscitation.
- Dofetilide can cause lethal ventricular dysrhythmias including torsade de pointes–type ventricular tachycardia resulting from prolongation of the QT interval. The QT interval should be less then 440 msec (500 msec in patients with abnormal conduction) to initiate dofetilide.
- Use with caution in renal and hepatic impaired patients. Dose must be reduced in renal impaired patients.

AGE-RELATED

- **Children:** Safety and efficacy of dofetilide in children under 18 yr have not been established.
- **Elderly:** Age-related renal impairment may warrant a reduction in dosage.

PREGNANCY/LACTATION-RELATED

- Pregnancy category C; no information on the presence of dofetilide in breast milk; breast-feeding while on dofetilide is not advised.

MONITORING

- **Baseline assessment:** Assess vital signs for stability if patients are in atrial fibrillation or flutter and for history of renal and liver disease.
- **Baseline diagnostic tests:** Perform a 12-lead ECG with rhythm strip to assess QT interval and document baseline rhythm.
- **Baseline lab work:** Biochemical profile including potassium and magnesium levels, BUN/creatinine, and liver enzymes. Hypokalemia and hypomagnesemia may exacerbate dysrhythmias.
- **Unstable atrial fibrillation or flutter:** Prepare patients for synchronized cardioversion according to Advanced Cardiac Life Support (ACLS) guidelines. Dofetilide may be used following stabilization to maintain normal sinus rhythm.
- **Continuous ECG:** Monitor for ventricular dysrhythmias and for prolongation of the QT interval.
- **Ongoing lab work:** Monitor serum creatinine, potassium, and magnesium levels for changes.
- **Patient education:** When using dofetilide outside the hospital, explain to take without regard to food. Advise that therapy compliance is essential and dosing instructions must be followed diligently. Warn to report dizziness, severe diarrhea, or other adverse effects. When outside the hospital, patients should have a 12-lead ECG at least every 3 mo to monitor for prolongation of the QT interval.

SERIOUS ADVERSE REACTIONS

- Chest pain, prolonged QT interval, ventricular dysrhythmias, bradycardia, heart block, dizziness.

OVERDOSE/TOXICITY

- Angioedema, bradycardia, cerebral ischemia, facial paralysis, torsade de pointes, second- or third-degree heart block.
- **Management:** Calculate creatinine clearance and reduce dose if warranted. Dose may need to be reduced by half in patients who experience QT prolongation. Ensure magnesium and potassium levels are normal.
- **GI decontamination:** No specific recommendations.

ANTIDOTE/DIALYSIS

- **Antidote:** No specific recommendations.
- **Dialysis:** No data are available on removal of dofetilide using hemodialysis, high-permeability hemodialysis, or peritoneal dialysis.

dolasetron

dol-a'-se-tron

Classes

Chemical: nonbenzamide
Therapeutic: antiemetic

Pregnancy Category: B

Trade Names

Prescription: Anzemet

Do not confuse Anzemet with Aldomet.

CLINICAL PHARMACOLOGY

Mechanism of Action

A 5-HT_3 (serotonin) receptor antagonist that acts centrally in the chemoreceptor trigger zone and peripherally at the vagal nerve terminals. **Therapeutic Effect:** Prevents nausea and vomiting.

PHARMACOKINETICS

Readily absorbed from the GI tract after PO administration. Protein binding: 69%-77%.

Metabolized in the liver. Primarily excreted in urine. Unknown if removed by hemodialysis. **Half-life:** 5-8 hr.

AVAILABILITY

Tablets: 50 mg, 100 mg.
Injection: 20 mg/mL in single use 0.625 mL amps, 0.625 mL fill in 2 mL Carpuject and 5-mL vials.

INDICATIONS AND DOSAGE

Prevention of chemotherapy-induced nausea and vomiting

PO

Adults: 100 mg within 1 hr of chemotherapy. **Children 2-16 yr:** 1.8 mg/kg within 1 hr of chemotherapy. Maximum: 100 mg.

IV

Adults, Children 1-16 yr: 1.8 mg/kg as a single dose 30 min before chemotherapy. Maximum: 100 mg.

Treatment or prevention of postoperative nausea or vomiting

PO

Adults: 100 mg within 2 hr of surgery. **Children 2-16 yr:** 1.2 mg/kg within 2 hr of surgery. Maximum: 100 mg.

IV

Adults: 12.5 mg 15 min before cessation of anesthesia or as soon as nausea occurs. **Children 2-16 yr:** 0.35 mg/kg 15 min before cessation of anesthesia or as soon as nausea occurs. Maximum: 12.5 mg.

OFF-LABEL USES

Radiation therapy induced nausea and vomiting

CONTRAINDICATIONS

Hypersensitivity to dolasetron; concomitant use with bepredil, levomethadyl, mesoridazine, pimozide, thioridazine, ziprasidone

INTERACTIONS

Drug: None known. **Herbal:** None known. **Food:** None known.

DIAGNOSTIC TEST EFFECTS

May transiently increase AST (SGOT) and ALT (SGPT) levels.

IV INCOMPATIBILITIES

No information available for Y-site administration.

SIDE-EFFECTS

Frequent (23%-5%): Headache, diarrhea, fatigue, dizziness (23%); blurred vision (9%); sedation (8%). **Occasional (5%-1%):** Fever, tachycardia, dyspepsia, pruritis (3%)

CRITICAL CARE CONSIDERATIONS

ADMINISTRATION/HANDLING

PO ALERT

- Do not cut, break, or chew film-coated tablets.
- For children 2-16 yr, injectable solution may be mixed in apple or apple-grape juice and given orally at a dosage of 1.8 mg/kg up to a maximum of 100 mg.

IV ALERT

- **Storage:** Store vials at room temperature.
- **Stability:** After dilution, store solution for up to 24 hr at room temperature or up to 48 hr if refrigerated.
- **Dilution:** Dilute the injection in 0.9% NaCl, D_5W, dextrose 5% in 0.45% NaCl, lactated Ringer's solution, D_5LR, or 10% mannitol injection to 50 mL.
- **IV push:** Administer by IV push as rapidly as 100 mg/30 sec.
- **IV intermittent infusion (piggyback):** Infuse over 15 min.

PRECAUTIONS

HEALTH-RELATED

- Use dolasetron cautiously in patients with congenital prolonged QT interval syndrome, hypokalemia, hypomagnesemia, or prolonged cardiac conduction intervals.
- Use dolasetron cautiously in patients taking diuretics with the potential to cause electrolyte disturbances, antidysrhythmics that may lead to prolonged QT interval, or high doses of anthracyclines.

AGE-RELATED

- **Children:** Safety and efficacy of dolasetron have not been established in children under 2 yr.
- **Elderly:** No age-related precautions have been noted.

PREGNANCY/LACTATION-RELATED

- Pregnancy category B; excretion in breast milk unknown; use caution in nursing mothers.

MONITORING

- **Baseline assessment:** Assess patients who experience severe vomiting for dehydration: dry mucous membranes, longitudinal furrows in the tongue, and poor skin turgor.
- **Baseline lab work:** Biochemical profile including potassium and magnesium levels; liver enzymes.

- **Therapeutic effect:** Assess for relief of nausea and vomiting.
- **Continuous ECG:** Monitor the ECG of high-risk patients: hypokalemia, hypomagnesemia, congenital QT syndrome, cumulative anthracycline therapy (*DOXOrubicin/Adriamycin), those with second- or third-degree heart block. Dolasetron should be discontinued for significant prolongation of conduction intervals.
- **Environment of care:** Maintain a quiet, supportive atmosphere. Offer emotional support and consider referral to a cancer support group for appropriate patients.
- **Patient education:** Instruct patients not to cut, break, or chew film-coated tablets. Advise postoperative patients to report nausea as soon as it occurs because prompt administration of the drug increases its effectiveness. Teach patients other methods of reducing nausea such as lying quietly and avoiding strong odors.

SERIOUS ADVERSE REACTIONS

- Prolonged PR, QTC, and ST (JT), bradycardia, and hypotension. May cause transient elevations in liver enzymes.

OVERDOSE/TOXICITY

- Second- or third-degree heart block, QT prolongation leading to torsade de pointes, other ventricular dysrhythmias, dizziness, or hypotension leading to shock.
- **Management:** Manage bradycardia, heart block, and torsade de pointes according to Advanced Cardiac Life Support (ACLS) guidelines. Bradycardia management includes atropine, *DOPamine, epinephrine, and transcutaneous cardiac pacing. Drug should be discontinued until patients stabilize. Resuscitate as necessary per ACLS guidelines.
- **GI decontamination:** No specific recommendations.

ANTIDOTE/DIALYSIS

- **Antidote:** No specific recommendations.
- **Dialysis:** No data are available regarding removal of dolasetron using hemodialysis, high-permeability hemodialysis, or peritoneal dialysis.

donepezil hydrochloride

doe-nep'-e-zil hye-droe-klor'-ide

Classes

Chemical: cholinesterase inhibitor, piperidine derivative
Therapeutic: antidementia agent, cholinergic

Pregnancy Category: C

Trade Names

Prescription: Aricept, Aricept ODT

Do not confuse Aricept with Aciphex or Ascriptin.

CLINICAL PHARMACOLOGY

Mechanism of Action

A cholinesterase inhibitor that inhibits the enzyme acetylcholinesterase, thus increasing the concentration of acetylcholine at cholinergic synapses and enhancing cholinergic function in the CNS. **Therapeutic Effect:** Slows the progression of Alzheimer's disease.

PHARMACOKINETICS

Well absorbed after PO administration. Protein binding: 96%. Extensively metabolized. Eliminated in urine and feces. **Half-life:** 70 hr.

AVAILABILITY

Tablets (Aricept): 5 mg, 10 mg.
Tablets (orally disintegrating [Aricept ODT]): 5 mg, 10 mg.

INDICATIONS AND DOSAGE

Alzheimer's disease

PO

Adults, Elderly: Initially, 5 mg/day at bedtime. May increase at 4- to 6 wk interval to 10 mg/day at bedtime.

OFF-LABEL USES

Treatment of attention-deficit/hyperactivity disorder, autism, behavioral syndromes in dementia

CONTRAINDICATIONS

History of hypersensitivity to donepezil or other piperidine derivatives

INTERACTIONS

Drug: **Anticholinergics:** May decrease the effect of anticholinergics. **Cholinergic agonists, neuromuscular blockers,**

succinylcholine: May increase the synergistic effects of these drugs. **Ketoconazole, quinidine:** May inhibit the metabolism of donepezil. **NSAIDs:** May increase gastric acid secretion of NSAIDs. **Herbal:** None known. **Food:** None known.

DIAGNOSTIC TEST EFFECTS

May increase blood glucose and serum creatine kinase and LDH concentrations. May decrease the serum potassium level.

SIDE-EFFECTS

Frequent (11%-8%) : Nausea, diarrhea, headache, insomnia, nonspecific pain, dizziness, fatigue. **Occasional (6%-3%):** Mild muscle cramps, fatigue, vomiting, anorexia, ecchymosis. **Rare (3%-2%):** Depression, abnormal dreams, weight loss, arthritis, somnolence, syncope, frequent urination

CRITICAL CARE CONSIDERATIONS

ADMINISTRATION/HANDLING

PO ALERT

- Give donepezil without regard to food.
- Donepezil may be given in the morning or evening; best results may be achieved if given at bedtime.

PRECAUTIONS

HEALTH-RELATED

- Use donepezil cautiously in patients with asthma, bladder outflow obstruction, chronic obstructive pulmonary disease (COPD), peptic ulcer disease, history of seizures, sick sinus syndrome, bradycardia, heart block, or other supraventricular conduction disturbances.
- Use the drug cautiously in patients taking NSAIDs concurrently.
- **Anesthesia:** Patients may have exaggerated effect to succinylcholine-like neuromuscular blocking agents.

AGE-RELATED

- **Children:** Safety and efficacy of donepezil have not been established in children.
- **Elderly:** No age-related precautions have been noted.

PREGNANCY/LACTATION-RELATED

- Pregnancy category C; unknown if excreted in breast milk; donepezil generally has no indication for nursing mothers.

MONITORING

- **Baseline assessment:** Obtain vital signs. Determine history of asthma, cardiac conduction disturbances, COPD, peptic ulcer disease, seizure disorder, or urinary obstruction. Assess for behavioral, cognitive, and functional deficits.
- **Behavioral changes:** Monitor behavioral, cognitive, and functional status.
- **Cholinergic reactions:** Assess for diaphoresis, dizziness, excessive salivation, facial warmth, abdominal cramps or discomfort, lacrimation, pallor, urinary urgency, diarrhea, headache, insomnia, and nausea.
- **Patient education:** Tell patients that donepezil may be taken with or without food. Instruct to report abdominal pain, diarrhea, excessive sweating or salivation, dizziness, or nausea and vomiting indicative of cholinergic reaction. Inform patients and families that donepezil is not a cure for Alzheimer's disease but may slow the progression of its symptoms. Refer patients' families to the local chapter of the Alzheimer's Association for a guide to available services.

SERIOUS ADVERSE REACTIONS

- Severe nausea and vomiting, hypotension, confusion, and muscle weakness.

OVERDOSE/TOXICITY

- **Cholinergic crisis:** Severe nausea, increased salivation, diaphoresis, bradycardia, hypotension, flushed skin, abdominal pain, respiratory depression, seizures, and cardiorespiratory collapse. Increasing muscle weakness may result in death if respiratory muscles are involved.
- **Management:** Atropine IV injection and benzodiazepines (e.g., lorazepam [Ativan], diazepam [Valium]) may be given for seizures, using support ventilation and oxygenation as needed. Care is done on a case-by-case basis.
- **GI decontamination:** No specific recommendations.

ANTIDOTE/DIALYSIS

- **Antidote:** Antidote is 1-2 mg IV atropine sulfate with subsequent doses based on therapeutic response.
- **Dialysis:** Donepezil is not likely to be removed by hemodialysis or peritoneal dialysis. No data are available on removal using high-permeability dialysis.

*DOPamine hydrochloride

doe'-pa-meen hye-droe-klor'-ide

Classes

Chemical: catecholamine, synthetic
Therapeutic: vasopressor, α- and ß-adrenergic sympathomimetic

Pregnancy Category: C

Do not confuse *DOPamine with *DOBUTamine or Dopram or Inotropin with Isoptin.

CLINICAL PHARMACOLOGY

Mechanism of Action

A sympathomimetic (adrenergic agonist) that stimulates adrenergic receptors. Effects are dose-dependent. Low dosages (less than 5 mcg/kg/min) stimulate dopaminergic receptors, causing renal vasodilation. Low to moderate dosages (10 mcg/kg/min or less) have a positive inotropic effect by direct action and release of norepinephrine. High dosages (greater than 10 mcg/kg/min) stimulate alpha-receptors. **Therapeutic Effect:** With low dosages, may increase renal blood flow, urine flow, and sodium excretion. With low to moderate dosages, increases myocardial contractility, stroke volume, and cardiac output. With high dosages, increases peripheral resistance, renal vasoconstriction, and systolic and diastolic BP.

PHARMACOKINETICS

Route	Onset	Peak	Duration
IV	1-2 min	N/A	Less than 10 min

Widely distributed. Does not cross blood-brain barrier. Metabolized in the liver, kidney, and plasma. Primarily excreted in urine. Not removed by hemodialysis. **Half-life:** 2 min.

AVAILABILITY

Injection: 40 mg/mL, 80 mg/mL, 160 mg/mL.
Injection (Premix with dextrose): 80 mg/100 mL, 160 mg/100 mL, 320 mg/100 mL.

INDICATIONS AND DOSAGE

Treatment and prevention of acute hypotension; shock (associated with cardiac decompensation, MI, open heart surgery, renal failure, or trauma), treatment of low cardiac output, treatment of heart failure

IV

Adults, Elderly: 2-5 mcg/kg/min up to 50 mcg/kg/min increased by 5-10 mcg/kg/min titrated to desired response. **Children:** 2-5 mcg/kg/min. Maximum: 50 mcg/kg/min. **Neonates.** 1-20 mcg/kg/min.

CONTRAINDICATIONS

Pheochromocytoma, sulfite sensitivity, uncorrected tachydysrhythmias, ventricular fibrillation, hypersensitivity to *DOPamine

INTERACTIONS

Drug: Beta-blockers: May decrease the effects of *DOPamine. **Digoxin:** May increase the risk of dysrhythmias. **Ergot alkaloids:** May increase vasoconstriction. **MAOIs:** May increase cardiac stimulation and vasopressor effects. **Tricyclic antidepressants:** May increase cardiovascular effects. **Herbal:** None known. **Food:** None known.

DIAGNOSTIC TEST EFFECTS

None known.

IV INCOMPATIBILITIES

Acyclovir (Zovirax), amphotericin B complex (Abelcet, Ambisome, Amphotec), cefepime (Maxipime), furosemide (Lasix), insulin, sodium bicarbonate

IV COMPATIBILITIES

Amiodarone (Cordarone), calcium chloride, diltiazem (Cardizem), *DOBUTamine (Dobutrex), enalapril (Vasotec), heparin, hydromorphone (Dilaudid), labetalol (Trandate), levofloxacin (Levaquin), lidocaine, lorazepam (Ativan), *methylPREDNIsolone (Solu-Medrol), midazolam (Versed), milrinone (Primacor), morphine, nicardipine (Cardene), nitroglycerin, norepinephrine (Levophed), piperacillin/tazobactam (Zosyn), potassium chloride, propofol (Diprivan), total parenteral nutrition (TPN)

SIDE-EFFECTS

Frequent: Headache, ectopic beats, tachycardia, anginal pain, palpitations, vasoconstriction, hypotension, nausea, vomiting, dyspnea, mydriasis. **Occasional:** Piloerection or goose bumps, bradycardia, widening of QRS complex.

CRITICAL CARE CONSIDERATIONS

ADMINISTRATION/HANDLING

IV ALERT

- **Hypovolemia:** Correct volume depletion/hypovolemia before administering *DOPamine. Volume replacement may occur simultaneously with *DOPamine infusion.

- **Discolored solutions:** Do not use solutions darker than slightly yellow or solutions that have discolored to brown or pink to purple because these discolorations indicate decomposition of the drug.
- **Prediluted solution:** *DOPamine is available prediluted in 250 or 500 mL of D_5W.
- **Dilution:** Dilute 200-400 mg ampule in 250-500 mL 0.9% NaCl, D_5W/0.45 NaCl, D_5W/0.45 NaCl, D_5W/lactated Ringer's or lactated Ringer's. Concentration is dependent on dosage and fluid requirements. A 200 mg/250 mL solution yields 800 mcg/mL; a 200 mg/500 mL solution yields 400 mcg/mL.
- **Maximum concentration:** Maximum concentration is 3.2 g/250 mL or 12.8 mg/mL (12,800 mcg/mL).
- **Stability:** *DOPamine is stable for 24 hr after dilution.
- **Administration:** Administer into large vein such as the antecubital or subclavian vein to prevent drug extravasation.
- **Infusion pump:** Use infusion pump to control flow rate.
- **Titration of dose:** Titrate dosage to the desired hemodynamic values or optimum urine flow, as prescribed.

***DOPAMINE DOSAGE (mcg/kg/min) CALCULATION CHART (400 mg/250 mL OR 1600 mcg/mL)**

	PATIENT WEIGHT (kg)										
Infusion Rate (mL/hour)	40	45	50	55	60	65	70	75	80	85	90
5	3.4	2.9	2.6	2.4	2.2	2.0	1.9	1.8	1.6	1.6	1.5
10	6.7	5.9	5.3	4.9	4.5	4.1	3.8	3.6	3.3	3.1	2.9
15	10	8.9	8	7.3	6.6	6.1	5.7	5.3	5	4.7	4.4
20	13.3	11.8	10.7	9.7	8.9	8.2	7.6	7.1	6.7	6.3	5.9
25	16.6	14.8	13.4	12.1	11.1	10.2	9.5	8.9	8.4	7.8	7.2
30	20	17.8	16	14.6	13.3	12.3	11.4	10.7	10	9.4	8.8
35	23.3	20.7	18.6	17	15.5	14.3	13.3	12.4	11.6	11	10.5
40	26.7	23.7	21.3	19.4	17.8	16.4	15.2	14.2	13.3	12.3	11.4
45	30	26.6	24	21.8	20	18.4	17.1	16	15	14.1	13.2
50	33.3	29.6	26.7	24.2	22.2	25	19	17.8	16.7	15.7	14.8
55	36.6	32.6	29.3	26.6	24.4	22.5	20.9	19.5	18.3	17.2	16.2
60	40	35.6	32	29.1	26.7	24.6	22.9	21.3	20	18.8	17.9
65	43.4	38.6	34.7	31.6	28.9	26.7	24.8	23.1	21.7	20.4	19.1

PRECAUTIONS

HEALTH-RELATED

- Use middle-range to high-dose *DOPamine cautiously in patients with ischemic heart disease or occlusive vascular disease to avoid myocardial or peripheral ischemia.
- Severe acidosis should be corrected before initiating therapy if possible. Catecholamines including *DOPamine may be inactive if the arterial blood gas pH is less than 7.15.

AGE-RELATED

- **Children:** Drug clearance is highly variable in neonates who are more sensitive to the vasoconstrictive effects of *DOPamine. Closely monitor IV insertion sites in children; gangrene due to extravasation has been reported.
- **Elderly:** Lower doses may be warranted due to age-related organ dysfunction. No age-related precautions have been noted.

PREGNANCY/LACTATION-RELATED

- Pregnancy category C; because *DOPamine is indicated only in life-threatening situations, chronic use would not be expected; no data are available regarding use in breast-feeding.

MONITORING

- **Baseline assessment:** Obtain vital signs and weigh the patient. Determine whether the patients have been on MAOI therapy within the last 2-3 wk. If patients have received MAOIs within this time frame, *DOPamine dosage should be reduced to one tenth of the usual dose.
- **Continuous ECG:** Initiate continuous cardiac monitoring to assess for dyshythmias.
- **Persistent hypotension:** Dosage is titrated based on BP and heart rate response. If tachycardia is noted when BP has not improved to desired range, consider switching to another vasopressor such as norepinephrine (Levophed) or phenylephrine (Neosynephrine).
- **Tachycardia:** Excessive tachycardia is undesirable in patients with history of cardiac ischemia. If tachycardia ensues, consider use of another medication or reduce dose, if possible.
- **Renal perfusion:** Measure urine output frequently. When *DOPamine dose is above 10 mcg/kg/min, urine output may be reduced, indicating renal perfusion may be compromised.
- **Extravasation:** If extravasation occurs, immediately infiltrate the affected tissue with 10-15 mL 0.9% NaCl solution containing 5-10 mg phentolamine mesylate (Regitine).
- **Unstable patients:** Monitor BP, heart rate, and respiration rate at least every 15 min during *DOPamine administration in unstable patients.
- **Hemodynamic monitoring:** Assess cardiac output, cardiac index, pulmonary

wedge pressure, central venous pressure and/or SVO_2 (mixed venous O_2 saturation) frequently.

- **Peripheral vasoconstriction:** Examine peripheral circulation by palpating pulses and noting the color and temperature of extremities; slow or temporarily stop the *DOPamine infusion.
- **Manage adverse effects:** Manage dysrhythmias, decreased peripheral circulation (marked by cold, pale, or mottled extremities), decreased urine output, or significant changes in BP or heart rate. Patients may require a volume infusion, dosage adjustment, or additional vasoactive medications to normalize hemodynamics and increase peripheral perfusion.
- **Abrupt discontinuation:** Taper *DOPamine dosage before discontinuing. Abrupt cessation of *DOPamine therapy may result in marked hypotension.
- **Patient education:** Tell patients to report chest pain or palpitations during the infusion or pain or burning at the IV site.

SERIOUS ADVERSE REACTIONS

- **Ventricular dysrhythmias:** High doses may produce ventricular dysrhythmias.
- **Peripheral arterial disease:** Patients with occlusive vascular disease are at high-risk for further compromise of circulation to the extremities, which may result in gangrene.
- **Extravasation:** Tissue necrosis with sloughing may occur with extravasation of IV solution. Manage with local IV site infusion of phentolamine (Regitine).

OVERDOSE/TOXICITY

- Tachycardia, ventricular dysrhythmias including ventricular tachycardia, hypertension, oliguria, anuria, cold extremities, decreased to absent peripheral pulses in cold extremities.
- Gravely ill patients may cease responding to *DOPamine and other medications when nearing death. BP changes should be used to differentiate overall deterioration from peripheral vasoconstriction. If BP is maintaining reasonable normalcy but extremities are cold with decreased pulses, peripheral vasoconstricition has ensued.
- **GI decontamination:** No specific recommendations.

ANTIDOTE/DIALYSIS

- **Antidote:** No specific antidote. Beta-blockers may be used to control ventricular dysrhythmias.
- **Dialysis:** *DOPamine is not removed by hemodialysis and is unlikely to be removed by peritoneal dialysis. No data are available on removal using high-permeability hemodialysis.

D

dornase alfa

door'-nace al'-fa

Classes

Chemical: recombinant human deoxyribonuclease I

Therapeutic: mucolytic

Pregnancy Category: B

Trade Names

Prescription: Pulmozyme

CLINICAL PHARMACOLOGY

Mechanism of Action

An enzyme that selectively splits and hydrolyzes DNA in sputum. **Therapeutic Effect:** Reduces sputum viscosity and elasticity.

PHARMACOKINETICS

Minimal absorption occurs via inhalation.

AVAILABILITY

Inhalation: 2.5 mg/2.5 mL ampules for nebulization.

INDICATIONS AND DOSAGE

To improve management of pulmonary function in patients with cystic fibrosis

Nebulization

Adults, Children older than 5 yr: 2.5 mg (1 ampule) once daily by recommended nebulizer. May increase to 2.5 mg twice daily.

CONTRAINDICATIONS

Sensitivity to dornase alfa, epoetin alfa, Chinese hamster ovary cell products, or any component of the product

INTERACTIONS

Drug: None known. **Herbal:** None known. **Food:** None known.

DIAGNOSTIC TEST EFFECTS

None known.

SIDE-EFFECTS

Frequent (greater than 10%): Pharyngitis, chest pain or discomfort, voice changes, rash. **Occasional (10%-3%):** Conjunctivitis, hoarseness

D

CRITICAL CARE CONSIDERATIONS

ADMINISTRATION/HANDLING

NEBULIZATION ALERT

- **Storage:** Refrigerate unopened ampules and protect them from light. Do not expose them to room temperature longer than 24 hr.
- **Do not mix:** Do not mix any other medications in the nebulizer with dornase alfa.

PRECAUTIONS

HEALTH-RELATED

- Dornase alfa should be used in conjunction with standard therapies for cystic fibrosis.
- Safety and efficacy of daily administration have not been demonstrated in patients for greater than 12 mo.
- Non–Food and Drug Administration approved indications include patients with chronic bronchitis and with atelectasis secondary to asthma and cystic fibrosis to help improve breathing.

AGE-RELATED

- **Children:** Use in children under 5 yr should be considered only for those who are at risk for pulmonary infection or may improve pulmonary function.
- **Elderly:** No age-related precautions have been noted.

PREGNANCY/LACTATION-RELATED

- Pregnancy category B; excretion into breast milk unknown; however, because serum levels of dornase have not been shown to increase above endogenous levels, little drug would be expected to be excreted into breast milk.

MONITORING

- **Baseline assessment:** Assess BP before administering dornase alfa. BP may rise during early therapy in patients with history of hypertension.
- **Baseline lab work:** Obtain ABG levels. Note CO_2 level on biochemical panel.
- **Therapeutic effect:** Assess for decreased viscosity of pulmonary secretions and relief of dyspnea and fatigue. Improvement in FVC increase to greater than 10% of predicted.
- **Patient education:** When using dornase alfa outside the hospital, instruct to refrigerate it and not to dilute or mix it with other drugs. Teach how to use and clean the nebulizer. Explain that hoarseness, chest pain, or sore throat may result during dornase alfa therapy. Encourage drinking plenty of fluids.

SERIOUS ADVERSE REACTIONS

- **Hypersensitivity:** Rash, fever, dyspnea, wheezing.
- **Respiratory:** Apnea, bronchiectasis, dyspnea, hemoptysis, laryngitis, sputum increase.

OVERDOSE/TOXICITY

- Persistent laryngitis, severe cough, chest pain, rash.
- **GI decontamination:** No specific recommendations.

ANTIDOTE/DIALYSIS

- **Antidote:** No specific recommendations.
- **Dialysis:** Dornase alfa is unlikely to be removed by hemodialysis, high-permeability hemodialysis, or peritoneal dialysis.

doxazosin mesylate 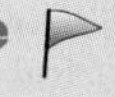

dox-ay'-zoe-sin mes'-il-ate

Classes

Chemical: quinazoline derivative
Therapeutic: antihypertensive, α1-adrenergic blocker

Pregnancy Category: C

Trade Names

Prescription: Cardura, Cardura XL

Do not confuse doxazosin with doxapram, doxepin, or *DOXOrubicin or Cardura with Cardene, Cordarone, Coumadin, K-Dur, or Ridaura.

CLINICAL PHARMACOLOGY

Mechanism of Action

An antihypertensive that selectively blocks $alpha_1$-adrenergic receptors, decreasing peripheral vascular resistance. Therapeutic Effect: Causes peripheral vasodilation and lowers BP. Also relaxes smooth muscle of bladder and prostate.

PHARMACOKINETICS

Route	Onset	Peak	Duration
PO	N/A	2-6 hr	24 hr

Well absorbed from the GI tract. Protein binding: 98%-99%. Metabolized in the liver. Primarily eliminated in feces. Not removed by hemodialysis. Half-life: 19-22 hr.

AVAILABILITY

Tablets: 1 mg, 2 mg, 4 mg, 8 mg.

INDICATIONS AND DOSAGE

Mild to moderate hypertension

PO

Adults: Initially, 1 mg once per day. May increase to a maximum of 16 mg/day. **Elderly:** Initially, 0.5 mg once per day.

Benign prostatic hyperplasia, alone or in combination with finasteride (Proscar)

PO

Adults, Elderly: Initially, 1 mg/day. May increase every 1-2 wk. Maximum: 8 mg/day.

PO, Extended Release

Adults, Elderly: 4 mg once daily with breakfast initially; increase every 3-4 wk to 4-8 mg/day.

CONTRAINDICATIONS

Hypersensitivity to doxazosin or other quinazolines

INTERACTIONS

Drug: **Estrogen, NSAIDs:** May decrease the effect of doxazosin. **Hypotension-producing medications, such as antihypertensives and diuretics:** May increase the effect of doxazosin. **Sildenafil, tadalafil, vardenafil:** May potentiate hypotensive effects. Herbal: None known. Food: None known.

DIAGNOSTIC TEST EFFECTS

None known.

SIDE-EFFECTS

Frequent (20%-10%): Dizziness (14%), asthenia, headache (16%); fatigue. Occasional (9%-3%): Nausea (4%); pharyngitis, rhinitis, pain in extremities, somnolence, edema (4%); hypotension (9%). Rare (3%-1%): Palpitations, diarrhea, constipation, dyspnea, myalgia, altered vision, nervousness

CRITICAL CARE CONSIDERATIONS

ADMINISTRATION/HANDLING

PO ALERT

- Give doxazosin without regard to food.
- Give first dose of doxazosin at bedtime. If the initial dose is given during the day, keep patients recumbent for 3-4 hr.
- Minimize syncope and hypotension. Initial dose should be 1 mg and then increased when response to smallest dose is known. Use of other antihypertensive agents must be done with great caution when using doxazosin.

PRECAUTIONS

HEALTH-RELATED

- Use doxazosin cautiously in patients with chronic renal failure or impaired hepatic function.
- Syncope may be noted not only with first dose, but with dosage increases and if patients resume doxazosin after not receiving it for several days.

AGE-RELATED

- **Children:** Safety and efficacy of doxazosin have not been established in children.
- **Elderly:** May be more sensitive to the hypotensive effects of doxazosin.

PREGNANCY/LACTATION-RELATED

- Pregnancy category C; may accumulate in breast milk; use caution in nursing mothers.

MONITORING

- **Baseline assessment:** Assess BP and heart rate immediately before each dose and every 15 to 30 min thereafter if hypotension or tachycardia is present. BP and heart rate may fluctuate.
- **First-dose syncope:** Monitor pulse frequently because first-dose syncope may be preceded by a rapid pulse rate.
- **Orthostatic hypotension:** Assist patients with ambulation following first dose or after dosage increases because dizziness is more likely.
- **Therapeutic effect:** Improvement in initiating and maintaining urine flow during voiding in males with benign prostatic hypertrophy. If used as an antihypertensive agent, BP reduction is the desired effect.
- **Patient education:** Advise that the full therapeutic effect of doxazosin may not appear for 3-4 wk. Explain that doxazosin may cause fainting or syncope. Warn to avoid performing tasks that require mental alertness or motor skills until response to the drug is known.

SERIOUS ADVERSE REACTIONS

- **First-dose syncope:** Hypotension with sudden loss of consciousness may occur 30-90 min following initial dose of 2 mg or greater, a too rapid increase in dosage, or addition of another antihypertensive agent to therapy. First-dose syncope may be preceded by tachycardia (heart rate of 120-160 beats/min).
- **Priapism:** Sustained, painful penile erection lasting several hours can occur. Patients

must seek emergency medical management to avoid permanent erectile dysfunction.

OVERDOSE/TOXICITY

- Fatigue, headache, hypotension, palpitations, edema, dizziness, dyspnea; rarely leukopenia, neutropenia.
- **Management:** Hypotension should be managed with fluid volume infusion and vasopressors, if needed.
- **GI decontamination:** No specific recommendations.

ANTIDOTE/DIALYSIS

- **Antidote:** For extreme hypotension, large doses of alpha-adrenergic agents including phenylephrine (Neosynephrine) and norepinephrine (Levophed) may be needed to overcome the alpha blockade included by doxazosin.
- **Dialysis:** Doxazosin is not removed by hemodialysis or peritoneal dialysis. No data are available on removal using high-permeability hemodialysis.

doxepin hydrochloride

See Antianxiety Agents (p. 890)

doxycycline

dox-i-sye′-kleen

Classes

Chemical: tetracycline derivative
Therapeutic: antibiotic

Pregnancy Category: D

Trade Names

Prescription: Adoxa, Atridox, Doryx, Doxy-100, Doxy Caps, Doxychel Hyclate, Doxycin ♣, Doxytab ♣, Monodox, Periostat, Vibramycin, Vibra-Tabs

Do not confuse doxycycline with Dicyclomine or doxylamine, or Monodox with Monopril.

CLINICAL PHARMACOLOGY

Mechanism of Action

A tetracycline antibiotic that inhibits bacterial protein synthesis by binding to ribosomes. **Therapeutic Effect:** Bacteriostatic.

PHARMACOKINETICS

Rapidly and almost completely absorbed after PO administration. Protein binding: greater than 90%. Metabolized in liver. Partially excreted in urine; partially eliminated in bile. **Half-life:** 15-24 hr.

AVAILABILITY

Capsules: 50 mg (Monodox), 100 mg (Doryx, Monodox, Vibramycin).
Oral suspension (Vibramycin): 25 mg/5 mL.
Syrup (Vibramycin): 50 mg/5 mL.
Tablets: 20 mg (Periostat), 50 mg (Adoxa), 75 mg (Adoxa), 100 mg (Adoxa, Vibra-Tabs), 150 mg (Adoxa, Vibra-Tabs).
Injection, powder for reconstitution (Doxy-100): 100 mg.

INDICATIONS AND DOSAGE

Respiratory, skin, and soft-tissue infections; urinary tract infections (UTIs); pelvic inflammatory disease (PID); brucellosis; trachoma; Rocky Mountain spotted fever; typhus; Q fever; rickettsia; severe acne (Adoxa); smallpox; psittacosis; ornithosis; granuloma inguinale; lymphogranuloma venereum; intestinal amebiasis (adjunctive treatment); prevention of rheumatic fever

PO

Adults, Elderly: Initially, 100 mg every 12 hr, then 100 mg/day as single dose or 50 mg every 12 hr for severe infections. **Children 8 yr and older and weighing less than 45 kg:** 2-4 mg/kg/day divided every 12-24 hr. Maximum: 200 mg/day. **Children 8 yr and older and weighing more than 45 kg:** Initially, 100 mg every 12 hr, then 100 mg/day as single dose or 50 mg every 12 hr for severe infections.

IV

Adults, Elderly: Initially, 200 mg as 1-2 infusions; then 100-200 mg/day in 1-2 divided doses. **Children 8 yr and older:** 2-4 mg/kg/day divided every 12-24 hr. Maximum: 200 mg/day.

Acute gonococcal infections (uncomplicated)

PO

Adults: Initially, 100 mg every 12 hr for 7 days or 300 mg once, then 300 mg in 1 hr; then 100 mg twice per day for 14 days.

Syphilis

PO, IV

Adults: 200 mg/day in divided doses for 14-28 days.

Traveler's diarrhea

PO

Adults, Elderly: 100 mg/day during a period of risk (up to 14 days) and for 2 days after returning home.

Periodontitis

PO

Adults: 20 mg twice per day.

OFF-LABEL USES

Treatment of atypical mycobacterial infections, gonorrhea, malaria, rheumatoid arthritis; prevention of Lyme disease; prevention or treatment of traveler's diarrhea.

CONTRAINDICATIONS

Children 8 yr and younger, hypersensitivity to tetracyclines or sulfites, last half of pregnancy, severe hepatic dysfunction

INTERACTIONS

Drug: **Antacids containing aluminum, calcium, or magnesium; laxatives containing magnesium:** Decrease doxycycline absorption. **Barbiturates, carbamazepine, phenytoin:** May decrease doxycycline blood concentrations. **Cholestyramine, colestipol:** May decrease doxycycline absorption. **Oral contraceptives:** May decrease the effects of oral contraceptives. **Oral iron preparations:** Impair absorption of doxycycline. **Herbal:** None known. **Food:** None known.

DIAGNOSTIC TEST EFFECTS

May increase BUN serum alkaline phosphatase, amylase, bilirubin, AST (SGOT), and ALT (SGPT) levels. May alter CBC.

IV INCOMPATIBILITIES

Allopurinol (Aloprim), heparin, piperacillin, and tazobactam (Zosyn)

IV COMPATIBILITIES

Amiodarone (Cordarone), diltiazem (Cardizem), hydromorphone (Dilaudid), magnesium sulfate, morphine, propofol (Diprivan), total parenteral nutrition (TPN)

SIDE-EFFECTS

Frequent: Anorexia, nausea, vomiting, diarrhea, dysphagia, possibly severe photosensitivity, uremia. **Occasional:** Rash, urticaria

CRITICAL CARE CONSIDERATIONS

ADMINISTRATION/HANDLING

PO ALERT

- Store capsules and tablets at room temperature. Store oral suspension for up to 2 wk at room temperature.
- Give doxycycline with food, milk, or a full glass of fluid.
- Give oral doxycycline 1-2 hr before or after antacids containing aluminum, calcium, or magnesium; laxatives containing magnesium; or oral iron preparations because these drugs may impair doxycycline absorption.

IM/SUBCUTANEOUS ALERT

- **Do not** administer doxycycline IM or subcutaneously.

IV ALERT

- **Storage:** Protect doxycycline from direct sunlight. Discard it if a precipitate forms.
- **First dilution:** Reconstitute each 100-mg vial with 10 mL of sterile water for injection to yield a concentration of 10 mg/mL.
- **Further dilution:** Further dilute each 100 mg with at least 100 mL of D_5W, 0.9% NaCl, or lactated Ringer's solution.
- **Stability:** After reconstitution, an IV piggyback infusion may be stored for up to 12 hr at room temperature or up to 72 hr if refrigerated.
- **Administration:** Give the intermittent IV (piggyback) infusion over 1-4 hr.
- **Evenly spaced doses:** Space doses evenly around the clock.

PRECAUTIONS

HEALTH-RELATED

- Use doxycycline cautiously in patients who cannot avoid sun or ultraviolet light exposure because such exposure may produce a severe photosensitivity reaction.
- Doxycycline can be used to treat anthrax due to bacillus anthracis, including inhalational anthrax (postexposure).

AGE-RELATED

- **Children:** Use is not recommended in children under 8 yr unless being treated for anthrax because doxycycline can cause permanent discoloration of the teeth.
- **Elderly:** No age-related precautions have been noted.

PREGNANCY/LACTATION-RELATED

- Pregnancy category D; excreted into breast milk; theoretical possibility for dental staining seems remote because serum levels in infant are undetectable.

MONITORING

- **Baseline assessment:** Investigate for a history of allergies, especially to tetracyclines or sulfites before beginning drug therapy.
- **Baseline lab work:** CBC with WBC differential to assess infection, perform appropriate cultures before administering

the drug, biochemical profile to assess liver function and glucose.

- **Ongoing lab work:** Monitor WBC count for decrease, positive cultures until bacterial growth resolves, blood cultures for superinfections, blood glucose for hypoglycemia (insulin requirements may decrease), and liver enzymes for elevation during therapy.
- **Superinfection:** Assess the oral cavity for white patches on the mucous membranes and tongue, abdominal pain or cramping, moderate to severe diarrhea, severe anal or genital pruritus or discharge, and severe mouth or tongue soreness.
- **Possible *Clostridium difficile* colitis:** Assess the pattern of daily bowel activity and stool consistency. Although mild GI effects may be tolerable, severe symptoms may indicate the onset of antibiotic-associated colitis.
- **Hand washing:** If *C. difficile* colitis develops, wash hands with antibacterial soap; alcohol-based foam is ineffective against *C. difficile* spores.
- **Evenly spaced doses:** Space doses evenly around the clock.
- **Intracranial hypertension:** Monitor for impaired level of consciousness.
- **Patient education:** When using doxycycline outside the hospital, instruct to continue taking doxycycline for the full course of therapy. Instruct not to take with antacids or iron products because they will reduce drug absorption. Encourage avoidance of overexposure to sun or ultraviolet light to prevent photosensitivity reactions.

SERIOUS ADVERSE REACTIONS

- **Benign intracranial hypertension:** Headache, visual changes; bulging fontanels in infants.
- **Hypersensitivity:** Patients with a history of allergies, especially to tetracyclines, are at increased risk for developing a severe hypersensitivity reaction marked by severe pruritus, angioedema, bronchospasm, and anaphylaxis.

OVERDOSE/TOXICITY

- Hepatoxicity, fatty degeneration of the liver, and pancreatitis occur rarely.
- **Superinfection:** Especially fungal (systemic candidiasis) and *C.difficile* colitis.
- **Manage *C. difficile* (antibiotic-associated) colitis:** Discontinue medication. Oral vancomycin (Vancocin) or metronidazole (Flagyl) are the most effective treatments for antibiotic-associated (pseudomembraous) colitis.
- **GI decontamination:** No specific recommendations.

ANTIDOTE/DIALYSIS

- **Antidote:** No specific recommendations.
- **Dialysis:** Doxycycline is not removed by hemodialysis or peritoneal dialysis. No data are available on removal using high-permeability hemodialysis.

dronabinol

droe-nab'-i-nol

DEA Schedule: II, III

Classes

Chemical: cannabinoid derivative

Therapeutic: antiemetic, appetite stimulant

Pregnancy Category: C

Trade Names

Prescription: Marinol

Do not confuse dronabinol with droperidol.

CLINICAL PHARMACOLOGY

Mechanism of Action

An antiemetic and appetite stimulant that may act by inhibiting vomiting control mechanisms in the medulla oblongata. Therapeutic Effect: Inhibits vomiting and stimulates appetite.

PHARMACOKINETICS

Well absorbed after PO administration. Protein binding: 97%. Undergoes first-pass metabolism. Is highly lipid soluble. Primarily excreted in feces. Half-life: 4 hr.

AVAILABILITY

Capsules (Gelatin [Marinol]): 2.5 mg, 5 mg, 10 mg.

INDICATIONS AND DOSAGE

Prevention of chemotherapy-induced nausea and vomiting

PO

Adults, Children: Initially, 5 mg/m^2 1-3 hr before chemotherapy, then every 2-4 hr after chemotherapy for total of 4-6 doses per day. May increase by 2.5 mg/m^2 up to 15 mg/m^2 per dose.

Appetite stimulant

PO

Adults: Initially, 2.5 mg twice per day (before lunch and dinner). Range: 2.5-20 mg/day.

OFF-LABEL USES

Postoperative nausea and vomiting

CONTRAINDICATIONS

Treatment of nausea and vomiting not caused by chemotherapy, hypersensitivity to sesame oil, dronabinol, or other tetrahydrocannabinol products

INTERACTIONS

Drug: **Alcohol, other CNS suppressants:** May increase CNS depression. **Herbal:** None known. **Food:** None known.

DIAGNOSTIC TEST EFFECTS

None known.

SIDE-EFFECTS

Frequent (24%-3%): Euphoria, dizziness, paranoid reaction, somnolence. **Occasional (3%-1%):** Asthenia, ataxia, confusion, abnormal thinking, depersonalization. **Rare (less than 1%):** Diarrhea, depression, nightmares, speech difficulties, headache, anxiety, tinnitus, flushed skin

CRITICAL CARE CONSIDERATIONS

ADMINISTRATION/HANDLING

PO ALERT

- Store in a cool environment in a well-closed container; protect from freezing.
- Patients and health care workers with substance abuse history or addictive tendencies may be tempted to abuse the drug for the cannabinoid high (easy laughing, heightened awareness, elation).

PRECAUTIONS

HEALTH-RELATED

- Use dronabinol cautiously in patients with history of substance abuse, heart disease, hypertension, depression, mania, or schizophrenia.

AGE-RELATED

- **Children:** Dronabinol is not recommended for use in children.
- **Elderly:** No age-related precautions have been noted.

PREGNANCY/LACTATION-RELATED

- Pregnancy category C; excreted in breast milk.

MONITORING

- **Baseline assessment:** Assess patients with severe vomiting for dehydration, including dry mucous membranes, low urine output, and poor skin turgor. Determine history of substance abuse or mental health problems.
- **Exacerbation of underlying mental health problems:** Observe closely for serious behavioral and mood reactions. Dronabinol is not recommended for patients with underlying mania, depression, or schizophrenia.
- **Tachycardia and hypotension:** Monitor BP and heart rate.
- **Nausea and vomiting:** If GI symptoms develop, or these symptoms worsen, dronabinol should be discontinued since it is ineffective.
- **Cannabinoid "high":** Note if easy laughing, elation, increased awareness are experienced; these effects may prompt abuse of dronabinol.
- **Patient education:** When using dronabinol outside the hospital to stimulate appetite, instruct taking it before lunch and dinner. Inform that relief from nausea or vomiting generally occurs within 15 min of drug administration. Urge avoidance of alcohol, barbiturates, and other CNS depressants while taking dronabinol and avoidance of tasks that require mental alertness or motor skills until response to the drug is known.

SERIOUS ADVERSE REACTIONS

- **Mild intoxication:** Increased sensory awareness (including taste, smell, and sound), altered time perception, reddened conjunctiva, dry mouth, palpitations, and tachycardia.
- **Moderate intoxication:** Memory impairment and urine retention.

OVERDOSE/TOXICITY

- **Severe intoxication:** Lethargy, decreased motor coordination, slurred speech, and orthostatic hypotension.
- **GI decontamination:** No specific recommendations.

ANTIDOTE/DIALYSIS

- **Antidote:** No specific recommendations.
- **Dialysis:** Dronabinol is unlikely to be removed by hemodialysis or peritoneal dialysis. No data are available on removal using high-permeability hemodialysis.

D

droperidol ⚑

droe-per'-i-dole

Classes

Chemical: butyrophenone derivative
Therapeutic: anesthesia adjunct, antiemetic, sedative

Pregnancy Category: C

Trade Names

Prescription: Inapsine

Do not confuse droperidol with dronabinol.

Combinations

Prescription: with fentanyl (Innovar)

CLINICAL PHARMACOLOGY

Mechanism of Action

A general anesthetic and antiemetic agent that antagonizes dopamine neurotransmission at synapses by blocking postsynaptic dopamine receptor sites; partially blocks adrenergic receptor binding sites. **Therapeutic Effect:** Produces tranquilization, antiemetic effect.

PHARMACOKINETICS

Onset of action occurs within 30 min. Well absorbed. Metabolized in liver. Excreted in urine and feces. **Half-life:** 2.3 hr.

AVAILABILITY

Injection: 2.5 mg/mL (Inapsine).

INDICATIONS AND DOSAGE

Preoperative

IM/IV

Adults, Elderly, Children 12 yr and older: 2.5-10 mg 30-60 min before induction of general anesthesia. **Children 2-12 yr:** 0.088-0.165 mg/kg.

Adjunct for induction of general anesthesia

IV

Adults, Elderly, Children 12 yr and older: 0.22-0.275 mg/kg. **Children 2-12 yr:** 0.088-0.165 mg/kg.

Adjunct for maintenance of general anesthesia

IV

Adults, Elderly: 1.25-2.5 mg.

Diagnostic procedures without general anesthesia

IM

Adults, Elderly: 2.5-10 mg 30-60 min before procedure. If needed, may give additional doses of 1.25-2.5 mg (usually by IV injection).

CONTRAINDICATIONS

Known or suspected QT prolongation, hypersensitivity to droperidol or any component of the formulation

INTERACTIONS

Drug: **CNS depressants:** May increase CNS depressant effect. **Class I, IA, or III antidysrhythmics, cisapride, cyclobenzaprine, phenothiazines, pimozide, quinolone antibiotics, tricylic antidepressants:** May increase risk of QT prolongation. **Hypotensive agents:** May increase hypotension. **Herbal:** None known. **Food:** None known.

SIDE-EFFECTS

Frequent: Mild to moderate hypotension. **Occasional:** Tachycardia, postoperative drowsiness, dizziness, chills, shivering. **Rare:** Postoperative nightmares, facial sweating, bronchospasm

CRITICAL CARE CONSIDERATIONS

ADMINISTRATION/HANDLING

DOSAGE ALERT

- Droperidol is intended for IV or IM use only.
- Dosage should be individualized to age, body weight, physical status, underlying diseases, type of anesthesia used, and type of surgical procedure.

PRECAUTIONS

HEALTH-RELATED

- Use droperidol with extreme caution in patients at risk for prolongation of the QT interval who do not have history of QT prolongation (a contraindication). Factors predisposing patients to QT prolongation include clinically significant bradycardia (heart rate less than 50 beats/min), any clinically significant heart disease, treatment with Class 1 (sodium channel agents) or Class 2 (beta-adrenergic blocking agents) antidysrhythmic agents, MAOIs, and other drugs that prolong the QT interval and electrolyte imbalance affecting dysrhythmias (especially hypokalemia and hypomagnesemia).
- Use with caution in patients with pheochromocytoma and impaired hepatic and renal function.

AGE-RELATED

- **Children:** Safety and efficacy of droperidol have not been established in children under 2 yr.

- **Elderly:** Age-related organ impairment (renal and liver) may prompt cautious use; a decreased dosage is recommended for elderly patients, who are more susceptible to extrapyramidal and anticholinergic effects, orthostatic hypotension, and sedation.

PREGNANCY/LACTATION-RELATED

- Pregnancy category C; has been used to promote analgesia for cesarean-section patients without affecting respiration of the newborn; excretion into breast milk unknown; use caution in nursing mothers. *Note:* Has been used as a continuous IV infusion for hyperemesis gravidarum during the second and third trimesters without apparent fetal harm.

MONITORING

- **Baseline assessment:** Assess for history of cardiac disease including dysrhythmias and renal or liver disease. Evaluate lab work for hypokalemia and hypomagnesemia.
- **Lab work:** Biochemical profile including renal (BUN, creatinine) and liver (AST [SGOT], ALT [SGPT], bilirubin, alkaline phosphatase) function tests, magnesium, calcium, and potassium levels.
- **Baseline diagnostic tests:** 12-lead ECG to evaluate for myocardial ischemia and dysrhythmias. Evaluate ECG for prolonged QT interval. Ensure heart rate is at least 50 beats/min prior to administering droperidol.
- **Resuscitation:** Ensure equipment needed for resuscitation is readily available.
- **Drug interactions:** Evaluate if drugs have been taken that may prolong the QT interval, including antihistamines, antidysrhythmic drugs, antimalarials, antidepressants, and neuroleptic drugs.
- **Cardiac effects:** Monitor ECG continuously following administration for prolongation of the QT interval, which may prompt torsades de pointes, a pulse ventricular tachycardia requiring immediate resuscitation. ECG should be monitored continuously for at least 3 hr following last dose.
- **EEG effects:** EEG may be delayed in returning to normal following surgery. For patients receiving serial EEGs or bispectral sedation monitoring, expect readings may be abnormal.
- **Behavioral effects:** Assess for hallucinations and restlessless. Shivering may ensue, which may further upset patients.
- **Patient education:** Instruct not to drink alcoholic beverages or take other CNS depressant drugs including antihistamines, analgesics, and sedatives for at least 24 hr after receiving droperidol. Warn not to engage in activities requiring mental alertness, including operating dangerous machinery or driving a motor vehicle, for 24 hr after receiving the drug.

SERIOUS ADVERSE REACTIONS

- **Prolonged QT syndrome:** May lead to torsades de pointes, which requires resuscitation. Do not manage torsades with standard antidysrhythmic agents used for ventricular tachycardia; these drugs may worsen the patient. Consider use of isoproterenol infusion, magnesium infusion, and defibrillation.

OVERDOSE/TOXICITY

- **Overdose:** Respiratory depression, apnea, hypotension, palpitations, syncope, bradycardia, prolonged QT syndrome, cardiac arrest, extrapyramidal involuntary muscle movements, neuroleptic malignant syndrome, and death. Epinephrine is contraindicated for hypotension, because it worsens hypotension. Treat extrapyramidal symptoms with benztropine (Cogentin) or *diphenhydrAMINE (Benadryl).
- **Neuroleptic malignant syndrome:** Fever, muscular rigidity, altered mental status, autonomic dysfunction including fever, tachycardia, tachypnea, hypertension, and hypotension. Extrapyramidal movements are often present including tremors, nystagmus, and dysarthria. Akinetic mutism and seizures have been reported. Signs and symptoms vary and are influenced by timing of the diagnosis and type of treatment. Muscle rigidity usually does not respond to anticholinergic treatment.
- **Management:** Immediate discontinuation of droperidol. No individual therapy or combination of therapies works for all patients. Dantrolene, bromocriptine, amantadine, carbidopa-levodopa, and levodopa have all had varying levels of success treating muscle relaxation and droperidol-induced dopaminergic blockade.
- **GI decontamination:** No specific recommendations.

ANTIDOTE/DIALYSIS

- **Antidote:** No specific recommendations.

- **Dialysis:** Droperidol is unlikely to be removed by hemodialysis or peritoneal dialysis. No data are available on removal by high-permeability hemodialysis.

D

drotrecogin alfa

droe-tre-koe'-jin al'-fa

Classes
Chemical: glycoprotein
Therapeutic: antisepsis syndrome agent

Pregnancy Category: C

Trade Names
Prescription: Xigris

Do not confuse Xigris with Xanax.

CLINICAL PHARMACOLOGY

Mechanism of Action

A recombinant form of human-activated protein C that exerts an antithrombotic effect by inhibiting Factors Va and VIIIa and may exert an indirect profibrinolytic effect by inhibiting plasminogen activator inhibitor-1 and limiting the generation of activated thrombin-activatable-fibrinolysis-inhibitor. The drug may also exert an antiinflammatory effect by inhibiting tumor necrosis factor (TNF) production by monocytes, by blocking leukocyte adhesion to selectins, and by limiting thrombin-induced inflammatory responses. **Therapeutic Effect:** Produces antiinflammatory, antithrombotic, and profibrinolytic effects.

PHARMACOKINETICS

Inactivated by endogenous plasma protease inhibitors. Clearance occurs within 2 hr of initiating infusion. **Half-life:** 1.6 hr.

AVAILABILITY

Powder for infusion: 5 mg, 20 mg.

INDICATIONS AND DOSAGE

Severe sepsis

IV Infusion

Adults, Elderly: 24 mcg/kg/hr for 96 hr. Immediately stop infusion if clinically significant bleeding is identified.

CONTRAINDICATIONS

Active internal bleeding, evidence of cerebral herniation, intracranial neoplasm or mass lesion, presence of an epidural catheter, recent (within the past 3 mo) hemorrhagic stroke, recent (within the past 2 mo) intracranial or intraspinal surgery or severe head trauma, trauma with an increased risk of life-threatening bleeding, or hypersensitivity to drotrecogin alfa

INTERACTIONS

Drug: None known. **Herbal:** None known. **Food:** None known.

DIAGNOSTIC TEST EFFECTS

May prolong aPTT.

IV INCOMPATIBILITIES

Do not mix drotrecogin alfa with other medications.

IV COMPATIBILITIES

Lactated Ringer's solution, 0.9% NaCl and dextrose are the only solutions that can be administered through the same line.

SIDE-EFFECTS

Bleeding (3.5%)

CRITICAL CARE CONSIDERATIONS

ADMINISTRATION/HANDLING

IV ALERT

- **Storage:** Store unreconstituted vials at room temperature. Drotrecogin alfa is preservative-free; when the vial is opened, it should be prepared into IV solution immediately.
- **First dilution:** Reconstitute the 5-mg and 20-mg vials by slowly adding 2.5 mL or 10 mL of sterile water for injection, respectively, to yield a concentration of 2 mg/mL. Swirl the vial gently to mix; do not shake or invert it.
- **Further dilution:** Add the reconstituted drug to an infusion bag containing 0.9% NaCl and dilute to a final concentration of 100 to 200 mcg/mL. Direct the stream to the side of the bag to minimize agitation. Invert the infusion bag to mix the solution.
- **Stability:** Start the infusion within 3 hr after reconstitution. Intravenous infusion must be finished within 12 hr of when IV solution has been prepared. If the infusion bag is not finished, it should be changed to avoid bacterial growth.
- **Infusion:** Administer the drug through a dedicated IV line or a dedicated lumen of a multilumen central venous catheter at a rate of 24 mcg/kg/hr for 96 hr.
- **Interrupted infusion:** If infusion is interrupted, restart at 24 mcg/kg/hr.

PRECAUTIONS

HEALTH-RELATED

- Use drotrecogin alfa cautiously in patients with chronic, severe hepatic disease, intracranial aneurysm, platelet count less than 30,000/mm^3, or prolonged prothrombin time and in those who have had GI bleeding within the past 6 wk.
- Use drotrecogin alfa cautiously in patients who are using heparin concurrently and in those who have had thrombolytic therapy within the past 3 days or anticoagulant or aspirin therapy within the past 7 days.
- Use caution when administering other drugs that affect hemostasis.

AGE-RELATED

- **Children:** Safety and efficacy of drotrecogin alfa have not been established in children.
- **Elderly:** Safety and efficacy of drotrecogin alfa have not been established in elderly.

PREGNANCY/LACTATION-RELATED

- Pregnancy category C; excretion into breast milk unknown.

MONITORING

- **Baseline assessment:** The following criteria must be met before initiating drotrecogin alfa therapy: age of at least 18 yr; weight less than 135 kg; no pregnancy or breast-feeding; three or more systemic inflammatory response (SIRS) criteria (fever, heart rate greater than 90 beats/min, respiratory rate greater than 20 breaths/min, increased WBC count); and at least one sepsis-induced organ or system failure (cardiovascular, hepatic, renal, respiratory, or unexplained metabolic acidosis). Patients ideally should not have a history of bleeding, an epidural catheter, or any spinal catheters in place because of risk for bleeding.
- **Baseline lab work:** CBC with WBC differential and platelet count, coagulation studies, and complete biochemical profile to assess renal and liver function, and blood glucose.
- **Bleeding:** Monitor closely for hemorrhagic complications.
- **Drug discontinuation:** Discontinue drotrecogin alfa for 2 hr before a major invasive or surgical procedure. May be reconsidered at 12 hr following a major invasive procedure or surgery.
- **Septic shock:** May require fluid resuscitation and vasopressors to manage shock-related hypotension.
- **Antibiotics:** Patients must continue to receive antibiotics if infection is present. Drotrecogin alfa targets systemic inflammatory response syndrome but has no bacteriocidal effects.
- **Patient education:** Inform that bleeding may occur for up to 28 days after treatment. Warn to report unusual bleeding to their health care provider immediately.

SERIOUS ADVERSE REACTIONS

- Bleeding (intrathoracic, retroperitoneal, GI, GU, intraabdominal, intracranial, intraspinal with epidural or spinal catheters in place) occurs in about 3.5% of patients.
- **Hypersensitivity:** Rash, pruritis, anaphylaxis; antibody development has been reported rarely

OVERDOSE/TOXICITY

- Severe bleeding.
- **Manage bleeding:** Stop the infusion. May require transfusion of packed RBCs, platelets, cryoprecipitate, fresh frozen plasma and desmopressin, tranexamic acid, and aminocaproic acid. Use prothrombin time, platelet count, and fibrinogen level to guide therapy. Consider protamine if heparin has been used.

ANTIDOTE/DIALYSIS

- **Antidote:** No specific recommendations.
- **Dialysis:** Drotrecogin alfa is unlikely to be removed using hemodialysis, high-permeability hemodialysis, or peritoneal dialysis.

dutasteride

doo-tas'-teer-ide

Classes

Chemical: 5-alpha reductase inhibitor
Therapeutic: hormone inhibitor, androgen inhibitor

Pregnancy Category: X

Trade Names

Prescription: Avodart

CLINICAL PHARMACOLOGY

Mechanism of Action

An androgen hormone inhibitor that inhibits 5-alpha reductase, an intracellular enzyme that converts testosterone into dihydrotestosterone (DHT) in the prostate gland, reducing the serum DHT level. **Therapeutic Effect:** Reduces size of the prostate gland.

PHARMACOKINETICS

Route	Onset	Peak	Duration
PO	30 days	N/A	5 wk

Moderately absorbed after PO administration. Widely distributed. Protein binding: 99%. Metabolized in the liver. Primarily excreted in feces. **Half-life:** Up to 5 wk.

AVAILABILITY

Capsule: 0.5 mg.

INDICATIONS AND DOSAGE

Benign prostatic hyperplasia (BPH)

PO

Adults, Elderly (men only): 0.5 mg once per day.

OFF-LABEL USES

Treatment of hair loss

CONTRAINDICATIONS

Females, physical handling of tablets by those who are or may be pregnant, hypersensitivity to dutasteride

INTERACTIONS

Drug: **Cimetidine, ciprofloxacin, diltiazem, ketoconazole, ritonavir, verapamil:** May increase dutasteride plasma concentrations. **Herbal:** None known. **Food:** None known.

DIAGNOSTIC TEST EFFECTS

Decreases the serum prostate-specific antigen (PSA) level

SIDE-EFFECTS

Occasional: Gynecomastia, sexual dysfunction (decreased libido, impotence, and decreased volume of ejaculate)

CRITICAL CARE CONSIDERATIONS

ADMINISTRATION/HANDLING

PO ALERT

- Do not break, crush, or open capsules.
- Give dutasteride without regard to food.

PRECAUTIONS

HEALTH-RELATED

- Use dutasteride cautiously in patients with hepatic impairment, preexisting sexual dysfunction (such as impotence and decreased libido), or obstructive uropathy.
- Males should not donate blood until at least 6 mo have passed following their last dose of dutasteride to prevent administration of dutasteride to a pregnant female transfusion recipient.
- **CYP3A4 inhibitors:** Patients receiving CYP3A4 inhibitors which include cimetidine, ciprofloxacin, diltiazem, ketoconazole, ritonavir, and verapamil, may have drug interactions if dutasteride is taken along with these medications.

AGE-RELATED

- **Children:** Safety and efficacy of dutasteride in children under 18 yr have not been established.
- **Elderly:** No dosage adjustment is needed.

PREGNANCY/LACTATION-RELATED

- Pregnancy category X.

MONITORING

- **Baseline assessment:** Assess for benign prostatic hyperplasia (BPH), including urinary hesitancy, postvoid dribbling, reduced force of urinary stream, and sensation of incomplete bladder emptying.
- **Baseline lab work:** Obtain serum PSA determinations before and periodically during therapy.
- **Urinary retention/hesitancy:** Monitor fluid intake and output.
- **Therapeutic effect:** Assess for improvement of BPH signs and symptoms.
- **Patient education:** Inform that dutasteride may cause impotence and decrease ejaculate volume. Explain that urinary flow may not improve for up to 6 mo after beginning treatment. Caution not to let women who are or may be pregnant handle dutasteride capsules. Explain the drug has a pregnancy risk category of X and carries the risk of causing anomalies in the male fetus.

SERIOUS ADVERSE REACTIONS

- Urinary retention, which may require urinary catheter insertion by a urologist if other health care providers are unable to pass the catheter past the enlarged prostate gland.

OVERDOSE/TOXICITY

- Rash, diarrhea, and abdominal pain.
- **GI decontamination:** No specific recommendations.

ANTIDOTE/DIALYSIS

- **Antidote:** No specific recommendations.
- **Dialysis:** Dutasteride is unlikely to be removed using hemodialysis, high-permeability hemodialysis, or peritoneal dialysis.

edrophonium chloride

ed-roe-foe'-nee-um klor'-ide

Classes

Chemical: cholinesterase inhibitor, quaternary ammonium derivative
Therapeutic: antidote, curare; cholinergic

Pregnancy Category: C

Trade Names

Prescription: Enlon, Reversol, Tensilon

Combinations

Prescription: with atropine (Enlon-Plus)

CLINICAL PHARMACOLOGY

Mechanism of Action

A parasympathetic, anticholinesterase agent that inhibits destruction of acetylcholine by acetylcholinesterase, thus causing accumulation of acetylcholine at cholinergic synapses. Results in an increase in cholinergic responses such as miosis, increased tonus of intestinal and skeletal muscles, bronchial and ureteral constriction, bradycardia, and increased salivary and sweat gland secretions. **Therapeutic Effect:** Diagnosis of myasthenia gravis.

PHARMACOKINETICS

Onset of action occurs within 30-60 sec and has duration of 10 min. Rapid absorption after IV administration. Exact method of metabolism is unknown. Rapidly excreted in urine. **Half-life:** 1.8 hr.

AVAILABILITY

Injection: 10 mg/mL (Enlon, Reversol, Tensilon).

INDICATIONS AND DOSAGE

Diagnosis of myasthenia gravis

IV

Adults, Elderly: 2 mg test dose over 15-30 sec. If no reaction in 45 sec, give additional dose of 8 mg. Test dose may be repeated after 30 min. **Children more than 34 kg:** Initially, 2 mg over 1 min. If no reaction in 45 sec, may repeat at a rate of 1 mg every 30-45 sec. Maximum cumulative dose: 10 mg. **Children less than 34 kg:** Initially, 1 mg over 1 min. If no reaction in 45 sec, may repeat at a rate of 1 mg every 30-45 sec. Maximum cumulative dose: 5 mg. **Infants:** 0.5 mg infused over 1 min.

IM/Subcutaneous

Adults, Elderly, Children: Initially, 10 mg as a single dose. If no cholinergic reaction occurs, give 2 mg 30 min later to rule out false-negative reaction. **Children more than 34 kg:** 5 mg as a single dose. **Children less than 34 kg:** 2 mg as a single dose. **Infants:** 0.5-1 mg as a single dose.

Neuromuscular blockade antagonism

IV

Adults, Elderly: 10 mg over 30-45 sec. May be repeated as needed until a cholinergic response is detected. Maximum: 40 mg.

IM

Children: 233 mcg/kg as a single dose. **Infants:** 145 mcg/kg as a single dose.

Dosage in renal impairment

Dose may need to be reduced in patients with chronic renal failure.

CONTRAINDICATIONS

Gastrointestinal or genitourinary (GU) obstruction, hypersensitivity to edrophonium, sulfites, or any component of the formulation

INTERACTIONS

Drug: **Atropine, nondepolarizing muscle relaxants, procainamide, quinidine:** May decrease the effects of edrophonium. **Succinylcholine, digoxin, IV acetazolamide, neostigmine, physostigmine.** May increase the effects of edrophonium. **Herbal:** None known. **Food:** None known.

DIAGNOSTIC TEST EFFECTS

May increase serum amylase, AST (SGOT) and ALT (SGPT) levels.

IV COMPATIBILITIES

Heparin, hydrocortisone, vitamin B complex with C

SIDE-EFFECTS

Frequent: Bradycardia, hypotension, increased salivation, intestinal secretions, lacrimation, nausea, vomiting, urinary urgency, hyperperistalsis, sweating. **Occasional:** Convulsions, dysphagia, diarrhea. **Rare:** Bronchoconstriction, cardiac arrest, central respiratory paralysis

CRITICAL CARE CONSIDERATIONS

ADMINISTRATION/HANDLING

IV ALERT

- **Preparation:** Atropine should always be readily available as an antagonist for treatment of cholinergic reactions. Intubation and controlled ventilation may also be required if cholinergic crisis occurs.

- **IV route alternatives:** Usually administered IV; however, if not possible, IM or subcutaneous may be used.

PRECAUTIONS

HEALTH-RELATED

- Use edrophonium with caution in patients with bronchial asthma, heart block, those receiving a cardiac glycoside or an anticholinesterase drug (e.g., neostigmine [Prostigmine]).
- **Tachycardias:** Edrophonium is used off label for termination of paroxysmal atrial tachycardia and to slow supraventricular tachycardia unresponsive to cardiac glycosides or adenosine.
- **Reversal agent:** Edrophonium may be used to reverse briefly nondepolarizing neuromuscular blocking agents (e.g., atracurium, pancuronium, vecuronium).

AGE-RELATED

- **Children:** No age-related precautions noted in children. Safety and efficacy of reversal of nondepolarizing neuromuscular blocking agents have not been established.
- **Elderly:** Age-related renal impairment may require adjustment.

PREGNANCY/LACTATION-RELATED

- Pregnancy category C; because it is ionized at physiologic pH, would not be expected to cross placenta in significant amounts or to be excreted into breast milk; may cause premature labor.

MONITORING

- **Baseline assessment:** Determine history of allergies, especially to edrophonium and sulfite. Ensure all anticholinesterase medications have been stopped 8 hr before procedure. Evaluate for history of apnea and mechanical obstructions of the intestines or urinary tract.
- **Baseline lab work:** Biochemical profile.
- **Cholinergic response:** Monitor for minimal or no cholinergic response.
- **Vital signs:** Monitor heart rate, respiratory rate, and BP.
- **Heart block:** Initiate continuous ECG monitoring to assess for first-, second-, or third-degree heart block.
- **Myasthenia gravis testing:** Monitor preinjection- and postinjection strength (cranial musculature is most useful).
- **Toxicity:** Monitor for bradycardia and respiratory distress.
- **Patient education:** Explain that anticholinesterase insensitivity may be developed for a period of time and should be carefully monitored by the physician. Instruct to report difficulty breathing, dizziness, muscle cramps and spasms, or vomiting. Reassure that the side effects of edrophonium will not last long because the effects of the drug are short-lived.

SERIOUS ADVERSE REACTIONS

- **Heart block:** Vagal stimulation slows conduction through the AV node.

OVERDOSE/TOXICITY

- **Cholinergic crisis:** Muscle weakness, nausea, vomiting, bradycardia, miosis, bronchospasm, and respiratory paralysis.
- **Management:** Endotracheal intubation or tracheostomy may be done as a precautionary measure if patients are undergoing anesthesia when being tested for myasthenia gravis. Ensure a patent airway, ventilation, adequate suctioning to manage secretions, IV fluids, and/or vasopressors to manage hypotension.
- **GI decontamination:** No specific recommendations.

ANTIDOTE/DIALYSIS

- **Antidote:** Atropine sulfate 0.4-0.5 mg IV will reverse most side effects; may be repeated every 3-10 min.
- **Dialysis:** No data are available on removal of edrophonium using hemodialysis, high-permeability hemodialysis, or peritoneal dialysis.

efalizumab

e-fa-li-zoo'-mab

Classes

Chemical: monoclonal antibody
Therapeutic: antipsoriatic, immunomodulatory agent

Pregnancy Category: C

Trade Names

Prescription: Raptiva

CLINICAL PHARMACOLOGY

Mechanism of Action

A monoclonal antibody that interferes with lymphocyte activation by binding to the lymphocyte antigen, inhibiting the adhesion of leukocytes to other cell types. **Therapeutic Effect:** Prevents the release of cytokines and the growth and migration of circulating total lymphocytes, predominant in psoriatic lesions.

PHARMACOKINETICS

Clearance is affected by body weight, not by gender or race, after subcutaneous injection. Serum concentration reaches steady state at 4 wk. Mean time to elimination: 25 days.

AVAILABILITY

Powder for injection: 150 mg, designed to deliver 125 mg/1.25 mL.

INDICATIONS AND DOSAGE

Psoriasis

Subcutaneous

Adults, Elderly: Initially, 0.7 mg/kg followed by weekly doses of 1 mg/kg. Maximum: 200 mg (single dose).

CONTRAINDICATIONS

Concurrent use of immunosuppressive agents, hypersensitivity to efalizumab or any murine or humanized monoclonal antibody preparation

INTERACTIONS

Drug: Immunosuppressive agents: Increase the risk of infection. **Live-virus vaccines:** Decrease the immune response. **Herbal:** None known. **Food:** None known.

DIAGNOSTIC TEST EFFECTS

May increase the lymphocyte count.

SIDE-EFFECTS

Frequent (32%-10%): Headache, chills, nausea, injection site pain. **Occasional (8%-7%):** Myalgia, flulike symptoms, fever. **Rare (4%):** Back pain, acne

CRITICAL CARE CONSIDERATIONS

ADMINISTRATION/HANDLING

SUBCUTANEOUS ALERT

- **Storage:** Refrigerate unopened vials. Reconstituted solution may be stored at room temperature for up to 8 hr.
- **Dissolution:** Swirl the vial gently to dissolve; do not shake because foaming will occur. Dissolution takes less than 5 min.
- **Injection:** Slowly inject 1.3 mL of sterile water for injection into the efalizumab vial using the provided prefilled diluent syringe.
- **Injection sites:** Administer into the abdomen, buttocks, thigh, or upper arm.

PRECAUTIONS

HEALTH-RELATED

- Use efalizumab cautiously in patients with asthma, chronic infections, a history of allergic reactions, or a history of malignancy.
- **Vaccines:** Acellular, live, and live attenuated vaccines should not be administered since safety and efficacy of use with vaccines have not been established.

AGE-RELATED

- **Children:** Efalizumab is not indicated for use in children.
- **Elderly:** Age-related increased incidence of infection requires cautious use in elderly.

PREGNANCY/LACTATION-RELATED

- Pregnancy category C; breast milk excretion unknown.

MONITORING

- **Baseline assessment:** Examine the skin before beginning efalizumab therapy; document the size, appearance, and location of psoriasis lesions.
- **Baseline lab work:** CBC, lymphocyte, and platelet counts before beginning therapy and periodically thereafter.
- **Therapeutic effect:** Document improvement or worsening of psoriasis lesions.
- **Drug discontinuation:** Patients who both respond and do not respond to efalizumab should be monitored closely for status of psoriasis following discontinuation of the drug.
- **Patient education:** When efalizumab will be used outside the hospital, teach patients and caregivers the proper sterile technique for preparing and injecting efalizumab. Advise that efalizumab increases the risk of developing an infection. Inform about the duration of efalizumab treatment and the required monitoring procedures. Instruct to report bleeding from the gums, bruising or petechiae of the skin, fever, or other signs of any infection to a health care provider. Instruct to inform all other physicians involved in their care of efalizumab use, especially if being managed for cancer. Advise not to undergo phototherapy treatments.

SERIOUS ADVERSE REACTIONS

- Hypersensitivity reaction, malignancies, serious infections including abscess, cellulitis, postoperative wound infection, and pneumonia.

OVERDOSE/TOXICITY

- Thrombocytopenia and worsening of psoriasis occur rarely.
- **Hemolytic anemia:** Immune mediated hemolytic anemia.
- **Psoriatic arthritis:** New onset or recurrent.
- **GI decontamination:** No specific recommendations.

ANTIDOTE/DIALYSIS

- **Antidote:** No specific recommendations.
- **Dialysis:** No data are available on removal of efalizumab using hemodialysis, high-permeability hemodialysis, or peritoneal dialysis.

E

efavirenz

See HIV Medications (p. 961)

eletriptan

See Triptans (p. 984)

emtricitabine

See HIV Medications (p. 961)

enalapril maleate

e-nal'-a-pril mal'-ee-ate

Classes

Chemical: angiotensin-converting enzyme (ACE) inhibitor, nonsulfhydryl
Therapeutic: antihypertensive

Pregnancy Category: C (1st trimester), D (2nd and 3rd trimesters)

Trade Names

Prescription: Enalaprilat, Enalaprit Novaplus, Vasotec

Combinations

Prescription: with diltiazem (Teczem); with felodipine (Lexxel); with hydrochlorothiazide (Vaseretic)

Do not confuse enalapril with Anafranil, Eldepryl, or ramipril.

CLINICAL PHARMACOLOGY

Mechanism of Action

This angiotensin-converting enzyme (ACE) inhibitor suppresses the renin-angiotensin-aldosterone system and prevents conversion of angiotensin I to angiotensin II, a potent vasoconstrictor; may inhibit angiotensin II at local vascular, renal sites. Decreases plasma angiotensin II, increases plasma renin activity, decreases aldosterone secretion. **Therapeutic Effect:** In hypertension, reduces peripheral arterial resistance. In congestive heart failure, increases cardiac output; decreases peripheral vascular resistance, BP, pulmonary capillary wedge pressure, heart size.

PHARMACOKINETICS

Route	Onset	Peak	Duration
PO	1 hr	4-6 hr	24 hr
IV	15 min	1-4 hr	6 hr

Readily absorbed from the GI tract (not affected by food). Protein binding: 50%-60%. Converted to active metabolite. Primarily excreted in urine. Removed by hemodialysis. **Half-life:** 11 hr (half-life is increased in those with impaired renal function).

AVAILABILITY

Tablets: 2.5 mg, 5 mg, 10 mg, 20 mg.
Injection: 1.25 mg/mL.

INDICATIONS AND DOSAGE

Hypertension alone or in combination with other antihypertensives

PO

Adults, Elderly: Initially, 2.5-5 mg/day. May increase at 1- to 2-wk intervals. Range: 10-40 mg/day in 1-2 divided doses. **Children:** 0.1 mg/kg/day in 1-2 divided doses. Maximum: 0.5 mg/kg/day. **Neonates:** 0.08 mg/kg every 24 hr.

IV

Adults, Elderly: 0.625-1.25 mg every 6 hr up to 5 mg every 6 hr. **Children, Neonates:** 5-10 mcg/kg/dose every 8-24 hr.

Adjunctive therapy for heart failure

PO

Adults, Elderly: Initially, 2.5-5 mg/day. Range: 5-20 mg/day in 2 divided doses.

Dosage in renal impairment

Dosage is modified based on creatinine clearance.

Creatinine Clearance	% Usual Dose every 12 hr
10-50 mL/min	75-100
Less than 10 mL/min	50

OFF-LABEL USES

Diabetic nephropathy, hypertension due to scleroderma renal crisis, hypertensive crisis, idiopathic edema, renal artery stenosis, rheumatoid arthritis, post-MI for prevention of ventricular failure

CONTRAINDICATIONS

History of angioedema from previous treatment with enalapril, enalaprilat, or other ACE inhibitors; pregnancy

INTERACTIONS

Drug: Alcohol, antihypertensives, diuretics: May increase the effects of enalapril. **Herbal:** None known. **Food:** None known.

DIAGNOSTIC TEST EFFECTS

May increase BUN and serum alkaline phosphatase, serum bilirubin, serum creatinine, serum potassium, AST (SGOT), and ALT (SGPT) levels. May decrease serum sodium levels. May cause positive antinuclear antibody (ANA) titer.

IV INCOMPATIBILITIES

Amphotericin B (Fungizone), amphotericin B complex (Abelcet, Ambisome, Amphotec), cefepime (Maxipime), phenytoin (Dilantin)

IV COMPATIBILITIES

Calcium gluconate, *DOBUTamine (Dobutrex), *DOPamine (Inotropin), fentanyl (Sublimaze), heparin, lidocaine, magnesium sulfate, morphine, nitroglycerin, potassium chloride, potassium phosphate, propofol (Diprivan)

SIDE-EFFECTS

Frequent (7%-5%): Headache, dizziness. **Occasional (3%-2%):** Orthostatic hypotension, fatigue, diarrhea, cough, syncope. **Rare (less than 2%):** Angina, abdominal pain, vomiting, nausea, rash, asthenia (loss of strength, energy), syncope

CRITICAL CARE CONSIDERATIONS

ADMINISTRATION/HANDLING

PO ALERT

- Give enalapril without regard to food.
- Tablets may be crushed if necessary.
- Store below 30°C (86°F) in a moisture-proof, tightly closed container.

IV ALERT

- **Storage:** Enalaprilat should be stored below 30°C (86°F).
- **Stability:** Stable for 24 hr at room temperature when mixed with IV diluents. Use only clear, colorless solutions.
- **IV diluents:** May be mixed with 5% dextrose, normal saline, dextrose 5% with normal saline, 5% dextrose with Ringer's lactate, Isolyte E.
- **Infusion:** Enalaprilat should be given as a slow IV infusion as provided or diluted with 50 mL of IV diluent.
- **IV piggyback:** Infuse over 10-15 min.
- **IV push:** Give undiluted over 5 min.

PRECAUTIONS

HEALTH-RELATED

- Use cautiously in patients with history of angioedema, aortic stenosis, hypertrophic cardiomyopathy, cerebrovascular or coronary insufficiency, hypovolemia, renal impairment, and sodium depletion.
- Use cautiously during surgery or in any setting where anesthesia is used and patients may become hypotensive.
- Use cautiously in patients who are receiving dialysis and diuretic therapy.

AGE-RELATED

- **Children:** Safety and efficacy of enalapril have not been established.
- **Elderly:** May be more susceptible to the hypotensive effects of enalapril, especially if also taking diuretics.

PREGNANCY/LACTATION-RELATED

- Pregnancy category C (first trimester), category D (second and third trimesters); ACE inhibitors can cause fetal and neonatal morbidity and death when administered to pregnant women; when pregnancy is detected, discontinue ACE inhibitors as soon as possible; detectable in breast milk in trace amounts; effect on nursing infant has not been determined; use with caution in nursing mothers.

MONITORING

- **Baseline assessment:** Assess BP immediately before each enalapril dose. BP may fluctuate during therapy.
- **Lab work:** Complete blood count (CBC) and blood chemistry before beginning enalapril therapy, then every 2 wk for 3 mo and periodically thereafter in patients with autoimmune disease, renal impairment, or who are taking drugs that affect immune or leukocyte responses.
- **Neutropenia:** Monitor WBC counts with CBC.
- **Dizziness:** Assist patients with ambulation if dizziness occurs. Encourage remaining recumbent following initial dosage.
- **Renal insufficiency:** Monitor for increased BUN, serum creatinine, and serum potassium levels.

- **Diarrhea:** Assess pattern of daily bowel activity and stool consistency.
- **Patient education:** Advise rising slowly from a lying to a sitting position and to permit legs to dangle from the bed momentarily before standing to reduce the hypotensive effect of enalapril. When using enalapril outside the hospital, explain that the full therapeutic effect of BP reduction may take several weeks to appear if using the oral preparation. Caution against noncompliance with drug therapy or skipping drug doses because this may produce severe, rebound hypertension. Urge limiting alcohol consumption while taking enalapril.
- **Significant side effects:** Warn to report diarrhea, difficulty breathing, excessive perspiration, vomiting, or swelling of the face, lips, or tongue.

SERIOUS ADVERSE REACTIONS

- **First dose syncope:** Excessive hypotension may occur in patients with heart failure and in those who are severely salt- or volume-depleted.
- **Angioedema:** Swelling of the face and lips and hyperkalemia occur rarely.
- **Agranulocytosis and neutropenia:** May be seen in patients with collagen vascular diseases, including scleroderma and systemic lupus erythematosus, and impaired renal function.
- **Nephrotic syndrome:** May be noted in those with history of renal disease.

OVERDOSE/TOXICITY

- **Hepatotoxicity:** Elevated liver enzymes, cholestatic jaundice.
- **Nephrotoxicity:** Oliguria, anuria, elevated BUN, and creatinine.
- **Cardiac effects:** Bradycardia, atrial fibrillation, chest pain, palpitations.
- **GI decontamination:** No specific recommendations.

ANTIDOTE/DIALYSIS

- **Antidote:** No specific recommendations.
- **Dialysis:** Enalapril is removed by hemodialysis and peritoneal dialysis and is likely to be removed by high-permeability hemodialysis. Hypersensitivity reactions have been reported in patients undergoing hemodialysis using high-flux dialysis membranes (e.g., AN69) when receiving enalapril and other ACE inhibitors. Consideration should be given to using another type of membrane for patients on ACE inhibitors.

enfuvirtide

en-fyoo'-vir-tide

Classes

Chemical: fusion inhibitor, HIV; polypeptide, synthetic
Therapeutic: antiretroviral

Pregnancy Category: B

Trade Names

Prescription: Fuzeon

Do not confuse Fuzeon with Furoxone.

CLINICAL PHARMACOLOGY

Mechanism of Action

A fusion inhibitor that interferes with the entry of HIV-1 into CD4+ cells by inhibiting the fusion of viral and cellular membranes. **Therapeutic Effect:** Impairs HIV replication, slowing the progression of HIV infection.

PHARMACOKINETICS

Comparable absorption when injected into subcutaneous tissue of abdomen, arm, or thigh. Protein binding: 92%. Undergoes catabolism to amino acids. **Half-life:** 3.8 hr.

AVAILABILITY

Powder for injection: 108-mg (approximately 90 mg/mL when reconstituted) vials.

INDICATIONS AND DOSAGE

HIV infection (in combination with other antiretrovirals)

Subcutaneous

Adults, Elderly: 90 mg (1 mL) twice per day. **Children 6-16 yr:** 2 mg/kg twice per day. Maximum 90 mg twice per day.

Pediatric Dosing Guidelines

Weight: kg (lb)	Dose: mg (mL)
11-15.5 (24-34)	27 (0.3)
15.6-20 (35-44)	36 (0.4)
20.1-24.5 (45-54)	45 (0.5)
24.6-29 (55-64)	54 (0.6)
29.1-33.5 (65-74)	63 (0.7)
33.6-38 (75-84)	72 (0.8)
38.1-42.5 (85-94)	81 (0.9)
Greater than 42.5 (greater than 94)	90 (1)

CONTRAINDICATIONS

Hypersensitivity to enfuvirtide

INTERACTIONS

Drug: None known. **Herbal:** None known. **Food:** None known.

DIAGNOSTIC TEST EFFECTS

May elevate blood glucose and serum amylase, creatine kinase (CK), lipase, triglyceride, AST (SGOT), and ALT (SGPT) levels. May decrease blood hemoglobin levels and WBC count.

SIDE-EFFECTS

Expected (98%): Local injection site reactions (pain, discomfort, induration, erythema, nodules, cysts, pruritus, ecchymosis). **Frequent (26%-16%):** Diarrhea, nausea, fatigue. **Occasional (11%-4%):** Insomnia, peripheral neuropathy, depression, cough, decreased appetite or weight loss, sinusitis, anxiety, asthenia, myalgia, cold sores. **Rare (3%-2%):** Constipation, influenza, upper abdominal pain, anorexia, conjunctivitis

CRITICAL CARE CONSIDERATIONS

ADMINISTRATION/HANDLING

SUBCUTANEOUS ALERT

- Store the drug at room temperature. Refrigerate the reconstituted solution and use it within 24 hr.
- Reconstitute the drug with 1.1 mL of sterile water for injection. Visually inspect the vial for particulate matter. The solution normally appears clear and colorless. Discard the unused portion. Bring the reconstituted solution to room temperature before injection.
- Administer the drug subcutaneously into the upper abdomen, anterior thigh, or arm. Rotate injection sites.

PRECAUTIONS

HEALTH-RELATED

- Studies have not been conducted for use in patients with liver and renal disease.
- **CYP 450 enzymes:** Enfuvirtide does not inhibit these enzymes.
- Enfuvirtide must be taken as part of a combination antiretroviral regimen. Use of the drug alone may lead to rapid development of virus resistant to enfurvirtide and possibly other drugs in the same class.

AGE-RELATED

- **Children:** Safety and efficacy of enfuvirtide have not been established in children 6 yr and younger.
- **Elderly:** No age-related precautions have been noted in the elderly.

PREGNANCY/LACTATION-RELATED

- Pregnancy category B; breast milk excretion unknown (breast-feeding not advised for women infected with HIV).

MONITORING

- **Baseline assessment:** Assess medication history, including which drugs have been most effective in controlling the HIV virus.
- **Baseline and ongoing lab work:** Liver function tests and serum triglyceride levels, before and periodically during enfuvirtide therapy.
- **Local injection site reactions:** Assess skin for local injection site reactions, which are fairly common.
- **Bacterial pneumonia:** Monitor for cough, fever, and respiratory distress. If seen, obtain a chest x-ray to help diagnose pneumonia.
- **Impending hypersensitivity reaction:** Observe for fatigue, nausea, chills, respiratory distress, vomiting, hypotension, and Guillain-Barre–like symptoms.
- **Insomnia:** Evaluate sleep patterns and monitor for insomnia.
- **Depression:** Monitor for depression related to chronic illness.
- **Patient education:** Advise continuing to take enfuvirtide for the full course of treatment when using drug outside the hospital. Warn that this drug may cause bacterial pneumonia and hypersensitivity reactions. Instruct seeking medical attention if cough with fever and rapid difficult breathing occurs. Inform that enfuvirtide is not a cure for HIV infection nor does it reduce the risk of transmitting HIV to others. Explain the need to continue practices to prevent transmission of HIV.

SERIOUS ADVERSE REACTIONS

- **Bacterial pneumonia:** Enfuvirtide use may potentiate bacterial pneumonia.

OVERDOSE/TOXICITY

- Hypersensitivity (rash, fever, chills, rigors, hypotension), thrombocytopenia, neutropenia, and renal insufficiency or failure may occur rarely.
- **GI decontamination:** No specific recommendations.

ANTIDOTE/DIALYSIS

- **Antidote:** No specific recommendations.
- **Dialysis:** It is unlikely that enfuvirtide is removed by hemodialysis, peritoneal dialysis, or high-permeability hemodialysis.

E

enoxaparin sodium

ee-nox-a-pa'-rin soe'-dee-um

Classes

Chemical: heparin derivative, depolymerized; low-molecular weight heparin
Therapeutic: anticoagulant

Pregnancy Category: B

Trade Names

Prescription: Clexane ♣, Klexane ♣, Lovenox

Do not confuse Lovenox with Lotronex.

CLINICAL PHARMACOLOGY

Mechanism of Action

A low-molecular-weight heparin that potentiates the action of antithrombin III and inactivates coagulation factor Xa. **Therapeutic Effect:** Produces anticoagulation. Does not significantly influence bleeding time, prothrombin time, or aPTT.

PHARMACOKINETICS

Route	Onset	Peak	Duration
Subcutaneous	N/A	3-5 hr	12 hr

Well absorbed after subcutaneous administration. Eliminated primarily in urine. Not removed by hemodialysis. **Half-life:** 4.5 hr.

AVAILABILITY

Injection: 30 mg/0.3 mL, 40 mg/0.4 mL, 60 mg/0.6 mL, 80 mg/0.8 mL, 100 mg/mL, 120 mg/0.8 mL, 150 mg/mL in prefilled syringes.

INDICATIONS AND DOSAGE

Prevention of deep vein thrombosis (DVT) after hip and knee surgery

Subcutaneous

Adults, Elderly: 30 mg twice per day, generally for 7-10 days.

Prevention of DVT after abdominal surgery

Subcutaneous

Adults, Elderly: 40 mg per day for 7-10 days.

Prevention of long-term DVT in nonsurgical acute illness

Subcutaneous

Adults, Elderly: 40 mg once per day for 3 wk.

Prevention of ischemic complications of unstable angina and non-Q-wave MI (with oral aspirin therapy)

Subcutaneous

Adults, Elderly: 1 mg/kg every 12 hr.

Acute DVT

Subcutaneous

Adults, Elderly: 1 mg/kg every 12 hr or 1.5 mg/kg once daily.

Usual pediatric dosage

Subcutaneous

Children: 0.5 mg/kg every 12 hr (prophylaxis); 1 mg/kg every 12 hr (treatment).

Dosage in renal impairment

Clearance of enoxaparin is decreased when creatinine clearance is less than 30 mL/min. Monitor patient and adjust dosage as necessary. When enoxaparin is used in abdominal, hip, or knee surgery or acute illness, the dosage in renal impairment is 30 mg once per day. When enoxaparin is used to treat DVT, angina, or MI the dosage in renal impairment is 1 mg/kg once per day.

OFF-LABEL USES

Prevention of DVT following general surgical procedures

CONTRAINDICATIONS

Active major bleeding; concurrent heparin therapy; hypersensitivity to enoxaparin, heparin, or pork products; thrombocytopenia associated with positive in vitro test for antiplatelet antibodies; heparin-induced thrombocytopenia (HIT)

INTERACTIONS

Drug: **Anticoagulants, platelet inhibitors:** May increase bleeding. **Herbal:** None known. **Food:** None known.

DIAGNOSTIC TEST EFFECTS

Increases (reversible) LDH, serum alkaline phosphatase, AST (SGOT), and ALT (SGPT) levels.

SIDE-EFFECTS

Occasional (4%-1%): Injection site hematoma, nausea, peripheral edema

CRITICAL CARE CONSIDERATIONS

ADMINISTRATION/HANDLING

SUBCUTANEOUS ALERT

- Store at room temperature. Parenteral form normally appears clear and colorless to pale yellow.
- Instruct patients to lie down before administering by deep subcutaneous injection.
- **Abdominal wall injection:** Inject between the left and right anterolateral and left and right posterolateral abdominal wall. Introduce entire length of needle (.5 inch) into

skinfold held between thumb and forefinger, holding skinfold during injection.

- **Initial postoperative dose:** Give initial dose as soon as possible after surgery but not more than 24 hr after surgery.
- **Dosage:** Enoxaparin cannot be used interchangeably (unit for unit) with heparin or other low molecular weight heparins, as they differ in their manufacturing process, molecular weight distribution, anti-Xa and anti-IIa activities and units.

IM ALERT

- **Do not give IM:** Do not mix with other injections or infusions.

PRECAUTIONS

HEALTH-RELATED

- **Heparin induced thrombocytopenia (HIT):** Use with extreme caution in patients with a history HIT/white clot syndrome, as some patients may develop the syndrome with enoxaparin.
- **Increased risk of bleeding:** Use enoxaparin cautiously in patients at high risk of bleeding with increased risk of hemorrhage including those with bacterial endocarditis, congenital or acquired bleeding disorders, hemorrhagic stroke, recent brain, spinal or ophthalmalogic surgery, those receiving platelet inhibitors, history of recent GI ulceration and hemorrhage, impaired renal function, or uncontrolled systemic hypertension.
- **Prosthetic heart valves:** Enoxaparin is not recommended for clot prevention in patients with prosthetic heart valves because the drug is not always effective in these patients. Pregnant women with prosthetic heart valves are at increased risk for thromboembolism.

AGE-RELATED

- **Children:** Safety and efficacy of enoxaparin have not been established in children.
- **Elderly:** May be more susceptible to bleeding, especially if renal impaired because of delayed elimination of the drug.

PREGNANCY/LACTATION-RELATED

- Pregnancy category B; reports of congenital anomalies and fetal death, cause-and-effect relationship has not been determined; excretion into breast milk unknown; use caution in nursing mothers.

MONITORING

- **Baseline assessment:** Determine history of HIT or other allergies, especially to heparin or pork products, and assess for risk for bleeding. Assess lower legs for deep vein thrombosis (redness, swelling, positive Homan's sign).
- **Baseline lab work:** Complete blood count (CBC) including platelet count and possibly coagulation studies if other antithrombotic agents are being taken and/or possible bleeding is a concern. Prothrombin time and PTT are relatively insensitive measures for ongoing monitoring of enoxaparin effects. Liver enzymes may be noted if the patient is high risk for MI, pulmonary emboli, or liver disease.
- **Ongoing lab work:** Periodically monitor CBC for anemia and thrombocytopenia, stool for occult blood, and coagulation studies if bleeding occurs. There is no need for daily monitoring in patients with normal presurgical coagulation parameters. Prothrombin time and PTT are relatively insensitive measures for ongoing monitoring of enoxaparin effects. Antifactor Xa may be used to monitor renal impaired patients or if bleeding occurs. Liver enzymes are increased by enoxaparin, so must be interpreted with care during differential diagnoses.
- **Therapeutic effect:** Enoxaparin will prevent incidence of DVT without causing bleeding.
- **Bleeding:** Assess for bleeding at injection or surgical sites, from gums, blood in stool, bruising, hematuria, petechiae, neurologic deterioration, deteriorated vision, or eye pain.
- **Epidural catheter for pain management:** Decision to use enoxaparin when patients have an indwelling epidural or spinal catheter should weigh risk of developing paralysis due to spinal bleeding against benefit of preventing deep vein thrombosis. Patients must be monitored closely for loss of sensation and movement in lower extremities if epidural or spinal catheter is in place.
- **Menstrual flow:** Female patients may have heavier than usual menstrual flow.
- **Patient education:** Tell patients that the usual length of therapy is 7-10 days. If therapy continues outside the hospital, instruct to report immediately bleeding from surgical site, black or red stool, coffee-ground vomitus, dark or red urine, red-speckled mucus from cough, chest pain, or dyspnea to a health care provider. Advise using an electric razor and soft toothbrush to prevent bleeding during

therapy. Advise not to take other medications, including OTC drugs (especially aspirin), without prior discussion with a health care provider.

SERIOUS ADVERSE REACTIONS

- **Spinal/epidural hematomas:** If spinal or epidural anesthesia or analgesia are used during surgery and/or indwelling catheters are inserted for postoperative pain management, patients receiving enoxaparin are at risk for developing an epidural or spinal hematoma which can result in long-term or permanent paralysis.
- **Mild to moderate bleeding:** Local ecchymoses, hemoptysis, blood in stool, progressive anemia, bleeding gums, thrombocytopenia.

OVERDOSE/TOXICITY

- Overdose may lead to bleeding complications, including major internal or external hemorrhage. Intracranial bleeding and intraocular bleeding may be experienced, which may lead to permanent impairment or blindness.
- **Management:** Administer protamine sulfate to reverse effects of enoxaparin. For neurologic deterioration indicative of stroke or chest pain indicative of possible acute MI, prompt action is necessary to help reduce the chance of permanent impairment. Administer blood products for severe anemia and hemorrhagic shock along with fluids and vasopressors if needed to maintain blood pressure. Severe anemia can prompt myocardial ischemia leading to acute MI or cerebral ischemia in high-risk patients with or without profound hypotension.
- **GI decontamination:** No specific recommendations.

ANTIDOTE/DIALYSIS

- **Antidote:** Protamine sulfate (1% solution) equal to the dose of enoxaparin injected. One mg protamine sulfate neutralizes 1 mg enoxaparin. A second dose of 0.5 mg protamine sulfate per 1 mg enoxaparin may be given if aPTT tested 2-4 hr after first injection remains prolonged. Antifactor Xa is superior to aPTT for monitoring effects of enoxaparin.
- **Dialysis:** Enoxaparin is not removed by hemodialysis and is unlikely to be removed by peritoneal dialysis. No data are available on removal using high-permeability hemodialysis.

entacapone

en-ta'-ka-pone

Classes

Chemical: catechol-*O*-methyl-tranferase (COMT) inhibitor, nitrocatechol
Therapeutic: antiparkinson's agent

Pregnancy Category: C

Trade Names

Prescription: Comtan

CLINICAL PHARMACOLOGY

Mechanism of Action

An antiparkinson agent that inhibits the enzyme, catechol-*O*-methyltransferase (COMT), potentiating dopamine activity and increasing the duration of action of levodopa. **Therapeutic Effect:** Decreases signs and symptoms of Parkinson's disease.

PHARMACOKINETICS

Rapidly absorbed after PO administration. Protein binding: 98%. Metabolized in the liver. Primarily eliminated by biliary excretion. Not removed by hemodialysis. **Half-life:** 2.4 hr.

AVAILABILITY

Tablets: 200 mg.

INDICATIONS AND DOSAGE

Adjunctive treatment of Parkinson's disease

PO

Adults, Elderly: 200 mg concomitantly with each dose of carbidopa and levodopa up to a maximum of 8 times per day (1600 mg).

CONTRAINDICATIONS

Hypersensitivity to entacapone, use within 14 days of MAOIs

INTERACTIONS

Drug: **Ampicillin, cholestyramine, erythromycin, probenecid:** May decrease the excretion of entacapone. **Bitolterol, *DOBUTamine, *DOPamine, epinephrine, isoetharine, isoproterenol, methyldopa, norepinephrine:** May increase the risk of dysrhythmias and changes in BP. **Nonselective MAOIs (including phenelzine):** May inhibit catecholamine metabolism. **Other CNS depressants:** May increase CNS depression. **Herbal:** None known. **Food:** None known.

DIAGNOSTIC TEST EFFECTS

None known.

SIDE-EFFECTS

Frequent (greater than 10%): Dyskinesia, nausea, dark yellow or orange urine and sweat, diarrhea. **Occasional (9%-3%):** Abdominal pain, vomiting, constipation, dry mouth, fatigue, back pain. **Rare (less than 2%):** Anxiety, somnolence, agitation, dyspepsia, flatulence, diaphoresis, asthenia, dyspnea

CRITICAL CARE CONSIDERATIONS

ADMINISTRATION/HANDLING

PO ALERT

- Always administer entacapone with carbidopa and levodopa.
- Give entacapone without regard to food.

PRECAUTIONS

HEALTH-RELATED

- Use entacapone cautiously in patients with hepatic or renal impairment, ongoing diarrhea, orthostatic hypotension, or syncope.

AGE-RELATED

- **Children:** Entacapone has no potential identified use in children.
- **Elderly:** No age-related precautions have been noted.

PREGNANCY/LACTATION-RELATED

- Pregnancy category C; use caution in nursing mothers.

MONITORING

- **Baseline assessment:** Obtain baseline vital signs, note BP. Assess for dyskinesic movements, muscle rigidity, gait alteration, and facial expression. Ensure patients are not receiving MAOIs.
- **Baseline lab work:** Biochemical profile, including liver enzymes, CPK, BUN, and creatinine.
- **Administer with carbidopa and levodopa:** Entacapone is used to prolong effects of other antiparkinsonian medications and is not intended for use as a sole agent.
- **Side effects:** Monitor for increased dyskinesia, diarrhea, hallucinations, confusion, orthostatic hypotension, fever, muscle pain, dark urine and jaundice, which may indicate intolerance of entacapone.
- **Dysrhythmias and hypertension:** Patients receiving catecholamine infusions should have continuous ECG monitoring and frequent BP measurements to identify enhanced effects of catecholamines when entacapone is given.
- **Therapeutic effect:** Assess for relief of symptoms, including improvement of mask-like facial expression, muscular rigidity, shuffling gait, and resting tremors of the hands and head.
- **Patient education:** When using entacapone outside the hospital, instruct to take entacapone with carbidopa and levodopa. Caution avoidance of tasks that require mental alertness or motor skills until response to the drug is known. Entacapone may cause sweat or urine to turn dark yellow or orange. Instruct to report an increase in uncontrolled movement of the hands, arms, legs, eyelids, face, mouth, or tongue.

SERIOUS ADVERSE REACTIONS

- Increased dyskinesia, persistent severe diarrhea, hallucinations, confusion, muscle pain, increased liver enzymes, jaundice, fever, hypotension.
- **Patients receiving catecholamine infusions:** Patients on *DOBUTamine, *DOPamine, epinephrine, isoproterenol, and norepinephrine are at increased risk of dysrhythmias and may experience hypertension with a relatively small dose of the infusions.

OVERDOSE/TOXICITY

- **Neuroleptic malignant-like syndrome:** A rare, unexpected, atypical reaction including elevated temperature, muscular rigidity, altered level of consciousness, elevated CPK, which should resolve when entacapone is discontinued.
- **Rhabdomyolysis:** Extreme elevation in CPK, myoglobinuria, brown- or rust-colored urine, muscle pain, acute renal failure.
- **Liver failure:** Elevated liver enzymes, jaundice, generalized third spaced fluid, ascites, and dark urine.
- **Management of muscle rigidity and fever:** Patients will benefit from rapid resolution of muscle rigidity using intravenous benzodiazepines (diazepam, lorazepam), antipyretics to control fever, and external cooling blanket. Neuromuscular blockade (drug-induced paralysis) has been used in extreme cases.
- **GI decontamination:** No specific recommendations.

ANTIDOTE/DIALYSIS

- **Antidote:** No specific recommendations.
- **Dialysis:** Hemodialysis, high-permeability hemodialysis, or peritoneal dialysis are not likely to effectively remove entacapone.

ephedrine

eh-fed'-rin

Classes

Chemical: catecholamine
Therapeutic: bronchodilator, decongestant, vasopressor

Pregnancy Category: C

E

Trade Names

Over the Counter: Pretz-D, Kondon's Nasal

Combinations

Prescription: with potassium iodide, phenobarbital, theophylline (Quadrinal), with *hydrOXYzine, theophylline (Hydrophed DF, Marax-DF); with guaifenesin (Broncholate, Ephex SR)

Do not confuse ephedrine with epinephrine.

CLINICAL PHARMACOLOGY

Mechanism of Action

An adrenergic agonist that stimulates alpha-adrenergic receptors causing vasoconstriction and pressor effects, $beta_1$-adrenergic receptors, resulting in cardiac stimulation, and $beta_2$-adrenergic receptors, resulting in bronchial dilation and vasodilation. **Therapeutic Effect:** Increases BP and pulse rate.

PHARMACOKINETICS

Well absorbed after nasal and parenteral absorption. Metabolized in liver. Excreted in urine. **Half-life:** 3-6 hr.

AVAILABILITY

Capsules: 25 mg.
Injection: 50 mg/mL.
Intranasal spray: 0.25% (Pretz-D).

INDICATIONS AND DOSAGE

Asthma

PO

Adults: 25-50 mg every 3-4 hr as needed. **Children:** 3 mg/kg/day in 4 divided doses.

Hypotension

IM

Adults. 25-50 mg as a single dose. Maximum 150 mg/day. **Children:** 0.2-0.3 mg/kg/dose every 4-6 hr.

IV

Adults: 5 mg/dose slow IV push as prevention. 10-25 mg/dose slow IV push repeated every 5-10 min as treatment. Maximum: 150 mg/day. **Children:** 0.2-0.3 mg/kg/dose slow IV push every 4-6 hr.

Subcutaneous

Adults: 25-50 every 4-6 hr. Maximum 150 mg/day. **Children:** 3 mg/kg/day every 4-6 hr.

Nasal congestion

PO

Adults: 25-50 mg every 6 hr as needed. **Children.** 3 mg/kg/day in 4 divided doses.

Nasal

Adults, Children 12 yr and older: 2-3 sprays into each nostril every 4 hr. **Children 6-12 yr:** 1-2 sprays into each nostril every 4 hr.

OFF-LABEL USES

Obesity, propofol-induced pain, radiocontrast media reactions

CONTRAINDICATIONS

Anesthesia with cyclopropane or halothane, diabetes (ephedrine injection), hypersensitivity to ephedrine or other sympathomimetic amines, hypertension or other cardiovascular disorders, pregnancy with maternal BP above 130/80, thyrotoxicosis

INTERACTIONS

Drug: Caffeine: May increase cardiac stimulation. **Cardiac glycosides, sympathomimetics, theophylline, general anesthetics:** May increase toxic cardiac stimulation. **Atropine, MAOIs, oxytocics, tricyclic antidepressants:** May increase cardiovascular effects. **Herbal: Ephedra, bitter orange, yohimbe:** May increase central nervous system (CNS) and cardiovascular stimulation and effects. **Food:** None known.

DIAGNOSTIC TEST EFFECTS

May result in false-positive amphetamine EMIT assay. Lactic acid serum values may be increased.

IV INCOMPATIBILITIES

Phenobarbital (Luminal), secobarbital (Seconal)

IV COMPATIBILITIES

Chloramphenicol, fenoldopam (Corlopam), lidocaine, metaraminol (Aramine), nafcillin (Unipen), penicillin G, propofol (Diprivan), tetracycline

SIDE-EFFECTS

Frequent: Hypertension, anxiety. **Occasional:** Nausea, vomiting, palpitations, tremor. **Nasal:** Burning, stinging, runny nose. **Rare:** Psychosis, decreased urination, necrosis at injection site from repeated injections

CRITICAL CARE CONSIDERATIONS

ADMINISTRATION/HANDLING

INTRANASAL ALERT

- **Administration:** Before using spray, clear nasal passages; blow nose gently. Keep head in the upright position and spray into each nostril. After using ephedrine, blow nose well 3-5 min.
- Do not administer more frequently than every 4 hr to avoid dependence.

IV ALERT

- **Storage:** Store at room temperature. Do not use if solution appears discolored or contains a precipitate.
- **IV push:** Inject by slow IV push. Not usually added to IV solutions. Drug is less potent but longer acting than epinephrine.

PRECAUTIONS

HEALTH-RELATED

- Use cautiously in patients with angina pectoris, diabetes, hyperthyroidism, chronic heart disease, history of hypertension, or prostatic hypertrophy; drug has a cumulative effect.
- Ephedrine has generally been replaced by more effective vasopressors and bronchodilators, but is sometimes used orally (off-label) to help manage chronic orthostatic hypotension unresponsive to other agents.
- Ephedrine should not be used to treat an overdose of phenothiazines (e.g., *chlorproMAZINE [Thorazine]) because profound hypotension and irreversible shock may ensue.

AGE-RELATED

- **Children:** No age-related precautions have been noted in children.
- **Elderly:** Use very cautiously because of age-related risk of heart attack and stroke. Not recommended for elderly.

PREGNANCY/LACTATION-RELATED

- Pregnancy category C; routinely used to treat or prevent maternal hypotension following spinal anesthesia; may cause fetal heart rate changes; excretion into breast milk unknown; one case report of adverse effects (excessive crying, irritability, and disturbed sleeping patterns) in a 3-month-old nursing infant whose mother consumed disoephedrine.

MONITORING

- **Baseline assessment:** Obtain vital signs; note heart rate and BP. Determine history of heart, brain, or peripheral ischemia, diabetes, thyroid disease, or enlarged prostate.
- **Baseline diagnostic tests:** Baseline 12-lead ECG to compare for changes when therapy ensues. IV ephedrine is more dangerous than other routes.
- **Tachycardia and hypertension:** Monitor continuous ECG, BP, and pulse. Assess for mental status changes which may indicate cerebral ischemia or impending stroke.
- **Myocardial ischemia:** Monitor ECG for ST depression or elevation (acute MI).
- **Renal ischemia:** Monitor for decreased urine output.
- **Therapeutic effect:** Assess for decreased congestion and bronchoconstriction or resolution of chronic hypotension.
- **Patient education:** Instruct patient to promptly report side effects including headaches, dizziness, and fast heart beat to a health care provider. Urge avoidance of excessive caffeine consumption from chocolate, cocoa, coffee, cola, or tea. Ephedrine may cause nervousness and wakefulness, so it should be taken at least 4-6 hr before bedtime. Instruct on proper use of the nasal spray. Advise not to use nasal spray for more than 3-5 days. Runny or stuffy nose may worsen and increase risk of developing side effects.

SERIOUS ADVERSE REACTIONS

- Disorientation, weakness, hyperventilation, hyperglycemia, headache, nausea, vomiting, and diarrhea.

OVERDOSE/TOXICITY

- **Sympathomimetic syndrome:** Hypertension, intracranial hemorrhage, seizures, anginal pain, hyperglycemia, and fatal dysrhythmias. Prolonged or excessive use may result in metabolic acidosis due to increased serum lactic acid concentrations.
- **Mangement:** Treat hypotension with IV fluids; vasopressors (e.g., *DOPamine [Intropin]) are contraindicated. Treat hypertension with phentolamine (Regitine) or nitroprusside (Nipride) and seizures with benzodiazepines (diazepam [Valium], lorazepam [Ativan]). Treat tachycardias with beta-blockers (propranolol [Inderal], metoprolol [Lopressor]), but monitor

closely for acute hypertension; response to beta-blockers is variable.

- **GI decontamination:** No specific recommendations.

ANTIDOTE/DIALYSIS

- **Antidote:** No specific recommendations. Ephedrine should be immediately discontinued if severe side effects occur.
- **Dialysis:** No data are available on removal of ephedrine using hemodialyis, high-permeability hemodialysis, or peritoneal dialysis.

E

epinephrine

ep-i-nef'-rin

Classes

Chemical: catecholamine

Therapeutic: antiglaucoma agent, bronchodilator, decongestant, vasopressor

Pregnancy Category: C

Trade Names

Prescription: Adrenalin, Adrenalin Topical, EpiPen, EpiPen 2-Pak, EpiPen Auto Injector, EpiPen Jr. Auto Injector, Sus-Phrine Injection

Over the Counter: Adrenalin, AsthmaHaler Mist, Asthma-Nefrin, microNefrin, Nephron, Primatene Mist, S-2

Combinations

Prescription: with etidocaine (Duranest with Epinephrine); with prilocaine (Citanest Forte); with lidocaine (Xylocaine with Epinephrine); with pilocarpine (E-Pilo Ophthalmic)

Do not confuse epinephrine with ephedrine.

CLINICAL PHARMACOLOGY

Mechanism of Action

A sympathomimetic, adrenergic agonist that stimulates alpha-adrenergic receptors, causing vasoconstriction and pressor effects; $beta_1$-adrenergic receptors, resulting in cardiac stimulation; and $beta_2$-adrenergic receptors, resulting in bronchial dilation and vasodilation. With ophthalmic form, increases outflow of aqueous humor from anterior eye chamber. **Therapeutic Effect:** Relaxes smooth muscle of the bronchial tree, produces cardiac stimulation, and dilates skeletal muscle vasculature. The ophthalmic form dilates pupils and constricts conjunctival blood vessels.

PHARMACOKINETICS

Route	Onset	Peak	Duration
IM	5-10 min	20 min	1-4 hr
Subcutaneous	5-10 min	20 min	1-4 hr
Inhalation	3-5 min	20 min	1-3 hr
Ophthalmic	1 hr	4-8 hr	12-24 hr

Well absorbed after parenteral administration; minimally absorbed after inhalation. Metabolized in the liver, other tissues, and sympathetic nerve endings. Excreted in urine. The ophthalmic form may be systemically absorbed as a result of drainage into nasal pharyngeal passages. Mydriasis occurs within several min and persists several hr; vasoconstriction occurs within 5 min, and lasts less than 1 hr.

AVAILABILITY

Injection (Adrenalin): 0.1 mg/mL, 1 mg/mL.
Injection: 0.3 mg/0.3 mL (EpiPen Auto Injector), 0.15 mg/0.3 mL (EpiPen Jr Auto-Injector, EpiPen 2-Pak).
Inhalation (aerosol [Primatene Mist]): 0.2 mg/inhalation.
Inhalation solution: 1%, 2.25%.
Ophthalmic solution (Epifrin): 0.5%, 1%, 2%.
Subcutaneous suspension (Sus-Phrine Injection): 5 mg/mL.
Topical solution (Adrenalin, Topical): 1:100.

INDICATIONS AND DOSAGE

Anaphylaxis

IM

Adults, Elderly: 0.3 mg (0.3 mL of 1:1000 solution). May repeat if anaphylaxis persists. **Children:** 0.15-0.3 mg or 0.01 mg/kg for patients weighing less than 30 kg. May repeat if anaphylaxis persists.

Asthma

Subcutaneous

Adults, Elderly: 0.2-0.5 mg (0.2-0.5 mL of 1:1000 solution) every 2 hr as needed. In severe attacks, may repeat every 20 min times 3 doses. **Children:** 0.01 mL/kg/dose (1:1000 solution). Maximum: 0.4-0.5 mL/dose. May repeat every 15-20 min for 3-4 doses or every 4 hr as needed.

Inhalation

Adults, Elderly, Children 4 yr and older: 1 inhalation, wait at least 1 min. May repeat once. Do not use again for at least 3 hr.

Cardiac arrest

IV

Adults, Elderly: Initially, 1 mg. May repeat every 3-5 min as needed. **Children:** Initially,

0.01 mg/kg (0.1 mL/kg of a 1:10,000 solution). May repeat every 3-5 min as needed.

Endotracheal

Children: 0.1 mg/kg (0.1 mL/kg of a 1:1000 solution. May repeat every 3-5 min as needed.

Hypersensitivity reaction

IM, Subcutaneous

Adults, Elderly: 0.3-0.5 mg every 15-20 min

Subcutaneous

Children: 0.01 mg/kg every 15 min for 2 doses, then every 4 hr. Maximum single dose: 0.5 mg.

Inhalation

Adults, Elderly, Children 4 yr and older: 1 inhalation, may repeat in at least 1 min. Give subsequent doses no sooner than 3 hr.

Nebulizer

Adults, Elderly, Children 4 yr and older: 1-3 deep inhalations. Give subsequent doses no sooner than 3 hr.

Glaucoma

Ophthalmic

Adults, Elderly: 1-2 drops 1-2 times per day.

OFF-LABEL USES

Systemic: Treatment of gingival or pulpal hemorrhage, priapism

Ophthalmic: Treatment of conjunctival congestion during surgery, secondary glaucoma

CONTRAINDICATIONS

Cardiac dysrhythmias, cerebrovascular insufficiency, hypertension, hyperthyroidism, ischemic heart disease, narrow-angle glaucoma, shock, hypersensitivity to epinephrine

INTERACTIONS

Drug: **Beta-blockers:** May decrease the effects of beta-blockers. **Digoxin, sympathomimetics:** May increase risk of dysrhythmias. **Ergonovine, methergine, oxytocin:** May increase vasoconstriction. **MAOIs, tricyclic antidepressants:** May increase cardiovascular effects. Herbal: None known. Food: None known.

DIAGNOSTIC TEST EFFECTS

May decrease serum potassium level.

IV INCOMPATIBILITIES

Ampicillin (Omnipen, Polycillin)

IV COMPATIBILITIES

Calcium chloride, calcium gluconate, diltiazem (Cardizem), *DOBUTamine (Dobutrex), *DOPamine (Intropin), fentanyl (Sublimaze), heparin, hydromorphone (Dilaudid), lorazepam (Ativan), midazolam (Versed), milrinone (Primacor), morphine, nitroglycerin, norepinephrine (Levophed), potassium chloride, propofol (Diprivan)

SIDE-EFFECTS

Frequent: **Systemic:** Tachycardia, palpitations, nervousness. **Ophthalmic:** Headache, eye irritation, watering of eyes. Occasional: **Systemic:** Dizziness, lightheadedness, facial flushing, headache, diaphoresis, increased BP, nausea, trembling, insomnia, vomiting, fatigue **Ophthalmic:** Blurred or decreased vision, eye pain. Rare: **Systemic:** Chest discomfort or pain, dysrhythmias, bronchospasm, dry mouth or throat

CRITICAL CARE CONSIDERATIONS

ADMINISTRATION/HANDLING

SUBCUTANEOUS ALERT

- **Preparation:** Shake ampule thoroughly.
- **Administration:** Use a tuberculin syringe for injection into lateral deltoid region. Massage injection site to minimize vasoconstriction effect.
- **Anaphylactic shock:** Epinephrine is often used with corticosteroids to manage shock. If patients do not respond to subcutaneous dosing, IV infusion may be warranted.

INTRACARDIAC ALERT

- **Last resort only:** Give intracardiac only if no other route is available during cardiopulmonary resuscitation. Most patients may be endotracheally intubated and epinephrine may be given via the endotracheal tube into the respiratory tract.

ENDOTRACHEAL ALERT

- **Dilution:** Dilute 2.5 mg (1:1000) epinephrine in 10 mL normal saline solution (2.5 mg/10 mL) in a 10-mL syringe.
- **Administration:** Administer 2-2.5 mg for adults in divided doses into endotracheal tube. Use a mechanical resuscitation device (AmbuBag) to give several rapid breaths to help disperse the medication in the respiratory mucosa. The action of 1 mg IV epinephrine may be attained using 2.5 mg via endotracheal tube.

IV ALERT

- **Storage:** Store parenteral forms at room temperature. Do not use if solution appears pink or brown or contains a precipitate.

- **IV push injection:** Dilute 1 mg of 1:1000 solution with 10 mL 0.9% NaCl to provide 1:10,000 solution; inject each dose over more than 1 min.
- **IV continuous infusion:** Further dilute IV injection with 250-500 mL D_5W. Begin at lowest dose and titrate upward to desired BP and/or heart rate response. Average dose is 1-10 mcg/min.
- Maximum concentration of continuous IV infusion is 64 mg/250 mL.

EPINEPHRINE INFUSION DOSAGE/RATE TABLE

Dose mcg/min	1 mg/500 mL (2 mcg/mL)			1 mg/250 mL (4 mcg/mL)		
	mcg/hr	mL/hr	mL/min	mcg/hr	mL/hr	mL/min
1	60	30	0.5	60	15	0.25
2	120	60	1	120	30	0.5
3	180	90	1.5	180	45	0.75
4	240	120	2	240	60	1
5	300	150	2.5	360	75	1.25
8	480	240	4	480	120	2
10	600	300	5	600	150	2.5

PRECAUTIONS

HEALTH-RELATED

- Use epinephrine cautiously in patients with angina pectoris, diabetes mellitus, hypoxia, MI, psychoneurotic disorders, tachycardia, or severe hepatic or renal impairment.
- **Anesthesia:** Epinephrine is contraindicated in patients receiving anesthesia with halogenated hydrocarbons or cyclopropane.
- Do not use epinephrine to manage overdosage of adrenergic-blocking agents (phenoxybenzamine [Dibenzyline]), phenothiazines (*chlorproMAZINE [Thorazine]), methotrimeprazine (Levodrome), as further hypotension and irreversible shock may result.

AGE-RELATED

- **Children:** No age-related precautions have been noted in children.
- **Elderly:** Use caution when administering to older patients suspected of underlying diabetes, cardiac, vascular, neurologic, or other disorder.

PREGNANCY/LACTATION-RELATED

- Pregnancy category C; excreted into breast milk; use caution in nursing mothers.

MONITORING

- **Baseline assessment:** Obtain vital signs; note heart rate and BP. Assess for cardiovascular disease. Patients with heart disease may not tolerate increases in heart rate and increased cardiac rhythm irritability.
- **Baseline lab work:** Biochemical profile including blood glucose and electrolyte levels. Arterial blood gases for patients with respiratory distress.
- **Baseline diagnostic tests:** Obtain baseline 12-lead ECG to record baseline rhythm and assess for myocardial ischemia.
- **Vital signs:** Monitor BP, respiratory rate, and heart rate at least every 5 min when using epinephrine in unstable patients or when using IV push during cardiopulmonary resuscitation.
- **Hemodynamic monitoring:** Epinephrine infusion should prompt an increase in cardiac output and cardiac index.
- **Dysrhythmias:** Use continuous ECG monitoring to monitor for tachycardias and increased ventricular irritability. Assess biochemical panel for hypokalemia, which increases cardiac irritability.
- **Chest discomfort:** If chest discomfort is experienced, obtain a repeat 12-lead ECG, compare to baseline 12-lead ECG and assess for myocardial ischemia.
- **Respiratory distress:** For patients receiving epinephrine for an allergic reaction, monitor respiratory rate, depth, and work of breathing to ensure appropriate ventilation. Assess breath sounds for crackles, rhonchi, and wheezing. Check arterial blood gases if breathing deteriorates.
- **Hyperglycemia:** Monitor blood glucose levels because epinephrine creates insulin resistance. If patients require an insulin infusion, monitor hourly blood glucose and adjust insulin infusion with epinephrine; insulin resistance increases as dose of epinephrine increases, and decreases when epinephrine decreases.
- **Therapeutic effect:** If used for hypotension or to manage bradycardia, assess for resolution of bradycardia (heart rate increase) and increase in BP.
- **Cardiopulmonary resuscitation:** Monitor ECG and the patient's condition constantly. Administer epinephrine according to current Advanced Cardiac Life Support (ACLS) guidelines.

- **Patient education:** When patients use epinephrine outside the hospital to manage allergic reactions, urge them to avoid consuming excessive amounts of caffeine derivatives such as chocolate, cocoa, coffee, cola, and tea following administration. Explain that they will feel a slight burning or stinging when the drug is initially administered. Instruct to immediately report any new symptoms such as dizziness, shortness of breath, and tachycardia because they may be signs of systemic absorption.

SERIOUS ADVERSE REACTIONS

- Excessive doses may cause acute hypertension, extreme hyperglycemia, ST segment depression indicative of cardiac ischemia, and increasing dyshythmias.

OVERDOSE/TOXICITY

- **Metabolic acidosis:** Prolonged or excessive use may result in metabolic acidosis resulting from increased serum lactic acid concentrations secondary to hypoperfusion during shock state. Metabolic acidosis may cause disorientation, fatigue, hyperventilation, headache, nausea, vomiting, and diarrhea.
- **Lethal dysrhythmias:** Patients *not* in cardiac arrest who receive 1:1000 or 1:10,000 concentrations of epinephrine IV push may quickly experience lethal ventricular dysrhythmias.
- **Ventricular fibrillation or pulseless ventricular tachycardia:** May be managed with IV Vasopressin as a first agent instead of IV epinephrine using current ACLS guidelines.
- **Too rapid injection:** May cause cerebrovascular hemorrhage, tachycardia, ventricular fibrillation, severe headache, hypertension, irreversible hypotension, pulmonary edema, papillary dilation, restlessness, death.
- **GI decontamination:** No specific recommendations.

ANTIDOTE/DIALYSIS

- **Antidote:** Dysrhythmias induced by epinephrine may resolve with beta-blocking agents (propranolol, metoprolol). Profound hyperglycemia is corrected with continuous insulin infusion.
- **Dialysis:** No data are available regarding removal of epinephrine using hemodialysis, high-permeability hemodialysis, or peritoneal dialysis.

eplerenone

e-pler'-en-one

Classes

Chemical: pregnene methyl ester
Therapeutic: selective aldosterone receptor antagonist

Pregnancy Category: B

Trade Names

Prescription: Inspra

CLINICAL PHARMACOLOGY

Mechanism of Action

An aldosterone receptor antagonist that binds to the mineralocorticoid receptors in the kidney, heart, blood vessels, and brain, blocking the binding of aldosterone. Therapeutic Effect: Reduces BP.

PHARMACOKINETICS

Absorption unaffected by food. Protein binding: 50%. No active metabolites. Excreted in the urine with a lesser amount eliminated in the feces. Not removed by hemodialysis. Half-life: 4-6 hr.

AVAILABILITY

Tablets: 25 mg, 50 mg.

INDICATIONS AND DOSAGE

Hypertension

PO

Adults, Elderly: 50 mg once per day. If 50 mg once per day produces an inadequate BP response, may increase dosage to 50 mg twice per day. If patient is concurrently receiving erythromycin, saquinavir, verapamil, or fluconazole (after 4 wk, maximum 50 mg/day), reduce initial dose to 25 mg once per day.

Heart failure following MI

PO

Adults, Elderly: Initially, 25 mg once per day. If tolerated, titrate up to 50 mg once per day within 4 wk.

CONTRAINDICATIONS

Concurrent use of potassium supplements or potassium-sparing diuretics (such as amiloride, spironolactone, and triamterene), or strong inhibitors of the cytochrome P450 3A4 enzyme system (including ketoconazole and itraconazole), creatinine clearance less than 50 mL/min, serum creatinine level greater than 2 mg/dL in males or 1.8 mg/dL in females, serum potassium level greater than 5.5 mEq/L, type 2 diabetes mellitus with microalbuminuria, hypersensitivity to eplerenone

INTERACTIONS

Drug: **Angiotensin-converting enzyme (ACE)/protease inhibitors, angiotensin II antagonists, erythromycin, fluconazole, itraconazole, saquinavir, verapamil:** Increase risk of hyperkalemia. Herbal: **St. John's wort:** Decreases eplerenone effectiveness. Food: **Grapefruit, grapefruit juice:** Produces small increase in serum potassium level.

DIAGNOSTIC TEST EFFECTS

May increase serum potassium level. May decrease serum sodium level.

SIDE-EFFECTS

Rare (3%-1%): Dizziness, diarrhea, cough, fatigue, flulike symptoms, abdominal pain, headache

CRITICAL CARE CONSIDERATIONS

ADMINISTRATION/HANDLING

PO ALERT

- Film-coated tablets should not be broken, crushed, or chewed.
- Grapefruit juice may induce mild hyperkalemia if taken with eplerenone.

PRECAUTIONS

HEALTH-RELATED

- Use eplerenone cautiously in patients with hyperkalemia, mild renal insufficiency, diabetes, or hepatic impairment.
- **Cytochrome P450 metabolism:** Eplerenone is metabolized via CYP3A4 and should not be used with strong inhibitors of CYP3A4 to avoid potentially toxic effects of eplerenone.

AGE-RELATED

- **Children:** Safety and efficacy of eplerenone have not been established in children.
- **Elderly:** No age-related precautions have been noted.

PREGNANCY/LACTATION-RELATED

- Pregnancy category B; excreted into breast milk of lactating rabbits; human information unknown.

MONITORING

- **Baseline assessment:** Obtain heart rate and BP immediately before each dose, in addition to regular monitoring.
- **Baseline lab work:** Biochemical profile with sodium and potassium levels, BUN and creatinine, liver enzymes, cholesterol, and triglycerides.
- **Ongoing lab work:** Monitor for hyperkalemia and hyponatremia, liver and renal dysfunction, and hyperlipidemia in patients with borderline high lipid levels when therapy was begun.
- **BP fluctuations:** Assess BP for hypertension or hypotension.
- **Hypotension:** If excessive reduction in BP occurs, place in the supine position with feet slightly elevated. Assist with ambulation if needed.
- **Hyperkalemia:** Monitor ECG continuously for tall, thin T waves, prolonged PR interval, ST depression, widened QRS complex, and loss of P waves.
- **Impending cardiac arrest:** Profound widening of QRS with loss of P waves indicates cardiac arrest from hyperkalemia will ensue if measures to lower potassium quickly are not initiated promptly.
- **Patient education:** When eplerenone is used outside the hospital, instruct to avoid tasks that require mental alertness or motor skills until response to the drug is known. Explain that eplerenone will have to be taken throughout life to control hypertension. Eplerenone has rarely caused gynecomastia and abnormal vaginal bleeding. Advise not to break, crush, or chew film-coated tablets. Caution against exercising outside during hot weather to avoid dehydration and hypotension.

SERIOUS ADVERSE REACTIONS

- **Hyperkalemia:** More common in patients with type 2 diabetes mellitus and microalbuminuria, indicative of probable renal insufficiency.
- **Hyponatremia:** May be seen alone or in association with hyperkalemia.
- **Hyperlipidemia:** Rare increases in cholesterol and triglycerides have been reported.

OVERDOSE/TOXICITY

- **Severe hyperkalemia:** Irritability, abdominal cramping, diarrhea, ascending weakness, paresthesias; irregular pulse, abdominal distention and cardiac standstill may occur when level is greater than 8.5 mEq/L.
- **Management of hyperkalemia:** Kayexelate may not work quickly enough to avoid severe dysrhythmias and low BP. IV calcium gluconate will counteract the neuromuscular and cardiac effects of hyperkalemia. IV glucose and insulin, IV

sodium bicarbonate and beta-2 agonists (albuterol) may be used to shift potassium back into the cells for a temporary reduction in potassium level.

- **Severe hyponatremia:** Neurologic symptoms occur when serum sodium has decreased to 120-125 mEq/L and include confusion, restlessness or lassitude, and personality changes. Muscle weakness commonly occurs. Seizures, coma, and permanent neurologic damage can occur if sodium level is below 115 mEq/L. Volume status affects other symptoms related to hyponatremia.
- **Management of hyponatremia:** Managed based on volume status and levels of other electrolytes. IV hypertonic (3%) saline is used if serum sodium is dangerously low or patients have extreme symptoms.
- **GI decontamination:** No specific recommendations.

ANTIDOTE/DIALYSIS

- **Antidote:** No specific recommendations. Manage hyperkalemia and hyponatremia according to current standard of care.
- **Dialysis:** Eplerenone is not removed by hemodialysis. No data are available on removal using high-permeability hemodialysis or peritoneal dialysis. Hemodialysis may be used for rapid removal of potassium for acute hyperkalemia that is not effectively managed using medications.

epoetin alfa

eh-poh'-ee-tin al'-fa

Classes

Chemical: amino acid glycoprotein
Therapeutic: hematopoietic agent

Pregnancy Category: C

Trade Names

Prescription: Epogen, Procrit

Do not confuse Epogen with Neupogen.

CLINICAL PHARMACOLOGY

Mechanism of Action

A glycoprotein that stimulates division and differentiation of erythroid progenitor cells in bone marrow. Therapeutic Effect: Induces erythropoiesis and releases reticulocytes from bone marrow.

PHARMACOKINETICS

Well absorbed after subcutaneous administration. Following administration, an increase in reticulocyte count occurs within 10 days, and increases in Hgb, Hct, and RBC count are seen within 2-6 wk. Half-life: 4-13 hr (IV); 13-28 hr (subcutaneous).

AVAILABILITY

Injection (Epogen, Procrit): 2000 units/mL, 3000 units/mL, 4000 units/mL, 10,000 units/mL, 20,000 units/mL, 40,000 units/mL.

INDICATIONS AND DOSAGE

Treatment of anemia in chemotherapy patients

IV, Subcutaneous

Adults, Elderly, Children: 150 units/kg/dose 3 times wk. Maximum: 1200 units/kg/wk.

Reduction of allogenic blood transfusions in elective surgery

Subcutaneous

Adults, Elderly: 300 units/kg/day 10 days before day of, and 4 days after surgery, or 600 units/kg once weekly 21, 14, 7 days before surgery, plus a fourth dose on the day of surgery.

Chronic renal failure

IV Bolus, Subcutaneous

Adults, Elderly: Initially, 50-100 units/kg 3 times per wk. Target Hct range: 30%-36%. Adjust dosage no earlier than 1-mo intervals unless prescribed. Decrease dosage if Hct is increasing and approaching 36%. Plan to withhold doses temporarily if Hct continues to rise and to reinstate lower dosage when Hct begins to decrease. If Hct increases by more than 4 points in 2 wk, monitor Hct twice a wk for 2-6 wk. Increase dose if Hct does not increase 5-6 points after 8 wk (with adequate iron stores) and if Hct is below target range. Maintenance: *For patients on dialysis:* 75 units/kg 3 times per wk. Range: 12.5-525 units/kg. *For patients not on dialysis:* 75-150 units/kg/wk.

HIV infection in patients treated with AZT

IV, Subcutaneous

Adults: Initially, 100 units/kg 3 times per wk for 8 wk; may increase by 50-100 units/kg 3 times per wk. Evaluate response every 4-8 wk thereafter. Adjust dosage by 50-100 units/kg 3 times per wk. If dosages larger than 300 units/kg 3 times per wk are not eliciting response, it is unlikely patient will respond. Maintenance: Titrate to maintain desired Hct.

OFF-LABEL USES
Anemia associated with frequent blood donations, anemia in critically ill patients, malignancy, management of hepatitis C, myelodysplastic syndromes

CONTRAINDICATIONS
History of sensitivity to epoetin alfa, mammalian cell-derived products, or human albumin; uncontrolled hypertension

E

INTERACTIONS
Drug: **Heparin:** An increase in RBC volume may enhance blood clotting. Heparin dosage may need to be increased. **Herbal:** None known. **Food:** None known.

DIAGNOSTIC TEST EFFECTS
May increase BUN, serum phosphorus, serum potassium, serum creatinine, serum uric acid, and sodium levels. May decrease bleeding time, iron concentration, and serum ferritin levels.

IV INCOMPATIBILITIES
Do not mix with other medications.

SIDE-EFFECTS
Patients receiving chemotherapy: **Frequent (20%-17%):** Fever, diarrhea, nausea, vomiting, edema. **Occasional (13%-11%):** Asthenia, shortness of breath, paresthesia. **Rare (5%-3%):** Dizziness, trunk pain

Patients with chronic renal failure: **Frequent (24%-11%):** Hypertension, headache, nausea, arthralgia. **Occasional (9%-7%):** Fatigue, edema, diarrhea, vomiting, chest pain, skin reactions at administration site, asthenia, dizziness

Patients with HIV infection treated with AZT: **Frequent (38%-15%):** Fever, fatigue, headache, cough, diarrhea, rash, nausea. **Occasional (14%-9%):** Shortness of breath, asthenia, skin reaction at injection site, dizziness

CRITICAL CARE CONSIDERATIONS

ADMINISTRATION/HANDLING

IV ALERT
- **Storage:** Refrigerate vials.
- **Preparation:** Avoid excessive agitation/shaking of vial, which can cause foaming. Vigorous shaking may denature medication, rendering it inactive.
- **Dilution:** Reconstitution is not necessary.
- **IV bolus:** May be given as an IV bolus.

SUBCUTANEOUS ALERT
- Use one dose per vial. Do not reenter vial. Discard unused portion.
- **Mixing:** May be mixed in a syringe with bacteriostatic 0.9% NaCl with benzyl alcohol 0.9% or bacteriostatic saline at a 1:1 ratio.
- **Benzyl alcohol:** Acts as a local anesthetic; may reduce injection site discomfort.

PRECAUTIONS

HEALTH-RELATED
- Use epoetin alfa cautiously in patients with a history of seizures and known porphyria (an impairment of erythrocyte formation in bone marrow).
- Patients receiving AZT who have serum erythropoietin levels greater than 500 milliunits are not likely to respond to therapy.
- Renal patients undergoing vascular access graft placement may require discontinuation of epoetin alfa 2 wk before surgery to avoid graft clotting.
- Epoetin alfa is not intended for use in anemias resulting from iron or folate deficiencies, hemolysis, or GI bleeding.

AGE-RELATED
- **Children:** Safety and efficacy of epoetin alfa have not been established in children 12 yr and younger.
- **Elderly:** May be at increased risk of age-related renal and cardiovascular complications, including hypertension and vascular occlusion.

PREGNANCY/LACTATION-RELATED
- Pregnancy category C; excretion into breast milk unknown; use caution in nursing mothers.

MONITORING
- **Baseline assessment:** Assess BP before administering epoetin; 80% of patients with chronic renal failure have hypertension. BP may rise during early therapy.
- **Baseline lab work:** CBC with differential and platelet counts; note Hct. Assess bleeding time. Assess serum iron level. Transferrin saturation should be greater than 20%; serum ferritin level should be greater than 100 ng/mL before and during therapy. Assess biochemical profile for all patients, including BUN, creatinine, potassium, and phosphorous levels to assess for renal insufficiency.
- **Ongoing lab work:** Monitor Hct level twice weekly until patients have stabilized in target Hct range and twice weekly for

2-6 wk following dosage adjustments. Reduce the dosage if the Hct level increases more than 4 points in 2 wk or if hematocrit is greater than 36% in renal patients or 40% in other patients.

- **Supplemental iron:** All patients will eventually need supplemental iron therapy.
- **Hypertension:** Monitor aggressively for increased BP; 25% of patients receiving epoetin alfa require antihypertensive therapy and dietary restrictions.
- **Infection masked by immunosuppression:** Monitor body temperature, especially in patients receiving chemotherapy or with HIV infection treated with zidovudine.
- **Chronic renal failure:** Monitor serum BUN and creatinine, phosphorus, potassium, and uric acid levels, especially in patients with chronic renal failure.
- **Patient education:** Stress that frequent blood tests are needed to determine correct dosage. Stress importance of compliance with diet, vitamin supplementation (folic acid, B_{12}) and iron supplementation. Instruct to report severe headache and chest pain because this may indicate impending cardiovascular crisis. Caution about avoiding potentially hazardous activities during the first 90 days of therapy because of increased potential for development of seizures in chronic renal failure patients.

SERIOUS ADVERSE REACTIONS

- **Neurologic:** Hypertensive encephalopathy and seizures occur rarely.
- **Hyperkalemia:** Occurs more frequently in patients with chronic renal failure; usually in those who are noncompliant with medications, dietary guidelines, and frequency of dialysis regimen.

OVERDOSE/TOXICITY

- **Polycythemia or erythrocytosis:** Excessively high hematocrit may be thrombogenic; thrombosis, cerebrovascular accident, transient ischemic attacks, and acute MI occur rarely.
- **Management:** Consider phlebotomy if hematocrit is greater than 45% or if the patient is symptomatic for vascular occlusion. Anticoagulation may be required.
- **GI decontamination:** No specific recommendations.

ANTIDOTE/DIALYSIS

- **Antidote:** No specific recommendations. Hypertension resolves with reduced dose or discontinuation of epoetin alfa. Anticoagulation may be effective for patients experiencing vascular occlusion.
- **Dialysis:** Epoetin alfa is not removed by hemodialysis or peritoneal dialysis. No data are available regarding removal using high permeability hemodialysis. Epoetin alfa may be given to dialysis patients via the venous line at the end of the dialysis procedure to reduce need for additional venous access or subcutaneous injections. Clotting of vascular access and artificial kidney during dialysis is possible; dialysis patients may require additional anticoagulation.

E

epoprostenol sodium, prostacyclin

e-poe-pros'-ten-ol soe'-dee-um, pros-tah-sie'-clin

Classes

Chemical: prostaglandin I2
Therapeutic: vasodilator

Pregnancy Category: B

Trade Names

Prescription: Flolan

CLINICAL PHARMACOLOGY

Mechanism of Action

An antihypertensive that directly dilates pulmonary and systemic arterial vascular beds and inhibits platelet aggregation. **Therapeutic Effect:** Reduces right and left ventricular afterload; increases cardiac output and stroke volume.

PHARMACOKINETICS

Extensively metabolized by rapid hydrolysis at neutral pH in blood and by enzymatic degradation. The metabolites are excreted in urine. **Half-life:** 3-5 min.

AVAILABILITY

Injection, powder for reconstitution: 0.5 mg, 1.5 mg.

INDICATIONS AND DOSAGE

Long-term treatment of New York Heart Association Class III and IV primary pulmonary hypertension

IV Infusion

Adults, Elderly: Procedure to determine dose range: Initially, 2 ng/kg/min, increased in increments of 2 ng/kg/min every 15 min until dose-limiting adverse effects occur. Chronic infusion: Start at 4 ng/kg/min less than the maximum dose rate tolerated during acute dose ranging (or half of the maximum rate if rate was less than 5 ng/kg/min).

OFF-LABEL USES

Cardiopulmonary bypass surgery; hemodialysis; pulmonary hypertension associated with acute respiratory distress syndrome, systemic lupus erythematosus, or congenital heart disease; neonatal pulmonary hypertension, refractory heart failure; severe community-acquired pneumonia

CONTRAINDICATIONS

Long-term use in patients with heart failure (severe ventricular systolic dysfunction), hypersensitivity to epoprostenol

INTERACTIONS

Drug: Acetate in dialysis fluids, other vasodilators: May increase hypotensive effect. **Anticoagulants, antiplatelets:** May increase the risk of bleeding. **Vasoconstrictors:** May decrease effects of epoprostenol.
Herbal: None known. **Food:** None known.

DIAGNOSTIC TEST EFFECTS

None known.

IV INCOMPATIBILITIES

Do not mix epoprostenol with other medications.

SIDE-EFFECTS

Frequent: Acute phase: Flushing (58%), headache (49%), nausea (32%), vomiting (32%), hypotension (16%), anxiety (11%), chest pain (11%), dizziness (8%). **Chronic phase:** (greater than 20%): Dyspnea, asthenia, dizziness, headache, chest pain, nausea, vomiting, palpitations, edema, jaw pain, tachycardia, flushing, myalgia, nonspecific muscle pain, paresthesia, diarrhea, anxiety, chills, fever, or flulike symptoms. **Occasional: Acute phase (5%-2%):** Bradycardia, abdominal pain, muscle pain, dyspnea, back pain. **Chronic phase (20%-10%):** Rash, depression, hypotension, pallor, syncope, bradycardia, ascites. **Rare: Acute phase:** Paresthesia. **Chronic phase (less than 2%):** Diaphoresis, dyspepsia, tachycardia

CRITICAL CARE CONSIDERATIONS

ADMINISTRATION/HANDLING

IV ALERT

- **Storage:** Store unopened vial at room temperature. Do not freeze.
- **Stability:** Reconstituted solutions are stable for up to 48 hr if refrigerated. Stable in pump reservoir for 8 hr. Use of cold pouches with frozen gel packs can extend reservoir life to 24 hr. Time stored in refrigerator and in pump reservoir must be included in the 48-hr refrigeration stability time.
- **Dilution:** Follow instructions of manufacturer for dilution to specific concentrations. Use only the diluent provided by the manufacturer.
- **Infusion:** Give as pump infusion only. Infuse epoprostenol continuously through an indwelling central venous catheter. May temporarily infuse through a peripheral vein if necessary. While in use, must not be exposed to direct sunlight or temperatures above 25°C (77°F).
- **Infusion interruptions:** Flow rate must not be interrupted for longer than 2-3 min to avoid rebound pulmonary hypertension.

EPOPROSTENOL INFUSION RATE TABLE (3000 ng/mL)

Weight (kg)	DOSE (ng/kg/min)								
	2	4	6	8	10	12	14	16	18
	Infusion Rates (mL/min)								
10	—	—	1.2	1.6	2	2.4	2.8	3.2	3.6
20	—	1.6	2.4	3.2	4	4.8	5.6	6.4	7.2
30	1.2	2.4	3.6	4.8	6	7.2	8.4	9.6	10.8
40	1.6	3.2	4.8	6.4	8	9.6	11.2	12.8	14.4
50	2	4	6	8	10	12	14	16	18
60	2.4	4.8	7.2	9.6	12	14.4	16.8	19.2	21.6
70	2.8	5.6	8.4	11.2	14	16.8	19.6	22.4	25.2
80	3.2	6.4	9.6	12.8	16	19.2	22.4	25.6	28.8
90	3.6	7.2	10.8	14.4	18	21.6	25.2	28.8	32.4
100	4	8	12	16	20	24	28	32	36
110	4.4	8.8	13.2	17.6	22	26.4	30.8	35.2	39.6

Note: Epoprostenol is administered in nanograms (ng) per kilogram (kg) per minute (min).

PRECAUTIONS

HEALTH-RELATED

- **Rebound pulmonary hypertension:** Avoid *any* interruption in the IV infusion; a short break in infusion may result in rebounding pulmonary hypertension.
- **Pulmonary edema:** Epoprostenol is not recommended for patients who develop pulmonary edema during acute dose-ranging.
- **Pulmonary venoocclusive disease:** Patients may develop thrombi in pulmonary vasculature.

AGE-RELATED

- **Children:** Safety for use in children has not been established. Some studies suggest children may tolerate higher doses than adults.

- **Elderly:** Use epoprostenol cautiously in elderly patients. Age-related organ dysfunction (cardiac, renal, liver), other diseases present, and medications may prompt concern about use.

PREGNANCY/LACTATION-RELATED

- Pregnancy category B; women with pulmonary hypertension should avoid pregnancy; unknown if excreted in breast milk.

MONITORING

- **Baseline assessment:** Obtain vital signs and assess for chest discomfort and respiratory distress. Before beginning therapy, ensure a backup infusion pump and IV infusion sets are available to avoid interruptions in therapy. A central venous catheter should be in place.
- **Lab work:** Biochemical profile including renal (BUN, creatinine) and liver (AST [SGOT], ALT [SGPT], bilirubin, alkaline phosphatase) function tests.
- **Dosage adjustment BP monitoring:** Monitor standing and supine BP for hypotension for several hours after a dosage adjustment. Assess for syncope.
- **Acute dose ranging:** Observe continuous ECG monitoring and perform frequent vital signs until response to the drug is known. Asymptomatic increases may be seen in pulmonary artery pressures with an increased cardiac output; dosage adjustment may be warranted if pulmonary artery pressure increase is observed.
- **Anticoagulation:** Patients should be anticoagulated to reduce the possibility of pulmonary thromboembolism unless contraindicated.
- **Therapeutic response:** Assess for decreased chest discomfort, less dyspnea, less fatigue; decreased pulmonary arterial pressures, pulmonary vascular resistance, and improved pulmonary function.
- **Patient education:** When preparing to discharge patients on epoprostenol infusion, teach how to reconstitute and administer epoprostenol using aseptic technique and how to care for the permanent central venous catheter. Instruct to report fever, pain, or redness at central catheter insertion site. Advise that brief interruptions in drug delivery may result in rapidly worsening symptoms. Explain that epoprostenol therapy will be necessary for a prolonged period, possibly years. Dosage adjustments should be made only after consulting with the health care provider monitoring the therapy.

SERIOUS ADVERSE REACTIONS

- Angina, MI, and thrombocytopenia occur rarely.
- **Abrupt withdrawal:** Stopping or significantly reducing the IV infusion may produce rebound pulmonary hypertension (dyspnea, dizziness, asthenia).

OVERDOSE/TOXICITY

- Hypotension, respiratory distress, hypoxemia, respiratory failure/arrest, death.
- **GI decontamination:** No specific recommendations.

ANTIDOTE/DIALYSIS

- **Antidote:** No specific recommendations.
- **Dialysis:** No data are available regarding removal of epoprostenol using hemodialysis, high-permeability dialysis, or peritoneal dialysis.

eprosartan mesylate

See Angiotensin II Receptor Antagonists (p. 889)

eptifibatide

ep-tih-fib'-ah-tide

Classes

Chemical: glycoprotein (GP) IIb/IIIa inhibitor

Therapeutic: antiplatelet agent

Pregnancy Category: B

Trade Names

Prescription: Integrilin

CLINICAL PHARMACOLOGY

Mechanism of Action

A glycoprotein IIb/IIIa inhibitor that rapidly inhibits platelet aggregation by preventing binding of fibrinogen to receptor sites on platelets. **Therapeutic Effect:** Prevents closure of treated coronary arteries. Also prevents acute cardiac ischemic complications.

PHARMACOKINETICS

Inhibition of platelet function (IV): 1 hr. Protein binding: 25%. Excreted in urine. Duration of action: 2-4 hr. **Half-life:** 2.5 hr.

AVAILABILITY

Injection solution: 0.75 mg/mL, 2 mg/mL.

E

INDICATIONS AND DOSAGE

Adjunct to percutaneous coronary intervention (PCI)

IV Bolus, IV Infusion

Adults, Elderly: 180 mcg/kg before PCI initiation, then continuous drip of 2 mcg/kg/min and a second 180 mcg/kg bolus 10 min after the first. Maximum: 15 mg/hr. Continue until hospital discharge or for up to 18-24 hr. Minimum 12 hr is recommended. Concurrent aspirin and heparin therapy is recommended.

Acute coronary syndrome

IV Bolus, IV Infusion

Adults, Elderly: 180 mcg/kg bolus then 2 mcg/kg/min until discharge or coronary artery bypass graft, up to 72 hr. Maximum: 15 mg/hr. Concurrent aspirin and heparin therapy is recommended.

Dosage in renal impairment

Creatinine clearance less than 50 mL/min or more than 2 mg/dL. Use 180 mcg/kg bolus (maximum 22.6 mg) and 1 mcg/kg/min infusion (maximum: 7.5 mg/hr).

CONTRAINDICATIONS

Active internal bleeding, AV malformation or aneurysm, history of cerebrovascular accident (CVA) within 2 yr or CVA with residual neurologic defect, history of vasculitis, intracranial neoplasm, oral anticoagulant use within last 7 days unless prothrombin time is less than 1.22 times the control, recent (6 wk or less) GI or gastrourinary bleeding, recent (6 wk or less) surgery or trauma, prior IV dextran use before or during percutaneous coronary intervention (PCI), severe uncontrolled hypertension, hypersensitivity to eptifibatide

INTERACTIONS

Drug: **Anticoagulants, heparin:** May increase the risk of hemorrhage. **Dextran, other platelet aggregation inhibitors (such as aspirin), thrombolytic agents:** May increase the risk of bleeding. **Herbal:** None known. **Food:** None known.

DIAGNOSTIC TEST EFFECTS

Increases aPTT, prothrombin time, and clotting time. Decreases platelet count.

IV INCOMPATIBILITIES

Administer in separate line; do not add other medications to infusion solution.

SIDE-EFFECTS

Occasional (less than 12%): Hypotension, minor bleeding (3%-12%)

CRITICAL CARE CONSIDERATIONS

ADMINISTRATION/HANDLING

IV ALERT

- **Storage:** Store vials in refrigerator.
- **Preparation:** Do not shake. Discard unused portions. Solution normally appears clear and is colorless. Discard if preparation contains any opaque particles.
- **IV bolus:** Withdraw bolus dose from 10-mL vial (2 mg/mL). Give IV bolus dose over 1-2 min.
- **IV infusion:** Withdraw from 100-mL vial (0.75 mg/mL). May give IV push and infusion undiluted.

EPTIFIBATIDE WEIGHT BASED DOSING TABLE

Patient Weight (kg)	Bolus Volume 0.75 mg/mL Vial 180 mcg/kg	Infusion Rate 0.75 mg/mL Vial 1 mcg/kg/min	Bolus Volume 2 mg/mL Vial 180 mcg/kg	Infusion Rate 2 mg/mL Vial 1 mcg/kg/min
47-53	12 mL	4 mL/hr	4.5 mL	1.5 mL/hr
54-59	13.3 mL	4.5 mL/hr	5 mL	1.8 mL/hr
60-65	15 mL	5 mL/hr	5.6 mL	1.9 mL/hr
66-71	16.4 mL	5.5 mL/hr	6.2 mL	2 mL/hr
72-78	18 mL	6 mL/hr	6.8 mL	2.3 mL/hr
79-84	19.4 mL	6.5 mL/hr	7.3 mL	2.5 mL/hr
85-90	21 mL	7 mL/hr	7.9 mL	2.7 mL/hr
91-96	22.6 mL	7.5 mL/hr	8.5 mL	2.8 mL/hr
97-103	24 mL	8 mL/hr	9 mL	3 mL/hr
104-109	25.2 mL	8.5 mL/hr	9.5 mL	3.2 mL/hr
110-115	27 mL	9 mL/hr	10.2 mL	3.4 mL/hr
116-121	28.5 mL	9.5 mL/hr	10.7 mL	3.5 mL/hr
More than 121	30 mL	10 mL/hr	11.3 mL	3.7 mL/hr

PRECAUTIONS

HEALTH-RELATED

- Use eptifibatide cautiously in patients who weigh less than 75 kg; who are older than 65 yr; have a history of GI disease; or who are receiving platelet inhibitors including aspirin, thrombin inhibitors including heparin, low molecular weight heparin, or thrombolytics. Aspirin is given as part of the current Advanced Cardiac Life Support (ACLS) guidelines for acute coronary syndrome and should not be withheld. Drug should should be given to patients receiving other GP IIB/IIIA inhibitors (abciximab [Reopro] or tirofiban [Aggrastat]), or have thrombocytopenia (less than 100,000 cells/mcL).
- Target activated clotting time (ACT) during percutaneous coronary interventions (PCI)

is 200-300 sec. Additional heparin boluses may be needed during the procedure, but heparin use is discouraged following PCI.
- Use cautiously in PCI (e.g., coronary angioplasty) patients less than 12 hr from the onset of symptoms of acute MI, PCI procedure lasting more than 70 min, and failed angioplasty.

AGE-RELATED
- **Children:** Safety and efficacy of eptifibatide have not been established in children.
- **Elderly:** Risk of major bleeding is increased.

PREGNANCY/LACTATION-RELATED
- Pregnancy category B; use caution in nursing mothers

MONITORING
- **Baseline assessment:** Assess bleeding potential, including history of bleeding, liver disease, blood dyscrasias, recent stroke, GI bleeding, cancer, hemodialysis patients, as drug is contraindicated. Assess for hypertension; drug is contraindicated in patients with systolic BP more than 220 mmHg and diastolic BP more than 110 mmHg.
- **Baseline lab work:** Obtain Hgb, Hct, and platelet count before treatment. If platelet count is less than 90,000/mm^3, obtain additional platelet counts routinely to avoid development of thrombocytopenia. Obtain ACT for patients undergoing PCI for acute coronary syndrome.
- **Bleeding:** Diligently monitor for bleeding, including arterial and venous puncture sites; all invasive sites; and in urine, stool, secretions, or emesis; for neurologic changes that may indicate intracranial bleeding. During infusion, avoid placement of invasive devices, including endotracheal tube, NG tube, and urinary catheter, if possible. Do not manipulate devices already in place.
- **Surgery:** Eptifibatide should be discontinued before any surgical procedure.
- **Other medications:** Do not administer additional drugs which may facilitate bleeding unless absolutely necessary. Aspirin is routinely given for patients with acute coronary syndromes in keeping with ACLS guidelines.
- **Patient education:** Instruct to report bleeding from invasive sites, chest pain, or dyspnea. Remind about the need to use an electric razor and soft toothbrush to prevent bleeding. Instruct to report black or red stool, dark or red urine, or red-speckled mucus from cough. Advise female patients that menstrual flow may be heavier than usual during infusion.

SERIOUS ADVERSE REACTIONS
- Minor to major bleeding complications may occur, most commonly at arterial access site for cardiac catheterization.

OVERDOSE/TOXICITY
- **Human toxicity:** Human study data not available. Animal studies revealed muscle weakness, decreased muscle tone, dyspnea, loss of righting reflex, ptosis, and development of abdominal and femoral petechiae.
- **Overdose:** Bleeding leading to hypovolemic/hemorrhagic shock, which can compromise coronary circulation leading to chest discomfort and acute MI.
- **GI decontamination:** No specific recommendations.

ANTIDOTE/DIALYSIS
- **Antidote:** No specific recommendations. Eptifibatide should be discontinued immediately if bleeding occurs; platelet inhibition should reverse quickly. Platelet transfusion may be required in thrombocytopenic patients.
- **Dialysis:** Eptifibatide is removed using hemodialysis and high-permeability hemodialysis. No data are available regarding removal by peritoneal dialysis.

ergotamine tartrate/ dihydroergotamine

er-got'-a-meen tar'-trate/die-hie-dro-er-got'-a-meen

Classes
Chemical: ergot alkaloid
Therapeutic: antimigraine agent

Pregnancy Category: X

Combinations
Prescription: with caffeine (Cafergot, Ercaf, Wigraine); with belladonna alkaloids, phenobarbital (Bellergal-S)

CLINICAL PHARMACOLOGY

Mechanism of Action
An ergotamine derivative and alpha-adrenergic blocker that directly stimulates vascular smooth muscle, resulting in peripheral and cerebral vasoconstriction. May also have antagonist effects on serotonin. **Therapeutic Effect:** Suppresses vascular headaches.

PHARMACOKINETICS

Slowly and incompletely absorbed from the GI tract; rapidly and extensively absorbed after rectal administration. Protein binding: greater than 90%. Undergoes extensive first-pass metabolism in the liver to active metabolite. Eliminated in feces by the biliary system. **Half-life:** 21 hr.

AVAILABILITY

Tablets (sublingual [Ergomar]): 2 mg.
Injection (DHE 45): 1 mg/mL.
Nasal spray (Migranal): 0.5 mg/spray.
Suppositories (ergotamine and caffeine): 2 mg, with 100 mg caffeine.

INDICATIONS AND DOSAGE

Vascular headaches

PO (Cafergot [fixed-combination of ergotamine and caffeine])

Adults, Elderly: 2 mg at onset of headache, then 1-2 mg every 30 min. Maximum: 6 mg/episode; 10 mg/wk.

PO, Sublingual

Children: 1 mg at onset of headache, then 1 mg every 30 min. Maximum: 3 mg/episode.

IV

Adults, Elderly: 1 mg at onset of headache; may repeat hourly. Maximum: 2 mg/day; 6 mg/wk.

Sublingual

Adults, Elderly: 1 tablet at onset of headache, then 1 tablet every 30 min. Maximum: 3 tablets/24 hr; 5 tablets/wk.

IM, Subcutaneous (dihydroergotamine)

Adults, Elderly: 1 mg at onset of headache; may repeat hourly. Maximum: 3 mg/day; 6 mg/wk.

Intranasal

Adults, Elderly: 1 spray (0.5 mg) into each nostril; may repeat in 15 min. Maximum: 4 sprays/day; 8 sprays/wk.

Rectal

Adults, Elderly: 1 suppository at onset of headache; may repeat dose in 1 hr. Maximum: 2 suppositories/episode; 5 suppositories/wk.

OFF-LABEL USES

Prevention of deep venous thrombosis, prevention and treatment of orthostatic hypotension, pulmonary thromboembolism

CONTRAINDICATIONS

Coronary artery disease, hypertension, impaired hepatic or renal function, malnutrition, peripheral vascular diseases (such as thromboangiitis obliterans, syphilitic arteritis, severe arteriosclerosis, thrombophlebitis, and Raynaud's disease), sepsis, severe pruritus, hypersensitivity to ergotamine, and concommitant use of CYP3A4 inhibitors, protease inhibitors, macrolide antibiotics, and azole antifungals

INTERACTIONS

Drug: **Beta-blockers, erythromycin:** May increase the risk of vasospasm. **Ergot alkaloids, systemic vasoconstrictors:** May increase pressor effect. **Macrolide antibiotics (erythromycin, clarithromycin, azithromycin), nitroglycerin:** May decrease the effects of these agents. **Herbal:** None known. **Food:** Grapefruit juice may increase effects.

DIAGNOSTIC TEST EFFECTS

None known.

SIDE-EFFECTS

Occasional (5%-2%): Cough, dizziness, pruritis, nausea, vomiting. **Rare (less than 2%):** Myalgia, fatigue, diarrhea, upper respiratory tract infection, dyspepsia

CRITICAL CARE CONSIDERATIONS

ADMINISTRATION/HANDLING

SUBLINGUAL ALERT

- Do not administer with water. Place the sublingual dihydroergotamine tablet under the tongue, let it dissolve, and instruct patients to swallow.

PO ALERT

- Do not administer with grapefruit juice.

SUBCUTANEOUS/IM ALERT

- **DHE 45 injection:** Clear, colorless solution in a single 1-mL ampule with 1 mg/mL ergotamine.
- **Maximum dose:** 1 mL should be injected in each dose. May be repeated with 1 hr between doses to a total of no more than 3 mL in 24 hr.

IV ALERT

- **IV push:** Slowly administer 1 mL dihydroergotamine (DHE 45) undiluted over 1 min.
- **Maximum dose:** May repeat dose once after at least 1 hr to a total of no more than 2 mL given IV in 24 hr.

NASAL ALERT

- **Storage:** Do not refrigerate the nasal form.
- **Stability:** Discard the drug within 8 hr of opening the container.
- Before administration, prime the pump by squeezing it four times.

PRECAUTIONS

HEALTH-RELATED

- Use ergotamine with caution in patients with suspected cardiac and/or peripheral vascular disease, including those with chest discomfort, dysrhythmias, transient ischemic attacks, intermittent claudication, diabetes, leg cramps, suspected renal or liver disease, and dehydration. Patients who manifest symptoms of any of these conditions warrant further differential diagnosis of those diseases.
- **Cytochrome P450 inhibitors:** Co-administration of ergotamine and potent CYP3A4 inhibitors is contraindicated. Serious and/or life-threatening peripheral ischemia has been reported with co-administration of CYP3A4 inhibitors including protease inhibitors and macrolide antibiotics. CYP3A4 inhibitors elevate serum levels of dihydroergotamine and increase risk of cerebral and peripheral arterial vasospasms resulting in ischemia and possible injury.
- Dihydroergotamine should not be given within 24 hr of patients receiving 5HT1 agonists (triptans [sumatriptan]), other ergot alkaloids, or methysergide.

AGE-RELATED

- **Children:** Safety and efficacy of ergotamine have not been established in children. May use in children of at least 6 yr only when unresponsive to other drugs.
- **Elderly:** Age-related occlusive peripheral vascular disease increases risk of peripheral vasoconstriction; elderly are at risk of age-related renal impairment.

PREGNANCY/LACTATION-RELATED

- Pregnancy category X; excreted into breast milk; has caused symptoms of ergotism (e.g., vomiting, diarrhea) in the infant; excessive dosage or prolonged administration may inhibit lactation.

MONITORING

- **Baseline assessment:** Determine history of cardiac, neurologic, peripheral vascular disease; renal or hepatic impairment. Carefully assess peripheral circulation, including temperature, sensation, movement, color, and strength of pulses in the extremities.
- **Pregnancy:** Determine pregnancy; ergotamine is contraindicated in pregnancy.
- **Lab work:** Biochemical profile including renal (BUN, creatinine) and liver (AST [SGOT], ALT [SGPT], bilirubin, alkaline phosphatase) function tests.
- **Migraine and cluster headaches:** Determine onset, location, and duration of the vascular headaches and possible precipitating factors.
- **Toxicity/overdose:** Monitor closely for evidence of ergotamine poisoning from prolonged administration or excessive dosage. If headaches worsen with treatment, patients may be toxic on ergotamine rather than unresponsive to treatment. Initiate continuous ECG and BP monitoring if toxicity is suspected, along with frequent neurological and peripheral vascular assessments.
- **Patient education:** When using ergotamine outside the hospital, instruct to take ergotamine at the first sign of a vascular headache. Instruct to report to a health care provider if the drug does not relieve headache or if palpitations or if irregular heartbeat, nausea or vomiting, numbness or tingling of the fingers and toes, pain or weakness of the extremities occurs. Warn female patients to avoid pregnancy during therapy and to report immediately if they become pregnant. Teach methods of contraception if needed.

SERIOUS ADVERSE REACTIONS

- Vasoconstriction of peripheral arteries and arterioles may result in localized edema and pruritus. Muscle pain will occur when walking and later, even at rest. Other rare effects include confusion, depression, drowsiness, seizures, and gangrene.

OVERDOSE/TOXICITY

- **Ergot alkaloid poisoning:** Prolonged administration or excessive ergotamine dosage may cause generalized vasospasms manifested as hypertension, hypotension, tachycardia, bradycardia, chest discomfort, angina, strokelike symptoms, seizures, limb ischemia, other end-organ damage (renal or intestinal), nausea, and vomiting; paresthesia; and muscle pain or weakness. Ergot-induced vasospasm can be present in some cases weeks after the last dose. Respiratory rate and temperature are not usually affected by ergotamine.
- **Severe headache:** Patients with migraine headaches are difficult to manage with ergot alkaloids because worsening headaches may be migraine or may be induced by ergotamine toxicity. Persistent, severe headaches may require diagnostic tests including arteriogram and/or MRI/MRA. Patients with ergot alkaloid poisoning treated with another ergot, a triptan, or a sympathomimetic will experience further

worsening of symptoms and may experience a stroke.

- **GI decontamination:** No specific recommendations.

ANTIDOTE/DIALYSIS

- **Antidote:** Cyproheptadine, alprostadil (prostaglandin E1) and epoprostenol (prostacyclin [Flolan]) may be attempted for ergot-induced vasospasms. If thrombosis occurs, antiplatelet agents (e.g., aspirin, GPIIb/IIIa inhibitors), anticoagulants, or thrombolytics may be warranted. Ergotamine-induced hypertension may require nitroprusside (Nipride) infusion. Calcium channel blockers or ACE inhibitors may be effective for moderately elevated BP.
- **Dialysis:** Ergotamine is removed using hemodialysis and high-permeability hemodialysis. No data are available on removal using peritoneal dialysis.

ertapenem

er-ta-pen'-em

Classes

Chemical: carbapenem
Therapeutic: antibiotic

Pregnancy Category: B

Trade Names

Prescription: Invanz

CLINICAL PHARMACOLOGY

Mechanism of Action

A carbapenem that penetrates the bacterial cell wall of microorganisms and binds to penicillin-binding proteins, inhibiting cell wall synthesis. **Therapeutic Effect:** Produces bacterial cell death.

PHARMACOKINETICS

Almost completely absorbed after IM administration. Protein binding: 85%-95%. Widely distributed. Primarily excreted in urine with smaller amount eliminated in feces. Removed by hemodialysis. **Half-life:** 4 hr.

AVAILABILITY

Injection powder for reconstitution: 1 g.

INDICATIONS AND DOSAGE

Intraabdominal infection

IV, IM

Adults, Elderly: 1 g/day for 5-14 days. **Children 13 yr and older:** 1 g/day for 5-14 days. **Children 3 mo-12 yr:** 15 mg/kg twice daily for 5-14 days. Maximum: not to exceed 1 g/day.

Skin and skin structure infection

IV, IM

Adults, Elderly: 1 g/day for 7-14 days. **Children 13 yr and older:** 1 g/day for 7-14 days. **Children 3 mo-12 yr:** 15 mg/kg twice daily for 7-14 days. Maximum: 1 g/day.

Pneumonia, urinary tract infection (complicated)

IV, IM

Adults, Elderly: 1 g/day for 10-14 days. **Children 13 yr and older:** 1 g/day for 10-14 days. **Children 3 mo-12 yr:** 15 mg/kg twice daily for 10-14 days. Maximum: 1 g/day.

Pelvic infection

IV, IM

Adults, Elderly: 1 g/day for 3-10 days. **Children 13 yr and older:** 1 g/day for 3-10 days. **Children 3 mo-12 yr:** 15 mg/kg twice daily for 3-10 days. Maximum: 1 g/day.

Diabetic foot infection (without osteomyelitis)

IV, IM

Adults, Elderly: 1 g once daily for up to 28 days. **Children 13 yr and older:** 1 g once daily for up to 28 days. **Children 3 mo-12 yr:** 15 mg/kg for up to 28 days. Maximum: 1 g/day.

Dosage in renal impairment

For adults and elderly patients with creatinine clearance less than 30 mL/min dosage is 500 mg once per day.

CONTRAINDICATIONS

History of hypersensitivity or anaphylaxis to ertapenem or beta-lactams (imipenem and cilastin, meropenem), hypersensitivity to amide-type local anesthetics (IM), meningitis (especially in children; drug has poor penetration to cerebrospinal fluid)

INTERACTIONS

Drug: Probenecid: Reduces renal excretion of ertapenem. **Herbal:** None known. **Food:** None known.

DIAGNOSTIC TEST EFFECTS

May increase serum alkaline phosphatase, AST (SGOT) and ALT (SGPT) levels. May decrease platelet count, blood Hct and Hgb levels, and serum potassium level.

IV INCOMPATIBILITIES

Do not mix or infuse ertapenem with any other medications. Do not use diluents or IV solutions containing dextrose.

IV COMPATIBILITIES

Sterile water for injection, 0.9% NaCl

SIDE-EFFECTS

Frequent (10%-6%): Diarrhea, nausea, headache. **Occasional (5%-2%):** Altered mental status, insomnia, rash, abdominal pain, constipation, vomiting, edema, fever. **Rare (less than 2%):** Dizziness, cough, oral candidiasis, anxiety, tachycardia, phlebitis at IV site

CRITICAL CARE CONSIDERATIONS

ADMINISTRATION/HANDLING

IV ALERT

- **Stability:** Reconstituted solution is stable for 6 hr at room temperature and 24 hr if refrigerated. The solution normally appears colorless to yellow; variations in color do not affect potency; discard if solution contains precipitate.
- **First dilution:** Dilute the 1-g vial with 10 mL of 0.9% NaCl or bacteriostatic water for injection. Shake well to dissolve.
- **Further dilution:** Further dilute with 50 mL of 0.9% NaCl.
- **Intermittent IV infusion:** Give by intermittent IV infusion (piggyback), not by IV push. Infuse over 20-30 min.

IM ALERT

- **Suspension preparation:** Reconstitute the lyophilized powder with 3.2 mL of 1% lidocaine injection without epinephrine. Shake the vial thoroughly.
- **Stability:** Administer the suspension IM within 1 hr after preparation. Suspension may not be given IV.
- **Administration:** To minimize discomfort, slowly inject the drug deep into the gluteus maximus rather than the lateral aspect of the thigh.

PRECAUTIONS

HEALTH-RELATED

- Use ertapenem cautiously in patients with CNS disorders (tumors or a history of seizures), impaired renal function, hypersensitivity to cephalosporins, penicillins, or other allergens.
- **Probenecid:** Use should be avoided in patients receiving ertapenem.

AGE-RELATED

- **Children:** Safety and efficacy of ertapenem have not been established in infants under 3 mo.
- **Elderly:** Age-related or advanced renal insufficiency may require dosage reduction.

PREGNANCY/LACTATION-RELATED

- Pregnancy category B; excreted into breast milk; bottle-feeding recommended during and for 5 days after therapy.

MONITORING

- **Baseline assessment:** Determine history of allergies, particularly to beta-lactams, cephalosporins, or penicillins before beginning ertapenem therapy. Determine history of seizures.
- **Baseline lab work:** Biochemical profile including BUN and creatinine, liver enzymes. Appropriate cultures to assess for sensitivity of the organism to ertapenem.
- **Rash or diarrhea:** Withhold ertapenem if rash or diarrhea occurs. Although a rash is a common side effect, it may also indicate hypersensitivity. Severe diarrhea with abdominal pain, blood or mucus in stools, and fever may indicate antibiotic-associated colitis. Evaluate hydration status.
- **IV site phlebitis:** Evaluate the IV site for signs of phlebitis, such as heat, pain, and red streaking over vein.
- **IM injections:** Check the IM injection site for pain and swelling. Inform patients that IM injections may cause discomfort.
- **Renal function:** Monitor intake and output, renal function test results, and urinalysis results.
- **Superinfection:** Assess for signs and symptoms of superinfection, such as anal or genital pruritus, black hairy tongue, changes in oral mucosa, diarrhea, increased fever, sore throat, and vomiting.
- ***Clostridium difficile*–associated diarrhea (CDAD):** Wash hands with soap and water if CDAD is present; *Clostridium* spores are not controlled by alcohol foam.
- **Seizures:** Evaluate mental status; observe for seizures and tremors.
- **Insomnia:** Assess sleep pattern for evidence of insomnia.
- **Evenly spaced doses:** Space doses evenly around the clock.
- **Patient education:** When using ertapenem outside the hospital, instruct to take it for the full course of treatment. Instruct to report diarrhea, rash, seizures, tremors, or any other new symptoms to a health care provider.

SERIOUS ADVERSE REACTIONS

- Abdominal distention, pain, chills, nervousness, dermatitis, septicemia, septic shock.

OVERDOSE/TOXICITY

- **Seizures:** Seen when higher than usual doses are used and in patients with brain lesions or a history of seizures, bacterial meningitis, or severe renal impairment.
- **Hypersensitivity:** Severe hypersensitivity reactions, including anaphylaxis, acute interstitial nephritis, and blood dyscrasias may occur.
- **Colitis:** Antibiotic-associated colitis and other superinfections may result from altered bacterial balance.
- **GI decontamination:** No specific recommendations.

ANTIDOTE/DIALYSIS

- **Antidote:** No specific recommendations.
- **Dialysis:** Patients on hemodialysis may need a supplemental dose if ertapenem is administered within 6 hr before treatment. Ertapenem is removed by hemodialysis and is likely to be removed by high-permeability hemodialysis. No data are available regarding removal by peritoneal dialysis.

erythromycin

er-ith-roe-mye'-sin

Classes

Chemical: macrolide derivative
Therapeutic: antibiotic

Pregnancy Category: B

Trade Names

Prescription: (A/T/S, Akne-Mycin, EES, Emgel, E-Mycin, Eryc, Eryc-125 ♣, Eryc-250 ♣, Erycette, EryDerm, Erygel, EryPed, Erymax, Ery-Tab, Erythra-Derm, Erythrocin, PCE Dispertab, Romycin, Roymicin, Staticin, Theramycin, Theramycin Z, T-Stat)

Combinations

Prescription: with sulfisoxazole (Pediazole); with benzoyl peroxide (Benzamycin)

Do not confuse erythromycin with azithromycin or Ethmozine or Eryc with Emcyt.

CLINICAL PHARMACOLOGY

Mechanism of Action

A macrolide that reversibly binds to bacterial ribosomes, inhibiting bacterial protein synthesis. **Therapeutic Effect:** Bacteriostatic.

PHARMACOKINETICS

Variably absorbed from the GI tract (depending on dosage form used). Protein binding: 70%-90%. Widely distributed. Metabolized in the liver. Primarily eliminated in feces by bile. Not removed by hemodialysis. **Half-life:** 1.4-2 hr (increased in impaired renal function).

AVAILABILITY

Topical gel (A/T/S, Emgel, Erygel): 2%.
Injection powder for reconstitution (Erythrocin): 500 mg, 1 g.
Ophthalmic ointment (Roymicin): 0.5%.
Oral suspension (EryPed, EES): 200 mg/5 mL, 400 mg/5 mL.
Topical ointment (Akne-Mycin): 2%.
Topical solution: 1.5% (Staticin), 2% (A/T/S, Erymax, EryDerm, Erythra-Derm, Romycin, Theramycin Z, T-Stat).
Topical swab (Erycette, T-Stat): 2%.
Tablets (chewable [Ery-Ped]): 200 mg.
Tablets: 250 mg (E-Mycin, Ery-Tab, Erythrocin), 333 mg (Ery-Tab, E-Mycin, PCE Dispertab), 400 mg (EES), 500 mg (E-Mycin, Ery-Tab, Erythrocin, PCE Dispertab).
Capsules (enteric-coated [Eryc]): 250 mg.

INDICATIONS AND DOSAGE

Mild to moderate infections of the upper and lower respiratory tract, pharyngitis, skin infections

PO

Adults, Elderly: 250 mg every 6 hr, 500 mg every 12 hr, or 333 mg every 8 hr. Maximum: 4 g/day. **Children:** 30-50 mg/kg/day in divided doses every 6-8 hr up to 60-100 mg/kg/day for severe infections. **Neonates:** 20-40 mg/kg/day in divided doses every 6-12 hr.

IV

Adults, Elderly, Children: 15-20 mg/kg/day in divided doses. Maximum: 4 g/day.

Preoperative intestinal antisepsis

PO

Adults, Elderly: 1 g at 1 PM, 2 PM, and 11 PM on day before surgery (with neomycin). **Children.** 20 mg/kg at 1 PM, 2 PM, and 11 PM on day before surgery (with neomycin).

Acne vulgaris

Topical

Adults: Apply thin layer to affected area twice per day.

Gonococcal ophthalmia neonatorum

Ophthalmic

Neonates: 0.5-2 cm no later than 1 hr after delivery.

OFF-LABEL USES

Systemic: Treatment of acne vulgaris, chancroid, *Campylobacter* enteritis, gastroparesis, Lyme disease
Topical: Treatment of minor bacterial skin infections

Ophthalmic: Treatment of blepharitis, conjunctivitis, keratitis, chlamydial trachoma

CONTRAINDICATIONS

Administration of fixed-combination product, Pediazole, to infants younger than 2 mo; history of hepatitis due to macrolides; hypersensitivity to erythromycin or other macrolides; preexisting hepatic disease.

INTERACTIONS

Drug: Buspirone, *cycloSPORINE, felodipine, lovastatin, simvastatin: May increase the blood concentration and toxicity of these drugs. **Carbamazepine:** May inhibit the metabolism of carbamazepine. **Chloramphenicol, clindamycin:** May decrease the effects of these drugs. **Hepatotoxic medications:** May increase the risk of hepatotoxicity. **Theophylline:** May increase the risk of theophylline toxicity. **Warfarin:** May increase warfarin's effects. **Herbal:** None known. **Food:** None known.

DIAGNOSTIC TEST EFFECTS

May increase serum alkaline phosphatase, bilirubin, AST (SGOT), and ALT (SGPT) levels.

IV INCOMPATIBILITIES

Fluconazole (Diflucan)

IV COMPATIBILITIES

Aminophylline, amiodarone (Cordarone), diltiazem (Cardizem), heparin, hydromorphone (Dilaudid), lidocaine, lorazepam (Ativan), magnesium sulfate, midazolam (Versed), morphine, multivitamins, potassium chloride, total parenteral nutrition (TPN)

SIDE-EFFECTS

Frequent: IV: Abdominal cramping or discomfort, phlebitis or thrombophlebitis. **Topical:** Dry skin (50%). **Occasional:** Nausea, vomiting, diarrhea, rash, urticaria. **Rare: Ophthalmic:** Sensitivity reaction with increased irritation, burning, itching, and inflammation. **Topical:** Urticaria

CRITICAL CARE CONSIDERATIONS

ADMINISTRATION/HANDLING

PO ALERT

- Give tablets or capsules with 8 oz of water.
- Make sure patients do not swallow chewable tablets whole.
- If patients have difficulty swallowing, sprinkle capsule contents in a teaspoonful of applesauce and follow with water.
- Store capsules and tablets at room temperature.
- Oral suspension is stable for 14 days at room temperature.
- **Erythromycin base or stearate:** Administer 1 hr before or 2 hr after a meal.
- **Erythromycin estolate and ethylsuccinate:** May be given without regard to food but are absorbed better when given on an empty stomach.

IV ALERT

- **Storage:** Store parenteral form at room temperature.
- **Stability:** Initial reconstituted solution in vial is stable for 24 hr at room temperature and 2 wk if refrigerated. Diluted IV solutions are stable for 8 hr at room temperature and 24 hr if refrigerated. Discard solution if a precipitate forms.
- **Reconstitution:** Reconstitute each 500-mg vial with 10 mL or each 1-g vial with 20 mL sterile water for injection without a preservative to provide a concentration of 50 mg/mL.
- **Further dilution:** Dilute with 100-250 mL D_5W or 0.9% NaCl.
- **Intermittent IV infusion (piggyback):** Administer over 20-60 min.
- **Continuous infusion:** Administer over 6-24 hr.

OPHTHALMIC ALERT

- **Administration:** Place a gloved finger on the lower eyelid and pull it out until a pocket is formed between the eye and the lower lid. Place 0.25-0.5 inch of ointment into the pocket. Close the eye for 1-2 min and roll the eyeball gently to increase the drug's distribution. Remove excess ointment around the eye with tissue.

PRECAUTIONS

HEALTH-RELATED

- Use erythromycin cautiously in patients with hepatic or renal dysfunction.
- **Cytochrome P450 enzyme inhibitors:** Coadministration of erythromycin and cytochrome P450 inhibitors results in elevated levels of the other medications.
- **Pediazole:** Use the combination drug (erythromycin and sulfisoxazole) cautiously in patients with impaired renal or hepatic function, severe allergies, bronchial asthma, or glucose-6-phosphate dehydrogenase deficiency.

E

AGE-RELATED

- **Children:** Pediazole should not be used in children under 2 mo.
- **Elderly:** No age-related precautions have been noted.

PREGNANCY/LACTATION-RELATED

- Pregnancy category B; excreted into breast milk; compatible with breast-feeding.

MONITORING

- **Baseline assessment:** Determine history of hepatitis or allergies to erythromycin or other macrolides before beginning drug therapy.
- **Baseline lab work:** Biochemical profile including BUN and creatinine, liver enzymes. Appropriate cultures to assess for sensitivity of the organism to erythromycin unless used to treat acne.
- **Rash or diarrhea:** Withhold erythromycin if rash or diarrhea occurs. Although a rash is a common side effect, it may also indicate hypersensitivity. Severe diarrhea with abdominal pain, blood or mucus in stools, and fever may indicate antibiotic-associated colitis. Evaluate hydration status.
- **IV site phlebitis:** Evaluate the IV site for signs of phlebitis, such as heat, pain, and red streaking over vein.
- **Renal function:** Monitor intake and output, renal function test results, and urinalysis results.
- **Superinfection:** Assess for signs and symptoms of superinfection, such as anal or genital pruritus, black hairy tongue, changes in oral mucosa, diarrhea, increased fever, sore throat, and vomiting.
- ***Clostridium difficile*–associated diarrhea (CDAD):** Wash hands with soap and water if CDAD is present; *Clostridium* spores are not controlled by alcohol foam.
- **Prolonged QT interval:** Rarely patients have a prolonged QT interval; if there is a history of dysrhythmias, monitor ECG for ventricular dysrhythmias.
- **Hearing loss:** Monitor for hearing loss; high dosages can cause hearing loss in patients with hepatic or renal dysfunction.
- **Evenly-spaced doses:** Space doses evenly around the clock.
- **Patient education:** When using erythromycin outside the hospital, instruct patients to take erythromycin for the full course of treatment. Tell patients to report diarrhea, rash, seizures, tremors, or any other new symptoms to a health care provider. Instruct patients to take the oral form of erythromycin with 8 oz of water 1 hr before or 2 hr after food or beverage. Instruct not to swallow chewable tablets whole. Advise spacing doses evenly around the clock and continuing erythromycin therapy for the full course of treatment. Instruct patients using ophthalmic erythromycin to report promptly burning, inflammation, or itching of the eye to a health care provider. Instruct patients using topical erythromycin to promptly report burning, excessive dryness, or itching skin to a health care provider. Inform patients being treated for acne that maximum improvement may take 3 mo and that erythromycin therapy may need to be continued for months or years. Advise to wait at least 1 hr before using other topical acne preparations containing abrasive or peeling agents, such as medicated soaps and cosmetics or aftershave containing alcohol.

SERIOUS ADVERSE REACTIONS

- Abdominal distention, pain, chills, nervousness, dermatitis, septicemia, septic shock, prolonged QT interval.

OVERDOSE/TOXICITY

- **Ototoxicity:** High doses can cause hearing loss in patients with hepatic or renal dysfunction.
- **Hepatotoxicity:** Elevated liver enzymes, hepatitis, jaundice. Anaphylaxis and hepatotoxicity occur rarely.
- **Dysrhythmias:** Prolonged QT interval leading to torsade de pointes and ventricular tachycardia occur rarely with the IV drug form.
- **Superinfections:** Antibiotic-associated colitis and other superinfections.
- **GI decontamination:** No specific recommendations.

ANTIDOTE/DIALYSIS

- **Antidote:** No specific recommendations.
- **Dialysis:** Erythromycin is not removed by hemodialysis or peritoneal dialysis. No data are available on removal using high-permeability hemodialysis.

escitalopram oxalate

es-sye-tal'-oh-pram ok'-sal-ate

Classes

Chemical: bicyclic phthalane derivative
Therapeutic: antidepressant, selective serotonin reuptake inhibitor (SSRI)

Pregnancy Category: C

Trade Names

Prescription: Cipralex ♣, Lexapro

CLINICAL PHARMACOLOGY

Mechanism of Action

A selective serotonin reuptake inhibitor that blocks the uptake of the neurotransmitter serotonin at neuronal presynaptic membranes, increasing its availability at postsynaptic receptor sites. **Therapeutic Effect:** Relieves depression.

PHARMACOKINETICS

Well absorbed after PO administration. Primarily metabolized in the liver. Primarily excreted in feces with a lesser amount eliminated in urine. **Half-life:** 35 hr.

AVAILABILITY

Oral Solution: 5 mg/5 mL.
Tablets: 5 mg, 10 mg, 20 mg.

INDICATIONS AND DOSAGE

Depression, general anxiety disorder (GAD)

PO

Adults: Initially, 10 mg once per day in the morning or evening. May increase to 20 mg after a minimum of 1 wk. **Elderly, Patients with hepatic impairment:** 10 mg/day.

OFF-LABEL USES

Mixed anxiety and depressive disorder

CONTRAINDICATIONS

Breast-feeding, use within 14 days of MAOIs, hypersensitivity to escitalopram

INTERACTIONS

Drug: Alcohol, other CNS suppressants: May increase CNS depression. **Antifungals, cimetidine, macrolide antibiotics:** May increase plasma level of escitalopram. **Lithium:** May increase lithium concentration and increase the risk of serotonin syndrome. **MAOIs:** May cause serotonin syndrome, marked by autonomic hyperactivity, coma, diaphoresis, excitement, hyperthermia, and rigidity, and neuroleptic malignant syndrome. **Metoprolol:** Increases plasma level of metoprolol. **Herbal: Ginkgo biloba, St. John's wort:** May increase the risk of serotonin syndrome. **Food:** None known.

DIAGNOSTIC TEST EFFECTS

May reduce serum sodium level.

SIDE-EFFECTS

Frequent (21%-11%): Nausea, dry mouth, somnolence, insomnia, diaphoresis. **Occasional (8%-4%):** Tremor, diarrhea, abnormal ejaculation, dyspepsia, fatigue, anxiety, vomiting, anorexia. **Rare (3%-2%):** Sinusitis, sexual dysfunction, menstrual disorder, abdominal pain, agitation, decreased libido

CRITICAL CARE CONSIDERATIONS

ADMINISTRATION/HANDLING

PO ALERT

- Give escitalopram without regard to food.
- Do not crush film-coated tablets.
- Make sure at least 14 days elapse between the use of MAOIs and escitalopram.

PRECAUTIONS

HEALTH-RELATED

- Use escitalopram cautiously in patients with hepatic or renal impairment; those with history of hypomania, mania, or seizures; those concurrently using CNS depressants.

AGE-RELATED

- **Children:** Safety and efficacy have not been established in children; escitalopram use may increase anticholinergic effects and hyperexcitability.
- **Elderly:** More sensitive to the anticholinergic effects, such as dry mouth; are more likely to experience confusion, dizziness, hyperexcitability, and sedation.

PREGNANCY/LACTATION-RELATED

- Pregnancy category C; excreted in human breast milk; reports of infants experiencing excessive somnolence, decreased feeding, and weight loss in association with breast-feeding from a citalopram-treated mother.

MONITORING

- **Baseline assessment:** Observe and record behavior, appearance, interest in the environment, mood, sleep pattern, and thought content.

- **Baseline lab work:** CBC and liver and renal function tests before and periodically during long-term therapy.
- **Suicidal patients:** Closely supervise suicidal patients during early therapy. As depression lessens, energy level generally improves, increasing the suicide potential.
- **Therapeutic effect:** Assess for improvement in appearance, behavior, level of interest, mood, and sleep pattern.
- **Patient education:** Caution against discontinuing escitalopram or increasing the dosage. Urge avoiding alcohol while taking escitalopram. Warn to avoid tasks that require mental alertness or motor skills until response to the drug is known.

SERIOUS ADVERSE REACTIONS

- Dizziness, drowsiness, tachycardia, somnolence, palpitations, persistent severe cough, confusion.

OVERDOSE/TOXICITY

- **Cardiac:** Dyshythmias, fatigue, dyspnea, respiratory distress.
- **Dysrhythmias/ECG changes:** Sinus tachycardia, prolonged PR interval, prolonged QT interval, widened QRS complex greater than 100 msec, right axis deviation.
- **Neurologic:** Seizures, severe somnolence, hallucinations, agitation, weakness, fever.
- **Antimuscarinic/anticholinergic effects:** Dilated pupils, blurred vision, tachycardia, hyperthermia, hypertension, decreased oral and bronchial secretions, dry skin, ileus, urinary retention, increased muscle tone, tremor.
- **GI decontamination:** Ensure airway protection prior to initiating activated charcoal or gastric lavage on those patients who present quickly following ingestion.

ANTIDOTE/DIALYSIS

- **Antidote:** No specific recommendations. Manage fever and muscle rigidity aggressively. Cyproheptadine, methysergide, propranol, benzodiazepines may all have some benefit if serotonin syndrome is present. *ChlorproMAZINE should be used cautiously if diagnosis of serotonin syndrome is not clear.
- **Dialysis:** No data are available regarding removal of escitalopram using hemodialysis, high-permeability hemodialysis, or peritoneal dialysis.

esmolol hydrochloride

ess'-moe-lol hye-droe-klor'-ide

Classes

Chemical: β1-adrenergic blocker, cardioselective

Therapeutic: antidysrhythmic, class II

Pregnancy Category: C

Trade Names

Prescription: Brevibloc

CLINICAL PHARMACOLOGY

Mechanism of Action

An antidysrhythmic that selectively blocks $beta_1$-adrenergic receptors. **Therapeutic Effect:** Slows sinus heart rate, decreases cardiac output, reducing BP.

PHARMACOKINETICS

Rapidly metabolized primarily by esterase in the cytosol of red blood cells. Protein binding: 55%. Less than 1%-2% excreted in urine. **Half-life:** 9 min.

AVAILABILITY

Injection: 10 mg/mL, 20 mg/mL, 250 mg/mL.

INDICATIONS AND DOSAGE

Dysrhythmias

IV

Adults, Elderly: Initially, loading dose of 500 mcg/kg/min for 1 min, followed by 50 mcg/kg/min for 4 min. If optimum response is not attained in 5 min, give second loading dose of 500 mcg/kg/min for 1 min, followed by infusion of 100 mcg/kg/min for 4 min. Additional loading doses can be given and infusion increased by 50 mcg/kg/min, up to 200 mcg/kg/min, for 4 min. Once desired response is attained, cease loading dose and increase infusion by no more than 25 mcg/kg/min. Interval between doses may be increased to 10 min. Infusion usually administered over 24-48 hr in most patients. Range: 50-200 mcg/kg/min, with average dose of 100 mcg/kg/min.

Intraoperative tachycardia or hypertension (immediate control)

IV

Adults, Elderly: Initially, 80 mg over 30 sec, then 150 mcg/kg/min infusion up to 300 mcg/kg/min.

CONTRAINDICATIONS

Cardiogenic shock, overt cardiac failure, second- and third-degree heart block, sinus bradycardia, hypersensitivity to esmolol

INTERACTIONS

Drug: **Insulin, oral hypoglycemics:** May mask symptoms of hypoglycemia and prolong hypoglycemic effect of these drugs. **MAOIs:** May cause significant hypertension. **Sympathomimetics, xanthines:** May mutually inhibit effects. **Herbal:** None known. **Food:** None known.

DIAGNOSTIC TEST EFFECTS

None known.

IV INCOMPATIBILITIES

Amphotericin B complex (Abelcet, Ambisome, Amphotec), furosemide (Lasix)

IV COMPATIBILITIES

Amiodarone (Cordarone), diltiazem (Cardizem), *DOPamine (Intropin), heparin, magnesium, midazolam (Versed), potassium chloride, propofol (Diprivan)

SIDE-EFFECTS

Frequent: Esmolol is generally well tolerated, with transient and mild side effects. Hypotension (systolic BP less than 90 mmHg) manifested as dizziness, nausea, diaphoresis, headache, cold extremities, fatigue. **Occasional:** Anxiety, drowsiness, flushed skin, vomiting, confusion, inflammation at injection site, fever

CRITICAL CARE CONSIDERATIONS

ADMINISTRATION/HANDLING

IV ALERT

- **IV infusion only:** Give esmolol by IV infusion into a large vein. Avoid butterfly needles and very small veins. *Do not administer esmolol by direct IV injection.*
- **Storage:** Store vials and premixed infusion at controlled room temperature. Use only clear and colorless to light yellow solution.
- **Stability:** After dilution, solution is stable for 24 hr. Discard solution if it is discolored or if precipitate forms.
- **Infusion:** Remove 20 mL from 500-mL container IV solution and dilute the prescribed amount of esmolol 250 mg/mL concentration in the remaining 480 mL of solution to provide a concentration of 10 mg/mL.
- **Maximum concentration:** 10 g/250 mL (40 mg/mL), which must be given into a large or central vein. Administer by controlled infusion device and titrate according to patient tolerance and response.
- **Loading dose:** Infuse IV loading dose over 1-2 min.

PRECAUTIONS

HEALTH-RELATED

- Use esmolol cautiously in patients with bronchial asthma, bronchitis, coronary artery disease, chronic obstructive pulmonary disease (COPD), diabetes mellitus, emphysema, heart failure, history of allergy, history of hypoglycemia, and impaired renal function.

AGE-RELATED

- **Children:** Safety and efficacy of esmolol have not been established in children.
- **Elderly:** May require reduced dose due to increased potential of heart block and heart failure.

PREGNANCY/LACTATION-RELATED

- Pregnancy category C; potential for hypotension and subsequent decreased uterine blood flow and fetal hypoxia should be considered; excretion into breast milk unknown; use caution in nursing mothers.

MONITORING

- **Baseline assessment:** Assess pulse and BP immediately before giving esmolol. If pulse is less than 60 beats/min or systolic BP is less than 90 mmHg, nurses should withhold the medication and contact the physician for further directions on dosing before beginning infusion. Another medication may be needed to reduce heart rate or BP (calcium channel blocker). Determine history of heart, respiratory, or kidney problems, hypoglycemia, or diabetes mellitus.
- **Bradycardia and heart block:** Monitor ECG continuously for decreased heart rate, prolonged PR interval, and dropped QRS complexes.
- **Hypotension:** Monitor BP at least every 15 min for systolic of less than 90 mmHg, which may result from decreasing heart rate or decreased strength of ventricular contraction, especially during the first 30 min of infusion. Observe for diaphoresis and dizziness indicative of hypotension.
- **Respiratory distress:** Monitor the respiratory rate, work of breathing and pulse oximetry (SpO_2), and heart rate, especially if there is a history of asthma, bronchitis, emphysema, or heart failure. Assess breath

sounds for increased wheezes, crackles, and rales if patients complain of dyspnea. Dose may need to be reduced.

- **Heart failure:** Assess pulse for slowing/bradycardia and decreased strength which indicate cardiac output may be reduced. Assess extremities for coldness. Evaluate for diaphoresis, fatigue, headache, and nausea.
- **IV morphine:** IV morphine increases esmolol steady state levels by 50%.
- **Succinylcholine:** Esmolol may prolong neuromuscular blockade induced by this drug.
- **Patient education:** Explain that BP and heart rate will be continuously monitored during esmolol therapy. Instruct to report immediately cold extremities, dizziness, faintness, or nausea.

SERIOUS ADVERSE REACTIONS

- **Hypoglycemia:** Esmolol may mask symptoms of hypoglycemia and potentiate insulin-induced hypoglycemia in diabetic patients.
- **Respiratory distress:** COPD patients dependent on bronchodilators may not tolerate esmolol without increasing doses of bronchodilators; because bronchodilators often cause tachycardia and increased BP, this may defeat the purpose of using esmolol to reduce heart rate or BP.
- **IV site induration:** Esmolol is very irritating to veins; use of small veins or infusion concentrations over more than 10 mg/mL may prompt phlebitis.
- **Abrupt withdrawal:** May cause angina, acute MI, and lethal ventricular dysrhythmias if not withdrawn gradually unless patients are toxic.

OVERDOSE/TOXICITY

- Profound hypotension, bradycardia, dizziness, syncope, drowsiness, breathing difficulty, nausea, vomiting, pallor, central cyanosis, bluish fingernails or palms of hands, somnolence, speech disorders, weakness, and seizures.
- **GI decontamination:** No specific recommendations.

ANTIDOTE/DIALYSIS

- **Antidote:** Once the esmolol infusion is off, *DOPamine or epinephrine infusions may be used to increase heart rate and help manage heart block and may help relieve respiratory distress. Atropine may be used for bradycardia but does not have catecholamine properties useful for overriding beta blockade. Unresponsive hypotension and bradycardia may be reversed by glucagon 5-10 mg IV over 30 sec, followed by a continuous infusion of 5 mg/hr, titrated down as patients improve.
- **Dialysis:** Esmolol is removed using hemodialysis and peritoneal dialysis and is likely to be removed using high-permeability hemodialysis.

esomeprazole

es-oh-mep'-rah-zole

Classes

Chemical: benzimidazole derivative

Therapeutic: antiulcer agent, gastrointestinal antisecretory agent

Pregnancy Category: B

Trade Names

Prescription: Nexium, Nexium IV

CLINICAL PHARMACOLOGY

Mechanism of Action

A proton pump inhibitor that is converted to active metabolites that irreversibly bind to and inhibit hydrogen-potassium adenosine triphosphates, an enzyme on the surface of gastric parietal cells. Inhibits hydrogen ion transport into gastric lumen. Therapeutic Effect: Increases gastric pH, reducing gastric acid production.

PHARMACOKINETICS

Well absorbed after oral administration. Protein binding: 97%. Extensively metabolized by the liver. Primarily excreted in urine. Half-life: 1-1.5 hr.

AVAILABILITY

Capsules (delayed release, Magnesium [Nexium]): 20 mg, 40 mg.

Powder for solution (sodium [Nexium IV]): 20 mg, 40 mg.

INDICATIONS AND DOSAGE

Erosive esophagitis

PO

Adults, Elderly: 20-40 mg once daily for 4-8 wk.

IV

Adults, Elderly: 20 or 40 mg once daily by IV injection over at least 3 min or IV infusion over 10-30 min.

To maintain healing of erosive esophagitis

PO

Adults, Elderly: 20 mg/day.

Gastroesophageal reflux disease (GERD), to reduce the risk of NSAID-induced gastric ulcer
PO
Adults, Elderly: 20 mg once per day for 4 wk.
Duodenal ulcer caused by *Helicobacter pylori*
PO
Adults, Elderly: 40 mg (esomeprazole) once per day, with amoxicillin 1000 mg and clarithromycin 500 mg twice per day for 10 days.

CONTRAINDICATIONS
Hypersensitivity to esomeprazole or other benzimidazoles

IV INCOMPATIBILITIES
Do not mix esomeprazole with any other medications through the same IV line or tubing.

INTERACTIONS
Drug: Digoxin, iron, ketoconazole: May decrease the concentration of digoxin, iron, and ketoconazole. **Herbal:** None known. **Food:** None known.

DIAGNOSTIC TEST EFFECTS
None known.

SIDE-EFFECTS
Frequent (7%): Headache. **Occasional (3%-2%):** Diarrhea, abdominal pain, nausea. **Rare (less than 2%):** Dizziness, asthenia or loss of strength, vomiting, constipation, rash, cough

CRITICAL CARE CONSIDERATIONS

ADMINISTRATION/HANDLING
PO ALERT
- Give 1 hr or more before eating.
- Do not crush or open capsules; instruct to swallow the capsule whole. If patients have difficulty swallowing, open the capsule and mix pellets with 1 tablespoon of applesauce. Instruct to swallow the spoonful without chewing.

PRECAUTIONS
HEALTH-RELATED
- Esomeprazole is often used in combination with other medications to help heal erosive esophagitis secondary to GERD (acid reflux), and as part of a drug regimen including clarithromycin and amoxicillin to eradicate *H. pylori* infection to reduce the risk of duodenal ulcer recurrence.

AGE-RELATED
- **Children:** Safety and efficacy of esomeprazole have not been established in children.
- **Elderly:** No age-related precautions have been noted.

PREGNANCY/LACTATION-RELATED
- Pregnancy category B; likely to be excreted into breast milk, use caution in nursing mothers (suppression of gastric acid secretion is potential effect in nursing infant, clinical significance unknown).

MONITORING
- **Baseline assessment:** Before giving esomeprazole, determine ability to swallow capsules whole or if capsule must be opened and mixed with food. Determine whether patients are on a regimen to eradicate *H. pylori* because this population is at risk for developing GI complications related to the antibiotics (clarithromycin and amoxicillin).
- **Therapeutic effect:** Evaluate for relief of GI symptoms including heartburn, gas, chest discomfort, abdominal pain, nausea, and diarrhea.
- **Superinfections:** If receiving antibiotics for *H. pylori*, assess the mouth for white patches on the mucous membranes or tongue, severe mouth or tongue soreness, and severe anal or genital pruritus or discharge.
- **Possible *Clostridium difficile* colitis:** Assess pattern of daily bowel activity and stool consistency. Although mild GI effects may be tolerable, severe symptoms including abdominal pain or cramping and moderate to severe diarrhea may indicate the onset of antibiotic-associated colitis, which can be confused with failure of treatment regimen for *H. pylori*.
- **Hand washing:** If patients are on antibiotics and develop *C. difficile* (antibiotic-associated) colitis, wash hands with antibacterial soap. Alcohol-based foam is ineffective against *C. difficile* spores.
- **Patient education:** Instruct to report if persistent headache occurs during esomeprazole therapy to a health care provider. Instruct to take esomeprazole 1 hr or more before eating. Teach patients who have difficulty swallowing to open the capsule, mix the pellets with 1 tablespoon of applesauce, and swallow the spoonful without chewing.

E

SERIOUS ADVERSE REACTIONS
- None life-threatening from esomeprazole but patients may have drug-specific side effects from clarithromycin or amoxicillin if used as part of *H. pylori* eradication.

OVERDOSE/TOXICITY
- Headache, diarrhea, nausea, vomiting, flatulence, abdominal pain, altered taste, dry mouth.
- **GI decontamination:** No specific recommendations.

ANTIDOTE/DIALYSIS
- **Antidote:** No specific recommendations.
- **Dialysis:** Esopmeprazole is unlikely to be removed by hemodialysis, high-permeability hemodialysis, or peritoneal dialysis.

estrapenem

See Antibiotics (p. 892)

etanercept

eh-tan'-er-sept

Classes
Chemical: recombinant human fusion protein
Therapeutic: disease-modifying antirheumatic drug (DMARD), immunomodulatory agent

Pregnancy Category: B

Trade Names
Prescription: Enbrel

CLINICAL PHARMACOLOGY
Mechanism of Action
A protein that binds to tumor necrosis factor (TNF), blocking its interaction with cell surface receptors. Elevated levels of TNF, which is involved in inflammatory and immune responses, are found in the synovial fluid of rheumatoid arthritis patients. **Therapeutic Effect:** Relieves symptoms of rheumatoid arthritis.

PHARMACOKINETICS
Well absorbed after subcutaneous administration. **Half-life:** 115 hr.

AVAILABILITY
Powder for injection: 25 mg.
Prefilled syringe: 50 mg.

INDICATIONS AND DOSAGE
Rheumatoid arthritis, psoriatic arthritis, ankylosing spondylitis
Subcutaneous
Adults, Elderly: 50 mg weekly. Maximum: 50 mg/wk.
Juvenile rheumatoid arthritis
Subcutaneous
Children 4-17 yr: 0.4 mg/kg (maximum: 25 mg dose) twice weekly given 72-96 hr apart. Alternative weekly dosing: 50 mg once weekly. Maximum: 25 mg/dose.
Plaque psoriasis
Subcutaneous
Adults, Elderly: 50 mg twice per wk (give 3-4 days apart) for 3 mo. Maintenance: 50 mg once per wk.

OFF-LABEL USES
Treatment of Crohn's disease, reactive arthritis

CONTRAINDICATIONS
Serious active infection or sepsis, hypersensitivity to etanercept

INTERACTIONS
Drug: Cyclophosphamide: May increase incidence of developing noncutaneous solid malignancies. **Herbal:** None known. **Food:** None known.

DIAGNOSTIC TEST EFFECTS
None known.

SIDE-EFFECTS
Frequent (37%): Injection site erythema, pruritus, pain, and swelling; abdominal pain (19%), vomiting (more common in children than adults). **Occasional (16%-4%):** Headache, rhinitis, dizziness, pharyngitis, cough, asthenia, abdominal pain, dyspepsia. **Rare (less than 3%):** Sinusitis, allergic reaction

CRITICAL CARE CONSIDERATIONS

ADMINISTRATION/HANDLING

SUBCUTANEOUS ALERT
- **Storage:** Refrigerate unopened vials. Do not freeze. Once reconstituted, the drug may be stored for up to 14 days if refrigerated at 2-8°C (36-46°F).
- **Reconstitution/dilution:** Reconstitute only with 1 mL sterile bacteriostatic water for injection (containing 0.9% benzyl alcohol). Do not use other diluents. Slowly inject the diluent into the vial. Some foaming will occur. To avoid

excessive foaming, slowly swirl the contents until the powder is dissolved (less than 5 min). Reconstituted solution normally appears clear and colorless. Discard the solution if it contains particles or becomes cloudy or discolored.

- **Before injection:** Withdraw all the solution into the syringe. The final volume should be approximately 1 mL. Do not add other medications to the solution or use a filter during reconstitution or administration.
- **Administration:** Inject the drug into the abdomen, thigh, or upper arm. Rotate injection sites. Administer each new injection at least 1 inch from an old site, avoiding tender, bruised, hard, or red areas.

PRECAUTIONS

HEALTH-RELATED

- Use etanercept cautiously in patients with a history of recurrent infections or illnesses that predispose to infection, such as diabetes mellitus.
- Patients should not receive live virus vaccines during treatment.
- Glucocorticoids, nonsteroidal antiinflammatory agents, and analgesics may be continued in juvenile rheumatoid arthritis patients.

AGE-RELATED

- **Children:** No age-related precautions in children 4 yr and older.
- **Elderly:** No age-related precautions have been noted.

PREGNANCY/LACTATION-RELATED

- Pregnancy category B; information on breast milk excretion is unknown; breastfeeding not advised.

MONITORING

- **Baseline assessment:** Assess the duration, location, onset, and type of inflammation or pain being experienced.
- **Baseline lab work:** CBC with WBC differential, erythrocyte sedimentation rate, and/or C-reactive protein level.
- **Therapeutic response:** Evaluate for improved grip strength, increased joint mobility, reduced joint tenderness, and relief of pain, stiffness, and swelling.
- **Varicella exposure:** If significant exposure to varicella virus (chicken pox) occurs during treatment, temporarily discontinue therapy and treat with varicella-zoster immune globulin.
- **Pancytopenia:** Monitor patients for persistent fever, bruising, bleeding.
- **Injection site reaction:** Assess injection sites for redness, pain, and hardness. Do not inject within 1 inch of a tender, reddened, or hardened site.
- **Patient education:** When using etanercept outside the hospital, teach patients and caregivers how to prepare and inject the drug as well as preferred injection sites. Reassure patients that injection site reactions generally occur in the first month of treatment and decrease in frequency with continued therapy. Caution against receiving live-virus vaccines during treatment. Instruct to report bleeding, bruising, pallor, or persistent fever to a health care provider. Instruct to report muscle weakness, visual changes, and abnormal sensation to a health care provider immediately.

SERIOUS ADVERSE REACTIONS

- **Infections:** Upper respiratory infections, pyelonephritis, cellulitis, osteomyelitis, wound infection, leg ulcer, septic arthritis, diarrhea, bronchitis, and pneumonia; infections occur in about one third of patients.
- **Malignancies:** Occurrence of new cancer.
- **Rare adverse effects:** Include heart failure, chest pain, hypertension, hypotension, cholecystitis, pancreatitis, GI hemorrhage, and dyspnea.

OVERDOSE/TOXICITY

- **Autoimmune antibodies:** Patients may develop autoimmune antibodies.
- **Central nervous system:** Rare cases of new onset transverse myelitis, optic neuritis, multiple sclerosis, and exacerbation or new onset of seizure disorders.
- **Pancytopenia:** Rare cases of aplastic anemia manifested by persistent fever, bleeding, bruising, pallor.
- **GI decontamination:** No specific recommendations.

ANTIDOTE/DIALYSIS

- **Antidote:** No specific recommendations.
- **Dialysis:** Etanercept is unlikely to be removed using hemodialysis, high-permeability hemodialysis, or peritoneal dialysis.

ethacrynic acid

See Diuretics (p. 956)

ethambutol

e-tham'-byoo-tole

Classes

Chemical: diisopropylethylene diamide derivative

Therapeutic: antituberculosis agent

Pregnancy Category: B

Trade Names

Prescription: Etibi ♣, Myambutol

Do not confuse ethambutol or Myambutol with Nembutal.

CLINICAL PHARMACOLOGY

Mechanism of Action

An isonicotinic acid derivative that interferes with RNA synthesis. **Therapeutic Effect:** Suppresses the multiplication of mycobacteria.

PHARMACOKINETICS

Rapidly and well absorbed from the GI tract. Protein binding: 20%-30%. Widely distributed. Metabolized in the liver. Primarily excreted in urine. Removed by hemodialysis. **Half-life:** 3-4 hr (increased in impaired renal function).

AVAILABILITY

Tablets: 100 mg, 400 mg.

INDICATIONS AND DOSAGE

Tuberculosis, other mycobacterial diseases

PO

Adults, Elderly: 15-25 mg/kg/day. Maximum: 1.6 g/dose. **Children at least 13 yr:** 15 mg/kg/day. Maximum: 1 g/day.

Dosage in renal impairment

Dosage interval is modified based on creatinine clearance.

Creatinine Clearance	Dosage Interval
10-50 mL/min	Every 24-36 hr
Less than 10 mL/min	Every 48 hr

OFF-LABEL USES

Treatment of atypical mycobacterial infections such as *Mycobacterium avium* complex (MAC)

CONTRAINDICATIONS

Optic neuritis, hypersensitivity to ethambutol

INTERACTIONS

Drug: **Neurotoxic medications:** May increase the risk of neurotoxicity. **Aluminum-containing products:** Decrease ethambutol concentration. **Herbal:** None known. **Food:** None known.

DIAGNOSTIC TEST EFFECTS

May increase serum uric acid levels.

SIDE-EFFECTS

Occasional: Acute gouty arthritis (chills, pain, swelling of joints with hot skin), confusion, abdominal pain, nausea, vomiting, anorexia, headache. **Rare:** Rash, fever, blurred vision, eye pain, red-green color blindness

CRITICAL CARE CONSIDERATIONS

ADMINISTRATION/HANDLING

PO ALERT

- Ethambutol should not be used as a sole agent to treat tuberculosis but given in combination with isoniazid or isoniazid and streptomycin for initial treatment or retreatment.
- Give ethambutol with food to decrease GI upset.

PRECAUTIONS

HEALTH-RELATED

- Use ethambutol cautiously in patients with cataracts, diabetic retinopathy, recurrent ocular inflammatory conditions, gout, or renal dysfunction.
- Ethambutol use is not recommended for children under 13 yr.

AGE-RELATED

- **Children:** Safety and efficacy of ethambutol have not been established in children under 13 yr.
- **Elderly:** Age-related renal impairment may require a dosage adjustment in the elderly.

PREGNANCY/LACTATION-RELATED

- Pregnancy category B; compatible with breast-feeding.

MONITORING

- **Baseline assessment:** Determine history of kidney and liver disease, problems with vision, gout, arthritis, nausea, and other GI problems to be better able to assess drug side effects. Assess the home situation so others exposed may be assessed and treated.
- **Baseline lab work:** CBC with differential, biochemical profile including renal and liver function, and uric acid results.
- **Infection control:** Report tuberculosis to the hospital infection control specialists and implement strict isolation. Family

members should be screened and managed by the public health department.

- **Vision changes:** Assess for altered color perception and decreased visual acuity. If vision changes occur, discontinue ethambutol.
- **Arthritis and gout:** Monitor serum uric acid levels. Assess for hot, painful, or swollen joints, especially in the ankle, big toe, or knee, indicative of gout.
- **Peripheral neuritis:** Assess for burning, numbness, or tingling of the extremities which may warrant discontinuing the drug.
- **Patient education:** Advise not to skip drug doses and to take ethambutol for the full course of therapy, which may be months or years. Warn to report visual problems immediately to a health care provider. Explain that visual effects are generally reversible after ethambutol is discontinued, but that in rare cases they may take up to a year to resolve or may become permanent. Advise to report promptly burning, numbness, or tingling of the feet or hands, as well as pain and swelling of joints.

SERIOUS ADVERSE REACTIONS

- Vision disturbances, movement disorders, arthritis, and gout.

OVERDOSE/TOXICITY

- **Nervous system:** Optic neuritis (more common with high-dosage or long-term ethambutol therapy), peripheral neuritis.
- **Hematology/immunology:** Rare thrombocytopenia and anaphylactoid reaction.
- **GI decontamination:** No specific recommendations.

ANTIDOTE/DIALYSIS

- **Antidote:** No specific recommendations.
- **Dialysis:** Ethambutol is removed by hemodialysis, high-permeability hemodialysis, and peritoneal dialysis.

ethosuximide

See Anticonvulsants (p. 903)

ethotoin

See Anticonvulsants (p. 903)

etodolac

See NSAIDs and Cox-2 Inhibitors (p. 976)

etomidate

e-tome'-i-date

Classes

Chemical: imidazole carboxylate, GABA mimetic

Therapeutic: hypnotic, anesthetic

Pregnancy Category: C

Trade Names

Prescription: Amidate

CLINICAL PHARMACOLOGY

Mechanism of Action

An ultra-short-acting hypnotic that appears to have gamma-aminobutyric acid (GABA)-like effects. **Therapeutic Effect:** Produces CNS hypnosis and anesthesia.

PHARMACOKINETICS

Hypnosis occurs within 1 min of intravenous injection. Rapidly metabolized in liver. Excreted in urine. **Half-life:** 75 min.

AVAILABILITY

Solution for Injection: 2 mg/mL.

INDICATIONS AND DOSAGE

Induction of general anesthesia

IV

Adults, Children older than 10 yr: 0.2 and 0.6 mg/kg of body weight, individualized in each case. The usual dose for induction in these patients 0.3 mg/kg, injected over a period of 30-60 sec.

CONTRAINDICATIONS

Hypersensitivity to etomidate

INTERACTIONS

Drug: None known. **Herbal:** None known. **Food:** None known.

DIAGNOSTIC TEST EFFECTS

May decrease plasma cortisol and aldosterone concentrations.

SIDE-EFFECTS

Frequent: Myoclonus, transient venous pain. **Occasional:** Nausea, vomiting. **Rare:** Hypertension, hypotension, tachycardia, bradycardia, dysrhythmias, hyperventilation, hypoventilation, apnea of short duration, laryngospasm, hiccups, snoring

CRITICAL CARE CONSIDERATIONS

ADMINISTRATION/HANDLING

IV ALERT

- **Not for prolonged infusion:** Because of the hazards of prolonged suppression of endogenous cortisol and aldosterone production, this formulation is not intended for administration by prolonged infusion.
- **IV only:** Only administer intravenously. Inject over 30-60 sec.
- **Anesthesia professionals:** Etomidate should be administered only by people specially trained in administration of general anesthetics.

PRECAUTIONS

HEALTH-RELATED

- Use etomidate cautiously in patients with severe cardiovascular disease, severe asthma, or marked hypotension.

AGE-RELATED

- **Children:** Safety and efficacy of etomidate have not been established in children under 10 yr.
- **Elderly:** May be more susceptible to adverse effects associated with etomidate.

PREGNANCY/LACTATION-RELATED

- Pregnancy category C; unknown if excreted in breast milk.

MONITORING

- **Baseline assessment:** Obtain BP and heart rate. Assess for respiratory distress if drug will be used for rapid sequence endotracheal intubation.
- **Lab work:** CBC with differential; biochemical profile in preparation for surgical or other procedures.
- **Diagnostic tests:** Chest x-ray to assess pulmonary status; 12-lead ECG to evaluate for dysrhythmias and myocardial ischemia.
- **Before anesthesia induction:** Monitor BP, heart rate, oxygen saturation, and respiratory rate.
- **Anesthesia induction:** Monitor the induction of anesthesia. Hypnosis occurs within 1 min of intravenous injection.
- **Skeletal muscle movements:** When used as a part of anesthesia for invasive procedures, ensure a neuromuscular blocking agent is also given to avoid unexpected skeletal muscle movements during the procedure.
- **Patient education:** Instruct to immediately report chest pain, shortness of breath, or irregular heartbeat to the health care provider administering the drug.

SERIOUS ADVERSE REACTIONS

- **Hypersensitivity:** One case of severe hypotension and tachycardia, judged to be anaphylaxis, has been reported.

OVERDOSE/TOXICITY

- Hypertension, hypotension, tachycardia, bradycardia, dysrhythmias, hyperventilation, hypoventilation, apnea of short duration, laryngospasm, hiccup, snoring.
- **GI decontamination:** No specific recommendations.

ANTIDOTE/DIALYSIS

- **Antidote:** No specific recommendations.
- **Dialysis:** No data are available on removal of etomidate by hemodialysis, high-permeability hemodialysis, or peritoneal dialysis.

exenatide 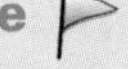

ex-en'-a-tide

Classes

Chemical: incretin mimetic
Therapeutic: antihyperglycemic

Pregnancy Category: C

Trade Names

Prescription: Byetta

CLINICAL PHARMACOLOGY

Mechanism of Action

An incretin mimetic agent that mimics the enhancement of glucose-dependent insulin secretion and several other antihyperglycemic actions of incretins. Incretins, such as glucagon-like peptide-1 (GLP-1), enhance glucose-dependent insulin secretion and exhibit other antihyperglycemic actions following release into circulation from the gut. **Therapeutic Effect:** Controls glucose levels in diabetic patients.

PHARMACOKINETICS

Following subcutaneous administration, exenatide reaches median peak plasma concentrations in 2.1 hr. Excreted in the kidney predominantly by glomerular filtration with subsequent proteolytic degradation. **Half-life:** 2.4 hr.

AVAILABILITY

Solution for subcutaneous injection (Byetta): 250 mcg/mL.

INDICATIONS AND DOSAGE

Type 2 diabetes mellitus, as an adjunct in patients taking metformin, a sulfonylurea, or a combination of metformin and a sulfonylurea but have not achieved adequate glycemic control

Subcutaneous

Adults, Elderly: Initially, 5 mcg administered twice daily 60 min before the morning and evening meals. The dose may be increased to 10 mcg twice daily after 1 mo of therapy.

CONTRAINDICATIONS

Hypersensitivity to exenatide or any component of the formulation

INTERACTIONS

Drug: Acetaminophen: May decrease the bioavailability of acetaminophen. **Lovastatin:** May decrease the bioavailability of lovastatin. **Orally administered drugs:** May reduce the extent and rate of absorption of orally administered drugs. **Herbal:** None known. **Food:** None known.

DIAGNOSTIC TEST EFFECTS

None known.

SIDE-EFFECTS

Frequent: Nausea (44%), vomiting (13%), diarrhea (13%), hypoglycemia (5%-35%). **Occasional:** Jittery feeling, dizziness, headache, dyspepsia. **Rare:** Weakness, decreased appetite, gastroesophageal reflux disease, hyperhidrosis

CRITICAL CARE CONSIDERATIONS

ADMINISTRATION/HANDLING

SUBCUTANEOUS ALERT

- **Storage:** Store unused pens in the original carton in the refrigerator. Protect from light. Do not freeze.
- **Stability:** Discard pen 30 days after first use, even if some drug remains in the pen.
- **Food:** Inject 60 min before morning and evening meals. Do not inject after meals.
- **Timing:** Medications dependent on threshold concentrations (e.g., antibiotics and contraceptives) should be taken at least 1 hr before injection of exenatide.
- **Injection site:** Administer in the thigh, abdomen, or upper arm.

PRECAUTIONS

HEALTH-RELATED

- Exenatide is not a substitute for insulin in patients requiring insulin and should not be used in patients with type 1 diabetes or for treatment of diabetic ketoacidosis (DKA).
- Not recommended for patients with end-stage renal disease, severe renal impairment, or severe gastrointestinal disease.
- Exenatide may slow gastric emptying, affecting absorption of orally administered medications; most significant if patients are taking a drug that requires rapid GI absorption.

AGE-RELATED

- **Children:** Safety and efficacy of exenatide have not been established in children.
- **Elderly:** No age-related precautions have been noted.

PREGNANCY/LACTATION-RELATED

- Pregnancy category C; unknown if excreted in human breast milk.

MONITORING

- **Baseline assessment:** Discuss lifestyle to determine the extent of emotional and learning needs regarding diabetes mellitus.
- **Baseline lab work:** Biochemical panel including blood glucose.
- **Blood glucose:** Monitor blood glucose level and food intake. Monitor more closely when conditions arise that alter blood glucose requirements including fever, increased activity, stress, or a surgical procedure. Some patients attain blood glucose control for the first time in the course of having diabetes when started on exenatide.
- **Hypoglycemia:** Assess for anxiety; cool, wet skin; diplopia; dizziness; headache; hunger; numbness in mouth; tachycardia, and tremors.
- **Hyperglycemia:** Assess for deep rapid breathing, dim vision, fatigue, nausea, polydipsia, polyphagia, polyuria, and vomiting.
- **Weight loss:** Monitor weight. Weight may be lost when started on the medication; weight gain is possible when medication is withdrawn.
- **Patient education:** Stress that prescribed diet is a principal part of treatment. Warn not to skip or delay meals. Teach signs and symptoms of hypoglycemia and hyperglycemia. Instruct to carry candy, sugar

packets, or other sugar supplements for immediate response to hypoglycemia. Urge wearing medical alert identification. Instruct to report to a health care provider when glucose demands are altered such as with fever, heavy physical activity, infection, stress, or trauma. Ensure follow-up instruction if patients or families do not thoroughly understand diabetes management or blood glucose-testing technique. Teach to wear sunscreen and protective eyewear to prevent the effects of light sensitivity.

E

SERIOUS ADVERSE REACTIONS

- **Hypoglycemia:** Jittery feeling, dizziness, headache, dyspepsia.
- **Medication withdrawal:** Patients may experience hyperglycemia.

OVERDOSE/TOXICITY

- **Acute hypoglycemia:** Nausea, severe vomiting, and rapidly decreasing blood glucose levels; possible tachycardia, diaphoresis, confusion, and seizures if hypoglycemia is not treated promptly.
- **GI decontamination:** No specific recommendations.

ANTIDOTE/DIALYSIS

- **Antidote:** 50% dextrose (D50) IV up to 25 mL (should be given based on blood glucose level) which may be repeated every 15 min until blood glucose normalizes; glucagon 1-2 mg IM is the recognized antidote. Oral carbohydrates (juice, soda, candy, glucose tablets) will help resolve hypoglycemia if patients are safely able to have PO food or fluids.
- **Dialysis:** No data are available on removal of exenatide by hemodialysis, high-permeability hemodialysis, or peritoneal dialysis.

ezetimibe

ez-et'-i-mibe

Classes

Chemical: substituted azetidinone

Therapeutic: selective cholesterol absorption inhibitor

Pregnancy Category: C

Trade Names

Prescription: Ezetrol ♣, Zetia

Combinations

Prescription: with simvastatin (Vytorin)

Do not confuse Zetia with Zestril.

CLINICAL PHARMACOLOGY

Mechanism of Action

An antihyperlipidemic that inhibits cholesterol absorption in the small intestine, leading to a decrease in the delivery of intestinal cholesterol to the liver. **Therapeutic Effect:** Reduces total serum cholesterol, LDL cholesterol, and triglyceride levels and increases HDL cholesterol concentration.

PHARMACOKINETICS

Poorly absorbed following oral administration. Protein binding: greater than 90%. Metabolized in the small intestine and liver. Excreted by the kidneys and bile. **Half-life:** 22 hr.

AVAILABILITY

Tablets: 10 mg.

INDICATIONS AND DOSAGE

Hypercholesterolemia

PO

Adults, Elderly: Initially, 10 mg once per day, given with or without food. If the patient is also receiving a bile acid sequestrant, give ezetimibe at least 2 hr before or at least 4 hr after the bile acid sequestrant.

Sitosterolemia

PO

Adults, Elderly: 10 mg/day.

CONTRAINDICATIONS

Concurrent use of an hydroxymethylglutaryl-CoA (HMG-CoA) reductase inhibitor (atorvastatin, fluvastatin, lovastatin, pravastatin, or simvastatin) in patients with active hepatic disease or unexplained persistent elevations in serum transaminase levels, moderate or severe hepatic insufficiency, hypersensitivity to ezetimibe

INTERACTIONS

Drug: Aluminum and magnesium-containing antacids, *cycloSPORINE, fenofibrate, gemfibrozil: Increase ezetimibe plasma concentration. **Cholestyramine resin:** Decreases drug effectiveness. **Herbal:** None known. **Food:** None known.

DIAGNOSTIC TEST EFFECTS

May increase serum alkaline phosphatase, serum bilirubin, AST (SGOT), and ALT (SGPT) levels.

SIDE-EFFECTS

Occasional (4%-3%): Back pain, diarrhea, arthralgia, sinusitis, abdominal pain. **Rare (2%):** Cough, pharyngitis, fatigue

CRITICAL CARE CONSIDERATIONS

ADMINISTRATION/HANDLING

PO ALERT

- Give ezetimibe without regard to food.

PRECAUTIONS

HEALTH-RELATED

- Use ezetimibe cautiously in patients with chronic renal failure, diabetes, hypothyroidism, liver function impairment, or obstructive liver disease.

AGE-RELATED

- **Children:** Safety and efficacy of ezetimibe have not been established in children 10 yr and younger.
- **Elderly:** Age-related mild hepatic impairment requires dosage adjustment. This drug is not recommended for use in elderly patients with moderate or severe hepatic impairment.

PREGNANCY/LACTATION-RELATED

- Pregnancy category C; human breast milk exposure unknown; up to half of exposure of maternal plasma in animal pups.

MONITORING

- **Baseline assessment:** Assess weight, waist circumference, BP, history of hyperglycemia, and other indicators for metabolic syndrome. Discuss current diet, exercise, and willingness to change dietary habits.
- **Baseline lab work:** CBC with differential, biochemical profile including blood glucose, lipid cholesterol and triglyceride levels, and liver function test results during initial therapy and periodically during treatment.
- **Drug discontinuation:** Discontinue treatment if liver enzyme levels are consistently greater than 3 times the normal limit.
- **Diarrhea:** Assess pattern of daily bowel activity and stool consistency.
- **Pain:** Evaluate for abdominal and back pain.
- **Therapeutic response:** Monitor for decreased serum cholesterol and triglyceride concentrations.
- **Patient education:** Teach dietary habits used to lower lipid levels, including low-fat and consistent carbohydrate diets. Explain importance of managing weight and blood glucose level if metabolic syndrome is present. Discuss increased risk of cardiac and peripheral vascular disease. Stress that periodic laboratory tests are an essential part of therapy. Caution against discontinuing ezetimibe without physician approval.

SERIOUS ADVERSE REACTIONS

- **Liver dysfunction:** Elevated liver enzymes.

OVERDOSE/TOXICITY

- Chest pain, dizziness, headache, abdominal pain, diarrhea, upper respiratory symptoms, muscle and joint discomfort.
- **GI decontamination:** No specific recommendations.

ANTIDOTE/DIALYSIS

- **Antidote:** No specific recommendations.
- **Dialysis:** Ezetimibe is unlikely to be removed using hemodialysis, high-permeability hemodialysis, or peritoneal dialysis.

E

factor IX complex

fak'-tor nine kom'-pleks

Classes
Chemical: human factor IX, blood modifier
Therapeutic: antihemorrhagic

Pregnancy Category: C

Trade Names
Prescription: Bebulin VH, Benefix, Immunine VH ♣, Konyne, Mononine, Profilnine SD, Propex T

F

CLINICAL PHARMACOLOGY

Mechanism of Action
A blood modifier that raises plasma levels of factor IX, restoring hemostasis in patients with factor IX deficiency. **Therapeutic Effect:** Increases blood-clotting factors II, VII, IX, and X.

PHARMACOKINETICS

Unknown absorption, metabolism, and elimination. **Half-life:** 18-36 hr.

AVAILABILITY

Injection: Number of units is indicated on each vial.

INDICATIONS AND DOSAGE

Reversal of anticoagulant effect of coumarin anticoagulants; bleeding caused by hemophilia B; bleeding in patients with hemophilia A who have factor VIII inhibitors
IV
Adults, Elderly, Children: Amount of factor IX required is individualized. Dosage depends on degree of deficiency, level of each factor desired, weight, and severity of bleeding.

CONTRAINDICATIONS

Sensitivity to factor IX complex or mouse protein

INTERACTIONS

Drug: **Aminocaproic acid:** May increase the risk of thrombosis. **Herbal:** None known. **Food:** None known.

DIAGNOSTIC TEST EFFECTS

None known.

IV INCOMPATIBILITIES

Do not mix with other medications.

SIDE-EFFECTS

Rare: Mild hypersensitivity reaction, marked by fever, chills, change in BP and pulse rate, rash, and urticaria

CRITICAL CARE CONSIDERATIONS

ADMINISTRATION/HANDLING

IV ALERT
- **Storage:** Store in refrigerator.
- **Stability:** Reconstituted solution is stable for 12 hr at room temperature; do not refrigerate.
- **Reconstitution:** Before reconstitution, warm diluent to room temperature. Gently agitate vial until powder is completely dissolved so that active components will not be removed when the solution is filtered during administration.
- **Administration:** Begin administration within 3 hr of reconstitution. Filter during administration. Administer by slow IV push or IV infusion. Infuse no faster than 3 mL/min. Too rapid an IV infusion may produce a change in BP and pulse rate, headache, flushing, and a tingling sensation.

PRECAUTIONS

HEALTH-RELATED
- Use factor IX complex cautiously in patients with hepatic impairment, recent surgery, or sensitivity to factor IX.

AGE-RELATED
- **Children:** Use with extreme caution in neonates because of high morbidity rate.
- **Elderly:** No age-related precautions have been noted.

PREGNANCY/LACTATION-RELATED
- Pregnancy category C; unknown if excreted in human breast milk.

MONITORING

- **Baseline assessment:** Assess the extent of existing bleeding, joint pain, overt bleeding or bruising, and swelling.
- **Baseline lab work:** CBC with differential, coagulation studies. Biochemical profile with liver function studies (AST [SGOT], ALT [SGPT], bilirubin, alkaline phosphatase).
- **Hypersensitivity reaction:** Monitor vital signs for fever, tachycardia, tachypnea, and hypotension. Assess for respiratory distress, muscle pain, or petechiae. Hematuria or change in vital signs warrants discontinuation of factor IX.
- **Bleeding:** Avoid administering other medications by the IM or subcutaneous route. Monitor coagulation studies closely.

Monitor IV site for oozing every 5-15 min for 1-2 hr after administration. Monitor for blood in secretions, urine, and stool.

- **Patient education:** Instruct to use an electric razor and soft toothbrush to prevent bleeding. Instruct to report black or red stool, coffee-ground emesis, dark or red urine, or red-speckled mucus from cough. Instruct to report if medication seems less effective because they may develop antibodies to factor IX. Caution against using OTC medications without prior discussion with a health care provider. Identification should be carried that indicates their condition or disease.

SERIOUS ADVERSE REACTIONS

- **Venous thrombosis and disseminated intravascular coagulation (DIC):** High risk for venous thrombosis and DIC during the postoperative period.
- **Transmitted viral hepatitis or HIV:** Risk of transmitting viral hepatitis and other viral diseases.

OVERDOSE/TOXICITY

- **Acute hypersensitivity reaction or anaphylactic reaction:** Hives, rash, redness along IV site, acute respiratory distress, flushing, tachycardia, tachypnea, hypotension, shock.
- **DIC:** Overt bleeding and covert clotting in the microvasculature. Lab results reveal elevated D-dimer, decreased fibrinogen, positive fibrin degradation products, decreased platelets, increased aPTT, increased prothrombin time, increased thrombin time.
- **GI decontamination:** No specific recommendations.

ANTIDOTE/DIALYSIS

- **Antidote:** No specific antidote. For thrombosis or DIC, anticoagulation with heparin may be warranted. Concurrent use of aminocaproic acid may increase risk of thrombosis.
- **Dialysis:** Factor IX complex is not removed by hemodialysis, high-permeability hemodialysis, or peritoneal dialysis.

famciclovir

See Antivirals (p. 937)

famotidine

fa-moe'-ti-deen

Classes

Chemical: thiazole derivative
Therapeutic: antiulcer agent

Pregnancy Category: B

Trade Names

Prescription: Pepcid, Pepcid RPD
Over the Counter: Mylanta AR, Pepcid AC

Combinations

Over the Counter: with calcium carbonate and magnesium hydroxide (Pepcid Complete)

CLINICAL PHARMACOLOGY

Mechanism of Action

An antiulcer agent and gastric acid secretion inhibitor that inhibits histamine action at H_2-histamine receptors of parietal cells. **Therapeutic Effect:** Inhibits gastric acid secretion when fasting, at night, or when stimulated by food, caffeine, or insulin.

PHARMACOKINETICS

Route	Onset	Peak	Duration
PO	1 hr	1-4 hr	10-12 hr
IV	1 hr	0.5-3 hr	10-12 hr

Rapidly, incompletely absorbed from the GI tract. Protein binding: 15%-20%. Partially metabolized in the liver. Primarily excreted in urine. Not removed by hemodialysis. **Half-life:** 2.5-3.5 hr (increased with impaired renal function).

AVAILABILITY

Oral suspension (Pepcid): 40 mg/5 mL.
Tablets: 10 mg (Pepcid AC), 20 mg (Pepcid, Pepcid AC), 40 mg (Pepcid).
Tablets (chewable [Pepcid AC]): 10 mg.
Capsules (Pepcid AC): 10 mg.
Injection (Pepcid): 10 mg/mL.

INDICATIONS AND DOSAGE

Acute treatment of duodenal and gastric ulcers

PO

Adults, Elderly, Children 12 yr and older: 40 mg/day at bedtime. **Children 1-16 yr:** 0.5 mg/kg/day at bedtime. Maximum: 40 mg/day.

Duodenal ulcer maintenance

PO

Adults, Elderly: 20 mg/day at bedtime.

Gastroesophageal reflux disease

PO

Adults, Elderly, Children 16 yr and older: 20 mg twice per day. **Children 1-16 yr:** 1 mg/kg/day in 2 divided doses. **Children 3 mo to 11 mo:** 0.5 mg/kg/dose twice per day. **Children younger than 3 mo:** 0.5 mg/kg/dose once per day.

Esophagitis

PO

Adults, Elderly, Children 16 yr and older: 2-40 mg twice per day.

Hypersecretory conditions

PO

Adults, Elderly, Children 12 yr and older: Initially, 20 mg every 6 hr. May increase up to 160 mg every 6 hr.

Acid indigestion, heartburn (over the counter)

PO

Adults, Elderly, Children 12 yr and older: 10-20 mg 15-60 min before eating. Maximum: 2 doses per day.

Usual parenteral dosage

IV

Adults, Elderly, Children 12 yr and older: 20 mg every 12 hr.

Dosage in renal impairment

Dosing frequency is modified based on creatinine clearance.

Creatinine Clearance	Dosing Frequency
10-50 mL/min	Every 24 hr
Less than 10 mL/min	Every 36-48 hr

OFF-LABEL USES

Autism, prevention of aspiration pneumonitis, *Heliobacter pylori* eradication

CONTRAINDICATIONS

Hypersensitivity to famotidine

INTERACTIONS

Drug: Antacids: May decrease the absorption of famotidine. **Ketoconazole:** May decrease the absorption of ketoconazole. **Herbal:** None known. **Food:** None known.

DIAGNOSTIC TEST EFFECTS

Interferes with skin tests using allergen extracts. May increase liver enzyme levels.

IV INCOMPATIBILITIES

Amphotericin B complex (Abelcet, Amphotec, Ambisome), cefepime (Maxipime), furosemide (Lasix), piperacillin/tazobactam (Zosyn)

IV COMPATIBILITIES

Calcium gluconate, *DOBUTamine (Dobutrex), *DOPamine (Intropin), heparin, hydromorphone (Dilaudid), insulin (regular), lidocaine, lorazepam (Ativan), magnesium sulfate, midazolam (Versed), morphine, nitroglycerin, norepinephrine (Levophed), potassium chloride, potassium phosphate, propofol (Diprivan), total parenteral nutrition (TPN)

SIDE-EFFECTS

Occasional (5%): Headache. **Rare (2% or less):** Constipation, diarrhea, dizziness

CRITICAL CARE CONSIDERATIONS

ADMINISTRATION/HANDLING

PO ALERT

- May give famotidine without regard to meals, but it is best given after meals or at bedtime.
- **Storage:** Store tablets and suspension at room temperature.
- **Oral suspension:** After reconstitution, oral suspension is stable for 30 days at room temperature. Shake suspension well before use.
- **Antacids:** Do not administer within 30 min to 1 hr of antacids.
- **Ketoconazole:** Give at least 2 hr after ketoconazole administration.

IV ALERT

- **Storage:** Refrigerate unreconstituted vials.
- **Stability:** After dilution, IV solution is stable for 48 hr at room temperature.
- **IV push:** Dilute 20 mg with 5-10 mL 0.9% NaCl, D_5W, $D_{10}W$, lactated Ringer's solution, or 5% sodium bicarbonate. Give push over 2 min. IV solution normally appears clear and is colorless.
- **Intermittent IV (piggyback) infusion:** Dilute with 50-100 mL D_5W, or 0.9% NaCl. Administer over 15-30 min.

PRECAUTIONS

HEALTH-RELATED

- Use famotidine cautiously in patients with impaired hepatic or renal function.

AGE-RELATED

- **Children:** No age-related precautions for children 1-16 yr. Safety and efficacy have not been established in children under 1 yr.
- **Elderly:** More likely to experience confusion, especially if renal or hepatic

impaired. Drug clearance may be reduced in elderly with renal disease.

PREGNANCY/LACTATION-RELATED

- Pregnancy category B; concentrated in breast milk (less than cimetidine or ranitidine); no problems reported with other H_2-histamine receptor antagonists; compatible with breast-feeding.

MONITORING

- **Baseline assessment:** Assess for abdominal pain and occult/frank blood in stool, gastric aspirate, or emesis.
- **Change in bowel activity:** Monitor bowel sounds, stool consistency; assess for constipation, diarrhea, and headache.
- **Neurologic changes:** Monitor for confusion, delirium, tremors, and anxiety, which may indicate toxicity.
- **Patient education:** When using famotidine outside the hospital, tell that famotidine can be taken without regard to meals but is most effective when taken after meals or at bedtime. Instruct to report headaches to a health care provider. Urge avoidance of substances that cause GI distress, including alcohol, aspirin, and coffee, during famotidine therapy. Common GI distress includes persistent acid indigestion, heartburn, or sour stomach. Patients should report if symptoms persist despite the medication.

SERIOUS ADVERSE REACTIONS

- Severe headache, confusion.

OVERDOSE/TOXICITY

- **Central anticholinergic syndrome:** Agitation, altered mental status, anxiety, ataxia, coma, delirium, dysarthria, extrapyramidal reactions, auditory and visual hallucinations, paranoia, psychosis, seizures, cardiopulmonary arrest.
- **GI decontamination:** No specific recommendations.

ANTIDOTE/DIALYSIS

- **Antidote:** No specific antidote. Manage symptoms according to accepted guidelines. Protect agitated patients from hurting themselves using sedation.
- **Dialysis:** Famotidine is not removed using hemodialysis or peritoneal dialysis. No data are available regarding removal using high-permeability hemodialysis dialysis.

felbamate

See Anticonvulsants (p. 903)

felodipine

See Calcium Channel Blockers (p. 950)

fenofibrate

fen-oh-fye'-brate

Classes

Chemical: fibric acid derivative
Therapeutic: antilipemic

Pregnancy Category: C

Trade Names

Prescription: Antara, Lipidil ♣, Lipidil Supra, Lipofen, Lofibra, Tricor, Triglide

Do not confuse Tricor with Tracleer.

CLINICAL PHARMACOLOGY

Mechanism of Action

An antihyperlipidemic that enhances synthesis of lipoprotein lipase and reduces triglyceride-rich lipoproteins and very low density lipoprotein (VLDLs). **Therapeutic Effect:** Increases VLDL catabolism and reduces total plasma triglyceride levels.

PHARMACOKINETICS

Well absorbed from the GI tract. Absorption increased when given with food. Protein binding: 99%. Rapidly metabolized in the liver to active metabolite. Excreted primarily in urine; lesser amount in feces. Not removed by hemodialysis. **Half-life:** 20 hr.

AVAILABILITY

Capsules: 43 mg (Antara), 50 mg (Lipofen), 67 mg (Lofibra), 87 mg (Antara), 100 mg (Lipofen), 130 mg (Antara), 134 mg (Lofibra), 150 mg (Lipofen), 200 mg (Lipidil Supra, Lofibra).
Tablets: 48 mg (Tricor), 50 mg (Triglide), 54 mg (Lofibra), 145 mg (Tricor), 160 mg (Lofibra, Triglide).

INDICATIONS AND DOSAGE

Hypertriglyceridemia

PO (Antara)

Adults, Elderly: 43-130 mg/day.

PO (Lofibra)

Adults, Elderly: 67-200 mg/day with meals.

PO (Tricor)

Adults, Elderly: 48-145 mg/day.

PO (Triglide)

Adults, Elderly: 50-160 mg/day.

Hypercholesterolemia

PO (Antara)

Adults, Elderly: 130 mg/day.

PO (Lofibra)

Adults, Elderly: 200 mg/day with meals.

PO (Tricor)

Adults, Elderly: 145 mg/day.

PO (Triglide)

Adults, Elderly: 160 mg/day.

CONTRAINDICATIONS

Gallbladder disease, severe renal or hepatic dysfunction (including primary biliary cirrhosis, unexplained persistent liver function abnormality), hypersensitivity to fenofibrate

INTERACTIONS

Drug: Anticoagulants: Potentiates effects of these drugs. **Bile acid sequestrants:** May impede fenofibrate absorption. ***CycloSPORINE:** Increases risk of nephrotoxicity. **HMG-CoA reductase inhibitors:** Increases risk of severe myopathy, rhabdomyolysis, and acute renal failure. **Herb:** None known. **Food: All foods:** Increase absorption of fenofibrate.

DIAGNOSTIC TEST EFFECTS

May increase BUN and serum CK, AST (SGOT), and ALT (SGPT), levels. May decrease blood Hgb and Hct levels, serum uric acid level, and WBC count.

SIDE-EFFECTS

Frequent (8%-4%): Pain, rash, headache, asthenia or fatigue, flu symptoms, dyspepsia, nausea or vomiting, rhinitis. **Occasional (3%-2%):** Diarrhea, abdominal pain, constipation, flatulence, arthralgia, decreased libido, dizziness, pruritus. **Rare (less than 2%):** Increased appetite, insomnia, polyuria, cough, blurred vision, eye floaters, earache

CRITICAL CARE CONSIDERATIONS

ADMINISTRATION/HANDLING

PO ALERT

- Give fenofibrate with meals.
- Administer fenofibrate 1 hr before or 4-6 hr after giving a bile acid sequestrant.

PRECAUTIONS

HEALTH-RELATED

- Use fenofibrate cautiously in patients who are receiving anticoagulant therapy, have a history of hepatic or renal disease, or consume substantial amounts of alcohol.

AGE-RELATED

- **Children:** Safety and efficacy of fenofibrate have not been established in children.
- **Elderly:** No age-related precautions have been noted.

PREGNANCY/LACTATION-RELATED

- Pregnancy category C; embryocidal and teratogenic in rats; no adequate and well-controlled studies in pregnant women; tumorigenicity seen in animal studies; avoid breast-feeding.

MONITORING

- **Baseline assessment:** Assess for possible gall bladder disease and liver and renal problems. Assess medications for use of oral coumarins; may require dose of anticoagulants reduced. Discern weight, waist circumference, BP, history of hyperglycemia, and other indicators for metabolic syndrome. Discuss current diet, exercise, and willingness to change dietary habits.
- **Baseline lab work:** CBC with differential; biochemical profile including serum cholesterol, triglyceride levels, and liver function test results, including serum ALT (SGPT) level during initial therapy and periodically during treatment.
- **Drug discontinuation:** Discontinue fenofibrate if liver enzyme levels are consistently greater than 3 times the normal limit or if myopathy or other signs of toxicity develop.
- **Other lipid-lowering agents:** Monitor patients also receiving HMG-CoA reductase inhibitors for myopathy, including muscle pain and weakness.
- **Therapeutic response:** Monitor serum CK, cholesterol, and triglyceride levels for a therapeutic response.
- **Patient education:** When using fenofibrate outside the hospital, advise that fenofibrate should be taken with food. Teach dietary habits used to best lower lipid levels, including low fat and consistent carbohydrate diets. Explain the importance of managing weight and blood glucose level if metabolic syndrome is present. Discuss increased risk of cardiac and peripheral vascular disease. Stress that periodic laboratory tests are an essential part of therapy. Instruct to report constipation, diarrhea, severe nausea, dizziness, insomnia, muscle pain, rash, or skin irritation to a health care provider.

SERIOUS ADVERSE REACTIONS

- **Gallbladder disease:** Fenofibrate may increase excretion of cholesterol into bile, leading to cholelithiasis.

OVERDOSE/TOXICITY

- **Hepatotoxicity:** Elevated liver enzymes, hepatitis, abdominal pain, jaundice.
- **Nephrotoxicity:** Elevated BUN, creatinine, low urine output, edema.
- **Myopathy:** Muscle pain and weakness, followed by generalized muscle pain with elevated creatine kinase (CK) levels.
- **Rhabdomyolysis:** Rare cases; can lead to acute renal failure. Markedly elevated serum creatine kinase and possible myoglobinuria indicate the condition may be present. Manage according to accepted guidelines, which include aggressive volume replacement, hemodialysis, or continuous hemofiltration (CVVH) to support patients during acute renal failure. Use of bicarbonate to induce alkaline diuresis or mannitol for osmotic diuresis has not been well studied. Hyperkalemia and hyperphosphatemia are commonly seen with rhabdomyolysis and may require aggressive management.
- **Pancreatitis:** Often associated with a common bile duct obstruction from gallstones or gallbladder sludge.
- **Hematologic:** Thrombocytopenia and agranulocytosis occur rarely.
- **GI decontamination:** No specific recommendations.

ANTIDOTE/DIALYSIS

- **Antidote:** No specific recommendations.
- **Dialysis:** Fenofibrate is not removed by hemodialysis and is unlikely to be removed by peritoneal dialysis. No data are available regarding removal using high-permeability hemodialysis.

fenoldopam mesylate 

feh-noll'-doh-pam mes'-sil-ate

Classes

Chemical: benzodiazepine derivative
Therapeutic: vasodilator

Pregnancy Category: B

Trade Names

Prescription: Corlopam

CLINICAL PHARMACOLOGY

Mechanism of Action

A rapid-acting vasodilator. An agonist for D_1-like dopamine receptors; also produces vasodilation in coronary, renal, mesenteric, and peripheral arteries. **Therapeutic Effect:** Reduces systolic and diastolic BP and increases heart rate.

PHARMACOKINETICS

After IV administration, metabolized in the liver. Primarily excreted in urine. Unknown if removed by hemodialysis. **Half-life:** Approximately 5 min.

AVAILABILITY

Injection: 10 mg/mL.

INDICATIONS AND DOSAGE

Short-term management of severe hypertension when rapid but quickly reversible emergency reduction of BP is clinically indicated, including malignant hypertension with deteriorating end-organ function

IV Infusion (continuous)

Adults, Elderly: Initially, 0.1 mcg/kg/min. May increase in increments of 0.05-0.1 mcg/kg/min until target BP is achieved. Usual length of treatment is 1-6 hr with tapering of dose every 15-30 min. Average rate: 0.25-0.5 mcg/kg/min. Maximum rate: 1.6 mcg/kg/min. **Children:** Initially, 0.2 mcg/kg/min. May increase increments of 0.3-0.5 mcg/kg/min every 20-30 min. Dosage greater than 0.8 mcg/kg/min have resulted in tachycardia with no additional benefit.

OFF-LABEL USES

Prevention of contrast media-induced nephrotoxicity

CONTRAINDICATIONS

Sensitivity to sulfites, hypersensitivity to fenoldopam

INTERACTIONS

Drug: **Beta-blockers:** May produce excessive hypotension. **Herbal:** None known. **Food:** None known.

DIAGNOSTIC TEST EFFECTS

May elevate BUN, blood glucose, serum LDH, and serum transaminase levels. May decrease serum potassium levels.

IV INCOMPATIBILITIES

Do not mix fenoldopam with other medications. Specific IV incompatibilities are not available.

SIDE-EFFECTS

Expected: Beta-blockers may cause unforeseen hypotension. **Occasional:** Headache (7%), flushing (3%), nausea (4%), hypotension (2%). **Rare (2% or less):** Nervousness or anxiety, vomiting, constipation, nasal congestion, diaphoresis, back pain

F

CRITICAL CARE CONSIDERATIONS

ADMINISTRATION/HANDLING

IV ALERT

- **Continuous infusion only:** Give fenoldopam only by continuous IV infusion; do not give as a bolus injection. Use an infusion pump and administer as an IV infusion at an initial rate of 0.1 mcg/kg/min.
- **Storage:** Store ampules at room temperature.
- **Stability:** Diluted solution is stable for 24 hr. Discard any solution not used within 24 hr.
- **Dilution:** Each 10 mg (1 mL) must be diluted with 250 mL 0.9% NaCl or D_5W to provide a concentration of 40 mcg/mL.

PRECAUTIONS

HEALTH-RELATED

- Use fenoldopam cautiously in patients with glaucoma, hypokalemia, hypotension, intraocular hypertension, sulfite sensitivity, or tachycardia.
- Has been used off-label for renal protection before studies with IV contrast/dye.

AGE-RELATED

- **Children:** Safety and efficacy of fenoldopam have not been established in children.
- **Elderly:** No age-related precautions have been noted.

PREGNANCY/LACTATION-RELATED

- Pregnancy category B; animal studies show no evidence of impaired fertility or fetal harm; no human data available; excreted into breast milk of rats; human information unknown.

MONITORING

- **Baseline assessment:** Obtain pulse and BP before therapy begins. Assess medication history, especially beta-blocker use. Determine whether asthmatic patients have a history of sulfite sensitivity.
- **Baseline lab work:** Biochemical panel, note potassium, BUN, and creatinine. Monitor for hypokalemia, BUN, and creatinine during the fenoldopam infusion.
- **Neurologic changes:** If patients are being managed for malignant hypertension, monitor for neurologic changes or signs of other end-organ damage.
- **Hypotension:** Diligently monitor BP during the infusion for hypotension to avoid a severe decrease in BP. Discontinue drug immediately if severe hypotension occurs.
- **Tachycardia:** Monitor ECG continuously for tachycardia, which may lead to angina, ischemic heart disease, acute MI, extrasystoles, or worsening heart failure. Cardiac problems may occur when average doses are administered.
- **Patient education:** Advise changing positions slowly to avoid orthostasis. Inform that they will likely require an oral antihypertensive when fenoldopam therapy has been completed.

SERIOUS ADVERSE REACTIONS

- **Excessive hypotension:** Occurs occasionally.
- **Allergic-type reaction:** Includes anaphylaxis and life-threatening asthmatic exacerbation; may occur in patients with sulfite sensitivity.
- **Hypokalemia:** May lead to ventricular dysrhythmias.
- **Elevated serum creatinine:** May indicate impending renal insufficiency.

OVERDOSE/TOXICITY

- **Cardiovascular:** Substantial tachycardia may lead to ischemic cardiac events, life-threatening dysrhythmias, or worsened heart failure. If symptoms occur, drug should be discontinued immediately. Drug half-life is short. Recovery should begin within 5-15 min.
- **GI decontamination:** No specific recommendations.

ANTIDOTE/DIALYSIS

- **Antidote:** No specific antidote. Give IV potassium for hypokalemia.
- **Dialysis:** Fenoldopam is unlikely to be removed using hemodialysis and is not removed by peritoneal dialysis. No data are available regarding removal using high-permeability hemodialysis.

fenoprofen calcium

See NSAIDs and Cox-2 Inhibitors (p. 976)

fentanyl

fen'-ta-nill

DEA Schedule: II

Classes

Chemical: opiate derivative, phenylpiperidine derivative
Therapeutic: narcotic analgesic

Pregnancy Category: C

Trade Names

Prescription: Injection: Sublimaze; Transdermal: Duragesic; Lozenge: Actiq

Combinations

Prescription: with droperidol (Innovar)

Do not confuse fentanyl with alfentanil.

CLINICAL PHARMACOLOGY

Mechanism of Action

An opioid agonist that binds to opioid receptors in the CNS, reducing stimuli from sensory nerve endings and inhibiting ascending pain pathways. **Therapeutic Effect:** Alters pain reception and increases the pain threshold.

PHARMACOKINETICS

Route	Onset	Peak	Duration
IV	1-2 min	3-5 min	0.5-1 hr
IM	7-15 min	20-30 min	1-2 hr
Transdermal	6-8 hr	24 hr	72 hr
Transmucosal	5-15 min	20-30 min	1-2 hr

Well absorbed after IM or topical administration. Transmucosal form absorbed through the buccal mucosa and GI tract. Protein binding: 80%-85%. Metabolized in the liver. Primarily eliminated by biliary system. **Half-life:** 2-4 hr IV; 17 hr transdermal; 6.6 hr transmucosal.

AVAILABILITY

Injection (Sublimaze): 50 mcg/mL.
Transdermal patch (Duragesic): 12 mcg/hr, 25 mcg/hr, 50 mcg/hr, 75 mcg/hr, 100 mcg/hr.
Transmucosal lozenges (Actiq): 200 mcg, 400 mcg, 600 mcg, 800 mcg, 1200 mcg, 1600 mcg.

INDICATIONS AND DOSAGE

Sedation in minor procedures, analgesia

IV, IM

Adults, Elderly, Children 12 yr and older: 0.5-1 mcg/kg/dose; may repeat in 30-60 min. **Children 1-11 yr:** 1-2 mcg/kg/dose. **Children younger than 1 yr:** 1-4 mcg/kg/dose.

Preoperative sedation, postoperative pain, adjunct to regional anesthesia

IV, IM

Adults, Elderly, Children 12 yr and older: 50-100 mcg/dose.

Adjunct to general anesthesia

IV

Adults, Elderly, Children 12 yr and older: 2-50 mcg/kg.

Usual transdermal dose

Adults, Elderly, Children 12 yr and older: Initially, 25 mcg/hr. May increase after 3 days.

Usual transmucosal dose

Adults, Children: 200-400 mcg for breakthrough cancer pain.

Usual epidural dose

Adults, Elderly: Bolus dose of 100 mcg, followed by continuous infusion of 10 mcg/mL concentration at 4-12 mL/hr.

Continuous analgesia

IV

Adults, Elderly, Children 1-12 yr: Bolus dose of 1-2 mcg/kg, followed by continuous infusion of 1 mcg/kg/hr. Range: 1-5 mcg/kg/hr. **Children younger than 1 yr:** Bolus dose of 1-2 mcg/kg, followed by continuous infusion of 0.5-1 mcg/kg/hr.

Dosage in renal impairment

Dosage is modified based on creatinine clearance.

Creatinine Clearance	Dosage
10-50 mL/min	75% of usual dose
Less than 10 mL/min	50% of usual dose

CONTRAINDICATIONS

Increased intracranial pressure, severe hepatic or renal impairment, severe respiratory depression, hypersensitivity to fentanyl

INTERACTIONS

Drug: **Benzodiazepines, CNS depressants:** May increase the risk of hypotension and respiratory depression. **Buprenorphine:** May decrease the effects of fentanyl.
Herbal: None known. **Food:** None known.

DIAGNOSTIC TEST EFFECTS

May increase serum amylase and lipase concentrations.

IV INCOMPATIBILITIES

Phenytoin (Dilantin)

IV COMPATIBILITIES

Atropine, bupivacaine (Marcaine, Sensorcaine), clonidine (Duraclon), diltiazem

(Cardizem), *diphenhydrAMINE (Benadryl), *DOBUTamine (Dobutrex), *DOPamine (Intropin), droperidol (Inapsine), heparin, hydromorphone (Dilaudid), ketorolac (Toradol), lorazepam (Ativan), metoclopramide (Reglan), midazolam (Versed), milrinone (Primacor), morphine, nitroglycerin, norepinephrine (Levophed), ondansetron (Zofran), potassium chloride, propofol (Diprivan)

SIDE-EFFECTS

Frequent: **IV:** Postoperative drowsiness, nausea, vomiting. **Transdermal (10%-3%):** Headache, pruritus, nausea, vomiting, diaphoresis, dyspnea, confusion, dizziness, somnolence, diarrhea, constipation, decreased appetite. Occasional: **IV:** Postoperative confusion, blurred vision, chills, orthostatic hypotension, constipation, difficulty urinating. **Transdermal (3%-1%):** Chest pain, dysrhythmias, erythema, pruritus, swelling of skin, syncope, agitation, tingling or burning of skin

F

CRITICAL CARE CONSIDERATIONS

ADMINISTRATION/HANDLING

EPIDURAL/REGIONAL ANESTHESIA/ ANALGESIA ALERT

- Fentanyl may be combined with a local anesthetic, such as bupivacaine, for added pain relief.

IV ALERT

- **Storage:** Store the parenteral form at room temperature.
- **Preparation:** Make sure resuscitative equipment and an opiate antagonist (naloxone 0.5 mcg/kg) is readily available before administering the drug.
- **IV push initial dose:** Give lowest possible dose by slow IV push, over 1-2 min, using a tuberculin syringe for children and patients who are high risk for respiratory depression.
- **IV infusion:** Too-rapid IV infusion increases severe adverse reactions, such as anaphylaxis, bronchospasm, laryngospasm, peripheral circulatory collapse, cardiac arrest, and skeletal and thoracic muscle rigidity, which may result in apnea.

TRANSDERMAL ALERT

- **Site selection:** Apply the patch to a flat, unirritated, nonhairy area of intact skin on the upper torso. Rotate application sites.
- **Skin preparation:** Clean the patch site before application using only water because soap and oils may irritate the skin.
- **Application:** Press patch firmly and evenly onto skin for 10-20 sec to ensure full contact with the skin, especially around the edges.
- **Disposal:** Carefully fold used patches in half so they adhere to themselves; discard in a designated container according to institutional policy.

TRANSMUCOSAL ALERT

- Have patients suck the lozenge vigorously.

PRECAUTIONS

HEALTH-RELATED

- Use fentanyl cautiously in patients with bradycardia, head injuries, altered LOC, hepatic, renal, and mild respiratory disease.
- **Contraindication for respiratory diseases:** Narcotic analgesics are contraindicated in patients with acute or severe bronchial asthma, if an upper airway obstruction or significant respiratory depression is present.
- **MAOIs:** Use fentanyl cautiously in patients who use MAOIs within 14 days of fentanyl administration.
- **Sedation and analgesia:** If sedation is needed for management of anxiety, agitation, or mechanical ventilation, give fentanyl before sedation to ensure pain relief rather than having sedation mask patient response to pain.

AGE-RELATED

- **Children:** Transdermal fentanyl is not recommended for children under 12 yr or children under 18 yr who weigh less than 50 kg. Neonates are more susceptible to respiratory depressant effects.
- **Elderly:** Age-related renal impairment may require a lower dosage; elderly are more susceptible to the drug's respiratory depressant effects.

PREGNANCY/LACTATION-RELATED

- Pregnancy category C (D if used for prolonged periods or at high dosages at term); excreted in breast milk.

MONITORING

- **Baseline assessment:** Obtain BP and respiratory rate. Assess duration, intensity, location, and type of pain experienced.

- **Respiratory depression:** Monitor BP, heart rate, respiratory rate, and oxygen saturation.
- **Bedridden patients:** Assist patients to cough, turn, and breathe deeply every 2 hr. If able to sit or get out of bed, assist with ambulation.
- **Therapeutic effect:** Assess for relief of pain. If patients cannot communicate, note tachycardia, hypertension, increased level of agitation, and grimacing, which may indicate pain is not relieved.
- **Combining forms of pain relief:** Pain management can be complex. Consider use of transdermal form to attain baseline pain relief and use small doses of IV form for breakthrough pain.
- **Patient education:** When using fentanyl outside the hospital, instruct to use fentanyl as directed to avoid an overdose. Explain that prolonged use of the drug may cause physical dependence and often causes tolerance. Teach proper application of the fentanyl transdermal patch. Instruct to discontinue fentanyl slowly after long-term use. Urge avoidance of alcohol during fentanyl therapy and consulting with a health care provider before taking other medications. Warn to avoid tasks requiring mental alertness or motor skills until response to the drug is known.

SERIOUS ADVERSE REACTIONS

- **Hypoxemia:** Decreased rate and depth of respirations may not be adequate to provide effective oxygen saturation and bradycardia may lead to decreased oxygen delivery. Low oxygen saturation can be a late sign of impending respiratory arrest in healthier patients with more ability to compensate for respiratory depression.
- **Tolerance:** Patients with severe pain or who use fentanyl repeatedly may develop a tolerance to the drug's analgesic effect.

OVERDOSE/TOXICITY

- Overdose or too rapid IV administration may cause severe respiratory depression and skeletal and thoracic muscle rigidity which may lead to apnea, laryngospasm, bronchospasm, hypotension, peripheral circulatory collapse indicated by cold and clammy skin, cyanosis, possible coma, and cardiac arrest.
- **GI decontamination:** No specific recommendations.

ANTIDOTE/DIALYSIS

- **Antidote:** Naloxone given IV is effective in reversing the effects of fentanyl and other opioid narcotics. May require repeated administration.
- **Dialysis:** Fentanyl is not removed using high-permeability hemodialysis and is unlikely to be removed with hemodialysis. No data are available regarding removal using peritoneal dialysis.

ferrous salts

fer'-us salts

Classes

Chemical: iron preparation
Therapeutic: hematinic

Pregnancy Category: A

Trade Names

Prescription: (ferrous fumarate) Feostat, Femiron, Ferro-Sequels, Nephro-Fer; (ferrous gluconate) Fergon; (ferrous sulfate) Fer-In-Sol, Fer-Iron, Slow-Fe

CLINICAL PHARMACOLOGY

Mechanism of Action

An enzymatic mineral that is as an essential component in the formation of Hgb, myoglobin, and enzymes. Promotes effective erythropoiesis and transport and utilization of oxygen (O_2). **Therapeutic Effect:** Prevents iron deficiency.

PHARMACOKINETICS

Absorbed in the duodenum and upper jejunum. Ten percent absorbed in patients with normal iron stores; increased to 20%-30% in those with inadequate iron stores. Primarily bound to serum transferrin. Excreted in urine, sweat, and sloughing of intestinal mucosa and by menses. **Half-life:** 6 hr.

AVAILABILITY

Ferrous fumarate

Tablets: 63 mg (20 mg elemental iron) (Femiron), 350 mg (115 mg elemental iron) (Nephro-Fer).
Tablets (chewable [Feostat]): 100 mg (33 mg elemental iron).
Tablets (time release [Ferro-Sequels]): 150 mg (50 mg elemental iron).

Ferrous gluconate

Tablets: 240 mg (27 mg elemental iron) (Fergon), 325 mg (36 mg elemental iron).

Ferrous sulfate

Tablets: 325 mg (65 mg elemental iron).
Tablets (time release [Slow FE]): 160 mg (50 mg elemental iron).

Elixir: 220 mg/5 mL (44 mg elemental iron per 5 mL).
Oral Drops (Fer-In-Sol, Fer-Iron): 75 mg/ 0.6 mL.

INDICATIONS AND DOSAGE

Iron deficiency anemia

PO (ferrous fumarate)
Adults, Elderly: 60-100 mg twice per day. **Children:** 3-6 mg/kg/day in 2-3 divided doses.
PO (ferrous gluconate)
Adults, Elderly: 60 mg 2-4 times per day. **Children:** 3-6 mg/kg/day in 2-3 divided doses.
PO (ferrous sulfate)
Adults, Elderly: 325 mg 2-4 times per day. **Children:** 3-6 mg/kg/day in 2-3 divided doses.
Dosage is expressed in terms of milligrams of elemental iron, degree of anemia, patient weight, and presence of any bleeding. Expect to use periodic hematologic determinations as guide to therapy.

Prevention of iron deficiency

PO (ferrous fumarate)
Adults, Elderly: 60-100 mg/day. **Children:** 1-2 mg/kg/day.
PO (ferrous gluconate)
Adults, Elderly: 60 mg/day. **Children:** 1-2 mg/kg/day.
PO (ferrous sulfate)
Adults, Elderly: 325 mg/day. **Children:** 1-2 mg/kg/day.

CONTRAINDICATIONS

Hemochromatosis, hemosiderosis, hemolytic anemias, peptic ulcer disease, regional enteritis, ulcerative colitis, hypersensitivity to ferrous salts

INTERACTIONS

Drug: Antacids, calcium supplements, pancreatin, pancrelipase: May decrease the absorption of ferrous fumarate, ferrous gluconate, and ferrous sulfate. **Etidronate, quinolones, tetracyclines:** May decrease the absorption of etidronate, quinolones, and tetracyclines. **Herbal:** None known. **Food:** **Eggs, milk:** Inhibit ferrous fumarate absorption.

DIAGNOSTIC TEST EFFECTS

May increase serum bilirubin and iron levels. May decrease serum calcium level. May obscure occult blood in stools.

SIDE-EFFECTS

Occasional: Mild, transient nausea. **Rare:** Heartburn, anorexia, constipation, diarrhea

CRITICAL CARE CONSIDERATIONS

ADMINISTRATION/HANDLING

PO ALERT

- Give ferrous salts between meals with water unless GI discomfort occurs; if so, give with meals. Eggs and milk inhibit drug absorption.
- Do not crush sustained-release form.
- Store all forms (tablets, capsules, suspension, and drops) at room temperature.
- Use a dropper or straw to administer the liquid preparation and allow the drug solution to drop on the back of the tongue to prevent transient mucous membrane and teeth staining.
- Avoid simultaneous administration of antacids or tetracycline.

PRECAUTIONS

HEALTH-RELATED

- Use cautiously in patients with bronchial asthma or iron hypersensitivity.

AGE-RELATED

- **Children:** No age-related precautions have been noted.
- **Elderly:** No age-related precautions have been noted.

PREGNANCY/LACTATION-RELATED

- Pregnancy category A; excreted in breast milk.

MONITORING

- **Baseline assessment:** Assess nutritional status and dietary intake.
- **Baseline lab work:** Monitor Hgb, reticulocyte count, ferritin and serum iron levels, and total iron-binding capacity before and during therapy.
- **GI symptoms:** Assess for constipation or diarrhea.
- **Therapeutic effect:** Evaluate for relief of iron deficiency symptoms including fatigue, headache, irritability, pallor, and paresthesias in extremities.
- **Patient education:** Inform that stools will darken in color. Ferrous salts should be taken after meals, or with food if GI discomfort occurs. Instruct not to take with milk or eggs. Instruct not to take within 2 hr of antacids because antacids prevent absorption.

SERIOUS ADVERSE REACTIONS

- **GI symptoms:** Large doses may aggravate existing GI tract disease, such as peptic ulcer disease, regional enteritis, and ulcerative colitis.

OVERDOSE/TOXICITY

- **Severe iron poisoning:** Occurs more often in children. Poisoning has five stages, which often overlap: GI symptoms, quiescence, shock, hepatotoxicity, and gut obstruction, which occurs 1-7 wk following ingestion. Manifested by severe epigastric pain, vomiting, diarrhea, followed by hyperventilation, altered mental status, pallor or cyanosis, and cardiovascular collapse. Metabolic acidosis is present. Not all patients are hepatotoxic, but it is a poor prognostic sign when present. Gut obstruction does not occur in all patients but is typically gastric outlet obstruction, which occurs at least 1 wk following ingestion. May also cause coagulopathy early and then 2-7 days postingestion.
- **Management:** Oxygen supplementation, airway/ventilatory support, cardiac monitoring, fluid volume replacement, and administration of deferoxamine once diagnosis is confirmed by elevated serum iron concentration or abdominal x-ray.
- **GI decontamination:** Activated charcoal has not been shown to be effective in absorbing iron. Syrup of ipecac is not recommended because of risk for aspiration and because differential diagnosis of GI symptoms is more difficult. Gastric lavage may be attempted if patients present within 1 hr of ingestion but has not been proven effective and carries serious risks.

ANTIDOTE/DIALYSIS

- **Antidote:** Deferoxamine is an iron chelating agent and should be given as soon as possible following ingestion to manage overdoses. Pregnant women may receive deferoxamine.
- **Dialysis:** Ferrous salts are unlikely to be removed by hemodialysis or peritoneal dialysis. No data are available on removal using high-permeability hemodialysis.

fexofenadine hydrochloride

See Antihistamines (p. 925)

filgrastim

fil-gra'-stim

Classes

Chemical: blood modifier, antineutropenic
Therapeutic: colony stimulating factor

Pregnancy Category: C

Trade Names

Prescription: Neupogen

Do not confuse Neupogen with Epogen or Nutramigen.

CLINICAL PHARMACOLOGY

Mechanism of Action

A biologic modifier that stimulates production, maturation, and activation of neutrophils to increase their migration and cytotoxicity. **Therapeutic Effect:** Decreases incidence of infection.

PHARMACOKINETICS

Readily absorbed after subcutaneous administration. Not removed by hemodialysis. **Half-life:** 3.5 hr.

AVAILABILITY

Injection: 300 mcg/mL, 480 mcg/0.8 mL, 600 mcg/mL.

INDICATIONS AND DOSAGE

Myelosuppression

IV or Subcutaneous Infusion, Subcutaneous Injection

Adults, Elderly: Initially, 5 mcg/kg/day. May increase by 5 mcg/kg for each chemotherapy cycle based on duration or severity of absolute neutrophil count nadir.

Bone marrow transplant

IV or Subcutaneous Infusion

Adults, Elderly, Children: 5-10 mcg/kg/day. Adjust dosage daily during period of neutrophil recovery based on neutrophil response.

Mobilization progenitor cells

IV or Subcutaneous Infusion

Adults: 10 mcg/kg/day beginning at least 4 days before first leukopheresis and continuing until last leukopheresis.

Chronic neutropenia, congenital neutropenia

Subcutaneous

Adults, Children: 6 mcg/kg/dose twice per day.

Idiopathic or cyclic neutropenia

Subcutaneous

Adults, Children: 5 mcg/kg/dose once per day.

OFF-LABEL USES

Treatment of AIDS-related neutropenia, drug-induced neutropenia, myelodysplastic syndrome

CONTRAINDICATIONS

Hypersensitivity to filgrastim or *E. coli*–derived proteins, 24 hr before or after cytotoxic chemotherapy, concurrent use of other drugs that may result in lowered platelet count

INTERACTIONS

Drug: None known. **Herbal:** None known. **Food:** None known.

DIAGNOSTIC TEST EFFECTS

May increase LDH concentrations, leukocyte alkaline phosphatase (LAP) scores, and serum alkaline phosphatase and uric acid levels.

IV INCOMPATIBILITIES

Amphotericin (Fungizone), cefepime (Maxipime), cefotaxime (Claforan), cefoxitin (Mefoxin), ceftizoxime (Cefizox), ceftriaxone (Rocephin), cefuroxime (Zinacef), clindamycin (Cleocin), dactinomycin (Cosmegen), etoposide (VePesid), fluorouracil, furosemide (Lasix), heparin, mannitol, *methylPREDNIsolone (Solu-Medrol), mitomycin (Mutamycin), prochlorperazine (Compazine), total parenteral nutrition (TPN)

IV COMPATIBILITIES

Bumetanide (Bumex), calcium gluconate, hydromorphone (Dilaudid), lorazepam (Ativan), morphine, potassium chloride

SIDE-EFFECTS

Frequent: Nausea or vomiting (57%), mild to severe bone pain (22%) that occurs more frequently with high-dose IV form and less frequently with low-dose subcutaneous form; alopecia (18%), diarrhea (14%), fever (12%), fatigue (11%). **Occasional (9%-5%):** Anorexia, dyspnea, headache, cough, rash. **Rare (less than 5%):** Psoriasis, hematuria or proteinuria, osteoporosis

CRITICAL CARE CONSIDERATIONS

ADMINISTRATION/HANDLING

IV ALERT

- **Storage:** Refrigerate vials. Do not allow to freeze. Do not expose to direct sunlight.
- **Stability:** Filgrastim is stable in a syringe for up to 24 hr at room temperature and up to 7 days if refrigerated. Diluted solutions must be refrigerated and used within 24 hr. Vial contents should appear clear and colorless.
- **Single dose only:** Use single-dose vial. Do not reenter vial.
- **Chemotherapy:** Begin filgrastim therapy at least 24 hr after last dose of chemotherapy; discontinue at least 24 hr before next dose of chemotherapy.
- **Bone marrow transplant:** Begin therapy at least 24 hr after bone marrow infusion.
- **Dilution:** Dilute with 10-50 mL D_5W to a concentration of 15 mcg/mL or higher. Do not shake. For a concentration from 5-14 mcg/mL, add 2 mL of 5% albumin to each 50 mL D_5W to provide a final concentration of 2 mg/mL. Do not dilute to a final concentration of less than 5 mcg/mL.
- **Before administration:** Flush IV line with D_5W before and after administration.
- **Intermittent infusion (piggyback):** Infuse over 15-30 min.
- **Continuous IV infusion:** Give a single dose over 4-24 hr.

SUBCUTANEOUS ALERT

- **Storage:** Store in refrigerator but remove before use to allow warming.
- **Prior to injection:** Ensure drug is room temperature. Aspirate syringe before injecting drug to avoid intraarterial administration.

PRECAUTIONS

HEALTH-RELATED

- Use filgrastim cautiously in patients with malignancy with myeloid characteristics (granulocyte colony–stimulating factor may act as a growth factor) and heart disease.

AGE-RELATED

- **Children:** Safety and efficacy of filgrastim in neonates and with autoimmune neutropenia of infancy have not been established. No age-related precautions have been noted for children 4 mo to 17 yr.
- **Elderly:** No age-related precautions have been noted.

PREGNANCY/LACTATION-RELATED

- Pregnancy category C; high doses caused fetal damage and death in rabbits; unknown if excreted in human breast milk.

MONITORING

- **Baseline assessment:** Obtain history of cancer and chemotherapy.
- **Baseline lab work:** CBC with platelet count and WBC differential before the start of filgrastim therapy and twice weekly thereafter. Biochemical profile including liver enzymes and uric acid.
- **Acute respiratory distress syndrome:** Monitor for tachypnea and increased work of breathing in septic patients.
- **Cardiac effects:** Continuous ECG monitoring on patients with preexisting cardiac conditions when therapy is initiated in the hospital. Cardiac events are rare but include dysrhythmias and acute MI.
- **Bone pain:** Manage bone pain with nonnarcotic analgesics unless mild pain control agents are ineffective.
- **Hypotension:** Monitor BP for a transient decrease.
- **Fever:** Febrile patients may be developing an infection.
- **Patient education:** Instruct to report chest pain, chills, fever, palpitations, or severe bone pain to a health care provider immediately. Instruct to avoid situations that might increase risk of an infectious disease, such as influenza.

SERIOUS ADVERSE REACTIONS

- **Hematologic:** Long-term administration occasionally produces chronic neutropenia, splenomegaly, thrombocytopenia, and anemia.
- **Cardiac:** MI and dysrhythmias occur rarely.
- **Cutaneous vasculitis:** Occurs rarely.
- **Acute respiratory distress syndrome:** May occur in patients with sepsis.

OVERDOSE/TOXICITY

- No specific information available other than serious reactions.
- **GI decontamination:** No specific recommendations.

ANTIDOTE/DIALYSIS

- **Antidote:** No specific recommendations.
- **Dialysis:** Filgrastim is not removed by hemodialysis and is unlikely to be removed using peritoneal dialysis. There are no data to support removal using high-permeability hemodialysis.

finasteride

fin-as'-tur-ide

Classes

Chemical: 5α-reductase inhibitor
Therapeutic: antiandrogen, hair-growth stimulant

Pregnancy Category: X

Trade Names

Prescription: Proscar, Propecia

Do not confuse Proscar with Posicor, ProSom, Prozac, or Psorcon.

CLINICAL PHARMACOLOGY

Mechanism of Action

An androgen hormone inhibitor that inhibits 5-alpha reductase, an intracellular enzyme that converts testosterone into dihydrotestosterone (DHT) in the prostate gland, resulting in a decreased serum DHT level. Therapeutic Effect: Reduces size of the prostate gland.

PHARMACOKINETICS

Route	Onset	Peak	Duration
PO	24 hr	1-2 days	14 days

Rapidly absorbed from the GI tract. Protein binding: 90%. Widely distributed. Metabolized in the liver. Half-life: 6-8 hr. Onset of clinical effect: 3-6 mo of continued therapy.

AVAILABILITY

Tablets: 1 mg (Propecia), 5 mg (Proscar).

INDICATIONS AND DOSAGE

Benign prostatic hyperplasia (BPH)

PO

Adults, Elderly: 5 mg once per day (for a minimum of 6 mo).

Hair loss

PO

Adults: 1 mg/day.

OFF-LABEL USES

Adjuvant monotherapy after radical prostatectomy in treatment of prostate cancer, female hirsutism

CONTRAINDICATIONS

Exposure to the patient's semen or handling of finasteride tablets by those who are or may be pregnant

INTERACTIONS

Drug: None known. Herbal: None known. Food: None known.

DIAGNOSTIC TEST EFFECTS

Decreases the serum prostate-specific antigen (PSA) level, even in patients with prostate cancer

SIDE-EFFECTS

Rare (4%-2%): Gynecomastia, sexual dysfunction (impotence, decreased libido, decreased volume of ejaculate)

CRITICAL CARE CONSIDERATIONS

ADMINISTRATION/HANDLING

PO ALERT

- Give finasteride without regard to food.
- Do not break or crush film-coated tablets.

PRECAUTIONS

HEALTH-RELATED

- Use finasteride cautiously in patients with hepatic impairment.
- Finasteride is not intended for female baldness.

AGE-RELATED

- **Children:** Finasteride is not indicated for use in children.
- **Elderly:** No dosage adjustment is required.

PREGNANCY/LACTATION-RELATED

- Pregnancy category X; not indicated for use in women; pregnant women should not handle crushed tablets

MONITORING

- **Baseline assessment:** Perform a digital rectal exam to assess for prostate enlargement. For baldness, document pattern of baldness.
- **Baseline lab work:** Biochemical profile including liver function tests before starting therapy. For prostate disease patients, prostate specific antigen (PSA) before and periodically during finasteride therapy.
- **Urinary retention:** Monitor fluid intake and output, especially in patients with prostate disease. Obstructive uropathy may be present (large residual urinary volume or severely diminished urinary flow).
- **Therapeutic effect:** Decreased PSA level, improved urinary flow; for balding patients, growth of new hair.
- **Patient education:** For patients with prostate enlargement, explain finasteride may cause impotence and decrease ejaculate volume. Stress the need to take the drug for at least 6 mo. Patients may not notice improved urinary flow even if the prostate gland shrinks. Inform that it is unknown if taking this drug decreases the need for prostate surgery. Warn patients not to let women who are or may be pregnant handle finasteride tablets or be exposed to their semen because of the potential risk to a male fetus.

SERIOUS ADVERSE REACTIONS

- Impotence.

OVERDOSE/TOXICITY

- Malformation of male external genitalia if male fetus is exposed to finasteride in utero.
- **GI decontamination:** No specific recommendations.

ANTIDOTE/DIALYSIS

- **Antidote:** No specific recommendations.
- **Dialysis:** Finasteride is unlikely to be removed by hemodialysis or peritoneal dialysis. No data are available regarding removal using high-permeability hemodialysis.

flecainide

See Antidysrhythmics (p. 919)

fluconazole

floo-con'-a-zole

Classes

Chemical: triazole derivative
Therapeutic: antifungal

Pregnancy Category: C

Trade Names

Prescription: Diflucan

Do not confuse Diflucan with diclofenac.

CLINICAL PHARMACOLOGY

Mechanism of Action

A fungistatic antifungal that interferes with cytochrome P-450, an enzyme necessary for ergosterol formation. **Therapeutic Effect:** Directly damages fungal membrane, altering its function.

PHARMACOKINETICS

Well absorbed from GI tract. Widely distributed, including to cerebrospinal fluid. Protein binding: 11%. Partially metabolized in liver. Excreted unchanged primarily in urine. Partially removed by hemodialysis. **Half-life:** 20-30 hr (increased in impaired renal function).

AVAILABILITY

Tablets: 50 mg, 100 mg, 150 mg, 200 mg.
Powder for oral suspension: 10 mg/mL, 40 mg/mL.
Injection: 2 mg/mL (in 100- or 200-mL containers).

INDICATIONS AND DOSAGE

Oropharyngeal candidiasis
PO, IV
Adults, Elderly: 200 mg once, then 100 mg/day for at least 14 days. **Children:** 6 mg/kg/day once, then 3 mg/kg/day.

Esophageal candidiasis
PO, IV
Adults, Elderly: 200 mg once, then 100 mg/day (up to 400 mg/day) for 21 days and at least 14 days following resolution of symptoms. **Children:** 6 mg/kg/day once, then 3 mg/kg/day (up to 12 mg/kg/day) for 21 days, and then for at least 14 days following resolution of symptoms.

Vaginal candidiasis
PO
Adults: 150 mg once.

Prevention of candidiasis in patients undergoing bone marrow transplantation
PO
Adults: 400 mg/day

Systemic candidiasis
PO, IV
Adults, Elderly: 400 mg once, then 200 mg/day (up to 400 mg/day) for at least 28 days and at least 14 days following resolution of symptoms. **Children:** 6-12 mg/kg/day.

Urinary candidiasis
PO, IV
Adults, Elderly: 50-200 mg/day.

Cryptococcal meningitis
PO, IV
Adults, Elderly: 400 mg once, then 200 mg/day (up to 800 mg/day) for 10-12 wk after CSF becomes negative (200 mg/day for suppression of relapse in patients with AIDS). **Children:** 12 mg/kg/day once, then 6-12 mg/kg/day (6 mg/kg/day for suppression of relapse in patients with AIDS).

Onychomycosis
PO
Adults: 150 mg/wk.

Dosage in renal impairment
After a loading dose of 400 mg, the daily dosage is based on creatinine clearance.

Creatinine Clearance	% of Recommended Dose
Greater than 50 mL/min	100
21-50 mL/min	50
11-20 mL/min	25
Dialysis	Dose after dialysis

OFF-LABEL USES

Treatment of coccidioidomycosis, cryptococcosis, fungal pneumonia, onychomycosis, ringworm of the hand, septicemia

CONTRAINDICATIONS

Hypersensitivity to fluconazole, concurrent use with cisapride (Propulsid); use very cautiously in those sensitive to other azoles (e.g., ketoconazole)

INTERACTIONS

Drug: *CycloSPORINE: High fluconazole doses increase *cycloSPORINE blood concentration. **Oral antidiabetics:** May increase blood concentration and effects of oral antidiabetics. **Phenytoin, warfarin:** May decrease the metabolism of these drugs. **Rifampin:** May increase fluconazole metabolism. **Herbal:** None known. **Food:** None known.

DIAGNOSTIC TEST EFFECTS

May increase serum alkaline phosphatase, serum bilirubin, AST (SGOT), and ALT (SGPT) levels.

IV INCOMPATIBILITIES

Amphotericin B (Fungizone), amphotericin B complex (Abelcet, Ambisome, Amphotec), ampicillin (Polycillin), calcium gluconate, cefotaxime (Claforan), ceftazidime (Fortaz), ceftriaxone (Rocephin), cefuroxime (Zinacef), chloramphenicol (Chloromycetin), clindamycin (Cleocin), co-trimoxazole (Bactrim), diazepam (Valium), digoxin (Lanoxin), erythromycin (Erythrocin), furosemide (Lasix), haloperidol (Haldol), *hydrOXYzine (Vistaril), imipenem and cilastatin (Primaxin), total parenteral nutrition (TPN)

IV COMPATIBILITIES

Diltiazem (Cardizem), *DOBUTamine (Dobutrex), *DOPamine (Intropin), heparin, lorazepam (Ativan), midazolam (Versed), propofol (Diprivan)

SIDE-EFFECTS

Occasional (4%-1%): Hypersensitivity reaction (including chills, fever, pruritus, and rash), dizziness, drowsiness, headache, constipation, diarrhea, nausea, vomiting, abdominal pain

CRITICAL CARE CONSIDERATIONS

ADMINISTRATION/HANDLING

PO ALERT

- Give fluconazole without regard to meals.
- PO and IV therapy are equally effective; IV therapy is used in patients who cannot swallow, do not tolerate the oral drug, or do not have an enteral tube.

IV ALERT

- **Storage:** Store the drug at room temperature. Do not remove from the outer wrap until ready to use.
- **Preparation:** Squeeze the inner bag to check for leaks. Do not use the parenteral form if the seal is not intact or if the solution is cloudy or discolored or contains a precipitate.
- **IV infusion:** Do not add another medication to the solution. Do not exceed a flow rate of 200 mg/hr.

PRECAUTIONS

HEALTH-RELATED

- Use fluconazole cautiously in patients with hepatic or renal impairment, hypersensitivity to other triazoles (such as itraconazole and terconazole), or hypersensitivity to imidazoles (such as butoconazole and ketoconazole).
- Diabetic patients on oral hypoglycemic agents are at higher risk for hypoglycemia while taking fluconazole.

AGE-RELATED

- **Children:** No age-related precautions have been noted in children.
- **Elderly:** Age-related renal impairment may require a dosage adjustment.

PREGNANCY/LACTATION-RELATED

- Pregnancy category C; excreted into breast milk in concentrations similar to plasma; not recommended in nursing mothers.

MONITORING

- **Baseline assessment:** Obtain history of use of antibiotics or other antifungal medications. Assess for cause of possible immunosuppression, including high stress level and use of immunosuppressive medications. Assess for history of liver dysfunction or risk factors such as substance abuse.
- **Baseline lab work:** Baseline CBC with WBC differential, biochemical profile including liver function tests, blood glucose and serum potassium level, appropriate cultures before initiating therapy, if possible.
- **Ongoing lab work:** CBC, liver and renal function test results, platelet count, and serum potassium levels.
- **Hypersensitivity reaction:** Assess for itching, rash, hives, chills, and fever. Advise to report these symptoms promptly to a health care provider.
- **Hypoglycemia:** Monitor blood glucose at least daily and as needed for symptoms of hypoglycemia (altered level of consciousness, tachycardia, diaphoresis) in patients also receiving oral hypoglycemic agents.
- **Side effects:** Monitor for headache, nausea, vomiting, diarrhea, and abdominal pain.
- **Sepsis:** Monitor for fever, tachycardia, and hypotension.
- **Therapeutic effect:** Observe for resolution of oral, esophageal, or vaginal candidiasis. Note resolution of sepsis in patients with systemic candidiasis. Note improvement in neurological status in patients with cryptococcal meningitis.
- **Patient education:** When using fluconazole outside the hospital, caution not to drive or use machinery until response to the drug is known. Instruct to report dark urine, pale stool; rash with or without itching; or yellow skin or eyes indicative of hepatotoxicity. Teach those with an oropharyngeal infection to perform good oral hygiene. Advise consultation with a health care provider before taking all other medications.

SERIOUS ADVERSE REACTIONS

- Rash, hepatitis, anaphylaxis, and blood dyscrasias including eosinophilia, thrombocytopenia, anemia, and leukopenia have been reported rarely.

OVERDOSE/TOXICITY

- **Hepatotoxicity:** Elevated liver enzymes (AST [SGOT], ALT [SGPT], alkaline phosphatase, bilirubin), right upper quadrant abdominal pain, ascites, jaundice, hypovolemia with edema, which can lead to associated renal failure and death. Fluconazole-induced liver damage is not

related to daily dose/duration of therapy and is usually reversible when the drug is discontinued, but has been fatal.
- **Dermatologic:** Rare exfoliative skin disorders, which have been fatal in immunocompromised patients (AIDS, malignancy).
- **GI decontamination:** No specific recommendations.

ANTIDOTE/DIALYSIS
- **Antidote:** No specific recommendations.
- **Dialysis:** Fluconazole is removed by hemodialysis and peritoneal dialysis and is likely to be removed by high-permeability hemodialysis.

flucytosine
See Antifungals (p. 922)

fludrocortisone acetate
floo-droe-kor′-tis-sone as′-e-tate

Classes
Chemical: mineralocorticoid, synthetic
Therapeutic: mineralocorticoid

Pregnancy Category: C

Trade Names
Prescription: Florinef Acetate

Do not confuse Florinef with Fioricet or Florinal.

CLINICAL PHARMACOLOGY
Mechanism of Action
A mineralocorticoid that acts at distal tubules. **Therapeutic Effect:** Increases potassium and hydrogen ion excretion. Replaces sodium loss and raises BP (with low dosages). Inhibits endogenous adrenal cortical secretion, thymic activity, and secretion of corticotropin by pituitary gland (with higher dosages).

PHARMACOKINETICS
Well absorbed from the GI tract. Protein binding: 42%. Widely distributed. Metabolized in the liver and kidney. Primarily excreted in urine. **Half-life:** 3.5 hr.

AVAILABILITY
Tablets: 0.1 mg.

INDICATIONS AND DOSAGE
Addison's disease
PO
Adults, Elderly: 0.05-0.1 mg/day. Range: 0.1 mg 3 times/wk to 0.2 mg/day. Administration with cortisone or hydrocortisone preferred.
Salt-losing adrenogenital syndrome
PO
Adults, Elderly: 0.1-0.2 mg/day.
Usual pediatric dosage
Children: 0.05-0.1 mg/day.

OFF-LABEL USES
Treatment of acidosis in renal tubular disorders, idiopathic orthostatic hypotension

CONTRAINDICATIONS
Heart failure, systemic fungal infection, hypersensitivity to fludrocortisone or other corticosteroids

INTERACTIONS
Drug: Digoxin: May increase the risk of digoxin toxicity caused by hypokalemia. **Hepatic enzyme inducers (such as phenytoin):** May increase the metabolism of fludrocortisone. **Hypokalemia-causing medications:** May increase the effects of fludrocortisone. **Sodium-containing medications:** May increase BP, incidence of edema, and serum sodium level. **Herbal:** None known. **Food:** None known.

DIAGNOSTIC TEST EFFECTS
May increase serum sodium level. May decrease Hct and serum potassium level.

SIDE-EFFECTS
Frequent: Increased appetite, exaggerated sense of well-being, abdominal distention, weight gain, insomnia, mood swings. **High dosages, prolonged therapy, too rapid withdrawal:** Increased susceptibility to infection with masked signs and symptoms, delayed wound healing, hypokalemia, hypocalcemia, GI distress, diarrhea or constipation, hypertension. **Occasional:** Headache, dizziness, menstrual difficulty or amenorrhea, gastric ulcer development. **Rare:** Hypersensitivity reaction

CRITICAL CARE CONSIDERATIONS

ADMINISTRATION/HANDLING
PO ALERT
- Give fludrocortisone with food or milk.

PRECAUTIONS

HEALTH-RELATED

- Use fludrocortisone cautiously in patients with edema, hypertension, or impaired renal function.

AGE-RELATED

- **Children:** Safety and efficacy of fludrocortisone have not been established in children. Fludrocortisone use in children may suppress growth and inhibit endogenous steroid production.
- **Elderly:** Effects of fludrocortisone use in the elderly are unknown.

PREGNANCY/LACTATION-RELATED

- Pregnancy category C; observe newborn for signs and symptoms of adrenocortical insufficiency; corticosteroids are found in breast milk; use caution in nursing mothers.

MONITORING

- **Baseline assessment:** Determine hypersensitivity to corticosteroids; measure height, weight, and vital signs. If diabetes mellitus is present, increase antidiabetic drug regime or consider IV insulin infusion to manage initially steroid-induced hyperglycemia. Assess if patients are receiving drugs that are affected by cortisone and adjust dosage. Obtain chest x-ray and ECG.
- **Baseline lab work:** Biochemical profile including blood glucose and serum electrolyte levels.
- **Infection:** Be alert for infection caused by reduced immune response, including fever, sore throat, and vague symptoms.
- **Weight gain/elevated BP:** Monitor for salt- and retention-induced weight gain, edema, and increases in BP.
- **Hypokalemia:** Monitor ECG for dysrhythmias induced by increased potassium excretion such as premature ventricular beats and ventricular and supraventricular tachycardias.
- **Electrolyte imbalance:** Monitor for hypocalcemia (muscle twitching, cramps, and positive Chvostek's or Trousseau's signs), or hypokalemia (ECG changes, nausea and vomiting, irritability, weakness and muscle cramps, numbness and tingling, especially in lower extremities).
- **Avoid adrenal insufficiency:** Wean fludrocortisone slowly to discontinue both aggressive short-term and prolonged therapy.
- **Sleep disturbance and emotional lability:** Assess sleep pattern and emotional status, fludrocortisone may cause sleeplessness, euphoria, high energy, or labile emotional state. Inform that fludrocortisone often causes mood swings.
- **Patient education:** Warn against abruptly discontinuing fludrocortisone or altering the dosage or schedule. Explain that the drug must be withdrawn gradually under medical supervision. Instruct to report continuing headaches, fever, muscle aches, sore throat, or sudden weight gain or swelling. Instruct to maintain careful personal hygiene and to avoid exposure to disease or trauma. Explain that severe stress, such as serious infection, surgery, or trauma may require an increase in the fludrocortisone dosage. Explain that steroids often cause mood swings ranging from euphoria to depression.

SERIOUS ADVERSE REACTIONS

- **Cushingoid appearance:** Long-term therapy may cause muscle wasting (especially in the arms and legs), osteoporosis, spontaneous fractures, amenorrhea, cataracts, glaucoma, peptic ulcer disease, and heart failure.
- **Abrupt withdrawal of drug:** After long-term therapy, may cause anorexia, nausea, fever, headache, joint pain, rebound inflammation, fatigue, weakness, lethargy, dizziness, and orthostatic hypotension.

OVERDOSE/TOXICITY

- **Severe behavioral changes:** Extreme euphoria, personality changes, severe depression, frank psychosis (more likely in patients with mental health history).
- **Cardiotoxicity:** Significant weight gain (over 15 lb), pitting edema, heart failure, difficulty breathing, hypertension, dysrhythmias.
- **Metabolic:** Hypokalemia, hypokalemic alkalosis, hypernatremia, seizures.
- **GI bleeding:** Hematemesis, bloody stools, expectoration of blood.
- **Severe infection:** Patients who have underlying infection or acquire a significant infection may develop fatal septic shock.
- **Musculoskeletal:** Muscle weakness, steroid-induced myopathy.
- **GI decontamination:** No specific recommendations.

ANTIDOTE/DIALYSIS

- **Antidote:** No specific recommendations.
- **Dialysis:** No data are available on removal of fludrocortisone using hemodialysis, high-permeability hemodialysis, or peritoneal dialysis.

flumazenil

floo-may'-zuh-nil

Classes

Chemical: imidazobenzodiazepine derivative

Therapeutic: benzodiazepine antagonist

Pregnancy Category: C

Trade Names

Prescription: Anexate ♣, Romazicon

CLINICAL PHARMACOLOGY

Mechanism of Action

An antidote that antagonizes the effect of benzodiazepines on the gamma-aminobutyric acid receptor complex in the CNS. **Therapeutic Effect:** Reverses sedative effect of benzodiazepines.

PHARMACOKINETICS

Route	Onset	Peak	Duration
IV	1-2 min	6-10 min	Less than 1 hr

Duration and degree of benzodiazepine reversal depend on dosage and plasma concentration. Protein binding: 50%. Metabolized by the liver; excreted in urine.

AVAILABILITY

Injection: 0.1 mg/mL.

INDICATIONS AND DOSAGE

Reversal of conscious sedation or general anesthesia

IV

Adults, Elderly: Initially, 0.2 mg (2 mL) over 15 sec; may repeat dose in 45 sec; then at 60-sec intervals. Maximum: 1 mg (10-mL) total dose. **Children, Neonates.** Initially, 0.01 mg/kg; may repeat in 45 sec, then at 60-sec intervals. Maximum: 0.2 mg single dose; 0.05 mg/kg or 1 mg cumulative dose.

Benzodiazepine overdose

IV

Adults, Elderly: Initially, 0.2 mg (2 mL) over 30 sec; if desired level of consciousness (LOC) is not achieved after 30 sec, 0.3 mg (3 mL) may be given over 30 sec. Further doses of 0.5 mg (5 mL) may be administered over 30 sec at 60-sec intervals. Maximum: 3 mg (30 mL) total dose.

Children, Neonates: Initially, 0.01 mg/kg; may repeat in 45 sec, then at 60-sec intervals. Maximum: 0.2-mg single dose; 1-mg cumulative dose.

CONTRAINDICATIONS

Anticholinergic signs (such as mydriasis, dry mucosa, and hypoperistalsis), dysrhythmias, cardiovascular collapse, history of hypersensitivity to flumazenil or benzodiazepines, patients with signs of serious cyclic antidepressant overdose (such as motor abnormalities), patients who have been given a benzodiazepine for control of a potentially life-threatening condition (such as control of status epilepticus or increased intracranial pressure [ICP]), not recommended for treatment of benzodiazepine dependence

INTERACTIONS

Drug: Tricyclic antidepressants: May produce seizures and dysrhythmias because flumazenil reverses the sedative effects of tricyclic antidepressants. **Herbal:** None known. **Food:** None known.

DIAGNOSTIC TEST EFFECTS

None known.

IV INCOMPATIBILITIES

No information available for Y-site administration.

IV COMPATIBILITIES

Aminophylline, cimetidine (Tagamet), *DOBUTamine (Dobutrex), *DOPamine (Intropin), famotidine (Pepcid), heparin, lidocaine, procainamide (Pronestyl), ranitidine (Zantac)

SIDE-EFFECTS

Frequent (11%-4%): Agitation, anxiety, dry mouth, dyspnea, insomnia, palpitations, tremors, headache, blurred vision, dizziness, ataxia, nausea, vomiting, pain at injection site, diaphoresis. **Occasional (3%-1%):** Fatigue, flushing, auditory disturbances, thrombophlebitis, rash. **Rare (less than 1%):** Urticaria, pruritus, hallucinations

CRITICAL CARE CONSIDERATIONS

ADMINISTRATION/HANDLING

IV ALERT

- **Storage:** Store the parenteral form at room temperature.
- **Stability:** Discard the injection 24 hr after it has been drawn into a syringe or mixed with any other IV solutions; also discard if it becomes discolored or contains particulate.

- **Compatibility:** Flumazenil is compatible with D_5W, lactated Ringer's solution, or 0.9% NaCl.
- **IV push:** Administer flumazenil over 15 sec for reversal of conscious sedation or general anesthesia or over 30 sec for benzodiazepine overdose. Inject the drug into a large vein through a free-flowing IV infusion because local injection produces pain and inflammation at the injection site.
- **Cleanse skin:** Rinse any spilled solution from the skin with cool water.
- If sedation recurs, give up to 1 mg (as 0.2 mg/min) as a single dose or up to 3 mg in 1 hr.

PRECAUTIONS

HEALTH-RELATED

- Use of flumazenil has been associated with occurrence of seizures in patients who are dependent on benzodiazepines or in patients with signs of tricyclic antidepressant overdose.
- Use flumazenil cautiously in patients with alcoholism, drug dependence, head injury, or hepatic impairment.

AGE-RELATED

- **Children:** Safety and efficacy of flumazenil have been established in children aged 1-17 yr for reversal of sedation. Not recommended for management of overdose or in the resuscitation of the newborn.
- **Elderly:** Benzodiazepine-induced sedation tends to be deeper and more prolonged, requiring careful monitoring.

PREGNANCY/LACTATION-RELATED

- Pregnancy category C; excretion into breast milk unknown; use caution in nursing mothers; not recommended during labor and delivery.

MONITORING

- **Baseline assessment:** Determine amount of benzodiazepines received. Perform a thorough neurologic assessment.
- **Baseline lab work:** Obtain ABG levels before and as needed during IV flumazenil administration if questions arise regarding respiratory status.
- **Hypoventilation and hypoxemia:** Maintain a patent airway and prepare to assist with ventilation if flumazenil does not fully reverse the respiratory depressant effects of the benzodiazepine. The effects of flumazenil may wear off before the effects of the benzodiazepine.
- **Vital signs:** Frequently monitor heart and respiratory rates, continuous ECG, and BP.
- **Following dosage:** Assess for hypoventilation, resedation, and respiratory depression. Closely monitor for return of unconsciousness or narcosis for at least 1 hr after patients are fully alert.
- **Resedation:** Declining neurologic status may be experienced after responding effectively to initial treatment with flumazenil. Resedation is more common in children aged 1-5 yr.
- **Patient education:** Encourage avoidance of tasks requiring mental alertness or motor skills until for least 24 hr after discharge. Instruct to avoid taking OTC drugs for 18-24 hr after discharge.

SERIOUS ADVERSE REACTIONS

- **Panic attack:** Flumazenil may cause a panic attack in patients with a panic disorder.
- **Benzodiazepine-dependent patients:** Use of flumazenil may prompt withdrawal symptoms in patients dependent on a benzodiazepine (diazepam, lorazepam).

OVERDOSE/TOXICITY

- **Toxic effects:** Seizures and dysrhythmias, the toxic effects of other drugs taken in overdose, especially tricyclic antidepressants, may emerge with reversal of sedative effect of benzodiazepines.
- **GI decontamination:** No specific recommendations.

ANTIDOTE/DIALYSIS

- **Antidote:** No specific recommendations.
- **Dialysis:** No data are available regarding removal of flumazenil using hemodialysis, high-permeability hemodialysis, or peritoneal dialysis.

flunisolide

See Bronchodilators (p. 947)

fluoxetine hydrochloride

floo-ox'-e-teen hye-droe-klor'-ide

Classes

Chemical: aryloxypropylamine
Therapeutic: antidepressant, selective serotonin reuptake inhibitor (SSRI)

Pregnancy Category: C

Trade Names

Prescription: Prozac, Prozac Weekly, Sarafem

Combinations

Prescription: with olanzapine (Symbyax)

Do not confuse fluoxetine with fluvastatin; Prozac with Prilosec, Proscar, or ProSom; or Sarafem with Serophene.

CLINICAL PHARMACOLOGY

Mechanism of Action

A psychotherapeutic agent that selectively inhibits serotonin uptake in the CNS, enhancing serotonergic function. Therapeutic Effect: Relieves depression; reduces obsessive-compulsive and bulimic behavior.

PHARMACOKINETICS

Well absorbed from the GI tract. Crosses the blood-brain barrier. Protein binding: 94%. Metabolized in the liver to active metabolite. Primarily excreted in urine. Not removed by hemodialysis. Half-life: 2-3 days; metabolite 7-9 days.

AVAILABILITY

Capsules: 10 mg (Prozac, Sarafem), 20 mg (Prozac, Sarafem), 40 mg (Prozac).
Capsules (delayed release [Prozac Weekly]): 90 mg.
Oral Solution (Prozac): 20 mg/5 mL.
Tablets (Prozac, Rapiflux): 10 mg, 20 mg.

INDICATIONS AND DOSAGE

Depression

PO

Adults: Initially, 20 mg each morning. If therapeutic improvement does not occur after 2 wk, gradually increase to maximum of 80 mg/day in 2 equally divided doses in morning and at noon. Prozac Weekly: 90 mg/wk, begin 7 days after last dose of 20 mg. **Elderly:** Initially, 10 mg/day. May increase by 10-20 mg every 2 wk. **Children 7-17 yr:** Initially, 5-10 mg/day. Titrate upward as needed. Usual dosage is 20 mg/day.

Panic disorder

PO

Adults, Elderly: Initially, 10 mg/day. May increase to 20 mg/day after 1 wk. Maximum: 60 mg/day.

Bulimia nervosa

PO

Adults: 60 mg each morning.

Obsessive-compulsive disorder (OCD)

PO

Adults, Elderly: 40-80 mg/day. **Children 7-18 yr:** Initially, 10 mg/day. May increase to 20 mg/day after 2 wk. Range: 10-80 mg/day.

Premenstrual dysphoric disorder

PO

Adults: 20 mg/day.

OFF-LABEL USES

Treatment of body dysmorphic disorder, fibromyalgia, hot flashes, posttraumatic stress disorder, Raynaud's phenomenon

CONTRAINDICATIONS

Use within 14 days of MAOIs, hypersensitivity to fluoxetine

INTERACTIONS

Drug: **Alcohol, other CNS depressants:** May increase CNS depression. **Highly protein-bound medications (including oral anticoagulants):** May increase adverse effects. **MAOIs:** May produce serotonin syndrome and neuroleptic malignant syndrome. **Phenytoin:** May increase phenytoin blood concentration and risk of toxicity. Herbal: **St. John's wort:** May increase fluoxetine's pharmacologic effects and risk of toxicity. Food: None known.

DIAGNOSTIC TEST EFFECTS

None known.

SIDE-EFFECTS

Frequent (more than 10%): Headache, asthenia, insomnia, anxiety, nervousness, somnolence, nausea, diarrhea, decreased appetite. Occasional (9%-2%): Dizziness, tremor, fatigue, vomiting, constipation, dry mouth, abdominal pain, nasal congestion, diaphoresis, rash. Rare (less than 2%): Flushed skin, lightheadedness, impaired concentration

CRITICAL CARE CONSIDERATIONS

ADMINISTRATION/HANDLING

PO ALERT

- Give fluoxetine with food or milk if GI distress occurs.
- Make sure at least 14 days elapse between the use of MAOIs and fluoxetine.
- Avoid administration at night.

F

PRECAUTIONS

HEALTH-RELATED

- Use fluoxetine cautiously in patients with cardiac dysfunction, diabetes, or seizure disorder and in patients at high risk for suicide.
- **Lower dosage:** May decrease dosage or frequency in patients with hepatic or renal impairment and in those who take multiple medications.
- **Cytochrome P450 inhibitors:** Patients taking other medications metabolized by cytochrome P4503A4 may have drug interactions. Medications include phenytoin, carbamazepine, haloperidol, clozapine, alprazolam, lithium, and trytophan.

AGE-RELATED

- **Children:** Safety and efficacy of fluoxetine in children under 8 yr in major depressive disorder and under 7 yr for obsessive-compulsive disorder (OCD) have not been established. Children may be more sensitive to behavioral side effects such as insomnia and restlessness.
- **Elderly:** No age-related precautions, but some elderly patients may require lower doses due to age-related organ impairments; may cause clinically significant hyponatremia.

PREGNANCY/LACTATION-RELATED

- Pregnancy category C; excreted into breast milk; use caution in nursing mothers.

MONITORING

- **Baseline assessment:** Assess for depression, suicidal ideation, and behavior patterns in OCD.
- **Baseline lab work:** CBC with differential, biochemical profile including liver and renal function tests before and periodically during long-term therapy.
- **Suicidal patients:** Closely supervise suicidal patients during early therapy. As depression lessens, energy level improves, increasing the suicide potential.
- **Therapeutic effect:** Assess for improved appearance, behavior, level of interest, mood, and sleep pattern before and during therapy.
- **Diarrhea:** Assess pattern of daily bowel activity and stool consistency.
- **Rash:** Examine skin for rash, which may signal an allergic reaction.
- **Liver dysfunction:** Monitor blood glucose level and serum alkaline phosphatase, bilirubin, sodium, AST (SGOT) and ALT (SGPT) levels.
- **Patient education:** Instruct to take the last dose of the drug before 4 PM to avoid insomnia. Caution against discontinuing fluoxetine abruptly. Inform that the drug's full therapeutic response may require 4 wk or more of therapy. Warn to avoid tasks that require mental alertness or motor skills until response to the drug is known. Urge avoidance of alcohol while taking fluoxetine.

SERIOUS ADVERSE REACTIONS

- **Rash and allergic reaction:** Systemic events possibly related to vasculitis and including lupuslike syndrome have developed in patients with rash.
- **Interaction with thioridazine:** May elevate thioridazine levels, which causes prolonged QT interval; prolonged QT syndrome may lead to torsades de pointes.

OVERDOSE/TOXICITY

- **Serotonin syndrome:** Altered cognition, abnormal behavior and possibly neuromuscular dysfunction (myoclonus, hyperreflexia, muscle rigidity, extreme tremor), which can lead to seizures, hyperthermia, coma, disseminated intravascular coagulation, hypotension, ventricular tachycardia, and metabolic acidosis. May occur when fluoxetine is given within 14 days of an MAOI (phenelzine [Nardil], tranylcypromine [Parnate]) or other seritoninergic medication. May occur when dose of fluoxetine is increased.
- **GI decontamination:** No specific recommendations.

ANTIDOTE/DIALYSIS

- **Antidote:** No specific antidote. Cyproheptadine is the most consistently effective antiserotoninergic agent in humans. *ChlorproMAZINE may be effective. Benzodiazepines may be used as adjunctive agents to control muscle rigidity.
- **Dialysis:** Fluoxetine is not removed using hemodialysis or peritoneal dialysis. No data are available on removal using high-permeability hemodialysis.

fluphenazine

See Antipsychotics (p. 934)

flurazepam hydrochloride

flure-az'-e-pam hye-droe-klor'-ide

DEA Schedule: IV

Classes
Chemical: benzodiazepine
Therapeutic: sedative/hypnotic

Pregnancy Category: X

Trade Names
Prescription: Apo-Flurazepam ♣, Dalmane

Do not confuse Dalmane with Dialume.

CLINICAL PHARMACOLOGY

Mechanism of Action
A benzodiazepine that enhances action of inhibitory neurotransmitter gamma-aminobutyric acid (GABA). **Therapeutic Effect:** Produces hypnotic effect due to CNS depression.

PHARMACOKINETICS

Route	Onset	Peak	Duration
PO	15-20 min	3-6 hr	7-8 hr

Well absorbed from the GI tract. Protein binding: 97%. Crosses the blood-brain barrier. Widely distributed. Metabolized in liver to active metabolite. Primarily excreted in urine. Not removed by hemodialysis. **Half-life:** 2.3 hr; metabolite: 40-114 hr.

AVAILABILITY

Capsules: 15 mg, 30 mg.

INDICATIONS AND DOSAGE

Insomnia
PO
Adults: 15-30 mg at bedtime. **Elderly, debilitated, liver disease, low serum albumin, Children 15 yr and older:** 15 mg at bedtime.

CONTRAINDICATIONS

Acute alcohol intoxication, acute angle-closure glaucoma, hypersensitivity to flurazepam or other benzodiazepines, pregnancy, or breast-feeding

INTERACTIONS

Drug: **Alcohol, CNS depressants:** May increase CNS depression. **Azole antifungals:** May increase flurazepam concentration and the potential for benzodiazepine toxicity. **Herbal:** **Kava kava, valerian:** May increase CNS depression. **St. John's wort:** May reduce flurazepam effectiveness. **Food:** None known.

DIAGNOSTIC TEST EFFECTS

None known.

SIDE-EFFECTS

Frequent: Drowsiness, dizziness, ataxia, sedation; morning drowsiness may occur initially. **Occasional:** GI disturbances, nervousness, blurred vision, dry mouth, headache, confusion, skin rash, irritability, slurred speech. **Rare:** Paradoxic CNS excitement or restlessness, particularly noted in elderly or debilitated

CRITICAL CARE CONSIDERATIONS

ADMINISTRATION/HANDLING

PO ALERT
- Give flurazepam without regard to meals.
- May empty capsules and mix with food.

PRECAUTIONS

HEALTH-RELATED
- Use cautiously in patients with impaired liver or renal function and in severely debilitated patients.
- Use cautiously in severely depressed patients who may be at increased risk of suicide.

AGE-RELATED
- **Children:** Safety and efficacy of flurazepam have not been established in children under 15 yr.
- **Elderly:** Use small initial doses with gradual dose increases to avoid ataxia or excessive sedation. Dosage may be limited to 15 mg to help prevent falls.

PREGNANCY/LACTATION-RELATED
- Pregnancy category X; administration to nursing mothers is not recommended.

MONITORING

- **Baseline assessment:** Assess BP, pulse, and respirations immediately before beginning flurazepam administration.
- **Baseline lab work:** Biochemical profile including BUN/creatinine and liver enzymes.
- **Prevent falls:** Raise bed rails and place the call bell within reach.
- **Promote sleep:** Provide an environment conducive to sleep.

- **Paradoxic reaction:** Assess for excitability, particularly during early therapy.
- **Therapeutic response:** Evaluate for a decrease in number of nocturnal awakenings and an increase in length of sleep.
- **Patient education:** Discuss that smoking reduces the drug's effectiveness. Caution against abruptly withdrawing the medication after long-term use to avoid possible withdrawal. Explain that flurazepam may be habit-forming, and that sleep may be disturbed 1-2 nights after discontinuing the drug. Urge avoidance of alcohol and other CNS depressants during therapy. Instruct female patients to report pregnancy or plans for pregnancy. Explain that flurazepam is pregnancy risk category X and the drug cannot be taken because of its risk factor.

SERIOUS ADVERSE REACTIONS

- **Abrupt or too-rapid withdrawal after long-term use:** May result in pronounced restlessness and irritability, insomnia, hand tremors, tachycardia, hypertension, abdominal or muscle cramps, vomiting, diaphoresis, and seizures.

OVERDOSE/TOXICITY

- **Severe sedation:** Overdose results in somnolence, confusion, diminished reflexes, ataxia, coma, and respiratory depression.
- **Paradoxic neuropsychiatric reaction:** Uncommon reaction of restlessness and agitation, which occurs more often in children and older adults.
- **Management:** Supportive care including providing a patent airway and ventilation, nasogastric tube to help protect against aspiration, IV fluids for hydration. Advanced Cardiac Life Support (ACLS) guidelines should be followed for other resuscitative efforts.
- **GI decontamination:** No specific recommendations.

ANTIDOTE/DIALYSIS

- **Antidote:** Flumazenil (Romazicon) may help to reverse drug effects. Naloxone (Narcan) may be tried in patients with respiratory depression unrelieved by flumazenil. May result in withdrawal symptoms in flurazepam-dependent patients.
- **Dialysis:** Flurazepam is not removed by hemodialysis and is unlikely to be removed by peritoneal dialysis. No data are available regarding removal using high-permeability hemodialysis.

flurbiprofen

See NSAIDs and Cox-2 Inhibitors (p. 976)

fluticasone propionate

flu-tic'-a-zone pro'-pee-o-nate

Classes

Chemical: corticosteroid, synthetic
Therapeutic: corticosteroid, inhaled; corticosteroid, systemic; corticosteroid, topical

Pregnancy Category: C

Trade Names

Prescription: Cutivate, Flonase, Flovent, Flovent Diskus, Flovent HFA, Flovent Rotadisk

Combinations

Prescription: with salmeterol (Advair Diskus)

CLINICAL PHARMACOLOGY

Mechanism of Action

A corticosteroid that controls the rate of protein synthesis, depresses migration of polymorphonuclear leukocytes, reverses capillary permeability, and stabilizes lysosomal membranes. **Therapeutic Effect:** Prevents or controls inflammation.

PHARMACOKINETICS

Inhalation/intranasal: Protein binding: 91%. Undergoes extensive first-pass metabolism in liver. Excreted in urine. **Half-life:** 3-7.8 hr. **Topical:** Amount absorbed depends on affected area and skin condition (absorption increased with fever, hydration, inflamed or denuded skin).

AVAILABILITY

Aerosol for oral inhalation (Flovent, Flovent HFA): 44 mcg/inhalation, 110 mcg/inhalation, 220 mcg/inhalation.
Powder for oral inhalation (Flovent Diskus): 50 mcg, 100 mcg, 250 mcg.
Intranasal spray (Flonase): 50 mcg/inhalation.
Topical cream (Cutivate): 0.05%.
Topical ointment (Cutivate): 0.005%.

INDICATIONS AND DOSAGE

Allergic rhinitis

Intranasal

Adults, Elderly: Initially, 200 mcg (2 sprays in each nostril once daily or 1 spray in each nostril every 12 hr). Maintenance: 1 spray in each nostril once daily. Maximum: 200 mcg/day. **Children 4 yr and**

older: Initially, 100 mcg (1 spray in each nostril once daily). Maximum: 200 mcg/day.

Relief of inflammation and pruritus associated with steroid-responsive disorders, such as contact dermatitis and eczema

Topical

Adults, Elderly, Children 3 mo and older: Apply sparingly to affected area once or twice per day.

Maintenance treatment for asthma for those previously treated with bronchodilators

Inhalation Powder (Flovent Diskus)

Adults, Elderly, Children 12 yr and older: Initially, 100 mcg every 12 hr. Maximum: 500 mcg/day.

Inhalation (Oral [Flovent])

Adults, Elderly, Children 12 yr and older: 88 mcg twice per day. Maximum: 440 mcg twice per day.

Maintenance treatment for asthma for those previously treated with inhaled steroids

Inhalation Powder (Flovent Diskus)

Adults, Elderly, Children 12 yr and older: Initially, 100-250 mcg every 12 hr. Maximum: 500 mcg every 12 hr.

Inhalation (Oral [Flovent])

Adults, Elderly, Children 12 yr and older: 88-220 mcg twice per day. Maximum: 440 mcg twice per day.

Maintenance treatment for asthma for those previously treated with oral steroids

Inhalation Powder (Flovent Diskus)

Adults, Elderly, Children 12 yr and older: 500-1000 mcg twice per day.

Inhalation (Oral [Flovent])

Adults, Elderly, Children 12 yr and older: 880 mcg twice per day.

CONTRAINDICATIONS

Primary treatment of status asthmaticus or other acute asthma episodes (inhalation); untreated localized infection of nasal mucosa, hypersensitivity to fluticasone or other corticosteroids

INTERACTIONS

Drug: ***BuPROPion:** May lower the seizure threshold. **Herbal:** None known. **Food:** None known.

DIAGNOSTIC TEST EFFECTS

May increase blood glucose level

SIDE-EFFECTS

Frequent: **Inhalation:** Throat irritation, hoarseness, dry mouth, cough, temporary wheezing, oropharyngeal candidiasis (particularly if mouth is not rinsed with water after each administration). **Intranasal:** Mild nasopharyngeal irritation; nasal burning, stinging, or dryness; rebound congestion; rhinorrhea; loss of taste. **Occasional:** **Inhalation:** Oral candidiasis. **Intranasal:** Nasal and pharyngeal candidiasis, headache. **Topical:** Skin burning, pruritus

CRITICAL CARE CONSIDERATIONS

ADMINISTRATION/HANDLING

INHALATION ALERT

- **Concomitant use with a bronchodilator inhaler:** If a bronchodilator inhaler is being used concomitantly with a steroid inhaler, the bronchodilator should be used several minutes before using the corticosteroid to help the steroid penetrate into the bronchial tree.
- **Administration:** Shake the container well. Exhale as completely as possible. Place the mouthpiece fully into the mouth. While holding the inhaler upright, inhale deeply and slowly while pressing the top of the canister. Hold the breath for as long as possible; then exhale slowly. Allow 1 min between inhalations to promote deeper bronchial penetration. Rinse the mouth with water immediately after inhalation to prevent mouth and throat dryness and oral candidiasis.
- **Flovent Diskus inhaler:** Should not be used with a spacer device. Never inhale into a Diskus or attempt to take the device apart. Always activate the Diskus in a level, horizontal position. *Keep it dry.* Never wash the mouthpiece or any part of the device. Discard after removal from moisture-protective overwrap pouch or when all blisters are used (indicator shows zero) in a maximum of 6 wk (50 mcg strength) or 2 mo (100 and 250 mcg strength).

INTRANASAL ALERT

- Clear the nasal passages before using fluticasone; may require use of a topical nasal decongestant 5-15 min before fluticasone use.
- **Preparation:** Tilt the head slightly forward. Insert spray tip up into the nostril, pointing toward inflamed nasal turbinates, away from the nasal septum.
- **Administration:** Spray the drug into the nostril while holding the other nostril closed; at the same time, inhale through the nose.

PRECAUTIONS

HEALTH-RELATED

- **Adrenal insufficiency:** Use fluticasone cautiously in patients with adrenal insufficiency. Withdrawal of drug or transitioning from systemic to inhaled steroids may prompt adrenal insufficiency.
- **Hyperglycemia:** Fluticasone is systemically absorbed and may increase blood glucose.
- **Latent infections:** May mask recurrent symptoms in patients with active quiescent pulmonary tuberculosis, other recently treated bacterial, fungal, or viral infection.
- **Candidiasis:** Fluticasone may cause fungal infections in the nasal passages, oral cavity, and pharynx, which may require treatment with antifungal medications.

AGE-RELATED

- **Children:** Safety and efficacy of fluticasone have not been established in children under 4 yr. Children 4 yr and older may experience growth suppression with prolonged or high doses.
- **Elderly:** No age-related precautions have been noted.

PREGNANCY/LACTATION-RELATED

- Pregnancy category C; no information on excretion into human breast milk.

MONITORING

- **Baseline assessment:** Determine history of asthma or rhinitis or of latent or recently treated infections. Examine nasal passages to ensure there are no ulcers or history of nosebleeds.
- **Baseline lab work:** CBC with WBC differential, biochemical panel including blood glucose level. Serum ACTH or corticotropin levels if adrenal insufficiency is suspected.
- **Acute asthma:** Fluticasone should not be used as a primary treatment. Monitor blood gases if patients are in respiratory distress. Monitor heart rate, rhythm and respiratory rates, depth, rhythm. Auscultate breath sounds for rales, rhonchi, and wheezing.
- **Therapeutic effect (inhaled/intranasal):** Expect to see improvement of symptoms within a few days and relief of symptoms within 3 wk. Prepare to discontinue the drug after 3 wk if no significant improvement.
- **Endocrine dysfunction:** Monitor blood glucose and electrolytes regularly to assess for hyperglycemia, hyperkalemia, and hyponatremia.
- **Infection:** Monitor for nasal, oropharyngeal, or respiratory infections, including candidiasis.
- **Growth disturbance:** Monitor growth in pediatric patients.
- **Patients using topical fluticasone:** Examine the affected area for a therapeutic response.
- **Patient education:** Inform that symptoms should improve in several days. Caution against discontinuing fluticasone abruptly or changing the dosage schedule. Explain that dosage must be tapered gradually under medical supervision. If receiving fluticasone by inhalation, urge patients to maintain fastidious oral hygiene. Instruct on how to rinse the mouth with water immediately after inhalation to prevent mouth or throat dryness and fungal infection. Remind to drink plenty of fluids to decrease the thickness of lung secretions. If a bronchodilator inhaler is being used concomitantly with a steroid inhaler, advise to use the bronchodilator several minutes before using the corticosteroid to help the steroid penetrate into the bronchial tree. If taking fluticasone intranasally, instruct on proper use of the nasal spray. Patients must clear the nasal passages before use. Advise to report nasal irritation or if symptoms, such as sneezing, fail to improve. If using topical fluticasone, instruct how to rub a thin film gently on the affected area. Stress the importance of using the drug only on the prescribed area and for no longer than prescribed. Warn to keep preparation away from the eyes.

SERIOUS ADVERSE REACTIONS

- **Acute hypersensitivity reaction:** Urticaria, angioedema, and severe bronchospasm.
- **Tapering or withdrawing systemic steroids from steroid-dependent patients:** Joint pain, muscle pain, lassitude, and depression commonly occur; avoid adrenal insufficiency using a slow taper. A transfer from systemic to local steroid therapy may unmask previously suppressed bronchial asthma condition.

OVERDOSE/TOXICITY

- Nausea, vomiting, headache, sore throat, cold symptoms, nasal congestion, diarrhea, upset stomach, flulike symptoms, unpleasant tastes, possible palpitations, edema, nervousness, shakiness.

- **Cushingoid appearance:** May appear in overdosed or extremely sensitive patients.
- **Eosinophilic conditions:** Elevated eosinophil count on WBC differential, vasculitic rash, worsening pulmonary symptoms, cardiac complications, or neuropathy.
- **GI decontamination:** No specific recommendations.

ANTIDOTE/DIALYSIS

- **Antidote:** No specific recommendations.
- **Dialysis:** Fluticasone is unlikely to be removed using hemodialysis, high-permeability hemodialysis, or peritoneal dialysis.

fluvastatin sodium

See Antihyperlipidemics (p. 928)

fluvoxamine maleate

See Antidepressants (p. 906)

fomepizole

foe-mep'-i-zoll

Classes
Chemical: pyrazole derivative
Therapeutic: antidote, ethylene glycol (antifreeze)

Pregnancy Category: C

Trade Names
Prescription: Antizol

CLINICAL PHARMACOLOGY

Mechanism of Action

An alcohol dehydrogenase inhibitor that inhibits the enzyme that catalyzes the metabolism of ethanol, ethylene glycol, and methanol to their toxic metabolites. **Therapeutic Effect:** Inhibits conversion of ethylene glycol and methanol into toxic metabolites.

PHARMACOKINETICS

Protein binding: low. Rapidly distributes to total body water after IV infusion. Extensively metabolized by the liver. Minimal excretion in the urine. Removed by hemodialysis. **Half-life:** 5 hr.

AVAILABILITY

Solution for injection: 1 g/mL (Antizol).

INDICATIONS AND DOSAGE

Ethylene glycol or methanol intoxication
IV infusion

Adults, Elderly: 15 mg/kg as loading dose, followed by 10 mg/kg every 12 hr for 4 doses, then 15 mg/kg every 12 hr until ethylene glycol or methanol concentrations are below 20 mg/dL. All doses should be administered as a slow IV infusion over 30 min.

Dosage in renal impairment

During hemodialysis. 15 mg/kg as a loading dose, followed by 10 mg/kg every 4 hr for 4 doses, then 15 mg/kg every 4 hr until ethylene glycol or methanol concentrations are below 20 mg/dL. **After hemodialysis.** If the time between the last dose and end of hemodialysis is less than 1 hr, do not give dose. If the time between is 1-3 hr, give 50% of next scheduled dose. If time is greater than 3 hr, give next scheduled dose.

OFF-LABEL USES

Butoxyethanol intoxication, diethylene glycol intoxication, ethanol sensitivity

CONTRAINDICATIONS

Hypersensitivity to fomepizole or other pyrazoles

INTERACTIONS

Drug: Alcohol: May reduce elimination of both drugs. **Herbal:** None known. **Food:** None known.

DIAGNOSTIC TEST EFFECTS

None known.

IV INCOMPATIBILITIES

No drug incompatibilities reported.

SIDE-EFFECTS

Frequent: Hypertriglyceridemia, headache, nausea, dizziness. **Occasional:** Abnormal sense of smell, nystagmus, visual disturbances, ringing in ears, agitation, seizures, anorexia, heartburn, anxiety, vertigo, lightheadedness, altered sense of awareness. **Rare:** Anuria, disseminated intravascular coagulopathy

CRITICAL CARE CONSIDERATIONS

ADMINISTRATION/HANDLING

IV ALERT

- **Storage:** Store unopened vial at room temperature. Do not freeze.

- **Stability:** Reconstituted solutions are stable for up to 24 hr; store refrigerated or at room temperature.
- **Dilution:** Dilute at least 100 mL of 0.9% NaCl or D_5W.
- **IV infusion only:** Administer fomepizole as a slow infusion over 30 min. Do not give undiluted or by bolus injection.
- **Dialysis:** Adjust fomepizole dose in dialysis patients.

PRECAUTIONS

F

HEALTH-RELATED

- Use cautiously in patients with liver disease or renal impairment.
- **Dialysis:** Should be considered in addition to fomepizole in cases of renal failure related to poisoning.
- **Cytochrome P450 inhibitors:** Fomepizole is metabolized by cytochrome P450. Other inhibitors of these enzymes may interact with fomepizole metabolism and lead to numerous drug interactions.

AGE-RELATED

- **Children:** Safety and efficacy of fomepizole have not been established in children.
- **Elderly:** Age-related renal impairment may require a dosage adjustment.

PREGNANCY/LACTATION-RELATED

- Pregnancy category C; unknown if excreted in breast milk; use with caution.

MONITORING

- **Baseline assessment:** Fomepizole is used primarily as an antidote for methanol or ethylene glycol poisoning. Obtain history and allergies. Assess for neurologic deterioration, respiratory distress, tachycardia, bradycardia, abdominal distention, bleeding, and other signs of poisoning. Obtain mental health history to assess for depression or suicidal ideation.
- **Lab work:** Biochemical panel including hepatic and renal function tests; complete blood count (CBC), and urinalysis before beginning therapy and routinely thereafter.
- **Diagnostic tests:** Assess chest x-ray and 12-lead ECG for respiratory or cardiac changes. Abdominal x-rays if abdomen is distended or painful.
- **Hemodialysis:** Should be considered for patients with high ethylene glycol or methanol concentrations (more than or equal to 50 mg/dL), metabolic acidosis, or renal failure.
- **Therapeutic response:** Obtain ongoing lab work including plasma/urinary ethylene glycol or methanol, urinary oxalate, plasma/urinary osmolality, renal/hepatic function, serum electrolytes, and arterial blood gases. Assess for resolution of visual disturbances and other symptoms of poisoning.
- **Vein irritation:** Monitor IV site for redness and irritation. Infusion time should be at least 30 min.
- **Patient education:** Teach that fomepizole is given to treat antifreeze or windshield-wiper fluid ingestion. If not treated, these poisons will cause kidney damage, eye damage, seizures, coma, and possibly death. Inform that common side effects of fomepizole are headache and nausea.

SERIOUS ADVERSE REACTIONS

- Mild allergic reactions including rash and eosinophilia occur rarely.
- Anuria and disseminated intravascular coagulation (DIC) have been reported, but it is not clear whether organ failure was due to fomepizole or underlying poisoning.

OVERDOSE/TOXICITY

- Fomepizole overdose may cause nausea, dizziness, and vertigo. Ethanol can also be used to manage methanol and ethylene glycol poisoning.
- **GI decontamination:** No specific recommendations.

ANTIDOTE/DIALYSIS

- **Antidote:** No specific recommendations.
- **Dialysis:** Fomepizole is removed by hemodialysis and is likely removed by high-permeability hemodialysis. There are no data on removal using peritoneal dialysis. When used with hemodialysis, if less than 6 hr have passed since last fomepizole dose, do not give the dose before dialysis treatment. If more than 6 hr have passed since last dose, give next scheduled dose before dialysis treatment. Give doses of fomepizole every 4 hr during hemodialysis.

fomivirsen sodium

foh-mih-ver'-sen soe'-dee-um

Classes

Chemical: antisense oligonucleotide
Therapeutic: antiviral

Pregnancy Category: C

Trade Names

Prescription: Vitravene

CLINICAL PHARMACOLOGY

Mechanism of Action

An antiviral that binds to messenger RNA, inhibiting the synthesis of viral proteins. **Therapeutic Effect:** Blocks replication of cytomegalovirus (CMV).

PHARMACOKINETICS

Minimal systemic absorption following intravitreal injection.

AVAILABILITY

Intravitreal Injection: 6.6 mg/mL.

INDICATIONS AND DOSAGE

CMV retinitis

Intravitreal injection

Adults: 330 mcg (0.05 mL) every other wk for 2 doses, then 330 mcg every 4 wk.

CONTRAINDICATIONS

Hypersensitivity to fomivirsen

INTERACTIONS

Drug: None significant. **Herbal:** None significant. **Food:** None significant.

DIAGNOSTIC TEST EFFECTS

May alter liver function test results and serum alkaline phosphatase level. May decrease blood Hgb levels and neutrophil and platelet counts.

SIDE-EFFECTS

Frequent (10%-5%): Fever, headache, nausea, diarrhea, vomiting, abdominal pain, anemia, uveitis, abnormal vision. **Occasional (5%-2%):** Chest pain, confusion, dizziness, depression, neuropathy, anorexia, weight loss, pancreatitis, dyspnea, cough

CRITICAL CARE CONSIDERATIONS

ADMINISTRATION/HANDLING

OPHTHALMIC ALERT

- **Intravitreal injection:** Fomivirsen is given by intravitreal injection (0.05 mL/eye) into the affected eye following application of standard topical and/or local anesthetics and antimicrobials using a 30-gauge needle on a low-volume (e.g., tuberculin) syringe.

PRECAUTIONS

HEALTH-RELATED

- Be aware that fomivirsen use should be avoided in patients who have received cidofovir within 2-4 wk of fomivirsen therapy.
- Use this drug cautiously in patients with increased intraocular pressure.

AGE-RELATED

- **Children:** Safety and efficacy of fomivirsen have not been established in children.
- **Elderly:** No age-related precautions have been established; an insufficient number of subjects over 65 yr have been studied.

PREGNANCY/LACTATION-RELATED

- Pregnancy category C; breast milk excretion unlikely.

MONITORING

- **Baseline assessment:** A comprehensive retinal exam including indirect ophthalmoscopy should be done. Differential diagnosis is made by assessment of appearance of the retina by a trained specialist.
- **After fomivirsen injection:** Evaluate light perception, optic nerve head perfusion, and intraocular pressure.
- **Extraocular CMV infection:** Monitor for other CMV infections including pneumonitis and colitis. Assess for CMV infection in the untreated eye if only one eye is undergoing treatment.
- **Patient education:** Inform that fomivirsen treats but does not cure CMV retinitis. Explain that regular eye exams and follow-up care will be required.

SERIOUS ADVERSE REACTIONS

- Decreased visual acuity, eye pain, increased intraocular pressure, retinal hemorrhage.

OVERDOSE/TOXICITY

- Abdominal pain, anemia, asthenia, diarrhea, fever, headache, pneumonia, rash, sepsis, sinusitis, systemic CMV.
- **GI decontamination:** No specific recommendations.

ANTIDOTE/DIALYSIS

- **Antidote:** No specific recommendations.
- **Dialysis:** No data are available regarding removal of fomivirsen by any mode of dialysis.

fondaparinux sodium 

fon-da-pa'-rin-ux soe'-dee-um

Classes

Chemical: pentasaccharide
Therapeutic: anticoagulant

Pregnancy Category: B

Trade Names

Prescription: Arixtra

CLINICAL PHARMACOLOGY

Mechanism of Action

A factor Xa inhibitor and pentasaccharide that selectively binds to antithrombin and increases its affinity for factor Xa, thereby inhibiting factor Xa and stopping the blood coagulation cascade. **Therapeutic Effect:** Indirectly prevents formation of thrombin and subsequently the fibrin clot.

PHARMACOKINETICS

Well absorbed after subcutaneous administration. Undergoes minimal, if any, metabolism. Highly bound to antithrombin III. Distributed mainly in blood and to a minor extent in extravascular fluid. Excreted unchanged in urine. Not removed by hemodialysis. **Half-life:** 17-21 hr (prolonged in patients with impaired renal function).

AVAILABILITY

Injection: 2.5 mg/0.5 mL prefilled syringe.

INDICATIONS AND DOSAGE

Prevention of venous thromboembolism

Subcutaneous

Adults: 2.5 mg once per day for 5-9 days after surgery. Initial dose should be given 6-8 hr after surgery. Dosage should be adjusted in the elderly and in those with renal impairment.

Treatment venous thromboembolism, pulmonary embolism

Subcutaneous

Adults, Elderly weighing greater than 100 kg: 10 mg once daily. **Adults, Elderly weighing 50-100 kg:** 7.5 mg once daily. **Adults, Elderly weighing less than 50 kg:** 5 mg once daily.

CONTRAINDICATIONS

Active major bleeding, bacterial endocarditis, body weight less than 50 kg, severe renal impairment (with creatinine clearance less than 30 mL/min), thrombocytopenia associated with antiplatelet antibody formation in the presence of fondaparinux, hypersensitivity to fondaparinux

INTERACTIONS

Drug: **Anticoagulants, platelet inhibitors:** May increase bleeding. **Herbal:** None known. **Food:** None known.

DIAGNOSTIC TEST EFFECTS

Increases reversible serum creatinine, AST (SGOT), and ALT (SGPT) levels. May decrease Hgb, Hct, and platelet count.

SIDE-EFFECTS

Occasional (14%): Fever. **Rare (4%-1%):** Injection site hematoma, nausea, peripheral edema

CRITICAL CARE CONSIDERATIONS

ADMINISTRATION/HANDLING

SUBCUTANEOUS ALERT

- **Storage:** Store at room temperature. The parenteral form normally appears clear and colorless. Discard if discoloration or particulate matter is noted.
- **Preparation:** Do not expel the air bubble from the prefilled syringe before injection to avoid expelling the drug.
- **Administration:** Pinch a fold of the skin at the injection site between the thumb and forefinger. Introduce the entire length of subcutaneous needle into the skinfold. Inject into fatty tissue between the left and right abdominal wall either anterolaterally or posterolaterally. Rotate injection sites to decrease tissue irritation and damage.
- **Not for IM injection:** Fondaparinux is not intended for IM injection.
- **Other anticoagulants:** Fonaparinux cannot be used interchangeably (unit for unit) with heparin, low molecular weight heparin, and heparinoids.

PRECAUTIONS

HEALTH-RELATED

- Use fondaparinux cautiously in the elderly and in patients with conditions associated with increased risk of hemorrhage, such as concurrent use of antiplatelet agents, GI ulceration, hemophilia, history of cerebrovascular accident, and severe uncontrolled hypertension; history of heparin-induced thrombocytopenia; impaired renal function; and indwelling epidural catheter or neuraxial anesthesia.
- **First postoperative injection:** Should be done at least 6 hr following surgery to avoid increased risk of major bleeding.

AGE-RELATED

- **Children:** Safety and efficacy of fondaparinux have not been established in children.
- **Elderly:** Age-related decreased renal function may increase the risk of bleeding.

PREGNANCY/LACTATION-RELATED

- Pregnancy category B; excreted in milk of lactating rats, but human studies are lacking; use caution in nursing mothers.

MONITORING

- **Baseline assessment:** Assess for history of bleeding, including bleeding and clotting disorders, heart attack, stroke, or risk factors for vascular disease. Assess if platelet count has decreased with heparin use (possible HIT).
- **Baseline lab work:** CBC; biochemical panel including BUN, creatinine, and liver enzymes. Coagulation studies may be done if history is unclear.
- **Ongoing lab work:** Periodically monitor CBC, biochemical profile and stool for occult blood. There is no need for daily monitoring in patients with normal presurgical coagulation parameters. Action of fondaparinux on factor Xa is not effectively measured by standard coagulation studies.
- **Bleeding:** Assess for bleeding, including bleeding at injection or surgical sites or from gums, blood in stool, unusual back pain, black or red stool, coffee ground vomitus, dark or red urine, bloody phlegm, ecchymosis, hematuria, and petechiae. If bleeding occurs during therapy, the drug should be discontinued regardless of coagulation study results (ineffective measurement for fondaparinux).
- **Hemorrhage:** Monitor for tachycardia, tachypnea, and hypotension, which may indicate bleeding.
- **Epidural catheter for pain management:** Decision to use fondaparinux in patients with an indwelling epidural or spinal catheter should weigh the risk of developing paralysis due to spinal bleeding against the benefit of preventing deep vein thrombosis. Patients must be monitored closely for loss of sensation and movement in lower extremities if an epidural or spinal catheter is in place.
- **Patient education:** Advise that the usual length of therapy is 5-9 days. Advise not to take other medications, including OTC drugs (especially aspirin and NSAIDs) before discussing with a health care provider. Instruct to report promptly severe or sudden headache, swelling in the feet or hands, unusual back pain, black or red stool, coffee ground vomitus, dark or red urine, bloody phlegm or unusual bleeding, bruising, chest pain, dyspnea, or weakness to a health care provider because these findings may indicate bleeding. Advise about use of an electric razor and soft toothbrush to prevent bleeding during therapy. Explain to female patients that menstrual flow may be heavier than usual.

SERIOUS ADVERSE REACTIONS

- **Spinal/epidural hematomas:** If spinal or epidural anesthesia or analgesia are used during surgery or indwelling catheters are inserted for postoperative pain management, patients receiving fondaparinux are at risk for developing an epidural or spinal hematoma which can result in long-term or permanent paralysis.
- **Mild to moderate bleeding:** Local ecchymoses, hemoptysis, blood in stool, progressive anemia, bleeding gums.
- **Thrombocytopenia:** Occurs rarely with fondaparinux.
- **Elevated liver enzymes:** Enzyme elevations are not clinically significant.

OVERDOSE/TOXICITY

- **Symptoms:** May lead to bleeding complications, including major internal or external hemorrhage. Patients may experience intracranial bleeding and intraocular bleeding, which may lead to permanent impairment or blindness.
- **Management:** Transfusion with fresh frozen plasma to help replenish factor Xa. For neurologic deterioration indicative of stroke or other signs of hemorrhage, prompt action is necessary to help reduce the chance of permanent impairment. Administer blood products for severe anemia and hemorrhagic shock, along with fluids and vasopressors if needed to maintain BP. Severe anemia can prompt myocardial ischemia leading to acute MI or cerebral ischemia in high risk patients with or without profound hypotension.
- **GI decontamination:** No specific recommendations.

ANTIDOTE/DIALYSIS

- **Antidote:** No specific recommendations.
- **Dialysis:** Fondaparinux is not removed using hemodialysis and is unlikely to be removed using peritoneal dialysis. No data are available on removal using high-permeability hemodialysis.

formoterol fumarate ⚑

See Bronchodilators (p. 947)

fosamprenavir calcium

See HIV Medications (p. 961)

foscarnet sodium

See Antivirals (p. 937)

F

fosfomycin tromethamine

fos-foe-mye'-sin troe-meth'-a-meen

Classes
Chemical: phosphoric acid derivative
Therapeutic: antibiotic

Pregnancy Category: B

Trade Names
Prescription: Monurol

Do not confuse Monurol with Monopril.

CLINICAL PHARMACOLOGY

Mechanism of Action
An antibiotic that prevents bacterial cell wall formation by inhibiting the synthesis of peptidoglycan. **Therapeutic Effect:** Bactericidal.

PHARMACOKINETICS

Rapidly absorbed following PO administration. Not bound to plasma proteins. Not metabolized. Partially excreted in urine; minimal elimination in feces. **Half-life:** 5.7 ± 2.8 hr.

AVAILABILITY

Powder for oral solution: 3 g.

INDICATIONS AND DOSAGE

Urinary tract infections (UTIs)
PO (Uncomplicated)
Females: 3 g mixed in 4 oz water as a single dose.
PO (Complicated)
Males. 3 g/day every 2-3 days for 3 doses.

OFF-LABEL USES

Serious UTI in men

CONTRAINDICATIONS

Hypersensitivity to fosfomycin tromethamine

INTERACTIONS

Drug: Metoclopramide: Lowers serum concentration and urinary excretion of fosfomycin. **Herbal:** None known. **Food:** None known.

DIAGNOSTIC TEST EFFECTS

May increase blood eosinophil count and serum alkaline phosphatase, bilirubin, AST (SGOT), and ALT (SGPT) levels. May alter platelet and WBC counts. May decrease blood Hct and Hgb levels.

SIDE-EFFECTS

Occasional (9%-3%): Diarrhea, nausea, headache, back pain. **Rare (less than 2%):** Dysmenorrhea, pharyngitis, abdominal pain, rash

CRITICAL CARE CONSIDERATIONS

ADMINISTRATION/HANDLING

PO ALERT

- Give fosfomycin without regard to food.
- Pour entire contents of a single dose sachet into 3-4 oz water; stir to dissolve; do not use hot water.
- Drug should be taken immediately after dissolving in water.

PRECAUTIONS

HEALTH-RELATED

- Fosfomycin is undergoing study as an antidote for dose-limiting ototoxicity and nephrotoxicity associated with cisplatin chemotherapy.

AGE-RELATED

- **Children:** Safety and efficacy of fosfomycin have not been established in children.
- **Elderly:** No age-related precautions have been noted.

PREGNANCY/LACTATION-RELATED

- Pregnancy category B; excretion into breast milk unknown.

MONITORING

- **Baseline assessment:** Assess for symptoms of bladder infection.
- **Baseline lab work:** Urine culture to identify organism.
- **Therapeutic effect:** Resolution of dysuria.
- **Patient education:** Instruct to always mix fosfomycin with water before consuming. Symptoms should improve within 2-3 days of treatment with fosfomycin.

SERIOUS ADVERSE REACTIONS

- **Liver dysfunction:** Elevated AST (SGOT), ALT (SGPT), bilirubin, and alkaline phosphatase levels.

OVERDOSE/TOXICITY

- No information on cases of overdose or toxicity.
- **GI decontamination:** No specific recommendations.

ANTIDOTE/DIALYSIS

- **Antidote:** No specific recommendations.
- **Dialysis:** Fosfomycin is removed by hemodialysis and is likely removed by high-permeability hemodialysis. No data are available on removal by peritoneal dialysis.

fosinopril

See ACE Inhibitors (p. 883)

fosphenytoin sodium

fos-fen'-i-toyn soe'-dee-um

Classes

Chemical: hydantoin
Therapeutic: anticonvulsant

Pregnancy Category: D

Trade Names

Prescription: Cerebyx

Do not confuse Cerebyx with Celebrex or Celexa.

CLINICAL PHARMACOLOGY

Mechanism of Action

A hydantoin anticonvulsant that stabilizes neuronal membranes by decreasing sodium and calcium ion influx into the neurons. Also decreases posttetanic potentiation and repetitive discharge. **Therapeutic Effect:** Decreases seizure activity.

PHARMACOKINETICS

Completely absorbed after IM administration. Protein binding: 95%-99%. Rapidly and completely hydrolyzed to phenytoin after IM or IV administration. Time of complete conversion to phenytoin: 4 hr after IM injection; 2 hr after IV infusion. **Half-life:** 8-15 min (for conversion to phenytoin).

AVAILABILITY

Injection: 75 mg/mL (equivalent to 50 mg/mL phenytoin).

INDICATIONS AND DOSAGE

Status epilepticus

IV

Adults: Loading dose: 15-20 mg phenytoin equivalent (PE)/kg infused at rate of 100-150 mg PE/min.

Nonemergent seizures

IV, IM

Adults: Loading dose: 10-20 mg PE/kg. Maintenance: 4-6 mg PE/kg/day.

Short term substitution for oral phenytoin

IV, IM

Adults: May substitute for oral phenytoin at same total daily dose.

CONTRAINDICATIONS

Adams-Stokes syndrome; hypersensitivity to fosphenytoin, ethotoin, phenytoin, mephenytoin; second- or third-degree AV block; severe bradycardia; SA block

INTERACTIONS

Drug: Alcohol, other CNS depressants: May increase CNS depression. **Amiodarone, anticoagulants, cimetidine, disulfiram, fluoxetine, isoniazid, sulfonamides:** May increase fosphenytoin blood concentration, effects, and risk of toxicity. **Antacids:** May decrease fosphenytoin absorption. **Fluconazole, ketoconazole, miconazole:** May increase fosphenytoin blood concentration. **Glucocorticoids:** May decrease the effects of glucocorticoids. **Lidocaine, propranolol:** May increase cardiac depressant effects. **Valproic acid:** May increase the blood concentration and decrease the metabolism of fosphenytoin. **Xanthines:** May increase the metabolism of xanthines. **Herbal:** None known. **Food:** None known.

DIAGNOSTIC TEST EFFECTS

May increase blood glucose, serum GGT, and serum alkaline phosphatase levels.

IV INCOMPATIBILITIES

Midazolam (Versed)

IV COMPATIBILITIES

Lorazepam (Ativan), phenobarbital, potassium chloride

SIDE-EFFECTS

Frequent: Dizziness, paresthesia, tinnitus, pruritus, headache, somnolence. **Occasional:** Morbilliform rash

CRITICAL CARE CONSIDERATIONS

ADMINISTRATION/HANDLING

IV ALERT

- **Fosphenytoin dosage/phenytoin equivalents:** Dose, concentration, and infusion rate of fosphenytoin are expressed in terms of phenytoin equivalents (PE); 150 mg fosphenytoin yields 100 mg phenytoin.

- **Storage:** Refrigerate unopened vials. Discard vials that contain particulate matter.
- **Stability:** Do not store the drug at room temperature for longer than 48 hr. After dilution, the solution is stable for 8 hr at room temperature or 24 hr if refrigerated.
- **Dilution:** Dilute the drug in D_5W or 0.9% NaCl to a concentration of 1.5-25 mg PE/mL.
- **IV infusion:** Administer at less than 150 mg PE/min to decrease the risk of hypotension and dysrhythmias.

F

IM ALERT

- **Storage:** Refrigerate unopened vials. Discard vials that contain particulate matter.
- **Stability:** Do not store the drug at room temperature for longer than 48 hr.

PRECAUTIONS

HEALTH-RELATED

- Use fosphenytoin cautiously in patients with hypoalbuminemia, hypotension, hepatic or renal disease, porphyria, those who are critically ill, or severe myocardial insufficiency.
- **Cytochrome P450 enzyme metabolism:** Fosphenytoin is metabolized by this hepatic enzyme pathway and fosphenytoin levels may increase when other CYP450 inhibiting medications are given concomitantly with fosphenytoin. There is potential for numerous drug interactions.

AGE-RELATED

- **Children:** Safety and efficacy of fosphenytoin have not been established in children.
- **Elderly:** May require lower, less frequent fosphenytoin dosing because of reduced clearance or lower albumin levels, which prompt increased unbound drug in the bloodstream.

PREGNANCY/LACTATION-RELATED

- Pregnancy category D; avoid pregnancy (serious congenital malformations); newborns whose mothers received fosphenytoin have experienced a severe bleeding disorder, which can be prevented by giving vitamin K to the mother before delivery and to the neonate after delivery; breast-feeding should be discontinued.

MONITORING

- **Baseline assessment:** Assess level of consciousness; review history of the seizure disorder: duration, frequency, and intensity of seizures. Obtain vital signs and medication (including anticonvulsant use) history.
- **Lab work:** Assess fosphenytoin blood level 2 hr after IV infusion or 4 hr after IM injection.
- **Seizures:** Initiate seizure precautions.
- **Infusion:** Monitor BP, continuous ECG, cardiac, and respiratory function during and for 10-20 min after the infusion. Discontinue the infusion if rash develops.
- **Dysrhythmias:** Interrupt or decrease the infusion rate if bradycardia, heart block, or hypotension occurs.
- **Rash:** Observe for rash; discontinue drug if rash appears; if rash is mild, drug may be tried again. If rash reappears or if initial rash is severe, drug should be permanently discontinued.
- **Plasma levels:** Therapeutic plasma level is 5-20 mcg/mL (usually 10 mcg/mL controls seizures); toxic plasma level is more than 20 mcg/mL. There is a narrow margin between therapeutic and toxic dosage. Assess after the infusion for ataxia, dizziness, or drowsiness.
- **Patient education:** Teach about seizures; explain patients' roles in seizure management. If noncompliance with therapy was a factor in causing acute seizures, try to resolve the reasons for noncompliance. Advise to always carry an identification card or wear an identification bracelet that displays their seizure disorder and anticonvulsant therapy. Caution to avoid performing tasks that require mental alertness or motor skills until response to the drug is known.

SERIOUS ADVERSE REACTIONS

- **Elevated fosphenytoin blood concentration:** May produce ataxia, nystagmus, diplopia, lethargy, slurred speech, nausea, vomiting, and hypotension.
- **Severe rash:** Bullous, purpuric, toxic epidermal necrolysis, lupus erythematosus, Stevens–Johnson syndrome.
- **Severe bleeding disorder:** Experienced by newborns of mothers who received fosphenytoin during pregnancy.

OVERDOSE/TOXICITY

- **Neurotoxicity:** As the drug level increases, extreme lethargy may progress to coma; hyperreflexia and tremors may progress to seizures.
- **Cardiotoxicity:** Bradycardia, heart block, hypotension, asystole, ventricular fibrillation, cardiac arrest.

- **Nephrotoxicity:** Renal failure patients may experience severe hyperphosphatemia with associated hypocalcemia from phosphates present in fosphenytoin.
- **Management:** Manage dysrhythmias according to current Advanced Cardiac Life Support (ACLS) guidelines. Measure ionized free calcium levels to guide treatment in phosphate toxicity.
- **GI decontamination:** No specific recommendations.

ANTIDOTE/DIALYSIS

- **Antidote:** No specific recommendations.
- **Dialysis:** Fosphenytoin is unlikely to be removed by hemodialysis or peritoneal dialysis. No data are available on removal using high-permeability hemodialysis.

frovatriptan

See Triptans (p. 984)

furosemide

fur-oh'-se-mide

Classes

Chemical: anthranilic acid derivative
Therapeutic: antihypertensive, diuretic, loop

Pregnancy Category: C, D (if used in pregnancy-induced hypertension)

Trade Names

Prescription: Apo-Furosemide ♣, Lasix

Do not confuse Lasix with Lidex, Luvox, or Luxiq or furosemide with Torsemide.

CLINICAL PHARMACOLOGY

Mechanism of Action

A loop diuretic that enhances excretion of sodium, chloride, and potassium by direct action at the ascending limb of the loop of Henle. **Therapeutic Effect:** Produces diuresis and lowers BP.

PHARMACOKINETICS

Route	Onset	Peak	Duration
PO	30-60 min	1-2 hr	6-8 hr
IV	5 min	20-60 min	2 hr
IM	30 min	N/A	N/A

Well absorbed from the GI tract. Protein binding: 91%-97%. Partially metabolized in the liver. Primarily excreted in urine (nonrenal clearance increases in severe renal impairment). Not removed by hemodialysis. **Half-life:** 30-90 min (increased in renal or hepatic impairment, and in neonates).

AVAILABILITY

Oral solution: 10 mg/mL, 40 mg/5 mL.
Tablets: 20 mg, 40 mg, 80 mg.
Injection: 10 mg/mL.

INDICATIONS AND DOSAGE

Edema, hypertension

PO

Adults, Elderly: Initially, 20-80 mg/dose; may increase by 20-40 mg/dose every 6-8 hr. May titrate up to 600 mg/day in severe edematous states. **Children:** 1-6 mg/kg/day in divided doses every 6-12 hr. **Neonates:** 1-4 mg/kg/dose 1-2 times per day.

IV, IM

Adults, Elderly: 20-40 mg/dose; may increase by 20 mg/dose every 1-2 hr. **Children:** 1-2 mg/kg/dose every 6-12 hr. **Neonates:** 1-2 mg/kg/dose every 12-24 hr.

IV Infusion

Adults, Elderly: Bolus of 0.1 mg/kg, followed by infusion of 0.1 mg/kg/hr; may double every 2 hr. Maximum: 0.4 mg/kg/hr. **Children:** 0.05 mg/kg/hr; titrate to desired effect.

OFF-LABEL USES

Hypercalcemia

CONTRAINDICATIONS

Anuria, hepatic coma, severe electrolyte depletion, hypersensitivity to furosemide

INTERACTIONS

Drug: Amphotericin B, nephrotoxic and ototoxic medications: May increase the risk of nephrotoxicity and ototoxicity. **Anticoagulants, heparin:** May decrease the effects of these drugs. **Lithium:** May increase the risk of lithium toxicity. **Other hypokalemia-causing medications:** May increase the risk of hypokalemia. **Probenecid:** May increase furosemide blood concentration. **Herbal:** None known. **Food:** None known.

DIAGNOSTIC TEST EFFECTS

May increase blood glucose, BUN, and serum uric acid levels. May decrease serum calcium, chloride, magnesium, potassium, and sodium levels.

IV INCOMPATIBILITIES

Ciprofloxacin (Cipro), diltiazem (Cardizem), *DOBUTamine (Dobutrex), *DOPamine

(Intropin), *DOXOrubicin (Adriamycin), droperidol (Inapsine), esmolol (Brevibloc), famotidine (Pepcid), filgrastim (Neupogen), fluconazole (Diflucan), gemcitabine (Gemzar), gentamicin (Garamycin), idarubicin (Idamycin), labetalol (Trandate), meperidine (Demerol), metoclopramide (Reglan), midazolam (Versed), milrinone (Primacor), *niCARdipine (Cardene), ondansetron (Zofran), quinidine, thiopental (Pentothal), vecuronium (Norcuron), *vinBLASTine (Velban), *vinCRISTine (Oncovin), vinorelbine (Navelbine)

IV COMPATIBILITIES

Aminophylline, amiodarone (Cordarone), bumetanide (Bumex), calcium gluconate, cimetidine (Tagamet), heparin, hydromorphone (Dilaudid), lidocaine, morphine, nitroglycerin, norepinephrine (Levophed), potassium chloride, propofol (Diprivan)

SIDE-EFFECTS

Expected: Increased urinary frequency and urine volume. **Frequent**: Nausea, dyspepsia, abdominal cramps, diarrhea or constipation, electrolyte disturbances. **Occasional**: Dizziness, lightheadedness, headache, blurred vision, paresthesia, photosensitivity, rash, fatigue, bladder spasm, restlessness, diaphoresis. **Rare**: Flank pain

CRITICAL CARE CONSIDERATIONS

ADMINISTRATION/HANDLING

PO ALERT

- Give furosemide with food to avoid GI upset, preferably with breakfast to help prevent nocturia.

IV ALERT

- **Storage:** Store at room temperature. Solution normally appears clear and colorless. Discard discolored solutions.
- **Dilution:** Furosemide is compatible with D_5W, 0.9% NaCl, and lactated Ringer's solution, but it may also be given undiluted.
- **IV push:** Administer each 40 mg or less by IV push over 1-2 min. Do not exceed an administration rate of 4 mg/min in patients with renal impairment.

IM ALERT

- **Pain:** Monitor for temporary pain at the injection site.

PRECAUTIONS

HEALTH-RELATED

- Use furosemide cautiously in patients with hepatic cirrhosis.

AGE-RELATED

- **Children:** Neonates may require less frequent doses because the drug's half-life is increased in this age group. May increase risk of patent ductus arteriosus in preterm infants with respiratory distress syndrome. Prolonged use in premature infants may result in nephrocalcinosis.
- **Elderly:** Age-related renal impairment may require a dosage adjustment. Elderly may be more sensitive to the electrolyte and hypotensive effects and are at increased risk for circulatory collapse and thromboembolic effects (PE, stroke).

PREGNANCY/LACTATION-RELATED

- Pregnancy category C; (D if used in pregnancy-induced hypertension). Cardiovascular disorders such as pulmonary edema, severe hypertension, or heart failure are probably the only valid indications for this drug during pregnancy. Furosemide has been used after the first trimester without causing fetal or newborn adverse effects; does not appear to alter amniotic fluid volume significantly. Maternal use during pregnancy has not been associated with toxic or teratogenic effects, although metabolic complications have been observed (hyponatremia, hyperuricemia). Reduces placental and/or maternal hepatic perfusion. Excreted into breast milk; no reports of adverse effects in nursing infants.

MONITORING

- **Baseline assessment:** Monitor vital signs for fever and hypotension before giving furosemide. Assess for edema, observe mucous membranes and skin turgor to determine hydration status. Evaluate mental status and muscle strength. Obtain the baseline weight.
- **Baseline lab work:** Biochemical profile to monitor for hypokalemia, hyperglycemia, liver disease, and renal dysfunction.
- **Fluid balance:** Begin monitoring fluid intake and output. Note extent of diuresis.
- **Effects of diuresis:** Monitor for hypotension, serum electrolyte levels for hypokalemia or hyponatremia, fluid intake and output, and weight for gain or loss.
- **Hypokalemia:** May result in cardiac dysrhythmias, altered mental status, muscle cramps, asthenia, and tremor.

- **Hyponatremia:** May result in clammy and cold skin, confusion, and thirst.
- **Patient education:** Advise to expect an increase in the frequency and volume of urination. Instruct to report promptly hearing abnormalities (ringing, roaring, or sense of fullness in the ears) or signs of an electrolyte imbalance (irregular heartbeat, muscle cramps or weakness, tremor) to a health care provider. Encourage consumption of foods high in potassium, including apricots, bananas, orange juice, potatoes, raisins, legumes, meat, and whole grains (such as cereals). Warn to avoid overexposure to sunlight and artificial lights, such as sun lamps, because sulfonamides promote sunburn.

SERIOUS ADVERSE REACTIONS

- **Volume and electrolyte depletion:** Vigorous diuresis leads to hypokalemia, hyponatremia, and dehydration. Sudden volume depletion increases risk of thrombosis, circulatory collapse, and sudden death. Acute hypotensive episodes may occur, sometimes several days after beginning therapy.
- Furosemide use can exacerbate hyperglycemia, systemic lupus erythematosus, gout, and pancreatitis.
- Blood dyscrasias have been reported.

OVERDOSE/TOXICITY

- **Ototoxicity:** Deafness, vertigo, or tinnitus may occur, especially in patients with severe renal impairment.
- **Dysrhythmias:** Hypokalemia may prompt ventricular dysrhythmias.
- **Cardiovascular collapse:** Results from blood volume reduction or dehydration; may prompt vascular thrombosis and embolization.
- **GI decontamination:** No specific recommendations.

ANTIDOTE/DIALYSIS

- **Antidote:** No specific recommendations.
- **Dialysis:** Furosemide is not removed by hemodialysis and is not likely to be removed by peritoneal dialysis. No data are available on removal using high-permeability hemodialysis.

gabapentin

ga-ba-pen'-tin

Classes
Chemical: cyclohexanacetic acid derivative
Therapeutic: anticonvulsant

Pregnancy Category: C

Trade Names
Prescription: Neurontin

Do not confuse Neurontin with Neoral or Noroxin.

G

CLINICAL PHARMACOLOGY

Mechanism of Action

An anticonvulsant and antineuralgic agent whose exact mechanism is unknown. May increase the synthesis or accumulation of gamma-aminobutyric acid by binding to as-yet-undefined receptor sites in brain tissue. **Therapeutic Effect:** Reduces seizure activity and neuropathic pain.

PHARMACOKINETICS

Well absorbed from the GI tract (not affected by food). Protein binding: less than 3%. Widely distributed. Crosses the blood-brain barrier. Primarily excreted unchanged in urine. Removed by hemodialysis. **Half-life:** 5-7 hr (increased in impaired renal function and the elderly).

AVAILABILITY

Capsules (Neurontin): 100 mg, 300 mg, 400 mg.
Oral solution (Neurontin): 250 mg/5 mL.
Tablets (Neurontin): 100 mg, 300 mg, 400 mg, 600 mg, 800 mg.

INDICATIONS AND DOSAGE

Adjunctive therapy for seizure control

PO

Adults, Elderly, Children older than 12 yr: Initially, 300 mg 3 times per day. May titrate dosage. Range: 900-1800 mg/day in 3 divided doses. Maximum: 3600 mg/day.
Children 3-12 yr: Initially, 10-15 mg/kg/day in 3 divided doses. May titrate up to 25-35 mg/kg/day (for children 5-12 yr) and 40 mg/kg/day (for children 3-4 yr). Maximum: 50 mg/kg/day.

Adjunctive therapy for neuropathic pain

PO

Adults, Elderly: Initially, 100 mg 3 times per day; may increase by 300 mg/day at weekly intervals. Maximum: 3600 mg/day in 3 divided doses. **Children.** Initially, 5 mg/kg/dose at bedtime, followed by 5 mg/kg/dose for 2 doses on day 2, then 5 mg/kg/dose for 3 doses on day 3. Range: 8-35 mg/kg/day in 3 divided doses.

Postherpetic neuralgia

PO

Adults, Elderly: 300 mg on day 1300 mg twice per day on day 2, and 300 mg 3 times per day on day 3. Titrate up to 1800 mg/day.

Dosage in renal impairment

Dosage and frequency are modified based on creatinine clearance:

Creatinine Clearance	Dosage
60 mL/min or higher	900-3600 mg/day in 3 divided doses
30-59 mL/min	400-1400 mg/day in 2 divided doses
16-29 mL/min	200-700 mg/day once daily
Less than 16 mL/min	100-300 mg/day once daily
Hemodialysis	125-300 mg after each 4-hr hemodialysis session

OFF-LABEL USES

Treatment of bipolar disorder, chronic pain, diabetic peripheral neuropathy, essential tremor, hot flashes, hyperhidrosis, migraines, psychiatric disorders (social phobia)

CONTRAINDICATIONS

Hypersensitivity to gabapentin.

INTERACTIONS

Drug: Antacids (aluminum- and magnesium-containing): May decrease gabapentin's effectiveness. **Herbal:** None known. **Food:** None known.

DIAGNOSTIC TEST EFFECTS

May decrease serum WBC count.

SIDE-EFFECTS

Frequent (19%-10%): Fatigue, somnolence, dizziness, ataxia. **Occasional (8%-3%):** Nystagmus, tremor, diplopia, rhinitis, weight gain. **Rare (less than 2%):** Nervousness, dysarthria, memory loss, dyspepsia, pharyngitis, myalgia

CRITICAL CARE CONSIDERATIONS

ADMINISTRATION/HANDLING

PO ALERT

- Gabapentin may be given with food to reduce GI upset.
- When discontinuing gabapentin or adding another anticonvulsant to the treatment

regimen, initiate changes over at least 1 wk to prevent loss of seizure control.
- The interval between drug doses should not exceed 12 hr.

PRECAUTIONS

HEALTH-RELATED

- Use gabapentin cautiously in patients with renal impairment.

AGE-RELATED

- **Children:** Safety and efficacy of gabapentin have not been established in children 3 yr and younger. Children 3-12 yr are more prone to behavior problems and hyperactivity associated with use of gabapentin.
- **Elderly:** Age-related renal impairment may require dosage adjustment.

PREGNANCY/LACTATION-RELATED

- Pregnancy category C; excreted in breast milk; use with caution.

MONITORING

- **Baseline assessment:** Assess level of consciousness; review history of the seizure disorder, including the onset, duration, frequency, intensity, and type of seizures. For small children, obtain weight and assess behavior.
- **Baseline lab work:** Biochemical panel to assess BUN and creatinine. Creatinine clearance may be obtained to assist in prescribing the appropriate dose.
- **Ongoing lab work:** Routine laboratory monitoring of serum gabapentin levels is not necessary for safe use. Drug may be used with other anticonvulsants without altering levels of other medications.
- **Seizures:** Initiate seizure precautions and other safety measures needed. Monitor seizure duration and frequency.
- **Patient education:** Instruct to take gabapentin only as prescribed. Caution not to discontine gabapentin abruptly to avoid increased seizure frequency. Patients should avoid tasks requiring mental alertness or motor skills until response to the drug is known. Urge avoidance of alcohol while taking gabapentin. Advise carrying an identification card or wearing an identification bracelet indicating they have a seizure disorder and receive anticonvulsant therapy.

SERIOUS ADVERSE REACTIONS

- **Abrupt withdrawal:** May increase seizure frequency.
- **Children 3-12 yr:** Emotional lability, aggressive behavior, hostility, hyperkinesia, thought disorders, which may require discontinuing medication.

OVERDOSE/TOXICITY

- **Tumorigenic potential:** Both animal and human studies revealed development of tumors, but incidence made it impossible to be certain of the cause-effect relationship.
- **Symptoms:** Diplopia, dizziness, slurred speech, drowsiness, lethargy, edema, and diarrhea.
- **GI decontamination:** No specific recommendations.

ANTIDOTE/DIALYSIS

- **Antidote:** No specific recommendations.
- **Dialysis:** Gabapentin is removed by hemodialysis and likely to be removed by high-permeability hemodialysis. No data are available on removal using peritoneal dialysis. Patients must receive gabapentin AFTER a dialysis treatment.

galantamine hydrobromide

ga-lan'-ta-meen hye-droe-broe'-mide

Classes

Chemical: benzazepine derivative, cholinesterase inhibitor

Therapeutic: acetylcholinesterase inhibitor

Pregnancy Category: B

Trade Names

Prescription: Razadyne, Razadyne ER, Razadyne IR, Reminyl

Do not confuse Razadyne with Rozerem.

CLINICAL PHARMACOLOGY

Mechanism of Action

A cholinesterase inhibitor that inhibits the enzyme acetylcholinesterase, thus increasing the concentration of acetylcholine at cholinergic synapses and enhancing cholinergic function in the CNS. **Therapeutic Effect:** Slows the progression of Alzheimer's disease.

PHARMACOKINETICS

Rapidly absorbed from the GI tract. Protein binding: 18%. Distributed to blood cells; binds to plasma proteins, mainly albumin. Metabolized in the liver. Excreted in urine. **Half-life:** 7 hr.

G

AVAILABILITY

Capsules (extended release [Razadyne ER]): 8 mg, 16 mg, 24 mg.
Oral solution (Razadyne): 4 mg/mL.
Tablets (Razadyne): 4 mg, 8 mg, 12 mg.

INDICATIONS AND DOSAGE

Alzheimer's disease

PO

Adults, Elderly: Initially, 4 mg twice per day (8 mg/day). After a minimum of 4 wk (if well tolerated), may increase to 8 mg twice per day (16 mg/day). After another 4 wk, may increase to 12 mg twice daily (24 mg/day). Range: 16-24 mg/day in 2 divided doses. Maximum: 32 mg/day.

PO (Extended Release)

Adults, Elderly: 8-24 mg/day as a single daily dose.

Dosage in renal impairment

For moderate impairment, maximum dosage is 16 mg/day. Drug is not recommended for patients with severe impairment.

CONTRAINDICATIONS

Hypersensitivity to galantamine hydrobromide

INTERACTIONS

Drug: Amitriptyline, fluoxetine, paroxetine: May increase galantamine concentrations. **Bethanechol, succinylcholine:** May interfere with the effects of these drugs. **Cimetidine, erythromycin, ketoconazole, paroxetine:** May increase the galantamine blood concentration. **Herbal:** None known. **Food:** None known.

DIAGNOSTIC TEST EFFECTS

None known.

SIDE-EFFECTS

Frequent (24%-5%): Nausea (13%-24%), vomiting, diarrhea, anorexia, weight loss. **Occasional (9%-4%):** Abdominal pain, insomnia, depression, headache, dizziness, fatigue, rhinitis. **Rare (less than 3%):** Tremors, constipation, confusion, cough, anxiety, urinary incontinence

CRITICAL CARE CONSIDERATIONS

ADMINISTRATION/HANDLING

PO ALERT

- Give galantamine with morning and evening meals.
- If galantamine therapy is interrupted for several days or longer, reinstitute therapy.

PRECAUTIONS

HEALTH-RELATED

- Use galantamine cautiously in patients with asthma, bladder outflow obstruction, chronic obstructive pulmonary disease, peptic ulcer disease, history of seizures, moderate to severe hepatic or renal impairment, or supraventricular conduction disturbances.
- Use galantamine cautiously in patients taking NSAIDs concurrently.

AGE-RELATED

- **Children:** Galantamine is not prescribed for children.
- **Elderly:** No age-related precautions have been noted in the elderly, but galantamine is not recommended for those with severe hepatic or renal impairment (creatinine clearance of less than 9 mL/min).

PREGNANCY/LACTATION-RELATED

- Pregnancy category B; unknown if excreted in breast milk; drug has no indication in pregnant women.

MONITORING

- **Baseline assessment:** Assess behavioral, cognitive, and functional deficits.
- **Baseline lab work:** Biochemical profile including liver and renal function tests.
- **Baseline diagnostic tests:** Obtain a 12-lead ECG to use for comparison in the future.
- **Therapeutic effect:** Monitor for improvement in behavioral, cognitive, and functional status.
- **Dysrhythmias:** Periodically assess the 12-lead ECG and rhythm strips of patients with underlying dysrhythmias.
- **GI distress:** Assess for nausea, vomiting, diarrhea, anorexia, and weight loss.
- **Patient education:** Instruct to take galantamine with morning and evening meals to reduce the risk of nausea. Advise avoidance of tasks that require mental alertness or motor skills until response to the drug is known. Instruct to report promptly excessive sweating, tearing, or salivation; depression; dizziness; excessive fatigue; muscle weakness; insomnia; or persistent GI disturbances to a health care provider. Inform patients and families that galantamine is not a cure for Alzheimer's disease but may slow the progression of its symptoms. Refer patients' families to the local chapter of the Alzheimer's Disease Association for a guide to available services.

SERIOUS ADVERSE REACTIONS

- Bradycardia, hypotension, blurred vision, urinary frequency or incontinence, sweating, confusion, agitation which may indicate onset of cholinergic crisis.

OVERDOSE/TOXICITY

- **Cholinergic crisis:** Increased salivation, lacrimation, severe nausea and vomiting, bradycardia, respiratory depression, hypotension, and increased muscle weakness.
- **Management:** Treatment usually consists of supportive measures for specific symptoms and use of anticholinergic drugs (atropine).
- **GI decontamination:** No specific recommendations.

ANTIDOTE/DIALYSIS

- **Antidote:** Anticholinergic medications such as atropine may be helpful in managing cholinergic crisis.
- **Dialysis:** No data are available on removal of galantamine by hemodialysis, high-permeability hemodialysis, or peritoneal dialysis.

ganciclovir sodium

gan-sye'-kloe-veer soe'-dee-um

Classes

Chemical: acyclic purine nucleoside analog
Therapeutic: antiviral

Pregnancy Category: C

Trade Names

Prescription: Cytovene, Vitrasert (ophthalmic)

Do not confuse Cytovene with Cytosar.

CLINICAL PHARMACOLOGY

Mechanism of Action

This synthetic nucleoside competes with viral DNA polymerase and is incorporated into growing viral DNA chains. **Therapeutic Effect:** Interferes with synthesis and replication of viral DNA.

PHARMACOKINETICS

Widely distributed. Protein binding: 1%-2%. Undergoes minimal metabolism. Excreted unchanged primarily in urine. Removed by hemodialysis. **Half-life:** 2.5-3.6 hr (increased in impaired renal function).

AVAILABILITY

Capsules (Cytovene): 250 mg, 500 mg.
Powder for injection (Cytovene): 500 mg.
Implant (Vitrasert): 4.5 mg.

INDICATIONS AND DOSAGE

Cytomegalovirus (CMV) retinitis

IV

Adults, Children 3 mo and older: 10 mg/kg/day in divided doses every 12 hr for 14-21 days, then 5 mg/kg/day as a single daily dose for 7 days or 6 mg/kg 5 days per wk.

Prevention of CMV disease in transplant patients

IV

Adults, Children: 10 mg/kg/day in divided doses every 12 hr for 7-14 days, then 5 mg/kg/day as a single daily dose.

Other CMV infections

PO

Adults: Maintenance: 1000 mg 3 times per day or 500 mg every 3 hr (6 times per day). **Children younger than 3 mo:** Maintenance: 30 mg/kg/dose PO every 8 hr.

IV

Adults: Initially, 10 mg/kg/day in divided doses every 12 hr for 14-21 days, then 5 mg/kg/day as a single daily dose. **Children younger than 3 mo:** Initially, 10 mg/kg/day in divided doses every 12 hr for 14-21 days, then 5 mg/kg/day as a single daily dose.

Intravitreal implant

Adults: 1 implant every 6-9 months with or without oral ganciclovir. 1-1.5 g PO 3 times daily. **Children 9 yr and older:** 1 implant every 6-9 months plus oral ganciclovir (30 mg/dose every 8 hr).

Adult dosage in renal impairment

Dosage and frequency are modified based on creatinine clearance.

CrCl	Induction Dosage	Maintenance Dosage	Oral
50-69 mL/min	2.5 mg/kg every 12 hr	2.5 mg/kg every 24 hr	1500 mg/day
25-49 mL/min	2.5 mg/kg every 24 hr	1.25 mg/kg every 24 hr	1000 mg/day
10-24 mL/min	1.25 mg/kg every 24 hr	0.625 mg/kg every 24 hr	500 mg/day
Less than 10 mL/min	1.25 mg/kg 3 times/wk	0.625 mg/kg 3 times/wk	500 mg 3 times/wk

OFF-LABEL USES

Treatment of other CMV infections, such as gastroenteritis, hepatitis, and pneumonitis

CONTRAINDICATIONS

Absolute neutrophil count less than 500/mm^3, platelet count less than 25,000/mm^3, hypersensitivity to acyclovir or ganciclovir, immunocompromised patients, patients with congenital or neonatal CMV disease

INTERACTIONS

Drug: Bone marrow depressants: May increase bone marrow depression. **Imipenem and cilastatin:** May increase the risk of seizures. **Zidovudine (AZT):** May increase the risk of hepatotoxicity. **Herbal:** None known. **Food:** None known.

G

DIAGNOSTIC TEST EFFECTS

May increase serum alkaline phosphatase, bilirubin, AST (SGOT), and ALT (SGPT) levels.

IV INCOMPATIBILITIES

Aldesleukin (Proleukin), amifostine (Ethyol), aztreonam (Azactam), cefepime (Maxipime), cytarabine (ARA-C), *DOXOrubicin (Adriamycin), fludarabine (Fludara), foscarnet (Foscavir), gemcitabine (Gemzar), ondansetron (Zofran), piperacillin and tazobactam (Zosyn), sargramostim (Leukine), total parenteral nutrition (TPN), vinorelbine (Navelbine)

IV COMPATIBILITIES

Amphotericin B, enalapril (Vasotec), filgrastim (Neupogen), fluconazole (Diflucan), propofol (Diprivan)

SIDE-EFFECTS

Frequent: Diarrhea (41%), fever (40%), leukopenia (30%-40%), nausea (25%), anemia (20%-25%), abdominal pain (17%), vomiting (13%). **Rare (4%-2%):** Diaphoresis, infection, paresthesia, flatulence, pruritus, headache, stomatitis, dyspepsia, phlebitis

CRITICAL CARE CONSIDERATIONS

ADMINISTRATION/HANDLING

PO ALERT

- Give ganciclovir with food.

IV ALERT

- **Storage:** Store vials at room temperature. Do not refrigerate.
- **Stability:** Reconstituted solution in the vial remains stable for 12 hr at room temperature. After dilution, refrigerate the solution and use within 24 hr. Discard the solution if precipitate forms or discoloration occurs.
- **Safety precautions:** Avoid inhaling the solution. Also avoid exposing the solution to the eyes, mucous membranes, or skin. Use latex gloves and safety glasses during preparation and handling of ganciclovir solution. If the solution comes in contact with mucous membranes or the skin, wash the affected area thoroughly with soap and water; if it comes in contact with the eyes, rinse the eyes thoroughly with plain water. Follow disposal guidelines for cytotoxic agents.
- **Reconstitution:** Reconstitute the 500-mg vial with 10 mL of sterile water for injection to provide a concentration of 50 mg/mL; do not use bacteriostatic water because it contains parabens, which is incompatible with ganciclovir.
- **Further dilution:** Further dilute with 100 mL of D_5W, 0.9% NaCl, lactated Ringer's, or any combination of these to provide a concentration of 5 mg/mL.
- **Controlled rate IV infusion only:** Do not give ganciclovir by IV push or rapid IV infusion because these routes increase the risk of ganciclovir toxicity. Administer only by IV infusion over 1 hr.
- **Infiltration:** Protect patients from infiltration because the high pH of this drug causes severe tissue irritation.
- **Phlebitis:** Use large veins to permit rapid dilution and dissemination of ganciclovir and to minimize the risk of phlebitis. Central venous ports tunneled under subcutaneous tissue may reduce catheter-associated infection.

PRECAUTIONS

HEALTH-RELATED

- Use ganciclovir cautiously in patients with impaired renal function, neutropenia, or thrombocytopenia.
- Ganciclovir should not be administered if the absolute neutrophil count is less than 500 cells/mm^3 or if the platelet count is less than 25,000 cells/mm^3.
- Ganciclovir is indicated for use ONLY in the treatment of cytomegalovirus (CMV) retinitis in immunocompromised patients and for prevention of CMV disease in transplant patients and those with advanced HIV infection at risk for CMV disease.

AGE-RELATED

- **Children:** Use ganciclovir cautiously in pediatric patients. The long-term safety of ganciclovir has not been determined because of the potential for causing

adverse reproductive and carcinogenic effects.
- **Elderly:** Age-related renal impairment may require a dosage adjustment.

PREGNANCY/LACTATION-RELATED
- Pregnancy category C; excretion into breast milk unknown; not recommended in nursing mothers because of potential for serious adverse reactions in the nursing infant; do not resume nursing for at least 72 hr after last dose of ganciclovir.

MONITORING
- **Baseline assessment:** Evaluate history of eye pain and vision problems.
- **Baseline lab work:** Evaluate CBC with WBC differential. Obtain specimens (blood, feces, throat culture, urine) for culture and sensitivity testing before giving ganciclovir. Test results support the differential diagnosis and rule out retinal infection as the result of hematogenous dissemination.
- **Hydration:** Monitor intake and output; provide adequate hydration (at least 1500 mL/24 hr).
- **Bone marrow suppression:** Evaluate hematology reports for a decreased platelet count, anemia, neutropenia, and thrombocytopenia, and patients for infection and fatigue.
- **Skin damage:** Assess infiltration, phlebitis, pruritus, and a rash.
- **Intravitreal implant:** Evaluate for altered vision in patients with an intravitreal implant.
- **Patient education:** Explain that frequent blood tests and eye exams are necessary during therapy to evaluate for toxicity. Stress the need to report promptly any new symptom to a health care provider. Inform that ganciclovir suppresses but does not cure CMV retinitis. Inform male patients that ganciclovir may temporarily or permanently inhibit sperm production. Urge use of barrier contraception during ganciclovir therapy and for 90 days afterward because of the drug's mutagenic potential. Tell female patients that ganciclovir use may suppress fertility. Advise use of effective contraception during therapy.

SERIOUS ADVERSE REACTIONS
- **Intraocular insertion:** Occasionally results in visual acuity loss, vitreous hemorrhage, and retinal detachment.
- **GI hemorrhage:** Occurs rarely.

OVERDOSE/TOXICITY
- **Hematologic toxicity:** Commonly occurs; leukopenia (granulocytopenia) in 30%-40% of patients and anemia in 20%-25%.
- **Overdose:** Anorexia, anemia, leukopenia, thrombocytopenia, bloody diarrhea, increased BUN and creatinine, elevated liver enzymes, testicular atrophy (long-term use), vomiting, possible death.
- **Management:** Treat symptoms per accepted management guidelines. Filgrastim (Neupogen) may be used to help maintain neutrophil count. Discontinue drug when neutrophils fall below 500 cells/mm^3 or platelets are below 25,000 cells/mm^3.
- **GI decontamination:** No specific recommendations.

ANTIDOTE/DIALYSIS
- **Antidote:** No specific recommendations.
- **Dialysis:** Ganciclovir is removed by hemodialysis and is likely removed by high-permeability hemodialysis. No data are available on removal using peritoneal dialysis.

gatifloxacin

ga-ti-flocks'-a-sin

Classes
Chemical: fluoroquinolone derivative
Therapeutic: antibiotic

Pregnancy Category: C

Trade Names
Prescription: Tequin, Tequin Teq-Paqs, Zymar

Do not confuse gatifloxacin with gemifloxacin.

CLINICAL PHARMACOLOGY
Mechanism of Action
A fluoroquinolone that inhibits two enzymes, topoisomerase II and IV, in susceptible microorganisms. **Therapeutic Effect:** Interferes with bacterial DNA replication. Prevents or delays resistance emergence. Bactericidal.

PHARMACOKINETICS
Well absorbed from the GI tract after PO administration. Protein binding: 20%. Widely distributed. Metabolized in liver. Primarily excreted in urine. **Half-life:** 7-14 hr.

AVAILABILITY

Tablets (Tequin, Tequin Teqpaq): 200 mg, 400 mg.
Injection (Tequin): 200-mg, 400-mg vials.
Ophthalmic solution (Zymar): 0.3%.

INDICATIONS AND DOSAGE

Chronic bronchitis, complicated urinary tract infections, pyelonephritis, skin infections

PO, IV

Adults, Elderly: 400 mg/day for 7-10 days (5 days for chronic bronchitis).

Sinusitis

PO, IV

Adults, Elderly: 400 mg/day for 10 days.

Pneumonia

PO, IV

Adults, Elderly: 400 mg/day for 7-14 days.

Cystitis

PO, IV

Adults, Elderly: 400 mg as a single dose or 200 mg/day for 3 days.

Urethral gonorrhea in men and women, endocervical and rectal gonorrhea in women

PO, IV

Adults, Elderly: 400 mg as a single dose.

Topical treatment of bacterial conjunctivitis due to susceptible strains of bacteria

Ophthalmic

Adults, Elderly, Children 1 yr and older: 1 drop every 2 hr while awake for 2 days, then 1 drop up to 4 times/day for days 3-7.

Dosage in renal impairment

Creatinine Clearance	Dosage
40 mL/min	400 mg/day
Less than 40 mL/min	Initially 400 mg/day then 200 mg/day
Hemodialysis	Initially 400 mg/day then 200 mg/day following hemodialysis
Peritoneal dialysis	Initially 400 mg/day then 200 mg/day

CONTRAINDICATIONS

Diabetic patients, hypersensitivity to gatifloxacin or other quinolones

INTERACTIONS

Drug: Aluminum and magnesium containing antacids, bismuth subsalicylate, digoxin, iron preparations: May decrease gatifloxacin plasma concentration and half-life. **Antipsychotics, class 1A and class III antidysrhythmics, erythromycin, tricyclic antidepressants:** May increase the risk of prolonged QTc interval and life-threatening dysrhythmias. **NSAIDs:** May increase the risk of CNS stimulation and seizures. **Probenecid:** May increase gatifloxacin plasma concentration and half-life.
Herbal: None known. **Food:** None known.

DIAGNOSTIC TEST EFFECTS

None known.

IV INCOMPATIBILITIES

Amphotericin (Fungizone), potassium phosphate

IV COMPATIBILITIES

Aminophylline, calcium gluconate, hydromorphone (Dilaudid), lidocaine, lorazepam (Ativan), magnesium sulfate, *methylPREDNISolone (Solu-Medrol), metoclopramide (Reglan), midazolam (Versed), morphine, nitroglycerin, potassium chloride, sodium phosphate

SIDE-EFFECTS

Occasional (8%-3%): Nausea, vaginitis, diarrhea, headache, dizziness. **Ophthalmic:** conjunctival irritation, increased tearing, corneal inflammation. **Rare (3%-0.1%):** Abdominal pain, constipation, dyspepsia, stomatitis, edema, insomnia, abnormal dreams, diaphoresis, altered taste, rash. **Ophthalmic:** corneal swelling, dry eye, eye pain, eyelid swelling, headache, red eye, reduced visual acuity, altered taste

CRITICAL CARE CONSIDERATIONS

ADMINISTRATION/HANDLING

PO ALERT

- Give gatifloxacin without regard to meals.
- Administer oral gatifloxacin 4 hr before giving antacids, buffered tablets or solutions, ferrous sulfate, or multivitamins.

OPHTHALMIC ALERT

- **Administration:** Tilt the head backward and look up. Gently pull the lower eyelid down until a pocket is formed. Hold dropper above the pocket, and without touching the eyelid or conjunctival sac, place drops into the center of the pocket. Close the eye; apply gentle digital pressure to the lacrimal sac at the inner canthus. Remove excess solution around the eye with a tissue.

IV ALERT

- **Prediluted:** Drug is available prediluted and ready for use.

- **Dilution:** Dilute 20-mL vial in 100 mL and 40 mL in 200 mL D_5W, 0.9% NaCl.
- **IV intermittent (piggyback) infusion:** Infuse over 60 min.
- **Controlled rate infusion only:** Do not give by rapid or bolus IV.

PRECAUTIONS

HEALTH-RELATED

- Use gatifloxacin cautiously in patients with cerebral atherosclerosis, diabetes mellitus, CNS disorders, liver or renal impairment, seizures, and those with a prolonged QT interval.
- **Prolonged QT interval:** Use cautiously in patients taking medications known to prolong the QT interval (e.g., erythromycin, tricyclic antidepressants, amiodarone, quinidine, procainamide, and sotalol), and in patients with uncorrected hypokalemia.
- **NSAIDs:** Concomitant administration with gatifloxacin may increase risks of CNS stimulation and seizures.

AGE-RELATED

- **Children:** Safety and efficacy of gatifloxacin have not been established in children. Juvenile animal studies revealed quinolones caused arthropathy and osteochondrotoxicity.
- **Elderly:** Age-related renal impairment may require dosage adjustment.

PREGNANCY/LACTATION-RELATED

- Pregnancy category C; breast milk excretion unknown.

MONITORING

- **Baseline assessment:** Determine history of hypersensitivity to gatifloxacin and quinolones before beginning drug therapy. Consider baseline 12-lead ECG to evaluate QT interval.
- **Baseline lab work:** Basic chemical profile including K+, BUN, and creatinine levels to evaluate renal function. Obtain culture of infected area prior to drug administration (wound, blood, sputum, urine). Obtain prothrombin time on patients receiving warfarin.
- **QT interval prolongation:** Observe continuous ECG readings for QT interval prolongation.
- **Superinfections:** Assess the mouth for white patches on the mucous membranes or tongue and for severe mouth or tongue soreness; assess for severe anal or genital pruritus or discharge.
- **Possible *Clostridium difficile* colitis:** Assess pattern of daily bowel activity and stool consistency. Although mild GI effects may be tolerable, severe symptoms including abdominal pain or cramping, and moderate to severe diarrhea may indicate the onset of antibiotic-associated colitis.
- **Hand washing:** If *C. difficile* (antibiotic-associated) colitis develops, wash hands with antibacterial soap. Alcohol-based foam is ineffective against *C. difficile* spores.
- **Nephrotoxicity:** Monitor intake and output and renal function test results to assess for nephrotoxicity.
- **Therapeutic response:** Observe patients receiving the ophthalmic form for a resolution of eye redness, drainage, and pain.
- **Blood glucose changes:** Assess for hyperglycemia and hypoglycemia, especially in patients with diabetes mellitus.
- **Side effects:** Evaluate for dizziness, headache, tremors, and visual problems. Assess for chest and joint pain.
- **Patient education:** When using gatifloxacin outside the hospital, advise not to skip drug doses and to take gatifloxacin for the full course of therapy. Gatifloxacin should be taken during meals with 8 oz of water. Patients should drink several glasses of water between meals. Warn not to take antacids within 4 hr of taking the medication, because antacids will reduce or destroy gatifloxacin's effectiveness. Urge avoidance of exposure to direct sunlight during therapy and for several days after treatment. Instruct on symptoms of hyperglycemia and hypoglycemia. Warn not to perform tasks that require mental alertness or motor skills until response to the drug is known.

SERIOUS ADVERSE REACTIONS

- **Pseudomembranous colitis/*C. difficile*–associated diarrhea (CDAD):** Severe abdominal pain and cramps, severe watery diarrhea, and fever may occur. Oral vancomycin (Vancocin) or metronidazole (Flagyl) are the most effective treatments for CDAD.
- **Superinfection:** Genital or anal pruritus, ulceration or changes in oral mucosa, and moderate to severe diarrhea may occur.
- **Hyperglycemia:** Marked elevation of blood glucose has been noted in both diabetic and nondiabetic patients.

- **Sensitization to ophthalmic form:** Ophthalmic form of gatifloxacin may contraindicate later systemic use of the drug.
- **Hypersensitivity:** Patients with a history of allergies, especially to penicillin, are at increased risk for developing a severe hypersensitivity reaction, marked by severe pruritus, angioedema, bronchospasm, and anaphylaxis.
- **Management of hypersensitivity:** May require treatment with epinephrine and other emergency measures including oxygen, endotracheal intubation, mechanical ventilation, IV fluids, IV antihistamines, corticosteroids, and vasopressors.

G

OVERDOSE/TOXICITY

- **Neurologic:** Seizures, increased intracranial pressure, confusion, depression, hallucinations, tremors, toxic psychosis, vomiting.
- **Ophthalmic:** Cataracts and other eye abnormalities.
- **Cardiac:** Prolonged QT syndrome, ventricular dysrhythmias, and torsades de pointes; more common when patients are receiving other antidysrhythmic drugs that prolong the QT interval (procainamide, quinidine, amiodarone, sotalol).
- **Blood glucose changes:** Hyperglycemia including hyperosmolar nonketotic syndrome and severe hypoglycemia.
- **Nephrotoxicity:** May occur, especially in patients with preexisting renal disease.
- **Superinfections:** Antibiotic-associated colitis (pseudomembranous colitis) and other superinfections may result from altered bacterial balance.
- **GI decontamination:** No specific recommendations.

ANTIDOTE/DIALYSIS

- **Antidote:** No specific recommendations.
- **Dialysis:** No data are available regarding removal of gatifloxacin using hemodialysis, peritoneal dialysis, or high-permeability hemodialysis. Pharmacokinetics indicate the drug is unlikely to be removed.

gemfibrozil

See Antihyperlipidemics (p. 928)

gemifloxacin mesylate

See Antibiotics (p. 892)

gentamicin sulfate

jen-ta-mye'-sin sul'-fate

Classes

Chemical: aminoglycoside
Therapeutic: antibiotic

Pregnancy Category: C

Trade Names

Prescription: Garamycin, Garamycin Ophthalmic, Garamycin Topical, Genoptic, Gentacidin, Gentak, Gentacidin, Ocu-Mycin

Combinations

Prescription: with *prednisoLONE (Pred-G)

CLINICAL PHARMACOLOGY

Mechanism of Action

An aminoglycoside antibiotic that irreversibly binds to the protein of bacterial ribosomes. **Therapeutic Effect:** Interferes with protein synthesis of susceptible microorganisms. Bactericidal.

PHARMACOKINETICS

Rapid, complete absorption after IM administration. Protein binding: less than 30%. Widely distributed (does not cross the blood-brain barrier, low concentrations in cerebrospinal fluid). Excreted unchanged in urine. Removed by hemodialysis. **Half-life:** 2-4 hr (increased in impaired renal function and neonates; decreased in cystic fibrosis and burn or febrile patients).

AVAILABILITY

Injection: 10 mg/mL, 40 mg/mL (Garamycin), 40 mg/50 mL—0.9%, 60 mg/50 mL—0.9%, 60 mg/100 mL—0.9%, 70 mg/50 mL—0.9%, 80 mg/50 mL—0.9%, 80 mg/100 mL—0.9%, 90 mg/100 mL—0.9%, 100 mg/50 mL—0.9%, 100 mg/100 mL—0.9%.
Ophthalmic solution (Garamycin Ophthalmic, Gentacidin, Genoptic, Gentak, Ocu-Mycin): 0.3%.
Ophthalmic ointment (Gentak): 0.3%.
Cream (Garamycin Topical): 0.1%.
Ointment: 0.1%.

INDICATIONS AND DOSAGE

Acute pelvic, bone, intraabdominal, joint, respiratory tract, burn wound, postoperative, and skin or skin-structure infections; complicated urinary tract infections; septicemia; meningitis

IV, IM

Adults, Elderly: Usual dosage, 3-6 mg/kg/day in divided doses every 8 hr or 4-6.6

mg/kg once per day. **Children 5-12 yr:** Usual dosage 2-2.5 mg/kg/dose every 8 hr. **Children younger than 5 yr:** Usual dosage, 2.5 mg/kg/dose every 8 hr. **Neonates:** Usual dosage 2.5 mg/kg/dose every 8-12 hr. Frequency is dependent on age: less than 28 wk, every 24-36 hr; 28-32 wk, every 18 hr; 33-42 wk, every 12 hr.

Hemodialysis

IV, IM

Adults, Elderly: 1 mg/kg/dose after dialysis. **Children:** 2 mg/kg/dose after dialysis.

Intrathecal

Adults: 4-8 mg/day. **Children 3 mo-12 yr:** 1 mg/day. **Neonates:** 1 mg/day.

Superficial eye infections

Ophthalmic Ointment

Adults, Elderly: Apply half-inch thin strip to conjunctiva 2-3 times per day.

Ophthalmic Solution

Adults, Elderly, Children: Usual dosage, 1-2 drops every 2-4 hr up to 2 drops/hr.

Superficial skin infections

Topical

Adults, Elderly: Usual dosage, apply 3-4 times/day.

Dosage in renal impairment

Creatinine clearance greater than 41-60 mL/min. Dosage interval every 12 hr.

Creatinine clearance 20-40 mL/min. Dosage interval every 24 hr.

Creatinine clearance less than 20 mL/min. Monitor levels to determine dosage interval.

OFF-LABEL USES

Topical: Prophylaxis of minor bacterial skin infections, treatment of dermal ulcer

CONTRAINDICATIONS

Hypersensitivity to gentamicin or other aminoglycosides (cross-sensitivity), or their components. Sulfite sensitivity may result in anaphylaxis, especially in asthmatic patients.

INTERACTIONS

Drug: Nephrotoxic medications, other aminoglycosides, ototoxic medications: May increase the risk of nephrotoxicity or ototoxicity. **Neuromuscular blockers:** May increase neuromuscular blockade. **Herbal:** None known. **Food:** None known.

DIAGNOSTIC TEST EFFECTS

May increase serum creatinine, serum bilirubin, BUN, serum LDH, AST (SGOT), and ALT (SGPT) levels. May decrease serum calcium, magnesium, potassium, and sodium concentrations. Therapeutic peak serum level is 6-10 mcg/mL and trough is 0.5-2 mcg/mL. Toxic peak serum level is greater than 10 mcg/mL, and trough is greater than 2 mcg/mL.

IV INCOMPATIBILITIES

Allopurinol (Aloprim), amphotericin B complex (Abelcet, AmBisome, Amphotec), furosemide (Lasix), heparin, hetastarch (Hespan), idarubicin (Idamycin), indomethacin (Indocin), propofol (Diprivan)

IV COMPATIBILITIES

Amiodarone (Cordarone), diltiazem (Cardizem), enalapril (Vasotec), filgrastim (Neupogen), hydromorphone (Dilaudid), insulin, lorazepam (Ativan), magnesium sulfate, midazolam (Versed), morphine, multivitamins, total parenteral nutrition (TPN)

SIDE-EFFECTS

Occasional: IM: Pain, induration. **IV:** Phlebitis, thrombophlebitis, hypersensitivity reactions (fever, pruritus, rash, urticaria). **Ophthalmic:** Burning, tearing, itching, blurred vision. **Topical:** Redness, itching. **Rare:** Alopecia, hypertension, weakness

CRITICAL CARE CONSIDERATIONS

ADMINISTRATION/HANDLING

IV ALERT

- **Storage:** Store vials at room temperature. Solution normally appears clear or slightly yellow.
- **Stability:** Intermittent IV infusion or IV piggyback solution is stable for 24 hr at room temperature. Discard the IV solution if a precipitate forms.
- **Dilution:** Dilute with 50 to 200 mL of D_5W or 0.9% NaCl. The amount of diluent for infants and children depends on individual needs. Gentamicin dosage is based on ideal body weight.
- **IV intermittent (piggyback) infusion:** Infuse over 30 to 60 min for adults and older children. Infuse over 60 to 120 min for infants and young children. Space parenteral doses evenly around the clock.

IM ALERT

- **Administration:** To minimize pain, administer the IM injection slowly and deep in the gluteus maximus rather than the lateral aspect of the thigh.

G

INTRATHECAL ALERT

- **Preparation:** Use only 2 mg/mL of the intrathecal preparation without preservative. Mix with 10% of the estimated CSF volume or NaCl. Use the intrathecal form immediately after preparation. Discard any unused portion.
- **Administration:** Give over 3 to 5 min.

OPHTHALMIC ALERT

- **Administration:** Place a gloved finger on the lower eyelid and pull it out until a pocket is formed between the eye and lower lid. Hold the dropper above the pocket and place the correct number of drops (or one quarter to one half inch of ointment) into the pocket. Close the eye gently. If administering ophthalmic solution, apply digital pressure to the lacrimal sac for 1-2 min to minimize drainage into the nose and throat, thereby reducing the risk of systemic effects. If applying ophthalmic ointment, close the eye for 1-2 min, and roll the eyeball to increase the drug's contact with the eye. Use tissue to remove excess solution or ointment around the eye.

PRECAUTIONS

HEALTH-RELATED

- **Neuromuscular disorders:** Use gentamicin cautiously in patients with neuromuscular disorders because of the potential for respiratory depression.
- Use gentamicin cautiously in patients with prior hearing loss, renal impairment, or vertigo.
- Cumulative gentamicin effects may occur with concurrent systemic administration and topical application to large areas.

AGE-RELATED

- **Children:** Use cautiously in neonates because their immature renal function increases gentamicin half-life and risk of toxicity.
- **Elderly:** Age-related renal impairment may require dosage adjustment.

PREGNANCY/LACTATION-RELATED

- Pregnancy category C; ototoxicity has not been reported as an effect of in utero exposure; eighth cranial nerve toxicity in the fetus is well known following exposure to other aminoglycosides and could potentially occur with gentamicin. Potentiation of magnesium sulfate-induced neuromuscular weakness in neonates has been reported; use caution during the last 32 hr of pregnancy; data on excretion into breast milk are lacking.

MONITORING

- **Baseline assessment:** Before giving gentamicin, determine history of allergies, especially to aminoglycosides, sulfites, and parabens (for topical and ophthalmic forms). Establish baseline hearing acuity before starting therapy and assess for dehydration.
- **Baseline lab work:** Biochemical panel including renal and liver function studies. Obtain appropriate cultures before drug administration. Urinalysis: monitor results for casts, RBCs, WBCs, and decreased specific gravity.
- **Fluid balance:** Monitor intake and output and urinalysis results as appropriate. Urge drinking fluids to maintain adequate hydration.
- **Ototoxicity and neurotoxicity:** Assess for hearing loss, headaches, lethargy, tremors, and visual disturbances.
- **Neuromuscular disorders:** If a disorder is present, assess for respiratory depression throughout treatment. Assess for decreased pulse oximetry readings, and decreased respiratory rate and depth.
- **IM sites:** Assess for pain and induration at the IM injection site.
- **IV infusion sites:** Evaluate for phlebitis (heat, pain, and red streaking over the vein).
- **Rash:** Inspect the skin for a rash, which may indicate hypersensitivity.
- **Peak and trough serum drug levels:** Monitor levels periodically to maintain the desired serum concentrations and to minimize the risk of toxicity.
- **Peak serum levels:** Therapeutic level is 6-10 mcg/mL; toxic level is greater than 10 mcg/mL.
- **Trough serum levels:** Therapeutic level is 0.5-2 mcg/mL; toxic level is greater than 2 mcg/mL.
- **Ophthalmic form:** Monitor the eyes for burning, itching, redness, and tearing.
- **Topical form:** Monitor for itching and reddened skin.
- **Superinfections:** Assess the mouth for white patches on the mucous membranes or tongue and for severe mouth or tongue soreness; assess for severe anal or genital pruritus or discharge (even with topical gentamicin).
- **Possible *Clostridium difficile* colitis:** Assess pattern of daily bowel activity and stool consistency. Although mild GI

effects may be tolerable, severe symptoms including abdominal pain, cramping, or moderate to severe diarrhea may indicate the onset of antibiotic-associated colitis.

- **Hand washing:** If *C. difficile* (antibiotic-associated) colitis develops, wash hands with antibacterial soap. Alcohol-based foam is ineffective against *C. difficile* spores.
- **Patient education:** Instruct to report promptly if any balance, hearing, urinary, or vision problems occur to a health care provider, even after gentamicin therapy is completed. Inform that IM injection may cause discomfort. Ophthalmic gentamicin may cause brief blurred vision, irritation, redness, or tearing after each dose; instruct to report if these symptoms persist. Instruct when using topical gentamicin to clean the affected area gently before applying the ointment and to report if itching or redness occurs to a health care provider.

SERIOUS ADVERSE REACTIONS

- **Superinfections:** Particularly fungal infections may result from bacterial imbalance regardless of which administration route is used.
- **Ophthalmic:** Application may cause paresthesia of conjunctiva or mydriasis.
- **Respiratory depression:** Decreased respiratory rate and depth.

OVERDOSE/TOXICITY

- **Nephrotoxicity:** Increased BUN and serum creatinine levels; decreased creatinine clearance; may be reversible if the drug is stopped at the first sign of symptoms.
- **Irreversible ototoxicity:** Tinnitus, dizziness, ringing or roaring in the ears, and diminished hearing.
- **Neurotoxicity:** Headache, dizziness, lethargy, tremor, and visual disturbances occur occasionally; risk increases with higher dosages or prolonged therapy and when the solution is applied directly to the mucosa.
- **GI decontamination:** No specific recommendations.

ANTIDOTE/DIALYSIS

- **Antidote:** No specific recommendations.
- **Dialysis:** Gentamicin is removed by hemodialysis, high-permeability hemodialysis, and peritoneal dialysis.

glatiramer

See Immunologics (p. 968)

*gliMEPIRide

glye-meh'-peer-ide

Classes

Chemical: sulfonylurea (second generation)
Therapeutic: antidiabetic, hypoglycemic

Pregnancy Category: C

Trade Names

Prescription: Amaryl

Combinations

Prescription: with rosiglitazone (Avandaryl)

Do not confuse *gliMEPIRide with *glipiZIDE or *glyBURIDE.

CLINICAL PHARMACOLOGY

Mechanism of Action

A second-generation sulfonylurea that promotes release of insulin from beta cells of the pancreas and increases insulin sensitivity at peripheral sites. **Therapeutic Effect:** Lowers blood glucose concentration.

PHARMACOKINETICS

Route	Onset	Peak	Duration
PO	2-3 hr	Unknown	24 hr

Completely absorbed from the GI tract. Protein binding: greater than 99%. Metabolized in the liver. Excreted in urine and eliminated in feces. **Half-life:** 5-9.2 hr.

AVAILABILITY

Tablets: 1 mg, 2 mg, 4 mg.

INDICATIONS AND DOSAGE

Diabetes mellitus

PO

Adults, Elderly: Initially 1-2 mg once per day, with breakfast or first main meal. Maintenance: 1-4 mg once per day. After dose of 2 mg is reached, dosage should be increased in increments of up to 2 mg every 1-2 wk, based on blood glucose response. Maximum: 8 mg/day.

Dosage in renal impairment (creatinine clearance less than 22 mL/min)

PO

Adults: 1 mg once per day.

CONTRAINDICATIONS

Diabetic complications, such as ketosis, acidosis, and diabetic coma; monotherapy for type 1 diabetes mellitus; severe hepatic or renal impairment; stress situations, including severe infection, trauma, and surgery; hypersensitivity to *gliMEPIRide; diabetic complications should be managed with insulin

G

INTERACTIONS

Drug: **Beta-blockers:** May increase the hypoglycemic effect of *gliMEPIRide and mask signs of hypoglycemia. **Cimetidine, ciprofloxacin, fluconazole, MAOIs, quinidine, ranitidine, large doses of salicylates:** May increase the effects of *gliMEPIRide. **Corticosteroids, lithium, thiazide diuretics:** May decrease the effects of *gliMEPIRide. **Oral anticoagulants:** May increase the effects of oral anticoagulants. **Herbal:** None known. **Food:** None known.

DIAGNOSTIC TEST EFFECTS

May increase BUN and LDH concentrations and serum alkaline phosphatase, creatinine, and AST (SGOT) levels.

SIDE-EFFECTS

Frequent: Altered taste sensation, dizziness, somnolence, weight gain, constipation, diarrhea, heartburn, nausea, vomiting, stomach fullness, headache. **Occasional:** Increased sensitivity of skin to sunlight, peeling of skin, itching, rash

CRITICAL CARE CONSIDERATIONS

ADMINISTRATION/HANDLING

PO ALERT

- Give *gliMEPIRide with breakfast or first main meal.
- **Transitioning to/from other oral hypoglycemic drugs:** No transition period is needed when transferring to/from any sulfonylurea agents.

PRECAUTIONS

HEALTH-RELATED

- Use *gliMEPIRide cautiously in patients with adrenal insufficiency, debilitation, hepatic disease, impaired renal function, intestinal obstruction, malnutrition, pituitary insufficiency, prolonged vomiting, severe diarrhea, or uncontrolled hyperthyroidism.
- **Increased risk of cardiovascular mortality:** Administration of oral hypoglycemic drugs has been reported to be associated with increased cardiovascular mortality compared with those treated with diet alone or diet and insulin.
- **Persistent hyperglycemia:** Consider adding metformin (Glucophage) to treatment regime if patient remains hyperglycemic at maximum doses of *gliMEPIRide. When hospitalized, oral agents may need to be discontinued and insulin used to control blood glucose.

AGE-RELATED

- **Children:** Safety and efficacy of *gliMEPIRide have not been established in children.
- **Elderly:** Hypoglycemia may be more difficult to recognize in the elderly; age-related renal impairment may increase sensitivity to glucose-lowering effect.

PREGNANCY/LACTATION-RELATED

- Pregnancy category C; inappropriate for use during pregnancy because of inadequacy of blood glucose control, potential for prolonged neonatal hypoglycemia, and risk of congenital abnormalities. Insulin is the drug of choice for control of blood sugars during pregnancy. Breast milk secretion is unknown; the potential for neonatal hypoglycemia dictates caution in nursing mothers.

MONITORING

- **Baseline assessment:** Assess risk factors for cardiovascular disease. Obtain weight and waist circumference.
- **Baseline lab work:** Check biochemical panel including blood glucose, BUN, creatinine, liver enzymes, cholesterol, and triglycerides. Obtain hemoglobin $A1_C$ to assess blood glucose control over the prior 6-8 wk.
- **Ongoing monitoring:** Monitor blood glucose level and food intake.
- **Hypoglycemia:** Assess for anxiety, confusion, diaphoresis, diplopia, dizziness, headache, hunger, tachycardia, and tremors.
- **Hyperglycemia:** Monitor for deep rapid breathing, dim vision, fatigue, nausea, polydipsia, polyphagia, polyuria, vomiting. Consider initiating an insulin infusion if blood glucose is consistently above 140 mg/dL. If insulin infusion is needed, *gliMEPIRide and all oral hypoglycemic agents should be discontinued.
- **Stress effects:** Monitor blood glucose more frequently if stress level increases because of deteriorating health status, fever, or a surgical or other invasive procedure.
- **Patient education:** Discuss lifestyle to determine extent of emotional and learning needs related to diabetes mellitus. Stress that a consistent carbohydrate diet

and regular exercise are principal parts of treatment. Overweight patients should be placed on a diet to facilitate weight loss. Warn not to skip or delay meals. Teach signs and symptoms of hypoglycemia and hyperglycemia. Instruct to carry glucose tablets, candy, or other sugar supplements for immediate response to hypoglycemia. Urge wearing medical alert identification indicating diabetes. Stress to consult a health care provider when glucose demands are altered (fever, heavy physical activity, infection, stress, or trauma). Encourage enrollment in outpatient diabetes education classes to enhance understanding of diabetes management. Have patients wear sunscreen and protective eyewear to abate light sensitivity.

SERIOUS ADVERSE REACTIONS

- GI hemorrhage, cholestatic hepatic jaundice, leukopenia, thrombocytopenia, pancytopenia, agranulocytosis, and aplastic or hemolytic anemia occur rarely.

OVERDOSE/TOXICITY

- **Overdose or insufficient food intake:** May produce hypoglycemia, especially with increased glucose demands during a stressful state.
- **GI decontamination:** No specific recommendations.

ANTIDOTE/DIALYSIS

- **Antidote:** Glucose tablets, honey, sugar, juice, 50% dextrose IV, glucagon IM to raise blood glucose level if hypoglycemic.
- **Dialysis:** *GliMEPIRide is unlikely to be removed by hemodialysis or peritoneal dialysis. No data are available on removal using high-permeability hemodialysis.

*glipiZIDE

See Antidiabetics (p. 911)

*glipiZIDE/metformin

See Antidiabetics (p. 911)

glucagon hydrochloride

gloo'-ka-gon hye-droe-klor'-ide

Classes

Chemical: polypeptide hormone
Therapeutic: antihypoglycemic

Pregnancy Category: B

Trade Names

Prescription: Glucagon

Trade Names

Prescription: GlucaGen, GlucaGen Diagnostic Kit, Glucagon, Glucagon Diagnostic Kit, Glucagon Emergency Kit

Do not confuse glucagon with Glaucon.

CLINICAL PHARMACOLOGY

Mechanism of Action

A glucose-elevating agent that promotes hepatic glycogenolysis, gluconeogenesis. Stimulates production of cyclic adenosine monophosphate (cAMP), which results in increased plasma glucose concentration, smooth muscle relaxation, and an inotropic myocardial effect. **Therapeutic Effect:** Increases plasma glucose level.

PHARMACOKINETICS

Onset of action occurs within 4-10 min following IM administration. Peak occurs in 5-20 min. Recovery from IM occurs within 12-32 min. **Half-life:** 8-18 min. IV onset of action is 1 min, with peak in 5-20 min; duration of action 9-25 min. Peak from subcutaneous administration occurs in 5-20 min.

AVAILABILITY

Powder for injection (GlucaGen, GlucaGen Diagnostic Kit, Glucagon, Glucagon Diagnostic Kit, Glucagon Emergency Kit): 1 mg.

INDICATIONS AND DOSAGE

Hypoglycemia

IV, IM, Subcutaneous

Adults, Elderly, Children weighing more than 20 kg: 0.5-1 mg. May give 1 or 2 additional doses if response is delayed. May repeat in 20 min as needed. **Children weighing 20 kg or less:** 0.5 mg. May repeat in 20 min as needed.

Diagnostic aid
IV, IM
Adults, Elderly: 0.25-2 mg 10 min before procedure.
Beta adrenergic blocker or calcium channel blocker overdose (unlabeled)
IV, IM
Adults, Elderly: 5-10 mg over 1 min, then infusion of 1-10 mg/hr.

OFF-LABEL USES
Treatment of esophageal obstruction due to foreign bodies, toxicity associated with beta-blockers or calcium channel blockers

G

CONTRAINDICATIONS
Hypersensitivity to glucagon or beef or pork proteins, known pheochromocytoma

INTERACTIONS
Drug: Anticoagulants: May increase the effects of these drugs. **Herbal:** None known. **Food:** None known.

DIAGNOSTIC TEST EFFECTS
May decrease serum potassium level.

IV INCOMPATIBILITIES
Do not mix glucagon with any other medications.

SIDE-EFFECTS
Occasional: Nausea, vomiting. **Rare:** Allergic reaction, such as urticaria, respiratory distress, and hypotension

CRITICAL CARE CONSIDERATIONS

ADMINISTRATION/HANDLING

IV, IM, SUBCUTANEOUS ALERT
- **Storage:** Store vials at room temperature.
- **Reconstitution (2 mg or less):** Mix powder with diluent (contains phenol) supplied by the manufacturer when preparing doses of 2 mg or less; solution is stable for 48 hr if refrigerated. For 1 mg glucagon/mL, mix the 1-mg vial with 1 mL diluent.
- **Beta blockade/calcium channel blockade overdose:** Reconstitute each 1 mg (1 unit) glucagon with 1 mL sterile water. The phenol based manufacturer's diluent should not be used because larger doses may prompt phenol toxicity. May further dilute reconstituted solution with D_5W or normal saline solution for a continuous infusion of 1-5 mg/hr.
- **Stability:** Do not use glucagon solution if cloudy or if solution contains particles.
- **Aspiration prevention:** Position patients on their side to avoid aspiration; both glucagon and hypoglycemia may produce nausea and vomiting.

PRECAUTIONS

HEALTH-RELATED
- Use glucagon cautiously in patients with a history suggestive of insulinoma (insulin-secreting tumor) or pheochromocytoma.

AGE-RELATED
- **Children:** Safety and efficacy of glucagon as a GI diagnostic aid have not been established in children.
- **Elderly:** Use with caution in elderly with cardiac disease if used to inhibit GI motility during diagnostic procedures. Smooth muscle relaxation may induce hypotension.

PREGNANCY/LACTATION-RELATED
- Pregnancy category B; excretion into breast milk unknown; use caution in nursing mothers.

MONITORING
- **Baseline assessment:** Assess for hypoglycemia, with point of care blood glucose meter and/or findings of confusion, unresponsiveness, seizures, tachycardia, hypotension and diaphoresis. If being used to manage beta-blocker or calcium blocker overdose, obtain 12-lead ECG.
- **Cardiac dysrhythmias:** Initiate continuous cardiac monitoring. Hypoglycemic patients and elderly may develop unstable tachycardias. Those overdosed with beta-blockers or calcium channel blockers may develop bradycardia and heart block.
- **Hypoglycemia or overdose:** Give glucagon immediately. Position patients on their side if unconscious or confused to help prevent aspiration in case emesis occurs.
- **Therapeutic effect:** Hypoglycemic patients should awaken in 5-20 min. If patients are given 1-2 additional doses with no response, give IV dextrose 50%. For GI diagnostic procedures, motility is reduced by smooth muscle relaxation induced by glucagon.
- **Dextrose 50%:** Have IV dextrose readily available in case hypoglycemic patients fail to awaken within 20 min.
- **Postprocedure:** After patients awaken or GI procedure is finished, give oral

carbohydrates to restore hepatic glycogen stores and prevent secondary hypoglycemia.

- **Allergic reaction:** Assess for hypotension, respiratory difficulty, and urticaria.
- **Patient education:** Teach patients and support system members to recognize, report, and act on symptoms of hypoglycemia, including anxiety, diaphoresis, difficulty concentrating, headache, hunger, nausea, nervousness, pale or cool skin, shakiness, unusual fatigue, weakness, and unconsciousness. Treat early signs of hypoglycemia with a simple sugar first, such as hard candy, honey, orange juice, sugar cubes, or table sugar dissolved in water or juice, followed by a protein source, such as cheese and crackers, half a sandwich, or a glass of milk. Hypoglycemic episodes should be reported to a health care provider to evaluate for drug dosage adjustment. Urge wearing a medical identification bracelet.

SERIOUS ADVERSE REACTIONS

- Persistent nausea and vomiting and hypokalemia, marked by severe weakness, decreased appetite, irregular heartbeat, and muscle cramps.

OVERDOSE/TOXICITY

- **Severe hyperglycemia:** May lead to ketoacidosis or hyperosmolar state if not immediately recognized; symptoms may include polydipsia, polyuria, abdominal pain, weakness, strokelike symptoms, tachypnea, tachycardia, muscle cramps, hypokalemia, and dysrhythmias.
- **Management:** Aggressive IV hydration to manage hypovolemia and insulin infusion to lower blood glucose.
- **GI decontamination:** No specific recommendations.

ANTIDOTE/DIALYSIS

- **Antidote:** If sudden hypertension and tachycardia occurs following injection, phentolamine (Regitine) 5-10 mg may be given IV. Insulin administration may be needed for acute overdose to manage hyperglycemia.
- **Dialysis:** Glucagon is unlikely to be removed by hemodialysis or peritoneal dialysis. No data are available on removal using high-permeability hemodialysis.

*glyBURIDE

See Antidiabetics (p. 911)

glycopyrrolate

glye-koe-pye'-roe-late

Classes

Chemical: quaternary ammonium derivative
Therapeutic: anticholinergic, antiulcer agent (adjunct), gastrointestinal

Pregnancy Category: B

Trade Names

Prescription: Robinul, Robinul Forte

Do not confuse Robinul with Reminyl.

G

CLINICAL PHARMACOLOGY

Mechanism of Action

A quaternary anticholinergic that inhibits action of acetylcholine at postganglionic parasympathetic sites in smooth muscle, secretory glands, and CNS. **Therapeutic Effect:** Reduces salivation and excessive secretions of respiratory tract; reduces gastric secretions and acidity.

PHARMACOKINETICS

Poorly and irregularly absorbed from GI tract after oral administration. Metabolized in the liver. Primarily excreted in urine. **Half-life:** 0.5-1.5 hr.

AVAILABILITY

Injection (Robinul): 0.2 mg/mL.
Tablets: Robinul, 1 mg; Robinul forte, 2 mg.

INDICATIONS AND DOSAGE

Preoperative inhibition of salivation and excessive respiratory tract secretions

IM

Adults, Elderly: 4 mcg/kg 30-60 min before procedure. **Children 2 yr and older:** 4 mcg/kg. **Children younger than 2 yr:** 4-9 mcg/kg.

To block effects of anticholinesterase agents

IV

Adults, Elderly: 0.2 mg for each 1 mg neostigmine or 5 mg pyridostigmine.

CONTRAINDICATIONS

Acute hemorrhage, myasthenia gravis, narrow-angle glaucoma, obstructive uropathy, paralytic ileus, tachycardia, ulcerative colitis, hypersensitivity to glycopyrrolate

INTERACTIONS

Drug: **Antacids, antidiarrheals:** May decrease the absorption of glycopyrrolate. **Ketoconazole:** May decrease the absorption of ketoconazole. **Other anticholinergics:** May increase the effects of glycopyrrolate. **Potassium chloride:** May increase the severity of GI lesions with the wax matrix formulation of potassium chloride. **Herbal:** None known. **Food:** None known.

DIAGNOSTIC TEST EFFECTS

May decrease serum uric acid levels.

IV INCOMPATIBILITIES

None known.

IV COMPATIBILITIES

*DiphenhydrAMINE (Benadryl), droperidol (Inapsine), hydromorphone (Dilaudid), *hydrOXYzine (Vistaril), lidocaine, midazolam (Versed), morphine, promethazine (Phenergan)

SIDE-EFFECTS

Frequent: Dry mouth, decreased sweating, constipation. **Occasional:** Blurred vision, gastric bloating, urinary hesitancy, somnolence (with high dosage), headache, intolerance to light, loss of taste, nervousness, flushing, insomnia, impotence, mental confusion or excitement (particularly in the elderly and children), temporary lightheadedness (with parenteral form), local irritation (with parenteral form). **Rare:** Dizziness, faintness

CRITICAL CARE CONSIDERATIONS

ADMINISTRATION/HANDLING

PO ALERT

- Antacids and antidiarrheals reduce effects of glycopyrrolate; antacids or antidiarrheals should not be taken within 1 hr of glycopyrrolate.

IV ALERT

- **Direct/IV push injection:** Administer undiluted through the tubing of a free-flowing compatible IV solution.
- **Reversal of neuromuscular blockade:** Glycopyrrolate injectable is given 0.2 mg (1 mL) for each 1 mg of neostigmine or 5 mg of pyridostigmine. To minimize cardiac side effects, the drugs may be administered simultaneously by IV injection and may be mixed in the same syringe.

IM ALERT

- Administer undiluted or diluted with D_5W, $D_{10}W$, or 0.9% NaCl.

PRECAUTIONS

HEALTH-RELATED

- Use glycopyrrolate cautiously in patients with autonomic neuropathy, heart failure, ulcerative colitis, fever, GI infections, hepatic or renal disease, hyperthyroidism, prostatic hypertrophy, or reflux esophagitis.
- Glycopyrrolate may produce drowsiness or blurred vision.

AGE-RELATED

- **Children:** Safety and efficacy of glycopyrrolate have not been established. Injectable form should not be used in children under 1 mo due to the benzyl alcohol content. Glycopyrrolate tablets are not recommended in children under 12 yr. Injectable drug is not recommended for management of peptic ulcer disease in children under 12 yr, or in children under 16 yr as a preanesthetic.
- **Elderly:** Should be used with caution because of age-related organ dysfunction. Decreased dose may be warranted.

PREGNANCY/LACTATION-RELATED

- Pregnancy category B; has been used before cesarean section to decrease gastric secretions. Quaternary structure results in limited placental transfer. Excretion into breast milk is unknown but should be minimal due to quaternary structure.

MONITORING

- **Baseline assessment:** Screen for myasthenia gravis, narrow-angle glaucoma, obstructive uropathy, tachydysrhythmias, and ulcerative colitis. Instruct patients to void before giving glycopyrrolate to reduce the risk of urinary retention.
- **Lab work:** Biochemical profile including renal (BUN, creatinine) and liver (AST [SGOT], ALT [SGPT], alkaline phosphatase) function tests.
- **Urinary retention:** Palpate bladder for distention, indicative of urine retention; monitor for low urine output.
- **Hyperdynamic state:** Monitor for hypertension, fever, and tachycardia.
- **Diarrhea:** May be an early sign of intestinal obstruction, especially in patients with an ileostomy or colostomy. Assess pattern of daily bowel activity and stool consistency; auscultate bowel sounds for peristalsis.
- **Dehydration:** Assess mucous membranes and skin turgor for hydration status. Provide adequate fluid intake.

- **Reversal of neuromuscular blockade:** Observe for spontaneous movements and return of spontaneous respirations. Assess for return of muscle strength.
- **Patient education:** Inform that glycopyrrolate use may cause dry mouth. Warn not to become overheated while exercising in hot weather to avoid heat stroke. Urge avoidance of hot baths and saunas. Warn to avoid tasks that require mental alertness or motor skills until response to the drug is known. Instruct not to take antacids or antidiarrheals within 1 hr of taking glycopyrrolate because these drugs decrease glycopyrrolate's effectiveness.

SERIOUS ADVERSE REACTIONS

- **Cardiopulmonary:** Tachycardia; palpitations; hot, dry, or flushed skin; increased respiratory rate; ECG abnormalities.
- **Gastrointestinal:** Absence of bowel sounds; nausea; vomiting.
- **Neurologic/behavioral:** Hyperthermia; CNS stimulation; agitation, restlessness, rambling speech, visual hallucinations, paranoid behavior, delusions, followed by depression.
- **Hypersensitivity:** Rash over face or upper trunk.

OVERDOSE/TOXICITY

- **Anticholinergic syndrome:** Agitation, delirium, dysarthria, extrapyramidal signs, psychosis, seizures, dry skin, mouth and axilla, flushing, hyperthermia, urinary retention, diminished bowel sounds, pupillary dilation, tachycardia, hypertension, peripheral vasodilation, dysrhythmias, cardiogenic shock, and cardiac arrest.
- **Curare-like syndrome:** Muscle weakness and paralysis have been reported with overdose of tablets.
- **Management:** Supportive care; maintenance of airway, supplemental oxygen, endotracheal intubation and mechanical ventilation for respiratory failure; IV fluid replacement to correct intravascular volume deficit; cardiac monitoring and bladder catheterization; lab work to detect rhabdomyolysis.
- **GI decontamination:** No specific recommendations.

ANTIDOTE/DIALYSIS

- **Antidote:** Physostigmine may be used in diagnosis of anticholinergic syndrome and to help manage neuropsychiatric symptoms but may induce bronchospasm, seizures, and severe cardiac conduction abnormalities.
- **Dialysis:** No data are available on removal using hemodialysis, high-permeability hemodialysis, or peritoneal dialysis.

granisetron hydrochloride

gra-ni'-se-tron hye-droe-klor'-ide

Classes

Chemical: carbazole derivative
Therapeutic: antiemetic

Pregnancy Category: B

Trade Names

Prescription: Kytril

CLINICAL PHARMACOLOGY

Mechanism of Action

A 5-HT_3 receptor antagonist that acts centrally in the chemoreceptor trigger zone or peripherally at the vagal nerve terminals. **Therapeutic Effect:** Prevents nausea and vomiting.

PHARMACOKINETICS

Route	Onset	Peak	Duration
IV	1-3 min	N/A	24 hr

Rapidly and widely distributed to tissues. Protein binding: 65%. Metabolized in the liver to active metabolite. Eliminated in urine and feces. **Half-life:** 5-9 hr (increased in the elderly).

AVAILABILITY

Oral Solution: 2 mg/10 mL.
Tablets: 1 mg.
Injection: 0.1 mg/mL, 1 mg/mL.

INDICATIONS AND DOSAGE

Prevention of chemotherapy-induced nausea and vomiting

PO

Adults, Elderly: 2 mg 1 hr before chemotherapy or 1 mg 1 hr before and 12 hr after chemotherapy.

IV

Adults, Elderly, Children 2 yr and older: 10 mcg/kg/dose (or 1 mg/dose) within 30 min of chemotherapy.

Prevention of radiation-induced nausea and vomiting

PO

Adults, Elderly: 2 mg once per day, given 1 hr before radiation therapy.

Postoperative nausea or vomiting
PO
Children 4 yr and older: 20-40 mcg/kg. Maximum: 1 mg. **Adults, Elderly:** 2 mg given as a single dose.
IV
Adults, Elderly: 1 mg as a single postoperative dose. **Children older than 4 yr:** 20-40 mcg/kg. Maximum: 1 mg.

OFF-LABEL USES
PO: Prophylaxis of nausea or vomiting associated with radiation therapy

CONTRAINDICATIONS
Hypersensitivity to granisetron hydrochloride

INTERACTIONS
Drug: Hepatic enzyme inducers: May decrease the effects of granisetron. **Herbal:** None known. **Food:** None known.

DIAGNOSTIC TEST EFFECTS
May increase AST (SGOT) and ALT (SGPT) levels.

IV INCOMPATIBILITIES
Amphotericin B (Fungizone)

IV COMPATIBILITIES
Allopurinol (Aloprim), bumetanide (Bumex), calcium gluconate, carboplatin (Paraplatin), cisplatin (Platinol), cyclophosphamide (Cytoxan), cytarabine (Ara-C), dacarbazine (DTIC-Dome), dexamethasone (Decadron), *diphenhydrAMINE (Benadryl), docetaxel (Taxotere), *DOXOrubicin (Adriamycin), etoposide (VePesid), gemcitabine (Gemzar), magnesium, mitoxantrone (Novantrone), paclitaxel (Taxol), potassium

SIDE-EFFECTS
Frequent (21%-14%): Headache, constipation, asthenia. **Occasional (8%-6%):** Diarrhea, abdominal pain. **Rare (less than 2%):** Altered taste, hypersensitivity reaction

CRITICAL CARE CONSIDERATIONS

ADMINISTRATION/HANDLING

PO ALERT
- Keep bottle of oral solution tightly closed; protect from light; and store in an upright position.
- Administer only on days of chemotherapy. Give oral granisetron within 1 hr before starting chemotherapy.

IV ALERT
- **Storage:** Store vials at room temperature.
- **Stability:** After dilution, the solution is stable for at least 24 hr at room temperature.
- **Preparation:** Solution normally appears clear and colorless; inspect for particles and discoloration. Administer granisetron undiluted or dilute it. Do not mix with other medications.
- **Undiluted drug IV push:** Give undiluted drug by IV push over 30 sec.
- **Diluted drug intermittent IV infusion:** Dilute with 20 to 50 mL 0.9% NaCl or D_5W. Administer within 30 min before starting chemotherapy. For IV piggyback, infuse over 5-20 min, depending on volume of diluent used.

PRECAUTIONS

HEALTH-RELATED
- Use granisetron cautiously in patients under 2 yr.

AGE-RELATED
- **Children:** Safety and efficacy of granisetron have not been established in children under 2 yr. Safety and efficacy have not been established for the prevention or treatment of postoperative nausea or vomiting in children.
- **Elderly:** No age-related precautions have been noted.

PREGNANCY/LACTATION-RELATED
- Pregnancy category B; breast milk excretion unknown.

MONITORING
- **Baseline assessment:** Assess for nausea and vomiting; auscultate bowel sounds before and during drug therapy.
- **Therapeutic effect:** Monitor for nausea and/or vomiting.
- **Headache:** Assess for headache.
- **Diarrhea or constipation:** Assess pattern of daily bowel activity and stool consistency.
- **Patient education:** Inform patients that granisetron is effective shortly after administration in preventing nausea and vomiting. Explain that the drug may affect the sense of taste temporarily. Teach other methods of reducing nausea and vomiting, such as lying quietly and avoiding strong odors.

SERIOUS ADVERSE REACTIONS
- Hypertension, dysrhythmias, CNS stimulation including extrapyramidal symptoms, rare hypersensitivity reaction, fever.

OVERDOSE/TOXICITY

- Agitation, delirium, bradycardia, heart block, extrapyramidal signs, psychosis, hyperthermia, diminished bowel sounds, tachycardia, hypertension.
- **GI decontamination:** No specific recommendations.

ANTIDOTE/DIALYSIS

- **Antidote:** No specific recommendations.
- **Dialysis:** No data are available on removal of granisetron using hemodialysis, high-permeability hemodialysis, or peritoneal dialysis.

griseofulvin

See Antifungals (p. 922)

guaifenesin

gwye-fen'-e-sin

Classes

Chemical: glyceryl derivative
Therapeutic: expectorant, mucolytic

Pregnancy Category: C

Trade Names

Prescription: Allfen, Amibid LA, Balminil Expectorant ♣, Drituss G, Duratuss G, Fenesin, Ganidin NR, GG 200 NR, Guaibid-LA, Guaifenex G, Guaifenex LA, Gua-SR, Guiadrine G-1200, Guiatuss, Humavent LA, Humibid LA, Humibid Pediatric, Iofen, Iophen NR, Liquidbid, Liquidbid 1200, Liquidbid LA, Mucinex, Mucobid-LA, Muco-Fen, Muco-Fen 1200, Muco-Fen 800, Organ-1 NR, Organidin NR, Pneumomist, Q-Bid LA, Respa-GF, Touro EX
Over the Counter: Anti-Tuss, Breonesin, Genatuss, Glytuss, Guiatuss, Hytuss, Hytuss 2X, Mytussin, Naldecon Senior EX, Robitussin

Combinations

Prescription: with codeine (Guiatussin AC); with dextromethorphan (Guaibid-DM); with hydrocodone (Hycotuss)

Do not confuse guaifenesin with guanfacine.

CLINICAL PHARMACOLOGY

Mechanism of Action

An expectorant that stimulates respiratory tract secretions by decreasing adhesiveness and viscosity of phlegm. **Therapeutic Effect:** Promotes removal of viscous mucus.

PHARMACOKINETICS

Well absorbed from the GI tract. Metabolized in the liver. Excreted in urine. **Half-life:** 1 hr.

AVAILABILITY

Tablets (GG 200 NR, Iofen, Organ-1 NR, Organidin NR): 200 mg.
Tablets (Extended-Release): 300 mg (Humibid Pediatric), 575 mg (Touro EX), 600 mg (Amibid LA, Fenesin, Guaibid-LA, Guaifenex LA, Gua-SR, Humavent LA, Humibid LA, Liquidbid, Liquidbid LA, Mucinex, Mucobid-L.A., Pneumomist, A-Bid LA, Respa-GF), 800 mg (Muco-Fen 800), 1000 mg (Allfen, Muco-Fen), 1200 mg (Duratuss G, Guaifenex G, Guiadrine G-1200, Liquidbid 1200, Muco-Fen 1200).
Syrup (Ganidin NR, Guiatuss, Iophen NR, Robitussin, Tussin): 100 mg/5 mL.

INDICATIONS AND DOSAGE

Expectorant

PO

Adults, Elderly, Children older than 12 yr: 200-400 mg every 4 hr. Maximum: 2.4 g/day. **Children 6-12 yr:** 100-200 mg every 4 hr. Maximum: 1.2 g/day. **Children 2-5 yr:** 50-100 mg every 4 hr. Maximum: 600 mg/day. **Children younger than 2 yr:** 25-50 mg in 6 divided doses.

PO (Extended Release)

Adults, Elderly, Children older than 12 yr: 600-1200 mg every 12 hr. Maximum: 2.4 g/day. **Children 6-12 yr:** 600 mg every 12 hr. Maximum: 1.2 g/day.

CONTRAINDICATIONS

Hypersensitivity to guaifenesin

INTERACTIONS

Drug: None known. **Herbal:** None known. **Food:** None known.

DIAGNOSTIC TEST EFFECTS

None known.

SIDE-EFFECTS

Rare: Dizziness, headache, rash, diarrhea, nausea, vomiting, abdominal pain

CRITICAL CARE CONSIDERATIONS

ADMINISTRATION/HANDLING

PO ALERT

- Store syrup, liquid, and capsules at room temperature.
- Give guaifenesin without regard to food.
- Do not crush or break extended-release capsules. Contents may be sprinkled on soft food and then swallowed without chewing or crushing. Give extended-release tablets at 12-hr intervals.

PRECAUTIONS

HEALTH-RELATED

- Use cautiously for persistent, unrelieved cough unless patient has had a chest x-ray to rule out pneumonia, chronic obstructive pulmonary disease (asthma, emphysema, chronic bronchitis), or heart failure, or sinus x-ray series to rule out sinus infection.

AGE-RELATED

- **Children:** Use guaifenesin cautiously in children under 2 yr with a persistent cough.
- **Elderly:** No age-related precautions have been noted.

PREGNANCY/LACTATION-RELATED

- Pregnancy category C; excretion into breast milk unknown.

MONITORING

- **Baseline assessment:** Assess the frequency, severity, and type of cough. Ask about a history of cigarette smoking, asthma, emphysema, and chronic bronchitis because guaifenesin is not recommended for coughs caused by these conditions.
- **Baseline lab work:** CBC with WBC differential, biochemical panel to assess for fluid/electrolyte imbalance.
- **Pulmonary hygiene:** Have patients begin deep-breathing and coughing exercises, particularly if pulmonary function is impaired.
- **Hydration:** Increase environmental humidity, encourage PO fluids or provide IV fluid intake to lower the viscosity of lung secretions.
- **Therapeutic effect:** Assess for onset of and continued cough relief.
- **Patient education:** Remind not to take guaifenesin for chronic cough. Caution avoidance of tasks requiring mental alertness or motor skills until response to the drug is known. Urge drinking plenty of fluids. Instruct to report promptly to a health care provider if the cough persists or is accompanied by fever, rash, headache, or sore throat.

SERIOUS ADVERSE REACTIONS

- Exacerbation of an acute infection underlying the cough. It is important to diagnose the cause of the cough before initiating guiafenesin for temporary cough relief.

OVERDOSE/TOXICITY

- Overdose may produce nausea and vomiting.
- **GI decontamination:** No specific recommendations.

ANTIDOTE/DIALYSIS

- **Antidote:** No specific recommendations.
- **Dialysis:** No data are available on removal of guaifenesin using hemodialysis, high-permeability hemodialysis, or peritoneal dialysis.

guanabenz acetate 

See Antihypertensives, Miscellaneous (p. 931)

guanethidine monosulfate

gwahn-eth'-i-deen mah-noe-sul'-fate

Classes

Chemical: guanidine derivative
Therapeutic: antihypertensive, postganglionic adrenergic neuron inhibitor

Pregnancy Category: C

Trade Names

Prescription: Ismelin

Do not confuse guanethidine with guanfacine.

CLINICAL PHARMACOLOGY

Mechanism of Action

An adrenergic blocker that inhibits the release of catecholamines produced by sympathetic nerve stimulation, thus suppressing peripheral sympathetic vasoconstriction. **Therapeutic Effect:** Decreases BP.

PHARMACOKINETICS

Absorption is highly variable among patients. Protein binding: 26%. Metabolized in liver. Excreted in urine and feces. Half-life: 5-10 days.

AVAILABILITY

Tablets: 10 mg, 25 mg (Ismelin).

INDICATIONS AND DOSAGE

Hypertension

PO

Adults: Initially, 10 mg/day. May increase in 10-25 mg increments at 5- to 7-day intervals. Maximum: 100 mg/day. Lower initial doses are recommended for the elderly.

OFF-LABEL USES

Treatment of anxiety, chronic angina pectoris, hypertrophic cardiomyopathy, MI, pheochromocytoma, syndrome of mitral valve prolapse, thyrotoxicosis, and tremors

CONTRAINDICATIONS

MAOI therapy within 1 wk, overt congestive heart failure, pheochromocytoma, hypersensitivity to guanethidine or any component of the formulation

INTERACTIONS

Drug: **Amphetamines, *chlorproMAZINE, diethylpropion, epinephrine, imipramine, methylphenidate, MAOIs, prochlorperazine, tricyclic antidepressants, zotepine:** May decrease antihypertensive effectiveness. **Etilefrine:** May increase etilefrine effects. **Norepinephrine, phenylephrine:** May cause hypertension and/or dysrhythmias. **Phenylpropanolamine, pseudoephedrine:** May cause a loss of BP control and possible hypertensive urgency. Herbal: **Licorice, Ma huang, yohimbine:** May decrease hypotensive effect of guanethidine. Food: None known.

DIAGNOSTIC TEST EFFECTS

None known.

SIDE-EFFECTS

Frequent: Bradycardia, dizziness, blurred vision, orthostatic hypotension, fluid retention. Occasional: Impotence, inhibition of ejaculation, nasal stuffiness. Rare: Apnea, hypertension, renal dysfunction

CRITICAL CARE CONSIDERATIONS

ADMINISTRATION/HANDLING

PO ALERT

- Give guanethidine with or without meals.

PRECAUTIONS

HEALTH-RELATED

- **Preoperative or patients receiving anesthesia:** Discontinue use 48-72 hr before surgery to avoid hypotension during anesthesia.
- Use cautiously in patients with asthma, cerebral vascular disease, coronary artery disease, history of peptic ulcer disease, recent myocardial infarction, orthostatic hypotension, renal impairment, or sexual dysfunction.

AGE-RELATED

- **Children:** Safety and efficacy of guanethidine have not been established in children.
- **Elderly:** Incidence of dizziness may be increased.

PREGNANCY/LACTATION-RELATED

- Pregnancy category C; excreted in breast milk in very small amounts; use with caution in nursing mothers.

MONITORING

- **Baseline assessment:** Obtain vital signs and note BP immediately before each dose administration, in addition to regular monitoring.
- **Baseline lab work:** Biochemical profile including renal function (BUN, creatinine). BNP level may be obtained to evaluate for heart failure.
- **Cardiac:** Monitor ECG for bradycardia and atrioventricular block. Instances of complete heart block have been noted.
- **Diarrhea:** Monitor for frequent, watery stools; fairly common and possibly severe with guanethidine.
- **Orthostatic/postural hypotension:** Ensure patients are well supported when sitting on edge of the bed, when getting out of bed, or when head of bed is raised.
- **Chest discomfort:** Monitor BP for hypotension and assess for shortness of breath or heaviness/pain in the chest.
- **Fluid retention:** Monitor intake and output, examine for dependent edema.
- **Patient education:** Warn that guanethidine may cause severe dizziness or fainting, especially in the morning. Hot weather, exercise, and alcohol may increase this effect. Rise slowly from sitting or lying position to decrease dizziness or faintness. Explain not to use nasal decongestants or OTC cold preparations (stimulants) before discussing with a health care provider. Suggest restricting salt and alcohol intake.

SERIOUS ADVERSE REACTIONS

- **Cardiovascular:** Dysrhythmias, angina, and pulmonary edema have been reported.
- Abrupt withdrawal may result in rebound hypertension with nervousness, agitation, anxiety, insomnia, hand tingling, tremor, flushing, and sweating.

OVERDOSE/TOXICITY

- **Symptoms:** Bradycardia, diarrhea, nausea, orthostatic hypotension, and shock.
- **Management:** Maintain patent airway, support ventilation, manage bradycardia with atropine, then catecholamine infusion if ineffective. Administer IV fluids for hypotension and vasopressors with alpha-agonist properties if IV fluids fail to increase BP.
- **GI decontamination:** No specific recommendations.

ANTIDOTE/DIALYSIS

- **Antidote:** Severe hypotension may respond to an alpha-adrenergic agonist (e.g., phenylephrine, norepinephrine) titrated to effect.
- **Dialysis:** No data are available on removal of guanethidine by hemodialysis, high-permeability hemodialysis, or peritoneal dialysis.

G

guanfacine

See Antihypertensives, Miscellaneous (p. 931)

haloperidol

ha-loe-per'-ih-dole

Classes

Chemical: butyrophenone derivative
Therapeutic: antipsychotic

Pregnancy Category: C

Trade Names

Prescription: Apo-Haloperidol ♣, Haldol, Haldol Decanoate, Novoperidol ♣

Do not confuse Haldol with Halcion, Halog, or Stadol.

CLINICAL PHARMACOLOGY

Mechanism of Action

An antipsychotic, antiemetic, and antidyskinetic agent that competitively blocks postsynaptic dopamine receptors, interrupts nerve impulse movement and increases turnover of dopamine in the brain. Has strong extrapyramidal and antiemetic effects; weak anticholinergic and sedative effects. **Therapeutic Effect:** Produces tranquilizing effect.

PHARMACOKINETICS

Readily absorbed from the GI tract. Protein binding: 90%. Extensively metabolized in the liver. Primarily excreted in urine. Not removed by hemodialysis. **Half-life:** 12-37 hr PO; 10-19 hr IV; 17-25 hr IM.

AVAILABILITY

Oral concentrate: 1 mg/mL, 2 mg/mL.
Tablets (Haldol): 0.5 mg, 1 mg, 2 mg, 5 mg, 10 mg, 20 mg.
Injection (lactate [Haldol]): 5 mg/mL.
Injection (decanoate [Haldol Decanoate]): 50 mg/mL, 100 mg/mL.

INDICATIONS AND DOSAGE

Acute psychosis, delirium

IV

Adults, Elderly: 0.5-50 mg at a rate of 5 mg/min. May repeat as needed.

Psychotic disorder

PO

Adults, Elderly: Initially, 0.5-5 mg, 2-3 times per day. Maximum: 100 mg/day.

Severe behavioral problems

PO

Children 3-12 yr, weighing 15-40 kg: 0.05-0.075 mg/kg/day. Initially, 0.5 mg/day. May increase by 0.5 mg/day every 5-7 days divided into 2-3 doses per day.

Tourette's syndrome

PO

Adults, Elderly: 6-15 mg/day. May increase by 2-mg increments as needed. Maintenance: 9 mg/day. **Children 3-12 yr, weighing 15-40 kg:** 0.05-0.075 mg/kg/day. Initially 0.5 mg/day. May increase by 0.5 mg/day every 5-7 days divided into 2-3 doses per day. Maximum: 6 mg/day.

OFF-LABEL USES

Treatment of Huntington's chorea, infantile autism, nausea or vomiting associated with cancer chemotherapy

CONTRAINDICATIONS

Angle-closure (narrow-angle) glaucoma, CNS depression, myelosuppression, Parkinson's disease, severe cardiac or hepatic disease, hypersensitivity to haloperidol

INTERACTIONS

Drug: **Alcohol, other CNS depressants:** May increase CNS depression. **Epinephrine:** May block alpha-adrenergic effects. **Extrapyramidal symptom-producing medications:** May increase extrapyramidal symptoms. **Lithium:** May increase neurologic toxicity. **Herbal:** None known. **Food:** None known.

DIAGNOSTIC TEST EFFECTS

None known. Therapeutic serum level is 0.2-1 mcg/mL; toxic serum level is greater than 1 mcg/mL.

IV INCOMPATIBILITIES

Allopurinol (Aloprim), amphotericin B complex (Abelcet, AmBisome, Amphotec), cefepime (Maxipime), fluconazole (Diflucan), foscarnet (Foscavir), heparin, nitroprusside (Nipride), piperacillin and tazobactam (Zosyn)

IV COMPATIBILITIES

*DOBUTamine (Dobutrex), *DOPamine (Intropin), fentanyl (Sublimaze), hydromorphone (Dilaudid), lidocaine, lorazepam (Ativan), midazolam (Versed), morphine, nitroglycerin, norepinephrine (Levophed), propofol (Diprivan)

SIDE-EFFECTS

Frequent: Blurred vision, constipation, orthostatic hypotension, dry mouth, swelling or soreness of female breasts, peripheral edema. **Occasional:** Allergic reaction, difficulty urinating, decreased thirst, dizziness, decreased sexual function, drowsiness, nausea, vomiting, photosensitivity, lethargy

H

CRITICAL CARE CONSIDERATIONS

ADMINISTRATION/HANDLING

PO ALERT

- Give haloperidol without regard to food.
- Crush scored tablets as needed.

IV ALERT

- **IV form:** *Only haloperidol lactate is given IV.*
- **Storage:** Store vials at room temperature. Protect them from freezing and light. Discard the solution if it becomes discolored or contains precipitate.
- **Undiluted IV push:** Haloperidol may be given undiluted by IV push at a rate of 5 mg/min. Flush with at least 2 mL 0.9% NaCl before and after administration.
- **Dilution:** Add the drug to 30-50 mL of most solutions; D_5W is preferred.
- **Intermittent (piggyback) IV:** Infuse IV piggyback over 30 min.
- **Continuous IV infusion:** Administer up to 25 mg/hr, titrating dosage to patient response.

IM ALERT

- **Preparation:** Prepare haloperidol decanoate IM injection using a 21-gauge needle. Do not exceed a volume of 3 mL per IM injection site.
- **IM injection:** Slowly inject the drug deep into the upper outer quadrant of the gluteus maximus. Keep patients recumbent for 30-60 min after administration to minimize hypotensive effects.

PRECAUTIONS

HEALTH-RELATED

- Use haloperidol cautiously in patients with cardiovascular disease, hepatic or renal dysfunction, or a history of seizures.

AGE-RELATED

- **Children:** Children are more susceptible to dystonias. Haloperidol use is not recommended for children under 3 yr.
- **Elderly:** A decreased dosage is recommended for elderly, who are more susceptible to extrapyramidal and anticholinergic effects, orthostatic hypotension, and sedation.

PREGNANCY/LACTATION-RELATED

- Pregnancy category C. Has been used for hyperemesis gravidarum, chorea gravidarum, and manic-depressive illness during pregnancy. Excreted into breast milk; effect on nursing infants unknown, but may be of concern.

MONITORING

- **Baseline assessment:** Assess appearance, behavior, emotional status, response to environment, speech pattern, and thought content.
- **Baseline lab work:** Biochemical panel including BUN, creatinine, and liver enzymes.
- **Suicidal patients:** Closely supervise suicidal patients during early therapy. As depression lessens, energy level improves, which increases the suicide potential.
- **Tardive dyskinesia:** Monitor for fine tongue movement, masklike facial expression, rigidity, and tremor.
- **Therapeutic response:** Observe for improvement in self-care, increased interest in surroundings and ability to concentrate, and relaxed facial expression.
- **Serum levels:** Monitor serum levels. Therapeutic serum level is 0.2-1.0 mcg/mL. Toxic serum level is greater than 1 mcg/mL.
- **Patient education:** Explain the drug's full therapeutic effect may take up to 6 wk to appear. Caution against abruptly discontinuing haloperidol after long-term use. Inform that drowsiness generally subsides with continued therapy. Recommend avoiding tasks that require mental alertness or motor skills until response to the drug is known. Urge avoidance of alcohol during haloperidol therapy. Instruct to report promptly occurrence of muscle stiffness to a health care provider. Urge avoidance of exposure to sunlight and any conditions that may cause dehydration or overheating because they may increase the risk of heat stroke. Suggest taking sips of tepid water or chewing sugarless gum to help relieve dry mouth.

SERIOUS ADVERSE REACTIONS

- **Extrapyramidal symptoms:** Appear to be dose-related and typically occur in the first few days of therapy. Marked drowsiness and lethargy, excessive salivation, and fixed stare occur frequently. Less common reactions include severe akathisia (motor restlessness) and acute dystonias (such as torticollis, opisthotonos, and oculogyric crisis).
- **Tardive dyskinesia:** Tongue protrusion, puffing of the cheeks, chewing or puckering of the mouth may occur during long-term

therapy or after discontinuing the drug and may be irreversible. Elderly female patients have a greater risk of developing this reaction.

OVERDOSE/TOXICITY

- **Neuroleptic malignant syndrome:** Fever, muscular rigidity, altered mental status, autonomic dysfunction including fever, tachycardia, tachypnea, hypertension, and hypotension. Extrapyramidal movements are often present including tremors, nystagmus, and dysarthria. Akinetic mutism and seizures have been reported. Signs and symptoms vary and are influenced by timing of the diagnosis and treatment type. Muscle rigidity usually does not respond to anticholinergic treatment.
- **Management:** Immediate discontinuation of haloperidol. No individual therapy or combination of therapies works for all patients. Dantrolene, bromocriptine, amantadine, carbidopa-levodopa, and levodopa have all had varying levels of success treating muscle relaxation and haloperidol-induced dopaminergic blockade.
- **GI decontamination:** No specific recommendations.

ANTIDOTE/DIALYSIS

- **Antidote:** No specific recommendations.
- **Dialysis:** Haloperidol is not removed by hemodialysis or peritoneal dialysis. No data are available regarding removal using high-permeability hemodialysis.

heparin sodium 

hep'-a-rin soe'-dee-um

Classes

Chemical: glycosaminoglycan, sulfated
Therapeutic: anticoagulant

Pregnancy Category: C

Trade Names

Prescription: Hepalean ♣, Heparin Leo ♣, Hep-Lock, Hep-Pak CVC

Do not confuse heparin with Hespan.

CLINICAL PHARMACOLOGY

Mechanism of Action

A blood modifier that interferes with blood coagulation by binding to antithrombin III, thereby inactivating thrombin (factor IIa) and interfering with conversion of fibrinogen to fibrin. **Therapeutic Effect:** Prevents further extension of existing thrombi or new clot formation. Has no effect on existing clots.

PHARMACOKINETICS

Well absorbed following subcutaneous administration. Protein binding: Very high. Metabolized in the liver. Removed from the circulation via uptake by the reticuloendothelial system. Primarily excreted in urine. Not removed by hemodialysis. **Half-life:** 1-6 hr.

AVAILABILITY

Injection: 10 units/mL (Hep-Lock), 100 units/mL, 1000 units/mL, 2500 units/mL, 5000 units/mL, 7500 units/mL, 10,000 units/mL, 20,000 units/mL, 25,000 units/500 mL infusion.

Injectable kit (Hep-Pak CVC): 20 units/mL, 100 units/mL.

INDICATIONS AND DOSAGE

Line flushing

IV

Adults, Elderly, Children: 100 units every 6-8 hr. **Infants weighing less than 10 kg:** 10 units every 6-8 hr.

Treatment of venous thrombosis, pulmonary embolism, peripheral arterial embolism, atrial fibrillation with embolism

Intermittent IV

Adults, Elderly: Initially, 10,000 units, then 50-70 units/kg (5000-10,000 units) every 4-6 hr. **Children 1 yr and older:** Initially, 50-100 units/kg, then 50-100 units every 4 hr.

IV Infusion

Adults, Elderly: Loading dose: 80 units/kg, then 18 units/kg/hr, with adjustments based on aPTT. Range: 10-30 units/kg/hr. **Children 1 yr and older:** Loading dose: 75 units/kg, then 20 units/kg/hr with adjustments based on aPTT. **Children younger than 1 yr:** Loading dose: 75 units/kg, then 28 units/kg/hr.

Prevention of venous thrombosis, pulmonary embolism, peripheral arterial embolism, atrial fibrillation with embolism

Subcutaneous

Adults, Elderly: 5000 units every 8-12 hr.

CONTRAINDICATIONS

Intracranial hemorrhage, severe hypotension, severe thrombocytopenia, subacute bacterial endocarditis, uncontrolled bleeding, heparin-induced thrombocytopenia, hypersensitivity to heparin

INTERACTIONS

Drug: **Antithyroid medications, cefoperazone, cefotetan, valproic acid:** May cause hypoprothrombinemia. **Other anticoagulants, platelet aggregation inhibitors, thrombolytics:** May increase the risk of bleeding. Herbal: **Feverfew, ginkgo biloba:** May have additive effect. Food: None known.

DIAGNOSTIC TEST EFFECTS

May increase free fatty acid, AST (SGOT), and ALT (SGPT) levels. May decrease serum cholesterol and triglyceride levels.

IV INCOMPATIBILITIES

Amiodarone (Cordarone), amphotericin B complex (Abelcet, AmBisome, Amphotec), ciprofloxacin (Cipro), dacarbazine (DTIC), diazepam (Valium), *DOBUTamine (Dobutrex), *DOXOrubicin (Adriamycin), droperidol (Inapsine), filgrastim (Neupogen), gentamicin (Garamycin), haloperidol (Haldol), idarubicin (Idamycin), labetalol (Trandate), *niCARdipine (Cardene), phenytoin (Dilantin), quinidine, tobramycin (Nebcin), vancomycin (Vancocin)

IV COMPATIBILITIES

Aminophylline, ampicillin/sulbactam (Unasyn), aztreonam (Azactam), calcium gluconate, cefazolin (Ancef), ceftazidime (Fortaz), ceftriaxone (Rocephin), digoxin (Lanoxin), diltiazem (Cardizem), *DOPamine (Intropin), enalapril (Vasotec), famotidine (Pepcid), fentanyl (Sublimaze), furosemide (Lasix), hydromorphone (Dilaudid), insulin, lidocaine, lorazepam (Ativan), magnesium sulfate, *methylPREDNISolone (Solu-Medrol), midazolam (Versed), milrinone (Primacor), morphine, nitroglycerin, norepinephrine (Levophed), oxytocin (Pitocin), piperacillin/tazobactam (Zosyn), procainamide (Pronestyl), propofol (Diprivan), total parenteral nutrition (TPN)

SIDE-EFFECTS

Occasional: Itching, burning (particularly on soles of feet) caused by vasospastic reaction. Rare: Pain, cyanosis of extremity 6-10 days after initial therapy lasting 4-6 hr; hypersensitivity reaction, including chills, fever, pruritus, urticaria, asthma, rhinitis, lacrimation, and headache

CRITICAL CARE CONSIDERATIONS

ADMINISTRATION/HANDLING

SUBCUTANEOUS ALERT

- **Low-dose therapy:** The subcutaneous route is used for low-dose therapy.
- **Preparation:** After withdrawing heparin from the vial, change the needle before injection to prevent leakage along the needle track.
- **Injection:** Inject the heparin dose above the iliac crest or in abdominal fat layer. Do not inject within 2 inches of umbilicus or scar tissue. Do **not** give by IM injection because it may cause pain, hematoma, ulceration, and erythema.

IV ALERT

- **Storage:** Store at room temperature.
- **Continuous IV therapy:** Preferred because intermittent IV therapy produces a higher incidence of bleeding abnormalities.
- **Dilution for continuous infusion:** Dilute IV infusion in isotonic sterile saline, D_5W, or lactated Ringer's solution. Invert IV bag at least 6 times to ensure mixing and to prevent pooling of the medication.
- **Controlled rate infusion:** Use constant-rate IV infusion pump.
- **Continuous renal replacement therapy (CRRT):** Mix heparin according to manufacturer's direction for continuous syringe infusion. Directions may vary with different manufacturers based on how the syringe pump delivers the drug.
- **Monitoring of coagulation studies:** Patients on full-dose heparin therapy must have access to blood vessels so that appropriate monitoring of coagulation studies can be performed.

PRECAUTIONS

HEALTH-RELATED

- Use heparin cautiously during menstruation in patients receiving IM injections and in those with peptic ulcer disease, recent invasive or surgical procedures, or severe hepatic or renal disease.

AGE-RELATED

- **Children:** No age-related precautions have been noted in children. The benzyl alcohol preservative may cause gasping syndrome in infants.
- **Elderly:** Are more susceptible to hemorrhage, and age-related decreased renal function may increase the risk of bleeding.

PREGNANCY/LACTATION-RELATED

- Pregnancy category C; does not cross the placenta. Has major advantages over oral anticoagulants as the treatment of choice during pregnancy. Is not excreted into breast milk due to its high molecular weight.

MONITORING

- **Baseline assessment:** Assess for history of bleeding and clotting disorders. Discern whether patients have had unusual bleeding or low platelets with past heparin infusions or subcutaneous therapy. Cross-check heparin dose with another nurse before administering.
- **Baseline lab work:** Determine the aPTT before administering heparin and at least every 24 hr after administration; weight-based IV heparin protocols may require more frequent aPTT monitoring to adjust rate of heparin infusion. Once stabilized, aPTT may be done every 24-48 hr for the first wk of subcutaneous heparin therapy or until the maintenance dose is established. Assess Hct, platelet count, AST (SGOT) and ALT (SGPT) levels, and stool and urine cultures for occult blood, regardless of route of administration.
- **Ongoing lab work for DVT prophylaxis:** Monitor aPTT 1-2 times weekly for 3-4 wk. In long-term therapy, monitor aPTT 1-2 times per mo.
- **Therapeutic aPTT level:** Monitor for fine tongue movement, masklike facial expression, rigidity, and tremor.
- **Therapeutic response:** Therapeutic heparin dosage produces an aPTT of 1.5-2.5 times normal.
- **Menstruating females:** Monitor for increase in amount of menstrual flow.
- **Bleeding:** Assess the gums for erythema and gingival bleeding, skin for ecchymosis or petechiae, and urine for hematuria. Examine for excessive bleeding from invasive sites, minor cuts, and scratches.
- **Internal bleeding:** Evaluate for abdominal, flank, back or thigh pain, decreasing BP, hypotension, tachycardia, and severe headache, which may be evidence of internal hemorrhage or stroke. Check peripheral pulses for loss of peripheral circulation, which may indicate compression of an artery by a hematoma.
- **Hematoma prevention:** Avoid giving other medications by IM route because of the potential for hematomas.
- **Converting to warfarin:** When converting to warfarin therapy, monitor the prothrombin time results. Prothrombin time will be 10%-20% higher while heparin is being given concurrently.
- **Patient education:** Instruct to use an electric razor and soft toothbrush to prevent bleeding during heparin therapy. Advise not to take other medications, including OTC drugs, before discussing with a health care provider. Instruct to report black or red stool, coffee-ground vomitus, dark or red urine, or red-speckled mucus from cough. Suggest carrying or wearing identification that identifies anticoagulant therapy. Advise informing the dentist and other physicians of heparin therapy.

SERIOUS ADVERSE REACTIONS

- **Heparin-induced thrombocytopenia (HIT):** Type II HIT occurs in 0.3%-3% of patients. Generally seen 5-14 days after starting heparin therapy. Decrease in platelet count ranges from mild to severe, sometimes leading to bleeding and/or clotting. Heparin must be discontinued immediately to avoid severe bleeding. Alternate anticoagulation should be initiated. Low molecular weight heparin (enoxaparin) also causes HIT and so is an ineffective alternative. Direct thrombin inhibitors (argatroban) may be used. If patients are receiving heparin for CRRT, patients may benefit from using trisodium citrate solution for regional anticoagulation in the dialyzer/filter, rather than using systemic anticoagulation.
- **Venous thromboembolism/deep vein thrombosis (DVT):** Occurs in about 50% of patients with HIT. Progressive, recurrent, or bilateral lower extremity DVTs may be seen with 25% of those patients developing pulmonary emboli.

OVERDOSE/TOXICITY

- **Bleeding:** Hemorrhagic complications often occur during nonoverdose situations using an appropriate dose of heparin. Bleeding ranges from local ecchymoses to major hemorrhage; occurs more frequently in high-dose therapy, intermittent IV infusion, and in women aged 60 yr and older. GI and GU tract bleeding are seen most commonly.
- **Unusual, occult bleeding:** Retroperitoneal hemorrhage manifested by back, flank, hip or thigh pain with declining hemoglobin; rectus sheath hematomas present as a painful abdominal mass, which is external to the rectus muscle; bilateral adrenal hemorrhage may present as abdominal pain, nausea, fever, hypotension, tachycardia, hypoglycemia, and anemia; spinal epidural hematoma presents as persistent severe back pain radiating in a dermatomal pattern, which occurs both spontaneously and with an indwelling epidural catheter.
- **Nonhemorrhagic toxicities:** Hyperkalemia, skin necrosis, and osteoporosis.
- **GI decontamination:** No specific recommendations.

H

ANTIDOTE/DIALYSIS

- **Antidote:** Protamine sulfate 1-1.5 mg IV for every 100 units heparin subcutaneous within 30 min of overdose, 0.5-0.75 mg for every 100 units heparin subcutaneous if within 30-60 min of overdose, 0.25-0.375 mg for every 100 units heparin subcutaneous if 2 hr have elapsed since overdose, 25-50 mg if heparin was given by IV infusion. Protamine should be given slowly over 1-3 min to avoid severe adverse reactions including hypotension and bradycardia.
- **Dialysis:** Heparin is not removed using hemodialysis or peritoneal dialysis. No data are available using high-permeability hemodialysis for removal.

H

hetastarch

het'-ah-starch

Classes
Chemical: synthetic colloid
Therapeutic: plasma volume expander

Pregnancy Category: C

Trade Names
Prescription: Hespan, Hextend

CLINICAL PHARMACOLOGY

Mechanism of Action
A plasma volume expander that exerts osmotic pull on tissue fluids. **Therapeutic Effect:** Reduces hemoconcentration and blood viscosity; increases circulating blood volume.

PHARMACOKINETICS

Smaller molecules, less than 50,000 molecular weight, rapidly excreted by kidneys; larger molecules, 50,000 molecular weight and greater, slowly degraded to smaller-sized molecules, then excreted. **Half-life:** 17 days. Duration: 24-36 hr.

AVAILABILITY

Injection (Hespan, Hextend): 6 g/100 mL 0.9% NaCl (500 mL infusion container)

INDICATIONS AND DOSAGE

Plasma volume expander
IV
Adults, Elderly: 500-1000 mL (30-60 g) per dose. Maximum total daily dose: 1.2 g/kg or 1500 mL (90 g). Maximum: 20 mL/kg/day. **Children:** 10 mL/kg/dose. Maximum total daily dose: 20 mL/kg.

Leukapheresis
IV
Adults, Elderly: 250-700 mL infused at a constant rate, usually 1:8 to venous whole blood.

CONTRAINDICATIONS

Anuria, oliguria, severe bleeding disorders, severe heart failure, hypersensitivity to hetastarch; contains lactate—not appropriate for use in patients with lactic acidosis

INTERACTIONS

Drug: None known. **Herbal:** None known. **Food:** None known.

DIAGNOSTIC TEST EFFECTS

May prolong bleeding, and clotting times, aPTT, and prothrombin time. May decrease Hct concentration. Hespan increases erythrocyte sedimentation rate (ESR).

IV INCOMPATIBILITIES

Amikacin (Amikin), ampicillin (Polycillin), cefazolin (Ancef, Kefzol), cefotaxime (Claforan), cefoxitin (Mefoxin), gentamicin (Garamycin), ranitidine (Zantac), tobramycin (Nebcin)

SIDE-EFFECTS

Rare: Allergic reaction resulting in vomiting, mild temperature elevation, chills, itching, submaxillary and parotid gland enlargement, peripheral edema of lower extremities, mild flulike symptoms, headache, muscle aches

CRITICAL CARE CONSIDERATIONS

ADMINISTRATION/HANDLING

IV ALERT

- **Storage:** Store solution at room temperature. Solution normally appears clear, pale yellow to amber. Do not use if discolored a deep turbid brown or if precipitate forms.
- **IV infusion only:** Administer only by IV infusion. Do not add drugs to IV line or mix with other IV fluids.
- **Acute hemorrhagic shock:** Administer at a rate approaching 1.2 g/kg/hr (20 mL/kg/hr). Use slower rates in burns and septic shock.
- **Hextend:** Contains lactate; excessive lactate may worsen acid-base imbalance in patients with acidosis.

PRECAUTIONS

HEALTH-RELATED

- Use hetastarch cautiously in patients with heart failure, hepatic disease, pulmonary edema, sodium-restricted diets, or thrombocytopenia.

AGE-RELATED

- **Children:** Safety and efficacy of hetastarch have not been established in children.
- **Elderly:** Age-related renal impairment may put elderly at risk for toxic reactions.

PREGNANCY/LACTATION-RELATED

- Pregnancy category C; use with caution in breast-feeding women.

MONITORING

- **Baseline assessment:** Assess vitals signs, including BP, and central venous pressure (CVP).
- **Baseline lab work:** Coagulation studies and CBC.
- **Rapid infusion:** Monitor CVP when giving by rapid infusion. If CVP rises precipitously, immediately discontinue the drug to prevent blood volume overload. Monitor for anuria, changes in intake to output ratio, and oliguria and for bleeding from surgical or trauma sites.
- **Fluid overload:** Monitor for peripheral and pulmonary edema, which may indicate impending heart failure. Assess lung sounds for crackles and wheezing.
- **Leukapheresis:** Monitor aPTT; Hct and Hgb; fluid intake and output; leukocyte and platelet counts; and prothrombin time.
- **Urine output:** Expect increased urine output in patients after hetastarch administration with oliguria.
- **Allergic reaction:** Assess for itching, periorbital edema, wheezing, and urticaria.
- **Patient education:** Instruct to use an electric razor and soft toothbrush to prevent bleeding. Warn to report black or red stool, coffee-ground vomitus, dark or red urine, or red-speckled mucus from cough.

SERIOUS ADVERSE REACTIONS

- **Anaphylactic reaction:** Periorbital edema, urticaria, and wheezing may occur.
- **Coagulopathies:** Disseminated intravascular coagulation (DIC) manifested by bleeding from invasive sites, gums, tarry stool, and hematuria.
- **Intracranial bleeding:** Deterioriated neurologic status, possible unilateral weakness or paralysis, dysarthria, and dysphagia.

OVERDOSE/TOXICITY

- **Fluid overload:** Increased BP and distended neck veins. Headache, weakness, blurred vision, behavioral changes, incoordination, and isolated muscle twitching may occur. Pulmonary edema may be manifested by rapid breathing, crackles, wheezing, and coughing.
- **Management:** Discontinue infusion immediately. Loop diuretics such as furosemide may be used to promote diuresis.
- **GI decontamination:** No specific recommendations.

ANTIDOTE/DIALYSIS

- **Antidote:** No specific recommendations.
- **Dialysis:** Hetastarch is not removed using hemodialysis. No data are available regarding removal using high-permeability hemodialysis or peritoneal dialysis.

H

*hydrALAZINE hydrochloride

hye-dral'-a-zeen hye-droe-klor'-ide

Classes

Chemical: phthalazine derivative
Therapeutic: antihypertensive, direct vasodilator

Pregnancy Category: C

Trade Names

Prescription: Apresoline, Novo-Hylazin

Combinations

Prescription: with hydrochlorothiazide (Apresazide); with hydrochlorothiazide, reserpine (Ser-Ap-Es)

Do not confuse *hydrALAZINE with *hydrOXYzine.

CLINICAL PHARMACOLOGY

Mechanism of Action

An antihypertensive with direct vasodilating effects on arterioles. **Therapeutic Effect:** Decreases BP and systemic resistance.

PHARMACOKINETICS

Route	Onset	Peak	Duration
PO	20-30 min	N/A	2-4 hr
IV	5-20 min	N/A	2-6 hr

Well absorbed from the GI tract. Widely distributed. Protein binding: 85%-90%. Metabolized in the liver to active metabolite. Primarily excreted in urine. Not removed by hemodialysis. **Half-life:** 3-7 hr (increased with impaired renal function).

AVAILABILITY

Tablets: 10 mg, 25 mg, 50 mg, 100 mg.
Injection: 20 mg/mL.

INDICATIONS AND DOSAGE

Moderate to severe hypertension

PO

Adults: Initially, 10 mg 4 times per day. May increase by 10-25 mg/dose every 2-5 days. Maximum: 300 mg/day. **Elderly:** Initially, 10 mg 2-3 times per day. May increase by 10-25 mg every 2-5 days. **Children:** Initially, 0.75-1 mg/kg/day in 2-4 divided doses, not to exceed 25 mg/dose. May increase over 3-4 wk. Maximum: 7.5 mg/kg/day (5 mg/kg/day in infants). Maximum daily dose: 200 mg.

IV, IM

Adults, Elderly: Initially, 10-20 mg/dose every 4-6 hr. May increase to 40 mg/dose. **Children:** Initially, 0.1-0.2 mg/kg/dose (maximum: 20 mg) every 4-6 hr, as needed, up to 1.7-3.5 mg/kg/day in divided doses every 4-6 hr.

Dosage in renal impairment

Dosage interval is based on creatinine clearance.

Creatinine Clearance	Dosage Interval
10-50 mL/min	Every 8 hr
Less than 10 mL/min	Every 12-24 hr

OFF-LABEL USES

Treatment of heart failure, hypertension secondary to eclampsia and preeclampsia, primary pulmonary hypertension.

CONTRAINDICATIONS

Rheumatic heart disease, hypersensitivity to *hydrALAZINE

INTERACTIONS

Drug: **Diuretics, other antihypertensives:** May increase hypotensive effect. **Herbal:** None known. **Food:** None known.

DIAGNOSTIC TEST EFFECTS

May produce positive direct Coombs' test.

IV INCOMPATIBILITIES

Aminophylline, ampicillin (Polycillin), furosemide (Lasix)

IV COMPATIBILITIES

*DOBUTamine (Dobutrex), heparin, hydrocortisone (Solu-Cortef), nitroglycerin, potassium

SIDE-EFFECTS

Frequent: Headache, palpitations, tachycardia (generally disappears in 7-10 days). **Occasional:** GI disturbance (nausea, vomiting, diarrhea), paraesthesia, fluid retention, peripheral edema, dizziness, flushed face, nasal congestion

CRITICAL CARE CONSIDERATIONS

ADMINISTRATION/HANDLING

PO ALERT

- *HydrALAZINE is best given with food or regularly spaced meals. Administration with food causes higher plasma *hydrALAZINE levels. PO is the preferred route for nonemergency use of the drug.
- Crush tablets if necessary.

IV ALERT

- **Storage:** Store at room temperature.
- Give undiluted if necessary.
- **IV push:** Give single dose over 1 min.

PRECAUTIONS

HEALTH-RELATED

- **Vascular compromise:** Use *hydrALAZINE cautiously in patients with systemic lupus erythematosus, cerebrovascular disease, increased intracranial pressure, congestive heart failure, history of chest discomfort, tachycardia, and impaired renal function.
- **Antipyridoxine effect:** If peripheral neuritis develops, patients should be started on pyridoxine; studies have shown *hydrALAZINE has an antipyridoxine effect. Pyridoxine deficiency may lead to seizures.

AGE-RELATED

- **Children:** No age-related precautions have been noted in children. Hematomas, leukopenia, petechial bleeding, and thrombocytopenia have occurred in newborns; these conditions resolve within 1-3 wk.
- **Elderly:** Age-related renal impairment may require dosage adjustment. Elderly are more sensitive to hypotensive effects.

PREGNANCY/LACTATION-RELATED

- Pregnancy category C; commonly used in pregnant women; excreted into breast milk; compatible with breast-feeding.

MONITORING

- **Baseline assessment:** Obtain BP and pulse immediately before each dose.

Screen for headache, palpitations, and tachycardia, which warrant closer monitoring. Assess for heart failure, peripheral edema of the hands and feet.

- **Baseline lab work:** Biochemical panel including BUN and creatinine. CBC and antinuclear antibody (ANA) levels.
- **Ongoing lab work:** CBC and ANA to assess for blood dyscrasias and lupus erythematosus.
- **Acute hypotension:** *HydrALAZINE IV is often used to quickly reduce very high BP and may result in hypotension following a dose. Ensure IV push dose is given over 1 full min. Drug may reduce pressor response of epinephrine.
- **Acute angina:** Myocardial stimulation by *hydrALAZINE may cause angina and ECG changes of acute MI. Monitor continuous ECG during administration.
- **Heart failure:** Hyperdynamic circulation created by the drug may increase venous return resulting in increased preload/myocardial workload; in others, systemic arterial dilation reduces afterload/resistance to ejection and improves cardiac output. Drug either exacerbates or relieves symptoms of heart failure.
- **Hemodynamic monitoring:** May cause increased pulmonary artery pressures if increases in preload override effects from decreased afterload.
- **Diarrhea:** Assess pattern of daily bowel activity and stool consistency if used daily.
- **Patient education:** Instruct to rise slowly from a lying to a sitting to standing position to avoid dizziness from orthostatic hypotension. Instruct those who are receiving high doses of *hydrALAZINE to report promptly chest discomfort, shortness of breath, dizziness, fever (lupuslike reaction), paresthesia, numbness, or tingling (peripheral neuritis) to a health care provider.

SERIOUS ADVERSE REACTIONS

- **Extreme vasodilation:** Severe orthostatic hypotension, skin flushing, severe headache, confusion, decreased level of consciousness, tachycardia, myocardial ischemia, and tachydysrhythmias may develop.
- **Management:** Reduced dosage usually relieves adverse effects. Occasionally, drug may have to be stopped and another antihypertensive initiated.

OVERDOSE/TOXICITY

- **Severe overdose:** Profound shock, tachycardia, myocardial infarction, rheumatoid syndrome, and toxic psychosis may occur.
- **Blood dyscrasias:** Anemia, leukopenia, agranulocytosis, and purpura.
- **Lupus erythematosus-like reaction:** High dosage may cause fever, tachycardia, facial rash, muscle and joint aches, splenomegaly, and glomerulonephritis.
- **Management:** Drug should be discontinued immediately for lupuslike reaction. Other symptoms should be managed per accepted Advanced Cardiac Life Support (ACLS) guidelines. Hypotension may be better managed by alpha-adrenergic-blocking agents (methoxamine [Vasoxyl] or phenylephrine [Neosynephrine]) to avoid further dysrhythmias. Beta-blocking agents (propranolol [Inderal] or metoprolol [Lopressor]) may best control tachycardia. Pyridoxine should relieve numbness, tingling, and paresthesia.
- **GI decontamination:** No specific recommendations.

ANTIDOTE/DIALYSIS

- **Antidote:** No specific recommendations.
- **Dialysis:** *HydrALAZINE is not removed by hemodialysis or peritoneal dialysis. No data are available on removal using high-permeability hemodialysis.

hydrochlorothiazide

hye-droe-klor-oh-thye'-a-zide

Classes

Chemical: sulfonamide derivative
Therapeutic: antihypertensive, diuretic, thiazide

Pregnancy Category: B, D (if used in pregnancy-induced hypertension)

Trade Names

Prescription: Apo-Hydro ♣, Aquazide H, Esidrix, Hydrodiuril, Microzide, Oretic

Combinations

Prescription: with angiotensin-converting inhibitors—quinapril (Accuretic); captopril (Acediur, Capozide); lisinopril (Prinzide, Zestoretic); benazepril (Lotensin HCT); moexipril (Uniretic); enalapril (Vaseretic); with spironolactone (Aldactazide, Spirozide); with methyldopa (Aldoril); with *hydrALAZINE (Apresazide); with reserpine (Aqwesine, Hydropres, Hydroserpine, Hydrotensin, Mallopres, Marpres, Unipres); with angiotensin II receptor blockers—irbesartan (Avalide), valsartan (Diovan HCT), losartan (Hyzaar); with *hydrALAZINE and reserpine (Cam-ap-es, H.H.R., Hyserp, Lo-Ten, Ser-A-Gen, Seralazide, Ser-Ap-Es, Serpex, Uni-Serp); with triamterene (Dyazide, Maxzide); with potassium (Esidrix-K); with guanethidine (Esimil); with beta-blockers—propranolol (Inderide), metoprolol (Lopressor HCT), labetolol (Normazide, Trandate-HCT), timolol: (Timolide), bisoprolol (Ziac); with amiloride (Moduretic)

CLINICAL PHARMACOLOGY

Mechanism of Action

A sulfonamide derivative that acts as a thiazide diuretic and antihypertensive. As a diuretic, blocks reabsorption of water, sodium, and potassium at the cortical diluting segment of the distal tubule. As an antihypertensive, reduces plasma, extracellular fluid volume, and peripheral vascular resistance by direct effect on blood vessels. **Therapeutic Effect:** Promotes diuresis; reduces BP.

PHARMACOKINETICS

Route	Onset	Peak	Duration
PO (diuretic)	2 hr	4-6 hr	6-12 hr

Variably absorbed from the GI tract. Primarily excreted unchanged in urine. Not removed by hemodialysis. **Half-life:** 5.6-14.8 hr.

AVAILABILITY

Capsules (Microzide): 12.5 mg.
Oral Solution: 50 mg/5 mL.
Tablets (Aquazide, Oretic): 25 mg, 50 mg, 100 mg.

INDICATIONS AND DOSAGE

Edema

PO

Adults, Elderly: 25-100 mg/day as a single or in divided doses. **Children at least 6 mo:** 2 mg/kg/day in 2 divided doses. Maximum: 200 mg. **Infants younger than 6 mo:** 2-4 mg/kg/day in 2 divided doses. Maximum: 37.5 mg/day.

Hypertension

PO

Adults, Elderly: Initially, 12.5-25 mg once daily. May increase up to 50 mg/day as a single or in divided doses. **Children at least 6 mo:** 2 mg/kg/day in 2 divided doses. Maximum: 200 mg. **Infants younger than 6 mo:** 2-4 mg/kg/day in 2 divided doses. Maximum: 37.5 mg/day.

OFF-LABEL USES

Treatment of diabetes insipidus, prevention of calcium-containing renal calculi

CONTRAINDICATIONS

Anuria; history of hypersensitivity to hydrochlorothiazide, other sulfonamides, or thiazide diuretics; renal decompensation

INTERACTIONS

Drug: **Cholestyramine, colestipol:** May decrease the absorption and effects of hydrochlorothiazide. **Digoxin:** May increase the risk of digoxin toxicity associated with hydrochlorothiazide-induced hypokalemia. **Lithium:** May increase the risk of lithium toxicity. **Herbal:** None known. **Food:** None known.

DIAGNOSTIC TEST EFFECTS

May increase blood glucose and serum cholesterol, LDL, bilirubin, calcium, creatinine, uric acid, and triglyceride levels. May decrease urinary calcium, and serum magnesium, potassium, and sodium levels.

SIDE-EFFECTS

Expected: Increase in urinary frequency and urine volume. **Frequent:** Potassium depletion. **Occasional:** Orthostatic hypotension, headache, GI disturbances, photosensitivity

CRITICAL CARE CONSIDERATIONS

ADMINISTRATION/HANDLING

PO ALERT

- Give hydrochlorothiazide with food or milk if GI upset occurs.
- Give preferably with breakfast to help prevent nocturia.
- Store at room temperature; protect from light and freezing.

PRECAUTIONS

HEALTH-RELATED

- Use hydrochlorothiazide cautiously in debilitated or elderly patients and in patients with diabetes mellitus, thyroid disorders, hepatic impairment, or severe renal disease.

AGE-RELATED

- **Children:** Jaundiced infants may be at risk for hyperbilirubinemia. No other age-related precautions have been noted in children.
- **Elderly:** May be more sensitive to electrolyte and hypotensive effects. Age-related renal impairment may require dosage adjustment.

PREGNANCY/LACTATION-RELATED

- Pregnancy category B (D if used in pregnancy-induced hypertension). First trimester use may increase risk of congenital defects; use in later trimesters does not seem to carry this risk. Therapy for preexisting hypertension can be continued throughout pregnancy with minimal risk. Initiating for simple edema not recommended. Few unequivocal indications for diuretic therapy in pregnancy except for pulmonary edema or congestive heart failure. Excreted into breast milk in small amounts; considered compatible with breast-feeding.

MONITORING

- **Baseline assessment:** Obtain vital signs and a baseline weight. Assess for hypotension before giving hydrochlorothiazide. Diuresis will further lower BP.
- **Baseline lab work:** Biochemical panel including serum sodium and potassium.
- **Dehydration:** Monitor intake and output. Evaluate for dry mucous membranes, poor skin turgor, constipation; check for improvement in peripheral edema, which is expected unless the patient is malnourished with low albumin.
- **Hypotension:** Low BP may indicate dehydration. Check for decreased weight, excessive fluid loss, and electrolyte imbalance.
- **Hyponatremia:** Evaluate for irritability, altered mental status, tremors, muscle spasms, cold and clammy skin, confusion, and thirst. Seizures may occur in severe cases. Initiate seizure precautions for sodium less than 115 meq/L.
- **Hypokalemia:** Assess for muscle weakness and cramps, soft flabby muscles, nausea, vomiting, weak irregular pulse, decreased bowel sounds, paralytic ileus, paresthesias, and decreased digitalis effect.
- **Hypokalemic ECG changes:** Dysrhythmias may ensue; ST depression, flattened T wave, ventricular premature beats leading to ventricular tachycardia, and torsades de pointes.
- **Patient education:** Explain to expect an increase in the frequency and volume of urination. Instruct on fall prevention and to change positions slowly and pause before standing to reduce hypotensive effects. Encourage consumption of foods high in potassium, including apricots, bananas, raisins, orange juice, potatoes, legumes, meat, and whole grains (such as cereals). Urge limited exposure to sunlight and ultraviolet rays to avoid a photosensitivity reaction.

SERIOUS ADVERSE REACTIONS

- **Hypokalemia:** Dysrhythmias including ventricular tachycardia.
- **Profound water and electrolyte depletion:** Vigorous diuresis may result in hypokalemia, hyponatremia, and dehydration.
- **Severe hypotension:** Acute hypotensive episodes may occur.
- **Hyperglycemia:** May occur during prolonged therapy. Dosage adjustment in antidiabetic/oral hypoglycemic drugs may be required.
- **Manage hypokalemia immediately:** Give IV potassium intermittent infusions (K+ boluses, K+ runs) not to exceed 20 meq/hr unless K+ level fails to normalize. Evaluate magnesium level if hypokalemia persists following treatment. Potassium is never administered IV push to avoid lethal dosing.

OVERDOSE/TOXICITY

- **Symptoms:** Lethargy and coma without changes in electrolytes or hydration.
- **Multisystem effects:** Pancreatitis, blood dyscrasias, pulmonary edema, allergic pneumonitis, and dermatologic reactions occur rarely.
- **Management:** Manage specific symptoms. Evaluate for dosage reduction.
- **GI decontamination:** No specific recommendations.

ANTIDOTE/DIALYSIS

- **Antidote:** No specific recommendations.
- **Dialysis:** Hydrochlorothiazide is not removed using hemodialysis and is unlikely to be removed using peritoneal dialysis. No data are available on removal using high-permeability hemodialysis.

hydrocodone group

hye-droe-koe'-done

DEA Schedule: III

Classes

Chemical: opiate derivative, phenanthrene derivative

Therapeutic: antitussive, narcotic analgesic

Pregnancy Category: B, D (if used for prolonged periods or at high doses at term)

Trade Names

Prescription: Hycodan

Do not confuse hydrocodone with hydromorphone.

Combinations

Prescription: Hydrocodone and acetaminophen (Anexsia, Bancap HC, Ceta-Plus, Co-Gesic, Hydrocet, Hydrogesic, Lorcet 10/650, Lorcet-HD Lorcet Plus, Lortab, Margesic H, Maxidone, Norco, Stagesic, Vicodin, Vicodin ES, Vicodin HP, Zydone); hydrocodone and aspirin (Damason-P); hydrocodone and chlorpheniramine (Tussionex); hydrocodone and guaifenesin (Codiclear DH, Hycosin, Hycotuss, Kwelcof, Pneumotussin, Vicoden Tuss, Vitussin); hydrocodone and homatropin (Hycodan and Hydromet, Hydropane, Tussigon); hydrocodone and ibuprofen (Vicoprofen); hydrocodone and pseudoephedrine (Detussin, Histussin D, P-V Tussin); hydrocodone, chlorpheniramine, phenylephrine, acetaminophen, and caffeine (Hycomine Compound)

CLINICAL PHARMACOLOGY

Mechanism of Action

Hydrocodone blocks pain perception in the cerebral cortex by binding to specific opiate receptors (mu and kappa) neuronal membranes of synapses. This binding results in a decreased synaptic chemical transmission throughout the CNS thus inhibiting the flow of pain sensations into the higher centers and causing analgesia. **Therapeutic Effect:** Alters perception of pain and produces analgesic effect.

PHARMACOKINETICS

Well absorbed. Metabolized in liver. Excreted in urine. **Half-life:** 3.3-4.4 hr.

AVAILABILITY

Hydrocodone acetaminophen

Capsules: hydrocodone bitartrate 5 mg and acetaminophen 500 mg (Bancap HC, Ceta-Plus, Hydrocet, Hydrogesic, Lorcet-HD, Margesic H, Stagesic).

Elixir: hydrocodone bitartrate 7.5 mg and acetaminophen 500 mg/15 mL (Lortab).

Tablets: hydrocodone bitartrate 2.5 mg and acetaminophen 500 mg (Lortab), hydrocodone bitartrate 5 mg and acetaminophen 325 mg (Norco), hydrocodone bitartrate 5 mg and acetaminophen 400 mg (Zydone), hydrocodone bitartrate 5 mg and acetaminophen 500 mg (Anexsia, Co-Gesic, Lortab 5/500, Vicodin), hydrocodone bitartrate 7.5 mg and acetaminophen 325 mg (Norco), hydrocodone bitartrate 5 mg and acetaminophen 400 mg (Zydone), hydrocodone bitartrate 7.5 mg and acetaminophen 500 mg (Lortab 7.5/500), hydrocodone bitartrate 7.5 mg and acetaminophen 650 mg (Anexsia, Lorcet Plus), hydrocodone bitartrate 7.5 mg and acetaminophen 750 mg (Vicodin ES), hydrocodone bitartrate 10 mg and acetaminophen 325 mg (Norco), hydrocodone bitartrate 5 mg and acetaminophen 400 mg (Zydone), hydrocodone bitartrate 10 mg and acetaminophen 500 mg (Lortab 10/500), hydrocodone bitartrate 10 mg and acetaminophen 650 mg (Lorcet 10/650), hydrocodone bitartrate 10 mg and acetaminophen 660 mg (Vicodin HP), hydrocodone bitartrate 10 mg and acetaminophen 750 mg (Maxicodone).

Hydrocodone and aspirin

Tablets: hydrocodone bitartrate 5 mg and aspirin 500 mg (Damason-P).

Hydrocodone and chlorpheniramine

Syrup, extended release: hydrocodone polistirex 10 mg and chlorpheniramine polistirex 8 mg/5 mL (Tussionex).

Hydrocodone and guaifenesin

Liquid: hydrocodone bitartrate 2.5 mg and guaifenesin 200 mg/5 mL (Pneumotussin), hydrocodone bitartrate 5 mg and guaifenesin 100 mg/5 mL (Codiclear DH, Hycosin, Hycotuss, Kwelcof, Vicodin Tuss, Vitussin).

Tablets: hydrocodone bitartrate 2.5 mg and guaifenesin 300 mg (Pneumotussin).

Hydrocodone and homatropine

Syrup: hydrocodone bitartrate 5 mg and homatropine methylbromide 1.5 mg/5 mL (Hycodan, Hydromet, Hydropane)

Tablets: hydrocodone bitartrate 5 mg and homatropine methylbromide 1.5 mg (Hycodan, Tussigon).

Hydrocodone and ibuprofen

Tablets: hydrocodone bitartrate 7.5 mg and aspirin 200 mg (Vicoprofen).

Hydrocodone and pseudoephedrine

Liquid: hydrocodone bitartrate 5 mg and pseudoephedrine 60 mg/5 mL (Detussin, Histussin D).

Tablets: hydrocodone bitartrate 5 mg and pseudoephedrine 60 mg (P-V Tussin).

Hydrocodone, chlorpheniramine, phenylephrine, acetaminophen, and caffeine

Tablets: hydrocodone bitartrate 5 mg, chlorpheniramine maleate 2 mg, phenylephrine hydrochloride 10 mg, acetaminophen 250 mg, and caffeine 30 mg (Hycomine Compound).

INDICATIONS AND DOSAGE

Analgesia

Hydrocodone and acetaminophen

PO

Adults, Children older than 13 yr or more than 50 kg: 5-10 mg every 4-6 hr. Maximum: 60 mg/day hydrocodone. Maximum dose of acetaminophen: 4 g/day. **Elderly:** 2.5-5 mg hydrocodone every 4-6 hr. Titrate dose to appropriate analgesic effect. Maximum: 4 g/day acetaminophen. **Children 2-13 yr or less than 50 kg:** 0.135 mg/kg/dose hydrocodone every 4-6 hr. Maximum: 6 doses/day of hydrocodone or maximum recommended dose of acetaminophen.

Hydrocodone and aspirin

PO

Adults: 2.5-10 mg every 4-6 hr. Maximum: 60 mg/day hydrocodone. **Elderly:** 2.5-5 mg hydrocodone every 4-6 hr. Titrate dose to appropriate analgesic effect. **Children 2-13 yr or less than 50 kg:** 0.135 mg/kg/dose hydrocodone every 4-6 hr.

Hydrocodone and chlorpheniramine

Adults, Elderly, Children 12 yr and older: 5 mL every 12 hr. Maximum: 10 mL/24 hr. **Children 6-12 yr:** 2.5 mL every 12 hr. Maximum: 5 mL/24 hr.

Hydrocodone and guaifenesin

Adults, Elderly: 5-15 mL every 4 hr. Maximum: 30 mL/24 hr. **Children 12 yr and older:** Codiclear DH, Hycotuss, Kwelcof, Maxi-Tuss: 5-10 mL every 4 hr; maximum: 4 doses/24 hr. Pneumotussin: 1-2 tablets or 10 mL every 4-6 hr; maximum: 4 doses/24 hr. **Children 6-12 yr:** Codiclear DH, Hycotuss, Kwelcof, Maxi-Tuss: 2.5 mL every 4 hr. Pneumotussin: 1 tablet or 5 mL every 4-6 hr; maximum: 4 doses/24 hr. **Children less than 6 yr:** Hydrocodone 0.3 mg/kg/day in 4 divided doses.

Hydrocodone and homatropine

Adults, Elderly: 10 mg (hydrocodone) every 4-6 hr. A single dose should not exceed 15 mg and not more frequently than every 4 hr. **Children:** 0.6 mg/kg/day (hydrocodone) in 3-4 divided doses. Do not administer more frequently than every 4 hr.

Hydrocodone and ibuprofen

Adults: 7.5-15 mg (hydrocodone) every 4-6 hr as needed for pain. Maximum: 5 tablets/day.

Hydrocodone and pseudoephedrine

Adults, Elderly: 5 mL 4 times/day. When using this combination, MAOI therapy is contraindicated.

Hydrocodone, chlorpheniramine, phenylephrine, acetaminophen, and caffeine

Adults, Elderly: 1 tablet every 4 hr up to 4 times/day. When using this combination, MAOIs are contraindicated. Also, drug combination is contraindicated in patients with heart disease, hypertension, diabetes, hyperthyroidism, increased intracranial pressure, and impaired ventilatory function.

CONTRAINDICATIONS

CNS depression, severe respiratory depression, hypersensitivity to hydrocodone, or any component of the formulation

INTERACTIONS

Drug: **Alcohol, central nervous system (CNS) depressants:** May increase CNS or respiratory depression, and hypotension. **CYP2D6 inhibitors (e.g., *chlorproMAZINE):** May decrease the effects of hydrocodone. **Hepatotoxic medications (e.g., phenytoin), liver enzyme inducers (e.g., cimetidine):** May increase risk of hepatotoxicity associated with acetaminophen with prolonged high dose or single toxic dose. **MAOIs, tricyclic antidepressants:** May increase effects of MAOIs and TCAs and hydrocodone. **Warfarin:** May increase the risk of bleeding with regular use. Herbal: None known. Food: None known.

DIAGNOSTIC TEST EFFECTS

None known.

SIDE-EFFECTS

Frequent: Dizziness, sedation, drowsiness, bradycardia. Occasional: Anxiety, dysphoria, euphoria, fear, lethargy, lightheadedness, malaise, mental clouding, mental impairment, mood changes, physiologic dependence, sedation, somnolence, constipation, bradycardia, heartburn, nausea, vomiting. Rare: Hypersensitivity reaction, rash

CRITICAL CARE CONSIDERATIONS

ADMINISTRATION/HANDLING

PO ALERT

- Give hydrocodone without regard to meals.
- Patients with mild to moderate pain who may be ambulatory are at higher risk for dizziness, hypotension, nausea, and vomiting more frequently than patients in the supine position or with severe pain.

H

PRECAUTIONS

HEALTH-RELATED

- Use hydrocodone cautiously in patients with hypersensitivity reactions to other phenanthrene derivative opioid agonists (morphine, hydrocodone, hydromorphone, levorphanol, oxycodone, oxymorphone).
- **Sulfite sensitivity:** Tablets with metabisulfite may cause allergic reactions.
- **Initial dosage reduction:** Reduce the initial dosage in those with hypothyroidism, concurrent CNS depressants, elderly, and debilitated.

AGE-RELATED

- **Children:** Children under 2 yr may be more susceptible to respiratory depression.
- **Elderly:** May be more susceptible to respiratory depression and paradoxic excitement.

PREGNANCY/LACTATION-RELATED

- Pregnancy category B (category D if used for prolonged periods or in high doses at term); withdrawal could theoretically occur in infants exposed in utero to prolonged maternal ingestion. Excretion into breast milk unknown; use caution in nursing mothers.

MONITORING

- **Baseline assessment:** Assess the duration, location, onset, and type of pain. Obtain vital signs before administering hydrocodone. If patients are being treated for cough, assess the frequency, severity, and type of cough.
- **Persistent pain:** The drug's effect is reduced if the full pain response recurs before the next dose. Instruct patients to report when pain begins to return. It is inappropriate to tell patients in pain that it is not yet time for medication. Medication should be provided at the proper frequency/dosage to keep patients comfortable.
- **Autonomic nervous system depression:** Monitor vital signs for bradycardia, hypotension, and bradypnea. If respiratory rate is consistently below 10 breaths/min or very shallow, pulse rate is consistently below 50 beats/min, and BP is consistently below 85 systolic, with difficulty awakening patients or keeping patients awake, consider reducing medication dose or frequency of administration unless end-of-life comfort care is being administered.
- **Ventilatory/oxygenation monitoring:** Monitor pulse oximetry (SpO_2) continuously on patients receiving high doses or continuous IV or epidural medication infusions. Use reading to augment assessment of ventilation and oxygenation, rather than *in place of* the assessment. Low readings may be corrected using supplemental oxygen and/or noninvasive positive pressure ventilation (bilevel positive airway pressure [BiPAP] or continuous positive airway pressure [CPAP]) on nonintubated/mechanically ventilated patients if drug dosage reduction results in patients experiencing severe pain.
- **Pulmonary hygiene:** Initiate deep breathing and coughing exercises, particularly in patients with impaired respiratory function.
- **Persistent coughing:** For patients being treated for a cough, auscultate the lungs for adventitious breath sounds and increase fluid intake and environmental humidity to decrease the viscosity of lung secretions.
- **Constipation:** Assess pattern of daily bowel activity and stool consistency, especially with long-term use.
- **Therapeutic response:** Assess for clinical improvement and record the onset of pain or cough relief.
- **Tolerance and drug dependence:** Monitor usage pattern for development of tolerance and assess for physical dependence.
- **Patient education:** Instruct to alert a health care provider when pain starts to return; drug is less effective if a full pain response recurs before the next dose. Explain that drug dependence and tolerance may occur with prolonged use of high dosages. Urge avoidance of alcohol during hydrocodone therapy. Warn to avoid tasks that require mental alertness and motor skills until response to the drug is known. Instruct patients to change positions slowly to avoid orthostatic hypotension.

SERIOUS ADVERSE REACTIONS

- **Drug tolerance:** Drug tolerance is common when managing chronic pain patients and requires increasing doses of medication or combinations of medications to provide pain relief.
- **Drug dependence:** Addiction to narcotics occurs infrequently compared with drug tolerance, but chronic pain patients are often viewed as addicted when tolerance

has occurred. Patients with cancer pain or other severe pain may require extraordinary doses to attain pain relief due to drug tolerance or low pain tolerance rather than addiction. Do not withhold medication from patients based on dosage norms when dealing with patients in severe, persistent pain.

- **Cumulative effect:** Drug may have a prolonged duration of action and cumulative effect in patients with hepatic or renal impairment.
- **Compromised ventilation:** Acute airway obstruction, apnea, dyspnea, and respiratory depression occur rarely and are usually dose related.

OVERDOSE/TOXICITY

- Cardiac arrest, circulatory collapse, coma, hypotension, hypoglycemic coma, ureteral spasm, urinary retention, vesical sphincter spasm, agranulocytosis, bleeding time prolonged, hemolytic anemia, iron deficiency anemia, occult blood loss, thrombocytopenia, hepatic necrosis, hepatitis, skeletal muscle rigidity, renal toxicity, renal tubular necrosis have been reported.
- **Ototoxicity:** Hearing impairment or loss have been reported with chronic overdose.
- **Management:** Maintain patent airway, endotracheally intubate and provide mechanical ventilation for respiratory failure. Manage cardiac arrest per Advanced Cardiac Life Support (ACLS) guidelines. Consider use of continuous renal replacement therapy for acute renal failure support. For severe bleeding, consider transfusion of packed red blood cells if anemia occurs. Support hepatic failure per current liver failure management guidelines.
- **GI decontamination:** No specific recommendations.

ANTIDOTE/DIALYSIS

- **Antidote:** Naloxone 0.4-2 mg IV, subcutaneous, or IM; may repeat if ineffective. Well absorbed IM and subcutaneously in noncirculatory impaired patients. Use with caution in patients with cardiovascular disease to avoid compromise if opiates rapidly displace from receptors. Hypertension, tachypnea, and return of extreme pain may immediately return causing extreme increases in myocardial oxygen consumption.
- **Dialysis:** No data are available on removal of hydrocodone using hemodialysis, high-permeability hemodialysis, or peritoneal dialysis.

hydrocortisone

hye-droe-kor'-ti-sone

Classes

Chemical: glucocorticoid
Therapeutic: corticosteroid, systemic; corticosteroid, topical; immunosuppression

Pregnancy Category: C, D(1st trimester)

Trade Names

Prescription: Acticort 100, Aeroseb-HC, A-HydroCort, Ala-Cort, Ala-Scalp HP, Anucort-HC, Anumed-HC, Anusol-HC, Anutone-HC, Caldecort, Cetacort, Colocort, Cortane, Cortaid, Cortate ♣, Cort-Dome High Potency, Cortef, Cortenema, Cortifoam, Cortizone-5, Cortizone-10, Cotacort, Emcort, Emo-Cort ♣, Gly-Cort, Hemorrhoidal HC, Hemril-30, Hemril-HC Uniserts, Hydrocortone, Hydrocortone Phosphate, Hytone, Instacort 10, Lacticare-HC, Locoid, Locoid Lipocream, Nupercainal Hydrocortisone Cream, Nutracort, Orabase HCA, Pandel, Penecort, Preparation H Hydrocortisone, Protocort, Proctocream-HC, Procto-Kit 1%, Procto-Kit 2.5%, Proctosert HC, Proctosol-HC, Proctozone HC, Rectasol-HC, Rederm, Scalp-Aid, Solu-Cortef, Texacort, West-Cort

Over-the-Counter: Cortizone, Cortaid, Lanacort-5, Gynecort Female Creme, Dermolate, Tegrin-HC

Combinations

Prescription: with chloramphenicol (Chloromycetin/HC suspension—ophthalmic); with neomycin and polymyxin B (Cortisporin Otic, Drotic, Otocort—otic); with neomycin, polymyxin B, and bacitracin (Cortisporin Ointment, Neotricin HC—ophthalmic); with oxytetracycline (Terra-Cortril—ophthalmic); with urea (Carmol HC)

CLINICAL PHARMACOLOGY

Mechanism of Action

An adrenocortical steroid that inhibits accumulation of inflammatory cells at inflammation sites, phagocytosis, lysosomal enzyme release and synthesis and release of mediators of inflammation. **Therapeutic Effect:** Prevents or suppresses cell-mediated immune reactions. Decreases or prevents tissue response to inflammatory process.

PHARMACOKINETICS

Route	Onset	Peak	Duration
IV	N/A	4-6 hr	8-12 hr

H

Well absorbed after IM administration. Widely distributed. Metabolized in the liver. **Half-life:** Plasma, 1.5-2 hr; biologic, 8-12 hr.

AVAILABILITY

Tablets (Cortef): 5 mg, 10 mg, 20 mg.
Oral suspension, cypionate (Cortef): 10 mg/5 mL
Cream (rectal): 1% (Nupercainal Hydrocortisone Cream, Cortizone-10, Preparation H Hydrocortisone, Proctocort, Procto-Kit 1%), 2.5% (Anusol-HC, Hemorrhoidal HC, Procto-Kit 2.5%, Proctosol-HC, Proctozone-HC).
Cream, butyrate (topical [Locoid, Locoid Lipocream]): 0.1%.
Cream, probutate (topical [Pandel]): 0.1%.
Cream, valerate (topical [Westcort]): 0.2%.
Cream (topical): 0.5% (Cortizone-5), 1% (Ala-Cort, Caldecort, Cortizone-10, Hycort, Hytone, Penecort), 2.5% (Hytone, Proctocream-HC).
Foam (rectal [Cortifoam]): 10%.
Gel (topical [Instacort 10]): 1%.
Lotion: 0.5% (Cetacort), 1% (Ala-Cort, Cetacort, Cortone, Lacticare-HC, Nutracort), 2.5% (Hytone, Lacticare-HC, Nutracort).
Ointment, butyrate (topical [Locoid]): 0.1%.
Ointment, valerate (topical [Westcort]): 0.2%.
Ointment (Topical): 0.5% (Cortizone-5), 1% (Anusol-HC, Cortaid, Cortizone-10, Hydrocortisone 1%, Hytone), 2.5% (Hytone).
Paste (topical [Orabase HCA]): 0.5%.
Solution (topical): 1% (Acticort 100, Gly-Cort, Penecort, Rederm, Scalp-Aid, Texacort), 2.5% (Texacort).
Solution, butyrate (topical [Locoid]): 0.1%.
Spray (topical [Aeroseb-HC]): 0.5%.
Suppositories: 25 mg (Anucort-HC, Anumed-HC, Anusol-HC, Anutone-HC, Cort-Dome High Potency, Hemorrhoidal HC, Hemril-HC, Proctosol-HC, Rectasol-HC), 30 mg (Emcort, Hemril-30, Protocort, Proctosert HC).
Suppositories (rectal [Colocort, Cortenema]): 100 mg/60 mL.
Injection (A-hydro-Cort, Solu-Cortef): 100 mg, 250 mg, 500 mg, 1 g.
Injectable solution, sodium phosphate (hydrocortone phosphate): 50 mg/mL.
Injectable suspension, acetate: 25 mg/mL, 50 mg/mL.

INDICATIONS AND DOSAGE

Acute adrenal insufficiency

IV

Adults, Elderly: 100 mg IV bolus; then 300 mg/day in divided doses every 8 hr. **Older children:** 1-2 mg/kg IV bolus; then 150-250 mg/day in divided doses every 6-8 hr. **Infants and young children:** 1-2 mg/kg/dose IV bolus; then 25-150 mg/day in divided doses every 6-8 hr.

Antiinflammation, immunosuppression

IV, IM

Adults, Elderly: 15-240 mg every 12 hr. **Children:** 1-5 mg/kg/day in divided doses every 12 hr, or 30-150 mg/m^2/day in divided doses every 12 hr or 1 every 24 hr.

PO

Adults, Elderly: 15-240 mg every 12 hr. **Children:** 2.5-10 mg/kg/day or 75-300 mg/m^2/day every 6-8 hr.

Physiologic replacement

PO

Adults, Elderly: 20-30 mg/day. **Children:** 0.5-0.75 mg/kg/day in divided doses every 8 hr or 20-25 mg/m^2/day.

IM

Children: 0.25-0.35 mg/kg/day as a single dose or 12-15 mg/m^2/day.

Status asthmaticus

IV

Adults, Elderly, Children: 1-2 mg/kg every 6 hr for 24 hr, then 0.5-7 mg/kg every 6 hr.

Shock

IV

Adults, Elderly, Children 12 yr and older: 500 mg-2 g every 2-6 hr. **Children younger than 12 yr:** 50 mg/kg. May repeat in 4 hr, then every 24 hr as needed.

Adjunctive treatment of ulcerative colitis

Rectal

Adults, Elderly: 100 mg at bedtime for 21 nights or until clinical and proctologic remission occurs (may require 2-3 mo of therapy).

Rectal (Cortifoam)

Adults, Elderly: 1 applicator 1-2 times per day for 2-3 wk, then every second day until therapy ends.

Topical

Adults, Elderly: Apply sparingly 2-4 times per day.

CONTRAINDICATIONS

Fungal, tuberculosis, or viral skin lesions; serious infections; hypersensitivity to hydrocortisone or sulfites

INTERACTIONS

Drug: Amphotericin: May increase hypokalemia. **Bupropion:** May lower the seizure threshold. **Digoxin:** May increase the risk of digoxin toxicity caused by hypokalemia. **Diuretics, insulin, oral hypoglycemics, potassium supplements:** May decrease the effects of these drugs. **Hepatic enzyme**

inducers: May decrease the effects of hydrocortisone. **Live-virus vaccines:** May decrease patients' antibody response to vaccine, increase vaccine side effects, and potentiate virus replication. **Herbal: Cat's claw, echinacea:** May decrease the effects of hydrocortisone because of immunostimulant properties. **Food:** May interfere with calcium absorption.

DIAGNOSTIC TEST EFFECTS

May increase blood glucose and serum lipid, amylase, and sodium levels. May decrease serum calcium, potassium, and thyroxine levels.

IV INCOMPATIBILITIES

Ciprofloxacin (Cipro), diazepam (Valium), idarubicin (Idamycin), midazolam (Versed), phenytoin (Dilantin)

IV COMPATIBILITIES

Aminophylline, amphotericin, calcium gluconate, cefepime (Maxipime), digoxin (Lanoxin), diltiazem (Cardizem), *diphenhydrAMINE (Benadryl), *DOPamine (Intropin), insulin, lidocaine, lorazepam (Ativan), magnesium sulfate, morphine, norepinephrine (Levophed), procainamide (Pronestyl), potassium chloride, propofol (Diprivan)

SIDE-EFFECTS

Frequent: Insomnia, heartburn, nervousness, abdominal distention, diaphoresis, acne, mood swings, increased appetite, facial flushing, delayed wound healing, increased susceptibility to infection, diarrhea or constipation. **Occasional:** Headache, edema, change in skin color, frequent urination. **Topical:** Itching, redness, irritation. **Rare:** Tachycardia, allergic reaction (such as rash and hives), psychological changes, hallucinations, depression. **Topical:** Allergic contact dermatitis, purpura. **Systemic:** Absorption more likely with use of occlusive dressings or extensive application in young children

CRITICAL CARE CONSIDERATIONS

ADMINISTRATION/HANDLING

IV ALERT

- **Storage of hydrocortisone sodium succinate (Solu-Cortef):** Store at room temperature. After reconstitution, store hydrocortisone sodium succinate solution at room temperature and use within 72 hr. Use immediately if further diluted with D_5W, 0.9% NaCl, or other compatible diluent.
- **Hydrocortisone sodium succinate IV push:** Dilute to 50 mg/mL; give over 3-5 min.
- **Hydrocortisone sodium succinate intermittent infusion:** Dilute to 1 mg/mL. Give over 20-30 min. Maximum dose is 8 g in 24 hr.
- **Hydrocortisone phosphate (Hydrocortone Phosphate):** May be given without mixing or dilution. For IV infusions, may be added to NS or dextrose solutions. Once reconstituted, must be used within 24 hr. Maximum dose is 1 g in 24 hr.

TOPICAL ALERT

- Gently cleanse area before applying drug.
- Apply sparingly and rub into area thoroughly. Use of occlusive dressings must be ordered with details of dressing application.

RECTAL ALERT

- **Hydrocortisone acetate rectal foam (Cortifoam):** Place patients in a left-side lying position with left leg extended and right leg flexed. Fill applicator with foam from aerosol container.
- **Administration:** Gently insert applicator tip into rectum, pointed slightly toward umbilicus, and slowly instill medication. Do not insert any part of the aerosol container into the rectum. Contents are under pressure and may cause injury.

PRECAUTIONS

HEALTH-RELATED

- **Relative contraindications:** Acute psychoses, chicken pox, heart failure, diabetes mellitus, diverticulosis, fresh intestinal anastomoses, hypertension, myasthenia gravis, ocular herpes simplex, osteoporosis, peptic ulcer disease (active or latent), tuberculosis (active or healed), pregnancy; history of psychosis, renal insufficiency, thromboembolic tendencies, or recent vaccination.
- Use hydrocortisone cautiously in patients with cirrhosis, hyperthyroidism, osteoporosis, seizure disorders, thrombophlebitis, or ulcerative colitis.

AGE-RELATED

- **Children:** Prolonged treatment or high dosages may decrease cortisol secretion and short-term growth rate in children.

H

- **Elderly:** May be more susceptible to developing hypertension or osteoporosis.

PREGNANCY/LACTATION-RELATED

- Pregnancy category C (D if used in first trimester); excreted in breast milk; could interfere with infant growth and endogenous corticosteroid production.

MONITORING

- **Baseline assessment:** Determine hypersensitivity to corticosteroids and sulfites. Obtain vital signs, height, and weight.
- **Baseline lab work:** CBC with WBC differential, biochemical panel including blood glucose (BG), serum electrolytes. If the patient is taking digoxin, obtain serum digoxin level. Cortisol level is used to diagnose adrenal insufficiency. Blood cultures to rule out systemic fungal infection (drug is contraindicated).
- **Baseline diagnostic tests:** Chest x-ray if pneumonia and/or respiratory failure is present (may result from asthma, chronic obstructive pulmonary disease exacerbation or acute respiratory distress syndrome).
- **Hyperglycemia:** If patients have diabetes mellitus or have become hyperglycemic during illness, a continuous insulin infusion may be needed to maintain normoglycemia. Critically ill patients may benefit from BG 80-110 mg/dL. Catecholamine infusions (norepinephrine [Levophed], *DOPamine, *DOBUTamine, epinephrine) create insulin resistance, further complicating BG management.
- **Ongoing lab work:** Biochemical panel including calcium, magnesium, and phosphates.
- **Hypokalemia:** Assess for muscle weakness and cramps, soft flabby muscles, nausea, vomiting, weak irregular pulse, decreased bowel sounds, paralytic ileus, paresthesias, decreased digitalis effect.
- **Hypokalemic ECG changes:** Dysrhythmias may ensue; ST depression, flattened T wave, ventricular premature beats leading to ventricular tachycardia, and torsades de pointes.
- **Hypocalcemia:** Assess for cramps, muscle twitching, tremors; seizures are possible. Elevated phosphorous levels and decreased magnesium levels may prompt hypocalcemia.
- **Fluid retention:** Examine for edema following start of steroid use.
- **Immunosuppression:** Monitor for signs of infection including fever and sore throat. Infections are masked by steroids because of reduced immune response. WBC count often increases in response to steroid use and becomes an unreliable indicator of infection.
- **Insomnia and mood swings:** Evaluate for ability to sleep and emotional status.
- **Taper dosage:** Hydrocortisone dosage must be slowly tapered to avoid relative adrenal insufficiency. *Never stop steroids abruptly.*
- **GI effects:** Assess for ileus, tarry stools, coffee ground GI secretions, GI bleeding, and diarrhea if patient has colitis.
- **Patient education:** Warn to report fever, muscle aches, sore throat, or sudden weight gain or swelling. Patients should consult with a health care provider before taking aspirin or other medications during hydrocortisone therapy. Urge avoidance of alcohol and limiting caffeine intake. Instruct to notify the dentist and other physicians of taking cortisone during therapy and for up to 1 yr after dosage is discontinued. Caution against overuse of joints injected with hydrocortisone for symptomatic relief. Explain that steroids often cause mood swings ranging from euphoria to depression. Instruct to apply topical hydrocortisone valerate (Westcort) after a bath or shower for best absorption. Patients should not cover affected area with plastic pants, tight diapers, or other coverings unless instructed otherwise by a health care provider. Warn about avoiding medication contact with the eyes.

SERIOUS ADVERSE REACTIONS

- **Long-term therapy:** May cause hypocalcemia, hypokalemia, muscle wasting (especially in arms and legs), osteoporosis, spontaneous fractures, amenorrhea, cataracts, glaucoma, peptic ulcer disease, and heart failure.
- **Abrupt discontinuation after long-term therapy:** If drug dosage is not tapered, may cause relative adrenal insufficiency with hyperkalemia, hyponatremia, anorexia, nausea, fever, headache, sudden severe joint pain, rebound inflammation, fatigue, weakness, lethargy, dizziness, and orthostatic hypotension.

OVERDOSE/TOXICITY

- **Cushing's syndrome:** "Moon face," fragile skin, "buffalo hump," GI bleeding, aseptic necrosis of joints, muscle wasting, and osteoporosis.
- **Steroid-induced psychosis:** Marked behavioral changes ranging from severe

mood swings to bizarre, psychotic behaviors.

- **Steroid-induced diabetes mellitus:** Persistent hyperglycemia that can lead to dehydration and hyperosmolar state with confusion, disorientation, hypotension, electrolyte imbalance, and abdominal pain.
- **Management:** Directed at respective symptoms. Tapering dosage to a lower level reduces medication side effects. With severe inflammatory disease, dosage reduction may not be tolerated by the patient. Best course of action is determined by weighing complications against benefits of hydrocortisone.
- **GI decontamination:** No specific recommendations.

ANTIDOTE/DIALYSIS

- **Antidote:** No specific recommendations.
- **Dialysis:** Hydrocortisone is unlikely to be removed by hemodialysis or peritoneal dialysis. No data are available on removal using high-permeability hemodialysis.

hydroflumethazide

See Diuretics (p. 956)

hydromorphone hydrochloride

hye-droe-mor'-fone hye-droe-klor'-ide

DEA Schedule: II

Classes

Chemical: opiate derivative, phenanthrene derivative

Therapeutic: antitussive, narcotic analgesic

Pregnancy Category: C, D (if used for prolonged periods or at high doses at term)

Trade Names

Prescription: Dilaudid, Dilaudid-5, Dilaudid HP, Hydromorph, Hydromorph Contin ♣, Hydrostat IR

Do not confuse hydromorphone with morphine or hydrocodone or Dilaudid with Dilantin.

CLINICAL PHARMACOLOGY

Mechanism of Action

An opioid agonist that binds to opioid receptors in the CNS, reducing the intensity of pain stimuli from sensory nerve endings. **Therapeutic Effect:** Alters the perception of and emotional response to pain; suppresses cough reflex.

PHARMACOKINETICS

Route	Onset	Peak	Duration
PO	15-30 min	30-60 min	4 hr
IV	10-15 min	15-30 min	2-3 hr
IM	15 min	60-90 min	4-5 hr
Subcutaneous	15 min	30-90 min	4 hr
Rectal	15-30 min	N/A	N/A

Well absorbed from the GI tract after IM administration. Widely distributed. Metabolized in the liver. Excreted in urine. **Half-life:** 1-3 hr.

AVAILABILITY

Liquid: 1 mg/mL (Dilaudid-5), 5 mg/5 mL (Dilaudid).
Tablets: 2 mg (Dilaudid, Hydrostat IR), 3 mg (Dilaudid, Hydrostat IR), 4 mg (Dilaudid), 8 mg (Dilaudid).
Injection: 1 mg/mL (Dilaudid), 2 mg/mL (Dilaudid), 4 mg/mL (Dilaudid), 10 mg/mL (Dilaudid HP).
Suppository (Dilaudid): 3 mg.

INDICATIONS AND DOSAGE

Analgesia

PO

Adults, Elderly, Children weighing 50 kg and more: 2-4 mg every 3-4 hr. Range: 2-8 mg/dose. **Children older than 6 mo and weighing less than 50 kg:** 0.03-0.08 mg/kg/dose every 3-4 hr.

IV

Adults, Elderly, Children weighing more than 50 kg: 0.2-0.6 mg every 2-3 hr. **Children weighing 50 kg or less:** 0.015 mg/kg/dose every 3-6 hr as needed.

Rectal

Adults, Elderly: 3-6 mg every 4-8 hr.

Patient-controlled analgesia (PCA)

IV

Adults, Elderly: 0.05-0.5 mg at 5-15 min lockout. Maximum (4 hr): 4-6 mg.

Epidural

Adults, Elderly: Bolus dose of 1-1.5 mg at rate of 0.04-0.4 mg/hr. Demand dose of 0.15 mg at 30 min lockout.

Cough

PO

Adults, Elderly, Children older than 12 yr: 1 mg every 3-4 hr. **Children 6-12 yr:** 0.5 mg every 3-4 hr.

CONTRAINDICATIONS

Obstetrical analgesia, acute bronchial asthma, diarrhea caused by poisoning until patient has been detoxified, pulmonary edema caused by an airway irritant, respiratory depression in the absence of resuscitative equipment, status asthmaticus, hypersensitivity to hydromorphone or other opiates

INTERACTIONS

Drug: **Alcohol, other CNS depressants:** May increase CNS or respiratory depression and hypotension. **MAOIs:** May produce a severe, sometimes fatal reaction; plan to administer one quarter of usual hydromorphone dose. **Herbal:** **St. John's wort:** May increase sedation. **Food:** None known.

DIAGNOSTIC TEST EFFECTS

May increase serum amylase and lipase concentrations.

IV INCOMPATIBILITIES

Amphotericin B complex (Abelcet, AmBisome, Amphotec), cefazolin (Ancef, Kefzol), diazepam (Valium), phenobarbital, phenytoin (Dilantin), total parenteral nutrition (TPN)

IV COMPATIBILITIES

Diltiazem (Cardizem), *diphenhydrAMINE (Benadryl), *DOBUTamine (Dobutrex), *DOPamine (Intropin), fentanyl (Sublimaze), furosemide (Lasix), heparin, lorazepam (Ativan), magnesium sulfate, metoclopramide (Reglan), midazolam (Versed), milrinone (Primacor), morphine, propofol (Diprivan)

SIDE-EFFECTS

Frequent: Somnolence, dizziness, hypotension (including orthostatic hypotension), decreased appetite. **Occasional:** Confusion, diaphoresis, facial flushing, urine retention, constipation, dry mouth, nausea, vomiting, headache, pain at injection site. **Rare:** Allergic reaction, depression

CRITICAL CARE CONSIDERATIONS

ADMINISTRATION/HANDLING

PO ALERT

- Give hydromorphone without regard to food.
- Crush tablets, as needed.
- Side effects occur infrequently when hydromorphone is administered orally as an antitussive.
- Ambulatory patients may be more prone to dizziness, hypotension, nausea, and vomiting than patients in the supine position and those in severe pain.

IM, SUBCUTANEOUS ALERT

- Use a short 25- to 30-gauge needle for subcutaneous injection.
- **Injection:** Administer the drug slowly; rotate injection sites.
- **Delayed absorption warning:** Patients with circulatory impairment are at increased risk for overdose because of delayed absorption of repeated injections.

IV ALERT

- **High concentration (10 mg/mL):** Should be used only in patients currently receiving high doses of another opioid agonist for severe, chronic pain caused by cancer or those who have developed a tolerance to high doses of other opioids.
- **Storage:** Store vials at room temperature; protect from light. A slight yellow discoloration of the parenteral form does not indicate a loss of potency.
- **IV push:** Hydromorphone may be given undiluted as IV push over 2-5 min, or it may be further diluted with 5 mL sterile water for injection or 0.9% NaCl.
- **Rapid IV administration:** Increases the risk of a severe anaphylactic reaction, marked by apnea, cardiac arrest, and circulatory collapse.

EPIDURAL ALERT

- Ensure preservative-free hydromorphone is used for epidural administration.
- **Possible hematoma:** All medications that may promote bleeding should be discontinued to ensure patients do not develop a hematoma. Pressure from the hematoma can lead to loss of sensation, weakness, or paralysis of legs.

RECTAL ALERT

- **Storage:** Refrigerate suppositories.
- **Administration:** Moisten the suppository with cold water before inserting it well into the rectum.

PRECAUTIONS

HEALTH-RELATED

- Use hydromorphone extremely cautiously in patients with acute alcoholism, anoxia, CNS depression, hypercapnia, respiratory depression or dysfunction, seizures, shock, or untreated myxedema.
- Use hydromorphone cautiously in patients with acute abdominal conditions,

Addison's disease, chronic obstructive pulmonary disease, hypothyroidism, hepatic impairment, increased intracranial pressure, benign prostatic hyperplasia, or urethral stricture.
- **Epidural administration:** Patients with epidural catheters should not receive heparin or any agents which promote bleeding while epidural is in place.

AGE-RELATED

- **Children:** Children under 2 yr may be more susceptible to respiratory depression.
- **Elderly:** May be more susceptible to respiratory depression and paradoxical excitement. Age-related benign prostatic hypertrophy obstruction or renal impairment may prompt urinary retention; dosage reduction is recommended.

PREGNANCY/LACTATION-RELATED

- Pregnancy category C (category D if used for prolonged periods or in high doses at term): Use during labor produces neonatal respiratory depression; not recommended for use during labor and delivery. Excretion into breast milk unknown; use caution in nursing mothers.

MONITORING

- **Baseline assessment:** Assess the duration, location, onset, and type of pain. Obtain vital signs before administering hydromorphone. If patients are being treated for cough, assess the frequency, severity, and type of cough.
- **Persistent pain:** The drug's effect is reduced if the full pain response recurs before the next dose. Instruct patients to report when pain begins to return. It is inappropriate to tell patients in pain that it is not yet time for medication. Medication should be provided at the proper frequency/dosage to keep patients comfortable.
- **Autonomic nervous system depression:** Monitor vital signs for bradycardia, hypotension, and bradypnea. If respiratory rate is consistently below 10 breaths/min or very shallow, pulse rate is consistently below 50 beats/min, and BP is consistently below 85 systolic, with difficulty awakening patients or keeping patients awake, consider reducing medication dose or frequency of administration unless patient is receiving end-of-life comfort care.
- **Ventilatory/oxygenation monitoring:** Monitor pulse oximetry (SpO_2) continuously on patients receiving high doses or continuous IV or epidural medication infusions. Use reading to augment assessment of ventilation and oxygenation, rather than *in place of* the assessment. Low readings may be corrected using supplemental oxygen and/or noninvasive positive pressure ventilation (bilevel positive airway pressure [BiPAP] or continuous positive airway pressure [CPAP]) on nonintubated/mechanically ventilated patients if drug dosage reduction results in patients experiencing severe pain.
- **Pulmonary hygiene:** Initiate deep breathing and coughing exercises, particularly in patients with impaired respiratory function.
- **Persistent coughing:** For patients being treated for a cough, auscultate the lungs for adventitious breath sounds and increase fluid intake and environmental humidity to decrease the viscosity of lung secretions.
- **Constipation:** Assess pattern of daily bowel activity and stool consistency, especially with long-term use.
- **Therapeutic response:** Assess for clinical improvement and record the onset of pain or cough relief.
- **Tolerance and drug dependence:** Monitor usage pattern for development of tolerance and assess for physical dependence.
- **Patient education:** Instruct to alert a health care provider when pain starts to return; drug is less effective if a full pain response recurs before the next dose. Explain that drug dependence and tolerance may occur with prolonged use of high dosages. Urge avoidance of alcohol during hydromorphone therapy. Warn to avoid tasks that require mental alertness and motor skills until response to the drug is known. Instruct to change positions slowly to avoid orthostatic hypotension.

SERIOUS ADVERSE REACTIONS

- **Drug tolerance:** Drug tolerance is common when managing chronic pain patients and requires increasing doses of medication or combinations of medications to provide pain relief.
- **Drug dependence:** Addiction to narcotics occurs infrequently compared with drug tolerance, but chronic pain patients are often viewed as addicted when tolerance has occurred. Patients with cancer pain or other severe pain may require

H

extraordinary doses to attain pain relief because of drug tolerance or low pain tolerance rather than addiction. Do not withhold medication from patients based on dosage norms when dealing with patients in severe, persistent pain.
- **Cumulative effect:** Drug may have a prolonged duration of action and cumulative effect in patients with hepatic or renal impairment.

OVERDOSE/TOXICITY
- **Symptoms:** Respiratory depression, difficulty awakening, disorientation, skeletal muscle flaccidity, cold or clammy skin, cyanosis, and extreme somnolence progressing to seizures, stupor, coma and death.
- **Death from "double effect":** Terminally ill patients sometimes require dosage of medication for pain relief that may be lethal. For patients who will not be resuscitated and have been informed of the potential complications of high-dose narcotic administration, if death ensues, the ethics principle of double effect makes it permissible for health care providers to administer potentially lethal doses of medication as long as the intent is pain relief rather than euthanasia.
- **Management:** Initiate Advanced Cardiac Life Support (ACLS) guidelines for respiratory depression and management of bradycardia and hypotension if present.
- **GI decontamination:** No specific recommendations.

ANTIDOTE/DIALYSIS
- **Antidote:** Naloxone 0.4-2 mg IV, subcutaneous or IM; may repeat if ineffective. Well absorbed IM and subcutaneously in noncirculatory impaired patients. Use with caution in patients with cardiovascular disease to avoid compromise if opiates rapidly displace from receptors. Hypertension, tachypnea, and return of extreme pain may immediately return, causing extreme increases in myocardial oxygen consumption.
- **Dialysis:** No data are available on removal of hydromorphone using hemodialysis, high-permeability hemodialysis, or peritoneal dialysis.

H

hydroxychloroquine sulfate

hye-drox-ee-klor'-oh-kwin sul'-fate

Classes
Chemical: 4-aminoquinoline derivative
Therapeutic: antimalarial, disease-modifying antirheumatic drug (DMARD)

Pregnancy Category: C

Trade Names
Prescription: Plaquenil

Do not confuse hydroxychloroquine with hydrocortisone or *hydrOXYzine.

CLINICAL PHARMACOLOGY
Mechanism of Action
An antimalarial and antirheumatic that concentrates in parasite acid vesicles, increasing the pH of the vesicles and interfering with parasite protein synthesis. Antirheumatic action may involve suppressing formation of antigens responsible for hypersensitivity reactions. **Therapeutic Effect:** Inhibits parasite growth.

PHARMACOKINETICS
Completely absorbed. Widely distributed in body tissues (eyes, kidneys, liver, lungs). Protein binding: 55%. Partially metabolized in liver. Partially excreted in urine. **Half-life:** 32 days (in plasma); 50 days (in blood).

AVAILABILITY
Tablets: 200 mg (155 mg base).

INDICATIONS AND DOSAGE
Treatment of acute attack of malaria (dosage in mg base)
PO

Dose	Times	Adults	Children
Initial	Day 1	620 mg	10 mg/kg
Second	6 hr later	310 mg	5 mg/kg
Third	Day 2	310 mg	5 mg/kg
Fourth	Day 3	310 mg	5 mg/kg

Suppression of malaria
PO

Adults: 310 mg base weekly on same day each wk, beginning 2 wk before entering an endemic area and continuing for 4-6 wk after leaving the area. **Children:** 5 mg base/kg/wk, beginning 2 wk before entering an endemic area and continuing for 4-6 wk after leaving the area. If therapy is not begun before exposure, administer a loading dose of 10 mg base/kg in 2 equally divided doses 6 hr apart, followed by the usual dosage regimen.

Rheumatoid arthritis

PO

Adults: Initially, 400-600 mg (310-465 mg base) daily for 5-10 days, gradually increased to optimum response level. Maintenance (usually within 4-12 wk): Dosage decreased by 50% and then continued at maintenance dose of 200-400 mg/day. Maximum effect may not be seen for several months.

Lupus erythematosus

PO

Adults: Initially 400 mg (310 mg base) once or twice per day for several weeks or months. Maintenance: 200-400 mg/day.

OFF-LABEL USES

Treatment of juvenile arthritis, sarcoid-associated hypercalcemia

CONTRAINDICATIONS

Hypersensitivity to hydroxychloroquine

INTERACTIONS

Drug: Aurothioglucose: May increase risk of blood dyscrasias. **Penicillamine:** May increase blood penicillamine concentration and the risk of hematologic, renal, or severe skin reactions. **Herbal:** None known. **Food:** None known.

DIAGNOSTIC TEST EFFECTS

None known.

SIDE-EFFECTS

Frequent: Mild, transient headache; anorexia; nausea; vomiting. **Occasional:** Visual disturbances, nervousness, fatigue, pruritus (especially of palms, soles, and scalp), irritability, personality changes, diarrhea. **Rare:** Stomatitis, dermatitis, impaired hearing

CRITICAL CARE CONSIDERATIONS

ADMINISTRATION/HANDLING

PO ALERT

- **Dosage:** 200 mg hydroxychloroquine equals 155 mg base.
- Give hydroxychloroquine with food for treatment of malaria.

PRECAUTIONS

HEALTH-RELATED

- Use hydroxychloroquine cautiously in patients with preexisting retinal or visual changes, glucose-6-phosphate dehydrogenase deficiency, hepatic disease, active or prior alcohol abuse.
- **Patients with psoriasis or porphyria:** Hydroxycholoquine may prompt a severe psoriasis attack or may exacerbate porphyria.
- **Lupus erythematosus and rheumatoid arthritis:** Prescribers should thoroughly familiarize themselves with all prescribing information before selecting the drug.
- **Malaria:** Certain strains of *Plasmodium falciparum* are resistant to hydroxychloroquine. Patients may require treatment with quinine or other forms of therapy.
- Not recommended for long-term use in children.

AGE-RELATED

- **Children:** Children are highly susceptible to hydroxychloroquine's toxic effects.
- **Elderly:** No age-related precautions are noted.

PREGNANCY/LACTATION-RELATED

- Pregnancy category C; excreted in breast milk; safe use during nursing has not been established.

MONITORING

- **Baseline assessment:** Screen for history of visual disturbances, history of psoriasis or porphyria, which may contraindicate use of hydroxychloroquine.
- **Baseline and ongoing lab work:** CBC, biochemical panel including K+ level and liver function tests.
- **Cranial nerve damage:** Monitor for visual disturbances and impaired hearing. If noted, drug should be discontinued.
- **Nausea and vomiting:** Administer drug with meals. Manage with antiemetic drug if symptoms persist.
- **Skin/mucous membrane irritation:** Assess buccal mucosa and skin, and check for pruritus.
- **Cardiac dysrhythmias:** Monitor for steadily prolonged QT interval and widening of QRS which may indicate cardiac toxicity.
- **Patient education:** Advise to continue taking hydroxychloroquine for the full course of treatment. Therapeutic response may not be evident for up to 6 mo. Instruct patients to report promptly any new symptoms, such

as decreased hearing, tinnitus, muscle weakness, and visual disturbances, to a health care provider.

SERIOUS ADVERSE REACTIONS

- **Prolonged therapy:** May result in peripheral neuritis, neuromyopathy, hypotension, QT prolongation and widened QRS, agranulocytosis, aplastic anemia, thrombocytopenia, seizures, and psychosis.

OVERDOSE/TOXICITY

- **Poisoning:** Hydroxychloroquine use is the most severe and frequent cause of poisoning by antimalarial drugs.
- **Overdose:** Tachypnea, visual disturbances, transient blindness, hypokalemia, hypotension, agitation, seizures, followed by cardiovascular collapse and death. Cardiac arrest is occasionally the first sign of overdose.
- **Visual or retinal changes:** Occurrence of any visual disturbance or retinal change (on eye exam) should prompt immediate discontinuation of the drug. Retinopathy may occur and may progress even after drug is discontinued.
- **Myopathy and neuropathy:** May occur in the absence of symptoms when poisoning is present.
- **Management:** Antidysrhythmic agents should be avoided; they may prompt lethal dysrhythmias. Widening of QRS and prolonged QT interval may be seen. Class 1A agents (quinidine, procainamide) are contraindicated, and lidocaine should not be used because it may precipitate seizures. Potassium administration for hypokalemia should be done sparingly to avoid rebound hyperkalemia as hydroxychloroquine is eliminated. Hypotension should be managed with IV fluids. Inotropes (epinephrine) may be used to augment contractility if IV fluids do not correct hypotension. Treatment of ventricular tachycardia and torsades de pointes is overdrive pacing.
- **GI decontamination:** No specific recommendations.

ANTIDOTE/DIALYSIS

- **Antidote:** No specific antidote. Studies indicate sodium bicarbonate may be effective in managing dysrhythmias rather than using antidysrhythmic drugs.
- **Dialysis:** No data are available regarding removal of hydroxychloroquine using hemodialysis, high-permeability hemodialysis, or peritoneal dialysis. These therapies are unlikely to be effective because of the large volume of drug distribution, relatively high protein binding, and long half-life.

*hydrOXYzine

See Antianxiety Agents (p. 890)

hyoscyamine

hye-oh-sye'-a-meen

Classes

Chemical: belladonna alkaloid
Therapeutic: anticholinergic, gastrointestinal

Pregnancy Category: C

Trade Names

Prescription: A-Spas S/L, Anaspaz, Cystospaz, Cystospaz-M, Donnamar, Hyosine, IV-Stat, Levbid, Levsin, Levsin S/L, Levsinex, Neosol, NuLev, Spasdel, Symax SL, Symax SR

Combinations

Prescription: with phenobarbital (Levsin PB)

Do not confuse Anaspaz with Anaprox.

CLINICAL PHARMACOLOGY

Mechanism of Action

A GI antispasmodic and anticholinergic agent that inhibits the action of acetylcholine at postganglionic (muscarinic) receptor sites. **Therapeutic Effect:** Decreases secretions (bronchial, salivary, sweat gland) and gastric juices and reduces motility of GI and urinary tract.

PHARMACOKINETICS

Completely absorbed following PO administration. Partially hydrolyzed. Majority of hyoscyamine dose is excreted unchanged in urine. Removed by hemodialysis. **Half-life:** 3-5 hr (immediate-release); 7 hr (sustained-release).

AVAILABILITY

Tablets (Anaspaz, Cystospaz, Levsin, Spacol): 0.125 mg.
Tablets (oral disintegrating [NuLev]): 0.125 mg.
Tablets (sublingual [Levsin S/L, Symax SL]): 0.125 mg.

Tablets (extended release [Levbid, Spacol T/S, Symax SR]): 0.375 mg.
Capsules (extended release [Cystospaz-M, Levsinex]): 0.375 mg.
Liquid (Hyosine, Spacol): 0.125 mg/5 mL.
Oral drops (Hyosine, Levsin): 0.125 mg/mL.
Oral solution (Hyosine, Levsin): 0.125 mg/5 mL

INDICATIONS AND DOSAGE

GI tract disorders

PO

Adults, Elderly, Children 12 yr and older: 0.125-0.25 mg every 4 hr as needed. Extended release: 0.375-0.75 mg every 12 hr. Maximum: 1.5 mg/day. **Children 2-11 yr:** 0.0625-0.125 mg every 4 hr as needed. Extended release: 0.375 mg every 12 hr. Maximum: 0.75 mg/day.

IV, IM

Adults, Elderly, Children 12 yr and older: 0.25-0.5 mg every 4 hr for 1-4 doses.

Hypermotility of lower urinary tract

PO, Sublingual

Adults, Elderly: 0.125-0.25 mg 4 times per day; or extended release 0.375 mg every 12 hr.

Infant colic

PO

Infants: Individualized drops dosed every 4 hr as needed.

CONTRAINDICATIONS

GI or GU obstruction, myasthenia gravis, myocardial ischemia, narrow-angle glaucoma, paralytic ileus, severe ulcerative colitis, hypersensitivity to hyoscyamine

INTERACTIONS

Drug: **Antacids, antidiarrheals:** May decrease the absorption of hyoscyamine. **Ketoconazole:** May decrease the absorption of this drug. **Other anticholinergics:** May increase the effects of hyoscyamine. **Potassium chloride:** May increase the severity of GI lesions with the matrix formulation of potassium chloride. **Herbal:** None known. **Food:** None known.

DIAGNOSTIC TEST EFFECTS

None known.

SIDE-EFFECTS

Frequent: Dry mouth (sometimes severe), decreased sweating, constipation. **Occasional:** Blurred vision; bloated feeling; urinary hesitancy; somnolence (with high dosage); headache; intolerance to light; loss of taste; nervousness; flushing; insomnia; impotence; mental confusion or excitement (particularly in the elderly and children); temporary lightheadedness (with parenteral form); local irritation (with parenteral form). **Rare:** Dizziness, faintness

CRITICAL CARE CONSIDERATIONS

ADMINISTRATION/HANDLING

PO ALERT

- Give hyoscyamine without regard to meals.
- May crush or chew tablets.
- Extended-release capsules should be swallowed whole.

IV, IM, SUBCUTANEOUS ALERT

- **Administration:** May give undiluted.
- Hyoscyamine may be used IV to improve radiologic visibility of the kidneys.

PRECAUTIONS

HEALTH-RELATED

- Use hyoscyamine cautiously in patients with autonomic neuropathy, cardiac dysrhythmias, heart failure, hypertension, hyperthyroidism, neuropathy, prostatic hyperplasia, or renal disease.
- **Heat prostration:** Use when patients are exposed to high temperatures is not recommended because decreased sweating may lead to hyperthermia and heat prostration.

AGE-RELATED

- **Children:** No age-related precautions noted; may be used to treat infant colic.
- **Elderly:** Males may be more prone to urinary retention.

PREGNANCY/LACTATION-RELATED

- Pregnancy category C; excreted in breast milk. Infants are sensitive to anticholinergics.

MONITORING

- **Baseline assessment:** Assess for symptoms of the problem prompting drug use. Instruct to void before giving hyoscyamine to reduce risk of urinary retention.
- **Paralytic ileus:** Assess pattern of daily bowel activity and stool consistency. Assess bowel sounds for peristalsis and mucous membranes and skin turgor for hydration status. Encourage adequate fluid intake.
- **Urinary retention:** Palpate bladder for distention; monitor urine output. Place urinary catheter if urine continues to be retained.

- **Hyperthermia:** Monitor for hyperthermia and fever.
- **Patient education:** Inform that dry mouth may occur during hyoscyamine therapy. Urge maintenance of good oral hygiene; lack of saliva may increase the risk of cavities. Warn to report promptly constipation, difficulty urinating, eye pain, or rash to a health care provider. Urge avoidance of hot baths and saunas. Caution to avoid tasks requiring mental alertness or motor skills until response to the drug is known.

SERIOUS ADVERSE REACTIONS

- **Anticholinergic effects:** Tachycardia, paralytic ileus, severe dry mouth affecting swallowing and speech, urinary retention, dysuria, rash, heat stroke, fever, hyperthermia, toxic psychosis, anhidrosis (absence of sweating).
- **Toxic psychosis:** Confusion, disorientation, hallucinations, memory impairment, and exacerbation of preexisting mental disorders.
- **Rhabdomyolysis:** May ensue in response to agitation combined with impaired thermoregulation.

OVERDOSE/TOXICITY

- **Anticholinergic syndrome:** Syndrome created by hyoscyamine blocking acetylcholine from binding to acetylcholine receptor sites. Manifested by anticholinergic effects including confusion, hallucination, incoherent speech and agitation with hyperthermia, tachycardia, ECG abnormalities, dry axillae, decreased bowel sounds, urinary retention, and psychosis (marked by agitation, restlessness, rambling speech, visual hallucinations, paranoid behavior, and delusions, followed by depression). Syndrome is rarely life-threatening.
- **Rash:** Rash over face or upper trunk may also be present.
- **Supportive care:** Maintenance of airway, supplemental oxygen, IV fluid replacement to correct intravascular volume deficit, cardiac monitoring, and bladder catheterization; lab work to detect rhabdomyolysis.
- **GI decontamination:** Use of oral activated charcoal is effective if implemented within several hours of ingestion.

ANTIDOTE/DIALYSIS

- **Antidote:** No specific recommendations. Physostigmine is sometimes used in diagnosis of anticholinergic syndrome and to help manage neuropsychiatric symptoms but may induce bronchospasm, seizures, and severe cardiac conduction abnormalities.
- **Dialysis:** No data are available on removal of hyoscyamine using hemodialysis, high-permeability hemodialysis, or peritoneal dialysis.

ibuprofen

eye-byoo-proe'-fen

Classes

Chemical: propionic acid derivative
Therapeutic: NSAID, antipyretic, nonnarcotic analgesic

Pregnancy Category: C, D (3rd trimester)

Trade Names

Prescription: Advil, Advil Pediatric, Apo-Ibuprofen ♣, Children's Advil, Ibu, Ibu-4, Ibu-6, Ibu-8, Ibu-Tab, Motrin
Over the Counter: Advil, Arthritis Foundation Pain Reliever, Children's Motrin, Ibuprin, Junior Advil, Junior Strength Motrin, Motrin IB, Nuprin, Pediacare Fever

Combinations

Prescription: with Hydrocodone (Vicoprofen); with oxycodone (Combunox)
Over the Counter: With pseudoephedrine (Sine-Aid IB, Motrin IB Sinus)

CLINICAL PHARMACOLOGY

Mechanism of Action

An NSAID that inhibits prostaglandin synthesis. Also produces vasodilation by acting centrally on the heat-regulating center of the hypothalamus. **Therapeutic Effect:** Produces analgesic and antiinflammatory effects and decreases fever.

PHARMACOKINETICS

Route	Onset	Peak	Duration
PO (analgesic)	30-60 min	2 hr	4-6 hr
PO (antirheumatic)	2 days	1-2 wk	N/A

Rapidly absorbed from the GI tract. Protein binding: greater than 90%. Metabolized in the liver. Primarily excreted in urine. Not removed by hemodialysis. **Half-life:** 2-4 hr.

AVAILABILITY

Caplets (Advil, Menadol, Motrin): 200 mg.
Capsules (Advil, Advil Migraine): 200 mg.
Gelcaps (Advil, Motrin IB): 200 mg.
Tablets: 200 mg (Advil, Motrin IB), 400 mg (Ibu, Ibu-4, Ibu-6, Ibu-8, Ibu-Tab, Motrin), 600 mg (Ibu, Ibu-4, Ibu-6, Ibu-8, Ibu-Tab, Motrin), 800 mg (Ibu, Ibu-4, Ibu-6, Ibu-8, Ibu-Tab, Motrin).
Tablets (chewable): 50 mg (Children's Advil, Children's Motrin), 100 mg (Junior Advil, Junior Strength Motrin).
Oral suspension (Advil, Children's Advil, Children's Motrin): 100 mg/5 mL.
Oral drops (Advil Pediatric, Infant Advil, Infant Motrin, Children's Motrin, Pediacare Fever): 40 mg/mL.

INDICATIONS AND DOSAGE

Acute or chronic rheumatoid arthritis, osteoarthritis, migraine pain, gouty arthritis

PO

Adults, Elderly: 400-800 mg 3-4 times per day. Maximum: 3.2 g/day.

Mild to moderate pain, primary dysmenorrhea

PO

Adults, Elderly: 200-400 mg every 4-6 hr as needed. Maximum: 1.2 g/day.

Fever, minor aches or pain

PO

Adults, Elderly: 200-400 mg every 4-6 hr. Maximum: 1.2 g/day. **Children 6 mo-12 yr:** 5-10 mg/kg/dose every 6-8 hr. Maximum: 4 doses/day.

Juvenile arthritis

PO

Children: 30-50 mg/kg/day in 3-4 divided doses. Maximum: 2.4 g/day.

OFF-LABEL USES

Treatment of psoriatic arthritis, vascular headaches

CONTRAINDICATIONS

Active peptic ulcer, chronic inflammation of GI tract; GI bleeding disorders or ulceration; third trimester of pregnancy; history of hypersensitivity to ibuprofen, aspirin, or NSAIDs

INTERACTIONS

Drug: Antihypertensives, diuretics: May decrease the effects of these drugs. **Aspirin, other salicylates:** May increase the risk of GI side effects such as bleeding. **Bone marrow depressants:** May increase the risk of hematologic reactions. **Heparin, oral anticoagulants, thrombolytics:** May increase the effects of these drugs. **Lithium:** May increase the blood concentration and risk of toxicity of lithium. **Methotrexate:** May increase the risk of methotrexate toxicity. **Probenecid:** May increase the ibuprofen blood concentration. **Herbal: Feverfew:** May decrease the effects of feverfew. **Ginkgo biloba, garlic, ginger, ginseng:** May increase the risk of bleeding. **Food:** None known.

I

DIAGNOSTIC TEST EFFECTS

May prolong bleeding time. May alter blood glucose level. May increase BUN level, and serum creatinine, potassium, AST (SGOT), and ALT (SGPT) levels. May decrease blood Hgb and Hct.

SIDE-EFFECTS

Occasional (9%-3%): Nausea with or without vomiting, dyspepsia, dizziness, rash. **Rare (less than 3%):** Diarrhea or constipation, flatulence, abdominal cramps or pain, pruritus

CRITICAL CARE CONSIDERATIONS

ADMINISTRATION/HANDLING

PO ALERT

- Do not crush or break enteric-coated tablets.
- Give ibuprofen with food, milk, or antacids if GI distress occurs.

PRECAUTIONS

HEALTH-RELATED

- Use ibuprofen cautiously in patients with heart failure, hypertension, dehydration, GI disease including GI bleeding or ulcers, and hepatic or renal impairment and in patients using anticoagulants concurrently.

AGE-RELATED

- **Children:** Safety and efficacy of ibuprofen have not been established in children under 6 mo.
- **Adults:** Use cautiously for more than 10 days to minimize the chance of toxicity.
- **Elderly:** GI bleeding or ulceration is more likely to cause serious complications and age-related renal impairment may increase the risk of hepatotoxicity or renal toxicity; a reduced dosage is recommended.

PREGNANCY/LACTATION-RELATED

- Pregnancy category C, or D if used in the third trimester or near delivery. Reduces amniotic fluid volume, constriction of the ductus arteriosus in third trimester; compatible with breast-feeding.

MONITORING

- **Baseline assessment:** Assess the duration, location, onset, and type of inflammation or pain. Inspect the arthritic joints for deformity, immobility, and skin condition.
- **Baseline and ongoing lab work:** Monitor CBC, platelet count, and biochemical panel including BUN, creatinine, serum alkaline phosphatase, bilirubin, AST (SGOT), and ALT (SGPT) levels.
- **Side effects:** Monitor for dyspepsia, headache, and a change in daily bowel activity and stool consistency.
- **Therapeutic response:** Evaluate for pain relief, improved grip strength, increased joint mobility, and decreased joint pain, tenderness, stiffness, and swelling.
- **Patient education:** Instruct to swallow enteric-coated tablets whole and not to crush or chew. Advise taking ibuprofen with food or milk if experiencing GI upset. Warn avoidance of alcohol and aspirin during ibuprofen therapy because these substances increase the risk of GI bleeding. Instruct to report a persistent headache, black stools, changes in vision, pruritus, rash, or weight gain.

SERIOUS ADVERSE REACTIONS

- **Long-term or high-dose use:** Rare reactions include peptic ulcer disease, GI bleeding, gastritis, a severe hepatic reaction (cholestasis, jaundice); severe hypersensitivity reaction, most often seen in patients with systemic lupus erythematosus or other collagen diseases.

OVERDOSE/TOXICITY

- **Overdose:** Hypotonia, muscle fasciculations, twitching, bone marrow suppression, metabolic acidosis, nausea, vomiting, diarrhea, GI bleeding, abdominal pain, volume depletion with secondary hypotension, tachycardia, pulmonary edema and acute respiratory distress syndrome, acute psychosis, seizures, and CNS depression following agitation.
- **Nephrotoxicity:** Elevated BUN, creatinine, dysuria, hematuria, proteinuria, oliguria or anuria, possible hyperkalemia and nephrotic syndrome.
- **GI decontamination:** No specific recommendations.

ANTIDOTE/DIALYSIS

- **Antidote:** No specific antidote. Treatment should be supportive and directed at symptoms.
- **Dialysis:** Ibuprofen is not removed by hemodialysis and is unlikely to be removed by peritoneal dialysis. No data are available on removal using high-permeability hemodialysis.

ibutilide fumarate

eye-byoo'-ti-lide foo'-ma-rate

Classes
Chemical: methanesulfonamide derivative
Therapeutic: antidysrhythmic, class III

Pregnancy Category: C

Trade Names
Prescription: Corvert

CLINICAL PHARMACOLOGY

Mechanism of Action
An antidysrhythmic that prolongs both atrial and ventricular action potential duration and increases the atrial and ventricular refractory period. Activates slow, inward current (mostly of sodium), produces mild slowing of sinus node rate and AV conduction, and causes dose-related prolongation of QT interval. **Therapeutic Effect:** Converts dysrhythmias to sinus rhythm.

PHARMACOKINETICS

After IV administration, highly distributed, rapidly cleared. Protein binding: 40%. Primarily excreted in urine as metabolite. **Half-life:** 2-12 hr (average: 6 hr).

AVAILABILITY

Injection: 0.1 mg/mL solution.

INDICATIONS AND DOSAGE

Rapid conversion of atrial fibrillation or flutter of recent onset to normal sinus rhythm
IV Infusion
Adults, Elderly weighing 60 kg and more: One vial (1 mg) given over 10 min. If dysrhythmia does not stop within 10 min after end of initial infusion, a second 1 mg/10-min infusion may be given. **Adults, Elderly weighing less than 60 kg:** 0.01 mg/kg given over 10 min. If dysrhythmia does not stop within 10 min after end of initial infusion, a second 0.01 mg/kg, 10-min infusion may be given.

CONTRAINDICATIONS

Hypersensitivity to ibutilide, QTc interval greater than 440 msec

INTERACTIONS

Drug: Class IA antidysrhythmics (disopyramide, moricizine, procainamide, quinidine), Class III antidysrhythmics (amiodarone, bretylium, sotalol): Do not give ibutilide with these drugs or give these drugs within 4 hr after infusing ibutilide. **H_1 receptor antagonists, phenothiazines, tricyclic and tetracyclic antidepressants:** May prolong QT interval. **Herbal:** None known. **Food:** None known.

DIAGNOSTIC TEST EFFECTS

None known.

IV INCOMPATIBILITIES

No information is available for Y-site administration.

SIDE-EFFECTS

Ibutilide is generally well tolerated. **Occasional:** Ventricular extrasystoles (5.1%), ventricular tachycardia (4.9%), headache (3.6%), hypotension, orthostatic hypotension (2%). **Rare:** Bundle-branch block, AV block, bradycardia, hypertension

CRITICAL CARE CONSIDERATIONS

ADMINISTRATION/HANDLING

IV ALERT

- **Patient preparation:** Lethal ventricular dysrhythmias may result from ibutilide administration. Have advanced cardiac life-support equipment, medications, and trained personnel on hand during and after administration.
- **Dilution:** Ibutilide is compatible with D_5W and 0.9% NaCl; may be stored in bags composed of polyvinyl chloride plastic and polyolefin bag admixtures.
- **Stability:** Admixtures with diluent are stable at room temperature for up to 24 hr or up to 48 hr if refrigerated.
- **Administration:** Give undiluted over 10 min or dilute in 50 mL solution.

PRECAUTIONS

HEALTH-RELATED

- Use ibutilide cautiously in patients with abnormal hepatic function or heart block.

AGE-RELATED

- **Children:** Safety and efficacy of ibutilide have not been established in children.
- **Elderly:** Age-related organ dysfunction may require dosage reduction; there are no firm age-related precautions.

PREGNANCY/LACTATION-RELATED

- Pregnancy category C; excretion into breast milk unknown; breast-feeding not recommended.

MONITORING

- **Baseline assessment:** For patients with atrial fibrillation lasting more than 3 days, administer an anticoagulant for at least 2 wk before ibutilide therapy is started.
- **Baseline lab work:** Biochemical panel including K+, magnesium, phosphate, and calcium levels.
- **Lethal dysrhythmias:** Monitor electrocardiogram (ECG) continuously during and after ibutilide administration. Ibutilide is proarrhythmic and may prompt sustained polymorphic ventricular tachycardia, ventricular fibrillation and may be fatal.
- **Continuous ECG:** Continue monitoring for at least 4 hr following the ibutilide infusion or until the QT interval has returned to baseline. Continue ECG monitoring if the patient develops first-, second-, or third-degree atrioventricular (AV) heart block; bradycardia; bundle branch block; premature ventricular contractions (PVCs); or runs of monomorphic ventricular tachycardia.
- **Hypotension:** Ventricular dysrhythmias and heart block may prompt hypotension. Prolonged atrial fibrillation and/or heart block may prompt heart failure in rare cases.
- **Ongoing lab work:** Monitor serum electrolyte levels for hypomagnesemia and hypokalemia which may exacerbate dysrhythmias. Low levels should be replaced as part of dysrhythmia management.
- **Patient education:** Explain that BP and ECG will be continuously monitored during therapy. Instruct to report immediately palpitations or other adverse reactions.

SERIOUS ADVERSE REACTIONS

- **Dysrhythmias:** Sustained polymorphic ventricular tachycardia, occasionally with QT prolongation (torsades de pointes) occurs rarely. Exaggerated prolongation of repolarization may occur. Existing dysrhythmias may worsen or new dysrhythmias may develop.

OVERDOSE/TOXICITY

- **Symptoms:** CNS toxicity, including CNS depression, rapid gasping breathing, and seizures.
- **Management:** If lethal dysrhythmias occur, discontinue drug immediately. Correct hypokalemia and/or hypomagnesemia if present. Failure to correct electrolyte imbalance may sabotage further resuscitation efforts. Manage dysrhythmias according to current Advanced Cardiac Life Support (ACLS) guidelines. Avoid use of Class 1 antidysrhythmic agents, as they may worsen dysrhythmias resulting from QT prolongation, such as torsades de pointes.
- **GI decontamination:** No specific recommendations.

ANTIDOTE/DIALYSIS

- **Antidote:** No specific recommendations.
- **Dialysis:** No data are available regarding removal using hemodialysis, high-permeability hemodialysis, or peritoneal dialysis.

imiglucerase

im-i-gloo'-ser-ase

Classes

Chemical: betaglucocerebrosidase derivative
Therapeutic: enzyme replacement

Pregnancy Category: C

Trade Names

Prescription: Cerezyme

Do not confuse Cerezyme with Cerebyx or Ceredase.

CLINICAL PHARMACOLOGY

Mechanism of Action

An enzyme analogue of the enzyme beta-glucocerebrosidase, which catalyzes hydrolysis of the glycolipid glucocerebroside to glucose and ceramide. **Therapeutic Effect:** Minimizes conditions associated with Gaucher's disease, such as anemia and bone disease.

PHARMACOKINETICS

Excreted in urine. **Half-life:** 3.6-10.4 min.

AVAILABILITY

Powder for injection: 212 units (equivalent to a withdrawal dose of 200 units), 424 units (equivalent to a withdrawal dose of 400 units).

INDICATIONS AND DOSAGE

Gaucher's disease

IV

Adults, Elderly, Children: Initially, 2.5 units/kg infused over 1-2 hr 3 times per wk up to 60 units/kg/wk. Maintenance: Progressive reduction in dosage while monitoring patient response.

CONTRAINDICATIONS

Hypersensitivity to imiglucerase

INTERACTIONS

Drug: None known. **Herbal:** None known. **Food:** None known.

DIAGNOSTIC TEST EFFECTS

None known.

IV INCOMPATIBILITIES

Do not mix imiglucerase with any solution other than 0.9% NaCl.

SIDE-EFFECTS

Frequent (3%): Headache. **Occasional (less than 3%-1%):** Nausea, abdominal discomfort, dizziness, pruritus, rash, small decrease in BP, urinary frequency

CRITICAL CARE CONSIDERATIONS

ADMINISTRATION/HANDLING

IV ALERT

- **Storage:** Refrigerate vials.
- **Stability:** Reconstituted solution is stable for 24 hr if refrigerated.
- **Reconstitution:** Reconstitute the 200-unit vial with 5.1 mL sterile water (or the 400-unit vial with 10.2 mL) to provide a concentration of 40 units/mL.
- **Further dilution:** Further dilute with 100 to 200 mL 0.9% NaCl.
- **IV intermittent infusion:** Infuse the solution over 1-2 hr. Imiglucerase is effective only via IV route.

PRECAUTIONS

HEALTH-RELATED

- Imiglucerase should be prescribed only by health care providers familiar with management of Gaucher's disease. Use with caution in patients who have had hypersensitivity reaction to aglucerase (Ceredase).
- **IgG antibodies:** Approximately 15% of patients who receive imiglucerase will develop antibodies within the first 12 mo; antibodies increase the probability of allergic reaction.
- **Pulmonary hypertension:** May be present in patients with Gaucher's disease regardless of whether imiglucerase is used.

AGE-RELATED

- **Children:** Safety and efficacy of imiglucerase have not been established in children under 2 yr.
- **Elderly:** No specific age-related precautions have been noted.

PREGNANCY/LACTATION-RELATED

- Pregnancy category C; use with caution in breast-feeding women; unknown if excreted in breast milk.

MONITORING

- **Baseline assessment:** Confirm diagnosis of type 1 Gaucher's disease resulting in one of the following conditions: moderate/severe anemia, thrombocytopenia, bone disease, hepatomegaly or splenomegaly. Assess that patients are prepared for costs of therapy, which can exceed $150,000 per year. Monitor weight before initial and each dose so dose can be calculated.
- **Baseline and ongoing lab work:** CBC with WBC differential and platelet count; biochemical panel including liver function tests; acid phosphatase (AP) and plasma glucocerebroside. Frequency is determined by patient response. Initially, testing may be every 3-6 mo as dose is being adjusted.
- **Baseline and periodic diagnostic tests:** MRI to assess liver and/or spleen size; standard x-rays to assess bone changes.
- **Therapeutic effect:** Assess for increased energy, reduced bleeding tendency. Spleen and liver size should decrease, joint deformities should lessen, bone pain should improve. Treatment is required for life.
- **Respiratory distress:** Episodes of respiratory distress may require placement of a pulmonary artery catheter to evaluate for pulmonary hypertension.
- **Common side effects:** Monitor for headache, pruritus, and rash. During infusion, patients may experience chills, diarrhea, dizziness, mild hypotension, peripheral edema, and tachycardia.

- **Patient education:** Instruct to report any side effects. Explain the need and schedule for any required follow-up tests.

SERIOUS ADVERSE REACTIONS

- **Development of IgG antibodies:** Increases probability of hypersensitivity reaction in the future.

OVERDOSE/TOXICITY

- **Hypersensitivity reactions:** Anaphylaxis, angioedema, respiratory distress, chest discomfort, flushing, hypotension, pruritis, rash, and urticaria.
- **Management:** Discontinue imiglucerase if hypersensitivity reaction occurs. Patients may continue to receive therapy at a reduced dose if pretreatment medications abate hypersensitivity response; antihistamines (*diphenhydrAMINE) and/or corticosteroids (hydrocortisone or dexamethasone) may be used as premedications.
- **GI decontamination:** No specific recommendations.

ANTIDOTE/DIALYSIS

- **Antidote:** No specific recommendations.
- **Dialysis:** Imiglucerase is unlikely to be removed using hemodialysis, high-permeability hemodialysis, or peritoneal dialysis.

imipenem/cilastatin sodium

i-mi-pen'-em/sye-la-stat'-in soe'-dee-um

Classes

Chemical: carbapenem, renal dipeptidase inhibitor (cilistatin), thienamycin derivative

Therapeutic: antibiotic

Pregnancy Category: C

Trade Names

Prescription: Primaxin IM, Primaxin IV

Do not confuse imipenem with imipramine.

CLINICAL PHARMACOLOGY

Mechanism of Action

A fixed-combination carbapenem. Imipenem penetrates the bacterial cell membrane and binds to penicillin-binding proteins, inhibiting cell wall synthesis. Cilastatin competitively inhibits the enzyme dehydropeptidase, preventing renal metabolism of imipenem. **Therapeutic Effect:** Produces bacterial cell death.

PHARMACOKINETICS

Readily absorbed after IM administration. Protein binding: 13%-21%. Widely distributed. Metabolized in the kidneys. Primarily excreted in urine. Removed by hemodialysis. **Half-life:** 1 hr (increased in impaired renal function).

AVAILABILITY

IV injection (Primaxin IV): 250 mg, 500 mg.

IM injection (Primaxin IM): 500 mg.

INDICATIONS AND DOSAGE

Serious respiratory tract, skin and skin structure, gynecologic, bone, joint, intraabdominal, nosocomial, and polymicrobic infections; urinary tract infections (UTIs); endocarditis; septicemia

IV

Adults, Elderly: 2-4 g/day in divided doses every 6 hr.

Mild to moderate respiratory tract, skin and skin-structure, gynecologic, bone, joint, intraabdominal, and polymicrobic infections; UTIs; endocarditis; septicemia

IV

Adults, Elderly: 1-2 g/day in divided doses every 6-8 hr. **Children older than 3 mo-12 yr:** 60-100 mg/kg/day in divided doses every 6 hr. Maximum: 4 g/day. **Children 1-3 mo:** 100 mg/kg/day in divided doses every 6 hr. **Children younger than 1 mo:** 20-25 mg/kg/dose every 8-12 hr.

IM

Adults, Elderly: 500-750 mg every 12 hr.

Dosage in renal impairment

Dosage and frequency are modified based on creatinine clearance and the severity of the infection.

	DAILY DOSAGE				
Creatinine Clearance	**1 g/day**	**1.5 g/day**	**2 g/day**	**3 g/day**	**4 g/day**
Less than or equal to 71 mL/min	Less than or equal to 70 kg: 250 mg every 6 hr 60 kg: 250 mg every 8 hr 40-50 kg: 125 mg every 6 hr 30 kg: 125 mg every 8 hr	Less than or equal to 70 kg: 500 mg every 8 hr 60 kg: 250 mg every 6 hr 50 kg: 250 mg every 6 hr 40 kg: 250 mg every 8 hr 30 kg: 125 mg every 6 hr	Less than or equal to 70 kg: 500 mg every 6 hr 60 kg: 500 mg every 8 hr 40-50 kg: 250 mg every 6 hr 30 kg: 250 mg every 8 hr	Less than or equal to 70 kg: 1 g every 8 hr 60 kg: 750 mg every 8 hr 50 kg: 500 mg every 6 hr 40 kg: 500 mg every 8 hr 30 kg: 250 mg every 6 hr	Less than or equal to 70 kg: 1 g every 6 hr 60 kg: 1 g every 8 hr 50 kg: 750 mg every 8 hr 40 kg: 500 mg every 6 hr 30 kg: 500 mg every 8 hr
41-70 mL/min	Less than or equal to 70 kg: 250 mg every 8 hr 50-60 kg: 125 mg every 6 hr 30-40 kg: 125 mg every 8 hr	Less than or equal to 70 kg: 250 mg every 6 hr 50-60 kg: 250 mg every 8 hr 40 kg: 125 mg every 6 hr 30 kg: 125 mg every 8 hr	Less than or equal to 70 kg: 500 mg every 8 hr 50-60 kg: 250 mg every 6 hr 40 kg: 250 mg every 8 hr 30 kg: 125 mg every 6 hr	Less than or equal to 70 kg: 500 mg every 6 hr 50-60 kg: 500 mg every 8 hr 40 kg: 250 mg every 6 hr 30 kg: 250 mg every 8 hr	Less than or equal to 60 kg: 750 mg every 8 hr 50 kg: 500 mg every 6 hr 40 kg: 500 mg every 8 hr 30 kg: 250 mg every 6 hr
21-40 mL/min	Less than or equal to 60 kg: 250 mg every 12 hr 50 kg: 125 mg every 8 hr 30-40 kg: 125 mg every 12 hr	Less than or equal to 60 kg: 250 mg every 8 hr 50 kg: 250 mg every 12 hr 30-40 kg: 125 mg every 8 hr	Less than or equal to 70 kg: 250 mg every 6 hr 50-60 kg: 250 mg every 8 hr 40 kg: 250 mg every 12 hr 30 kg: 125 mg every 8 hr	Less than or equal to 60 kg: 500 mg every 8 hr 50 kg: 250 mg every 6 hr 30-40 kg: 250 mg every 8 hr	Less than or equal to 70 kg: 500 mg every 6 hr 50-60 kg: 500 mg every 8 hr 40 kg: 250 mg every 6 hr 30 kg: 250 mg every 8 hr
6-20 mL/min	Less than or equal to 70 kg: 250 mg every 12 hr 30-60 kg: 125 mg every 12 hr	Less than or equal to 50 kg: 250 mg every 12 hr 30-40 kg: 125 mg every 12 hr	Less than or equal to 40 kg: 250 mg every 12 hr 30 kg: 125 mg every 12 hr	Less than or equal to 60 kg: 500 mg every 12 hr 30-50 kg: 250 mg every 12 hr	Less than or equal to 40 kg: 500 mg every 12 hr 30-40 kg: 250 mg every 12 hr

CONTRAINDICATIONS

IM: Severe shock or heart block, hypersensitivity to imipenem cilastatin sodium or local anesthetics of the amide type. **IV:** Patients with meningitis.

INTERACTIONS

Drug: Ganciclovir: May cause seizures. **Herbal:** None known. **Food:** None known.

DIAGNOSTIC TEST EFFECTS

May increase BUN level and serum alkaline phosphatase, bilirubin, creatinine, LDH, AST (SGOT) and ALT (SGPT) levels. May decrease Hct and Hgb levels.

IV INCOMPATIBILITIES

Allopurinol (Aloprim), amphotericin B complex (Abelcet, AmBisome, Amphotec), fluconazole (Diflucan)

IV COMPATIBILITIES

Diltiazem (Cardizem), insulin, propofol (Diprivan), total parenteral nutrition (TPN)

SIDE-EFFECTS

Occasional (3%-2%): Diarrhea, nausea, vomiting, phlebitis. **Rare (2%-1%):** Rash, pain at IM injection site

CRITICAL CARE CONSIDERATIONS

ADMINISTRATION/HANDLING

IV ALERT

- **Storage:** Store dry powder at controlled room temperature.
- **Reconstitution:** Dilute each 250- or 500-mg vial with 100 mL D_5W or 0.9% NaCl. The solution normally appears colorless to yellow; discard it if it turns brown or contains a precipitate.
- **Stability:** Reconstituted solution is stable for 4 hr at room temperature and 24 hr if refrigerated.
- **IV intermittent infusion:** Give by IV piggyback infusion, not by IV push. Infuse over 20 to 30 min (over 40 to 60 min for the 1-g dose). Observe patients during the initial 30 min of first infusion for hypersensitivity reaction.

IM ALERT

- **Reconstitution:** Reconstitute 500-mg vial with 2 mL of 1% lidocaine HCl injection without epinephrine, and the 750-mg vial with 3 mL of 1% lidocaine.
- **Stability:** Administer suspension within 1 hr of preparation.
- **Preparation:** Do not mix suspension with any other medications.
- **Administration:** Slowly inject deep into the large gluteus maximus (buttock) muscle rather than the lateral aspect of the thigh to minimize discomfort.

PRECAUTIONS

HEALTH-RELATED

- Use imipenem and cilastatin cautiously in patients with a history of seizures, renal impairment, or sensitivity to penicillins.
- **Hemodialysis patients:** Not recommended for patients with a creatinine clearance of less than 5 mL/min unless hemodialysis in done within 48 hr to reduce the possibility of seizures.

AGE-RELATED

- **Children:** Drug may be used safely in children. Use preservative-free solutions for reconstitution of neonatal doses.
- **Elderly:** Age-related renal impairment may require a dosage adjustment.

PREGNANCY/LACTATION-RELATED

- Pregnancy category C; unknown if excreted in breast milk.

MONITORING

- **Baseline assessment:** Determine history of allergies, particularly to betalactams, cephalosporins, or penicillins, before beginning drug therapy. Determine history of seizures.
- **Baseline lab work:** CBC with WBC differential. Biochemical profile including K+, BUN, and creatinine levels to evaluate renal function and liver enzymes. Obtain culture of infected area before drug administration (wound, blood, sputum, urine, CSF) as appropriate.
- **Injection site reaction:** Evaluate for injection site pain or phlebitis as evidenced by heat, pain, and red streaking over the vein.
- **Superinfections:** Assess the mouth for white patches on the mucous membranes or tongue and for severe mouth or tongue soreness; assess for severe anal or genital pruritus or discharge.
- **Possible *Clostridium difficile* colitis:** Monitor BUN, creatinine, and potassium levels if the patient manifests myalgia or brown urine indicative of myoglobinuria. Urinalysis is used to diagnose myoglobinuria.
- **Handwashing:** If *C. difficile* (antibiotic-associated) colitis develops, wash hands with antibacterial soap. Alcohol-based foam is ineffective against *C. difficile* spores.

- **Nephrotoxicity:** Monitor intake and output and renal function test results to assess for nephrotoxicity.
- **Evenly spaced doses:** Space doses evenly around the clock and continue administration of imipenem-cilastatin for the full course of treatment. Advise patients to continue dosage regime if treatment will continue outside the hospital.
- **Seizures:** Observe for seizures and tremors.
- **Patient education:** When using imipenem-cilastatin outside the hospital, advise to immediately report severe diarrhea and to avoid taking antidiarrheals until directed to do so. Instruct to promptly report troublesome or serious adverse reactions, including infusion site pain, redness, or swelling; nausea or vomiting, or rash or itching to a health care provider.

SERIOUS ADVERSE REACTIONS

- **Hypersensitivity:** Patients with a history of allergies, especially to betalactams, cephalosporins, or penicillin, are at increased risk for developing a hypersensitivity reaction marked by severe pruritus, angioedema, bronchospasm, and anaphylaxis.
- **Management of hypersensitivity:** May require treatment with epinephrine and other emergency measures including oxygen, endotracheal intubation, mechanical ventilation, IV fluids, IV antihistamines, corticosteroids, and vasopressors.
- **Serum sickness–like reaction:** Stevens-Johnson syndrome, erythema multiforme, rashes, other skin lesions, accompanied by arthralgia/arthritis with or without fever.
- **Seizures:** Rare; reported primarily in renal failure patients not treated with reduced doses or when hemodialysis was not provided within 48 hr of dosing.

OVERDOSE/TOXICITY

- **Nephrotoxicity:** May occur, especially in patients with preexisting renal disease.
- **Superinfections:** Antibiotic-associated colitis (pseudomembranous colitis) and other superinfections may result from altered bacterial balance.
- **Management of *C. difficile* (antibiotic-associated) colitis:** Discontinue medication. Oral vancomycin (Vancocin) or metronidazole (Flagyl) are the most effective treatments for antibiotic-associated (pseudomembranous) colitis.
- **GI decontamination:** No specific recommendations.

ANTIDOTE/DIALYSIS

- **Antidote:** No specific recommendations.
- **Dialysis:** Imipenem is removed by hemodialysis and peritoneal dialysis and is likely removed using high-permeability hemodialysis.

imipramine

im-ip'-ra-meen

Classes

Chemical: dibenzazepine derivative, tertiary amine

Therapeutic: antidepressant, tricyclic, anti-incontinence agent

Pregnancy Category: D

Trade Names

Prescription: Apo-Imipramine ♣, Tofranil, Tofranil PM

Do not confuse imipramine with desipramine or imipenem.

CLINICAL PHARMACOLOGY

Mechanism of Action

A tricyclic antidepressant, antibulimic, anticataplectic, antinarcoleptic, antineuralgic, antineuritic, and antipanic agent that blocks the reuptake of neurotransmitters, such as norepinephrine and serotonin, at presynaptic membranes, increasing their concentration at postsynaptic receptor sites. **Therapeutic Effect:** Relieves depression and controls nocturnal enuresis.

PHARMACOKINETICS

Rapidly, well absorbed following PO administration. Protein binding: More than 90%. Metabolized in liver, with first-pass effect. Excreted in urine as metabolites. **Half-life:** 6-18 hr.

AVAILABILITY

Tablets (Tofranil): 10 mg, 25 mg, 50 mg.
Capsules (Tofranil-PM): 75 mg, 100 mg, 125 mg, 150 mg.

INDICATIONS AND DOSAGE

Depression

PO

Adults: Initially, 75-100 mg/day in 3-4 divided doses. May gradually increase to 300 mg/day then reduce dosage to effective maintenance level 50-150 mg/day. **Elderly:** Initially, 10-25 mg/day at bedtime. May increase by 10-25 mg every 3-7 days. Range: 50-150 mg/day. **Children:** 1.5 mg/kg/day. May increase by 1 mg/kg every 3-4 days. Maximum: 5 mg/kg/day in 1-4 divided doses.

Enuresis

PO

Children older than 6 yr: Initially, 10-25 mg at bedtime. May increase by 25 mg/day after 1 wk. Maximum: 75 mg for children older than 12 yr, 50 mg for children 6-12 yr.

OFF-LABEL USES

Treatment of attention-deficit/hyperactivity disorder, cataplexy associated with narcolepsy, neurogenic pain, panic disorder

CONTRAINDICATIONS

Acute recovery period after MI, use within 14 days of MAOIs, hypersensitivity to imipramine

I

INTERACTIONS

Drug: Alcohol, other CNS depressants: May increase the hypotensive effects and CNS and respiratory depression caused by imipramine. **Antithyroid agents:** May increase the risk of agranulocytosis. **Cimetidine:** May increase imipramine blood concentration and risk of toxicity. **Clonidine, guanadrel:** May decrease the effects of these drugs. **Gatifloxacin, grepafloxacin, moxifloxacin, sparfloxacin, type Ia and type III antidysrhythmic drugs:** May prolong the QTc interval. **MAOIs:** May increase the risk of neuroleptic malignant syndrome, hyperpyrexia, hypertensive crisis, and seizures. **Phenothiazines:** May increase the anticholinergic and sedative effects of imipramine. **Phenytoin, rifampin, carbamazepine:** May decrease the imipramine blood concentration. **Sympathomimetics:** May increase the risk of cardiac effects. **Fluoxetine, quinine, paroxetine, ritonavir, ropinorole, delavirdine, quinidine:** May increase effects of imipramine. **Herbal: Ginkgo biloba:** May decrease seizure threshold. **St. John's wort:** May increase imipramine's pharmacologic effects and risk of toxicity. **Food:** None known.

DIAGNOSTIC TEST EFFECTS

May alter blood glucose levels and ECG readings. Therapeutic serum drug level is 225-300 ng/mL; toxic serum drug level is greater than 500 ng/mL.

SIDE-EFFECTS

Frequent: Somnolence, fatigue, dry mouth, blurred vision, constipation, delayed micturition, orthostatic hypotension, diaphoresis, impaired concentration, increased appetite, urine retention, photosensitivity. **Occasional:** GI disturbances (nausea, metallic taste). **Rare:** Paradoxical reactions, (agitation, restlessness, nightmares, insomnia), extrapyramidal symptoms (particularly fine hand tremor).

CRITICAL CARE CONSIDERATIONS

ADMINISTRATION/HANDLING

PO ALERT

- Give imipramine with food or milk if GI distress occurs.
- Do not crush or break film-coated tablets.
- Make sure at least 14 days elapse between the use of MAOIs and imipramine.

PRECAUTIONS

HEALTH-RELATED

- Use imipramine cautiously in patients with cardiac disease, diabetes mellitus, glaucoma, hiatal hernia, history of seizures, history of urinary obstruction or retention, hyperthyroidism, increased intraocular pressure (IOP), benign prostatic hyperplasia, renal or hepatic disease, or schizophrenia.
- **Cytochrome P450 metabolism:** Imipramine is metabolized by cytochrome P450 2D6, which may prompt numerous drug interactions.

AGE-RELATED

- **Children:** Imipramine is not recommended for children under 6 yr.
- **Elderly:** Administer a lower dosage due to increased risk for drug toxicity.

PREGNANCY/LACTATION-RELATED

- Pregnancy category D; likely to be excreted in human breast milk; use with caution.

MONITORING

- **Baseline assessment:** Observe and document the patient's appearance, behavior, interest in the environment, mood, and sleep pattern.
- **Baseline and ongoing lab work:** CBC and biochemical profile including blood glucose, liver enzymes, and renal function tests before and periodically during long-term therapy.
- **Baseline diagnostic tests:** Baseline 12-lead ECG if patient is at risk for dysrhythmias. Children and patients with conduction defects have higher incidence of dysrhythmias.

- **Suicidal patients:** Closely supervise patients at risk for suicide during early therapy. As depression lessens, energy level improves, increasing the likelihood of suicide attempts.
- **Therapeutic response:** Assess for improved appearance, behavior, level of interest, mood, and sleep pattern.
- **Cardiac effects:** Monitor for tachycardia/tachydysrhythmias and hypotension.
- **Serum drug levels:** Monitor serum drug levels. Therapeutic level is 225-300 ng/mL for imipramine. Toxic level is greater than 500 ng/mL.
- **Urinary retention:** Palpate the bladder for distention unrelieved by attempts to void.
- **Patient education:** Inform patients they will develop a tolerance to the drug's anticholinergic, hypotensive, and sedative effects during early therapy. Patients develop sensitivity to sunlight, making it easy to get sunburned. Urge to report any visual disturbances. Warn to avoid tasks that require alertness or motor skills until response to the drug is known. Caution against abruptly discontinuing imipramine. Inform that the full therapeutic effect may not be evident for 2 to 3 wk. Some improvement may be seen 2-5 days after starting therapy. Advise to change positions slowly to prevent dizziness.

SERIOUS ADVERSE REACTIONS

- **Abrupt withdrawal:** Abrupt discontinuation after prolonged therapy may produce headache, malaise, nausea, vomiting, and vivid dreams.
- Blood dyscrasias and cholestatic jaundice occur rarely.

OVERDOSE/TOXICITY

- **Cardiac:** Dysrhythmias, fatigue, dyspnea
- **Dysrhythmias/ECG changes:** Sinus tachycardia, prolonged PR interval, prolonged QT interval, widened QRS complex greater than 100 msec, right axis deviation (positive deflection) of terminal QRS complex in lead AVR greater than 3 mm.
- **Neurologic:** Seizures, severe somnolence, hallucinations, agitation, weakness, fever.
- **Antimuscarinic effects:** Dilated pupils, blurred vision, tachycardia, hyperthermia, hypertension, decreased oral and bronchial secretions, dry skin, ileus, urinary retention, increased muscle tone, tremor.
- **Toxicity:** Symptoms occur within the first 2 hr of ingestion or not at all. Should be screened by the ECG and serum and/or urine TCA levels.
- **GI decontamination:** Activated charcoal binds TCAs effectively and if used should be given in one dose within the first few hours of ingestion; the risks of using ipecac to induce vomiting outweighs the benefits; adding gastric lavage to activated charcoal may enhance removal effects if done within the first hr of ingestion.

ANTIDOTE/DIALYSIS

- **Antidote:** No specific antidote, but overdose may be managed as follows:
- **Serum alkalization/ventilator driven:** Ventilator driven hyperventilation with intravenous saline to raise the pH to 7.50-7.55 to induce respiratory alkalosis.
- **Sodium bicarbonate therapy:** Sodium bicarbonate intravenous infusion with initial bolus of 1-2 meq/kg until clinical improvement is noted or blood pH is 7.50-7.55 (induced metabolic alkalosis). Higher blood pH may be deleterious to the patient. IV potassium supplementation may be needed to correct hypokalemia which results from use of bicarbonate infusion.
- **Fluid volume expansion:** IV fluid infusion is used to manage hypotension. Vasopressors are used only when patients do not respond to fluid therapy.
- **Seizures:** May respond spontaneously; if persistent, benzodiazepines (lorazepam, diazepam) may be used; phenobarbital or propofol may be used if other medications fail.
- **Dialysis:** Imipramine is not removed by hemodialysis or peritoneal dialysis. No data are available on removal using high-permeability hemodialysis.

immune globulin (Human)

i-myoon' glob'-yoo-lin

Classes

Chemical: human immune globulin derivative

Therapeutic: antiinflammatory

Pregnancy Category: C

Trade Names

Prescription: Baygam, Carimune, Gamimune N 5%, Gamimune N 10%, Gammagard S/D, Gammar-P-IV, Gamunex, Iveegam EN, Octagam, Panglobulin, Polygam S/D, Sandoglobulin, Vivaglobin

Do not confuse Sandoglobulin with Sandimmune or Sandostatin.

CLINICAL PHARMACOLOGY

Mechanism of Action

An immune serum that increases antibody titer and antigen-antibody reaction. **Therapeutic Effect:** Provides passive immunity against infection; induces rapid increase in platelet count; produces antiinflammatory effect.

PHARMACOKINETICS

Evenly distributed between intravascular and extravascular space. **Half-life:** 21-23 days.

AVAILABILITY

Injection solution: 5% (Gamimune N 5%, Octagam), 10% (Gamimune N 10%, Gammagard, Gamunex).
Injection powder for reconstitution: 0.5 g (Iveegam EN), 1 g (Carimune, Gammar-P-IV, Iveegam EN, Panglobulin, Sandoglobulin), 2.5 g (Gammar-P-IV, Gammagard S/D, Iveegam EN, Polygam S/D, Sandoglobulin), 3 g (Carimune, Panglobulin, Sandoglobulin), 5 g (Gammar-P-IV, Gammagard S/D, Iveegam EN, Polygam S/D, Sandoglobulin), 6 g (Carimune, Panglobulin, Sandoglobulin), 10 g (Gammar-P-IV, Gammagard S/D, Polygam S/D, Sandoglobulin), 12 g (Carimune, Panglobulin, Sandoglobulin).
Subcutaneous injection formulation (Vivaglobin): 160 mg/mL.

INDICATIONS AND DOSAGE

Primary immunodeficiency syndrome

IV

Adults, Elderly, Children: 200-400 mg/kg once monthly.

Subcutaneous

Adults, Elderly: 100-200 mg/kg once weekly.

Idiopathic thrombocytopenic purpura (ITP)

IV

Adults, Elderly, Children: 400 mg/kg/day for 5 days, or 1000 mg/kg/day for 1-2 days.

Kawasaki disease

IV

Adults, Elderly, Children: 2 g/kg as a single dose, or 400 mg/kg/day for 4 days.

Chronic lymphocytic leukemia

IV

Adults, Elderly, Children: 400 mg/kg every 3 wk.

Bone marrow transplant

IV

Adults, Elderly, Children: 400-500 mg/kg/dose every wk for 12 wk, then every mo.

OFF-LABEL USES

Control and prevention of infections in infants and children with immunosuppression due to AIDS or AIDS-related complex; prevention of acute infections in immunosuppressed patients; prevention and treatment of infections in high-risk, preterm, low-birth-weight neonates; treatment of chronic inflammatory demyelinating polyneuropathies and multiple sclerosis

CONTRAINDICATIONS

Allergies to immune globulin (human), gamma globulin, thimerosal, or anti-IgA antibodies; isolated IgA deficiency

INTERACTIONS

Drug: Live-virus vaccines: May increase vaccine side effects, potentiate virus replication, and decrease antibody response to the vaccine. **Herbal:** None known. **Food:** None known.

DIAGNOSTIC TEST EFFECTS

None known.

IV INCOMPATIBILITIES

Do not mix IV immune globulin (IVIG) with any other medications.

SIDE-EFFECTS

Frequent: Tachycardia, backache, headache, arthralgia, myalgia. **Occasional:** Fatigue, wheezing, injection site rash or pain, leg cramps, urticaria, bluish lips and nailbeds, lightheadedness

CRITICAL CARE CONSIDERATIONS

ADMINISTRATION/HANDLING

IV ALERT

- **Storage:** Refer to individual IV preparations for storage requirements and information about stability after reconstitution.
- **Reconstitution:** Reconstitute IGIV only with the diluent provided by the manufacturer. Discard partially used or turbid preparations. When reconstitution is performed outside a sterile laminar flow hood, infusion should begin within 2 hr of reconstitution.
- **Preparation:** Administer IVIG by infusion only through separate tubing. Avoid mixing IVIG with other medications or IV infusion fluids.

- **IV infusion:** Infusion rate varies among products. Monitor BP and vital signs diligently during and immediately after IV administration.
- **Hypotension:** A precipitous fall in BP may indicate an anaphylactic reaction. Stop the infusion immediately if anaphylaxis is suspected. Keep epinephrine readily available.

PRECAUTIONS

HEALTH-RELATED

- **High risk for renal failure:** Use IVIG cautiously in patients with cardiovascular disease, diabetes mellitus, history of thrombosis, impaired renal function, sepsis, or volume depletion and in those who use nephrotoxic drugs concurrently. IVIG products should be administered using the minimal concentration at the minimal possible infusion rate to help prevent nephrotoxicity.
- **Sucrose as a stabilizer:** IVIG products containing sucrose as a stabilizer are more likely to cause acute renal failure in high risk patients.

AGE-RELATED

- **Children:** No age-related precautions have been noted.
- **Elderly:** Age-related renal function and other organ dysfunction place elderly at much higher risk for acute renal failure. Use with extreme caution.

PREGNANCY/LACTATION-RELATED

- Pregnancy category C; safety for use in breast-feeding has not been established.

MONITORING

- **Baseline assessment:** Assess for dehydration. Ensure patients are well hydrated before giving IVIG. Examine arms to identify the largest vein. Use of larger veins (e.g., antecubital) is recommended to reduce infusion site discomfort.
- **Baseline lab work:** CBC with WBC differential and platelet count; biochemical panel including blood glucose level, BUN, and creatinine.
- **Hypersensitivity:** Control infusion rate carefully. A too-rapid infusion increases the risk of a precipitous drop in BP and an anaphylactic reaction, marked by chest tightness, chills, diaphoresis, facial flushing, fever, nausea, and vomiting. Stop the infusion temporarily for anaphylaxis. Assess closely during the infusion, especially in the first hr.
- **Hypotension:** Monitor for tachycardia and hypotension continuously, which may indicate onset of anaphylaxis.
- **Aseptic meningitis:** Assess for decreased mental status, headache, nausea, and nuchal rigidity. May begin 2-48 hr after receiving infusion.
- **Thrombocytopenia:** Monitor platelet count of those treated for ITP.
- **Minimum serum level:** Serum IgG level should be greater than or equal to 300 mg/dL following infusion.
- **Patient education:** Explain the rationale for IVIG therapy. Inform to expect a rapid response to therapy, which will last 1-3 mo. Instruct to report promptly dyspnea, decreased urine output, fluid retention, edema, or sudden weight gain to a health care provider.

SERIOUS ADVERSE REACTIONS

- **Hypersensitivity reaction:** Anxiety, arthralgia, dizziness, flushing, myalgia, palpitations, and pruritus, occur rarely.
- **Anaphylactic reactions:** Rare, but the incidence increases with repeated injections of IVIG. Keep epinephrine readily available.
- **Aseptic meningitis syndrome:** Somnolence, severe headache, fever, nausea, vomiting, nuchal rigidity, photophobia and ocular pain with eye movements. Seen most often with 2-g doses. May begin 2-48 hr after receiving treatment.
- **Thrombosis:** Seen more commonly in patients with diabetes, cardiovascular disease, cerebrovascular disease, and hypertension.

OVERDOSE/TOXICITY

- **Anaphylaxis:** Chest tightness, chills, diaphoresis, dizziness, facial flushing, nausea, vomiting, fever, and hypotension.
- **Nephrotoxicity:** Acute renal failure, osmotic nephrosis, and death.
- **Management:** Reduce infusion rate for any discomfort. If patients experience fluid overload, manage with diuretics (e.g., furosemide [Lasix]). Consider premedication with hydrocortisone 1-2 mg/kg 30 min before start of infusion, or use of acetaminophen and *diphenhydrAMINE (Benadryl) for patients who do not tolerate infusions. Selection of another brand of IVIG sometimes resolves intolerance. Manage anaphylaxis immediately with epinephrine, *diphenhydrAMINE, corticosteroids, and endotracheal intubation if needed to maintain airway/ventilation, oxygen, IV fluid infusion, and vasopressors.

- **GI decontamination:** No specific recommendations.

ANTIDOTE/DIALYSIS
- **Antidote:** No specific recommendations.
- **Dialysis:** IVIG is unlikely to be removed by hemodialysis or peritoneal dialysis. No data are available on removal using high-permeability hemodialysis.

inamrinone lactate

in-am'-ri-nohn lack'-tate

Classes
Chemical: bipyridine derivative
Therapeutic: cardiac inotropic agent

Pregnancy Category: C

Trade Names
Prescription: Inamrinone

Do not confuse inamrinone with amiodarone.

CLINICAL PHARMACOLOGY
Mechanism of Action
A positive inotropic agent that inhibits myocardial cyclic adenosine monophosphate (cAMP) phosphodiesterase activity and directly stimulates cardiac contractility. Peripheral vasodilation reduces both preload and afterload. **Therapeutic Effect:** Reduces preload and afterload; increases cardiac output.

PHARMACOKINETICS
Onset is 2-5 min, peak is 10 min, duration is 30 min (low dose) to 2 hr (high dose). Protein binding: 10-49%. Partially metabolized in liver. Excreted in urine as both inamrinone and its metabolites. **Half-life:** 3-6 hr (half-life increased with congestive heart failure).

AVAILABILITY
Injection: 5 mg/mL (Inamrinone).

INDICATIONS AND DOSAGE
Short-term management of intractable heart failure
IV infusion (continuous)
Adults: Initially, 0.75 mg/kg loading dose over 2-3 min followed by a maintenance infusion of 5-10 mcg/kg/min. A bolus dose of 0.75 mg/kg may be given 30 min after the initiation of therapy. Use within 24 hr and do not dilute with solutions that contain dextrose. Maximum: 10 mg/kg/day.

CONTRAINDICATIONS
Severe aortic or pulmonic valvular disease; hypersensitivity to inamrinone or bisulfites.

INTERACTIONS
Drug: Digitalis: May increase the inotropic effects. **Diuretics:** May cause hypovolemia and decrease filling pressure. **Herbal:** None known. **Food:** None known.

DIAGNOSTIC TEST EFFECTS
None known.

IV INCOMPATIBILITIES
Furosemide (Lasix), D_5W

SIDE-EFFECTS
Occasional: Dysrhythmia, nausea, hypotension, thrombocytopenia. **Rare:** Fever, vomiting, abdominal pain, anorexia, chest pain, decreased tear production, hepatotoxicity, burning at the site of injection, hypersensitivity to inamrinone

CRITICAL CARE CONSIDERATIONS

ADMINISTRATION/HANDLING
IV ALERT
- **Storage:** Store unopened vials at room temperature. Do not freeze. Store reconstituted solution at room temperature. Reconstituted solutions should be used within 24 hr.
- **Dilution:** *Use saline-based solution only.* May not be diluted or reconstituted with dextrose solutions (chemically incompatible). Give IV bolus dose undiluted. Follow instructions of manufacturer for dilution to specific concentrations.
- **Furosemide (Lasix):** Do not administer furosemide in IV lines containing inamrinone; combination will result in an immediate precipitate.

UNDILUTED INAMRINONE LOADING DOSE (0.75 mg/kg)

Weight (kg)	30	40	50	60	70	80	90	100
mL undiluted inamrinone	4.5	6	7.5	9	10.5	12	13.5	15

INAMRINONE CONTINUOUS IV INFUSION (RATE mL/hr OF 2.5 mg/mL SOLUTION)

Weight (kg)	30	40	50	60	70	80	90	100
2.5 mcg/kg/min	2	2.5	3	3.5	4	5	5.5	6
5 mcg/kg/min	4	5	6	7	8	10	11	12
7.5 mcg/kg/min	5	7	9	11	13	14	16	18
10 mcg/kg/min	7	10	12	14	17	19	22	24

PRECAUTIONS

HEALTH-RELATED

- **Hypovolemia:** Use cautiously in patients with hypovolemia.
- **Ventricular dysrhythmias:** Use cautiously in patients with premature ventricular contractions (PVCs) or runs of ventricular tachycardia.
- **Acute MI:** Not recommended for use in acute phase of myocardial infarction because of lack of clinical trials to date.
- **Atrial fibrillation/flutter:** May increase ventricular rate response in atrial fibrillation/flutter. Premedication with digitalis (digitalization) is recommended.
- **Long-term use:** May result in increased risk of death, especially in New York Health Association class IV heart failure patients.

AGE-RELATED

- **Children:** Safety of inamrinone in children has not been established but drug has been used successfully. Elimination half-life is shorter in children.
- **Elderly:** May be more sensitive to the drug's hypotensive effects. Age-related renal impairment may require dosage adjustment.

PREGNANCY/LACTATION-RELATED

- Pregnancy category C; unknown if excreted in breast milk; safety has not been established for breast-feeding women.

MONITORING

- **Baseline assessment:** Obtain BP and heart rate immediately before each intermittent inamrinone dose, in addition to regular BP monitoring. Monitor BP hourly and as needed for instability during continuous infusion.
- **Baseline lab work:** Biochemical profile including potassium, calcium, magnesium, BUN, creatinine, and liver enzymes (AST [SGOT], ALT [SGPT], alkaline phosphatase). B type natriuretic peptide (BNP) level to assess heart failure. CBC including platelet count. Correct electrolyte abnormalities or hypovolemia prior to use. Dehydrated patients are at increased risk for hypotension.
- **Baseline diagnostic tests:** 12-lead ECG and echocardiogram to assess for dysrhythmias, myocardial ischemia, and heart failure.
- **Hemodynamic:** Monitor cardiac index (CI), stroke volume (SV), systemic vascular resistance (SVR), pulmonary vascular resistance (PVR), BP, and heart rate. Cardiac index and SV should increase, SVR and PVR should decrease.
- **Cardiac:** Continuous ECG for dysrhythmias, tachycardia, and ST depression or elevation. Drug should be discontinued for severe tachycardia, dysrhythmias, or ST changes.
- **Ongoing monitoring:** Platelet count, fluid status, and liver and renal function.
- **Patient education:** Teach to report any dizziness or trouble swallowing. Explain that inamrinone is for short-term therapy.

SERIOUS ADVERSE REACTIONS

- **Hypersensitivity reaction:** Interstitial shadowing and vascular pulmonary densities on chest x-ray, hypoxemia, pleuritis, pericarditis, myositis.

OVERDOSE/TOXICITY

- Overdose may cause severe hypotension and ventricular dysrhythmias.
- Thrombocytopenia, liver enzyme elevation, ascites, and elevated BUN and creatinine.
- **Management:** Discontinue infusion if significant thrombocytopenia (platelets less than 60,000), liver enzyme elevation, increased BUN/creatinine occurs. Give IV fluids and vasopressors for hypotension. Manage dysrhythmias according to Advanced Cardiac Life Support (ACLS) guidelines.
- **GI decontamination:** No specific recommendations.

ANTIDOTE/DIALYSIS

- **Antidote:** No specific recommendations.
- **Dialysis:** Inamrinone lactate is unlikely to be removed by hemodialysis, and is not removed by peritoneal dialysis. No data are available on removal using high-permeability hemodialysis.

indapamide

See Diuretics (p. 956)

indinavir

See HIV Medications (p. 961)

indomethacin

in-doe-meth'-a-sin

Classes

Chemical: indole acetic acid derivative
Therapeutic: NSAID, antipyretic, nonnarcotic analgesic

Pregnancy Category: C, D (3rd trimester)

Trade Names

Prescription: Apo-Indomethacin ♣, Indocin, Indocin IV, Indocin SR, Indo-Lemmon, Novomethacin ♣

Do not confuse Indocin with Imodium or Vicodin.

CLINICAL PHARMACOLOGY

Mechanism of Action

An NSAID that produces analgesic and antiinflammatory effects by inhibiting prostaglandin synthesis. Also increases the sensitivity of the premature ductus to the dilating effects of prostaglandins. **Therapeutic Effect:** Reduces the inflammatory response and intensity of pain. Closure of the patent ductus arteriosus.

PHARMACOKINETICS

Rectal absorption more rapid than oral administration. Protein binding: 99%. Metabolized in liver. Excreted in urine. **Half-life:** 4.5 hr.

AVAILABILITY

Capsules (Indocin): 25 mg, 50 mg.
Capsules (sustained release [Indocin SR]): 75 mg.
Oral suspension (Indocin): 25 mg/5 mL.
Powder for injection (Indocin IV): 1 mg.
Suppositories: 50 mg.

INDICATIONS AND DOSAGE

Moderate to severe rheumatoid arthritis, osteoarthritis, ankylosing spondylitis

PO

Adults, Elderly: Initially, 25 mg 2-3 times per day; increased by 25-50 mg/wk up to 150-200 mg/day. Or 75 mg/day (extended-release) up to 75 mg twice per day. **Children:** 1-2 mg/kg/day. Maximum: 150-200 mg/day.

Acute gouty arthritis

PO

Adults, Elderly: 50 mg 3 times per day.

Acute shoulder pain

PO

Adults, Elderly: 75-150 mg/day in 3-4 divided doses.

Usual rectal dosage

Adults, Elderly: 50 mg 4 times per day. **Children:** Initially, 1.5-2.5 mg/kg/day, increased up to 4 mg/kg/day. Maximum: 150-200 mg/day.

Patent ductus arteriosus

IV

Neonates: Initially, 0.2 mg/kg. Subsequent doses are based on age, as follows: **Neonates older than 7 days:** 0.25 mg/kg every 12-24 hr for second and third doses. **Neonates 2-7 days:** 0.2 mg/kg for second and third doses. **Neonates less than 48 hr:** 0.1 mg/kg for second and third doses.

OFF-LABEL USES

Treatment of fever due to malignancy, pericarditis, psoriatic arthritis, rheumatic complications associated with Paget's disease of bone, vascular headache

CONTRAINDICATIONS

Active GI bleeding or ulcerations; hypersensitivity to aspirin, indomethacin, or other NSAIDs; renal impairment, thrombocytopenia; third trimester of pregnancy

INTERACTIONS

Drug: Aminoglycosides: May increase the blood concentration of these drugs in neonates. **Antihypertensives, diuretics:** May decrease the effects of these drugs. **Aspirin, other salicylates:** May increase the risk of GI side effects such as bleeding. **Bone marrow depressants:** May increase the risk of hematologic reactions. **Heparin, oral anticoagulants, thrombolytics:** May increase the effects of these drugs. **Lithium:** May increase the blood concentration and risk of toxicity of lithium. **Methotrexate:** May increase the risk of methotrexate toxicity. **Probenecid:** May increase the indomethacin blood concentration. **Triamterene:** May potentiate acute renal failure. Do not give concurrently. **Herbal: Feverfew:** May decrease the effects of feverfew. **Ginkgo biloba:** May increase the risk of bleeding. **Food:** None known.

DIAGNOSTIC TEST EFFECTS

May prolong bleeding time. May alter blood glucose level. May increase BUN level, and serum creatinine, potassium, AST (SGOT), and ALT (SGPT) levels. May decrease serum sodium level and platelet count.

IV INCOMPATIBILITIES

Amino acid injection, calcium gluconate, cimetidine (Tagamet), *DOBUTamine (Dobutrex), *DOPamine (Intropin), gentamicin (Garamycin), tobramycin (Nebcin)

IV COMPATIBILITIES

Insulin, potassium

SIDE-EFFECTS

Frequent (12%-3%): Headache, nausea, vomiting, dyspepsia, dizziness. **Occasional (less than 3%):** Depression, tinnitus, diaphoresis, somnolence, constipation, diarrhea, bleeding disturbances in patent ductus arteriosus. **Rare:** Hypertension, confusion, urticaria, pruritus, rash, blurred vision

CRITICAL CARE CONSIDERATIONS

ADMINISTRATION/HANDLING

PO ALERT

- Give indomethacin after meals or with food or antacids.
- Do not crush extended-release capsules.

IV ALERT

- **Neonatal patients with patent ductus arteriosus:** IV injection is the preferred route. The drug may also be given orally, by NG tube, or rectally. Administer no more than 3 doses at 12- to 24-hr intervals.
- **Reconstitution:** Add 1 or 2 mL preservative-free sterile water for injection or 0.9% NaCl to the 1-mg vial to provide a concentration of 1 mg or 0.5 mg/mL, respectively. Do not dilute the solution any further.
- **Administration:** Give solution IV over 5-10 sec immediately after reconstitution. The solution normally appears clear; discard if cloudy or contains precipitate. Discard any unused portion.

RECTAL ALERT

- May refrigerate soft suppositories for 30 min or run cold water over the foil wrapper.
- **Administration:** Moisten suppository with cold water before inserting into rectum.

PRECAUTIONS

HEALTH-RELATED

- Use indomethacin cautiously in patients with cardiac dysfunction, hypertension, epilepsy, or hepatic or renal impairment, and in those receiving anticoagulant therapy concurrently.

AGE-RELATED

- **Children:** Safety and efficacy of indomethacin have not been established in children under 14 yr. However, drug is used in infants for closure of patent ductus arteriosus.
- **Elderly:** Age-related renal impairment may prompt dosage adjustment.

PREGNANCY/LACTATION-RELATED

- Pregnancy category C, D if used in the third trimester. Crosses placenta. Excreted in breast milk.

MONITORING

- **Baseline assessment:** Assess the duration, location, onset, and type of inflammation or pain. Inspect the arthritic joints for deformity, immobility, and skin condition. Assess baseline heart sounds in neonates with patent ductus arteriosus. Note the location, intensity, quality, and timing of murmurs.
- **Baseline and ongoing lab work:** CBC, platelet count, and biochemical panel including BUN, creatinine, serum alkaline phosphatase, bilirubin, AST (SGOT), and ALT (SGPT) levels.
- **Side effects:** Monitor for dyspepsia, headache, and a change in daily bowel activity and stool consistency.
- **Therapeutic response:** Evaluate for pain relief; improved grip strength; increased joint mobility; and decreased joint pain, tenderness, stiffness, and swelling.
- **Infection:** Indomethacin use may mask signs of infection.
- **Neonatal patients:** Monitor BP, ECG, heart rate, platelet count, serum sodium, and blood glucose levels and urine output. Auscultate heart sounds to detect the presence of changes in a murmur.
- **Patient education:** Instruct to swallow enteric-coated tablets whole and not to crush or chew. Advise taking indomethacin with food or milk if experiencing GI upset. Warn to avoid alcohol and aspirin during indomethacin therapy because these substances increase the risk of GI bleeding. Instruct to report a persistent headache, black stools, changes in vision, pruritus, rash, or weight gain.

SERIOUS ADVERSE REACTIONS

- **GI effects:** Paralytic ileus and ulceration of the esophagus, stomach, duodenum, or

I

small intestine leading to GI bleeding may occur.

- **Renal insufficiency:** Patients with impaired renal function may develop hyperkalemia and worsening of renal impairment.
- **Neuropsychiatric:** Indomethacin use may aggravate epilepsy, parkinsonism, and depression or other psychiatric disturbances.
- **Ocular effects:** Corneal deposits and retinal disturbance including macular damage may occur with prolonged therapy.

OVERDOSE/TOXICITY

- **Symptoms:** Hypotonia, muscle fasciculations, twitching, bone marrow suppression, metabolic acidosis, nausea, vomiting, diarrhea, GI bleeding, abdominal pain, volume depletion with secondary hypotension, tachycardia, pulmonary edema and acute respiratory distress syndrome, acute psychosis, seizures, CNS depression following agitation.
- **Nephrotoxicity:** Elevated BUN, creatinine, dysuria, hematuria, proteinuria, oliguria or anuria, possible hyperkalemia and nephrotic syndrome.
- **Patients with patent ductus arteriosus:** Metabolic acidosis or alkalosis, apnea, and bradycardia occur rarely.
- **GI decontamination:** No specific recommendations.

ANTIDOTE/DIALYSIS

- **Antidote:** No specific antidote recommended. Treatment should be supportive and directed at symptoms.
- **Dialysis:** Indomethacin is unlikely to be removed by peritoneal dialysis, and is not removed by hemodialysis. No data are available on removal using high-permeability hemodialysis.

infliximab

in-flix'-i-mab

Classes

Chemical: monoclonal antibody
Therapeutic: tumor necrosis factor α (TNF-α) antibody

Pregnancy Category: B

Trade Names

Prescription: Remicade

Do not confuse Remicade with Reminyl.

CLINICAL PHARMACOLOGY

Mechanism of Action

A monoclonal antibody that binds to tumor necrosis factor (TNF), inhibiting functional activity of TNF. Reduces infiltration of inflammatory cells. **Therapeutic Effect:** Decreases inflamed areas of the intestine.

PHARMACOKINETICS

Route	Onset	Peak	Duration
IV (Crohn's disease)	1-2 wk	N/A	8-48 wk
IV (Rheumatoid arthritis [RA])	3-7 days	N/A	6-12 wk

Absorbed into the GI tissue; primarily distributed in the vascular compartment. **Half-life:** 9.5 days.

AVAILABILITY

Powder for injection: 100 mg.

INDICATIONS AND DOSAGE

Crohn's disease (moderate to severe ulcerative colitis), psoriatic arthritis

IV Infusion

Adults, Elderly: Initially, 5 mg/kg at wk 0, 2, and 6. Maintenance: 5 mg/kg every 8 wk thereafter. May increase to 10 mg/kg in patients who initially respond but then lose control.

Ankylosing spondylitis

IV Infusion

Adults, Elderly: Initially, 5 mg/kg at wk 0, 2, and 6. Maintenance: 5 mg/kg every 6 wk thereafter.

Fistulizing Crohn's disease

IV Infusion

Adults, Elderly: Initially, 5 mg/kg at wk 0, 2, 6, then 5 mg/kg every 8 wk. May increase to 10 mg/kg if patient initially responds but then loses response.

Rheumatoid arthritis (RA)

IV Infusion

Adults, Elderly: Initially 3 mg/kg; followed by additional doses at wk 2 and 6, then every 8 wk.

OFF-LABEL USES

Heart failure, juvenile arthritis, psoriasis, reactive arthritis, sciatica

CONTRAINDICATIONS

Sensitivity to infliximab or murine proteins, sepsis, serious active infection, doses greater than 5 mg/kg in patients with heart failure (New York Heart Association class III or IV)

INTERACTIONS

Drug: Immunosuppressants: May reduce frequency of infusion reactions and antibodies to infliximab. **Live vaccines:** May decrease immune response. **Herbal:** None known. **Food:** None known.

DIAGNOSTIC TEST EFFECTS
None known.

IV INCOMPATIBILITIES
Do not infuse infliximab in the same IV line with other agents.

SIDE-EFFECTS
Frequent (22%-10%): Headache, nausea, fatigue, fever, diarrhea, abdominal pain, infusion reactions. **Occasional (9%-5%):** Pharyngitis, vomiting, pain, dizziness, bronchitis, rash, rhinitis, cough, pruritus, sinusitis, myalgia, back pain. **Rare (4%-1%):** Hypotension or hypertension, paresthesia, anxiety, depression, insomnia, diarrhea, urinary tract infection

CRITICAL CARE CONSIDERATIONS

ADMINISTRATION/HANDLING

IV ALERT
- **Storage:** Refrigerate vials. Infliximab is a protein.
- **Reconstitution:** Reconstitute each vial with 10 mL sterile water for injection, using a 21-gauge or smaller needle. Direct the stream of sterile water to the glass wall of the vial. Swirl the vial gently to dissolve the contents. Do not shake. Allow solution to stand for 5 min. The solution may develop a few translucent particles; do not use if opaque or foreign particles form. Solution should appear colorless to light yellow and opalescent; do not use if discolored.
- **Further dilution:** Withdraw/waste the volume of 0.9% NaCl from a 250-mL bag that is equal to the volume of reconstituted solution to be injected into the 250-mL bag (approximately 10 mL). Total dose to be infused should equal 250 mL. Slowly add reconstituted infliximab to the 250-mL infusion bag. Gently mix. Infusion concentration should range between 0.4 and 4 mg/mL.
- **IV intermittent infusion:** Administer IV infusion over 2 hr, using a set with a low-protein-binding filter.
- **Stability:** Begin infusion within 3 hr of reconstitution. Solution is preservative-free.

PRECAUTIONS

HEALTH-RELATED
- **Heart failure:** Infliximab is contraindicated in patients with moderate to severe (New York Heart Association class III/IV) heart failure.
- **Infection:** Use infliximab cautiously in patients with a history of recurrent infections. Fatal tuberculosis and invasive fungal infections (histoplasmosis, listeriosis, and pneumocystosis) have occurred during therapy.

AGE-RELATED
- **Children:** Safety and efficacy of infliximab have not been established in children.
- **Elderly:** Use infliximab cautiously because of a higher rate of infection in elderly.

PREGNANCY/LACTATION-RELATED
- Pregnancy category B; breast milk excretion unknown; nursing not recommended.

MONITORING
- **Baseline assessment:** Assess bowel habits and pattern of diarrhea. Obtain vital signs. Assess hydration status by examining for dry mucous membranes, poor skin turgor, and low urine output indicative of dehydration.
- **Baseline lab work:** CBC with WBC differential, erythrocyte sedimentation rate (ESR), and urinalysis. Tuberculosis skin test.
- **Baseline diagnostic tests:** Chest x-ray to assess for pneumonia, heart failure, or latent pulmonary infections.
- **Infection:** Assess for fever and elevated WBC count.
- **Heart failure:** Monitor for shortness of breath, weight gain, edema, pulmonary edema, decreased activity tolerance, especially if patients have a history of mild heart failure.
- **Crohn's disease:** Evaluate Crohn's patients' abdominal pain, C-reactive protein, and stool frequency.
- **Rheumatoid arthritis:** Evaluate arthritic patients' C-reactive protein and any decrease in pain, stiffness, and swollen joints.
- **Patient education:** Explain the need for follow-up lab work, such as erythrocyte sedimentation rate (ESR), C-reactive protein measurement, and urinalysis. Instruct the need to report signs of infection to a health care provider promptly. Instruct patients with rheumatoid arthritis to report increase in pain, stiffness, or swelling of joints. Tell patients with Crohn's disease to report changes in stool

color, consistency, or elimination pattern to a health care provider promptly.

SERIOUS ADVERSE REACTIONS

- Hypersensitivity reaction, development of human antichimeric antibody, which increases probability of an infusion reaction.

OVERDOSE/TOXICITY

- **Cardiotoxicity:** Shortness of breath, dyspnea, edema, pulmonary edema, or chest discomfort indicative of heart failure.
- **Lupuslike syndrome:** Fever, pleuritic pain, and pleural effusion may occur. Syndrome usually resolves within 10 days of when infusion is discontinued.
- **Management:** Discontinue infusion immediately for serious reactions/toxicity with signs of instability including tachycardia and hypotension. Administer acetaminophen, antihistamines, corticosteroids, and epinephrine as indicated. Use *DOPamine for hypotension and heart failure. *DOBUTamine may also be used for heart failure.
- **GI decontamination:** No specific recommendations.

ANTIDOTE/DIALYSIS

- **Antidote:** No specific recommendations.
- **Dialysis:** Infliximab is unlikely to be removed by hemodialysis, high-permeability hemodialysis, or peritoneal dialysis.

insulin group

in'-su-lin

Classes

Chemical: exogenous insulin
Therapeutic: antidiabetic, hypoglycemic

Pregnancy Category: B

Trade Names

Prescription: Rapid Acting—Insulin Aspart (*NovoLOG), Insulin Glulisine (Apidra), Insulin [inhaled (Exubera)], Insulin Lispro (*HumaLOG) **Prescription:** Regular Short Acting—*HumuLIN R, *NovoLIN R **Prescription:** Intermediate Acting—NPH (*HumuLIN N, *NovoLIN N, NPH Iletin II) **Prescription:** Lente—*HumuLIN L, Lente Iletin II, *NovoLIN L **Prescription:** Long-Acting—Insulin Glargine (Lantus Ultralente), Insulin Detemir (Levemir) **Prescription:** Intermediate- and short-acting mixtures—*HumuLIN 50/50, *HumuLIN 70/30, *HumaLOG Mix 75/25, *HumaLOG Mix 50/50, *NovoLIN 70/30, *NovoLOG Mix 70/30

CLINICAL PHARMACOLOGY

Mechanism of Action

An exogenous insulin that facilitates passage of glucose, potassium, and magnesium across the cellular membranes of skeletal and cardiac muscle and adipose tissue. Controls storage and metabolism of carbohydrates, protein, and fats. Promotes conversion of glucose to glycogen in the liver. **Therapeutic Effect:** Controls glucose levels in diabetic patients.

PHARMACOKINETICS

Drug Form	Onset (hr)	Peak (hr)	Duration (hr)
Glulisine	0.25	1	3-4
Lispro	0.25	0.5-1.5	4-5
Insulin aspart	0.25	1-3	3-5
Regular	0.5-1	2-4	5-7
Inhaled	0.5-1	2-4	5-7
NPH	1-2	6-14	24+
Lente	1-3	6-14	24+
Insulin glargine	3-4	N/A	24
Insulin detemir	3-4	6-8	6-23

AVAILABILITY

Rapid acting: Apidra, Exubera, *HumuLIN R, *NovoLIN R, *NovoLOG, *HumaLOG.
Intermediate acting: *HumuLIN L, *NovoLIN L, Lente Iletin II, *HumuLIN N, *NovoLIN N, NPH Illetin II.
Long acting: Lantus Ultralente, Levemir.
Intermediate- and short-acting mixtures: *HumuLIN 50/50, *HumuLIN 70/30, *HumaLOG Mix 75/25, *HumaLOG Mix 50/50, *NovoLIN 70/30, *NovoLOG Mix 70/30.

INDICATIONS AND DOSAGE

Treatment of insulin-dependent type 1 diabetes mellitus and non–insulin-dependent type 2 diabetes mellitus when diet or weight control has failed to maintain satisfactory blood glucose levels or in event of fever, infection, pregnancy, surgery, or trauma or severe endocrine, hepatic, or renal dysfunction; emergency treatment of ketoacidosis (regular insulin); to promote passage of glucose across cell membrane in hyperalimentation (regular insulin); to facilitate intracellular shift of potassium in hyperkalemia (regular insulin)

Subcutaneous

Adults, Elderly, Children: 0.5-1 unit/kg/day. **Adolescents (during growth spurt):** 0.8-1.2 unit/kg/day.

Inhalation

Adults, Elderly: 0.05 mg/kg 3 times daily within 10 min of meals

CONTRAINDICATIONS

Hypersensitivity or insulin resistance may require change of type or species source of insulin

INTERACTIONS

Alert: Regular human insulin and digoxin are physically compatible for 3 hr in 0.9% NaCl. In D_5W, a slight haze develops within 1 hr. Do not allow digoxin and insulin to come in contact with each other in an IV for more than 15 min. Drug: **Alcohol:** May increase the effects of insulin. **Beta-adrenergic blockers:** May increase the risk of hyperglycemia or hypoglycemia; may mask signs and prolong periods of hypoglycemia. **Glucocorticoids, thiazide diuretics:** May increase blood glucose level. Herbal: None known. Food: **Increased carbohydrates:** Requires increased doses of insulin. One unit of insulin is needed to cover 15 g of carbohydrates in the majority of diabetic patients.

DIAGNOSTIC TEST EFFECTS

May decrease serum magnesium, phosphate, and potassium concentrations.

IV INCOMPATIBILITIES

Diltiazem (Cardizem), *DOPamine (Intropin), nafcillin (Nafcil)

IV COMPATIBILITIES

Amiodarone (Cordarone), ampicillin/sulbactam (Unasyn), cefazolin (Ancef), cimetidine (Tagamet), digoxin ([Lanoxin], in 0.9% NaCl physically compatible for 3 hr; in D_5W, a slight haze develops within 1 hr), *DOBUTamine (Dobutrex), famotidine (Pepcid), gentamicin, heparin, magnesium sulfate, metoclopramide (Reglan), midazolam (Versed), milrinone (Primacor), morphine, nitroglycerin, potassium chloride, propofol (Diprivan), vancomycin (Vancocin)

SIDE-EFFECTS

Occasional: Localized redness, swelling, and itching caused by improper injection technique or allergy to cleansing solution or insulin. Infrequent: Somogyi effect, including rebound hyperglycemia with chronically excessive insulin dosages; systemic allergic reaction, marked by rash, angioedema, and anaphylaxis; lipodystrophy or depression at injection site due to breakdown of adipose tissue; lipohypertrophy or accumulation of subcutaneous tissue at injection site due to inadequate site rotation. Rare: Insulin resistance (resistance to exogenous insulin) is uncommon in the normal-sized general population; insulin resistance occurs commonly in the critically ill and is more common in obese patients

CRITICAL CARE CONSIDERATIONS

ADMINISTRATION/HANDLING

SUBCUTANEOUS ALERT

- **Dosage:** Insulin doses are individualized and monitored. Adjust dosage to achieve premeal and bedtime glucose levels of 80-120 mg/dL.
- **Storage:** Store currently used insulin at room temperature; avoid extreme temperatures and direct sunlight. Store extra vials in refrigerator. Discard unused vials if not used for several wk.
- **Preparation:** Warm the drug to room temperature; do not give cold insulin. Roll the drug vial gently between hands; do not shake. Regular insulin normally appears clear.
- **Basal insulin:** A long-acting insulin without peak action (e.g., glargine, detemir) or with peak action (e.g., isophane, NPH, or lente) should be used to provide coverage for metabolism. Basal insulin should not be withheld for patients who are not eating because metabolism continues with or without food consumption.
- **Mealtime/prandial insulin:** Administer scheduled mealtime regular insulin approximately 30 min before a meal. Insulin lispro, aspart, and glulisine may be given 15 min before to 15 min after meals. Check the blood glucose before administration.
- **Supplemental insulin:** Premeal blood glucose readings will determine whether supplemental insulin dosage will be required in addition to prandial insulin. Supplemental insulin may be drawn into the same syringe or dialed into a multidose insulin pen so only one injection is required to deliver both prandial and supplemental insulin.
- **Mixing insulin:** Always draw regular insulin first when insulin is mixed. Mixtures must be administered at once because binding can occur within 5 min. *HumaLOG may be mixed with *HumuLIN N and *HumuLIN L.
- **Injection sites:** Give subcutaneous injections in the abdomen, buttocks, thigh, upper arm, or upper back if there is

I

adequate adipose tissue. Maintain a careful record of rotated injection sites.

- **Prefilled syringes:** Are stable for 1 wk when refrigerated, including mixtures once they have stabilized; NPH/Regular stabilizes after 15 min while Lente/Regular stabilizes after 24 hr. Prefilled syringes should be stored in the vertical or oblique position to avoid plugging. The plunger should be pulled back slightly and the syringe rocked to remix the solution before injection.

IV ALERT (FOR REGULAR INSULIN)

- **Regular insulin only:** Regular insulin is the only insulin that may be given IV. Give all other types of insulin subcutaneously only. Use only if solution is clear.
- **Continuous IV insulin infusion:** Insulin infusion can be mixed using 250 units of regular insulin in 250 mL normal saline solution (1 unit/mL) or 125 units in 250 mL normal saline (0.5 units/mL).
- **IV push regular insulin:** May give undiluted.

PRECAUTIONS

HEALTH-RELATED

- Insulin dosage may require careful adjustment when patients undergo increased stress. Stress creates insulin resistance. As patients improve, insulin dosage may need to be decreased because stress level decreases during recovery. Continuous IV insulin infusion is the most accurate means of controlling blood glucose in the critically ill.

AGE-RELATED

- **Children:** No age-related precautions have been noted in children.
- **Elderly:** Decreased vision and shakiness in the elderly may lead to inaccurate insulin self-dosing. Newer insulin pens with dial-in, large numbers may make insulin dosing easier for elderly.

PREGNANCY/LACTATION-RELATED

- Pregnancy category B. Insulin requirements of pregnant diabetic patients are often decreased in the first half and increased in the latter half of pregnancy. Elevated blood glucose levels are associated with congenital abnormalities. Does not pass into breast milk.

MONITORING

- **Baseline assessment:** Obtain vital signs, height, weight, and waist circumference. Discuss lifestyle to determine diabetes management learning needs. Assess cardiovascular risk factors.
- **Baseline lab work:** Biochemical panel including blood glucose, BUN and creatinine, and a lipid profile (cholesterols, triglycerides). Hemoglobin $A1_C$ should be drawn to determine blood glucose control over the past 6 wk. Urinalysis to monitor for albuminuria or proteinuria, an early sign of renal damage due to complications of chronic hyperglycemia.
- **Ongoing blood glucose:** Check blood glucose levels before every meal and at bedtime if patients are eating, hourly if patients are on an insulin infusion.
- **Hypoglycemia:** Monitor all patients for diaphoresis, tachycardia, dysrhythmias, and restlessness. Patients may become confused, nauseated, dizzy, hungry, or agitated or have a headache when blood glucose level is low (below 60 mg/dL). Severe hypoglycemia may result in obtundation, seizures, and cardiac arrest.
- **Hyperglycemia:** Assess for polydipsia, polyphagia, polyuria, deep and rapid breathing (Kussmaul's respirations), dim vision, fatigue, nausea, and abdominal pain. Patients may become acutely dehydrated and manifest symptoms of hypovolemic shock. Hyperglycemic patients may require aggressive use of IV fluids to assist in rehydration in combination with an insulin infusion.
- **Insulin requirements:** Recognize conditions that increase blood glucose, such as fever, increased activity, stress, or a surgical procedure. Recent studies have validated that keeping blood glucose 80-110 mg/dL is associated with marked reduction morbidity and mortality in the critically ill.
- **Patient education:** Make sure patients are adept at drawing up the prescribed dosage of insulin and the proper injection technique. Ensure they can perform self-testing for blood glucose at the prescribed intervals. Stress that the regimen of exercise, good hygiene (including foot care), prescribed diet, and weight control is an integral part of treatment. Warn to avoid smoking and not to skip or delay meals. Explain the signs and symptoms of hypoglycemia and hyperglycemia. Advise to carry candy, sugar packets, or other sugar supplements for immediate response to hypoglycemia and to wear medical alert identification indicating presence of diabetes. Stress to promptly report alterations in glucose demands, such as with fever, heavy physical activity, infection, stress, and trauma,

to a health care provider skilled in blood glucose management. Instruct to inform dentists, other physicians, or surgeons of insulin therapy before any treatment is given.

SERIOUS ADVERSE REACTIONS

- **Hypoglycemia:** May occur during illness when insulin dose is fluctuating, with decreased or delayed food intake, with excessive exercise, and in those with brittle diabetes.
- **Diabetic ketoacidosis:** May result in a type 1 diabetic from stress, illness, omission of insulin dose, or long-term poor insulin control. Hyperosmolar nonketotic syndrome may result from unmanaged hyperglycemia in a type 2 diabetic.
- **Hyperosmolar nonketotic syndrome:** May result from unmanaged hyperglycemia in a type 2 diabetic.

OVERDOSE/TOXICITY

- **Severe hypoglycemia:** Seizures, dysrhythmias, tachycardia, diaphoresis, unresponsiveness, hypotension, coma, hypokalemia, cardiac arrest.
- **GI decontamination:** No specific recommendations.

ANTIDOTE/DIALYSIS

- **Antidote:** 50% dextrose (D50) IV up to 25 mg (should be given based on blood glucose level), which may be repeated every 15 min until blood glucose normalizes; Glucagon 1-2 mg IM is the recognized antidote. Oral carbohydrates (juice, soda, candy, glucose tablets) will help resolve hypoglycemia if the patient is able to safely have PO food/fluids.
- **Dialysis:** Insulin is not removed by hemodialysis or peritoneal dialysis. No data are available on removal by high-permeability hemodialysis.

interferon alfa-2a, Recombinant

in-ter-feer'-on

Classes

Chemical: biological response modifier
Therapeutic: immunosuppressive

Pregnancy Category: C

Trade Names

Prescription: Roferon-A

Do not confuse interferon alfa-2a with interferon alfa-2b.

CLINICAL PHARMACOLOGY

Mechanism of Action

A biological response modifier that inhibits viral replication in virus-infected cells, suppresses cell proliferation, increases phagocytic action of macrophage, and augments specific lymphocytic cell toxicity. Therapeutic Effect: Prevents rapid growth of malignant cells; inhibits hepatitis virus.

PHARMACOKINETICS

Well absorbed after IM and subcutaneous administration. Undergoes proteolytic degradation during reabsorption in kidneys. Half-life: 3.7-8.5 hr.

AVAILABILITY

Injection, vial: 18 million units/mL.

Injection (prefilled syringe): 3 million units/0.5 mL, 6 million units/0.5 mL, 9 million units/0.5 mL.

Injection (single-dose vial): 36 million units/mL.

INDICATIONS AND DOSAGE

Hairy cell leukemia

IM, Subcutaneous

Adults: Initially, 3 million units/day for 16-24 wk. Maintenance: 3 million units 3 times per wk. Do not use 36-million-unit vial.

Chronic myelogenous leukemia

IM, Subcutaneous

Adults: 9 million units/day. Continue treatment until worsening of disease.

Melanoma

IM, Subcutaneous

Adults, Elderly: 12 million units/m^2 3 times per wk for 3 mo or 3 million units 3 times per wk.

AIDS-related Kaposi's sarcoma

IM, Subcutaneous

Adults: Initially, 36 million units/day for 10-12 wk, may give 3 million units on day 1, 9 million units on day 2, 18 million units on day 3, then 36 million units/day for remaining of 10-12 wk. Maintenance: 36 million units/day 3 times per wk.

Chronic hepatitis C

IM, Subcutaneous

Adults, Elderly: 6 million units 3 times per wk for 3 mo, then 3 million units 3 times per wk for 9 mo, or 3 million units 3 times per wk for 12 mo.

OFF-LABEL USES

Treatment of active, chronic hepatitis; bladder or renal carcinoma; malignant melanoma; multiple myeloma; mycosis fungoides; non-Hodgkin's lymphoma

CONTRAINDICATIONS

Autoimmune hepatitis, hypersensitivity to interferon alfa-2a or any of its components (contains benzyl alcohol)

INTERACTIONS

Drug: **Bone marrow depressants:** May have increase myelosuppression. **Captopril, enalopril, enaloprilat:** May increase risk of granulocytopenia. Herbal: None known. Food: None known.

DIAGNOSTIC TEST EFFECTS

May increase serum LDH, alkaline phosphatase, AST (SGOT), and ALT (SGPT) levels. May decrease Hct, blood Hgb level, and leukocyte and platelet counts.

SIDE-EFFECTS

Frequent (greater than 20%): Flulike symptoms, nausea, vomiting, cough, dyspnea, hypotension, edema, chest pain, dizziness, diarrhea, weight loss, altered taste, abdominal discomfort, confusion, paresthesia, depression, visual and sleep disturbances, diaphoresis, lethargy. Occasional (20%-5%): Alopecia (partial), rash, dry throat or skin, pruritus, flatulence, constipation, hypertension, palpitations, sinusitis. Rare (less than 5%): Hot flashes, hypermotility, Raynaud's syndrome, bronchospasm, earache, ecchymosis

CRITICAL CARE CONSIDERATIONS

ADMINISTRATION/HANDLING

IM, SUBCUTANOUS ALERT

- **Storage:** Refrigerate vials.
- **Preparation:** Do not shake vials. The solution normally appears colorless; do not use if it contains precipitate or becomes discolored.
- **High risk for bleeding:** Subcutaneous administration is preferred for thrombocytopenic patients and other patients at risk for bleeding.
- **Dosage:** Individualized based on clinical response and tolerance of adverse effects. When used in combination therapy, consult specific protocols for optimum dosage and sequence of drug administration. If severe adverse reactions occur, modify the dosage or temporarily discontinue the drug.

PRECAUTIONS

HEALTH-RELATED

- Use interferon alfa-2a cautiously in patients with heart disease, lung disease chronic obstructive pulmonary disease, type 1 diabetes mellitus, hypercoagulability, history of thrombophlebitis or pulmonary embolism, hepatic or renal impairment, myelosuppression, or seizure disorders.
- May cause depression or suicidal behavior or worsen psychiatric disorders.
- May aggravate psoriasis.

AGE-RELATED

- **Children:** Safety and efficacy of interferon alfa-2a have not been established in children.
- **Elderly:** More prone to cardiotoxicity and neurotoxicity. Age-related renal impairment may require cautious use of interferon alfa-2a in the elderly.

PREGNANCY/LACTATION-RELATED

- Pregnancy category C; discontinue breastfeeding.

MONITORING

- **Baseline assessment:** Obtain history of disease process and treatments, both current and in the past. Obtain eye exam for those with hypertension and diabetes mellitus; 12-lead ECG for patients with heart disease.
- **Baseline lab work:** Urinalysis, CBC, platelet count, BUN level, and serum alkaline phosphatase, creatinine, AST (SGOT), and ALT (SGPT) levels, before and routinely during therapy.
- **Infection:** Monitor for fever, weakness, chills.
- **Hyperglycemia:** Monitor for increased blood glucose regularly in patients with and without diabetes mellitus.
- **Cardiac effects:** Monitor for dysrhythmias, tachycardia, hypotension, chest discomfort, and ECG changes indicative of cardiac ischemia.
- **Hydration:** Encourage PO fluids or provide IV hydration, particularly during early therapy.
- **Patient education:** Inform that the therapeutic effects may take 1-3 mo to appear. Advise that flulike symptoms tend to diminish with continued therapy. Caution avoidance of tasks that require mental alertness or motor skills until response to the drug is known. Instruct to report if nausea or vomiting continues after discharge from the hospital. Urge avoidance of alcohol during therapy. Instruct female patients on the use of effective contraception during therapy and to report promptly if pregnancy is suspected.

SERIOUS ADVERSE REACTIONS

- **Persistent fever:** May indicate occult infection; thorough workup should be initiated to locate infection.
- **Visual changes:** Eye exam may reveal retinal hemorrhages, cottonwool spots, retinal artery or vein obstruction.
- **Bleeding:** Thrombocytopenia may prompt bleeding. Interferon alpha-2a should be discontinued if platelet count is less than 25,000/mm^3.
- **Hypothyroidism:** Fatigue, weight gain, depression, activity intolerance.
- **Hypersensitivity:** Shortness of breath, wheezing, flushing, generalized redness, itching.

OVERDOSE/TOXICITY

- **Hematologic:** Thrombocytopenia, neutropenia, anemia, and aplastic anemia.
- **Neurotoxicity:** Decreased mental status, coma, obtundation, CVA/stroke, dizziness, impaired memory, agitation, mania, psychosis.
- **Cardiotoxicity:** Chest discomfort, myocardial ischemia, pulmonary edema, rare MI, dysrhythmias, tachycardia, hypotension.
- **Pulmonary toxicity:** Noncardiogenic pulmonary edema, pulmonary infiltrates.
- **Management:** Drug should be discontinued for hypersensitivity reaction, severe depression or psychosis, bone marrow suppression that persists after dosage reduction, extreme liver enzyme elevation, or pulmonary infiltrates or diminished pulmonary function tests.
- **GI decontamination:** No specific recommendations.

ANTIDOTE/DIALYSIS

- **Antidote:** No specific recommendations.
- **Dialysis:** Interferons are not removed by hemodialysis or peritoneal dialysis. No data are available on removal by high-permeability hemodialysis.

interferon alfa-2b

in-ter-feer'-on

Classes

Chemical: biological response modifier
Therapeutic: immunosuppressive

Pregnancy Category: X

Trade Names

Prescription: Intron-A, ribavirin (Rebetron)

Do not confuse interferon alfa-2b with interferon alfa-2a.

CLINICAL PHARMACOLOGY

Mechanism of Action

A biological response modifier that inhibits viral replication in virus-infected cells, suppresses cell proliferation, increases phagocytic action of macrophages, and augments specific cytotoxicity of lymphocytes for target cells. **Therapeutic Effect:** Prevents rapid growth of malignant cells; inhibits hepatitis virus.

PHARMACOKINETICS

Well absorbed after IM and subcutaneous administration. Undergoes proteolytic degradation during reabsorption in kidneys. **Half-life:** 2-3 hr.

AVAILABILITY

Injection (multidose vial): 6 million units/mL, 10 million units/mL.
Injection (single-dose vial powder for reconstitution): 3 million units, 5 million units, 10 million units, 18 million units, 25 million units, 50 million units.
Injection (prefilled solution): 3 million units/0.2 mL, 5 million units/0.2 mL, 10 million units/0.2 mL.

INDICATIONS AND DOSAGE

Hairy cell leukemia

IM, Subcutaneous

Adults: 2 million units/m^2 3 times per wk. If severe adverse reactions occur, modify dose or temporarily discontinue drug.

Condyloma acuminatum

Intralesional

Adults: 1 million units/lesion 3 times per wk for 3 wk. Use only 10-million-unit vial and reconstitute with no more than 1 mL diluent. Maximum: 5 lesions per treatment.

AIDS-related Kaposi's sarcoma

IM, Subcutaneous

Adults: 30 million units/m^2 3 times per wk. Use only 50-million-unit vials. If severe adverse reactions occur, modify dose or temporarily discontinue drug.

Chronic hepatitis C

IM, Subcutaneous

Adults: 3 million units 3 times per wk for up to 16 wk. For patients who tolerate therapy and whose ALT (SGPT) level normalizes at 16 wk, therapy may be extended for up to 18-24 mo.

Chronic hepatitis B

IM, Subcutaneous

Adults: 30-35 million units weekly, either as 5 million units/day or 10 million units 3 times per wk for 16 wk.

Malignant melanoma

IV

Adults: Initially, 20 million units/m^2 for 5 consecutive days 5 times weekly for 4 wk. Then maintenance: 10 million units IM or subcutaneously 3 times per wk for 48 wk.

Follicular lymphoma

Subcutaneous

Adults: 5 million units 3 times per wk for up to 18 mo.

OFF-LABEL USES

Treatment of bladder, cervical, or renal carcinoma; chronic myelocytic leukemia; laryngeal papillomatosis; multiple myeloma; mycosis fungoides

CONTRAINDICATIONS

Autoimmune hepatitis, impaired hepatic function, hypersensitivity to interferon alfa-2b, immunosuppressed organ transplant patients

INTERACTIONS

Drug: Bone marrow depressants: May increase myelosuppression. **Ribavirin:** May worsen mental depression, anger, and hostility. **Herbal:** None known. **Food:** None known.

DIAGNOSTIC TEST EFFECTS

May increase prothrombin time, aPTT, and serum LDH, alkaline phosphatase, AST (SGOT), and ALT (SGPT) levels. May decrease blood Hgb level, Hct, and leukocyte and platelet counts.

IV INCOMPATIBILITIES

Do not mix with other medications for Y-site administration.

SIDE-EFFECTS

Frequent: Flulike symptoms, rash (only in patients with hairy cell leukemia and Kaposi's sarcoma). **Patients with Kaposi's sarcoma:** All previously mentioned side effects plus depression, dyspepsia, dry mouth or thirst, alopecia, rigors. **Occasional:** Dizziness, pruritus, dry skin, dermatitis, altered taste. **Rare:** Confusion, leg cramps, back pain, gingivitis, flushing, tremor, nervousness, eye pain

CRITICAL CARE CONSIDERATIONS

ADMINISTRATION/HANDLING

IV ALERT

- **Combination therapy:** Rebetol (Rebetron) capsules may be used with Intron-A injection for the treatment of chronic hepatitis C.
- **Interferon alfa-2b recombinant solution for injection:** Not recommended for IV administration.
- **Storage:** Refrigerate unopened powder vials.
- **Stability:** Powder vials remain stable for 7 days at room temperature.
- **Powder vial reconstitution:** Prepare the solution immediately before use. Reconstitute with the diluent provided by the manufacturer. Withdraw the desired dose and further dilute with 100 mL 0.9% NaCl to provide final concentration of at least 10 million units/100 mL.
- **Dosage:** Individualized by clinical response and tolerance of adverse effects. When used in combination therapy, consult specific protocols for optimum dosage and sequence of drug administration. Side effects are dose related.
- **Malignant melanoma:** Interferon alfa-2b recombinant solution for injection is *not* recommended of IV administration and should not be used for the induction phase of malignant melanoma.

IM, SUBCUTANEOUS ALERT

- **High risk for bleeding:** Subcutaneous administration is preferred for thrombocytopenic patients (platelet count less than 50,000/m^3) and other patients at risk for bleeding.
- **Dosage:** Individualized based on clinical response and tolerance of adverse effects. When used in combination therapy, consult specific protocols for optimum dosage and sequence of drug administration. If severe adverse reactions occur, modify the dosage or temporarily discontinue the drug.
- **Hairy cell leukemia reconstitution:** Add 1 mL bacteriostatic water for injection to each 3 million-unit vial to provide a concentration of 3 million units/mL, or add 1 mL to each 5 million-unit vial, 2 mL to each 10 million-unit vial, or 5 mL to each 25 million-unit vial to provide a concentration of 5 million units/mL. The 50 million unit strength is NOT to be used for treatment of hairy cell leukemia.
- **Condylomata acuminate reconstitution:** Reconstitute each 10 million-unit vial with 1 mL bacteriostatic water for injection to provide a concentration of 10 million units/mL. Use a tuberculin syringe with a 25- or 26-gauge needle.

- **AIDS-related Kaposi's sarcoma reconstitution:** Reconstitute each 50 million-unit vial with 1 mL bacteriostatic water for injection to provide a concentration of 50 million units/mL.
- Give inteferon alpha-2b in the evening with acetaminophen to help alleviate side effects.
- **Preparation:** Agitate the vial gently and withdraw the solution with a sterile syringe.

PRECAUTIONS

HEALTH-RELATED

- **Packaging alert:** Interferon alfa-2b, recombinant is packaged as (1) powder for reconstitution/injection; (2) solution for injection; (3) solution in prefilled, multidose cartridges in a multidose pen device for subcutaneous injection. Not all dosage forms and strengths are appropriate for all indications.
- Use interferon alfa-2b cautiously in patients with heart disease, lung disease chronic obstructive pulmonary disease, type 1 diabetes mellitus, hypercoagulability, history of thrombophlebitis or pulmonary embolism; hepatic or renal impairment, myelosuppression, or seizure disorders.
- May cause depression or suicidal behavior or worsen psychiatric disorders.
- May aggravate psoriasis in affected patients.

AGE-RELATED

- **Children:** Safety and efficacy of interferon alfa-2b have not been established in children.
- **Elderly:** More prone to cardiotoxicity and neurotoxicity. Age-related renal impairment may require cautious use of interferon alfa-2b in the elderly.

PREGNANCY/LACTATION-RELATED

- Pregnancy category X; discontinue breast-feeding.

MONITORING

- **Baseline assessment:** Obtain history of disease process and treatments, both current and in the past. Obtain eye exam for those with hypertension and diabetes mellitus; 12-lead ECG for patients with heart disease.
- **Baseline lab work:** Urinalysis, CBC, platelet count, BUN level, and serum alkaline phosphatase, creatinine, AST (SGOT), and ALT (SGPT) levels, before and routinely during therapy.
- **Infection:** Monitor for fever, weakness, chills.
- **Hyperglycemia:** Monitor for increased blood glucose regularly in patients with and without diabetes mellitus.
- **Cardiac effects:** Monitor for dysrhythmias, tachycardia, hypotension, chest discomfort, and ECG changes indicative of cardiac ischemia.
- **Hydration:** Encourage PO fluids or provide IV hydration, particularly during early therapy.
- **Patient education:** Inform patients the therapeutic effects may take 1-3 mo to appear. Advise that flulike symptoms tend to diminish with continued therapy. Caution patients to avoid tasks that require mental alertness or motor skills until response to the drug is known. Instruct to report if nausea or vomiting continues after discharge from the hospital. Urge avoidance of alcohol during therapy. Caution to avoid receiving immunizations without prior approval from a health care provider and to avoid coming in contact with people who have recently received a live-virus vaccine since interferon alfa-2b lowers resistance. Instruct female patients on the use of effective contraception during therapy and to report promptly if pregnancy is suspected.

SERIOUS ADVERSE REACTIONS

- **Persistent fever:** May indicate occult infection; thorough workup should be initiated to locate infection.
- **Visual changes:** Eye exam may reveal retinal hemorrhages, cottonwool spots, retinal artery or vein obstruction.
- **Bleeding:** Thrombocytopenia may prompt bleeding. Interferon alpha-2a should be discontinued if platelet count is less than 25,000/mm^3.
- **Hypothyroidism:** Fatigue, weight gain, depression, activity intolerance.
- **Hypersensitivity:** Shortness of breath, wheezing, flushing, generalized redness, itching.

OVERDOSE/TOXICITY

- **Hematologic:** Thrombocytopenia, neutropenia, anemia, and aplastic anemia.
- **Neurotoxicity:** Decreased mental status, coma, obtundation, cerebral vascular accident (CVA)/stroke, dizziness, impaired memory, agitation, mania, psychosis.
- **Cardiotoxicity:** Chest discomfort, myocardial ischemia, pulmonary edema, rare

MI, dysrhythmias, tachycardia, and hypotension.
- **Pulmonary toxicity:** Noncardiogenic pulmonary edema, pulmonary infiltrates.
- **Management:** Drug should be discontinued for hypersensitivity reaction, severe depression or psychosis, bone marrow suppression that persists after dosage reduction, extreme liver enzyme elevation, or pulmonary infiltrates or diminished pulmonary function tests.
- **GI decontamination:** No specific recommendations.

ANTIDOTE/DIALYSIS
- **Antidote:** No specific recommendations.
- **Dialysis:** Interferons are not removed by hemodialysis or peritoneal dialysis. No data are available on removal by high-permeability hemodialysis.

interferon alfa-n3

See Immunologics (p. 968)

interferon alfacon-1

See Immunologics (p. 968)

interferon beta-1a

See Immunologics (p. 968)

interferon beta-1b

See Immunologics (p. 968)

interferon gamma-1b

See Immunologics (p. 968)

ipratropium bromide

See Bronchodilators (p. 947)

irbesartan

See Angiotensin II Receptor Antagonists (p. 889)

iron dextran

iron dex'-tran

Classes

Chemical: ferric hydroxide complexed with dextran

Therapeutic: hematinic

Pregnancy Category: C

Trade Names

Prescription: InFeD, Dexferrum, Dexiron ♣

CLINICAL PHARMACOLOGY

Mechanism of Action

A trace element and essential component in the formation of Hgb. Necessary for effective erythropoiesis and transport and use of oxygen. Serves as cofactor of several essential enzymes. **Therapeutic Effect:** Replenishes Hgb and depleted iron stores.

PHARMACOKINETICS

Readily absorbed after IM administration. Most absorption occurs within 72 hr; remainder within 3-4 wk. Bound to protein to form hemosiderin, ferritin, or transferrin. No physiologic system of elimination. Small amounts lost daily in shedding of skin, hair, and nails, and in feces, urine, and perspiration. **Half-life:** 5-20 hr.

AVAILABILITY

Injection (DexFerrum, Infed): 50 mg/mL.

INDICATIONS AND DOSAGE

Iron deficiency anemia (no blood loss)

Dosage is expressed in terms of milligrams of elemental iron and based on degree of anemia, patient weight, and presence of any bleeding. Expect to use periodic hematologic determinations as guide to therapy.

IV, IM

Adults, Elderly: Mg iron dose = 0.0442 [desired Hgb − observed Hgb] × lean body weight (kg) + (0.26 × lean body weight)

Iron replacement secondary to blood loss

IV, IM

Adults, Elderly: Replacement iron (mg) = blood loss (mL) × Hct.

Maximum daily dosages

Adults weighing more than 50 kg: 100 mg. **Children weighing 10-50 kg:** 100 mg. **Children weighing 5 kg to less than 10 kg:** 50 mg. **Infants weighing less than 5 kg:** 25 mg.

CONTRAINDICATIONS

All anemias except iron deficiency anemia, including pernicious, aplastic, normocytic, and refractory; hypersensitivity to iron dextran

INTERACTIONS

Drug: None known. **Herbal:** None known. **Food:** None known.

DIAGNOSTIC TEST EFFECTS

None known.

IV INCOMPATIBILITIES

No information available via Y-site administration.

SIDE-EFFECTS

Frequent: Allergic reaction (such as rash and itching), backache, myalgia, chills, dizziness, headache, fever, nausea, vomiting, flushed skin, pain or redness at injection site, brown discoloration of skin, metallic taste

CRITICAL CARE CONSIDERATIONS

ADMINISTRATION/HANDLING

IV ALERT

- **Oral iron supplements:** Discontinue oral iron before administering iron dextran. Excessive iron intake may produce excessive iron storage (hemosiderosis).
- **Test dose:** A test dose is generally given before the full dose; stay with the patient for several min after injection of a test dose because of the potential for anaphylactic reaction.
- **Storage:** Store at room temperature.
- **Preparation:** May give undiluted or dilute in 0.9% NaCl for infusion.
- **IV intermittent infusion:** Do not exceed an administration rate of 50 mg/min (1 mL/min). A too-rapid IV rate may produce flushing, chest pain, shock, hypotension, and tachycardia.
- **Following IV infusion:** Keep patients recumbent for 30-45 min after IV administration to minimize orthostatic hypotension.

IM ALERT

- **Oral iron supplements:** Discontinue oral iron before administering iron dextran. Excessive iron intake may produce excessive iron storage (hemosiderosis).
- **Preparation:** Draw up medication with one needle; use new needle for injection to minimize skin staining.
- **Administration:** Use Z-track technique by displacing subcutaneous tissue lateral to injection site before inserting needle to minimize skin staining. Administer deep into upper outer quadrant of buttock only.

PRECAUTIONS

HEALTH-RELATED

- Use iron dextran extremely cautiously in patients with serious hepatic impairment.
- Use cautiously in patients with bronchial asthma, a history of allergies, or rheumatoid arthritis.

AGE-RELATED

- **Children:** Not recommended for infants under 4 mo.
- **Elderly:** No age-related precautions have been noted.

PREGNANCY/LACTATION-RELATED

- Pregnancy category C; excreted in breast milk; use only if absolutely necessary.

MONITORING

- **Baseline assessment:** Assess for adequate muscle mass before injecting medication. Discontinue oral iron supplements because excessive iron may produce excessive iron storage, called hemosiderosis.
- **Baseline lab work:** Serum iron studies including serum ferritin level and serum transferrin saturation; complete blood count (CBC) to assess anemia.
- **Ongoing lab work:** Monitor serum ferritin level.
- **Test dose:** Administer test dose and wait at least 1 hr before administering additional iron dextran.
- **Postural hypotension:** Keep patients lying down after treatment.
- **Rheumatoid arthritis:** Acute exacerbation of joint pain and swelling in patients with rheumatoid arthritis and iron deficiency anemia may occur.
- **Inguinal lymphadenopathy:** Groin lymph nodes may become swollen and painful when using IM injection.
- **IM injection site:** Monitor the IM site for abscess formation, atrophy, brownish skin color, necrosis, and swelling. Evaluate for inflammation, pain, and soreness.
- **IV site:** Examine IV site for phlebitis.
- **Patient education:** Explain that pain and brown staining of the skin may occur at the injection site. Caution not to take oral iron while receiving iron injections. Discuss that stools may become black

during iron therapy, but this effect is harmless unless accompanied by abdominal cramping or pain with red streaking or sticky consistency of stool. Instruct to promptly report abdominal cramping or pain, back pain, fever, headache, or red streaking or a sticky consistency of stool to a health care provider. Suggest chewing gum, hard candy, and good oral hygiene to prevent or reduce metallic taste.

SERIOUS ADVERSE REACTIONS

- **Anaphylaxis:** Rare occurrence during the first few min after injection. May cause death. Allergic reactions are often delayed and may be more common with specific batches/lot numbers of the drug. Patients who tolerated the test dose are still susceptible to anaphylaxis.
- **Immunologic:** Leukocytosis and lymphadenopathy occur rarely. Arthritis may be reactivated.
- **Management:** Discontinue iron dextran. Provide epinephrine, benadryl, maintain patent airway, use endotracheal intubation as needed, support ventilation, and resuscitate as needed. Provide fluid infusion to help support BP.

OVERDOSE/TOXICITY

- **Overdose:** Usually produces no acute toxicity but may result in hemosiderosis (excessive iron storage). Excess iron increases risk for infection.
- **Iron toxicity:** Severe toxicity increases vasodilation and venous pooling, decreases circulating blood volume, increases peripheral vascular resistance, decreases cardiac output, resulting in shock and metabolic acidosis.
- **GI decontamination:** No specific recommendations.

ANTIDOTE/DIALYSIS

- **Antidote:** Deferoxamine is an iron-chelating agent used to manage iron toxicity. Deferoxamine has been shown to remove intracellular iron effectively. Provide IV hydration to help abate acute renal failure if deferoxamine is used. Metabolic acidosis is a reliable marker of cellular iron toxicity in need of treatment.
- **Dialysis:** Iron dextran is unlikely to be removed by hemodialysis or peritoneal dialysis and is not removed by high-permeability hemodialysis.

iron sucrose

iron sue'-crose

Classes

Chemical: ferric hydroxide complexed with sucrose
Therapeutic: hematinic

Pregnancy Category: B

Trade Names

Prescription: Venofer

CLINICAL PHARMACOLOGY

Mechanism of Action

A trace element that is an essential component in the formation of Hgb. It is necessary for effective erythropoiesis and oxygen transport capacity of blood, as well as transport and use of oxygen, and serves as cofactor of several essential enzymes. **Therapeutic Effect:** Replenishes body iron stores in patients who have iron deficiency anemia.

PHARMACOKINETICS

Distributed mainly in blood and to some extent in extravascular fluid. Iron sucrose is dissociated into iron and sucrose by the reticuloendothelial system. The sucrose component is eliminated mainly by urinary excretion. **Half-life:** 6 hr.

AVAILABILITY

Injection: 20 mg/mL or 100 mg elemental iron in 5-mL single-dose vial.

INDICATIONS AND DOSAGE

Iron deficiency anemia

IV

Dosage is expressed in terms of milligrams of elemental iron. **Adults, Elderly:** 5 mL iron sucrose or 100 mg elemental iron, delivered during dialysis; administer 1-3 times per wk to total dose of 1000 mg in 10 doses. Give no more than 3 times per wk.

OFF-LABEL USES

Treatment of dystrophic epidermolysis bullosa

CONTRAINDICATIONS

All anemias except iron deficiency anemia, including pernicious, aplastic, normocytic, and refractory anemia; evidence of iron overload; hypersensitivity to iron sucrose

INTERACTIONS

Drug: Oral iron preparations: May reduce the absorption of these preparations. **Herbal:** None known. **Food:** None known.

DIAGNOSTIC TEST EFFECTS

Increases Hgb and Hct, serum ferritin level, and serum transferrin saturation.

IV INCOMPATIBILITIES

Do not mix with other medications or add to parenteral nutrition solution for IV infusion.

SIDE-EFFECTS

Frequent (36%-23%): Hypotension, leg cramps, diarrhea

CRITICAL CARE CONSIDERATIONS

ADMINISTRATION/HANDLING

IV ALERT

- **Storage:** Store at room temperature.
- **Test dose:** Optional with iron sucrose.
- **Direct IV injection/push:** May be given as undiluted, slow IV injection.
- **Dialysis line IV injection:** Administer into the dialysis line at a rate of 1 mL, or 20 mg iron, undiluted solution per min. Allow 5 min per vial; do not exceed 1 vial per injection.
- **Dialysis line IV infusion:** Dilute each vial in a maximum of 100 mL 0.9% NaCl immediately before infusion. Administer into dialysis line at a rate of 100 mg iron over at least 15 min during hemodialysis to reduce the risk of hypotensive episodes.

PRECAUTIONS

HEALTH-RELATED

- Use iron sucrose cautiously in patients with cardiac dysfunction, bronchial asthma, history of allergies, or hepatic or renal impairment.
- Drug should not be used in patients with suspected tissue iron overload. May result in hemosiderosis (excessive tissue iron storage). Excess iron increases risk for infection.

AGE-RELATED

- **Children:** Safety and efficacy of iron sucrose have not been established in children.
- **Elderly:** Age-related organ dysfunction may warrant a reduced dose.

PREGNANCY/LACTATION-RELATED

- Pregnancy category B; safety for use in breast-feeding has not been established.

MONITORING

- **Baseline assessment:** Assess amount of oral iron supplementation. Ensure anemia has been diagnosed appropriately as iron deficiency-related.
- **Baseline lab work:** CBC including Hgb and Hct, serum ferritin level, and serum transferrin saturation.
- **Ongoing lab work:** Obtain serum iron levels 48 hr after iron sucrose administration.
- **Dialysis access:** Make sure dialysis access is patent before preparing drug.
- **Optional test dose:** Administer test dose and wait at least 1 hr before administering additional iron sucrose.
- **Postural hypotension:** Keep patients lying down after treatment.
- **Rheumatoid arthritis:** Acute exacerbation of joint pain and swelling in patients with rheumatoid arthritis may occur.
- **Patient education:** Instruct to expect follow-up blood tests to monitor the results of treatment. Hct, Hgb, serum ferritin, and serum transferrin levels are monitored monthly, then every 2-3 mo. Explain that iron sucrose is administered during dialysis. Instruct to report leg cramps or diarrhea.

SERIOUS ADVERSE REACTIONS

- **Too rapid IV administration:** May produce severe hypotension, headache, vomiting, nausea, dizziness, paresthesia, abdominal and muscle pain, edema, and cardiovascular collapse.
- **Anaphylaxis:** Rare occurrence during the first few min after injection. May cause death. Allergic reactions are often delayed and may be more common with specific batches/lot numbers of the drug. Patients who tolerate the test dose are still susceptible to anaphylaxis.
- **Management:** Discontinue iron sucrose. Provide epinephrine, benadryl, maintain patent airway, use endotracheal intubation as needed, support ventilation, and resuscitate as needed. Provide fluid infusion along with vasopressors to help support BP.

OVERDOSE/TOXICITY

- **Overdose:** Abdominal and muscle pain, bleeding in the GI tract and lungs, cardiovascular collapse, diarrhea, edema, headache, hemosiderosis, hypotension, joint aches, nausea, vomiting, and sedation.
- **Management:** Discontinue iron sucrose; resuscitate if indicated.
- **GI decontamination:** No specific recommendations.

ANTIDOTE/DIALYSIS

- **Antidote:** Deferoxamine is an iron-chelating agent used to manage iron toxicity. Deferoxamine has been shown to remove intracellular iron effectively. Metabolic acidosis is a reliable marker of cellular iron toxicity in need of treatment.
- **Dialysis:** Iron sucrose is unlikely to be removed by hemodialysis, high-permeability hemodialysis, or peritoneal dialysis.

isocarboxazid

See Antidepressants (p. 906)

isoetharine

See Bronchodilators (p. 947)

isoniazid

eye-soe-nye'-a-zid

Classes

Chemical: isonicotinic acid derivative
Therapeutic: antituberculosis agent

Pregnancy Category: C

Trade Names

Prescription: *INH:* Isotamine ♣, Nydrazid, PMS Isoniazid ♣

Combinations

Prescription: with rifampin (Rifamate); with rifampin, pyrazinamide (Rifater)

CLINICAL PHARMACOLOGY

Mechanism of Action

An isonicotinic acid derivative that inhibits mycolic acid synthesis and causes disruption of the bacterial cell wall and loss of acid-fast properties in susceptible mycobacteria. Active only during bacterial cell division. **Therapeutic Effect:** Bactericidal against actively growing intracelleluar and extracellular susceptible mycobacteria.

PHARMACOKINETICS

Readily absorbed from the GI tract. Protein binding: 10%-15%. Widely distributed (including to cerebrospinal fluid). Metabolized in the liver. Primarily excreted in urine. Removed by hemodialysis. **Half-life:** 0.5-5 hr.

AVAILABILITY

Tablets: 100 mg, 300 mg.
Syrup: 50 mg/5 mL.
Injection (Nydrazid): 100 mg/mL.

INDICATIONS AND DOSAGE

Tuberculosis (in combination with one or more antituberculars)

PO, IM

Adults, Elderly: 5 mg/kg/day as a single dose. Maximum 300 mg/day. **Children:** 10-15 mg/kg/day in 1-2 divided doses. Maximum 300 mg/day.

Prevention of tuberculosis (+PPD skin test)

PO, IM

Adults, Elderly: 300 mg/day as a single dose. **Children:** 10-20 mg/kg/day in 1-2 divided doses for 9 mo. Maximum 300 mg/day.

CONTRAINDICATIONS

Acute hepatic disease, history of hypersensitivity reactions or hepatic injury with previous isoniazid therapy

INTERACTIONS

Drug: **Alcohol:** May increase isoniazid metabolism and the risk of hepatotoxicity. **Carbamazepine, phenytoin:** May increase the toxicity of these drugs. **Disulfiram:** May increase CNS effects. **Hepatotoxic medications:** May increase the risk of hepatotoxicity. **Itraconazole:** May decrease itraconazole concentration. **Ketoconazole:** May decrease ketoconazole blood concentration. **Levodopa:** May decrease levodopa concentration. **Herbal:** None known. **Food:** **Tyramine-containing foods:** May cause a hypertensive crisis.

DIAGNOSTIC TEST EFFECTS

May increase serum bilirubin, AST (SGOT), and ALT (SGPT) levels.

SIDE-EFFECTS

Frequent: Nausea, vomiting, diarrhea, abdominal pain. **Rare:** Pain at injection site, hypersensitivity reaction

CRITICAL CARE CONSIDERATIONS

ADMINISTRATION/HANDLING

PO ALERT

- Give isoniazid 1 hr before or 2 hr after a meal. Drug may be given with food to decrease GI upset, but this will delay absorption.

- Administer isoniazid at least 1 hr before antacids, especially those containing aluminum.

PRECAUTIONS

HEALTH-RELATED

- Use isoniazid cautiously in alcoholic patients with chronic hepatic disease or severe renal impairment and patients with hypersensitivity to nicotinic acid or other chemically related medications because of the risk of cross-sensitivity.

AGE-RELATED

- **Children:** No age-related precautions have been noted.
- **Elderly:** Are more susceptible to developing hepatitis.

PREGNANCY/LACTATION-RELATED

- Pregnancy category C. The American Thoracic Society recommends use of isoniazid for tuberculosis during pregnancy. Excreted in breast milk; women can safely breast-feed their infants while taking isoniazid if the infant is periodically examined for signs and symptoms of peripheral neuritis or hepatitis.

MONITORING

- **Baseline assessment:** Determine history of hypersensitivity reactions, hepatic injury from isoniazid, a sensitivity to nicotinic acid or chemically related medications before starting drug therapy.
- **Baseline lab work:** Biochemical profile including liver enzymes. Ensure that appropriate specimens are obtained for culture and sensitivity testing before beginning therapy.
- **Ongoing lab work:** Monitor liver function tests.
- **Hepatitis:** Assess for symptoms of hepatitis including anorexia, dark urine, fatigue, jaundice, nausea, vomiting, and weakness. Withhold the drug if hepatitis is present.
- **Peripheral neuropathy:** Assess for burning, numbness, and tingling of the extremities. Patients at risk for neuropathy, including alcoholics, those with chronic hepatic disease, diabetics, the elderly, and malnourished individuals, may receive pyridoxine prophylactically.
- **Hypersensitivity:** Assess for signs and symptoms of a hypersensitivity reaction, including fever and skin eruptions.
- **Patient education:** Instruct to take isoniazid 1 hr before or 2 hr after a meal. Drug may be taken with food if GI upset occurs. Advise not to skip doses and to continue taking isoniazid for the full course of therapy (6-24 mo). Urge avoidance of alcohol consumption during treatment. Caution not to take other medications, including antacids, without prior approval by a health care provider. Explain that isoniazid should be taken at least 1 hr before taking an antacid. Instruct to report promptly new symptoms, including dark urine, fatigue, nausea or vomiting, visual problems, numbness or tingling of the extremities, and jaundice to a health care provider. Warn to avoid foods containing tyramine including aged cheeses, sauerkraut, smoked fish, and tuna. These foods may trigger a headache, a "hot flash," lightheadedness, pounding heartbeat, and red or itching skin. Instruct to report these reactions to a health care provider. Provide a list of tyramine-containing foods.

SERIOUS ADVERSE REACTIONS

- **Mild/moderate neurologic effects:** Optic neuritis, ataxia, lightheadeness, nystagmus, and paresthesias.
- **Peripheral neuropathy:** A side effect of long-term INH therapy. Risk of this neuropathy is increased by malnutrition, pregnancy, diabetes, alcoholism, and slow acetylator status. Doses of INH greater than 6 mg/kg/day place patients at greater risk for peripheral neuropathy.

OVERDOSE/TOXICITY

- **Neurotoxicity:** Refractory seizures, coma, and metabolic/lactic acidosis. Seizures may result in rhabdomyolysis. Respiratory depression may be associated with seizures. Psychosis, cerebellar syndrome, and either aflexia or hyperreflexia may be present. Persistent seizures result from pyridoxine deficiency. Pyridoxine should be taken throughout INH therapy to help prevent neurotoxicity and peripheral neuropathy.
- **Hepatotoxicity:** Elevated liver enzymes, digestive problems, fatigue, jaundice. Elevation of liver enzymes is seen 2 wk to 6 mo after starting INH.
- **Management:** Supportive care including maintaining patent airway, monitoring for cardiovascular collapse, and securing IV access for fluid volume replacement. Sodium bicarbonate may be used to manage metabolic acidosis if seizures are being aggressively treated. Metabolic acidosis results from persistent seizures.

- **GI decontamination:** Ipecac syrup should never be administered for INH overdose. Activated charcoal adsorbs INH well.

ANTIDOTE/DIALYSIS

- **Antidote:** Pyridoxine is the drug of choice for managing INH-induced seizures. Benzodiazepines or barbiturates may be used while 5 g of pyridoxine (or 70 mg/kg in children) is obtained to effectively manage seizures. Phenytoin may be ineffective in managing INH-induced seizures.
- **Dialysis:** Isoniazid is not removed by hemodialysis, high permeability hemodialysis, or peritoneal dialysis. Pyridoxine is removed by hemodialysis, and those patients are at higher risk for developing neurotoxicity.

isoproterenol hydrochloride

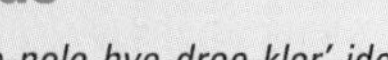

eye-soe-proe-ter'-e-nole hye-droe-klor'-ide

Classes

Chemical: catecholamine, synthetic

Therapeutic: antiasthmatic, bronchodilator, sympathomimetic, vasopressor, ß-adrenergic agonist

Pregnancy Category: C

Trade Names

Prescription: Isuprel

Combinations

Prescription: with phenylephrine (Duo-Medihaler)

CLINICAL PHARMACOLOGY

Mechanism of Action

A sympathomimetic (adrenergic agonist) that stimulates $beta_1$ and $beta_2$ adrenergic receptors. Therapeutic Effect: Increases myocardial contractility, stroke volume, cardiac output.

PHARMACOKINETICS

Readily absorbed. Metabolized in liver. Primarily excreted in urine. Half-life: 2.5-5 min.

AVAILABILITY

Injection: 0.02 mg/mL (Isuprel).

INDICATIONS AND DOSAGE

Dysrhythmias

IV Bolus

Adults, Elderly: Dose range: 0.01-0.2 mg (0.5-10 mL of diluted solution).

IV Infusion

Adults, Elderly: Initially, 5 mcg/min (1.25 mL/min of diluted solution, 1 mg/250 mL). Subsequent dose range: 2-20 mcg/min. **Children:** 0.05-2 mcg/kg/min.

Shock

IV Infusion

Adults, Elderly: Rate of 0.05-0.2 mcg/kg/min (0.25-2.5 mL of 1:500,000 dilution); rate of infusion based on clinical response (heart rate, central venous pressure, systemic BP, urine flow measurements).

CONTRAINDICATIONS

Tachycardia due to digitalis toxicity, preexisting dysrhythmias, angina, precordial distress, hypersensitivity to isoproterenol or any component of the formulation

INTERACTIONS

Drug: **Beta-blockers:** May antagonize the effects of isoproterenol. **Digoxin:** May increase the risk of dysrhythmias. **Tricyclic antidepressants:** May increase cardiovascular effects. Herbal: **Ma huang, yohimbe, ephedra:** May increase CNS stimulation. Food: None known.

DIAGNOSTIC TEST EFFECTS

Decreases serum potassium levels

IV INCOMPATIBILITIES

None known.

SIDE-EFFECTS

Frequent: Palpitations, tachycardia, restlessness, nervousness, tremor, insomnia, anxiety. Occasional: Increased sweating, headache, nausea, flushed skin, dizziness, coughing

CRITICAL CARE CONSIDERATIONS

ADMINISTRATION/HANDLING

IV ALERT

- **Storage:** Store at controlled room temperature (59°-86°F). Do not use if solution is pink to brown, contains a precipitate, or appears cloudy.
- **IV push reconstitution:** Dilute 0.2 mg (1 mL) of 1:5 000 solution to a volume of 10 mL 0.9% NaCl or D_5W.
- **Administer IV push:** Inject at a rate of 1 mL/min. Regulate by ECG monitoring.
- **IV infusion dilution:** Dilute 0.2-2 mg (1-10 mL) of 1:5000 solution in 500 mL D_5W to provide a solution of 0.4-4 mcg/mL.

- **Rate of IV infusion:** Determined by heart rate, central venous pressure, systemic BP, and urine output.
- **Controlled infusion:** Use infusion pump or microdrip (60 drops/mL) to administer drug. If ECG changes occur, heart rate exceeds 110 beats/min, or premature beats occur, reduce rate of infusion or temporarily stop infusion.

ISOPROTERENOL INFUSION DOSAGE/RATE (1 mg IN 250 mL D_5W)

DOSE		RATE	
mcg/min	mcg/hr	mL/min	mL/hr
2	120	0.5	30
5	300	1.25	75
10	600	2.5	150
25	1500	6.25	375

PRECAUTIONS

HEALTH-RELATED

- Use cautiously in patients with hypersensitivity to sulfites, hypertension, coronary artery disease, impaired renal function, hyperthyroidism, diabetes mellitus, prostatic hypertrophy, or glaucoma, or those who are elderly or debilitated.

AGE-RELATED

- **Children:** Safety and efficacy of isoproterenol have not been established in children.
- **Elderly:** May exhibit decreased therapeutic response (less increase in heart rate, less peripheral vasodilation).

PREGNANCY/LACTATION-RELATED

- Pregnancy category C. No reports linking isoproterenol with congenital defects have been located. Excretion into breast milk unknown; use caution in nursing mothers.

MONITORING

- **Baseline assessment:** Assess the need for use of isoproterenol; drug is no longer a first-line drug for management of bradycardia. Drug is used for low heart rate in patients who are unresponsive to atropine bolus, continuous IV infusion of *DOPamine or epinephrine or when transcutaneous cardiac pacing is not available or is ineffective. Drug is not routinely used for patients with angina or baseline tachycardia, when used for management cardiogenic shock, asthma, for diagnosis of mitral regurgitation, and beta-adrenergic blocker overdose.
- **Baseline lab work:** Biochemical profile including cardiac enzymes. B-type natriuretic peptide (BNP) level to assess heart failure.
- **Baseline diagnostic tests:** Obtain 12-lead ECG to use for comparison if patients experience ST changes indicative of myocardial ischemia (depression) or infarction (elevation), or chest discomfort while isoproterenol is infusing.
- **Cardiac ischemia:** Monitor ECG continuously for tachycardia, ST segment depression or elevation, indicative of ischemia or acute MI.
- **Bradycardia in heart transplant patients:** Transplanted hearts are not connected to the recipient's nervous system. Atropine blocks the slowing action of the vagus nerve, which has no effect on a transplanted heart. Heart rate must be increased using circulating catecholamines.
- **Hypotension:** Bradycardia, heart block, and heart failure prompt hypotension. Other medications should be used before using isoproterenol because drug markedly increases myocardial oxygen demand.
- **Oliguria:** Bradycardia, heart failure, and cardiogenic shock patients may have decreased urine output.
- **Refractory torsades de pointes:** Torsades results from prolonged QT syndrome. Isoproterenol use may shorten QT interval and abate the dysrhythmia when other strategies fail.
- **Patient education:** Instruct to report pain or burning at the IV site, chest pain, or palpitations during the infusion.

SERIOUS ADVERSE REACTIONS

- **Excessive sympathomimetic stimulation:** May cause palpitations, extrasystoles, tachycardia, chest pain, slight increase in BP followed by a substantial decrease, chills, sweating, and blanching of skin.
- **Ventricular dysrhythmias:** May occur if heart rate is above 130 beats/min.
- **Parotid gland swelling:** May occur with prolonged use.

OVERDOSE/TOXICITY

- **Acute myocardial infarction:** Chest discomfort, shortness of breath, ST segment elevation in at least two contiguous ECG leads, nausea, vomiting.
- **Management:** Stop or significantly reduce the rate of infusion. Resuscitate as needed according to Advanced Cardiac Life Support (ACLS) guidelines.
- **GI decontamination:** No specific recommendations.

ANTIDOTE/DIALYSIS

- **Antidote:** Beta-adrenergic blockers (e.g., metoprolol, propranolol) may block the effects, but slowing or stopping the infusion may be the safest option for patients having chest discomfort including an acute MI. The original need for isoproterenol may make use of beta-adrenergic blockade extremely dangerous.
- **Dialysis:** No data are available regarding removal of isoproterenol by hemodialysis, high-permeability hemodialysis, or peritoneal dialysis.

isosorbide dinitrate/ isosorbide mononitrate

eye-soe-sore'-bide dye-nye'-trate/eye-soe-soré-bide mon-oe-nye'-trate

I

Classes

Chemical: nitrate, organic
Therapeutic: antianginal

Pregnancy Category: C

Trade Names

Prescription: (isosorbide dinitrate) Dilatrate, Dilatrate-SR, ISDN, Isochron, Isordil, Isordil Tembids, Isordil Titradose, Sorbitrate **Prescription:** (isosorbide mononitrate) Imdur, ISMO, Monoket

Do not confuse Isordil with Isuprel or Plendil, or Imdur with Inderal or K-Dur.

CLINICAL PHARMACOLOGY

Mechanism of Action

A nitrate that stimulates intracellular cyclic guanosine monophosphate. Therapeutic Effect: Relaxes vascular smooth muscle of both arterial and venous vasculature. Decreases preload and afterload.

PHARMACOKINETICS

Route	Onset	Peak	Duration
Dinitrate			
Sublingual	2-10 min	15-45 min	1-2 hr
Oral (Chewable)	2-3 min	5 min	2 hr
Oral	40-60 min	N/A	4-6 hr
Oral (sustained release)	30 min	N/A	12 hr
Mononitrate			
Oral (extended release)	45-60 min	120 min	5-12 hr

Dinitrate is poorly absorbed and metabolized in the liver to its active metabolite isosorbide mononitrate. Mononitrate is well absorbed after PO administration. Excreted in urine and feces. Half-life: Dinitrate, 1-4 hr; mononitrate, 4 hr.

AVAILABILITY

Capsules (sustained release [Dilatrate, Isordil Tembids]): 40 mg.
Tablets: 5 mg (ISDN, Isordil, Isordil Titradose), 10 mg (ISDN, ISMO, Isordil, Isordil Titradose, Monoket), 20 mg (ISDN, ISMO, Isordil, Isordil Titradose, Monoket), 30 mg (ISDN, Isordil, Isordil Titradose), 40 mg (ISDN, Isordil, Isordil Titradose).
Tablets (chewable [Sorbitrate]): 5 mg, 10 mg.
Tablets (extended release [Imdur]): 30 mg, 60 mg, 120 mg.
Tablets (sublingual [Isordil]): 2.5 mg, 5 mg.

INDICATIONS AND DOSAGE

Angina

PO (isosorbide dinitrate)

Adults, Elderly: 5-40 mg 4 times per day. Sustained-release: 40 mg every 8-12 hr.

PO (isosorbide mononitrate)

Adults, Elderly: 5-20 mg twice per day given 7 hr apart. Sustained release: Initially 30-60 mg/day in morning as a single dose. May increase dose at 3-day intervals. Maximum: 240 mg/day.

OFF-LABEL USES

Heart failure, dysphagia, pain relief, relief of esophageal spasm with gastroesophageal reflux

CONTRAINDICATIONS

Closed-angle glaucoma; GI hypermotility or malabsorption (extended-release tablets); head trauma; hypersensitivity to nitrates; increased intracranial pressure; orthostatic hypotension; severe anemia (extended-release tablets); concurrent use with sildenafil, tadalafil, or verdenafil

INTERACTIONS

Drug: **Alcohol, antihypertensives, vasodilators, PDE-5 inhibitors (sildenafil, tadalafil, verdenafil):** May increase risk of orthostatic hypotension. Herbal: None known. Food: None known.

DIAGNOSTIC TEST EFFECTS

May increase urine catecholamine and urine vanillylmandelic acid levels.

SIDE-EFFECTS

Frequent: Burning and tingling at oral point of dissolution (sublingual), headache (possibly severe) occurs mostly in early therapy, diminishes rapidly in intensity, and usually disappears during continued treatment, transient flushing of face and neck, dizziness (especially if patient is standing immobile or is in a warm environment), weakness, orthostatic hypotension, nausea, vomiting, restlessness. **Occasional:** GI upset, blurred vision, dry mouth

CRITICAL CARE CONSIDERATIONS

ADMINISTRATION/HANDLING

PO ALERT

- Best if taken on an empty stomach; however, administer isosorbide with meals if the patient experiences a headache.
- Original, basic tablet form may be crushed.
- Do not crush or break extended-release or chewable tablet forms.

SUBLINGUAL ALERT

- Do not crush or chew sublingual tablets.
- Dissolve tablets under tongue without swallowing.

PRECAUTIONS

HEALTH-RELATED

- Use isosorbide cautiously in patients with acute MI, blood volume depletion from therapy, glaucoma (contraindicated in closed-angle glaucoma), hepatic or renal disease, or systolic BP less than 90 mmHg.

AGE-RELATED

- **Children:** Safety and efficacy of isosorbide have not been established in children.
- **Elderly:** May be more sensitive to the hypotensive effects. Age-related renal dysfunction may require cautious use.

PREGNANCY/LACTATION-RELATED

- Pregnancy category C; excretion into breast milk unknown; use caution in nursing mothers.

MONITORING

- **Baseline assessment:** Record onset, characteristics, radiation, location, intensity, duration, and precipitating factors (e.g., exertion and emotional stress) of angina.
- **Baseline lab work:** Biochemical profile including cardiac enzymes. B-type natriuretic peptide (BNP) level if heart failure is present.
- **Baseline diagnostic tests:** 12-lead ECG to use for comparison. Chest x-ray if history of heart failure is present.
- **Anginal pain:** Document the number of anginal episodes and correlate with heart rate and BP readings at time angina is present.
- **Patient education:** Teach to take sublingual tablets while sitting or lying down to avoid orthostatic hypotension. Explain that extended-release, sublingual, or sustained-release forms should not be chewed or crushed. Instruct to dissolve sublingual tablets under the tongue, not to swallow. Explain that isosorbide should be taken at the first sign or symptom of angina. If angina is not relieved within 5 min, patients should dissolve a second tablet under the tongue and then repeat the dosage 5 min later if pain is not relieved. Caution not to take more than 3 tablets within 15-30 min. Instruct to seek immediate emergency medical assistance if chest discomfort persists. Advise that after anginal pain is completely relieved, any remaining sublingual tablet should be expelled from under the tongue. Advise taking medication with meals if headache occurs when drug is taken without food. Patients should not alternate brands of isosorbide taken to ensure consistent effects. Urge avoidance of alcohol during isosorbide therapy because alcohol intensifies hypotensive effects. BP can drop significantly if alcohol is consumed within a short time of taking isosorbide.

SERIOUS ADVERSE REACTIONS

- Isosorbide administration may cause severe orthostatic hypotension manifested by fainting, pulselessness, cold or clammy skin, and diaphoresis.
- Tolerance may occur with repeated, prolonged therapy, but may not occur with the extended-release form. Minor tolerance may be seen with intermittent use of sublingual tablets.
- Methemoglobinemia is possible.

OVERDOSE/TOXICITY

- **Symptoms:** Confusion, hypotension, visual disturbances, headache, dry mouth, flushing, heart block, tachycardia, reflex paradoxic bradycardia, constrictive pericarditis, paralysis or paresis secondary to decreased cerebral perfusion, and cardiac arrest.

- **Management:** Discontinue isosorbide if dry mouth or visual disturbances occur. Administer IV fluids. Epinephrine and *DOPamine are contraindicated. Support ventilation, maintain patent airway. If methemoglobinemia is present, methylene blue should be infused IV. Resuscitate as needed using Advanced Cardiac Life Support (ACLS) guidelines.
- **GI decontamination:** No specific recommendations.

ANTIDOTE/DIALYSIS

- **Antidote:** No specific antidote. Alpha adrenergic agonists (e.g., phenylephrine [Neosynephrine] or methoxamine [Vasoxyl]) may be required to manage refractory hypotension.
- **Dialysis:** Isosorbide dinitrate is not removed by hemodialysis or peritoneal dialysis; no data are available on removal using high-permeability hemodialysis. Isosorbide mononitrate is removed by hemodialysis and is likely removed by high-permeability hemodialysis; it is not removed by peritoneal dialysis.

isradipine

See Calcium Channel Blockers (p. 950)

itraconazole

it-ra-con'-a-zol

Classes

Chemical: triazole derivative
Therapeutic: antifungal

Pregnancy Category: C

Trade Names

Prescription: Sporanox

Do not confuse Sporanox with Suprax.

CLINICAL PHARMACOLOGY

Mechanism of Action

A fungistatic antifungal that inhibits the synthesis of ergosterol, a vital component of fungal cell formation. Therapeutic Effect: Damages the fungal cell membrane, altering its function.

PHARMACOKINETICS

Moderately absorbed from the GI tract. Absorption is increased if the drug is taken with food. Protein binding: 99%. Widely distributed, primarily in the fatty tissue, liver, and kidneys. Metabolized in the liver to active metabolite. Primarily excreted in urine. Not removed by hemodialysis. Half-life: 21 hr; metabolite, 12 hr.

AVAILABILITY

Capsules: 100 mg.
Oral Solution: 10 mg/mL.
Injection: 10 mg/mL (25-mL ampule).

INDICATIONS AND DOSAGE

Blastomycosis, histoplasmosis

PO

Adults, Elderly: Initially, 200 mg once per day. Maximum: 400 mg/day in 2 divided doses.

IV

Adults, Elderly: 200 mg twice per day for 4 doses, then 200 mg once per day.

Aspergillosis

PO

Adults, Elderly: 600 mg/day in 3 divided doses for 3-4 days, then 200-400 mg/day in 2 divided doses × 3 mo for life-threatening infections; 200 mg/day for non-life-threatening infections.

IV

Adults, Elderly: 200 mg twice per day for 4 doses, then 200 mg once per day × 3 mo.

Esophageal candidiasis

PO

Adults, Elderly: Swish 100-200 mg (10-20 mL) in mouth for several sec, then swallow. Maximum: 200 mg/day.

Oropharyngeal candidiasis

PO

Adults, Elderly: 200 mg (10 mL) oral solution, swish and swallow once per day for 7-14 days.

Febrile neutropenia

IV

Adults, Elderly: 200 mg twice per day for 4 doses, then 200 mg for up to 14 days. Then give PO 200 mg twice per day until neutropenia resolves.

Onychomycosis (fingernail)

PO

Adults, Elderly: 200 mg twice per day for 7 days, off for 21 days, repeat 200 mg twice per day for 7 days.

Onychomycosis (toenail)

PO

Adults, Elderly: 200 mg once daily for 12 wk.

OFF-LABEL USES

Suppression of histoplasmosis; treatment of disseminated sporotrichosis, fungal pneumonia and septicemia, or ringworm of the hand

CONTRAINDICATIONS

Hypersensitivity to itraconazole, fluconazole, ketoconazole, or miconazole; coadministration with cisapride, oral midazolam, pimozide, quinidine, lovastatin, simvastatin, triazolam; ergot alkaloids; heart failure (if treating onychomycosis); pregnant women or those considering pregnancy (if treating onychomycosis)

INTERACTIONS

Drug: **Antacids, didanosine, H_2 antagonists:** May decrease itraconazole absorption. ***BusPIRone, *cycloSPORINE, digoxin, lovastatin, simvastatin:** May increase blood concentration of these drugs. **Oral anticoagulants:** May increase the effect of oral anticoagulants. **Phenytoin, rifampin:** May decrease itraconazole blood concentration. Herbal: None known. Food: **Grapefruit, grapefruit juice:** May alter itraconazole absorption.

DIAGNOSTIC TEST EFFECTS

May increase serum LDH serum alkaline phosphatase, serum bilirubin, AST (SGOT), and ALT (SGPT) levels. May decrease serum potassium level.

IV INCOMPATIBILITIES

Alert: Dilution compatibility of itraconazole with any solution other than 0.9% NaCl is unknown. Do not mix with D_5W or lactated Ringer's solution. Not for IV bolus administration. Do not administer any medication in same bag or through same IV line as itraconazole.

SIDE-EFFECTS

Frequent (11%-9%): Nausea, rash. Occasional (5%-3%): Vomiting, headache, diarrhea, hypertension, peripheral edema, Occasional fatigue, fever. Rare (2% or less): Abdominal pain, dizziness, anorexia, pruritus

CRITICAL CARE CONSIDERATIONS

ADMINISTRATION/HANDLING

PO ALERT

- Give capsules with food to increase absorption.
- Give oral solution on an empty stomach.
- Grapefruit juice may increase drug absorption and should be avoided.
- Give doses larger than 200 mg in 2 divided doses.

IV ALERT

- **Storage:** Store ampules at room temperature. Do not freeze.
- **Preparation:** Use only the components provided by the manufacturer. Do not dilute the drug with any other diluent. Add the full contents of the ampule (250 mg/10 mL) to the infusion bag provided (50 mL of 0.9% NaCl) and mix gently.
- **IV infusion:** Infuse the drug over 60 min using the extension line and infusion set provided.
- **Following infusion:** Flush the infusion set with 15 to 20 mL of 0.9% NaCl over 30 sec to 15 min, and discard the entire infusion line.
- Give doses larger than 200 mg in 2 divided doses.

PRECAUTIONS

HEALTH-RELATED

- Use itraconazole cautiously in patients with achlorhydria or hypochlorhydria, hepatitis, HIV infection, or impaired hepatic function.
- **Cytochrome P450 metabolism:** Itraconazole is metabolized by the CYP3A4 isoenzyme system which may result in numerous drug interactions. Itraconazole inhibits the enzyme as do the drugs that cause interactions, which can lead to prolonged QT syndrome, torsades de pointes, and cardiac arrest. Coadministration is contraindicated with cisapride (Propulsid), dofetilide (Tikosyn), hydroxymethylglutyral-CoA reductase inhibitors (e.g., lovastatin [Mevacor], simvastatin [Zocor]), oral midazolam (Versed), pimozide (Orap), quinidine, and triazolam (Halcion).

AGE-RELATED

- **Children:** Safety and efficacy of itraconazole have not been established in children.
- **Elderly:** Age-related renal impairment may require a lower dosage.

PREGNANCY/LACTATION-RELATED

- Pregnancy category C; excreted into breast milk; do not administer to nursing mothers.

MONITORING

- **Baseline assessment:** Obtain vital signs and assess history of illness. Determine history of allergies before giving the drug.

- **Baseline lab work:** Biochemical profile including liver function tests. Closely monitor liver function test results in patients with preexisting hepatic dysfunction.
- **Liver dysfunction:** Assess for liver enzyme elevation, fatigue, nausea, flulike symptoms, jaundice, and edema.
- **Patient education:** Instruct to take itraconazole capsules and itraconazole oral solution with food if GI distress is experienced. Explain that therapy will continue for at least 3 mo and until laboratory tests and overall condition indicate the infection is controlled. Warn to report promptly decreased appetite, dark urine, nausea, vomiting, pale stools, unusual fatigue, or yellow skin to a health care provider. Caution to avoid grapefruit and grapefruit juice because they may alter itraconazole absorption.

SERIOUS ADVERSE REACTIONS

- Reactions to itraconazole alone are difficult to discern because of multiple medical conditions and numerous medication interactions.
- **Hypersensitivity:** Allergic reactions have been reported.

OVERDOSE/TOXICITY

- **Hepatitis:** Anorexia, abdominal pain, unusual fatigue or weakness, jaundiced skin or sclera, and dark urine.
- **Exfoliative dermatitis:** Rash may signal onset of Stevens–Johnson syndrome.
- **Heart failure:** Dyspnea, activity intolerance, edema, crackles auscultated in lung fields, elevated B-type natriuretic peptide (BNP) level, infiltrates on chest x-ray.
- **Management:** Discontinue itraconazole. Manage symptoms per accepted guidelines.
- **GI decontamination:** No specific recommendations.

ANTIDOTE/DIALYSIS

- **Antidote:** No specific recommendations.
- **Dialysis:** Itraconazole is not removed by hemodialysis and is unlikely to be removed by peritoneal dialysis. No data are available on removal by high-permeability hemodialysis.

kanamycin sulfate

kan-a-mye'-sin sul'-fate

Classes

Chemical: aminoglycoside
Therapeutic: antibiotic

Pregnancy Category: D

Trade Names

Prescription: Kantrex

CLINICAL PHARMACOLOGY

Mechanism of Action

An aminoglycoside antibiotic that irreversibly binds to protein on bacterial ribosomes. **Therapeutic Effect:** Interferes with protein synthesis of susceptible microorganisms.

PHARMACOKINETICS

Negligible amounts are absorbed through intact intestinal mucosa. Protein binding: 0%-3%. Minimally metabolized in liver. Partially excreted in feces; 81%-94% eliminated in urine. Removed by hemodialysis. **Half-life:** approximately 2 hr.

AVAILABILITY

Injection: 1 g/3 mL.

INDICATIONS AND DOSAGE

Short-term treatment of serious infections

IV

Adults: 15 mg/kg/day divided every 8-12 hr (based on ideal body weight).

IM

Adults, Children: 15 mg/kg/day in 2 divided dosages administered at equally divided intervals (7.5 mg/kg every 12 hr). If continuously high blood levels are desired, the daily dose of 15 mg/kg may be given in equally divided doses every 6-8 hr (based on ideal body weight).

Dosage in renal impairment

Dosage and frequency are modified based on the degree of renal impairment and serum drug concentration. Based on creatinine clearance:

50-80 mL/min: Administer 60%-90% of dose or give every 8-12 hr.
10-50 mL/min: Administer 30%-70% of dose or give every 12 hr.
Less than 10 mL/min: Administer 20%-30% of dose or give every 24-48 hr.

CONTRAINDICATIONS

Hypersensitivity to kanamycin sulfate, other aminoglycosides (cross-sensitivity), or their components; long-term therapy; pregnancy

INTERACTIONS

Drug: Beta-lactam antibiotics: May result in mutual inactivation. **Nephrotoxic medications, other aminoglycosides, ototoxic medications:** May increase the risk of nephrotoxicity or ototoxicity. **Neuromuscular blockers:** May increase neuromuscular blockade. **Herbal:** None significant. **Food:** None significant.

DIAGNOSTIC TEST EFFECTS

Concomitant cephalosporin therapy may elevate creatinine determinations

SIDE-EFFECTS

Occasional: Hypersensitivity reactions (fever, pruritus, rash, urticaria). **Rare:** Headache

CRITICAL CARE CONSIDERATIONS

ADMINISTRATION/HANDLING

IM ALERT

- **Administration:** Kanamycin is most frequently given IM.

IV ALERT

- **Storage:** Discard partially used vials after 48 hr.
- **Dilution:** Up to 500 mg must be diluted with a minimum of 100 mL IV fluid for infusion. Kanamycin may not be premixed with other medications.
- **Infusion:** Infuse using a separate IV line. Ensure drug does not mix with other antibiotics if multiple intermittent infusions (piggybacks) are Y-site connected into a main IV solution line.

PRECAUTIONS

HEALTH-RELATED

- **Sulfites:** Kanamycin contains sulfites. Use cautiously in patients with asthma.
- **Superinfection:** Use extreme caution if therapy is required more than 7 days. Superinfection may occur from overgrowth of nonsusceptible organisms.
- **Malabsorption syndrome:** Increased fecal fat, decrease in serum carotene and xylose absorption may occur with prolonged therapy.

AGE-RELATED

- **Children:** Use with extreme caution in premature infants and neonates. Immature kidney function will prolong half-life. Rarely used IV in infants. Use with caution in children.

K

- **Elderly:** Age-related renal impairment may place elderly at higher risk for ototoxicity which can lead to permanent deafness and acute renal failure. Longer intervals between doses may reduce complications more than reduced dosage.

PREGNANCY/LACTATION-RELATED

- Pregnancy category D. Unavailable for irrigating solution. Eigth cranial nerve toxicity in the fetus has been reported. Excreted into breast milk in low concentrations; poor oral availability reduces potential for ototoxicity for the infant; compatible with breast-feeding.

MONITORING

- **Baseline assessment:** Assess for hypersensitivity to kanamycin, sulfites, or other aminoglycosides. Assess for history of kidney disease and hearing loss.
- **Baseline lab work:** Biochemical profile including BUN/creatinine, calcium, and magnesium. Levels of sodium, potassium, calcium, and magnesium may decrease.
- **Baseline diagnostic tests:** Consider auditory/hearing testing for comparison if ototoxicity is suspected during use.
- **Neuromuscular blockade:** Avoid concurrent use if possible to avoid potentiating neuromuscular blockade, causing severe respiratory depression.
- **Oliguria:** Monitor urine output closely. If output is less than 0.5 mL/kg, BUN and creatinine should be remeasured and checked for elevation to rule out acute renal failure. Ensure patients are well hydrated during therapy.
- **Hearing loss:** Monitor for progressive hearing loss/deafness.
- **Peak and trough serum drug levels:** Peak concentrations should not exceed 30 mcg/mL; trough should not exceed 5 mcg/mL.
- **Vestibular signs:** Assess for dizziness, especially when position is changed, and ataxia when walking. May indicate vestibular toxicity.
- **Superinfections:** Assess the mouth for white patches on the mucous membranes or tongue and for severe mouth or tongue soreness; assess for severe anal or genital pruritus or discharge.
- **Possible *Clostridium difficile* colitis:** Assess pattern of daily bowel activity and stool consistency. Although mild GI effects may be tolerable, severe symptoms including abdominal pain or cramping and moderate to severe diarrhea may indicate the onset of antibiotic-associated colitis.
- **Hand washing:** If *C. difficile* (antibiotic-associated) colitis develops, wash hands with antibacterial soap. Alcohol-based foam is ineffective against *C. difficile* spores.
- **Evenly space doses:** Space doses evenly around the clock. If drug is used outside the hospital, instruct to continue taking kanamycin for the full course of treatment.
- **IM injection site:** Evaluate the IM injection site for induration and tenderness.
- **Patient education:** Instruct to promptly report difficulty hearing.

SERIOUS ADVERSE REACTIONS

- **Hypersensitivity:** Patients with a history of allergies, especially to aminoglycosides, are at increased risk for developing a severe hypersensitivity reaction marked by severe pruritus, angioedema, bronchospasm, and anaphylaxis.
- **Management of hypersensitivity:** May require treatment with epinephrine and other emergency measures including oxygen, endotracheal intubation, mechanical ventilation, IV fluids, IV antihistamines, corticosteroids, and vasopressors.
- **Respiratory depression:** May potentiate neuromuscular blocking agents (doxacurium, succinylcholine), including drugs not primarily used for neuromuscular blockade (streptomycin, clindamycin) to cause severe respiratory depression and apnea. Calcium salts or neostigmine may reverse neuromuscular blockade and improve respiratory function.

OVERDOSE/TOXICITY

- **Nephrotoxicity:** Increased BUN and creatinine, decreased urine output, anuria, possible hyperkalemia, fluid overload indicative of acute renal failure. Renal failure is often reversible.
- **Ototoxicity:** Difficulty hearing and/or tinnitus, which can lead to permanent deafness.
- **Management:** Drug dose should be reduced, drug dosing interval increased, or drug discontinued. Consider exchange transfusion in the newborn.
- **GI decontamination:** No specific recommendations.

ANTIDOTE/DIALYSIS

- **Antidote:** No specific antidote. Complexation with ticarcillin may work as effectively as hemodialysis to manage overdose and toxicity.
- **Dialysis:** Kanamycin is removed by hemodialyis, peritoneal dialysis, and likely removed by using high-permeability hemodialysis.

kaolin (with pectin)

See Antidiarrheals (p. 917)

ketamine hydrochloride

keet'-a-meen hye-droe-klor'-ide

Classes

Chemical: cyclohexanone hydrochloride
Therapeutic: general anesthetic, analgesic, nonbarbiturate

Pregnancy Category: D

Trade Names

Prescription: Ketalar

CLINICAL PHARMACOLOGY

Mechanism of Action

A rapidly acting general anesthetic that selectively blocks afferent impulses and interacts with CNS transmitter systems. **Therapeutic Effect:** Produces an anesthetic state characterized by profound analgesia and normal pharyngeal-laryngeal reflexes.

PHARMACOKINETICS

Route	Onset	Peak	Duration
IM (anesthetic)	3-4 min	N/A	12-25 min
IM (analgesic)	10-15 min	N/A	15-30 min
IV (anesthetic)	30 sec	N/A	5-10 min

Rapidly distributed. Metabolized in the liver. Primarily excreted in urine. **Half-life:** Distribution: 10-15 min, elimination: 2-3 hr.

AVAILABILITY

Injection: 10 mg/mL, 50 mg/mL, 100 mg/mL.

INDICATIONS AND DOSAGE

Induction and maintenance of general anesthesia (especially when cardiovascular depression is to be avoided), sedation, analgesia

IV

Adults, Elderly: 1-4.5 mg/kg. Usual induction dose: 1-2 mg/kg. **Children.** 0.5-2 mg/kg. Usual induction dose: 1-2 mg/kg.

IM

Adults, Elderly: 3-8 mg/kg. **Children.** 3-7 mg/kg.

CONTRAINDICATIONS

Aneurysms, angina, heart failure, elevated intracranial pressure (ICP), hypertension, psychotic disorders, thyrotoxicosis, hypersensitivity to ketamine

INTERACTIONS

Drug: Antihypertensives, CNS depressants: May increase the risk of hypotension and respiratory depression. **Herbal:** None known. **Food:** None known.

DIAGNOSTIC TEST EFFECTS

May increase intraocular pressure (IOP).

IV INCOMPATIBILITIES

No information available for Y-site administration.

IV COMPATIBILITIES

Bupivacaine (Marcaine), clonidine (Duraclon), fentanyl (Sublimaze), lidocaine, morphine, propofol (Diprivan)

SIDE-EFFECTS

Frequent: Increased BP and pulse rate; emergence reaction (marked by dreamlike state, delirium, hallucinations, and vivid imagery and occasionally accompanied by confusion, excitement, and irrational behavior; lasts from few hours to 24 hr after ketamine administration). **Occasional:** Pain at injection site. **Rare:** Rash

CRITICAL CARE CONSIDERATIONS

ADMINISTRATION/HANDLING

IV ALERT

- **IV push:** Give ketamine by IV push when used to induce anesthesia. Dilute the 100 mg/mL vial of ketamine with an equal volume of sterile water for injection, D_5W, or 0.9% NaCl.
- **IV push maintenance dose:** Administer maintenance dose by IV push slowly at a rate of 0.5 mg/kg/min over 60 sec. A too-rapid IV administration may result in severe hypotension and respiratory depression.
- **Maintenance IV infusion:** Dilute the 50-mg/mL vial (10 mL) or 100-mg/mL vial (5 mL) of ketamine with 250-500 mL D_5W or 0.9% NaCl to provide a concentration of 1-2 mg/mL.

IM ALERT

- Use the 10-mg/mL vial of ketamine. Do not dilute the 10-mg/mL vial.

PRECAUTIONS

HEALTH-RELATED

- Use ketamine cautiously in intoxicated or chronic alcoholic patients, in those with a full stomach, gastroesophageal reflux disease, or hepatic impairment.

K

AGE-RELATED

- **Children:** No age-related precautions; low incidence of emergence reaction in children under 16 yr.
- **Elderly:** No age-related precautions have been noted; low incidence of emergence reaction.

PREGNANCY/LACTATION-RELATED

- Pregnancy category D; breast-feeding is not recommended until drug has fully cleared the patient's body (at least 24 hr).

MONITORING

- **Baseline assessment:** Anesthesiologist should obtain history including medication allergies and past problems with anesthesia. Obtain vital signs before giving ketamine. Have resuscitative equipment and oxygen available.
- **Baseline lab work:** CBC and biochemical profile including renal and hepatic studies. Coagulation studies are done on patients prior to surgery.
- **Baseline diagnostic tests:** If surgery is scheduled, chest x-ray and 12-lead ECG are generally used to help assess preoperative risk factors.
- **Potential for hypotension respiratory depression:** Monitor vital signs every 3-5 min during and after ketamine administration until patients have recovered. Observe rate and depth of respirations and work of breathing.
- **Emergence reaction:** Assess for an emergence reaction, with psychologic and behavioral symptoms that vary in intensity.
- **Anesthesia recovery care:** Minimize verbal, tactile, and visual stimulation during the recovery period.
- **Patient education:** Warn to avoid performing tasks requiring mental alertness or motor skills for 24 hr after anesthesia has been discontinued.

SERIOUS ADVERSE REACTIONS

- **Emergence reaction:** Psychologic symptoms include pleasant to disturbing dreams, hallucinations, delirium, excitement, and irrational behavior.
- **Management:** Administer a barbiturate or hypnotic for emergence reactions. Use of diazepam during induction and maintenance of anesthesia may reduce incidence of emergence reactions.

OVERDOSE/TOXICITY

- **Hypotension/respiratory depression:** Continuous or repeated intermittent infusion may result in extreme somnolence and circulatory or respiratory depression. Too-rapid IV administration may produce severe hypotension, respiratory depression, and irregular muscle movements.
- **Management:** Supportive care to maintain patent airway and ventilation, with IV fluids and possibly vasopressors to manage hypotension.
- **GI decontamination:** No specific recommendations.

ANTIDOTE/DIALYSIS

- **Antidote:** No specific recommendations.
- **Dialysis:** Ketamine is not removed by hemodialysis and is unlikely to be removed by peritoneal dialysis. No data are available on removal using high-permeability hemodialysis.

ketoconazole

kee-toe-kon'-na-zole

Classes

Chemical: imidazole derivative
Therapeutic: antifungal

Pregnancy Category: C

Trade Names

Prescription: Nizoral, Nizoral Topical
Over the Counter: Nizoral AD

Do not confuse Nizoral with Nasarel.

CLINICAL PHARMACOLOGY

Mechanism of Action

A fungistatic antifungal that inhibits the synthesis of ergosterol, a vital component of fungal cell formation. Therapeutic Effect: Damages the fungal cell membrane, altering its function.

PHARMACOKINETICS

Well absorbed from GI tract following PO administration. Protein binding: 93%-96%. Metabolized in liver. Primarily excreted in bile with minimal elimination in urine. Negligible systemic absorption following topical absorption. Ketoconazole is not detected in plasma after shampooing or topical administration. Half-life: 2-8 hr.

AVAILABILITY

Tablets (Nizoral): 200 mg.
Cream (Nizoral Topical): 2%.
Shampoo (Nizoral AD): 1%.

INDICATIONS AND DOSAGE

Histoplasmosis, blastomycosis, systemic candidiasis, chronic mucocutaneous candidiasis, coccidioidomycosis, paracoccidioidomycosis, chromomycosis, seborrheic dermatitis, tinea corporis, tinea capitis, tinea manus, tinea cruris, tinea pedis, tinea unguium (onychomycosis), oral thrush, candiduria

PO

Adults, Elderly: 200-400 mg/day as a single daily dose. **Children:** 3.3-6.6 mg/kg/day as a single dose. Continue for 1-2 wk for candidiasis, 4 wk for dermatologic infections, and up to 6 mo for other systemic mycotic infections. Maximum: 800 mg/day in 2 divided doses.

Topical

Adults, Elderly: Apply to affected area 1-2 times per day for 2-4 wk.

Shampoo

Adults, Elderly: Use twice weekly for 4 wk, allowing at least 3 days between shampooing. Use intermittently to maintain control.

OFF-LABEL USES

Systemic: Treatment of fungal pneumonia, prostate cancer, septicemia

CONTRAINDICATIONS

Hypersensitivity to ketoconazole; coadministration with terfenadine, astenuzole, or cisapride or ergot derivatives

INTERACTIONS

Drug: **Alcohol, hepatotoxic medications:** May increase hepatotoxicity of ketoconazole. **Antacids, anticholinergics, H_2 antagonists, omeprazole:** May decrease ketoconazole absorption. ***CycloSPORINE, lovastatin, simvastatin:** May increase blood concentration and risk of toxicity of these drugs. **Isoniazid, rifampin:** May decrease blood concentration of ketoconazole. Herbal: **Echinacea:** May have additive hepatotoxic effects. Food: None known.

DIAGNOSTIC TEST EFFECTS

May increase serum alkaline phosphatase, serum bilirubin, AST (SGOT), and ALT (SGPT) levels. May decrease serum corticosteroid and testosterone concentrations.

SIDE-EFFECTS

Occasional (10%-3%): Nausea, vomiting.
Rare (less than 2%): Abdominal pain, diarrhea, headache, dizziness, photophobia, pruritus. **Topical:** itching, burning, irritation

CRITICAL CARE CONSIDERATIONS

ADMINISTRATION/HANDLING

PO ALERT

- Give ketoconazole with food to minimize GI irritation.
- Tablets may be crushed.
- Ketoconazole requires acidity; give antacids and other medications used to reduce gastric acidity (anticholinergics, H_2 blockers, or omeprazole) at least 2 hr after administering the drug.

TOPICAL ALERT

- Apply and rub gently into the affected and surrounding area.

SHAMPOO ALERT

- Apply to wet hair, massage for 1 min, rinse thoroughly, reapply for 3 min, then rinse.

PRECAUTIONS

HEALTH-RELATED

- Use ketoconazole cautiously in patients with hepatic impairment.
- **Terfenadine, astemizole, cisapride:** Coadministration of ketoconazole with these drugs is contraindicated; combination may induce prolonged QT syndrome, ventricular tachycardia, torsades de pointes, and death.
- **Cytochrome P450 enzyme inhibitor:** Ketoconazole is a potent inhibitor of the cytochrome P450 3A4 enzyme system, which prompts the need to adjust dosage of many other medications metabolized by this pathway.

AGE-RELATED

- **Children:** Safety and efficacy of ketoconazole have not been established in children.
- **Elderly:** Age-related hepatic and bone marrow impairment warrants close monitoring of liver function studies and CBC.

PREGNANCY/LACTATION-RELATED

- Pregnancy category C. Has been used, apparently without harm, for the treatment of vaginal candidiasis during pregnancy. Not detected in plasma with chronic shampoo use. Unknown whether cream is absorbed. Oral ketoconazole probably excreted in breast milk; use in breast-feeding not recommended

K

MONITORING

- **Baseline assessment:** Assess history of infection. Obtain vital signs. Describe symptoms of the fungal infection.
- **Baseline lab work:** CBC with WBC differential and platelet count. Biochemical profile including liver enzymes (AST [SGOT], ALT [SGPT], alkaline phosphatase). Perform a culture or histologic test for accurate diagnosis of the causative organism.
- **Hepatotoxicity:** Monitor for dark urine, pale stools, jaundice, fatigue, and GI effects (anorexia, nausea, vomiting) unrelieved by giving drug with food.
- **Bone marrow suppression:** Monitor CBC for thrombocytopenia, anemia, and leukopenia.
- **GI effects:** Assess for diarrhea; provide hydration and antidiarrheal medication.
- **Dizziness:** Assess dizziness; provide assistance and institute safety precautions.
- **Sensitivity:** Evaluate skin for a rash, pruritus, and urticaria.
- **Topical ketoconazole:** Check skin for localized burning, itching, and irritation.
- **Patient education:** Explain that prolonged therapy over weeks or months is usually necessary. Instruct not to miss a dose and to continue therapy for as long as directed. Recommend avoidance of alcohol to minimize the risk of liver damage. Caution to avoid tasks that require mental alertness or motor skills until response to the drug is known. Instruct to take antacids or antiulcer medications at least 2 hr after taking ketoconazole. Explain the need to report immediately dark urine, pale stools, yellow skin or eyes, increased irritation (with topical use), or other new symptoms to a health care provider. Patients should avoid drug contact with the eyes and keep the skin clean and dry. Drug should be rubbed well into affected areas. Light clothing should be worn for ventilation. Encourage separation of personal items that come in direct contact with the affected area from items others will handle. Instruct patients to use the shampoo initially twice weekly for 4 wk and to wait at least 3 days between shampooing. Explain that further use will be based on the response to initial treatment.

SERIOUS ADVERSE REACTIONS

- Anaphylaxis occurs rarely.

OVERDOSE/TOXICITY

- **Hematologic toxicity:** Thrombocytopenia, hemolytic anemia, and leucopenia.
- **Hepatotoxicity:** May occur within 1 wk to several mo after starting therapy.
- **GI decontamination:** No specific recommendations.

ANTIDOTE/DIALYSIS

- **Antidote:** No specific recommendations.
- **Dialysis:** Ketoconazole is not removed by hemodialysis or peritoneal dialysis. No data are available on removal using high-permeability hemodialysis.

ketoprofen

See NSAIDs and Cox-2 Inhibitors (p. 976)

ketorolac tromethamine

kee-toe-role'-ak troe-meth'-a-meen

Classes

Chemical: acetic acid derivative
Therapeutic: NSAID, antipyretic, nonnarcotic analgesic

Pregnancy Category: C, D (3rd trimester)

Trade Names

Prescription: Acular, Acular LS, Acular PF, Toradol, Toradol IM, Toradol IV/IM

Do not confuse Acular with Acthar or Ocular.

CLINICAL PHARMACOLOGY

Mechanism of Action

An NSAID that inhibits prostaglandin synthesis and reduces prostaglandin levels in the aqueous humor. **Therapeutic Effect:** Relieves pain stimulus and reduces intraocular inflammation.

PHARMACOKINETICS

Route	Onset	Peak	Duration
PO	30 min	3 hr	5-6 hr
IV/IM	30 min	1-2 hr	4-6 hr

Readily absorbed from the GI tract, after IM administration. Protein binding: 99%. Largely metabolized in the liver. Primarily excreted in urine. Unlikely to be removed by hemodialysis. **Half-life:** 3.8-6.3 hr (increased with impaired renal function and in the elderly).

AVAILABILITY

Tablets (Toradol): 10 mg.

Injection (Toradol, Toradol IM, Toradol IV/IM): 15 mg/mL, 30 mg/mL.
Ophthalmic Solution: 0.4% (Acular LS), 0.5% (Acular, Acular PF).

INDICATIONS AND DOSAGE

Short-term relief of mild to moderate pain (multiple doses)

PO

Adults, Elderly: 20 mg followed by 10 mg every 4-6 hr. Maximum: 40 mg/24 hr. **Children:** 0.25 mg/kg every 6 hr.

IV, IM

Adults younger than 65 yr: 30 mg every 6 hr. Maximum: 120 mg/24 hr. **Adults 65 yr and older, those with renal impairment, those weighing less than 50 kg:** 15 mg every 6 hr. Maximum: 60 mg/24 hr. **Children 2-16 yr:** 0.5 mg/kg, then 0.25-1 mg/kg every 6 hr up to 48 hr. Maximum: 90 mg/day.

Short-term relief of mild to moderate pain (single dose)

IV

Adults younger than 65 yr, Children 17 yr and older, and weighing more than 50 kg: 30 mg. **Adults 65 yr and older, with renal impairment, or weighing less than 50 kg:** 15 mg. **Children 2-16 yr:** 0.5 mg/kg. Maximum: 15 mg.

IM

Adults younger than 65 yr, Children 17 yr and older, and weighing more than 50 kg: 60 mg. **Adults 65 yr and older, with renal impairment, or weighing less than 50 kg:** 30 mg. **Children 2-16 yr.** 1 mg/kg. Maximum: 30 kg.

Allergic conjunctivitis

Ophthalmic

Adults, Elderly, Children 3 yr and older: 1 drop 4 times per day.

Cataract extraction

Ophthalmic

Adults, Elderly: 1 drop 4 times per day. Begin 24 hr after surgery and continue for 2 wk.

Refractive surgery

Ophthalmic

Adults, Elderly: 1 drop 4 times per day for 3 days.

OFF-LABEL USES

Prevention or treatment of ocular inflammation (ophthalmic form)

CONTRAINDICATIONS

Active peptic ulcer disease; chronic inflammation of GI tract; GI bleeding or ulceration; history of hypersensitivity to ketorolac, aspirin, or NSAIDs; perioperative pain following Coronary artery bypass graft (bypass) surgery; pregnancy (third trimester)

INTERACTIONS

Drug: Antihypertensives, diuretics: May decrease the effects of these drugs. **Aspirin, other salicylates:** May increase the risk of GI side effects such as bleeding. **Bone marrow depressants:** May increase the risk of hematologic reactions. **Heparin, oral anticoagulants, thrombolytics:** May increase the effects of these drugs. **Lithium:** May increase the blood concentration and risk of toxicity of lithium. **Methotrexate:** May increase the risk of methotrexate toxicity. **Probenecid:** May increase ketorolac blood concentration. **Herbal: Feverfew:** May decrease the effects of feverfew. **Ginkgo biloba:** May increase the risk of bleeding. **Food:** None known.

DIAGNOSTIC TEST EFFECTS

May prolong bleeding time. May increase liver function test results.

IV INCOMPATIBILITIES

Promethazine (Phenergan)

IV COMPATIBILITIES

Fentanyl (Sublimaze), hydromorphone (Dilaudid), morphine, nalbuphine (Nubain)

SIDE-EFFECTS

Frequent (17%-12%): Headache, nausea, abdominal cramps or pain, dyspepsia. **Occasional (9%-3%):** Diarrhea. **Ophthalmic:** Transient stinging and burning. **Rare (3%-1%):** Constipation, vomiting, flatulence, stomatitis, dizziness. **Ophthalmic:** Ocular irritation, allergic reactions, superficial ocular infection, keratitis

CRITICAL CARE CONSIDERATIONS

ADMINISTRATION/HANDLING

DOSAGE ALERT

- Ketorolac should not be administered by any route or combination of routes for more than 5 days. Drug may be given as a single dose, on a schedule, or as needed for pain.

PO ALERT

- Give ketorolac with food, milk, or antacids if the patient experiences GI distress.

IV ALERT

- **IV push:** Administer ketorolac undiluted by IV push over at least 15 sec.

K

IM ALERT

- **Injection:** Slowly inject drug deeply and into a large muscle mass.

OPHTHALMIC ALERT

- **Instillation:** Pull out the lower eyelid with a gloved finger, forming a pocket between the eye and lower lid. Hold the dropper above the pocket, and place appropriate number of drops in the pocket. Gently close the eye; apply digital pressure to the lacrimal sac for 1 to 2 min to minimize post-nasal drainage, thus reducing risk of absorption causing systemic effects. Remove excess solution with a tissue.

PRECAUTIONS

HEALTH-RELATED

- Use ketorolac cautiously in patients with a history of GI tract disease, hepatic or renal impairment, or a predisposition to fluid retention.

K

AGE-RELATED

- **Children:** Safety and efficacy of ketorolac have not been established in children under 16 yr; doses of 0.5 mg/kg have been used successfully.
- **Elderly:** GI bleeding or ulceration is more likely to cause serious complications; age-related renal impairment may increase the risk of renal toxicity or hepatotoxicity; a decreased dosage is recommended.

PREGNANCY/LACTATION-RELATED

- Pregnancy category C (D if used in third trimester); excreted into breast milk; not recommended in lactation

MONITORING

- **Baseline assessment:** Assess the duration, location, onset, and type of pain.
- **Baseline lab work:** CBC, biochemical profile including renal (BUN, creatinine) and liver function tests (AST [SGOT], ALT [SGPT], alkaline phosphatase, bilirubin), prothrombin time, aPTT.
- **GI effects:** Monitor for dyspepsia, nausea, coffee ground emesis/NG secretions.
- **Nephrotoxicity/hepatotoxicity:** Monitor liver and renal function tests and urine output.
- **Bleeding:** Monitor for bleeding, which may also occur with ophthalmic use if systemic absorption occurs.
- **Therapeutic response:** Assess for decreased pain, tenderness, improved grip strength, increased joint mobility, and less stiffness and swelling.
- **Patient education:** Instruct to take ketorolac with food or milk if GI upset occurs. Instruct not to administer ketorolac ophthalmic solution while wearing soft contact lenses. Transient burning and stinging may occur after instillation. Recommend avoidance of alcohol and aspirin, which increase possibility of bleeding during oral or ophthalmic ketorolac therapy. Warn to avoid tasks requiring mental alertness or motor skills until response to the drug is known. Instruct female patients to report if they are or plan to become pregnant.

SERIOUS ADVERSE REACTIONS

- **GI effects:** Peptic ulcer disease, GI bleeding, gastritis.
- **Hypersensitivity reaction:** Fever, chills, joint pain, rash, itching.

OVERDOSE/TOXICITY

- **Overdose:** Hypotonia, muscle fasciculations, twitching, bone marrow suppression, metabolic acidosis, nausea, vomiting, diarrhea, GI bleeding, abdominal pain, volume depletion with secondary hypotension, tachycardia, pulmonary edema and acute respiratory distress syndrome, acute psychosis, seizures, CNS depression following agitation.
- **Nephrotoxicity:** Dysuria, hematuria, proteinuria, nephrotic syndrome, elevated BUN and creatinine.
- **Hepatotoxicity:** Cholestasis, jaundice, elevated liver enzymes.
- **GI decontamination:** No specific recommendations.

ANTIDOTE/DIALYSIS

- **Antidote:** No specific antidote. Treatment should be supportive and directed at symptoms.
- **Dialysis:** Ketorolac is unlikely to be removed by hemodialysis or peritoneal dialysis. No data are available on removal using high-permeability hemodialysis.

labetalol hydrochloride

la-bet'-a-lole hye-droe-klor'-ide

Classes

Chemical: α-adrenergic blocker, peripheral; β-adrenergic blocker, nonselective
Therapeutic: antihypertensive

Pregnancy Category: C, D (2nd and 3rd trimesters)

Trade Names

Prescription: Normodyne, Trandate

Combinations

Prescription: with hydrochlorothiazide (Normozide, Trandate HCT)

Do not confuse Trandate with tramadol or Trental.

CLINICAL PHARMACOLOGY

Mechanism of Action

An antihypertensive that blocks $alpha_1$-, $beta_1$-, and $beta_2$-(large doses) adrenergic receptor sites. Large doses increase airway resistance. Therapeutic Effect: Slows sinus heart rate; decreases peripheral vascular resistance, cardiac output, and BP.

PHARMACOKINETICS

Route	Onset	Peak	Duration
PO	0.5-2 hr	2-4 hr	8-12 hr
IV	2-5 min	5-15 min	2-4 hr

Completely absorbed from the GI tract. Protein binding: 50%. Undergoes first-pass metabolism. Metabolized in the liver. Primarily excreted in urine. Not removed by hemodialysis. Half-life: PO, 6-8 hr; IV, 5.5 hr.

AVAILABILITY

Tablets (Normodyne, Trandate): 100 mg, 200 mg, 300 mg.
Injection (Trandate): 5 mg/mL.

INDICATIONS AND DOSAGE

Hypertension

PO

Adults: Initially, 100 mg twice per day adjusted in increments of 100 mg twice per day every 2-3 days. Maintenance: 200-400 mg twice per day. **Elderly:** Initially, 100 mg 1-2 times per day. May increase weekly or biweekly.

Severe hypertension, hypertensive emergency

IV

Adults: Initially, 20 mg over 2 min. Additional doses of 20-80 mg may be given at 10-min intervals, up to total dose of 300 mg.

IV Infusion

Adults: Initially, 2 mg/min up to total dose of 300 mg.

PO (after IV therapy)

Adults: Initially 200 mg; then 200-400 mg in 6-12 hr. Increase dose at 1-day intervals to desired level.

OFF-LABEL USES

Control of hypertension during surgery, treatment of chronic angina pectoris

CONTRAINDICATIONS

Bronchial asthma, cardiogenic shock, overt cardiac failure, second- or third-degree heart block, severe bradycardia, uncontrolled heart failure, other conditions associated with severe and prolonged hypotension, hypersensitivity to labetalol

INTERACTIONS

Drug: **Diuretics, other antihypertensives:** May increase hypotensive effect. **Insulin, oral hypoglycemics:** May mask symptoms of hypoglycemia and prolong hypoglycemic effect of these drugs. **MAOIs:** May produce hypertension. **Sympathomimetics, xanthines:** May mutually inhibit effects. Herbal: None known. Food: None known.

DIAGNOSTIC TEST EFFECTS

May increase serum antinuclear antibody titer and BUN, serum LDH, lipoprotein, alkaline phosphatase, bilirubin, creatinine, potassium, triglyceride, uric acid, AST (SGOT), and ALT (SGPT) levels.

IV INCOMPATIBILITIES

Amphotericin B complex (Abelcet, AmBisome, Amphotec), ceftriaxone (Rocephin), furosemide (Lasix), heparin, nafcillin (Nafcil), thiopental

IV COMPATIBILITIES

Aminophylline, amiodarone (Cordarone), calcium gluconate, diltiazem (Cardizem), *DOBUTamine (Dobutrex), *DOPamine (Intropin), enalapril (Vasotec), fentanyl (Sublimaze), hydromorphone (Dilaudid), lidocaine, lorazepam (Ativan), magnesium sulfate, midazolam (Versed), milrinone (Primacor), morphine, nitroglycerin, norepinephrine (Levophed), potassium chloride, potassium phosphate, propofol (Diprivan)

SIDE-EFFECTS

Frequent: Drowsiness, difficulty sleeping, unusual fatigue or weakness, diminished sexual ability, transient scalp tingling, dizziness (9%-20%). Occasional: Dizziness, dyspnea, peripheral edema, depression, anxiety, constipation, diarrhea, nasal congestion, nausea, vomiting, abdominal discomfort. Rare: Altered taste, dry eyes, increased urination, paresthesia

CRITICAL CARE CONSIDERATIONS

ADMINISTRATION/HANDLING

PO ALERT

- Give labetalol without regard to food.
- Crush tablets if necessary.

IV ALERT

- **Storage:** Store at room temperature.
- **Stability:** After dilution, IV solution is stable for 24 hr. Solution normally appears clear and colorless to light yellow; discard solution if precipitate forms or discoloration occurs.
- **IV push:** May be given undiluted. Give over 2 min at 10-min intervals.
- **Dilution, IV infusion:** Dilute 200 mg in 160 mL dextrose 5% in water, 0.9% NaCl, lactated Ringer's solution, or any combination of these solutions to provide a concentration of 1 mg/mL.
- **Preparation:** Place patients in a supine position during IV administration.
- **Continuous IV infusion:** Administer at 2 mg/min (2 mL/min or 120 mL/hr) initially. Adjust rate according to BP. Monitor BP immediately before and every 5 to 10 min during IV administration. Maximum effect occurs within 5 min.
- **Following IV administration:** Keep patients supine for 3 hr after receiving the medication; hypotension is likely if patients stand within 3 hr following drug administration.

PRECAUTIONS

HEALTH-RELATED

- Use labetalol very cautiously in patients with liver disease, heart failure, diabetes mellitus or history of hypoglycemia; use cautiously in those with coronary artery disease, bronchitis, chronic obstructive pulmonary disease (COPD) (chronic bronchitis, emphysema), history of allergy, pheochromocytoma, and impaired renal function.
- **Pheochromocytoma:** Labetalol may effectively lower BP, which then may lead to paradoxic hypertension.

AGE-RELATED

- **Children:** Safety and efficacy of labetalol have not been established in children.
- **Elderly:** Age-related peripheral vascular disease may increase susceptibility to decreased peripheral circulation.

PREGNANCY/LACTATION-RELATED

- Pregnancy category C (D if used in second or third trimester). A similar drug, atenolol, is frequently used in the third trimester for treatment of hypertension (many studies of efficacy and safety of atenolol in pregnancy-induced hypertension). Long-term use has been associated with intrauterine growth retardation. Only a small amount of drug appears in breast milk (0.004% of dose); unlikely to be therapeutically significant.

MONITORING

- **Baseline assessment:** Determine history of heart, respiratory or kidney disease; hypoglycemia; or diabetes mellitus. Assess heart rate and BP immediately before giving labetalol. If heart rate is less than 60 beats/min or systolic BP is less than 90 mmHg, medication should be withheld. Physicians should consider another medication to reduce BP.
- **Baseline lab work:** Biochemical profile including liver and renal function tests. B-type natriuretic peptide (BNP) level if patient may have heart failure.
- **Baseline diagnostic tests:** 12-lead ECG to assess for ST depression and dysrhythmias. Chest x-ray if history of lung disease is present.
- **Cardiac effects:** Monitor continuous ECG for dysrhythmias. Assess for bradycardia, heart block, an irregular rate, and hypotension.
- **Hypotension:** Lower BP gradually to avoid cerebral ischemia or infarction, optic nerve infarction, angina, and myocardial ischemia (ST depression) or infarction (ST elevation).
- **Heart failure:** Evaluate for distended neck veins, dyspnea (on exertion or lying down), night cough, and peripheral edema. Monitor intake, output, and weight. An increase in weight or a decrease in urine output may indicate heart failure. Assist with ambulation if dizziness occurs.
- **Patient education:** Caution against discontinuing the drug without prior discussion with a health care provider. Explain stopping the drug abruptly may precipitate heart failure. Stress that compliance with

the therapy regimen is essential to control dysrhythmias and hypertension. Recommend avoidance of tasks requiring mental alertness or motor skills until response to the drug is known. Instruct to report promptly excessive fatigue, headache, prolonged dizziness, shortness of breath, or weight gain to a health care provider. Advise not to take nasal decongestants and OTC cold preparations, especially those containing stimulants, without prior discussion with a health care provider.

SERIOUS ADVERSE REACTIONS

- **Heart failure:** Labetolol administration may precipitate or aggravate heart failure due to reduced contractility.
- **Abrupt withdrawal:** May precipitate ischemic heart disease producing sweating, palpitations, headache, and tremor.
- **Hypoglycemia:** May mask acute hypoglycemia (tachycardia, BP changes), especially in patients with diabetes.
- **Respiratory distress:** COPD patients dependent on bronchodilators may not tolerate labetalol without increasing doses of bronchodilators; because bronchodilators often cause tachycardia and increased BP, this may defeat the purpose of using labetalol to reduce BP.

OVERDOSE/TOXICITY

- Profound hypotension, bradycardia, dizziness, syncope, drowsiness, breathing difficulty, nausea, vomiting, pallor, central cyanosis, bluish fingernails or palms of hands, somnolence, speech disorders, weakness, and seizures.
- **GI decontamination:** No specific recommendations.

ANTIDOTE/DIALYSIS

- **Antidote:** Once the labetalol infusion is off, *DOPamine or epinephrine infusions may be used to increase heart rate and help manage heart block and may possibly help relieve respiratory distress. Norepinephrine (Levophed) infusion may help increase BP. Atropine may be used for bradycardia but does not have catecholamine properties useful for overriding beta blockade. Unresponsive hypotension and bradycardia may be reversed by glucagon 5-10 mg IV over 30 sec, followed by a continuous infusion of 5 mg/hr, titrated down as patient improves.
- **Dialysis:** Labetalol is not removed by hemodialysis or peritoneal dialysis. No data are available on removal using high-permeability hemodialysis.

lactulose

lak'-tyoo-lose

Classes

Chemical: disaccharide lactose analog
Therapeutic: ammonia detoxicant, laxative

Pregnancy Category: B

Trade Names

Prescription: Acilac ♣, Apo-Lactulose ♣, Cholac, Constilac, Constulose, Enulose, Generlac, Kristalose

Do not confuse Cholac with diclofenac, or lactulose with lactose.

CLINICAL PHARMACOLOGY

Mechanism of Action

A lactose derivative that retains ammonia in the colon and decreases serum ammonia concentration, producing osmotic effect. Therapeutic Effect: Promotes increased peristalsis and bowel evacuation, which expels ammonia from the colon.

PHARMACOKINETICS

Route	Onset	Peak	Duration
PO	24-48 hr	N/A	N/A
Rectal	30-60 min	N/A	N/A

Poorly absorbed from the GI tract. Acts in the colon. Primarily excreted in feces.

AVAILABILITY

Syrup: 10 g/15 mL.
Packets: 10 g, 20 g.

INDICATIONS AND DOSAGE

Constipation

PO

Adults, Elderly: 15-30 mL (10-20 g)/day in 3-4 divided doses, up to 60 mL (40 g)/day. **Children:** 40-90 mL/day in 3-4 divided doses. **Infants:** 2.5-10 mL/day in 3-4 divided doses.

Portal-systemic encephalopathy

PO

Adults, Elderly: Initially, 30-45 mL every hr. Then, 30-45 mL (20-30 g) 3-4 times per day. Adjust dose every 1-2 days to produce 2-3 soft stools per day.

Rectal (as retention enema)

Adults, Elderly: 300 mL with 700 mL water or saline solution; patient should retain 30-60 min. Repeat every 4-6 hr. If evacuation occurs too promptly, repeat immediately.

CONTRAINDICATIONS
Galactosemia, patients on a galactose-free diet, vomiting, hypersensitivity to lactulose

INTERACTIONS
Drug: **Oral medication:** May decrease transit time of concurrently administered oral medications, decreasing lactulose absorption. Herbal: None known. Food: None known.

DIAGNOSTIC TEST EFFECTS
May decrease serum potassium level.

SIDE-EFFECTS
Occasional: Abdominal cramping, flatulence, increased thirst, abdominal discomfort. Rare: Nausea, vomiting

CRITICAL CARE CONSIDERATIONS

ADMINISTRATION/HANDLING

PO ALERT
- Store solution at room temperature. Solution normally appears pale yellow to yellow in color and viscous in consistency. Cloudy, darkened solution does not indicate potency loss.
- Drink juice, milk, or water with each dose to aid in stool softening and increase palatability.

RECTAL ALERT
- **Preparation:** Lubricate anus with petroleum jelly before applicator insertion.
- **Administration:** Insert applicator carefully, to prevent damage to the rectal wall, with nozzle toward navel. Squeeze container until entire dose has been expelled. Retain liquid until definite lower abdominal cramping is felt.

PRECAUTIONS

HEALTH-RELATED
- Use lactulose cautiously in patients with diabetes mellitus because of presence of galactose and lactose in the medication.

AGE-RELATED
- **Children:** Lactulose should be avoided in children under 6 yr; young children are usually unable to describe symptoms.
- **Elderly:** No age-related precautions have been noted.

PREGNANCY/LACTATION-RELATED
- Pregnancy category B; unknown if excreted in breast milk.

MONITORING
- **Baseline assessment:** Assess abdomen for tenderness, rigidity, and presence of bowel sounds. Determine date of last bowel movement, including amount and consistency. Assess mental status, including signs of a high ammonia level, such as jaundice and asterixis.
- **Baseline lab work:** Biochemical profile including liver enzymes and ammonia level.
- **Dehydration:** Provide IV fluid hydration and/or encourage patients to maintain adequate fluid intake. Monitor serum electrolyte levels in patients with excessive, frequent, or prolonged use of lactulose.
- **Bowel evacuation:** Assess bowel sounds for degree of peristalsis. Assess pattern of daily bowel activity, stool consistency; record time(s) of evacuation. Monitor for abdominal pain and bloating.
- **Liver disease:** When patients are near coma or comatose, at risk for aspiration, or endoscopic exams interfere with oral dosing, Cephulac may be given as a retention enema using a rectal balloon catheter. Obtain serum ammonia levels every 2-3 days, looking for a reduction. Assess mental status; watch for signs of reduced ammonia level, such as increased wakefulness or lessening of asterixis. Patients should have 2-3 soft stools daily. Oral medication should be initiated as soon as possible.
- **Patient education:** Instruct patients receiving lactulose rectally to retain the liquid until cramping is felt. Evacuation occurs in 24 to 48 hr of the initial dose of Chronulac. Advise on measures to promote defecation, such as increasing fluid intake, exercising, and eating a high-fiber diet.

SERIOUS ADVERSE REACTIONS
- **Laxative dependence:** Long-term use may result in chronic constipation and loss of normal bowel function.
- **Hyperglycemia:** Diabetics may experience elevated blood glucose from high sugar content of lactulose.

OVERDOSE/TOXICITY
- **Diarrhea:** Indicates overdose; severe diarrhea may lead to fluid and electrolyte imbalance (hypokalemia, hypernatremia), dysrhythmias, weakness, confusion, and hypotension.
- **Management:** Symptom specific support. Provide IV hydration, replace electrolytes as needed. Monitor and manage dysrhythmias per Advanced Cardiac Life Support

(ACLS) guidelines. Protect patients from self-injury.
- **GI decontamination:** No specific recommendations.

ANTIDOTE/DIALYSIS
- **Antidote:** No specific recommendations.
- **Dialysis:** Lactulose is unlikely to be removed using hemodialysis, peritoneal dialysis, or high-permeability hemodialysis.

lamivudine
See HIV Medications (p. 961)

lamotrigine
la-moe'-trih-jeen

Classes
Chemical: phenyltriazine derivative
Therapeutic: anticonvulsant

Pregnancy Category: C

Trade Names
Prescription: Lamictal, Lamictal CD

Do not confuse lamotrigine with lamivudine.

CLINICAL PHARMACOLOGY
Mechanism of Action
An anticonvulsant for which the exact mechanism is unknown. May block voltage-sensitive sodium channels, thus stabilizing neuronal membranes and regulating presynaptic transmitter release of excitatory amino acids. **Therapeutic Effect:** Reduces seizure activity.

PHARMACOKINETICS
Rapidly absorbed from the GI tract. Protein binding: 55%. Metabolized primarily by glucuronic acid conjugation. Excreted in the urine. **Half-life:** 13-30 hr.

AVAILABILITY
Tablets: 25 mg, 100 mg, 150 mg, 200 mg.
Tablets (chewable): 2 mg, 5 mg, 25 mg.

INDICATIONS AND DOSAGE
Seizure control in patients receiving enzyme-inducing antiepileptic drug (EIAEDs) but not valproic acid
PO

Adults, Elderly, Children older than 12 yr: Recommended as add-on therapy: 50 mg once per day for 2 wk, followed by 100 mg/day in 2 divided doses for 2 wk. Maintenance: Dosage may be increased by 100 mg/day every wk, up to 300-500 mg/day in 2 divided doses. **Children 2-12 yr:** 0.6 mg/kg/day in 2 divided doses for 2 wk, then 1.2 mg/kg/day in 2 divided doses for wk 3 and 4. Maintenance: 5-15 mg/kg/day. Maximum: 400 mg/day.

Seizure control in patients receiving combination therapy of EIAEDs and valproic acid
PO

Adults, Elderly, Children older than 12 yr: 25 mg every other day for 2 wk, followed by 25 mg once per day for 2 wk. Maintenance: Dosage may be increased by 25-50 mg/day every 1-2 wk, up to 150 mg/day in 2 divided doses. **Children 2-12 yr:** 0.15 mg/kg/day in 2 divided doses for 2 wk, then 0.3 mg/kg/day in 2 divided doses for wk 3 and 4. Maintenance: 1-5 mg/kg/day in 2 divided doses. Maximum: 200 mg/day.

Conversion to monotherapy for patients receiving EIAEDs
PO

Adults, Elderly, Children 16 yr and older: 500 mg/day in 2 divided doses. Titrate to desired dose while maintaining EIAED at fixed level, then withdraw EIAED by 20% each wk over a 4-wk period.

Conversion to monotherapy for patients receiving valproic acid
PO

Adults, Elderly, Children 16 yr and older: Titrate lamotrigine to 200 mg/day, maintaining valproic acid dose. Maintain lamotrigine dose and decrease valproic acid to 500 mg/day, no greater than 500 mg/day/wk, then maintain 500 mg/day for 1 wk. Increase lamotrigine to 300 mg/day and decrease valproic acid to 250 mg/day. Maintain for 1 wk, then discontinue valproic acid and increase lamotrigine by 100 mg/day each wk until maintenance dose of 500 mg/day reached.

Bipolar disorder in patients receiving EIAEDs
PO

Adults, Elderly: 50 mg/day for 2 wk, then 100 mg/day for 2 wk, then 200 mg/day for 1 wk, then 300 mg/day for 1 wk, then up to usual maintenance dose 400 mg/day in divided doses.

Bipolar disorder in patients receiving valproic acid
PO

Adults, Elderly: 25 mg/day every other day for 2 wk, then 25 mg/day for 2 wk, then

L

50 mg/day for 1 wk, then 100 mg/day. Usual maintenance dose with valproic acid: 100 mg/day.

Discontinuation therapy

Adults, Children older than 12 yr: A dosage reduction of approximately 50% per wk over at least 2 wk is recommended.

CONTRAINDICATIONS

Hypersensitivity to lamotrigine or any component of the product

INTERACTIONS

Drug: Carbamazepine, phenobarbital, phenytoin, primidone, valproic acid: Decrease lamotrigine blood concentration. **Carbamazepine, valproic acid:** May increase serum levels of these drugs. **Herbal:** None known. **Food:** None known.

DIAGNOSTIC TEST EFFECTS

None known.

SIDE-EFFECTS

Frequent: Dizziness (38%), diplopia (28%), headache (29%), ataxia (22%), nausea (19%), blurred vision (16%), somnolence, rhinitis (14%). **Occasional (10%-5%):** Rash, pharyngitis, vomiting, cough, flulike symptoms, diarrhea, dysmenorrhea, fever, insomnia, dyspepsia. **Rare:** Constipation, tremor, anxiety, pruritus, vaginitis, hypersensitivity reaction

L

CRITICAL CARE CONSIDERATIONS

ADMINISTRATION/HANDLING

PO ALERT

- Give lamotrigine without regard to food.
- Reduce lamotrigine dosage to less than half the normal dosage with concurrent use of valproic acid.

PRECAUTIONS

HEALTH-RELATED

- Use lamotrigine cautiously in patients with cardiac, hepatic, or renal impairment.
- Decreased dosage may be effective in patients with significant renal impairment.

AGE-RELATED

- **Children:** Use of lamotrigine in children under 16 yr is limited to those with seizures resulting from Lennox-Gastaut syndrome or in patients with partial seizures.
- **Elderly:** Age-related organ dysfunction may warrant starting at the lowest possible dosage.

PREGNANCY/LACTATION-RELATED

- Pregnancy category C; passes into breast milk; effects on infants exposed by this route are unknown.

MONITORING

- **Baseline assessment:** Assess LOC and review the drug history, including use of other anticonvulsants; history of the seizure disorder, including duration, frequency, intensity, onset, and type of seizure; and other medical conditions such as renal impairment. Baseline eye exam.
- **Baseline lab work:** CBC with WBC differential and platelet count.
- **Seizure precautions:** Provide patients with a quiet, dark environment and institute safety precautions.
- **Rash:** Discontinue drug if rash occurs.
- **Dizziness:** Assist patients with ambulation if ataxia or dizziness is present.
- **Therapeutic effect:** Assess for decrease in frequency and intensity of seizures.
- **Visual changes:** Assess for headache and visual abnormalities.
- **Patient education:** Instruct to take lamotrigine only as prescribed and not to discontinue abruptly after long-term therapy. Strict maintenance of drug therapy is essential for seizure control. Advise to avoid alcohol and tasks that require mental alertness or motor skills until response to the drug is known. Remind to report promptly fever, rash, or swollen glands to a health care provider. Instruct to avoid exposure to sunlight and artificial light because lamotrigine may cause a photosensitivity reaction. Advise carrying an identification card or wearing an identification bracelet displaying the seizure disorder and anticonvulsant therapy.

SERIOUS ADVERSE REACTIONS

- **Abrupt withdrawal:** May increase seizure frequency.
- **Blood dyscrasias:** Neutropenia, leukopenia, anemia, thrombocytopenia, pancytopenia, and aplastic anemia have been reported rarely.
- **Hypersensitivity reactions:** Some life-threatening and fatal reactions have occurred, some with associated multiorgan dysfunction syndrome. Fever and lymphadenopathy may be present without a rash.
- **Ocular toxicity:** Long-term use may result in visual changes due to binding of lamotrigine to melanin in the eye.

OVERDOSE/TOXICITY

- **Serious rashes:** Rashes including toxic epidermal necrolysis and Stevens–Johnson syndrome are seen at least twice as often in children aged under 16 yr than in adults. Most cases are seen 2-8 wk after beginning treatment; rare cases have been reported more than 6 mo after the start of treatment.
- **Management:** Discontinue drug at the first sign that a rash is developing.
- **GI decontamination:** No specific recommendations.

ANTIDOTE/DIALYSIS

- **Antidote:** No specific recommendations.
- **Dialysis:** Lamotrigine is not removed by hemodialysis and is unlikely to be removed by peritoneal dialysis. No data are available on removal using high-permeability hemodialysis.

lansoprazole

See Acid Secretion Inhibitors (p. 884)

laronidase

lah-ron'-ih-daze

Classes

Chemical: enzyme derivative, α-L-iduronidase

Therapeutic: enzyme replacement, lysosomal hydrolase

Pregnancy Category: B

Trade Names

Prescription: Aldurazyme

CLINICAL PHARMACOLOGY

Mechanism of Action

An enzyme that increases the catabolism of glycosaminoglycans in those with a deficiency of the lysosomal enzymes required for glycosaminoglycan catabolism. **Therapeutic Effect:** Prevents glycosaminoglycans from causing widespread cellular, tissue, and organ dysfunction.

PHARMACOKINETICS

Half-life: 1.5-3.6 hr.

AVAILABILITY

Injection: 2.9 mg/5 mL.

INDICATIONS AND DOSAGE

Mucopolysaccharidosis

IV

Adults, Elderly: 0.58 mg/kg infused once per wk.

CONTRAINDICATIONS

Hypersensitivity to laronidase

INTERACTIONS

Drug: None known. **Herbal:** None known. **Food:** None known.

DIAGNOSTIC TEST EFFECTS

None known.

SIDE-EFFECTS

Frequent (36%-18%): Infusion-related reactions, such as facial flushing, rash, fever, and headache. **Occasional (9%):** Cough, bronchospasm, urticaria, pruritus, angioedema, dependent edema, hypotension, hyperreflexia

CRITICAL CARE CONSIDERATIONS

ADMINISTRATION/HANDLING

IV ALERT

- **Storage:** Refrigerate vials.
- **Stability:** Once reconstituted, the solution should ideally be used immediately. Solution may be refrigerated for no longer than 36 hr from the time of preparation to completion of administration.
- **Premedication:** Pretreat patients with antipyretics and antihistamines as prescribed 60 min before starting the IV infusion.
- **Dilution:** Dilute with 0.1% albumin (human) in 0.9% NaCl. Take care not to shake the solution. Administer using a 0.2 micrometer filter.
- **Infusion volume:** Total volume of the infusion is determined by patient weight. Patients who weigh 20 kg or less should receive a total volume of 100 mL. Patients who weigh more than 20 kg should receive a total volume of 250 mL.
- **IV infusion:** Begin the infusion at a rate of 10 mcg/kg/hr, and increase it in 15-min increments to 20 mcg/kg/hr, then 50 mcg/kg/hr, and then 100 mcg/kg/hr during the first hr. Give the remainder of the infusion at 200 mcg/kg/hr over 2-3 hr for a total infusion time of 3-4 hr.

PRECAUTIONS

HEALTH-RELATED

- Infusion-related hypersensitivity reactions are common and may be severe; use with caution in patients with preexisting airway obstruction.

L

AGE-RELATED

- **Children:** Safety and efficacy of laronidase have not been established in children under 5 yr.
- **Elderly:** Age-related heart disease may make management of infusion reactions more difficult.

PREGNANCY/LACTATION-RELATED

- Pregnancy category B; breast-feeding is not recommended.

MONITORING

- **Baseline assessment:** Assess for history of airway/breathing difficulties. Pretreat patients with antipyretics and antihistamines 60 min before starting the IV infusion.
- **Baseline lab work:** CBC with WBC differential.
- **Baseline diagnostic tests:** 12-lead ECG to assess for heart disease.
- **Infusion-related reactions:** Closely monitor for infusion-related reactions including facial flushing, fever, tachycardia, increased work of breathing, tachypnea, and hypertension. Slowing the infusion rate, temporarily stopping the infusion, or administering additional antipyretics and antihistamines may ameliorate such reactions.
- **Patient education:** Instruct patients and/or parents to report side effects immediately. Urge to ask about the registry program that has been established for patients with mucopolysaccharidosis (MPSI) to monitor and evaluate treatments.

SERIOUS ADVERSE REACTIONS

- Upper respiratory tract infection occurs commonly.

OVERDOSE/TOXICITY

- **Anaphylactic reactions:** Angioedema, severe bronchospasm, and dyspnea, fever, and chills occur rarely.
- **Management:** Use epinephrine with great caution because many MPSI patients have heart disease. Maintain patent airway with endotracheal intubation, as needed. Provide manual or mechanical ventilation. Manage hypotension with IV fluids and vasopressors if needed. Reconsider trying infusion again carefully, weighing benefits against risks. Probability of another reaction is significant.
- **GI decontamination:** No specific recommendations.

ANTIDOTE/DIALYSIS

- **Antidote:** No specific recommendations.
- **Dialysis:** Laronidase is unlikely to be removed by hemodialysis. No data are available on removal using high-permeability hemodialysis or peritoneal dialysis.

lepirudin

leh-puh-roo'-din

Classes

Chemical: hirudin derivative, thrombin inhibitor

Therapeutic: anticoagulant

Pregnancy Category: B

Trade Names

Prescription: Refludan

CLINICAL PHARMACOLOGY

Mechanism of Action

An anticoagulant that inhibits thrombogenic action of thrombin (independent of antithrombin II and not inhibited by platelet factor 4). One molecule of lepirudin binds to one molecule of thrombin. **Therapeutic Effect:** Produces dose-dependent increases in aPTT.

PHARMACOKINETICS

Distributed primarily in extracellular fluid. Primarily eliminated by the kidneys. **Half-life:** 1.3 hr (increased in impaired renal function).

AVAILABILITY

Powder for injection: 50 mg.

INDICATIONS AND DOSAGE

Heparin-induced thrombocytopenia and associated thromboembolic disease to prevent further thromboembolic complications

IV, IV Infusion

Adults, Elderly: 0.2-0.4 mg/kg (44 mg maximum), IV slowly over 15-20 sec, followed by IV infusion of 0.1-0.15 mg/kg/hr for 2-10 days or longer.

Dosage in renal impairment (less than 60 mL/min creatinine clearance)

Initial dose is decreased to 0.2 mg/kg, with infusion rate adjusted based on creatinine clearance.

Creatinine Clearance (mL/min)	Infusion Rate (mg/kg/hr)
45-60	0.075
30-44	0.045
15-29	0.0225

CONTRAINDICATIONS

Hypersensitivity to lepirudin, active major bleeding

INTERACTIONS

Drug: **Platelet aggregation inhibitors, thrombolytics, warfarin:** May increase the risk of bleeding complications. Herbal: **Ginkgo biloba:** May increase the risk of bleeding. Food: None known.

DIAGNOSTIC TEST EFFECTS

Increases aPTT and thrombin time.

IV INCOMPATIBILITIES

Do not mix with other medications.

SIDE-EFFECTS

Frequent (14%-5%): Bleeding from gums, puncture sites, or wounds; hematuria; fever; and GI and rectal bleeding. Occasional (3%-1%): Epistaxis; allergic reaction, such as rash and pruritus; vaginal bleeding

CRITICAL CARE CONSIDERATIONS

ADMINISTRATION/HANDLING

IV ALERT

- **Storage:** Store unreconstituted vials at room temperature.
- **Stability:** Reconstituted solution should be used immediately, but the IV infusion is stable for up to 24 hr at room temperature.
- **Reconstitution:** Add 1 mL sterile water for injection or 0.9% NaCl to 50-mg vial and shake gently; reconstitution normally produces a clear, colorless solution. Do not use if solution is cloudy.
- **IV push dilution/administration:** Further dilute by transferring to syringe and adding sufficient sterile water for injection, 0.9% NaCl, or D_5W to produce a concentration of 5 mg/mL. Give IV push over 15-20 sec.
- **IV infusion dilution/administration:** Add contents of 2 vials (100 mg) to 250 or 500 mL 0.9% NaCl or D_5W, providing a concentration of 0.4 or 0.2 mg/mL, respectively. Adjust IV infusion based on aPTT or patient body weight.
- **Dosage adjustment:** Adjust dose according to aPTT ratio with target range of 1.5 to 2.5 normal. Give initial dose as soon as possible after surgery but not more than 24 hr after surgery.
- For patients weighing more than 110 kg, maximum initial dose is 44 mg, with maximum rate of 16.5 mg/hr.

PRECAUTIONS

HEALTH-RELATED

- Use lepirudin cautiously in patients with conditions associated with increased risk of bleeding, such as bacterial endocarditis, cerebrovascular accident, hemorrhagic diathesis, intracerebral surgery, recent major bleeding, recent major surgery, and severe hypertension, severe hepatic or renal impairment, or stroke.

AGE-RELATED

- **Children:** Safety and efficacy of lepirudin have not been established in children.
- **Elderly:** Age-related renal impairment may require dosage adjustment.

PREGNANCY/LACTATION-RELATED

- Pregnancy category B; use caution in nursing mothers.

MONITORING

- **Baseline assessment:** Determine past history of bleeding and allergy to hirudins. Assess initial heart rate and BP.
- **Baseline lab work:** CBC, including platelet count; aPTT and thrombin time; biochemical profile including BUN, serum alkaline phosphatase, creatinine, AST (SGOT), and ALT (SGPT) levels, to assess hepatic and renal function.
- **Ongoing lab work:** Monitor the aPTT diligently. Assess Hct; platelet count; renal function studies; BUN, serum creatinine, AST (SGOT) and ALT (SGPT) levels; and stool and urine specimen for occult blood.
- **Bleeding:** Assess for tachycardia, abdominal or back pain, hypotension, and severe headache, indicative of possible hemorrhage. Assess gums for erythema and gingival bleeding, skin for ecchymosis or petechiae, and for hematuria. Examine for excessive bleeding from minor cuts and scratches.
- **Female patients:** Monitor for increase in amount of menstrual flow.
- **Patient education:** Instruct to report promptly unusual bleeding, breathing difficulty, bruising, dizziness, edema, fever, itching, lightheadedness, bleeding from surgical site, black or red stool, coffee-ground vomitus, dark or red urine, red-speckled mucus from cough, chest pain, dyspnea, or rash to a health care provider. Instruct to use an electric razor and soft toothbrush to help prevent bleeding during lepirudin therapy. Advise not taking other medications, including OTC drugs (especially aspirin), without prior discussion

L

with a health care provider. Tell female patients that menstrual flow may be heavier than usual.

SERIOUS ADVERSE REACTIONS

- **Intracranial bleeding:** Occurs rarely. Concommitant use with thrombolytics increases probability of intracranial bleeding.
- **Antihirudin antibody formation:** Occurs in 40% of patients receiving lepirudin, which may increase the drug's anticoagulant effects. No data have revealed antibodies may lead to neutralization of lepirudin.
- **Cardiac effects:** Pericardial effusion and ventricular fibrillation. If patient has coronary artery disease or heart failure, anemia from bleeding may lead to acute myocardial ischemia or infarction.

OVERDOSE/TOXICITY

- **Bleeding:** Excessively high aPTT with possible bleeding from any high-risk site identified during patient's history or that may not have been identified.
- **Management of bleeding:** Immediately stop infusion and prepare for blood transfusion if hemoglobin and hematocrit are rapidly decreasing. Manage hypovolemic shock with IV fluids and vasopressors if packed RBCs are not quickly available.
- **Hepatotoxicity:** Abnormal hepatic function occurs in 6% of patients.
- **Nephrotoxicity:** Elevated BUN, creatinine, nausea, abdominal pain, oliguria.
- **GI decontamination:** No specific recommendations.

ANTIDOTE/DIALYSIS

- **Antidote:** No specific recommendations.
- **Dialysis:** Lepirudin is removed by hemodialysis and high-permeability hemodialysis. No data are available on removal by peritoneal dialysis.

levalbuterol

lee-val-byoo'-ter-ole

Classes

Chemical: β_2-adrenergic stimulant
Therapeutic: bronchodilator

Pregnancy Category: C

Trade Names

Prescription: Xopenex, Xopenex HFA

Do not confuse Xopenex with Xanax.

CLINICAL PHARMACOLOGY

Mechanism of Action

A sympathomimetic that stimulates beta$_2$-adrenergic receptors in the lungs resulting in relaxation of bronchial smooth muscle. **Therapeutic Effect:** Relieves bronchospasm and reduces airway resistance.

PHARMACOKINETICS

Route	Onset	Peak	Duration
Inhalation	10-17 min	1.5 hr	5-6 hr

Metabolized in the liver to inactive metabolite. **Half-life:** 3.3-4 hr.

AVAILABILITY

Inhalation aerosol: 45 mcg/activation.
Solution for nebulization: 0.31 in 3-mL vials, 0.63 mg in 3-mL vials, 1.25 mg in 3-mL vials.

INDICATIONS AND DOSAGE

Treatment and prevention of bronchospasm

Inhalation

Adults, Elderly, Children 4 yr and older: 1-2 inhalations every 6-8 hr.

Nebulization

Adults, Elderly, Children 12 yr and older: Initially, 0.63 mg 3 times per day 6-8 hr apart. May increase to 1.25 mg 3 times per day with dose monitoring. **Children 3-11 yr.** Initially 0.31 mg 3 times per day. Maximum: 0.63 mg 3 times per day

CONTRAINDICATIONS

History of hypersensitivity to levalbuterol or sympathomimetics

INTERACTIONS

Drug: **Beta-blockers:** Antagonize the effects of levalbuterol. **Digoxin:** May increase the risk of dysrhythmias. **MAOIs, tricyclic antidepressants:** May potentiate cardiovascular effects. **Herbal:** None known. **Food:** None known.

DIAGNOSTIC TEST EFFECTS

May increase serum potassium level.

SIDE-EFFECTS

Frequent: Tremor, nervousness, headache, throat dryness and irritation. **Occasional:** Cough, bronchial irritation. **Rare:** Somnolence, diarrhea, dry mouth, flushing, diaphoresis, anorexia

CRITICAL CARE CONSIDERATIONS

ADMINISTRATION/HANDLING

NEBULIZATION ALERT

- **Storage:** Store at room temperature. Protect the solution from light and excessive heat.
- **Stability:** Use the solution within 2 wk of opening the foil. Discard the solution if it is not colorless.
- **Dilution:** Do not dilute the solution. Do not mix levalbuterol with other medications.
- **Nebulization:** Administer levalbuterol over 5-15 min.

PRECAUTIONS

HEALTH-RELATED

- Use levalbuterol cautiously in patients with cardiovascular disorders (such as dysrhythmias), diabetes mellitus, hypertension, or seizures.

AGE-RELATED

- **Children:** Safety and efficacy of levalbuterol have not been established in children under 6 yr.
- **Elderly:** A lower initial dosage is recommended for the elderly.

PREGNANCY/LACTATION-RELATED

- Pregnancy category C; unknown if excreted in breast milk.

MONITORING

- **Baseline assessment:** Auscultate breath sounds before and after treatment. Obtain pulse oximetry (SpO_2) reading, heart and respiratory rates.
- **Baseline lab work:** Biochemical profile with potassium, magnesium, and calcium levels. Arterial blood gases (ABG) to assess for CO_2 retention.
- **Baseline diagnostic tests:** Chest x-ray to assess for lung disease and 12-lead ECG to assess for heart disease.
- **Ongoing monitoring:** Monitor heart rate, pulse quality, respiratory rate, depth, rhythm, and work of breathing. Auscultate breath sounds for crackles and wheezing, signs of bronchoconstriction.
- **Dysrhythmias:** Continuous ECG monitoring and serum potassium.
- **Patient education:** Advise to rinse mouth with water immediately after inhalation to prevent mouth and throat dryness. Encourage to drink plenty of fluids to decrease the thickness of lung secretions. Warn to notify the physician if they experience chest pain, dizziness, headache, palpitations, tachycardia, or tremors. Urge avoidance of excessive use of caffeinated products such as chocolate, cocoa, cola, coffee, and tea.

SERIOUS ADVERSE REACTIONS

- **Excessive use:** May lead to decreased bronchodilating effectiveness and severe paradoxical bronchoconstriction.
- **Immediate hypersensitivity reactions:** Urticaria, angioedema, bronchospasm, and rash, followed by anaphylaxis immediately following administration.
- **Management:** Hypersensitivity should be managed with epinephrine if patients are assessed to be able to tolerate epinephrine. If patients are hypertensive and have dysrhythmias, epinephrine must be used with caution.

OVERDOSE/TOXICITY

- Fatalities have been reported in asthmatics using excessive doses.
- **Cardiovascular effects:** Tachycardia, hypertension, and/or hypotension, nervousness, pallor, diaphoresis, shortness of breath, prolonged QT interval, ST segment depression, chest discomfort, premature ventricular contractions, and supraventricular tachycardia.
- **Electrolyte imbalance:** Hypokalemia and hyperglycemia with tremors, agitation, vomiting, hypomagnesemia, and hypophosphatemia.
- **Management:** Supplemental oxygen, IV fluids, and supportive therapies for changes in vital signs. Manage hypokalemia with potassium boluses and hyperglycemia with an insulin infusion if needed to control blood glucose.
- **GI decontamination:** No specific recommendations.

ANTIDOTE/DIALYSIS

- **Antidote:** Short acting beta-adrenergic blocking agents (esmolol) may be used to control tachycardia after other therapies have been attempted.
- **Dialysis:** Levalbuterol is not removed by hemodialysis and is not likely to be removed by peritoneal dialysis. No data are available on removal using high-permeability hemodialysis.

levetiracetam

lev-a-tear-as'-e-tam

Classes
Chemical: pyrrolidone derivative
Therapeutic: anticonvulsant

Pregnancy Category: C

Trade Names
Prescription: Keppra

Do not confuse Keppra with Kaletra.

CLINICAL PHARMACOLOGY

Mechanism of Action
An anticonvulsant that inhibits burst firing without affecting normal neuronal excitability. **Therapeutic Effect:** Prevents seizure activity.

PHARMACOKINETICS

Rapidly and almost completely absorbed through the GI tract. Protein binding: less than 10%. Insignificant amount metabolized in liver. Excreted in urine. Removed by hemodialysis. **Half-life:** 7 hr.

AVAILABILITY

Oral solution: 100 mg/mL.
Tablets: 250 mg, 500 mg, 750 mg.

INDICATIONS AND DOSAGE

Partial-onset seizures
PO
Adults, Elderly. Initially, 500 mg every 12 hr. May increase by 1000 mg/day every 2 wk. Maximum: 3000 mg/day. **Children 4-16 yr:** 10-20 mg/kg/day in 2 divided doses. May increase at weekly intervals by 10-20 mg/kg. Maximum: 60 mg/kg.

Dosage in renal impairment
Dosage is modified based on creatinine clearance.

Creatinine Clearance (mL/min)	Dosage
Higher than 80 mL/min	500-1500 mg every 12 hr
50-80 mL/min	500-1000 mg every 12 hr
30-50 mL/min	250-750 mg every 12 hr
Less than 30 mL/min	250-500 mg every 12 hr
End-stage renal disease using dialysis	500-1000 mg every 24 hr, after dialysis, a 250- to 500-mg supplemental dose is recommended

CONTRAINDICATIONS

Hypersensitivity to levetiracetam

INTERACTIONS

Drug: None known. **Herbal: Ginkgo biloba:** May decrease anticonvulsant effectiveness.
Food: None known.

DIAGNOSTIC TEST EFFECTS

May increase blood Hgb level, Hct, and RBC and WBC counts.

SIDE-EFFECTS

Frequent (15%-10%): Somnolence, asthenia, headache, infection, vomiting (up to 15%). **Occasional (9%-3%):** Dizziness, pharyngitis, pain, depression, nervousness, vertigo, rhinitis, anorexia. **Rare (less than 3%):** Amnesia, anxiety, emotional lability, cough, sinusitis, anorexia, diplopia

CRITICAL CARE CONSIDERATIONS

ADMINISTRATION/HANDLING

PO ALERT
- Store at controlled room temperature.

PRECAUTIONS

HEALTH-RELATED
- Use levetiracetam cautiously in patients with renal impairment.

AGE-RELATED
- **Children:** Safety and efficacy of levetiracetam have not been established in children under 16 yr.
- **Elderly:** Age-related renal impairment may prompt a dosage adjustment.

PREGNANCY/LACTATION-RELATED
- Pregnancy category C; developmental toxicity in animals; excretion into breast milk unknown.

MONITORING

- **Baseline assessment:** Assess LOC and review the history of the seizure disorder, including the duration, frequency, and intensity of seizures. Initiate seizure precautions. Assess for hypersensitivity to levetiracetam.
- **Baseline lab work:** Biochemical profile including BUN and serum creatinine levels to assess renal function.
- **Ongoing lab work:** Monitor renal function test results.
- **Therapeutic effect:** Assess for a decrease in the frequency or intensity of seizures. Observe for recurrence of seizures.
- **Dizziness:** Assist with ambulation if dizziness occurs.

- **Somnolence:** Excessive sleepiness is common after initiating therapy.
- **Patient education:** Caution against discontinuing levetiracetam therapy abruptly to avoid recurrent seizures. Explain strict maintenance of drug therapy is essential for seizure control. Inform that dizziness and somnolence usually diminish with continued therapy. Warn to avoid tasks requiring mental alertness or motor skills until response to the drug is known. Recommend always carrying an identification card or wearing an identification bracelet that displays the seizure disorder and anticonvulsant therapy.

SERIOUS ADVERSE REACTIONS

- **Withdrawal seizures:** If levetiracetam is withdrawn too quickly, seizures may recur.

OVERDOSE/TOXICITY

- **Hematologic:** Anemia, neutropenia.
- **GI decontamination:** No specific recommendations.

ANTIDOTE/DIALYSIS

- **Antidote:** No specific recommendations.
- **Dialysis:** Levetiracetam is removed by hemodialysis and is likely to be removed by high-permeability hemodialysis. No data are available on removal using peritoneal dialysis.

levofloxacin

lee-voe-flox'-a-sin

Classes

Chemical: fluoroquinolone derivative
Therapeutic: antibiotic

Pregnancy Category: C

Trade Names

Prescription: Iquix, Levaquin, Levaquin Leva-Pak, Quixin

CLINICAL PHARMACOLOGY

Mechanism of Action

A fluoroquinolone that inhibits the DNA enzyme gyrase in susceptible microorganisms, interfering with bacterial cell replication and repair. **Therapeutic Effect:** Bactericidal.

PHARMACOKINETICS

Well absorbed after both PO and IV administration. Protein binding: 38%. Penetrates rapidly and extensively into leukocytes, epithelial cells, and macrophages. Lung concentrations are 2-5 times higher than those of plasma. Eliminated unchanged in the urine. Unlikeky to be removed by hemodialysis. **Half-life:** 6-8 hr.

AVAILABILITY

Oral Solution: 25 mg/mL.
Tablets (Levaquin, Levaquin Leva-Pak): 250 mg, 500 mg, 750 mg.
Injection (Levaquin): 500-mg/20-mL vials.
Premixed solution (Levaquin): 25 mg/mL, 250 mg/50 mL, 500 mg/100 mL, 750 mg/150 mL.
Ophthalmic solution: 0.5% (Iquix), 1.5% (Quixin).

INDICATIONS AND DOSAGE

Bacterial sinusitis

PO

Adults, Elderly: 500 mg once daily for 10 days or 750 mg once daily for 5 days.

Bronchitis

PO, IV

Adults, Elderly: 500 mg every 24 hr for 7 days.

Community-acquired pneumonia

PO

Adults, Elderly: 750 mg/day for 5 days or 500 mg for 7-14 days.

Pneumonia, nosocomial

PO, IV

Adults, Elderly: 750 mg every 24 hr for 7-14 days.

Acute maxillary sinusitis

PO, IV

Adults, Elderly: 500 mg every 24 hr for 10-14 days.

Skin and skin-structure infections

PO, IV

Adults, Elderly: Uncomplicated: 500 mg every 24 hr for 7-10 days. Complicated: 750 mg every 24 hr for 7-14 days.

Prostatitis

IV, PO

Adults, Elderly: 500 mg every 24 hr for 28 days.

Uncomplicated urinary tract infections (UTI)

IV, PO

Adults, Elderly: 250 mg every 24 hr for 3 days.

UTIs, acute pyelonephritis

PO, IV

Adults, Elderly: 250 mg every 24 hr for 10 days.

Bacterial conjunctivitis

Ophthalmic

Adults, Elderly, Children 1 yr and older: 1-2 drops every 2 hr for 2 days (up to 8 times per day), then 1-2 drops every 4 hr for 5 days.

Corneal ulcer
Ophthalmic
Adults, Elderly, Children older than 5 yr: Days 1-3: Instill 1-2 drops every 30 min to 2 hr while awake and 4-6 hr after retiring. Days 4 through completion: 1-2 drops every 1-4 hr while awake.

Dosage in renal impairment
For chronic bronchitis, community acquired pneumonia, sinusitis, uncomplicated skin and skin structure infections, and chronic prostatitis, dosage and frequency are modified based on creatinine clearance.

Creatinine Clearance	Dosage
50-80 mL/min	No change
20-49 mL/min	500 mg initially, then 250 mg every 24 hr
10-19 mL/min	500 mg initially, then 250 mg every 48 hr
Dialysis	500 mg initially, then 250 mg every 48 hr

For nosocomial pneumonia, complicated skin infections, sinusitis, community-acquired pneumonia, dosage and frequency are modified based on creatinine clearance.

Creatinine Clearance	Dosage
Greater than 50 mL/min	No change
20-49 mL/min	750 mg given once, then 750 mg every 48 hr
10-19 mL/min	750 mg given once, then 500 mg every 48 hr
Hemodialysis (HD)/ Continuous ambulatory peritoneal dialysis (CAPD)	750 mg given once, then 500 mg every 48 hr

For UTIs and pyelonephritis, dosage and frequency are modified based on creatinine clearance.

Creatinine Clearance	Dosage
20 mL/min	No change
10-19 mL/min	250 mg initially, then 250 mg every 48 hr

OFF-LABEL USES
Anthrax, gonorrhea, pelvic inflammatory disease (PID)

CONTRAINDICATIONS
Hypersensitivity to levofloxacin, other fluoroquinolones, or nalidixic acid

INTERACTIONS
Drug: Antacids, iron preparations, sucralfate, zinc: Decrease levofloxacin absorption. **NSAIDs:** May increase the risk of CNS stimulation or seizures. **Herbal:** None known. **Food:** None known.

DIAGNOSTIC TEST EFFECTS
May alter blood glucose levels.

IV INCOMPATIBILITIES
Furosemide (Lasix), heparin, insulin, nitroglycerin, propofol (Diprivan)

IV COMPATIBILITIES
Aminophylline, *DOBUTamine (Dobutrex), *DOPamine (Intropin), fentanyl (Sublimaze), lidocaine, lorazepam (Ativan), morphine

SIDE-EFFECTS
Occasional (3%-1%): Diarrhea, nausea, abdominal pain, dizziness, drowsiness, headache, lightheadedness. **Ophthalmic:** Local burning or discomfort, margin crusting, crystals or scales, foreign body sensation, ocular itching, altered taste. **Rare (less than 1%):** Flatulence; altered taste; pain; inflammation or swelling in calves, hands, or shoulder; chest pain; difficulty breathing; palpitations; edema; tendon pain. **Ophthalmic:** Corneal staining, keratitis, allergic reaction, eyelid swelling, tearing, reduced visual acuity

CRITICAL CARE CONSIDERATIONS

ADMINISTRATION/HANDLING

PO ALERT
- Give levofloxacin without regard to food.
- Do not administer antacids (containing aluminum or magnesium), sucralfate, iron preparations, or multivitamins containing zinc within 2 hr of levofloxacin to avoid significantly reduced levofloxacin absorption.
- Provide citrus fruits and cranberry juice to acidify urine.

IV ALERT
- **Preparation:** Levofloxacin is available in single-dose 20-mL (500-mg) vials and as a premixed (with D_5W), ready-to-infuse solution.
- **IV dilution:** For infusion using the single-dose vial, withdraw the desired amount (10 mL for 250 mg, 20 mL for 500 mg). Dilute each 10 mL (250 mg) with at least 40 mL 0.9% NaCl or D_5W.
- **Administration:** Administer the drug slowly over at least 60 min.

OPHTHALMIC ALERT
- **Administration:** Pull out the lower eyelid with a gloved finger until a pocket is formed between the eye and lower lid.

Hold the dropper above the pocket, and place the correct number of drops into the pocket. Close the eye gently. Apply digital pressure to the lacrimal sac for 1-2 min to minimize drainage of the medication into the nose and throat, reducing the risk of systemic effects.

PRECAUTIONS

HEALTH-RELATED

- Use levofloxacin cautiously in patients with bradycardia, cardiomyopathy, hypokalemia, hypomagnesemia, impaired renal function, seizure disorder, or suspected CNS disorder.

AGE-RELATED

- **Children:** Safety and efficacy of levofloxacin have not been established in children.
- **Elderly:** Age-related renal impairment may require a dosage adjustment.

PREGNANCY/LACTATION-RELATED

- Pregnancy category C; excretion into breast milk unknown. Due to the potential for arthropathy and osteochondrosis, use extreme caution in nursing mothers.

MONITORING

- **Baseline assessment:** Determine history of hypersensitivity to levofloxacin or other fluoroquinolones before beginning drug therapy.
- **Baseline lab work:** Biochemical profile including blood glucose, liver and renal function tests; CBC including WBC differential and platelet count; obtain necessary cultures prior to dosing.
- **Ongoing lab work:** Monitor blood glucose levels and liver and renal function test results. Hyperglycemia, elevated liver enzymes, and elevated BUN and creatinine may signal adverse effects.
- **Hypersensitivity:** Assess for hypersensitivity reactions and manage immediately (photosensitivity, pruritus, skin rash, and urticaria).
- **Superinfections:** Assess the mouth for white patches on the mucous membranes or tongue and for severe mouth or tongue soreness; assess for severe anal or genital pruritus or discharge.
- **Possible *Clostridium difficile* colitis:** Assess pattern of daily bowel activity and stool consistency. Although mild GI effects may be tolerable, severe symptoms including abdominal pain or cramping, or moderate to severe diarrhea may indicate the onset of antibiotic-associated colitis.
- **Hand washing:** If *C. difficile* (antibiotic-associated) colitis develops, wash hands with antibacterial soap. Alcohol-based foam is ineffective against *C. difficile* spores.
- **Nephrotoxicity:** Monitor intake and output and renal function test results to assess for nephrotoxicity.
- **Nausea:** Provide symptomatic relief for nausea. Evaluate food tolerance and change in taste sensation.
- **Therapeutic response:** Observe patients receiving the ophthalmic form for a resolution of eye redness, drainage, and pain.
- **Side effects:** Evaluate for dizziness, headache, tremors, and visual problems. Assess for chest and joint pain.
- **Patient education:** When using levofloxacin outside the hospital, advise not to skip drug doses and to take levofloxacin for the full course of therapy. Encourage to drink 6-8 glasses of fluid per day, including citrus and cranberry juices to acidify urine. Warn not to take antacids within 2 hr of taking the medication; antacids reduce or destroy levofloxacin's effectiveness. Urge avoidance of exposure to direct sunlight during therapy and for several days after treatment. Instruct on symptoms of hyperglycemia and hypoglycemia. Warn not to perform tasks that require mental alertness or motor skills until response to the drug is known.

SERIOUS ADVERSE REACTIONS

- **Pseudomembranous colitis/*C. difficile*–associated diarrhea (CDAD):** Severe abdominal pain and cramps, severe watery diarrhea, and fever may occur. Oral vancomycin (Vancocin) or metronidazole (Flagyl) are the most effective treatments for CDAD.
- **Superinfection:** Genital or anal pruritus, ulceration or changes in oral mucosa, and moderate to severe diarrhea may occur.
- **Hyperglycemia:** Marked elevation of blood glucose has been noted in both diabetic and nondiabetic patients.
- **Sensitization to ophthalmic form:** May contraindicate later systemic use of levofloxacin.
- **Management of hypersensitivity:** Discontinue levofloxacin immediately. May require treatment with epinephrine and other emergency measures including oxygen, endotracheal intubation, mechanical ventilation, IV fluids, IV antihistamines, corticosteroids, and vasopressors.

L

OVERDOSE/TOXICITY

- **Neurological:** Seizures, increased intracranial pressure, confusion, depression, hallucinations, tremors, toxic psychosis, vomiting.
- **Cardiac:** Prolonged QT syndrome, ventricular dysrhythmias, torsades de pointes; more common when patients are receiving other antidysrhythmic drugs that prolong the QT interval (procainamide, quinidine, amiodarone, sotalol).
- **Nephrotoxicity:** May occur, especially in patients with preexisting renal disease.
- **Dermatologic:** Toxic epidermal necrolysis, Stevens–Johnson syndrome.
- **Hematologic:** Hemolytic anemia.
- **Tendon rupture:** Pain, inflammation, and rupture of tendons in the shoulder, hand, and Achilles tendon.
- **GI decontamination:** No specific recommendations.

ANTIDOTE/DIALYSIS

- **Antidote:** No specific recommendations.
- **Dialysis:** Levofloxacin is unlikely to be removed by hemodialysis or peritoneal dialysis. Levofloxacin is unlikely to be removed by high-permeability hemodialysis.

levorphanol

See Opioid Analgesics (p. 980)

levothyroxine sodium

lee-voe-thye-rox'-een soe'-dee-um

Classes

Chemical: synthetic levo isomer of thyroxine (T_4)
Therapeutic: thyroid hormone

Pregnancy Category: A

Trade Names

Prescription: Levo-T, Levothroid, Levoxine, Synthroid, Levoxyl

Combinations

Prescription: with liothyronine (Euthroid, Thyrolar)

Do not confuse levothyroxine with liothyronine.

CLINICAL PHARMACOLOGY

Mechanism of Action

A synthetic isomer of thyroxine involved in normal metabolism, growth, and development, especially of the CNS in infants. Possesses catabolic and anabolic effects. Therapeutic Effect: Increases basal metabolic rate, enhances gluconeogenesis, and stimulates protein synthesis.

PHARMACOKINETICS

Variable, incomplete absorption from the GI tract. Protein binding: greater than 99%. Widely distributed. Deiodinated in peripheral tissues, minimal metabolism in the liver. Eliminated by biliary excretion. Half-life: 6-7 days.

AVAILABILITY

Tablets (Levo-T, Levothroid, Levoxyl, Synthroid, Unithroid): 0.025 mg, 0.05 mg, 0.075 mg, 0.088 mg, 0.1 mg, 0.112 mg, 0.125 mg, 0.137 mg, 0.15 mg, 0.175 mg, 0.2 mg, 0.3 mg.
Injection (Synthroid): 200 mcg, 500 mcg.

INDICATIONS AND DOSAGE

Hypothyroidism

PO

Adults, Elderly, Children older than 12 yr, growth and puberty complete: 1.7 mcg/kg/day as single daily dose. Usual maintenance: 100-200 mcg/day. **Children older than 12 yr, growth and puberty incomplete:** 2-3 mcg/kg/day. **Children 6-12 yr:** 4-5 mcg/kg/day. **Children 1-5 yr:** 5-6 mcg/kg/day. **Children 6-12 mo:** 6-8 mcg/kg/day. **Children 3-6 mo:** 8-10 mcg/kg/day. **Children younger than 3 mo:** 10-15 mcg/kg/day.

Myxedema coma

IV

Adults, Elderly: Initially, 200-500 mcg. Second day: 100-300 mcg/day. Maintenance: 75-100 mcg/day.

Pituitary thyroid stimulating hormone suppression

PO

Adults, Elderly: Doses greater than 2 mcg/kg/day usually required to suppress thyroid stimulating hormone (TSH) below 0.1 milliunits/L.

CONTRAINDICATIONS

Hypersensitivity to levothyroxine tablet components, such as tartrazine; allergy to aspirin; lactose intolerance; MI and thyrotoxicosis uncomplicated by hypothyroidism; treatment of obesity

INTERACTIONS

Drug: Cholestyramine, colestipol: May decrease the absorption of levothyroxine. **Estrogens:** May cause a decrease in serum-free thyroxine concentration. **Oral anticoagulants:** May alter the effects of oral anticoagulants. **Sympathomimetics:** May increase the risk of coronary insufficiency and the effects of levothyroxine. **Herbal:** None known. **Food:** None known.

DIAGNOSTIC TEST EFFECTS

None known.

IV INCOMPATIBILITIES

Do not use or mix with other IV solutions.

SIDE-EFFECTS

Occasional: Reversible hair loss at the start of therapy (in children). **Rare:** Dry skin, GI intolerance, rash, hives, pseudotumor cerebri or severe headache in children

CRITICAL CARE CONSIDERATIONS

ADMINISTRATION/HANDLING

PO ALERT

- Begin therapy with small doses and increase the dosage gradually.
- Administer before breakfast to prevent insomnia. Give at same time each day to maintain hormone levels.
- Tablets may be crushed.
- Do not use different brands of levothyroxine interchangeably because of problems with bioequivalence among manufacturers.

IV ALERT

- **Storage:** Store vials at room temperature.
- **Reconstitution:** Reconstitute 200- or 500-mcg vial with 5 mL 0.9% NaCl to provide a concentration of 40 or 100 mcg/mL, respectively; shake until clear.
- **Stability:** Use immediately and discard unused portion.
- **Administration:** Give each 100 mcg or less over 1 min.

PRECAUTIONS

HEALTH-RELATED

- Use levothyroxine cautiously in patients with angina pectoris, adrenal insufficiency, diabetes insipidus, hypopituitarism, hypertension, or other cardiovascular disease.
- Levothyroxine therapy may intensify symptoms of adrenal insufficiency, diabetes insipidus, diabetes mellitus, and hypopituitarism.

AGE-RELATED

- **Children:** No age-related precautions have been noted in children. Use caution in interpreting thyroid function tests in neonates.
- **Elderly:** May be more sensitive to thyroid effects. Individualized dosages are recommended.

PREGNANCY/LACTATION-RELATED

- Pregnancy category A. Little or no transplacental passage at physiologic serum concentrations. Excreted into breast milk in low concentrations (inadequate to protect a hypothyroid infant; too low to interfere with neonatal thyroid screening programs).

MONITORING

- **Baseline assessment:** Determine hypersensitivity to aspirin, lactose, or tartrazine. Obtain weight and vital signs. Determine history of adrenal insufficiency. Administer adrenocortical steroids before thyroid therapy in patients with coexisting hypoadrenalism and hypothyroidism.
- **Baseline lab work:** Biochemical profile, thyroid function tests (free T4, TSH) and adrenal function tests (cortisol level).
- **Baseline diagnostic tests:** 12-lead ECG to assess for myocardial ischemia.
- **Tachycardia:** Monitor continuous ECG for rapid heart rate and dysrhythmias. Assess for nervousness and tremors.
- **Increased appetite:** Evaluate food intake and weigh daily.
- **Insomnia:** Evaluate sleep pattern. Dosage may have to be reduced if patients are unable to sleep while taking medication.
- **Patient education:** Caution against discontinuing levothyroxine. Explain that replacement therapy for hypothyroidism is lifelong. Stress that follow-up office visits and thyroid function tests are essential. Instruct to take the drug at the same time each day, preferably in the morning. Teach how to monitor the pulse for rate and rhythm and instruct on promptly reporting a change in rhythm or a pulse rate of 100 beats/min or more to a health care provider. Instruct not to change brands of the drug. Emphasize the importance of prompt reporting of chest pain, insomnia, nervousness, tremors, or weight loss. Advise pediatric patients and caregivers that children may experience reversible hair loss or increased aggressiveness during

L

the first few mo of therapy. Explain that full therapeutic effects of the drug may take 1-3 wk to appear.

SERIOUS ADVERSE REACTIONS

- **Withdrawal of medication:** Hypothyroidism including fatigue, somnolence, weakness, depression, hypothermia, weight gain, myxedema. Corticosteroids are required concomitantly to prevent acute adrenal insufficiency.

OVERDOSE/TOXICITY

- **Hyperthyroidism/thyrotoxicosis:** Fever, hypoglycemia, tachycardia, dehydration, palpitations, chest pain, tremors, nervousness, hypertension, headache, diarrhea, insomnia, heart failure, and menstrual irregularities.
- **Management:** Digitalis or other positive inotropic medication may be used to manage heart failure. Tachycardia and chest discomfort may be controlled using Advanced Cardiac Life Support (ACLS) guidelines. Provide IV hydration, control of fever.
- **GI decontamination:** No specific recommendations.

ANTIDOTE/DIALYSIS

- **Antidote:** Beta-adrenergic blockers (propranolol, metoprolol, esmolol) may be used to control tachycardia and hypertension.
- **Dialysis:** Levothyroxine is unlikely to be removed using hemodialysis or peritoneal dialysis. No data are available on removal using high-permeability hemodialysis.

lidocaine hydrochloride

lye'-doe-kane hye-droe-klor'-ide

Classes

Chemical: amide derivative
Therapeutic: antidysrhythmic, class IB

Pregnancy Category: B

Trade Names

Prescription: Anestacaine, Anestacon, Ela-Max, Ela-Max Plus, Laryng-O-Jet Spray, L-Caine, Lida Mantle, Lidoderm, Lidoject 1, Lidoject 2, LidoSite, LMX 4, LMX 4 with Tegaderm, LMX 5, Truxacaine, UAD Caine, Xylocaine, Xylocaine 10% Oral, Xylocaine Dental Cartridges, Xylocaine HCl For Spinal, Xylocaine Jelly, Xylocaine-MPF, Xylocaine Topical, Xylocaine Viscous

CLINICAL PHARMACOLOGY

Mechanism of Action

An amide anesthetic that inhibits conduction of nerve impulses. **Therapeutic Effect:** Causes temporary loss of feeling and sensation. Also an antidysrhythmic that decreases depolarization, automaticity, excitability of the ventricle during diastole by direct action. **Therapeutic Effect:** Inhibits ventricular dysrhythmias.

PHARMACOKINETICS

Route	Onset	Peak	Duration
IV	30-90 sec	N/A	10-20 min
Local anesthetic	3-5 min	N/A	30-60 min

Completely absorbed after IM administration. Protein binding: 60%-80%. Widely distributed. Metabolized in the liver. Primarily excreted in urine. Not removed by hemodialysis. **Half-life:** 1-2 hr.

AVAILABILITY

Injection (for continuous infusion [Xylocaine]): 4% w/v (40 mg/mL), 10% w/v (100 mg/mL), 20% w/v (200 mg/mL).
Injection (with dextrose for continuous infusion): 0.1% w/v (1 mg/mL), 0.2% w/v (2 mg/mL), 0.4% w/v 4 mg/mL), 0.8% (8 mg/mL).
Injection (for direct injection [Xylocaine]): 1% w/v (10 mg/mL), 2% w/v (20 mg/mL).
Injectable solution: 0.5% (Xylocaine HCl), 1% (Anestacaine, L-Caine, Lidoject 1, Truxacaine, UAD Caine, Xylocaine HCl, Xylocaine-MPF), 1.5% (Xylocaine HCl, Xylocaine-MPF), 2% (Anestacaine, Lidoject 2, Truxacaine, Xylocaine Dental Cartridges, Xylocaine HCl, Xylocaine-MPF), 4% (Xylocaine HCl, Xylocaine-MPF), 10% (Xylocaine), 20% (Xylocaine).
Ointment (Xylocaine Topical): 5%.
Cream: 3% (Lida Mantle), 4% (Ela-Max, Ela-Max Plus, LMX 4, LMX 4 with Tegaderm), 5% (LMX 5).
Gel (Anestacon, Xylocaine Jelly, Xylocaine Topical): 2%.
Topical spray (Xylocaine 10% Oral): 10%.
Topical solution: 2% (Xylocaine Viscous), 4% (Xylocaine Topical).
Topical film (Lidoderm): 5%.
Topical lotion (Lida Mantle): 3%.
Dermal patch (Lidoderm): 5%.
Kit (Laryng-O-Jet Spray): 4%.

INDICATIONS AND DOSAGE

Rapid control of acute ventricular dysrhythmias after an MI, cardiac catheterization, cardiac surgery, or digitalis-induced ventricular dysrhythmias

IM

Adults, Elderly: 300 mg (or 4.3 mg/kg). May repeat in 60-90 min.

IV

Adults, Elderly: Initially, 50-100 mg (0.7-1.4 mg/kg) IV bolus at rate of 25-50 mg/min. May repeat in 5 min. Give no more than 200-300 mg in 1 hr. Maintenance: 20-50 mcg/kg/min (1-4 mg/min) as IV infusion.
Children, Infants: Initially, 0.5-1 mg/kg IV bolus (maximum 100 mg bolus); may repeat but total dose not to exceed 3-5 mg/kg. Maintenance: 10-50 mcg/kg/min as IV infusion.

Dental or surgical procedures, childbirth

Infiltration, nerve block

Adults: Local anesthetic dosage varies with procedure, degree of anesthesia, vascularity, duration. Maximum dose: 4.5 mg/kg. Do not repeat within 2 hr.

Local skin disorders (minor burns, insect bites, prickly heat, skin manifestations of chicken pox, abrasions), and mucous membrane disorders (local anesthesia of oral, nasal, and laryngeal mucous membranes; local anesthesia of respiratory, urinary tract; relief of discomfort of pruritus ani, hemorrhoids, pruritus vulvae)

Topical

Adults, Elderly: Apply to affected areas as needed.

Treatment of shingles-related skin pain

Topical (Dermal patch)

Adults, Elderly: Apply to intact skin over most painful area (up to 3 applications once for up to 12 hr in a 24-hr period).

CONTRAINDICATIONS

Adams-Stokes syndrome, hypersensitivity to lidocaine or amide-type local anesthetics, septicemia (spinal anesthesia), supraventricular dysrhythmias, Wolff-Parkinson-White syndrome

INTERACTIONS

Drug: Anticonvulsants: May increase cardiac depressant effects. **Beta-adrenergic blockers:** May increase risk of toxicity. **Local anesthetics:** Amount absorbed from all formulations may be increased. **Other antidysrhythmics:** May increase cardiac effects. **Herbal:** None known. **Food:** None known.

DIAGNOSTIC TEST EFFECTS

IM lidocaine may increase creatine kinase (CK) level (used to diagnose acute MI). Therapeutic serum level is 1.5 to 6 mcg/mL; toxic serum level is greater than 6 mcg/mL.

IV INCOMPATIBILITIES

Amphotericin B complex (Abelcet, AmBisome, Amphotec), thiopental

IV COMPATIBILITIES

Aminophylline, amiodarone (Cordarone), calcium gluconate, digoxin (Lanoxin), diltiazem (Cardizem), *DOBUTamine (Dobutrex), *DOPamine (Intropin), enalapril (Vasotec), furosemide (Lasix), heparin, insulin, nitroglycerin, potassium chloride

SIDE-EFFECTS

CNS effects are generally dose-related and of short duration. **Occasional: IM:** Pain at injection site, hypotension, constipation, nausea, vomiting, dizziness, tremor, confusion, drowsiness. **Topical:** Burning, stinging, tenderness at application site. **Rare: Generally with high dose:** Drowsiness; dizziness; disorientation; lightheadedness; tremors; apprehension; euphoria; sensation of heat, cold, or numbness; blurred or double vision; ringing or roaring in ears (tinnitus); nausea

CRITICAL CARE CONSIDERATIONS

ADMINISTRATION/HANDLING

GENERAL ALERT

- **Possible cardiopulmonary instability:** Keep resuscitative equipment and drugs, including O_2, readily available when administering lidocaine by any route.

IM ALERT

- **Preparation:** Use 10% (100 mg/mL) and clearly identify that the lidocaine preparation is for IM use.
- **Injection:** Give in the deltoid muscle because the blood level will be significantly higher than if the injection is given in gluteus muscle or lateral thigh.

IV ALERT

- Use only lidocaine without preservative.
- **Labeling:** Clearly mark drug container with "for IV use."
- **Storage:** Store at room temperature.
- **IV push:** Use 1% (10 mg/mL) or 2% (20 mg/mL).

L

- **IV injection:** IV push at rate of 25-50 mg/min.
- **IV infusion preparation:** Prepare solution by adding 1 g to 1 L D_5W to provide concentration of 1 mg/mL (0.1%).
- **Commercially available IV preparation:** Premixed IV solutions of 0.2%, 0.4%, and 0.8% are available for IV infusion. Maximum concentration is 4 g/250 mL.
- **Administer for IV infusion:** Infuse at 1-4 mg/min with a volume control IV set.

TOPICAL ALERT

- Topical form is not for ophthalmic use.
- **Skin disorders:** Apply directly to affected area or put on a gauze or bandage, which is then applied to the skin.
- **Mucous membranes:** Apply to desired area according to manufacturer's insert.
- **Lowest dose:** Administer the lowest dosage possible that still provides anesthesia.

LIDOCAINE CONTINUOUS INFUSION

DOSE	1 g/250 mL (4 mg/mL)		4 g/500 mL (8 mg/mL)	
mg/min	mL/hr	mg/hr	mL/hr	mg/hr
1	15	60	7.5	60
2	30	120	15	120
3	45	180	22.5	180
4	60	240	30	240

L

PRECAUTIONS

HEALTH-RELATED

- Use cautiously in patients with atrial fibrillation, bradycardia, heart block, hypovolemia, liver disease, marked hypoxia, and severe respiratory depression.

AGE-RELATED

- **Children:** Safety for IV use in children has not been established. No age-related precautions noted for topical form.
- **Elderly:** Lidocaine dose and rate of infusion should be reduced for age-related renal impairment. Elderly are more sensitive to the adverse effects of lidocaine.

PREGNANCY/LACTATION-RELATED

- Pregnancy category B; unknown if excreted in human breast milk.

MONITORING

- **Baseline assessment:** Determine hypersensitivity to amide anesthetics and lidocaine before beginning drug therapy. Obtain vital signs.
- **Baseline lab work:** Biochemical panel including potassium, magnesium, and calcium to rule out electrolyte imbalance as the cause of dysrhythmias.
- **Baseline diagnostic tests:** 12-lead ECG for diagnosis of dysrhythmias and to evaluate for myocardial ischemia.
- **Cardiac:** Monitor ECG continuously during and following lidocaine administration for dysrhythmias, including bradycardia, prolongation of the PR interval or QRS complex.
- **Heart failure:** Monitor cardiopulmonary assessment closely for increased rales or rhonchi in breath sounds, shortness of breath, diminished pulse quality, neck vein distention, hypotension, or dependent edema.
- **Drug serum levels:** Evaluate serum drug levels. Therapeutic blood level is 1.5-6 mcg/mL; toxic serum level is greater than 6 mcg/mL.
- **Lidocaine by all routes:** Monitor level of consciousness and vital signs. Drowsiness may signal high lidocaine blood levels.
- **Patient education:** Ensure that patients receiving lidocaine as a local anesthetic understand the experience of the loss of feeling or sensation. Affected areas require protection until anesthetic wears off. Warn not to chew gum, drink, or eat for 1 hr after oral mucous membrane lidocaine application. The swallowing reflex may be impaired, increasing risk of aspiration, and numbness of tongue or buccal mucosa may lead to trauma.

SERIOUS ADVERSE REACTIONS

- **Malignant hyperthermia.**
- **Methemoglobinemia:** Abnormal hemoglobin that occurs following topical application of lidocaine for teething discomfort and laryngeal anesthetic spray. This hemoglobin does not carry oxygen, which prompts oxygen deficit at the cellular level, manifested by respiratory distress and cyanosis. Condition is managed using IV methylene blue infusion.
- **Hypersensitivity/anaphylaxis:** Rash, urticaria, laryngeal edema, respiratory distress, flushing with tachycardia, and hypertension followed by hypotension and cardiovascular collapse.

OVERDOSE/TOXICITY

- **CNS toxicity:** Occurs most often with regional anesthesia use, progressing rapidly from mild side effects to tremors, somnolence, seizures, vomiting, and respiratory depression. CNS stimulation may be managed with benzodiazepines (diazepam

[Valium] or lorazepam [Ativan]), short-acting barbiturates (thiopental [Pentothal]) or, if anesthetized, neuromuscular blocking agents (succinylcholine, vecuronium).

- **Cardiovascular toxicity:** High dosage by any route may produce cardiovascular depression, bradycardia, hypotension, dysrhythmias, heart block, cardiovascular collapse, and cardiac arrest. Manage patients according to Advanced Cardiac Life Support (ACLS) guidelines.
- **GI decontamination:** No specific recommendations.

ANTIDOTE/DIALYSIS

- **Antidote:** No specific recommendations.
- **Dialysis:** Lidocaine is not removed by hemodialysis and is unlikely to be removed by peritoneal dialysis. No data are available on removal by high-permeability hemodialysis.

linezolid

lih-neh'-zoe-lid

Classes

Chemical: oxazolidinone derivative
Therapeutic: antibiotic

Pregnancy Category: C

Trade Names

Prescription: Zyvox, Zyvoxam ♣

Do not confuse Zyvox with Zovirax.

CLINICAL PHARMACOLOGY

Mechanism of Action

An oxalodinone antiinfective that binds to a site on bacterial 23S ribosomal RNA, preventing the formation of a complex that is essential for bacterial translation. **Therapeutic Effect:** Bacteriostatic against enterococci and staphylococci; bactericidal against streptococci.

PHARMACOKINETICS

Rapidly and extensively absorbed after PO administration. Protein binding: 31%. Metabolized in the liver by oxidation. Excreted in urine. **Half-life:** 4-5.4 hr.

AVAILABILITY

Powder for oral suspension: 100 mg/5 mL.
Tablets: 400 mg, 600 mg.
Injection: 2 mg/mL in 100-mL, 200-mL, 300-mL bags.

INDICATIONS AND DOSAGE

Vancomycin-resistant infections (VRE)

PO, IV

Adults, Elderly, Children older than 11 yr: 600 mg every 12 hr for 14-28 days. **Children 11 yr and younger:** 10 mg/kg every 8-12 hr for 14-28 days.

Pneumonia, complicated skin and skin structure infections

PO, IV

Adults, Elderly, Children older than 11 yr: 600 mg every 12 hr for 10-14 days. **Children 11 yr and younger:** 10 mg/kg every 8 hr for 10-14 days.

Uncomplicated skin and skin structure infections

PO

Adults, Elderly: 400 mg every 12 hr for 10-14 days. **Children older than 11 yr:** 600 mg every 12 hr for 10-14 days. **Children 5-11 yr:** 10 mg/kg/dose every 12 hr for 10-14 days. **Children younger than 5 yr:** 10 mg/kg every 8 hr for 10-14 days.

Complicated skin and skin structure infections

PO

Adults, Elderly: 600 mg every 12 hr for 10-14 days. **Children younger than 12 yr:** 10 mg/kg every 8 hr for 10-14 days.

Usual neonate dosage

PO, IV

Neonates: 10 mg/kg/dose every 8-12 hr.

CONTRAINDICATIONS

Hypersensitivity to linezolid

INTERACTIONS

Drug: **Adrenergic agents (sympathomimetics):** Increase the effects of linezolid. **MAOIs:** Decrease the effects of MAOIs. **Herbal:** None known. **Food:** **Tyramine-containing foods and beverages:** Excessive amounts may cause significant hypertension.

DIAGNOSTIC TEST EFFECTS

May decrease blood Hgb, platelet count, WBC count, and ALT (SGPT) levels.

IV INCOMPATIBILITIES

Amphotericin B complex (Abelcet, AmBisome, Amphotec), *chlorproMAZINE (Thorazine), co-trimoxazole (Bactrim), diazepam (Valium), erythromycin (Erythrocin), pentamidine (Pentam IV), phenytoin (Dilantin), total parenteral nutrition (TPN)

SIDE-EFFECTS

Occasional (5%-2%): Diarrhea, nausea, headache. **Rare (less than 2%):** Altered taste, vaginal candidiasis, fungal infection, dizziness, tongue discoloration

CRITICAL CARE CONSIDERATIONS

ADMINISTRATION/HANDLING

PO ALERT

- Give linezolid without regard to food.
- Use the oral suspension within 21 days of reconstitution.

IV ALERT

- **Dedicated IV line:** Do not mix linezolid with other medications. If the same line is used to administer another drug, flush with compatible fluid (D_5W, 0.9% NaCl, lactated Ringer's).
- **Storage:** Store drug at room temperature and protect from light. A yellow color does not affect potency.
- **Infusion:** Infuse drug over 30-120 min.

PRECAUTIONS

HEALTH-RELATED

- Use linezolid cautiously in patients with carcinoid syndrome, pheochromocytoma, severe renal or hepatic impairment, uncontrolled hypertension, or untreated hyperthyroidism.
- **Resistant organisms:** Careful consideration should be given to alternative antibiotics before initiating linezolid to avoid developing resistant organisms. Drug should be reserved as an alternative for patients who have developed antibiotic resistance including those with VRE or methicillin-resistant *Staphylococcus aureus*.
- **MAOI effects:** Linezolid is a nonselective inhibitor of monoamine oxidase; use with caution with medications that may increase BP such as pseudoephedrine, phenylalanine, *DOPamine, and epinephrine.

AGE-RELATED

- **Children:** Safety and efficacy of linezolid have not been established in children.
- **Elderly:** No age-related precautions have been noted in the elderly.

PREGNANCY/LACTATION-RELATED

- Pregnancy category C; breast milk excretion unknown.

MONITORING

- **Baseline assessment:** Before giving linezolid, determine history of allergies, especially to linezolid or any of its components. Assess for dehydration.
- **Baseline lab work:** Biochemical panel including renal and liver function studies. Obtain appropriate cultures prior to drug administration. CBC with WBC differential and platelet count.
- **Fluid balance:** Monitor intake and output and urinalysis results as appropriate. Urge patients to drink fluids to maintain adequate hydration.
- **Optic and peripheral neurotoxicity:** Assess for numbness, tingling, headaches, lethargy, tremors, and visual disturbances.
- **IV infusion sites:** Evaluate for phlebitis (heat, pain, and red streaking over the vein).
- **Rash:** Inspect the skin for a rash, which may indicate hypersensitivity.
- **Superinfections:** Assess the mouth for white patches on the mucous membranes or tongue, for severe mouth or tongue soreness, and for severe anal or genital pruritus or discharge.
- **Possible *Clostridium difficile* colitis:** Assess pattern of daily bowel activity and stool consistency. Although mild GI effects may be tolerable, severe symptoms including abdominal pain or cramping, or moderate to severe diarrhea may indicate the onset of antibiotic-associated colitis.
- **Hand washing:** If *C. difficile* (antibiotic-associated) colitis develops, wash hands with antibacterial soap. Alcohol-based foam is ineffective against *C. difficile* spores.
- **Patient education:** Advise avoidance of excessive amounts of tyramine-containing foods (such as aged cheese and red wine) as these foods may cause severe reactions including diaphoresis, neck stiffness, palpitations, and severe headache. Provide a list of these foods. Instruct to discuss taking over-the-counter medications when taking linezolid; serotonin reuptake inhibitors, cold and allergy medications may have deleterious effects when taken concomitantly with linezolid.

SERIOUS ADVERSE REACTIONS

- Antibiotic-associated colitis and other superinfections may result from altered bacterial balance.
- **Hypertension:** May result from excessive intake of tyramine-containing foods.

OVERDOSE/TOXICITY

- **Bone marrow suppression:** Anemia, leukopenia, thrombocytopenia, and myelosuppression occur rarely.

- **Nephrotoxicity:** Increased BUN and serum creatinine levels; decreased creatinine clearance; may be reversible if the drug is stopped at the first sign of symptoms.
- **Neurotoxicity:** Headache, numbness, tingling, dizziness, lethargy, tremor, and visual disturbances occur occasionally; risk increases with higher dosages or prolonged therapy.
- **Management:** Toxic effects are generally reversible when linezolid dosing is stopped.
- **GI decontamination:** No specific recommendations.

ANTIDOTE/DIALYSIS

- **Antidote:** No specific recommendations.
- **Dialysis:** Linezolid is removed by hemodialysis and high-permeability hemodialysis. No data are available on removal by peritoneal dialysis.

liothyronine

lye-oh-thye'-roe-neen

Classes

Chemical: synthetic triiodothyronine (T_3)
Therapeutic: thyroid hormone

Pregnancy Category: A

Trade Names

Prescription: Cytomel, Triostat

Combinations

Prescription: with levothyroxine (Euthroid, Thyrolar)

Do not confuse liothyronine with levothyroxine.

CLINICAL PHARMACOLOGY

Mechanism of Action

A synthetic form of triiodothyronine (T_3), a thyroid hormone involved in normal metabolism, growth, and development, especially of the CNS in infants. Possesses catabolic and anabolic effects. **Therapeutic Effect:** Increases basal metabolic rate, enhances gluconeogenesis, and stimulates protein synthesis.

PHARMACOKINETICS

Almost completely absorbed following PO administration. Absorption is reduced to 43% in heart failure patients. Not firmly bound to serum protein. Excreted in urine. **Half-life:** 25 hr.

AVAILABILITY

Tablets (Cytomel): 5 mcg, 25 mcg, 50 mcg.
Injection (Triostat): 10 mcg/mL.

INDICATIONS AND DOSAGE

Hypothyroidism

PO

Adults, Elderly: Initially, 25 mcg/day. May increase in increments of 12.5-25 mcg/day every 1-2 wk. Maximum: 100 mcg/day. **Children:** Initially, 5 mcg/day. May increase by 5 mcg/day every 3-4 wk. Maintenance: 100 mcg/day (children older than 3 yr); 50 mcg/day (children 1-3 yr); 20 mcg/day (infants).

Myxedema

PO

Adults, Elderly: Initially, 5 mcg/day. Increase by 5-10 mcg every 1-2 wk (after 25 mcg/day has been reached, may increase in 12.5-mcg increments). Maintenance: 50-100 mcg/day.

Nontoxic goiter

PO

Adults, Elderly: Initially, 5 mcg/day. Increase by 5-10 mcg/day every 1-2 wk. When 25 mcg/day has been reached, may increase by 12.5-25 mcg/day every 1-2 wk. Maintenance: 75 mcg/day. **Children:** 5 mcg/day. May increase by 5 mcg every 1-2 wk. Maintenance: 15-20 mcg/day.

Congenital hypothyroidism

PO

Children: Initially, 5 mcg/day. Increase by 5 mcg/day every 3-4 days. Maintenance: Full adult dosage (children older than 3 yr); 50 mcg/day (children 1-3 yr); 20 mcg/day (infants).

T_3 suppression test

PO

Adults, Elderly: 75-100 mcg/day for 7 days; then repeat I^{131} thyroid uptake test.

Myxedema coma, precoma

IV

Adults, Elderly: Initially 25-50 mcg (10-20 mcg in patients with cardiovascular disease). Total dose at least 65 mcg/day.

CONTRAINDICATIONS

MI and thyrotoxicosis uncomplicated by hypothyroidism; obesity, uncorrected adrenal cortical insufficiency; hypersensitivity to liothyronine

INTERACTIONS

Drug: **Cholestyramine, colestipol:** May decrease the absorption of liothyronine. **Oral anticoagulants:** May alter the effects of these drugs. **Sympathomimetics:** May

L

increase the risk of coronary insufficiency and the effects of liothyronine. **Herbal:** None known. **Food:** None known.

DIAGNOSTIC TEST EFFECTS

None known.

SIDE-EFFECTS

Occasional: Reversible hair loss at start of therapy (in children). **Rare:** Dry skin, GI intolerance, rash, hives, pseudotumor cerebri or severe headache in children

CRITICAL CARE CONSIDERATIONS

ADMINISTRATION/HANDLING

PO ALERT

- Initial and subsequent dosages are based on clinical status and response.
- Do not use different brands of liothyronine interchangeably because of problems with bioequivalence among manufacturers.

IV ALERT

- **Storage:** Refrigerate until administration. Discard drug not used.
- **Dilution:** May be given undiluted.
- **Intermittent IV dosing:** Administer IV dose over 4 hr; space doses no longer than 12 hr apart.

PRECAUTIONS

HEALTH-RELATED

- Use liothyronine cautiously in patients with adrenal insufficiency, cardiovascular disease, coronary artery disease, diabetes insipidus, or diabetes mellitus.

AGE-RELATED

- **Children:** No age-related precautions. Use caution in interpreting thyroid function test results in neonates.
- **Elderly:** May be more sensitive to thyroid effects. Individualized dosages are recommended.

PREGNANCY/LACTATION-RELATED

- Pregnancy category A. Little or no transplacental passage at physiologic serum concentrations. Excreted into breast milk in low concentrations (inadequate to protect a hypothyroid infant; too low to interfere with neonatal screening programs).

MONITORING

- **Baseline assessment:** Obtain weight and vital signs. Determine hypersensitivity to aspirin or tartrazine. Liothyronine therapy may intensify the signs and symptoms of adrenal insufficiency, diabetes insipidus, diabetes mellitus, and hypopituitarism.
- **Baseline lab work:** Ensure patients have been tested for hypoadrenalism. Biochemical profile including a baseline blood glucose level.
- **Concomitant use of steroids:** Administer adrenocortical steroids before thyroid therapy in patients with coexisting hypoadrenalism and hypothyroidism.
- **Tachycardia:** Monitor heart rate and rhythm. Tachycardia may indicate dosage of medication is too high.
- **CNS stimulation:** Assess for nervousness, tremors, poor appetite, and insomnia, which may indicate dosage is too high.
- **Hypoglycemia:** Monitor for tremors, tachycardia, diaphoresis, and confusion.
- **Patient education:** Caution against discontinuing liothyronine. Explain that replacement therapy for hypothyroidism is lifelong. Stress follow-up office visits and thyroid function tests are essential. Instruct to take the drug at the same time each day, preferably in the morning. Teach how to monitor the pulse. Advise to report promptly a change in rhythm, a marked increase in rate, or a pulse of 100 beats/min or more to a health care provider. Warn not to change brands of the drug. Remind to report promptly chest pain, insomnia, nervousness, tremors, or weight loss. Explain to pediatric patients and caregivers that children may experience reversible hair loss or increased aggressiveness during the first few mo of therapy.

SERIOUS ADVERSE REACTIONS

- Cardiac dysrhythmias occur rarely.
- **Hyperthyroidism:** Excessive dosage may mimic hyperthyroidism, including weight loss, palpitations, increased appetite, tremors, nervousness, tachycardia, hypertension, headache, insomnia, and menstrual irregularities.

OVERDOSE/TOXICITY

- **Thyroid storm:** Overdose mimics thyrotoxicosis including angina pectoris, chest discomfort, diarrhea, heart failure, irritability, nervousness, tachycardia, possible acute MI, diaphoresis, and headache.
- **Management:** Discontinue medication temporarily. Initiate supportive care including maintaining patent airway, ventilation, and administering oxygen. Beta-adrenergic

blockers (propranolol, metoprolol) may effectively control tachycardia. Heart failure may be managed with digoxin or inodilators such as milrinone.
- **GI decontamination:** No specific recommendations.

ANTIDOTE/DIALYSIS
- **Antidote:** No specific recommendations.
- **Dialysis:** No data are available on removal of liothyronine using hemodialysis, high-permeability hemodialysis, or peritoneal dialysis.

lisinopril

ly-sin'-oh-pril

Classes
Chemical: angiotensin-converting enzyme (ACE) inhibitor, nonsulfhydryl
Therapeutic: antihypertensive

Pregnancy Category: C (1st trimester), D (2nd and 3rd trimesters)

Trade Names
Prescription: Prinivil, Zestril

Combinations
Prescription: with hydrochlorothiazide (Prinzide, Zestoretic)

Do not confuse lisinopril with fosinopril; Prinivil with Desyrel, Plendil, Proventil, or Restoril; Fibsol with Lioresal; or Zestril with Zostrix. Do not confuse lisinopril's combination form Zestoretic with Prilosec.

CLINICAL PHARMACOLOGY
Mechanism of Action
This ACE inhibitor suppresses the renin-angiotensin-aldosterone system and prevents conversion of angiotensin I to angiotensin II, a potent vasoconstrictor; may also inhibit angiotensin II at local vascular and renal sites. Decreases plasma angiotensin II, increases plasma renin activity, and decreases aldosterone secretion. **Therapeutic Effect:** Reduces peripheral arterial resistance, BP, afterload, pulmonary capillary wedge pressure (preload), and pulmonary vascular resistance. In those with heart failure, also decreases heart size, increases cardiac output, and exercise tolerance time.

PHARMACOKINETICS

Route	Onset	Peak	Duration
PO	1 hr	6 hr	24 hr

Incompletely absorbed from the GI tract. Protein binding: 25%. Primarily excreted unchanged in urine. Removed by hemodialysis. **Half-life:** 12 hr (prolonged with impaired renal function).

AVAILABILITY
Tablets (Prinivil, Zestril): 2.5 mg, 5 mg, 10 mg, 20 mg, 30 mg, 40 mg.

INDICATIONS AND DOSAGE
Hypertension (used alone)
PO

Adults: Initially, 10 mg/day. May increase by 5-10 mcg/day at 1- to 2-wk intervals. Maximum: 80 mg/day. **Elderly:** Initially, 2.5-5 mg/day. May increase by 2.5-5 mg/day at 1- to 2-wk intervals. Maximum: 80 mg/day.

Hypertension (used in combination with other antihypertensives)
PO

Adults: Initially, 2.5-5 mg/day titrated to patient needs.

Adjunctive therapy for management of heart failure
PO

Adults, Elderly: Initially, 2.5-5 mg/day. May increase by no more than 10 mg/day at intervals of at least 2 wk. Maintenance: 5-40 mg/day. Maximum: 80 mg/day.

Improve survival in patients after MI
PO

Adults, Elderly: Initially, 5 mg; 5 mg after 24 hr, 10 mg after 48 hr; then 10 mg/day for 6 wk. For patients with low systolic BP, give 2.5-mg/day for 3 days, then 2.5–5 mg/day.

Dosage in renal impairment
Titrate to patient's needs after giving the following initial dose:

Creatinine Clearance	Initital Dose
10-30 mL/min	5 mg/day
Less than 10 mL/min	2.5 mg/day

OFF-LABEL USES
Treatment of hypertension or renal crises with scleroderma

CONTRAINDICATIONS
History of angioedema from previous treatment with lisinopril or other ACE inhibitors

INTERACTIONS
Drug: **Alcohol, diuretics, hypotensive agents:** May increase the effects of lisinopril. **Lithium:** May increase lithium blood concentration and risk of toxicity. **NSAIDs:** May decrease the effects of lisinopril.

Potassium-sparing diuretics, potassium supplements: May cause hyperkalemia. **Herbal:** None known. **Food:** None known.

DIAGNOSTIC TEST EFFECTS

May increase BUN, serum alkaline phosphatase, serum bilirubin, serum creatinine, serum potassium, AST (SGOT), and ALT (SGPT) levels. May decrease serum sodium levels. May cause positive antinuclear antibodies titer.

SIDE-EFFECTS

Frequent (12%-5%): Headache, dizziness, postural hypotension. **Occasional (4%-2%):** Chest discomfort, fatigue, rash, abdominal pain, nausea, diarrhea, upper respiratory infection. **Rare (1% or less):** Palpitations, tachycardia, peripheral edema, insomnia, paresthesia, confusion, constipation, dry mouth, muscle cramps

CRITICAL CARE CONSIDERATIONS

ADMINISTRATION/HANDLING

PO ALERT

- Give lisinopril without regard to food.
- Tablets may be crushed if necessary.
- Discontinue diuretics 2-3 days before beginning lisinopril therapy.

PRECAUTIONS

HEALTH-RELATED

- Use cautiously in patients with cerebrovascular or coronary insufficiency, hypovolemia, renal impairment, severe congestive heart failure, and sodium depletion.
- Use cautiously in patients on dialysis or diuretic therapy.

AGE-RELATED

- **Children:** Safety and efficacy of lisinopril have not been established in children under 6 yr.
- **Elderly:** May be more sensitive to the hypotensive effects of lisinopril.

PREGNANCY/LACTATION-RELATED

- Pregnancy category C (first trimester), category D (second and third trimesters). ACE inhibitors can cause fetal and neonatal morbidity and death when administered to pregnant women; when pregnancy is detected, discontinue ACE inhibitors as soon as possible. Detectable in breast milk in trace amounts; a newborn would receive less than 0.1% of the mg/kg maternal dose; effect on nursing infant has not been determined.

MONITORING

- **Baseline assessment:** Assess heart rate and BP immediately before each lisinopril dose and regularly throughout therapy. Be alert to fluctuations in heart rate and BP.
- **Baseline and ongoing lab work:** CBC with WBC differential; biochemical panel including BUN, creatinine, and potassium levels. Perform before beginning lisinopril therapy, then every 2 wk for the next 3 mo; periodically thereafter in patients with autoimmune disease, renal impairment, or patients who are taking drugs that affect immune response or leukocyte count.
- **Hypotension:** If hypotension occurs, place in the supine position with legs elevated. Chest discomfort may accompany hypotension; if not resolved by lying flat, may require treatment with nitroglycerin if systolic BP is at least 90 mmHg.
- **Cardiac ischemia:** Monitor ECG continuously for ST segment depression or elevation in patients new to lisinopril with history of chest discomfort or MI.
- **Dependent edema:** Examine for edema of extremities, ankles, and sacrum.
- **Fluid retention:** Auscultate the lungs for rales. Monitor intake and output and daily weights. Edema and fluid retention may indicate worsening heart failure or renal insufficiency.
- **Constipation:** Assess pattern of bowel activity and stool consistency.
- **Fall prevention:** Assist with ambulation if dizziness occurs.
- **Cough:** Assess cough. If persistent and severe, may warrant discontinuation of therapy.
- **Hydration:** Offer fluids frequently or administer IV fluids to maintain hydration. Hypotension is common in volume-depleted patients.
- **Angioedema or allergic reaction:** Examine the skin for swelling of face, lips, tongue, pruritus, rash, respiratory distress, or any sign of adverse reaction to medication; patients receiving ACE inhibitors are more likely to have these reactions because the drugs impact inflammatory mediators.
- **Surgery/anesthesia:** If patients become hypotensive during a procedure, the blocked angiotensin II impairs BP compensation, prompting the need for correction of hypovolemia with IV fluid boluses.

- **Patient education:** Advise to rise slowly from lying to sitting position and to pause momentarily before standing to help abate orthostatic hypotension. Urge limiting consumption of alcohol while taking lisinopril. Instruct to report promptly diarrhea or vomiting (may lead to dehydration and low BP); difficulty breathing; excessive perspiration; swelling of the face, lips, or tongue to a health care provider.

SERIOUS ADVERSE REACTIONS

- **Excessive hypotension:** "First-dose syncope" may occur in patients with heart failure and severe salt and volume depletion.
- **Angioedema:** Swelling of face and lips; when involving the tongue, lips, and larynx may require subcutaneous epinephrine 1:1000 solution (0.3-0.5 mL) with possible endotracheal intubation to maintain patent airway.
- **Hyperkalemia:** Occurs rarely and may be associated with renal insufficiency.

OVERDOSE/TOXICITY

- **Bone marrow suppression:** Agranulocytosis and neutropenia may be noted in patients with collagen vascular disease (e.g., scleroderma and systemic lupus erythematosus) and impaired renal function.
- **Nephrotic syndrome:** May be noted in patients with history of renal disease.
- **GI decontamination:** No specific recommendations.

ANTIDOTE/DIALYSIS

- **Antidote:** No specific recommendations.
- **Dialysis:** Hypersensitivity-type reactions have been noted in patients undergoing hemodialysis using high flux dialysis membranes (e.g., AN69) when receiving lisinopril and other ACE inhibitors. Consideration should be given to using another type of dialysis membrane for patients on ACE inhibitors. Lisinopril is removed by hemodialysis and is likely to be removed by high permeability hemodialysis. No data are available on removal by peritoneal dialysis.

lithium carbonate/lithium citrate

See Antipsychotics (p. 934)

lomefloxacin hydrochloride

See Antibiotics (p. 892)

loperamide hydrochloride

loe-per'-a-mide hye-droe-klor'-ide

Classes

Chemical: piperidine derivative
Therapeutic: antidiarrheal

Pregnancy Category: C

Trade Names

Prescription: Imodium
Over the Counter: Diarr-Eze ♣, Imodium A-D, Loperacap ♣, Maalox Anti-Diarrheal

Combinations

Over the Counter: with simethicone (Imodium Advanced)

Do not confuse Imodium with Indocin or Ionamin.

L

CLINICAL PHARMACOLOGY

Mechanism of Action

An antidiarrheal that directly affects the intestinal wall muscles. **Therapeutic Effect:** Slows intestinal motility and prolongs transit time of intestinal contents by reducing fecal volume, diminishing loss of fluid and electrolytes, and increasing viscosity and bulk of stool.

PHARMACOKINETICS

Poorly absorbed from the GI tract. Protein binding: 97%. Metabolized in the liver. Eliminated primarily in feces. **Half-life:** 9.1-14.4 hr.

AVAILABILITY

Capsules: 2 mg.
Liquid: 1 mg/5 mL.
Tablets: 2 mg.

INDICATIONS AND DOSAGE

Acute diarrhea

PO (capsules)

Adults, Elderly: Initially, 4 mg; then 2 mg after each unformed stool. Maximum: 16 mg/day. **Children 9-12 yr, weighing more than 30 kg:** Initially, 2 mg 3 times per day for 24 hr. **Children 6-8 yr, weighing 20-30 kg:** Initially, 2 mg twice per day for 24 hr. **Children 2-5 yr, weighing 13-20 kg:** Initially, 1 mg 3 times per day for 24 hr. Maintenance: 1 mg/10 kg only after loose stool.

Chronic diarrhea

PO

Adults, Elderly: Initially, 4 mg; then 2 mg after each unformed stool until diarrhea is controlled. **Children:** 0.08-0.24 mg/kg/day in 2-3 divided doses. Maximum: 2 mg/dose.

Travelers diarrhea

PO

Adults, Elderly: Initially, 4 mg; then 2 mg after each loose bowel movement (LBM). Maximum: 8 mg/day for 2 days. **Children 9-11 yr (or 60-95 lb):** Initially, 2 mg; then 1 mg after each LBM. Maximum: 6 mg/day for 2 days. **Children 6-8 yr (or 48-59 lb):** Initially, 2 mg; then 1 mg after each LBM. Maximum: 4 mg/day for 2 days. **Children 2-5 yr (or 42-47 lb):** Initially, 1 mg; then 1 mg after each LBM. Maximum: 3 mg/day.

CONTRAINDICATIONS

Acute ulcerative colitis (may produce toxic megacolon), diarrhea associated with pseudomembranous enterocolitis due to broad-spectrum antibiotics or to organisms that invade intestinal mucosa (such as *Escherichia coli*, shigella, and salmonella), patients who must avoid constipation, hypersensitivity to loperamide hydrochloride

INTERACTIONS

Drug: Opioid (narcotic) analgesics: May increase the risk of constipation. **Herbal:** None known. **Food:** None known.

DIAGNOSTIC TEST EFFECTS

None known.

SIDE-EFFECTS

Rare: Dry mouth, somnolence, abdominal discomfort, allergic reaction (such as rash and itching)

CRITICAL CARE CONSIDERATIONS

ADMINISTRATION/HANDLING

ORAL LIQUID ALERT

- When administering loperamide to children, use the accompanying plastic dropper to measure the liquid.

PRECAUTIONS

HEALTH-RELATED

- Use loperamide cautiously in patients with fluid and electrolyte depletion or hepatic impairment. If clinical improvement is not seen in 48 hr, loperamide should be discontinued and cause of diarrhea should be further evaluated. Patients with hepatic dysfunction should be monitored closely for CNS toxicity.
- **Toxic megacolon:** Loperamide may induce megacolon if patients have ulcerative colitis or antibiotic-induced *Clostridium difficile* colitis (CDAD).
- **Acute dysentery:** Loperamide should not be used if patients have bloody diarrhea with high fever.

AGE-RELATED

- **Children:** Loperamide use is not recommended in children under 6 yr. Infants under 3 mo are more susceptible to CNS effects.
- **Elderly:** Loperamide use may mask dehydration and electrolyte depletion.

PREGNANCY/LACTATION-RELATED

- Pregnancy category C; unknown if excreted in breast milk; compatible with breast-feeding.

MONITORING

- **Baseline assessment:** Do not administer if bloody diarrhea or a temperature greater than 101°F is present. Determine history of ulcerative colitis.
- **Baseline lab work:** Stool specimens for culture and sensitivity and for ova and parasites if infectious diarrhea is suspected.
- **Hydration:** Provide IV fluid hydration and encourage the patient to maintain adequate fluid intake.
- **Ileus:** Assess bowel sounds for peristalsis. If bowel sounds are absent, abdomen is distended or painful, or fever occurs, discontinue drug.
- **Therapeutic effect:** Monitor for resolution of diarrhea.
- **Patient education:** Caution not to exceed the recommended dosage. Explain that loperamide may cause dry mouth. Urge avoidance of alcohol during loperamide therapy. Instruct to avoid tasks that require mental alertness or motor skills until response to the drug is known. If using loperamide outside the hospital, instruct to report if abdominal distention and pain, diarrhea that does not stop within 3 days, or fever occurs.

SERIOUS ADVERSE REACTIONS

- **Hypersensitivity:** Skin rash, pruritis.
- **Toxic megacolon:** Abdominal distention, absence of bowel sounds, abdominal pain, constipation, fever.

OVERDOSE/TOXICITY

- **CNS depression:** Altered mental status, disorientation, lethargy, confusion.
- **GI effects:** Severe nausea and vomiting, constipation, GI irritation.
- **GI decontamination:** Activated charcoal is used to treat loperamide toxicity.

ANTIDOTE/DIALYSIS

- **Antidote:** Naloxone may be used to try to reverse symptoms of an overdose.
- **Dialysis:** No data are available on removal using hemodialysis, high-permeability hemodialysis, or peritoneal dialysis.

lopinavir; ritonavir

See HIV Medications (p. 961)

loracarbef

See Antibiotics (p. 892)

loratadine

See Antihistamines (p. 925)

lorazepam

lor-a'-ze-pam

DEA Schedules: IV

Classes

Chemical: benzodiazepine

Therapeutic: anticonvulsant, anxiolytic, sedative/hypnotic

Pregnancy Category: D

Trade Names

Prescription: Apo-Lorazepam ♣, Ativan, Lorazepam Intensol, Novo-Lorazem ♣

Do not confuse lorazepam with Alprazolam.

CLINICAL PHARMACOLOGY

Mechanism of Action

A benzodiazepine that enhances the action of the inhibitory neurotransmitter gamma-aminobutyric acid in the CNS, affecting memory, as well as motor, sensory, and cognitive function. **Therapeutic Effect:** Produces anxiolytic, anticonvulsant, sedative, muscle relaxant, and antiemetic effects.

PHARMACOKINETICS

Route	Onset	Peak	Duration
PO	20-30 min	60-90 min	6-8 hr
IV	Less than 5 min	15-20 min	6-8 hr
IM	45-60 min	2 hr	6-8 hr

Well absorbed after PO and IM administration. Protein binding: 85%. Widely distributed. Metabolized in the liver. Primarily excreted in urine. Not removed by hemodialysis. **Half-life:** 12 hr.

AVAILABILITY

Tablets (Ativan): 0.5 mg, 1 mg, 2 mg.
Injection (Ativan): 2 mg/mL, 4 mg/mL.
Oral solution (Lorazepam Intensol): 2 mg/mL.

INDICATIONS AND DOSAGE

Anxiety

PO

Adults: 1-10 mg/day in 2-3 divided doses. Average: 2-6 mg/day. **Elderly:** Initially, 0.5-1 mg/day. May increase gradually. Range: 0.5-4 mg.

IV

Adults, Elderly: 0.02-0.06 mg/kg every 2-6 hr.

IV Infusion

Adults, Elderly: 0.01-0.1 mg/kg/hr.

PO, IV

Children: 0.05 mg/kg/dose every 4-8 hr. Range: 0.02-0.1 mg/kg. Maximum: 2 mg/dose.

Insomnia due to anxiety

PO

Adults: 2-4 mg at bedtime. **Elderly:** 0.5-1 mg at bedtime.

Preoperative sedation

IV

Adults, Elderly: 0.044 mg/kg 15-20 min before surgery. Maximum total dose: 2 mg.

IM

Adults, Elderly: 0.05 mg/kg 2 hr before procedure. Maximum total dose: 4 mg.

Status epilepticus

IV

Adults, Elderly: 4 mg over 2-5 min. May repeat in 10-15 min. Maximum: 8 mg in 12-hr period. **Children:** 0.1 mg/kg over 2-5 min. May give second dose of 0.05 mg/kg in 15-20 min. Maximum: 4 mg. **Neonates:** 0.05 mg/kg. May repeat in 10-15 min.

OFF-LABEL USES

Treatment of alcohol withdrawal, panic disorders, skeletal muscle spasms, chemotherapy-induced nausea or vomiting, tension headache,

L

tremors; adjunctive treatment before endoscopic procedures (diminishes patient recall)

CONTRAINDICATIONS

Angle-closure glaucoma, preexisting CNS depression, severe hypotension, severe uncontrolled pain, hypersensitivity to lorazepam

INTERACTIONS

Drug: **Alcohol, other CNS depressants:** May increase CNS depression. Herbal: **Kava kava, valerian:** May increase CNS depression. Food: None known.

DIAGNOSTIC TEST EFFECTS

None known. Therapeutic serum drug level is 50-240 ng/mL; toxic serum drug level is unknown.

IV INCOMPATIBILITIES

Aldesleukin (Proleukin), aztreonam (Azactam), idarubicin (Idamycin), ondansetron (Zofran), sufentanil (Sufenta)

IV COMPATIBILITIES

Bumetanide (Bumex), cefepime (Maxipime), diltiazem (Cardizem), *DOBUTamine (Dobutrex), *DOPamine (Intropin), heparin, labetalol (Normodyne, Trandate), milrinone (Primacor), norepinephrine (Levophed), piperacillin and tazobactam (Zosyn), potassium, propofol (Diprivan)

SIDE-EFFECTS

Frequent: Somnolence (initially in the morning), ataxia, confusion. Occasional: Blurred vision, slurred speech, hypotension, headache. Rare: Paradoxic CNS restlessness or excitement in elderly or debilitated

CRITICAL CARE CONSIDERATIONS

ADMINISTRATION/HANDLING

PO ALERT

- Give lorazepam with food.
- Crush tablets as needed.

IV ALERT

- **Storage:** Refrigerate; do not freeze the parenteral form. Do not use the solution if discolored or contains a precipitate.
- **IV push dilution:** Dilute with an equal volume of sterile water for injection, 0.9% NaCl, or D_5W.
- **Further dilution:** For IV infusion, inject IV push solution in adequate amount of D_5W or NaCl to a concentration of 0.1 mg/mL or 0.2 mg/mL. Solution is very viscous. Crystallization may occur from propylene glycol preservative, particularly when mixed in saline solution. Prepare amount of infusion to last for a maximum of 12 hr. Use only freshly prepared solutions.
- **Prefilled syringe dilution:** Remove air from a half-filled syringe, aspirate an equal volume of diluent, pull the plunger back slightly to allow for mixing, and gently invert the syringe several times; do not shake vigorously.
- **IV push:** Give by IV push into the tubing of a free-flowing IV infusion of 0.9% NaCl or D_5W at a rate not exceeding 2 mg/min. Keep patients recumbent after administration to reduce the hypotensive effects.
- **IV infusion:** Start with a small dose in elderly and children; increase gradually as needed for desired effect. Keep patients supine during continuous infusion.

IM ALERT

- Inject deep into a large muscle mass, such as gluteus maximus.

PRECAUTIONS

HEALTH-RELATED

- Use lorazepam cautiously in neonates; in patients with pulmonary, hepatic, or renal impairment; and in those using other CNS depressants concurrently.

AGE-RELATED

- **Children:** Safety and efficacy of lorazepam have not been established in children under 12 yr but drug has been used successfully to treat status epilepticus in neonates, infants, and children.
- **Elderly:** Age-related organ impairment may require a dosage reduction. Give small doses initially and to increase dosage gradually to avoid ataxia and excessive sedation.

PREGNANCY/LACTATION-RELATED

- Pregnancy category D (other benzodiazepines associated with cleft lip, cleft palate, microcephaly, pyloric stenosis); neonatal withdrawal, hypotonia. Excreted into breast milk in low quantities; effect on infant unknown.

MONITORING

- **Baseline assessment:** Assess for autonomic responses (cold and clammy hands and diaphoresis) and motor responses (agitation, trembling, and tension). Monitor BP, heart rate, respiratory rate.

- **Baseline lab work:** CBC with WBC differential, platelet count. Biochemical profile with BUN, creatinine, and liver function studies. For long-term therapy, perform tests periodically.
- **Paradoxic reactions:** Assess for paradoxic CNS reactions (increased agitation), particularly early in therapy.
- **Pain management:** Assess for pain in patients who are unable to communicate well. Patients in pain are sometimes given large doses of sedatives to control restlessness due to pain.
- **Respiratory status:** Assess for patent airway, secretions control, and effective breathing, especially following seizures and when dosage is increased.
- **Therapeutic response:** Assess for a calm facial expression, decreased restlessness, and insomnia when used to control agitation; resolution of seizures when used for status epilepticus or other seizures.
- **Drug levels:** Monitor serum drug levels. Therapeutic level for lorazepam is 50-240 ng/mL; toxic level remains unknown.
- **Patient education:** Caution not to stop taking lorazepam abruptly after long-term therapy. Inform that drowsiness usually disappears with continued therapy. Warn to avoid tasks that require mental alertness or motor skills until response to the drug is known. Urge avoidance of smoking, drinking alcoholic beverages, and taking other CNS depressants. Explain that smoking reduces the effectiveness of lorazepam; alcohol and CNS depressants increase sedation. Urge female patients on long-term therapy to use effective contraception during therapy and to report immediately pregnancy or suspected pregnancy to a health care provider.

SERIOUS ADVERSE REACTIONS

- **Abrupt or too-rapid withdrawal:** May result in pronounced restlessness, irritability, insomnia, hand tremor, abdominal or muscle cramps, diaphoresis, vomiting, and seizures.
- **Paradoxic reactions:** Some patients are intolerant of benzodiazepines and respond to the drug with increased agitation rather than sedation.

OVERDOSE/TOXICITY

- **Symptoms:** Somnolence, confusion, diminished reflexes, hypotension, and coma.
- **Management:** Ensure patent airway with endotracheal intubation if necessary, along with mechanical ventilation. Support BP with fluids and vasopressors if needed. Administer benzodiazepine antidote flumazenil. Forced diuresis and osmotic diuretics (e.g., mannitol) may facilitate elimination.
- **GI decontamination:** No specific recommendations.

ANTIDOTE/DIALYSIS

- **Antidote:** Cautiously use flumazenil (Romazicon) 0.2 mg (2 mL) over 30 sec; may repeat after 30 sec with 0.3 mg (3 mL) over 30 sec. Further doses may be given up to 0.5 mg (5 mL) up to a total of 3 mg (30 mL). Flumazenil reverses CNS depressive effects. Naloxone (Narcan) should be considered in addition to flumazenil if patients have significant respiratory depression.
- **Dialysis:** Lorazepam is not removed by hemodialysis and is unlikely to be removed by peritoneal dialysis. No data are available on removal using high-permeability hemodilalysis.

L

losartan potassium

lo-sar'-tan poe-tass'-ee-um

Classes

Chemical: angiotensin II receptor antagonist

Therapeutic: antihypertensive

Pregnancy Category: C, D (2nd and 3rd trimesters)

Trade Names

Prescription: Cozaar

Combinations

Prescription: with hydrochlorothiazide (Hyzaar)

Do not confuse Cozaar with Zocor.

CLINICAL PHARMACOLOGY

Mechanism of Action

An angiotensin II receptor, type AT_1, antagonist that blocks vasoconstrictor and aldosterone-secreting effects of angiotensin II, inhibiting the binding of angiotensin II to the AT_1 receptors. **Therapeutic Effect:** Causes vasodilation, decreases peripheral resistance, and decreases BP.

PHARMACOKINETICS

Route	Onset	Peak	Duration
PO	N/A	6 hr	24 hr

Well absorbed after PO administration. Protein binding: 98%. Undergoes first-pass metabolism in the liver to active metabolites. Excreted in urine and via the biliary system. Not removed by hemodialysis. **Half-life:** 2 hr, metabolite: 6-9 hr.

AVAILABILITY

Tablets: 25 mg, 50 mg, 100 mg.

INDICATIONS AND DOSAGE

Hypertension

PO

Adults, Elderly: Initially, 50 mg once per day. Maximum: May be given once or twice per day, with total daily doses ranging from 25 to 100 mg.

Nephropathy

PO

Adults, Elderly: Initially, 50 mg/day. May increase to 100 mg/day based on BP response.

Stroke reduction

PO

Adults, Elderly: 50 mg/day. Maximum: 100 mg/day.

Hypertension in patients with impaired hepatic function

PO

Adults, Elderly: Initially, 25 mg/day.

OFF-LABEL USES

Heart failure, erythrocytosis

CONTRAINDICATIONS

Hypersensitivity to losartan potassium or any components of the product

INTERACTIONS

Drug: Cimetidine: May increase the effects of losartan. **Ketoconazole, fluconazole, troleandomycin:** May decrease the effects of losartan. **Lithium:** May increase lithium blood concentration and risk of lithium toxicity. **Phenobarbital, rifampin:** May decrease the effects of losartan. **Herbal:** None known. **Food: Grapefruit, grapefruit juice:** May alter the absorption of losartan.

DIAGNOSTIC TEST EFFECTS

May increase BUN, serum alkaline phosphatase, serum bilirubin, serum creatinine, AST (SGOT), and ALT (SGPT) levels. May decrease blood Hgb and Hct levels.

SIDE-EFFECTS

Frequent (8%): Upper respiratory tract infection. **Occasional (4%-2%):** Dizziness, diarrhea, cough. **Rare (1% or less):** Insomnia, dyspepsia, heartburn, back and leg pain, muscle cramps, myalgia, nasal congestion, sinusitis

CRITICAL CARE CONSIDERATIONS

ADMINISTRATION/HANDLING

PO ALERT

- Give losartan without regard to food.
- Do not crush or break tablets.

PRECAUTIONS

HEALTH-RELATED

- Use cautiously in patients with hepatic or renal impairment or renal arterial stenosis.
- **Cytochrome P450 metabolism:** Losartan is a potent inhibitor of CYP3A4 and CYP2A9, which effects metabolism of other medications metabolized through this enzyme pathway.

AGE-RELATED

- **Children:** Safety and efficacy of losartan have not been established in children.
- **Elderly:** No age-related precautions have been noted.

PREGNANCY/LACTATION-RELATED

- Pregnancy category C (D if used in second or third trimesters).

MONITORING

- **Baseline assessment:** Assess heart rate and BP immediately before each losartan dose and regularly throughout therapy. Assess for dehydration.
- **Lab work:** CBC with WBC differential; biochemical panel including BUN, creatinine, potassium levels, and liver function tests.
- **Hypotension:** If hypotension occurs, place patients in the supine position with legs elevated. Reassess hydration. Chest discomfort may accompany hypotension; if not resolved by lying flat, may require treatment with nitroglycerin if systolic BP is at least 90 mmHg.
- **Cardiac ischemia:** Monitor ECG continuously for ST segment depression or

elevation in patients new to losartan with history of chest discomfort or MI.
- **Dependent edema:** Examine for edema of extremities, ankles, and sacrum.
- **Fluid retention:** Auscultate the lungs for rales. Monitor intake and output and daily weights. Edema and fluid retention may indicate worsening heart failure or renal insufficiency.
- **Fall prevention:** Assist with ambulation if dizziness occurs.
- **Cough:** Assess cough. If persistent and severe, may warrant discontinuation of therapy.
- **Hydration:** Offer fluids frequently or administer IV fluids to maintain hydration. Hypotension is common in volume-depleted patients.
- **Surgery/anesthesia:** If patients become hypotensive during a procedure, the blocked angiotensin II impairs BP compensation, prompting the need for correction of hypovolemia with IV fluid boluses.
- **Patient education:** Advise to rise slowly from lying to sitting position and to pause momentarily before standing to help abate orthostatic hypotension. Urge limiting consumption of alcohol while taking losartan. Instruct to report promptly diarrhea or vomiting (may lead to dehydration and low BP), difficulty breathing, excessive perspiration, and swelling of the face, lips, or tongue to a health care provider. Warn to avoid tasks that require mental alertness or motor skills until response to the drug is known. Emphasize the need to report chest pain or signs of infection, including fever and sore throat. Recommend avoiding cold preparations or nasal decongestants while on losartan therapy. Caution against abruptly discontinuing the drug. Stress to female patients the need to report pregnancy or suspected pregnancy immediately to a health care provider.

SERIOUS ADVERSE REACTIONS
- **Excessive hypotension:** May occur in patients with heart failure and severe salt- and volume-depletion.
- **Angioedema:** Swelling of face and lips, when involving the tongue, lips, and larynx may require subcutaneous epinephrine 1:1000 solution (0.3-0.5 mL) with possible endotracheal intubation to maintain patent airway.
- **Hyperkalemia:** Occurs rarely and may be associated with renal insufficiency.

OVERDOSE/TOXICITY
- **Hepatotoxicity:** Abdominal pain, jaundice, fluid retention, edema, elevated liver enzymes.
- **Cardiovascular:** Overdosage may manifest as hypotension and tachycardia due to vasodilation. Bradycardia occurs less often.
- **GI decontamination:** No specific recommendations.

ANTIDOTE/DIALYSIS
- **Antidote:** No specific recommendations.
- **Dialysis:** Losartan is not removed by hemodialysis, high-permeability hemodialysis, or peritoneal dialysis.

lovastatin

loe'-va-sta-tin

Classes
Chemical: substituted hexahydronaphthalene
Therapeutic: hydroxy methyl glutary (HMG)-CoA reductase inhibitor, antilipemic hydroxymethylglutanyl (HMG)

Pregnancy Category: X

Trade Names
Prescription: Altocor, Mevacor

Combinations
Prescription: With niacin extended release (Advicor)

Do not confuse lovastatin with Leustatin or Livostin, or Mevacor with Mivacron.

CLINICAL PHARMACOLOGY
Mechanism of Action
An antihyperlipidemic that inhibits HMG-CoA reductase, the enzyme that catalyzes the early step in cholesterol synthesis. **Therapeutic Effect:** Decreases LDL cholesterol, very low density lipoprotein (VLDL) cholesterol, plasma triglycerides; increases HDL cholesterol.

PHARMACOKINETICS

Route	Onset	Peak	Duration
PO	3 days	4-6 wk	4-6 wk

Incompletely absorbed from the GI tract (increased on empty stomach). Protein binding: 95%. Hydrolyzed in the liver to active metabolite. Primarily eliminated in feces.

Unlikely to be removed by hemodialysis. **Half-life:** 1.1-1.7 hr.

AVAILABILITY

Tablets (Mevacor): 10 mg, 20 mg, 40 mg. **Tablets (extended-release [Altocor]):** 20 mg, 40 mg, 60 mg.

INDICATIONS AND DOSAGE

Atherosclerosis, coronary artery disease

PO

Adults, Elderly: Initially, 20 mg/day. Maintenance: 10-80 mg once daily or in 2 divided doses. Maximum: 80 mg/day.

Hypercholesterolemia

PO

Adults, Elderly: Initially, 20 mg/day. Maintenance: 10-80 mg once daily or in 2 divided doses. Maximum: 80 mg/day.

PO (Extended Release)

Adults, Elderly: Initially, 20-60 mg once daily at bedtime. Maintenance: 10-60 mg once daily at bedtime.

Heterozygous familial hypercholesterolemia

PO

Children 10-17 yr: Initially, 10 mg/day. May increase to 20 mg/day after 8 wk and 40 mg/day after 16 wk if needed.

CONTRAINDICATIONS

Active liver disease, pregnancy, unexplained elevated liver function tests, hypersensitivity to lovastatin

INTERACTIONS

Drug: *CyclosPORINE, erythromycin, gemfibrozil, immunosuppressants, niacin: Increases the risk of acute renal failure and rhabdomyolysis. **Erythromycin, itraconazole, ketoconazole:** May increase lovastatin blood concentration causing severe muscle inflammation, myalgia, and weakness. **Herbal:** None known. **Food: Grapefruit juice:** Large amounts of grapefruit juice may increase risk of side effects, such as myalgia and weakness.

DIAGNOSTIC TEST EFFECTS

May increase serum creatine kinase and serum transaminase concentrations.

SIDE-EFFECTS

Frequent (9%-5%): Generally well tolerated. Side effects usually mild and transient. Headache, flatulence, diarrhea, abdominal pain or cramps, rash, and pruritus. **Occasional (4%-3%):** Nausea, vomiting, constipation, dyspepsia. **Rare (2%-1%):** Dizziness, heartburn, myalgia, blurred vision, eye irritation

CRITICAL CARE CONSIDERATIONS

ADMINISTRATION/HANDLING

PO ALERT

- Give lovastatin with meals.
- Caution patients against drinking more than a quart of grapefruit juice daily.

PRECAUTIONS

HEALTH-RELATED

- Use cautiously in patients with a history of heavy or chronic alcohol use, hepatic insufficiency, and renal impairment.
- **Serious illness:** Drug should be temporarily withheld or discontinued in acutely ill patients to avoid increased probability of development of a myopathy.
- **Increased probability of myopathy:** Increased when used concomitantly with CYP3A4 inhibitors including *cyclosPORINE, erthyromycin, fibric acid derivatives, immunosuppressive drugs, niacin, and azole antifungal agents.
- **Cytochrome P450 metabolism:** Lovastatin is a substrate for CYP3A4. Potent inhibitors of CYP3A4 can increase the level of lovastatin and other HMG CoA reductase inhibitors ("statins"), which increases probability of myopathy.

AGE-RELATED

- **Children:** Safety and efficacy of lovastatin have not been established in children.
- **Elderly:** No age-related precautions have been noted.

PREGNANCY/LACTATION-RELATED

- Pregnancy category X (may produce skeletal malformations). Excretion into breast milk unknown, contraindicated in nursing mothers.

MONITORING

- **Baseline assessment:** Determine pregnancy before beginning lovastatin therapy. Assess dietary habits and willingness to modify high fat diet.
- **Lab work:** Assess baseline serum cholesterol, triglyceride levels and liver function test results. Monitor cholesterol and triglycerides for therapeutic response and liver enzymes every 12 wk after initial therapy and each time dosage is adjusted. Semiannual monitoring may be appropriate for patients on fixed doses with good response. Periodic laboratory tests are an essential part of ongoing therapy.

- **Common side effects:** Constipation, abdominal pain, dyspepsia, flatulence. May require symptom specific management to control.
- **Myalgias:** CPK level may be measured for patients with unexplained myalgias. Assess for malaise, muscle cramping, or weakness. Urine will appear brown if myoglobin is present.
- **Renal failure:** Monitor BUN, creatinine, and potassium levels if patients manifest myalgia or brown urine indicative of myoglobinuria. Urinalysis is used to diagnose myoglobinuria.
- **CNS toxicity:** Evaluate for blurred vision, dizziness, and headache.
- **Hypersensitivity:** Assess for pruritus and rash.
- **Therapeutic effect:** Monitor for reduced serum cholesterol and triglyceride levels.
- **Diet instruction:** Patients must follow the prescribed diet because diet is an important part of lowering cholesterol and triglycerides.
- **Patient education:** When therapy is continued outside the hospital, warn not to take other medications without physician approval. Instruct to take lovastatin with meals. Stress that the prescribed diet and periodic laboratory tests are essential parts of therapy. Urge avoidance of consuming grapefruit juice during lovastatin therapy. Instruct to promptly report changes in the color of stool or urine, muscle weakness, myalgia, severe gastric upset, unusual bruising, vision changes, and yellowing of eyes or skin to a health care provider.

SERIOUS ADVERSE REACTIONS

- **Musculoskeletal pain:** Myopathy, arthralgia, myalgia, which may indicate impending rhabdomyolysis.
- **Renal failure:** Acute renal failure ensues when rhabdomyolysis is present.
- **Liver failure:** Liver enzyme elevation indicative of impending liver failure.

OVERDOSE/TOXICITY

- **CNS toxicity:** Optic nerve degeneration, perivascular hemorrhage, and edema with fibrin deposits, and necrosis of small vessels.
- **Ophthalmic:** Possible cataract development.
- **Rhabdomyolysis:** Rare cases; can lead to acute renal failure. Markedly elevated serum creatine kinase and possible myoglobinuria indicate the condition may be present. Should be managed according to accepted guidelines, which include aggressive volume replacement, hemodialysis, or continuous hemofiltration to support patients during acute renal failure. Use of bicarbonate to induce alkaline diuresis or mannitol for osmotic diuresis has not been well studied. Hyperkalemia and hyperphosphatemia are commonly seen with rhabdomyolysis and may require aggressive management.
- **Hypocalcemia:** Must be managed cautiously with rhabdomyolysis because calcium infusion may increase the deposition of calcium in the injured muscles.
- **Discontinuation:** Lovastatin should be discontinued if patient develops myopathy and/or rhabdomyolysis.
- **GI decontamination:** No specific recommendations.

ANTIDOTE/DIALYSIS

- **Antidote:** No specific recommendations.
- **Dialysis:** Lovastatin is unlikely to be removed by hemodialysis or peritoneal dialysis. No data is available on removal by high-permeability hemodialysis.

loxapine

See Antipsychotics (p. 934)

lymphocyte immune globulin

See Immunologics (p. 968)

magnesium salicylate

See Salicylates (p. 982)

magnesium salts

mag-nee'-zhum

Classes

Chemical: divalent cation

Therapeutic: antacid, antidysrhythmic, electrolyte supplement, laxative, uterine relaxant

Pregnancy Category: B

Trade Names

Over the Counter: (magnesium chloride) Mag-Delay SR, Slow-Mag; (magnesium citrate) Citrate of Magnesia; (magnesium hydroxide) Phillips Milk of Magnesia; (magnesium oxide) Mag-Ox 400, Uro-Mag; (magnesium protein complex) Mg-PLUS; (magnesium sulfate) Epsom salt, magnesium sulfate injection, Sulfamag

Do not confuse magnesium sulfate with manganese sulfate.

CLINICAL PHARMACOLOGY

Mechanism of Action

M

An antacid, laxative, electrolyte, and anticonvulsant. As an antacid, acts in the stomach to neutralize gastric acid. **Therapeutic Effect:** Increases pH.

As a laxative, has an osmotic effect, primarily in the small intestine, and draws water into the intestinal lumen. **Therapeutic Effect:** Produces distention and promotes peristalsis and bowel evacuation.

As a systemic dietary supplement and electrolyte replacement, is found primarily in intracellular fluids and is essential for enzyme activity, nerve conduction, and muscle contraction.

As an anticonvulsant, blocks neuromuscular transmission and the amount of acetylcholine released at the motor end plate. **Therapeutic Effect:** Controls seizure. Maintains and restores magnesium levels.

PHARMACOKINETICS

Antacid, laxative: Minimal absorption through the intestine. Absorbed dose primarily excreted in urine. Systemic: Widely distributed. Primarily excreted in urine.

AVAILABILITY

Magnesium chloride

Tablets (Mag Delay SR, Slo-Mag): 64 mg.

Magnesium citrate

Oral solution (Citrate of Magnesia): 290 mg/5 mL.

Magnesium hydroxide

Oral liquid (Phillips Milk of Magnesia): 400 mg/5 mL, 800 mg/5 mL.

Tablets (chewable [Phillips Milk of Magnesia]): 311 mg.

Magnesium oxide

Tablets (Mag-Ox 400): 400 mg.

Capsules (Uro-Mag): 140 mg.

Magnesium sulfate

Premix infusion solution: 10 mg/mL, 20 mg/mL, 40 mg/mL, 80 mg/mL.

Injection: 125 mg/mL, 500 mg/mL.

INDICATIONS AND DOSAGE

Hypomagnesemia

IV, IM

Adults, Elderly: 1-12 g/day in divided doses. **Children:** 25-50 mg/kg/dose every 4-6 hr for 3-4 doses. Maximum: 2 g (single dose). **Neonates:** 25-50 mg/kg/dose every 8-12 hr for 2-3 doses.

Hypertension, seizures

IV, IM (magnesium sulfate)

Children: 20-100 mg/kg/dose every 4-6 hr as needed. Maximum: 200 mg/kg/dose.

IV

Adults: Initially 4 g (20% solution) over 20 min, then 1-4 g/hr by continuous infusion.

Dysrhythmias

IV (magnesium sulfate)

Adults, Elderly: Initially 1-2 g over 5-20 min, then infusion of 0.5-1 g/hr.

Constipation

PO (magnesium sulfate)

Adults, Elderly, Children 12 yr and older: 10-30 g/day in divided doses. **Children 6-11 yr:** 5-10 g/day in divided doses. **Children 2-5 yr:** 2.5-5 g/kg/day in divided doses.

PO (magnesium hydroxide)

Adults, Elderly, Children 12 yr and older: 6-8 tablets or 30-60 mL/day. **Children 6-11 yr:** 3-4 tablets or 15-30 mL/day. **Children 2-5 yr:** 1-2 tablets or 5-15 mL/day.

Hyperacidity

PO (magnesium hydroxide)

Adults, Elderly: 2-4 tablets or 5-15 mL as needed up to 4 times per day. **Children 7-14 yr:** 1 tablet or 2.5-5 mL as needed up to 4 times per day.

Magnesium deficiency

PO (magnesium oxide)

Adults, Elderly: 1-2 tablets 2-3 times per day with food. **Adults, Elderly:** (Uro-Mag) 4-5 capsules daily with food.

Dietary supplement

PO (magnesium chloride)

Adults, Elderly: 2 tablets daily.

Cathartic

PO (magnesium citrate)

Adults, Elderly, Children 12 yr and older: 120-300 mL. **Children 6-11 yr:** 100-150 mL. **Children younger than 6 yr:** 0.5 mL/kg up to maximum of 200 mL every 4-6 hr until stool is cleared.

OFF-LABEL USES

Magnesium sulfate: Premature labor, torsades de pointes, acute asthma, MI, tocolysis

CONTRAINDICATIONS

Antacid: Appendicitis or symptoms of appendicitis, ileostomy, intestinal obstruction, severe renal impairment

Laxative: Appendicitis, heart failure, colostomy, hypersensitivity to magnesium sulfate, ileostomy, intestinal obstruction, undiagnosed rectal bleeding

Systemic: Heart block, myocardial damage, renal failure

INTERACTIONS

Drug: **Antacid: Ketoconazole, tetracyclines:** May decrease the absorption of ketoconazole and tetracyclines. **Antacid, laxative: Digoxin, oral anticoagulants, phenothiazines:** May decrease the effects of these drugs. **Tetracyclines:** May form nonabsorbable complex with tetracyclines. **Systemic (dietary supplement, electrolyte replacement): Calcium:** May neutralize the effects of magnesium. **CNS depression-producing medications:** May increase CNS depression. **Digoxin:** May cause changes in cardiac conduction or heart block with digoxin. **Herbal:** None known. **Food:** None known.

DIAGNOSTIC TEST EFFECTS

Antacid: May increase gastrin production and pH.

Laxative: May decrease serum potassium level.

Systemic (dietary supplement, electrolyte replacement): None known.

IV INCOMPATIBILITIES

Amphotericin B complex (Abelcet, AmBisome, Amphotec), cefepime (Maxipime)

IV COMPATIBILITIES

Amikacin (Amikin), cefazolin (Ancef), ciprofloxacin (Cipro), *DOBUTamine (Dobutrex), enalapril (Vasotec), gentamicin, heparin, hydromorphone (Dilaudid), insulin, milrinone (Primacor), morphine, piperacillin/tazobactam (Zosyn), potassium chloride, propofol (Diprivan), tobramycin (Nebcin), vancomycin (Vancocin)

SIDE-EFFECTS

Frequent: Antacid: Chalky taste, diarrhea, laxative effect. **Occasional: Antacid:** Nausea, vomiting, stomach cramps. **Antacid, laxative:** With prolonged use or large doses in renal impairment, possible hypermagnesemia, marked by dizziness, irregular heartbeat, mental changes, fatigue, and weakness. **Laxative:** Cramping, diarrhea, increased thirst, flatulence. **Systemic (dietary supplement, electrolyte replacement):** Reduced respiratory rate, decreased reflexes, flushing, hypotension, decreased heart rate

CRITICAL CARE CONSIDERATIONS

ADMINISTRATION/HANDLING

PO (ANTACID) ALERT

- Antacids may be given up to 4 times per day.
- Chew chewable tablets thoroughly before swallowing and follow by a full glass of water.
- Shake suspension well before use.

PO (LAXATIVE) ALERT

- Drink 8 oz liquid with each dose to prevent dehydration.
- Follow dose with citrus carbonated beverage or fruit juice to improve flavor.
- Refrigerate citrate of magnesia to retain potency and improve palatability.
- Take tablets at bedtime.

IV ALERT

- **Storage:** Store at room temperature.
- **Dilution:** Solution must be diluted to avoid exceeding 200 mg/mL concentration.
- **Infusion:** Do not exceed magnesium sulfate concentration of 200 mg/mL (20%). Do not exceed infusion rate of 150 mg/min.
- **Maximum:** 2 g/hr to avoid hypotension or 4 g/hr *only in emergencies* (seizures, eclampsia).

IM ALERT

- **Elderly:** Use 250 mg/mL (25%) or 500 mg/mL (50%) magnesium sulfate concentration.

PRECAUTIONS

HEALTH-RELATED

- Use magnesium antacids cautiously in patients with chronic diarrhea, colostomy,

M

diverticulitis, ulcerative colitis, or undiagnosed GI or rectal bleeding.
- **Laxative form:** Use cautiously in patients with diabetes mellitus and in those on a low-salt diet because some magnesium supplements contain sugar or sodium.
- **Parenteral:** When magnesium is given for systemic use, use cautiously in patients with severe renal impairment.

AGE-RELATED
- **Children:** Use magnesium cautiously in children under 6 yr. Safety is unknown.
- **Elderly:** Are at increased risk for developing magnesium deficiency because of decreased magnesium absorption, other medications they may be taking, and poor diet.

PREGNANCY/LACTATION-RELATED
- Pregnancy category B; compatible with breast-feeding.

MONITORING
- **Baseline assessment:** Determine sensitivity to magnesium. Assess for GI pain noting duration, quality, location, and causative and exacerbative factors. If magnesium is being taken as a laxative, assess the amount, color, and consistency of the stool. Evaluate recent pattern of daily bowel activity and evaluate the bowel sounds for peristalsis. Assess for history of recent abdominal surgery, nausea, vomiting, and weight loss.
- **Baseline lab work:** Biochemical panel including BUN, serum creatinine, and magnesium levels if using magnesium systemically.
- **Gastric effects:** Assess patients taking magnesium antacids for relief of gastric distress.
- **Renal insufficiency:** Monitor renal function in patients taking magnesium antacids, especially if dosing is long-term or frequent.
- **Laxative form:** Monitor patients taking the laxative form for constipation or diarrhea; ensure adequate fluid intake is maintained.
- **Systemic form:** Monitor continuous ECG for resolution of dysrhythmias; check BUN, serum creatinine, and magnesium levels.
- **CNS depression:** Test patellar reflexes before giving repeat parenteral doses of systemic magnesium to assess for CNS depression. Suppressed reflexes may indicate impending respiratory arrest. Ensure patellar reflexes are present and respiratory rate is greater than 16 breaths/min before giving each parenteral dose.
- **Seizures:** Provide seizure precautions for patients taking systemic magnesium.
- **Patient education:** Instruct to take magnesium antacids at least 2 hr before or 2 hr after other medications. Reinforce that magnesium antacids should not be taken for longer than 2 wk. Instruct patients with peptic ulcer disease to take magnesium antacids 1 and 3 hr after meals and at bedtime for 4 to 6 wk. Teach how to chew tablets thoroughly followed by a glass of water and to shake suspensions well. Warn that repeat dosing or taking large doses of magnesium antacids may have a laxative effect. Instruct patients taking magnesium laxatives to drink a full glass (8 oz) of liquid to aid stool softening. Explain that magnesium laxatives are for short-term use only. Warn to stop taking a magnesium laxative if abdominal pain, nausea, or vomiting occurs. Warn patients taking systemic magnesium to promptly report signs of hypermagnesemia including confusion, cramping, dizziness, irregular heartbeat, lightheadedness, or unusual fatigue or weakness to a health care provider.

SERIOUS ADVERSE REACTIONS
- Magnesium as an antacid or laxative has no known serious reactions.
- Systemic use of magnesium may produce prolonged PR interval and widening of QRS interval.

OVERDOSE/TOXICITY
- **Toxicity:** Loss of deep tendon reflexes, heart block, respiratory paralysis, hypotension, and cardiac arrest.
- **Management:** Reverse toxicity with calcium gluconate and physostigmine. Provide endotracheal intubation and mechanical ventilation if needed to support oxygenation. Dopamine may be used to manage hypotension.
- **GI decontamination:** No specific recommendations.

ANTIDOTE/DIALYSIS
- **Antidote:** The antidote for toxicity is 10-20 mL 10% calcium gluconate (5-10 mEq of calcium) and should reverse respiratory depression and heart block. Physostigmine 0.5-1 mg subcutaneously should help relieve respiratory paralysis.
- **Dialysis:** Magnesium is removed by hemodialysis, peritoneal dialysis, and high-permeability hemodialysis.

mannitol

man'-i-tall

Classes

Chemical: hexahydric alcohol
Therapeutic: antiglaucoma agent; diuretic, osmotic; genitourinary irrigant

Pregnancy Category: C

Trade Names

Prescription: Osmitrol, Resectisol

CLINICAL PHARMACOLOGY

Mechanism of Action

An osmotic diuretic, antiglaucoma, and antihemolytic agent that elevates osmotic pressure of the glomerular filtrate, inhibiting tubular reabsorption of water and electrolytes, resulting in increased flow of water into interstitial fluid and plasma. **Therapeutic Effect:** Produces diuresis; reduces intraocular pressure (IOP); reduces intracranial pressure (ICP) and cerebral edema.

PHARMACOKINETICS

Route	Onset	Peak	Duration
IV (diuresis)	15-30 min	N/A	2-8 hr
IV (reduced ICP)	15-30 min	N/A	3-8 hr
IV (reduced IOP)	N/A	30-60 min	4-8 hr

Remains in extracellular fluid. Primarily excreted in urine. Removed by hemodialysis. **Half-life:** 60-90 min.

AVAILABILITY

Injection (Osmitrol): 5%, 10%, 15%, 20%, 25%.
Irrigation solution (Resectisol): 5%.

INDICATIONS AND DOSAGE

ICP

IV

Adults, Elderly: 0.25-1 g/kg every 6-8 hr. Maximum: 6 g/24 hr. **Children:** 0.25-1 g/kg as needed. Maximum: 2 g/kg/dose.

IOP

IV

Adults, Elderly: 1.5-2 g/kg as a 15%-20% solution. Maximum: 6 g/24 hr. **Children:** 1-2 g/kg. Maximum: 2 g/kg/dose.

Renal impairment, oliguria

IV

Adults, Elderly: Use test dose. 300-400 mg/kg or up to 100 g given as a single dose. **Children:** 0.25-2 g/kg. Maximum: 6 g/kg/24 hr.

Toxicity, poisoning

IV

Adults, Elderly: Continuous infusion as a 5%-20% solution. **Children:** Up to 2 g/kg as 5%-10% solution.

CONTRAINDICATIONS

Dehydration, intracranial bleeding, severe pulmonary edema and congestion; severe renal disease (anuria), increasing oliguria and azotemia, hypersensitivity to mannitol

INTERACTIONS

Drug: **Digoxin:** May increase the risk of digoxin toxicity associated with mannitol-induced hypokalemia. **Herbal:** None known. **Food:** None known.

DIAGNOSTIC TEST EFFECTS

May decrease serum phosphate, potassium, and sodium levels.

IV INCOMPATIBILITIES

Cefepime (Maxipime), *DOXOrubicin liposomal (Doxil), filgrastim (Neupogen)

IV COMPATIBILITIES

Cisplatin (Platinol), ondansetron (Zofran), propofol (Diprivan)

SIDE-EFFECTS

Frequent: Dry mouth, thirst. **Occasional:** Blurred vision, increased urinary frequency and urine volume, headache, arm pain, backache, nausea, vomiting, urticaria, dizziness, hypotension or hypertension, tachycardia, fever, angina-like chest pain

CRITICAL CARE CONSIDERATIONS

ADMINISTRATION/HANDLING

IV ALERT

- **Test dose:** For patients with suspected renal insufficiency or marked oliguria, a test dose should be given. The test dose is 12.5 g for adults (200 mg/kg for children) over 3-5 min to produce a urine flow of at least 30 to 50 mL/hr (1 mL/kg/hr for children) over 2-3 hr.
- **Test dose for oliguria:** IV push over 3-5 min.
- **Test dose for cerebral edema or elevated ICP:** IV infusion over 20-30 min. Maximum concentration is 25%.
- **Storage:** Store mannitol at room temperature. If the solution crystallizes, warm the bottle in hot water and shake vigorously at

M

intervals. Do not use solution if crystals remain after the warming procedure.

- **Preparation:** Assess the IV site for patency before administering each dose. Pain and thrombosis are noted with extravasation. Cool the solution to body temperature before administration following warming procedure.
- **Filter:** Use an inline filter (less than 5 microns) for drug concentrations greater than 20%.
- **Additives:** Do not add potassium chloride or sodium chloride to mannitol with a concentration of 20% or greater.
- **Whole blood:** Do not add mannitol to whole blood for transfusion.

PRECAUTIONS

HEALTH-RELATED

- Use cautiously in patients with heart failure or renal insufficiency or failure.

AGE-RELATED

- **Children:** Safety and efficacy of mannitol have not been established in children under 12 yr.
- **Elderly:** Age-related renal impairment may require cautious use.

PREGNANCY/LACTATION-RELATED

- Pregnancy category C; use caution with breast-feeding.

MONITORING

- **Baseline assessment:** Monitor vital signs, especially for hypotension before giving mannitol. Evaluate for edema and assess mucous membranes and skin turgor to determine hydration status. Obtain baseline weight.
- **Baseline lab work:** Biochemical profile including BUN and creatinine. B-type natriuretic peptide (BNP) level to evaluate for heart failure. Monitor serum electrolyte levels and liver function test results.
- **Diuresis:** Begin monitoring intake and output. Monitor urine output to ascertain level of therapeutic response. Monitor BUN, serum electrolyte levels, and liver function test results. Weigh daily.
- **Seizures:** Initiate seizure precautions on patients with severe electrolyte imbalance.
- **Cardiac:** Monitor for dysrhythmias if fluid or electrolyte imbalances are present.
- **Fluid/electrolyte imbalance:** Hypokalemia may result in cardiac dysrhythmias, altered mental status, muscle cramps, nausea and vomiting, tachycardia, tremor, and weakness; hyperkalemia may result in dysrhythmias, colic, diarrhea, and muscle twitching followed by paralysis or weakness; hyponatremia may result in cold and clammy skin, confusion, drowsiness, and thirst.
- **Patient education:** Advise to expect an increase in the frequency and volume of urination. Explain mannitol may cause dry mouth. Instruct to weigh on the same scale daily if chronic fluid retention is a problem.

SERIOUS ADVERSE REACTIONS

- **Heart failure:** Circulatory overload may produce pulmonary edema.

OVERDOSE/TOXICITY

- **Fluid and electrolyte imbalance:** May occur from rapid administration of large doses or inadequate urine output resulting in overexpansion of extracellular fluid. Excessive diuresis may produce hypokalemia and hyponatremia. Fluid loss in excess of electrolyte excretion may produce hypernatremia and hyperkalemia. Severe electrolyte imbalance may prompt seizures.
- **Management:** Discontinue drug. Provide IV hydration for dehydrated patients. Replace electrolytes as needed. Manage other symptoms per accepted guidelines if they arise.
- **GI decontamination:** No specific recommendations.

ANTIDOTE/DIALYSIS

- **Antidote:** No specific recommendations.
- **Dialysis:** Mannitol is removed by hemodialysis, peritoneal dialysis, and is likely to be removed by high-permeability hemodialysis.

maprotiline

See Antidepressants (p. 906)

meclizine hydrochloride

mek'-li-zeen hye-droe-klor'-ide

Classes

Chemical: piperazine derivative
Therapeutic: antihistamine, antivertigo agent

Pregnancy Category: B

Trade Names

Prescription: Antivert, Meclicot, Meni-D
Over the Counter: Bonamine ♣, Bonine

Do not confuse Antivert with Axert.

CLINICAL PHARMACOLOGY

Mechanism of Action

An anticholinergic that reduces labyrinthine excitability and diminishes vestibular stimulation of the labyrinth, affecting the chemoreceptor trigger zone. **Therapeutic Effect:** Reduces nausea, vomiting, and vertigo.

PHARMACOKINETICS

Route	Onset	Peak	Duration
PO	30-60 min	N/A	12-24 hr

Well absorbed from the GI tract. Widely distributed. Metabolized in the liver. Primarily excreted in urine. **Half-life:** 6 hr.

AVAILABILITY

Tablets (Antivert, Meclicot, Meni-D): 12.5 mg, 25 mg, 50 mg.
Tablets (Chewable [Bonine]): 25 mg.

INDICATIONS AND DOSAGE

Motion sickness

PO

Adults, Elderly, Children 12 yr and older: 12.5-25 mg 1 hr before travel. May repeat every 12-24 hr. May require a dose of 50 mg.

Vertigo

PO

Adults, Elderly, Children 12 yr and older: 25-100 mg/day in divided doses, as needed.

CONTRAINDICATIONS

Hypersensitivity to meclizine

INTERACTIONS

Drug: Alcohol, anticholinergic medications: May increase CNS depressant effect.
Herbal: None known. **Food:** None known.

DIAGNOSTIC TEST EFFECTS

May produce false-negative results in antigen skin testing unless meclizine is discontinued 4 days before testing.

SIDE-EFFECTS

Frequent: Drowsiness. **Occasional:** Blurred vision; dry mouth, nose, or throat

CRITICAL CARE CONSIDERATIONS

ADMINISTRATION/HANDLING

PO ALERT

- Give meclizine without regard to food.
- Crush scored tablets if needed.

PRECAUTIONS

HEALTH-RELATED

- Use meclizine cautiously in patients with angle-closure glaucoma or obstructive diseases of the GI or GU tract.

AGE-RELATED

- **Children:** Meclizine is not recommended in children under 12 yr. May be more sensitive to the drug's anticholinergic effects, such as dry mouth.
- **Elderly:** Elderly patients (over 60 yr) are at increased risk for developing agitation, disorientation, dizziness, sedation, hypotension, confusion, and psychotic-like symptoms. May be more sensitive to anticholinergic effects.

PREGNANCY/LACTATION-RELATED

- Pregnancy category B; used for treatment of nausea and vomiting during pregnancy. Excretion into breast milk unknown.

MONITORING

- **Baseline assessment:** Assess hydration status, especially in elderly, who are at increased risk for hypotension. Assess history of dizziness, nausea, and vomiting.
- **Baseline lab work:** Biochemical panel to assess for fluid and electrolyte imbalance in patients who are vomiting. Repeat testing if vomiting persists.
- **Diagnostic tests:** If meclizine is ineffective, consider MRI/MRA of the brain to rule out other conditions including stroke, aneurysm, and tumors.
- **Paradoxic reactions:** Monitor children closely for paradoxic reactions.
- **Dehydration:** Assess mucous membranes and skin turgor to evaluate hydration status.
- **Patient education:** Inform that meclizine commonly causes dizziness, drowsiness, and dry mouth. Explain that coffee or tea may help reduce drowsiness. Reassure that they will probably develop a tolerance to the drug's sedative effect. Advise avoidance of tasks that require mental alertness or motor skills until response to the drug is known. Urge avoidance of alcohol during meclizine therapy. Sips of water and chewing gum may help relieve dry mouth.

SERIOUS ADVERSE REACTIONS

- **Hypersensitivity reaction:** Eczema, pruritus, rash, cardiac disturbances, and photosensitivity may occur.
- **Paradoxic reaction:** Children are more likely to have paradoxic reactions including

M

restlessness, insomnia, euphoria, nervousness, and tremors.

OVERDOSE/TOXICITY

- **CNS depression:** Sedation, apnea, cardiovascular collapse, or death.
- **Anticholinergic syndrome:** Hallucinations, tremor, seizures, tachycardia, hypertension, delayed gastric emptying, decreased peristalsis, urinary retention, possible rhabdomyolysis in severe cases (due to seizures and hyperthermia).
- Overdose in children may result in hallucinations, seizures, and death.
- **Sodium bicarbonate therapy:** Sodium bicarbonate intravenous infusion with initial bolus of 1-2 mEq/kg until clinical improvement is noted or blood pH is 7.50-7.55 (induced metabolic alkalosis). Higher blood pH may be deleterious to patients. IV potassium supplementation may be needed to correct hypokalemia which results from use of bicarbonate infusion.
- **Fluid volume expansion:** IV fluid infusion is used to manage hypotension. Vasopressors are used only when patients do not respond to fluid therapy.
- **Serum alkalization/ventilator driven:** Ventilator driven hyperventilation with intravenous saline to raise the pH to 7.50-7.55 to induce respiratory alkalosis.
- **Seizures:** May respond spontaneously; if persistent, benzodiazepines (lorazepam, diazepam) may be used; phenobarbital or propofol may be used if other medications fail.
- **GI decontamination:** Activated charcoal binds meclizine effectively and if used should be given in one dose within the first few hr of ingestion; the risks of using ipecac to induce vomiting outweigh the benefits; adding gastric lavage to activated charcoal may enhance removal effects if done within the first hr of ingestion.

ANTIDOTE/DIALYSIS

- **Antidote:** No specific recommendations.
- **Dialysis:** Meclizine is unlikely to be removed by hemodialysis, peritoneal dialysis, or high-permeability hemodialysis.

mefanomic acid

See NSAIDs and Cox-2 Inhibitors (p. 976)

M

meloxicam

mel-ox'-i-kam

Classes

Chemical: oxicam derivative
Therapeutic: NSAID, antipyretic, nonnarcotic analgesic

Pregnancy Category: C, D (3rd trimester)

Trade Names

Prescription: Mobic, Mobicox ♣

CLINICAL PHARMACOLOGY

Mechanism of Action

An NSAID that produces analgesic and antiinflammatory effects by inhibiting prostaglandin synthesis. **Therapeutic Effect:** Reduces the inflammatory response and intensity of pain.

PHARMACOKINETICS

Route	Onset	Peak	Duration
PO (analgesic)	30 min	4-5 hr	N/A

Well absorbed after PO administration. Protein binding: 99%. Metabolized in the liver. Eliminated in urine and feces. Not removed by hemodialysis. **Half-life:** 15-20 hr.

AVAILABILITY

Tablets: 7.5 mg, 15 mg.
Oral Suspension: 7.5 mg/5 mL.

INDICATIONS AND DOSAGE

Osteoarthritis, rheumatoid arthritis

PO

Adults: Initially, 7.5 mg/day. Maximum: 15 mg/day.

Juvenile rheumatoid arthritis

PO

Children 2 yr and older: 0.125 mg/kg once per day. Maximum: 7.5 mg.

OFF-LABEL USES

Ankylosing spondylitis

CONTRAINDICATIONS

Aspirin-induced nasal polyps associated with bronchospasm, hypersensitivity to meloxicam

INTERACTIONS

Drug: Aspirin: May increase the risk of epigastric distress, such as heartburn and indigestion. **Lithium:** May increase the plasma concentration and risk of toxicity of lithium. **Herbal: Ginkgo biloba:** May increase the risk of bleeding. **Food:** None known.

DIAGNOSTIC TEST EFFECTS

May increase serum creatinine, AST (SGOT), and ALT (SGPT) levels.

SIDE-EFFECTS

Frequent (9%-7%): Dyspepsia, headache, diarrhea, nausea. **Occasional (4%-3%):** Dizziness, insomnia, rash, pruritus, flatulence, constipation, vomiting. **Rare (less than 2%):** Somnolence, urticaria, photosensitivity, tinnitus

CRITICAL CARE CONSIDERATIONS

ADMINISTRATION/HANDLING

PO ALERT

- Give meloxicam without regard to food.

PRECAUTIONS

HEALTH-RELATED

- Use meloxicam cautiously in patients with asthma, heart failure, hypertension, dehydration, hemostatic disease, hepatic or renal impairment, or a history of GI disorders (peptic ulcer disease) and in those using anticoagulants concurrently.

AGE-RELATED

- **Children:** Safety and efficacy of meloxicam have not been established in children.
- **Elderly:** Age-related renal impairment and increased susceptibility to GI toxicity may prompt a dosage adjustment.

PREGNANCY/LACTATION-RELATED

- Pregnancy category C (D if used in third trimester or near delivery). Animal studies document both teratogenic and nonteratogenic (premature patent ductus arteriosus [PDA] closure) in animals. No studies in humans. No human studies on breast milk excretion; in rats, milk concentrations are twice that of plasma.

MONITORING

- **Baseline assessment:** Assess duration, location, onset, and type of inflammation or pain. Inspect arthritic joints for deformity, immobility, and skin condition.
- **Baseline lab work:** CBC with differential, biochemical panel including BUN, creatinine, alkaline phosphatase, bilirubin, AST (SGOT), and ALT (SGPT) levels.
- **Therapeutic response:** Note improved grip strength, increased joint mobility, and decreased pain, tenderness, stiffness, and swelling.
- **Patient education:** Instruct to take meloxicam with food or milk to reduce GI upset. Reinforce reporting chest pain, difficulty breathing, palpitations, peripheral edema, persistent abdominal cramps or pain, a rash, ringing in the ears, severe nausea or vomiting, or unusual bleeding or ecchymosis to a health care provider immediately. Warn to avoid tasks that require mental alertness or motor skills until response to the drug is known. Instruct female patients to inform the health care provider if they suspect pregnancy or plan to become pregnant.

SERIOUS ADVERSE REACTIONS

- **GI effects:** Include peptic ulcer disease, GI bleeding, gastritis.
- **Hypersensitivity:** Bronchospasm, angioedema.

OVERDOSE/TOXICITY

- **Symptoms:** Hypotonia, muscle fasciculations, twitching, bone marrow suppression, metabolic acidosis, nausea, vomiting, diarrhea, GI bleeding, abdominal pain, volume depletion with secondary hypotension, tachycardia, pulmonary edema and acute respiratory distress syndrome, acute psychosis, seizures, and CNS depression following agitation.
- **Management:** Provide oxygen therapy and maintain patent airway; may require endotracheal intubation and mechanical ventilation. Benzodiazepines and barbiturates may be used for seizures. Hypotension should be managed with IV fluids and then vasopressors if needed. Liver failure may be severe and eventually warrant liver transplantation. Blood transfusions may be needed for GI bleeding.
- **Nephrotoxicity:** Hematuria, dysuria, proteinuria.
- **Hepatotoxicity:** Elevated liver enzymes, abdominal pain, jaundice, edema.
- **GI decontamination:** Activated charcoal in either single or multiple doses may be effective but may interfere with endoscopy if patient is GI bleeding.

ANTIDOTE/DIALYSIS

- **Antidote:** No specific recommendations.
- **Dialysis:** Meloxicam is not removed by whemodialysis and is unlikely to be removed by high-permeability hemodialysis or peritoneal dialysis.

M

memantine hydrochloride

mem-an'-teen hye-droe-klor'-ide

Classes
Chemical: adamantane derivative, tricyclic amine
Therapeutic: antidementia agent

Pregnancy Category: B

Trade Names
Prescription: Ebixa ♣, Namenda

CLINICAL PHARMACOLOGY

Mechanism of Action
A neurotransmitter inhibitor that decreases the effects of glutamate, the principal excitatory neurotransmitter in the brain. Persistent CNS excitation by glutamate is thought to cause the symptoms of Alzheimer's disease. **Therapeutic Effect:** May reduce clinical deterioration in moderate to severe Alzheimer's disease.

PHARMACOKINETICS

Rapidly and completely absorbed after PO administration. Protein binding: 45%. Undergoes little metabolism; most of the dose is excreted unchanged in urine. **Half-life:** 60-80 hr.

M

AVAILABILITY

Tablets: 5 mg, 10 mg.
Oral Solution: 2 mg/mL.

INDICATIONS AND DOSAGE

Alzheimer's disease
PO
Adults, Elderly: Initially, 5 mg once per day. May increase dosage at intervals of at least 1 wk in 5-mg increments to 10 mg/day (5 mg twice per day), then 15 mg/day (5 mg and 10 mg as separate doses), and finally 20 mg/day (10 mg twice per day). Target dose: 20 mg/day.

CONTRAINDICATIONS

Hypersensitivity to memantine

INTERACTIONS

Drug: **Carbonic anhydrase inhibitors, sodium bicarbonate:** May decrease the renal elimination of memantine up to 80%. **Cimetidine, hydrochlorothiazide, nicotine, quinidine, ranitidine:** May alter plasma levels of both memantine and precipitant drugs. **Herbal:** None known. **Food:** None known.

DIAGNOSTIC TEST EFFECTS

None known.

SIDE-EFFECTS

Occasional (7%-4%): Dizziness, headache, confusion, constipation, hypertension, cough. **Rare (3%-2%):** Back pain, nausea, fatigue, anxiety, peripheral edema, arthralgia, insomnia.

CRITICAL CARE CONSIDERATIONS

ADMINISTRATION/HANDLING

PO ALERT
- Give memantine without regard to food.

PRECAUTIONS

HEALTH-RELATED
- Use memantine cautiously in patients with moderate to severe renal impairment.

AGE-RELATED
- **Children:** Memantine is not prescribed for use in children.
- **Elderly:** No age-related precautions have been noted; memantine is not recommended for elderly with severe renal impairment (creatinine clearance less than 9 mL/min).

PREGNANCY/LACTATION-RELATED
- Pregnancy category B; breast milk excretion unknown.

MONITORING

- **Baseline assessment:** Evaluate behavioral, cognitive, and functional deficits.
- **Baseline lab work:** Biochemical panel including BUN and creatinine levels.
- **Therapeutic effects:** Monitor for improvement in behavioral, cognitive, and functional status.
- **Urine pH:** Monitor urine pH because alkaline urine may lead to an accumulation of the drug with a possible increase in side effects.
- **Hydration:** Ensure patients are well hydrated; monitor intake and urine output.
- **Patient education:** Caution against abruptly discontinuing memantine or adjusting the drug dosage. If therapy is interrupted for several days, instruct to restart the drug at the lowest dose and increase the dosage at intervals of at least 1 wk to the most recent dose. Urge adequate fluid intake. Inform patients and family that memantine is not a cure for Alzheimer's disease but may slow the progression of its symptoms. Refer support system members to the local chapter of the Alzheimer's Disease Association.

SERIOUS ADVERSE REACTIONS
- None known.

OVERDOSE/TOXICITY
- **Nephrotoxicity:** Hematuria, oliguria, abdominal discomfort, nausea, vomiting, psychosis, restlessness, stupor.
- **GI decontamination:** No specific recommendations.

ANTIDOTE/DIALYSIS
- **Antidote:** No specific recommendations.
- **Dialysis:** No data are available on removal of memantine using hemodialysis, high-permeability hemodialysis, or peritoneal dialysis.

meperidine hydrochloride

me-per'-i-deen hye-droe-klor'-ide

DEA Schedule: II

Classes
Chemical: opiate derivative, phenylpiperidine derivative
Therapeutic: narcotic analgesic

Pregnancy Category: C, D

Trade Names
Prescription: Demerol

Combinations
Prescription: with promethazine (Mepergan)

Do not confuse Demerol with Demulen or Dymelor, or morphine with meperidine.

CLINICAL PHARMACOLOGY

Mechanism of Action
An opioid agonist that binds to opioid receptors in the CNS. **Therapeutic Effect:** Alters the perception of and emotional response to pain.

PHARMACOKINETICS

Route	Onset	Peak	Duration
PO	15 min	60 min	2-4 hr
IV	Less than 5 min	5-7 min	2-3 hr
IM	10-15 min	30-50 min	2-4 hr
Subcutaneous	10-15 min	30-50 min	2-4 hr

Variably absorbed from the GI tract; well absorbed after IM administration. Protein binding: 60%-80%. Widely distributed. Metabolized in the liver to active metabolite. Primarily excreted in urine. Not removed by hemodialysis. **Half-life:** 2.4-4 hr; metabolite 15-30 hr (increased in hepatic impairment and disease).

AVAILABILITY

Syrup: 50 mg/5 mL.
Tablets: 50 mg, 100 mg.
Injection: 10 mg/mL, 25 mg/mL, 50 mg/mL, 75 mg/mL, 100 mg/mL.

INDICATIONS AND DOSAGE

Analgesia
PO, IM, Subcutaneous
Adults, Elderly: 50-150 mg every 3-4 hr.
Children: 1-1.5 mg/kg every 3-4 hr. Do not exceed single dose of 100 mg.
Patient-controlled analgesia (PCA)
IV
Adults: Loading dose: 50-100 mg. Intermittent bolus: 5-25 mg. Lockout interval: 10-20 min. Continuous infusion: 5-40 mg/hr. Maximum (4 hr): 200-300 mg.
Dosage in renal impairment
Dosage is based on creatinine clearance.

Creatinine Clearance	Dosage
10-50 mL/min	75% of usual dose
Less than 10 mL/min	50% of usual dose

CONTRAINDICATIONS

Delivery of premature infant, diarrhea due to poisoning, use within 14 days of MAOIs, hypersensitivity to meperidine

INTERACTIONS

Drug: **Alcohol, other CNS depressants:** May increase CNS or respiratory depression and hypotension. **MAOIs:** May produce a severe, sometimes fatal reaction. Meperidine use is contraindicated. **Herbal:** **Kava kava, valerian:** May increase CNS depression. **St. John's wort:** May increase sedation. **Food:** None known.

DIAGNOSTIC TEST EFFECTS

May increase serum amylase and lipase levels. Therapeutic serum level is 100-550 ng/mL; toxic serum level is greater than 1000 ng/mL.

IV INCOMPATIBILITIES

Allopurinol (Aloprim), amphotericin B complex (Abelcet, AmBisome, Amphotec), cefepime (Maxipime), cefoperazone (Cefobid), *DOXOrubicin liposomal (Doxil), furosemide (Lasix), idarubicin (Idamycin), nafcillin (Nafcil)

M

IV COMPATIBILITIES

Atropine, bumetanide (Bumex), diltiazem (Cardizem), *diphenhydrAMINE (Benadryl), *DOBUTamine (Dobutrex), *DOPamine (Intropin), glycopyrrolate (Robinul), heparin, *hydrOXYzine (Vistaril), insulin, lidocaine, magnesium, midazolam (Versed), oxytocin (Pitocin), potassium, total parenteral nutrition (TPN)

SIDE-EFFECTS

Frequent: Sedation, hypotension (including orthostatic hypotension), diaphoresis, facial flushing, dizziness, nausea, vomiting, constipation. **Occasional:** Confusion, dysrhythmias, tremors, urine retention, abdominal pain, dry mouth, headache, irritation at injection site, euphoria, dysphoria. **Rare:** Allergic reaction (rash, pruritus), insomnia

CRITICAL CARE CONSIDERATIONS

ADMINISTRATION/HANDLING

PO ALERT

- Give meperidine without regard to food.
- Dilute syrup form in a glass of water to prevent an anesthetic effect on mucous membranes.

IV ALERT

- **Storage:** Store vials at room temperature.
- **Preparation:** Place patients in a recumbent position before administering parenteral meperidine.
- **IV push injection:** Give meperidine by very slow IV push over 2-3 min; may be given undiluted. Rapid IV administration increases risk of severe anaphylactic reaction, marked by apnea, cardiac arrest, and circulatory collapse.
- **IV dilution:** Meperidine may be diluted in D_5W, Ringer's solution, lactated Ringer's solution, a dextrose-saline combination (such as 2.5%, 5%, or 10% dextrose and 0.45% or 0.9% NaCl), or Molar (M/6) sodium lactate injection for IV injection or infusion.

IM/SUBCUTANEOUS ALERT

- **IM versus subcutaneous injection:** IM route is preferred over subcutaneous because subcutaneous injection can produce induration, local irritation, and pain.
- **IM injection:** Inject the drug slowly.
- **High risk for overdose:** Patients with circulatory impairment are at increased risk for overdose because of delayed absorption of repeated injections.

PRECAUTIONS

HEALTH-RELATED

- **Very cautious use:** Use cautiously in patients with acute bronchial asthma, those with airway obstruction, and patients with noncardiogenic pulmonary edema caused by chemical respiratory irritants.
- Use meperidine cautiously in elderly or debilitated patients and in patients with acute abdominal conditions, chronic obstructive pulmonary disease, cor pulmonale, glaucoma, head injuries, history of seizures, increased intracranial pressure, hepatic or renal impairment, respiratory abnormalities, or supraventricular tachycardia.
- **Renal impairment:** Use cautiously in patients with renal impairment because meperidine's metabolite normeperidine may increase and cause seizures, tremors, and twitching.
- **Side effects:** Meperidine's side effects are dependent on dosage and route of administration. IM administration increases risk of overdose if drug is not properly absorbed.
- Meperidine is potentiated by anesthetics (general), alcohol, antacids, anticholinergics (glycopyrrolate), cimetidine (Tagamet), tricyclic antidepressants (amitriptyline [Elavil]), isoniazid, neostigmine (Prostigmine), neuromuscular blocking agents (succinylcholine), oral contraceptives, other narcotics, and phenothiazines (promethazine [Phenergan]).
- **Protease inhibitors:** Antiretroviral drugs may increase risk of seizures and dysrhythmias.
- **Ambulatory patients/mild to moderate pain:** Patients may be more prone to dizziness, nausea, and vomiting than those placed supine or in severe pain.

AGE-RELATED

- **Children:** The neonate may develop respiratory depression if the mother receives meperidine during labor. Children under 2 yr are more susceptible to the drug's respiratory depressant effects. Children are more prone to develop paradoxic excitement.
- **Elderly:** Elderly are more susceptible to confusion, agitation, and the drug's respiratory depressant effects. Age-related

renal impairment may increase the risk of urinary retention.

PREGNANCY/LACTATION-RELATED

- Pregnancy category C (category D if used for prolonged periods or in high doses at term). Use during labor may produce neonatal respiratory depression. Compatible with breast-feeding; mothers should try to wait 4-6 hr after receiving dose to breast-feed, if possible

MONITORING

- **Baseline assessment:** Assess the duration, location, onset, and type of pain. Assess history of use of pain medications, including whether patients have had effective pain control from meperidine in the past. Obtain vital signs before giving meperidine. Withhold the drug if the respiratory rate is 10 breaths/min or less in adults or 15 breaths/min or less in children.
- **Baseline lab work:** Biochemical panel including renal function tests (BUN, creatinine) and liver function studies (AST [SGOT], ALT [SGPT], alkaline phosphatase, bilirubin).
- **Lesser pain relief:** Meperidine's effects are reduced if a full pain response recurs before the next dose.
- **Hypotension and respiratory depression:** Monitor vital signs for 15-30 min after an IM or subcutaneous dose and for 5-10 min after an IV dose. Note decreased BP, as decreasing pulse or lessening pulse amplitude.
- **Pain/sedation scale:** Monitor level of pain and sedation using appropriate pain and sedation scales.
- **Constipation:** Assess pattern of daily bowel activity and stool consistency.
- **Urinary retention:** Evaluate for adequate urination. Palpate bladder if patients are not voiding in adequate amounts (0.5-1 mL/kg/hr).
- **Respiratory depression:** Initiate deep-breathing and coughing exercises, particularly in patients with impaired respiratory function.
- **Serum drug levels:** Monitor serum drug levels. Therapeutic level is 100 to 550 ng/mL. Toxic level is greater than 1000 ng/mL.
- **Patient education:** Instruct to ask for meperidine before pain fully returns, within prescribed intervals and to use the drug the same way at home. Inform that injection may cause discomfort. Caution that drug dependence and tolerance may occur with prolonged use of high doses. Warn to avoid tasks that require mental alertness or motor skills until response to the drug is known. Instruct on changing positions slowly to avoid orthostatic hypotension. Advise to increase fluid intake and consumption of high-fiber foods to prevent constipation. Urge the avoidance of alcohol and other CNS depressants while taking meperidine.

SERIOUS ADVERSE REACTIONS

- **Paralytic ileus/bowel obstruction:** Too-frequent use may result in ileus or obstipation.
- **Tolerance and dependence:** Patients who use meperidine repeatedly may develop a tolerance to the drug's analgesic effect and physical dependence.
- **Withdrawal:** Patients who become physically dependent on the medication will experience withdrawal if meperidine is withheld.

OVERDOSE/TOXICITY

- **Symptoms:** Cold or clammy skin, confusion, seizures, decreased BP, restlessness, pinpoint pupils, bradycardia, respiratory depression, cyanosis, decreased LOC, extreme somnolence, stupor, coma, severe weakness, and skeletal muscle flaccidity.
- **Management:** Administer antidote naloxone and provide supportive care, which may include endotracheal intubation, mechanical ventilation, management of hypotension with fluids and vasopressors unless bradycardic. Manage bradycardia according to Advanced Cardiac Life Support (ACLS) guidelines (atropine IV, *DOPamine infusion).
- **Normeperidine toxicity:** Seizures, tremors, jerking, shaky hands.
- **GI decontamination:** Patients suspected of/who have concealed large amounts of drugs by ingesting packages (called "body packers") can be detected using a contrast enhanced upper GI series with small bowel follow through if initial GI radiograph is negative. Body packers may benefit from whole bowel irrigation. Simple ingestions may benefit from a single dose of activated charcoal.

ANTIDOTE/DIALYSIS

- **Antidote:** Naloxone IV, with dose calculation based on the likelihood of drug dependence. If patients initially respond but then experience resedation, rebolus with naloxone or begin continuous

M

naloxone infusion starting at two thirds of the initial reversal dose hourly titrated to effect. Nalmefene (Revex) may reverse toxic effects.

- **Dialysis:** Meperidine is not removed by hemodialysis or high-permeability hemodialysis and is unlikely to be removed by peritoneal dialysis. The metabolite normeperidine is removed by high-permeability hemodialysis; there are no data available on removal of normeperidine by hemodialysis or peritoneal dialysis.

mephenytoin

See Anticonvulsants (p. 903)

meprobamate

See Antianxiety Agents (p. 890)

meropenem

See Antibiotics (p. 892)

mesalamine/5 aminosalicylic acid/5-ASA

mez-al'-a-meen/five ah-meen'-oh-sal-ih-sil-ik as'-id

Classes

Chemical: 5-amino derivative of salicylic acid

Therapeutic: gastrointestinal antiinflammatory

Pregnancy Category: B

Trade Names

Prescription: Asacol, Mesasal ♣, Pentasa, Rowasa, Salofalk ♣

Do not confuse Asacol with Os-Cal.

CLINICAL PHARMACOLOGY

Mechanism of Action

A salicylic acid derivative that locally inhibits arachidonic acid metabolite production, which is increased in patients with chronic inflammatory bowel disease. **Therapeutic Effect:** Blocks prostaglandin production and diminishes inflammation in the colon.

PHARMACOKINETICS

Poorly absorbed from the colon. Moderately absorbed from the GI tract. Metabolized in the liver to active metabolite. Unabsorbed portion eliminated in feces; absorbed portion excreted in urine. Unknown if removed by hemodialysis. **Half-life:** 0.5-1.5 hr; metabolite, 5-10 hr.

AVAILABILITY

Tablets (delayed release [Asacol]): 400 mg.
Capsules (controlled release [Pentasa]): 250 mg.
Rectal suspension (Rowasa): 4 g/60 mL.
Suppositories (Canasa): 500 mg, 1 g.

INDICATIONS AND DOSAGE

Treatment of ulcerative colitis

PO (capsule)

Adults, Elderly: 1 g 4 times per day. **Children:** 50 mg/kg/day divided every 6-12 hr. Not recommended for use in children.

PO (tablet)

Adults, Elderly: 800 mg 3 times per day. **Children:** 50 mg/kg/day divided every 8-12 hr. Not recommended for use in children.

Maintenance of remission in ulcerative colitis

PO (capsule)

Adults, Elderly: 1 g 4 times per day.

PO (tablet)

Adults, Elderly: 1.6 g/day in divided doses.

Distal ulcerative colitis, proctosigmoiditis, proctitis

Rectal (retention enema)

Adults, Elderly: 60 mL (4 g) at bedtime; retained overnight for approximately 8 hr for 3-6 wk.

Rectal (500 mg suppository)

Adults, Elderly: Twice per day for 3 wk. May increase to 3 times per day.

Rectal (1000-mg suppository)

Adults, Elderly: Once daily at bedtime. Continue therapy for 3-6 wk.

CONTRAINDICATIONS

Hypersensitivity to mesalamine, sulfa-based products, sulfites, sulfasalazine, or salicylates; Canasa suppository is contraindicated in those allergic to saturated vegetable fatty acid esters (contained in the suppository)

INTERACTIONS

Drug: Anticoagulants: May increase the risk of bleeding. **Azathioprine, 6-MP:** May increase the risk of myelosuppression. **Varicella virus vaccine:** May increase the risk of developing Reye's syndrome. **Herbal:** None known. **Food:** Mesalamine levels are decreased when taken with food.

DIAGNOSTIC TEST EFFECTS

May increase BUN, serum alkaline phosphatase, creatinine, AST (SGOT), and ALT (SGPT) levels.

SIDE-EFFECTS

Mesalamine is generally well tolerated, with only mild and transient effects. **Frequent (greater than 6%): PO:** Abdominal cramps or pain, diarrhea, dizziness, headache, nausea, vomiting, rhinitis, unusual fatigue. **Rectal:** Abdominal or stomach cramps, flatulence, headache, nausea. **Occasional (6%-2%): PO:** Decreased appetite, back or joint pain, flatulence, acne. **Rare (less than 2%): Rectal:** Anal irritation

CRITICAL CARE CONSIDERATIONS

ADMINISTRATION/HANDLING

PO ALERT

- Store at room temperature.
- Swallow whole; do not break outer coating of tablet.
- Give mesalamine without regard to food.

RECTAL ALERT

- Store at room temperature.
- Shake enema suspension bottle well.
- **Preparation:** Instruct patients to lie on the left side with lower leg extended, upper leg flexed forward, or to assume the knee-chest position.
- **Administration:** Insert applicator tip into rectum, pointing toward umbilicus. Squeeze bottle steadily until contents are emptied. Retain the enema for as long as tolerable, preferably for a minimum of 8 hr.

PRECAUTIONS

HEALTH-RELATED

- Use mesalamine cautiously in patients with preexisting renal disease or sulfasalazine sensitivity.
- Mesalamine suspension enema contains metabisulfite, which may cause allergic reactions.

AGE-RELATED

- **Children:** Safety and efficacy of mesalamine have not been established in children.
- **Elderly:** Age-related renal impairment may require cautious use.

PREGNANCY/LACTATION-RELATED

- Pregnancy category B; has produced adverse effects in a nursing infant and should be used with caution during breast-feeding. Observe nursing infant closely for changes in stool consistency.

MONITORING

- **Baseline assessment:** Before administering mesalamine, ask about allergy to sulfa-based products. Obtain history of GI symptoms.
- **Baseline lab work:** Biochemical profile including BUN, serum alkaline phosphatase, creatinine, AST (SGOT), and ALT (SGPT) levels.
- **Hydration:** Provide adequate IV and/or PO fluid intake.
- **GI effects:** Assess bowel sounds for level of peristalsis. Evaluate for abdominal disturbances.
- **Bowel habits:** Assess pattern of daily bowel activity and stool consistency and record time of evacuation.
- **Rash:** Assess skin for rash and urticaria.
- **Discontinue drug:** Discontinue mesalamine if cramping, diarrhea, fever, or rash occur.
- **Patient education:** Warn to avoid tasks that require mental alertness or motor skills until response to the drug is known. Inform that mesalamine may discolor urine yellow-brown. Explain that mesalamine suppositories stain fabrics.

SERIOUS ADVERSE REACTIONS

- **Sulfite sensitivity:** May occur in susceptible patients manifested by cramping, headache, diarrhea, fever, rash, hives, itching, and wheezing. Discontinue drug immediately.
- **Management:** Epinephrine is the drug of choice for management of acute allergic reaction, even though epinephrine injection contains small amounts of sulfites. Alternate drugs may be ineffective.

OVERDOSE/TOXICITY

- Hepatitis, pancreatitis, and pericarditis occur rarely with oral forms; diarrhea, vomiting.
- **GI decontamination:** No specific recommendations.

ANTIDOTE/DIALYSIS

- **Antidote:** No specific recommendations.
- **Dialysis:** No data are available on removal of mesalamine using hemodialysis, high-permeability hemodialysis, or peritoneal dialysis.

mesoridazine besylate

See Antipsychotics (p. 934)

metaproterenol sulfate

See Beta-Adrenergic Blockers (p. 943)

metformin hydrochloride

met-for'-min hye-droe-klor'-ide

Classes

Chemical: biguanide
Therapeutic: antidiabetic, hypoglycemic

Pregnancy Category: B

Trade Names

Prescription: Fortamet, Glucophage, Glucophage XL, Glumetza, Glycon ♣, Riomet

Combinations

Prescription: with rosiglitazone (Avandamet); with *glyBURIDE (Glucovance)

M

CLINICAL PHARMACOLOGY

Mechanism of Action

An antihyperglycemic that decreases hepatic production of glucose. Decreases absorption of glucose and improves insulin sensitivity. **Therapeutic Effect:** Improves glycemic control, stabilizes or decreases body weight, and improves lipid profile.

PHARMACOKINETICS

Slowly, incompletely absorbed after oral administration. Food delays or decreases the extent of absorption. Protein binding: Negligible. Primarily distributed to intestinal mucosa and salivary glands. Primarily excreted unchanged in urine. Removed by hemodialysis. **Half-life:** 6 hr.

AVAILABILITY

Oral solution (Riomet): 100 mg/mL.
Tablets (Glucophage): 500 mg, 850 mg, 1000 mg.
Tablets (extended release): 500 mg (Fortamet, Glucophage XL, Glumetza), 750 mg (Glucophage XL), 1000 mg (Fortamet, Glumetza).

INDICATIONS AND DOSAGE

Diabetes mellitus

PO (Immediate-Release Tablets, Solution)

Adults, Elderly: Initially, 500 mg twice per day or 850 mg once daily. Maintenance: 1-2.55 g/day in 2-3 divided doses. Maximum: 2500 mg/day. **Children 10-16 yr:** Initially, 500 mg twice per day. Maintenance: Titrate in 500-mg increments weekly. Maximum: 2000 mg/day.

PO (Extended-Release Tablets [Glucophage XL])

Adults, Elderly: Initially, 500 mg once daily. Maintenance: 1-2 g daily. Maximum: 2000 mg/day.

PO (Extended-Release Tablets [Fortamet, Glumetza])

Adults, Elderly: 500 mg-1g once daily. Maintenance: 1-2.5 g once daily. Maximum: 2500 mg/day.

OFF-LABEL USES

Treatment of HIV liopodystrophy syndrome, metabolic complications of AIDS, polycystic ovary syndrome, prediabetes, weight reduction

CONTRAINDICATIONS

Acute heart failure, MI, cardiovascular collapse, renal disease (creatinine 1.5 in males, 1.4 in females) or dysfunction, respiratory failure, septicemia, hypersensitivity to metformin, metabolic acidosis, iodinated contrast media (withhold for 48 hr after contrast recieved)

INTERACTIONS

Drug: **Alcohol, amiloride, cimetidine, digoxin, furosemide, morphine, nifedipine, procainamide, quinidine, quinine, ranitidine, triamterene, trimethoprim, vancomycin:** Increases metformin blood concentration. **Furosemide, hypoglycemia-causing medications:** May require a decrease in metformin dosage. **Iodinated contrast studies:** May cause acute renal failure and increased risk of lactic acidosis, especially in those with prior renal insufficiency. **Herbal:** None known. **Food:** None known.

DIAGNOSTIC TEST EFFECTS

None known.

SIDE-EFFECTS

Occasional (up to 30%): GI disturbances (including diarrhea, nausea, vomiting, abdominal bloating, flatulence, and anorexia) that are transient and resolve spontaneously during therapy. **Rare (3%-1%):** Unpleasant or metallic taste that resolves spontaneously during therapy

CRITICAL CARE CONSIDERATIONS

ADMINISTRATION/HANDLING

PO ALERT

- Give metformin with meals.
- Do not crush film-coated tablets.
- Do not crush extended release capsules or attempt to open capsules.
- Metformin should be withheld 1-24 hr before procedure in patients undergoing studies with IV iodinated contrast and those undergoing major surgery to help avoid nephrotoxicity. Metformin should be withheld for 48 hr following the procedure and reinstituted only after renal function is confirmed to be normal.

PRECAUTIONS

HEALTH-RELATED

- **Lactic acidosis:** A rare but potentially fatal consequence of metformin therapy. Withhold metformin in patients with conditions that may predispose to lactic acidosis, such as hypotension, shock, dehydration, hypoperfusion, hypoxemia, impaired hepatic function, impaired renal function, impaired heart function, cardiovascular disease; heart failure, and sepsis.
- **Severe illness:** Patients with diabetes who become seriously ill may not be able to be safely maintained on metformin. Insulin or insulin infusion may be needed to control blood glucose. Continued use of metformin should be done cautiously when patients undergo stressful diseases involving diarrhea, high fever, infection, malnutrition, hyperthyroidism or hypothyroidism, gastroparesis, and vomiting.
- **Hypoglycemia:** Higher-risk patients include debilitated, elderly, anorexic, alcoholic, or malnourished patients; those taking sulfonylureas (e.g., *glipiZIDE, *glyBURIDE) to help lower blood glucose.
- **Hypoxic states:** Use cautiously in patients at risk for hypoxia including those with heart and/or vascular disease, acute MI, chronic respiratory difficulty.

AGE-RELATED

- **Children:** Safety and efficacy of metformin have not been established in children under 10 yr.
- **Elderly:** Age-related renal impairment or peripheral vascular disease may require decreased dosage or discontinuation of drug.

PREGNANCY/LACTATION-RELATED

- Pregnancy category B; breast milk excretion unknown.

MONITORING

- **Baseline assessment:** Evaluate blood glucose control. Evaluate symptoms of diabetes. Inform patients of the potential advantages and risks of metformin therapy and of alternative modes of treatment.
- **Baseline lab work:** Assess CBC with WBC differential; biochemical panel with fasting glucose, BUN, creatinine, AST (SGOT), ALT (SPGT), alkaline phosphatase, bilirubin, CPK, LDH, total cholesterol, triglycerides and folic acid; B-type natriuretic peptide (BNP) to evaluate heart failure; glucose tolerance test, hemoglobin $A1_C$ before beginning metformin therapy and annually thereafter.
- **Sulfonylureas and hypoglycemia:** Assess those concurrently taking oral sulfonylureas for symptoms of hypoglycemia including anxiety, cool wet skin, diplopia, dizziness, headache, hunger, numbness in mouth, tachycardia, and tremors.
- **Lactic acidosis:** Monitor for drowsiness, extreme fatigue, muscle aches, and unexplained hyperventilation. Obtain arterial blood gas, serum ketones, and serum lactate level. Check urine for ketones.
- **Toxic drug level:** Patients with lactic acidosis have metformin levels greater than 5 mcg/mL.
- **"Sick days":** Be alert to conditions that may induce stress and increase blood glucose levels such as an invasive procedure (cardiac catheterization, endoscopy, arteriogram) or major surgical procedure.
- **GI effects:** Monitor for diarrhea, flatulence, nausea, and vomiting. Patients new to metformin experience GI side effects. If effects persist for more than 3 wk, instruct patients to report promptly problems to a health care provider. Drug may need to be discontinued if patients become dehydrated and/or malnourished.
- **Patient education:** Instruct to report symptoms of lactic acidosis such as drowsiness, extreme fatigue, muscle aches, and unexplained hyperventilation, and to discontinue metformin immediately. Stress that a controlled, consistent carbohydrate diet is a principal part of treatment along with exercise. Overweight patients should be encouraged to lose weight. Warn not to skip or delay meals. Explain that diabetes mellitus requires

M

lifelong control. Urge avoidance of alcohol. Instruct to report diarrhea, easy bleeding or bruising, change in color of stool or urine, headache, nausea, persistent rash, and vomiting.

SERIOUS ADVERSE REACTIONS

- **Lactic acidosis:** Rare but fatal complication in 50% of cases; characterized by increased anion gap, blood lactate levels (greater than 5 mmol/L), decreased blood pH, and electrolyte imbalances. Symptoms may be subtle (malaise, myalgia, abdominal pain) but progress to unexplained hyperventilation, somnolence, shock, acute pulmonary edema, acute MI, and acute renal failure. Should be suspected in diabetic patients with metabolic acidosis without ketonuria and ketonemia.

OVERDOSE/TOXICITY

- **Nephrotoxicity:** Elevated BUN and creatinine, oliguria, abdominal pain, edema, malaise, nausea, vomiting.
- **Cardiotoxicity:** Heart failure, shock, hypotension, acute MI.
- **Anemia:** Caused by vitamin B_{12} deficiency; quickly reverses by discontinuation of metformin.
- **GI decontamination:** No specific recommendations.

M

ANTIDOTE/DIALYSIS

- **Antidote:** Prompt hemodialysis in a hospital setting is recommended to remove metformin.
- **Dialysis:** Metformin is removed by hemodialysis and is likely to be removed by high-permeability hemodialysis. No data are available on removal using peritoneal dialysis.

methadone hydrochloride 

meth'-a-done hye-droe-klor'-ide

DEA Schedule: II

Classes

Chemical: diphenylheptane derivative, opiate derivative

Therapeutic: narcotic analgesic

Pregnancy Category: B, D

Trade Names

Prescription: Dolophine, Metadol ♣, Methadone Intensol, Methadose

CLINICAL PHARMACOLOGY

Mechanism of Action

An opioid agonist that binds with opioid receptors in the CNS. **Therapeutic Effect:** Alters the perception of and emotional response to pain; reduces withdrawal symptoms from other opioid drugs.

PHARMACOKINETICS

Route	Onset	Peak	Duration
Oral	0.5-1 hr	2-4 hr	6-8 hr
IM	10-20 min	1-2 hr	4-5 hr
IV	15 min	15-30 min	3-4 hr

Well absorbed after IM injection. Protein binding: 80%-85%. Metabolized in the liver. Primarily excreted in urine. Not removed by hemodialysis. **Half-life:** 15-25 hr.

AVAILABILITY

Oral concentrate (Methadone Intensol, Methadose): 10 mg/mL.
Oral solution: 5 mg/5 mL, 10 mg/5 mL.
Tablets (Dolophine, Methadose): 5 mg, 10 mg.
Tablets (dispersible [Methadose]): 40 mg.
Injection (Dolophine): 10 mg/mL.

INDICATIONS AND DOSAGE

Analgesia

PO

Adults, Elderly: Initially, 2.5-10 mg every 3-4 hr. **Children:** 0.1-0.2 mg/kg every 6 hr as needed. Maximum: 10 mg/dose.

IV, IM, Subcutaneous

Adults, Elderly: Initially 2.5-10 mg every 3-4 hr.

Narcotic addiction

IM, PO

Adults, Elderly: 15-40 mg once daily or as needed. Reduce dose at 1- to 2-day intervals based on patient response. Maintenance: Individualized.

CONTRAINDICATIONS

Hypersensitivity to methadone or other narcotics

INTERACTIONS

Drug: Alcohol, other CNS depressants: May increase CNS or respiratory depression and hypotension. **MAOIs:** May produce a severe, sometimes fatal reaction; plan to administer one quarter of usual methadone dose. **Herbal: Valerian:** May increase CNS depression. **Food:** None known.

DIAGNOSTIC TEST EFFECTS

May increase serum amylase and lipase levels.

SIDE-EFFECTS

Frequent: Sedation, decreased BP (including orthostatic hypotension), diaphoresis, facial flushing, constipation, dizziness, nausea, vomiting. **Occasional:** Confusion, urine retention, palpitations, abdominal cramps, visual changes, dry mouth, headache, decreased appetite, anxiety, insomnia. **Rare:** Allergic reaction (rash, pruritus)

CRITICAL CARE CONSIDERATIONS

ADMINISTRATION/HANDLING

PO ALERT

- **Potency:** Oral methadone is one-half as potent as parenteral methadone.
- Give methadone without regard to food.
- Dilute syrup in a glass of water to prevent an anesthetic effect on mucous membranes.
- **Detoxification:** Methadone used for treatment of a narcotics addiction may be dispensed only by approved hospital pharmacies, approved community pharmacies, and maintenance programs approved by the Food and Drug Administration (FDA) and the state authority.
- **Analgesia:** Methadone used for pain management may be dispensed by any licensed hospital pharmacy.

IM, SUBCUTANEOUS ALERT

- IM route is preferred over subcutaneous route; subcutaneous route may produce induration, local irritation, and pain.
- Do not use solution if it appears cloudy or contains a precipitate.
- **Preparation:** Place patients in the recumbent position before giving parenteral methadone.
- **Administration:** Inject the drug slowly.
- **High risk for overdose:** Patients with circulatory impairment are at increased risk for overdose because of delayed absorption of repeated injections.
- **Detoxification:** Methadone used for treatment of a narcotics addiction may be dispensed only by approved hospital pharmacies, approved community pharmacies and maintenance programs approved by the FDA and the state authority.
- **Analgesia:** Methadone used for pain management may be dispensed by any licensed hospital pharmacy.

PRECAUTIONS

HEALTH-RELATED

- **Very cautious use:** Patients with acute bronchial asthma, those with airway obstruction, and in patients with noncardiogenic pulmonary edema caused by chemical respiratory irritants.
- Use methadone extremely cautiously in patients in labor, during delivery of a premature infant, in patients with acute abdominal conditions, cor pulmonale, history of seizures, impaired hepatic or renal function, increased intracranial pressure, respiratory abnormalities, or supraventricular tachycardia.
- Use methadone cautiously in debilitated or elderly patients and those with diarrhea due to poisoning.
- Drug is potentiated by: anesthetics (general), alcohol, antacids, anticholinergics (glycopyrrolate), cimetidine (Tagamet), tricyclic antidepressants (amitriptyline [Elavil]), isoniazid, neostigmine (Prostigmine), neuromuscular blocking agents (succinylcholine), oral contraceptives, other narcotics, and phenothiazines (promethazine [Phenergan]).
- **Ambulatory patients/mild to moderate pain:** Patients may be more prone to dizziness, nausea, and vomiting than those placed supine or in severe pain.

AGE-RELATED

- **Children:** Neonates may develop respiratory depression if mothers receive meperidine during labor. Children under 2 yr are more susceptible to the drug's respiratory depressant effects. Children are more prone to develop paradoxic excitement. Methadone is not recommended for use as an analgesic in children.
- **Elderly:** Elderly are more susceptible to confusion, agitation, and the drug's respiratory depressant effects. Age-related renal impairment may increase the risk of urinary retention.

PREGNANCY/LACTATION-RELATED

- Pregnancy category B (category D if used for prolonged periods or in high doses at term); compatible with breast-feeding if mother consumes no more than 20 mg/24 hr.

MONITORING

- **Baseline assessment:** If used as an analgesic, assess the duration, location, onset, and type of pain. Assess history of use of narcotics, including if patients have had effective pain or addiction control from methadone in the past. Obtain vital signs before giving methadone. Withhold the drug if respiratory rate is 10 breaths/min or less in an adult or 15 breaths/min or less in a child.
- **Baseline lab work:** Biochemical panel including renal function tests (BUN, creatinine) and liver function studies (AST [SGOT], ALT [SGPT], alkaline phosphatase, bilirubin).
- **Lesser pain relief:** Methadone's effects are reduced if a full pain response recurs before the next dose.
- **Hypotension and respiratory depression:** Monitor vital signs for 15 to 30 min after an IM or subcutaneous dose. Note decreased BP, as decreasing pulse or lessening pulse amplitude.
- **Pain/sedation scale:** Monitor level of pain and sedation using appropriate pain and sedation scales.
- **Constipation:** Assess pattern of daily bowel activity and stool consistency.
- **Urinary retention:** Evaluate for adequate urination. Palpate bladder if patients are not voiding in adequate amounts (0.5-1 mL/kg/hr).
- **Respiratory depression:** Initiate deep breathing and coughing exercises, particularly in patients with impaired respiratory function.
- **Detoxification:** Provide support to the patient in a detoxification program. Monitor for withdrawal symptoms.
- **Patient education:** Caution against abruptly discontinuing methadone after prolonged use. Inform that methadone may cause dizziness and dry mouth. Warn to avoid tasks that require mental alertness or motor skills until response to the drug is known. Urge avoidance of alcohol and CNS depressants during methadone therapy.

SERIOUS ADVERSE REACTIONS

- **Paralytic ileus/bowel obstruction:** Too-frequent use may result in ileus or obstipation.
- **Tolerance and dependence:** Patients who use methadone over time may develop a tolerance to the drug's analgesic effect and physical dependence.
- **Withdrawal:** Patients who become physically dependent on methadone will experience withdrawal if drug is withheld.

OVERDOSE/TOXICITY

- **Symptoms:** Cold or clammy skin, confusion, seizures, decreased BP, restlessness, pinpoint pupils, bradycardia, respiratory depression, cyanosis, decreased LOC, extreme somnolence, stupor, coma, severe weakness, and skeletal muscle flaccidity.
- **Management:** Administer antidote naloxone and provide supportive care which may include endotracheal intubation, mechanical ventilation, management of hypotension with fluids, and vasopressors unless bradycardic. Manage bradycardia according to Advanced Cardiac Life Support (ACLS) guidelines (atropine IV, *DOPamine infusion).
- **GI decontamination:** No specific recommendations.

ANTIDOTE/DIALYSIS

- **Antidote:** Naloxone IV, with dose calculation based on the likelihood of drug dependence. If patients initially respond but then experience resedation, rebolus with naloxone or begin continuous naloxone infusion starting at two thirds of the initial reversal dose hourly titrated to effect.
- **Dialysis:** Methadone is not removed by hemodialysis or peritoneal dialysis. No data are available on removal using high-permeability hemodialysis.

M

methimazole

meth-im'-a-zole

Classes

Chemical: thioimidazole derivative
Therapeutic: antithyroid agent

Pregnancy Category: D

Trade Names

Prescription: Tapazole

CLINICAL PHARMACOLOGY

Mechanism of Action

A thiomidazole derivative that inhibits synthesis of thyroid hormone by interfering with the incorporation of iodine into tyrosyl residues. **Therapeutic Effect:** Effectively treats hyperthyroidism by decreasing thyroid hormone levels.

PHARMACOKINETICS

Rapid absorption following PO administration. Protein binding: Not significant. Widely distributed throughout the body. Metabolized in liver. Excreted in urine. **Half-life:** 5-6 hr.

AVAILABILITY

Tablets: 5 mg, 10 mg, 20 mg.

INDICATIONS AND DOSAGE

Hyperthyroidism

PO

Adults, Elderly: Initially, 15-60 mg/day in 3 divided doses 8 hr apart. Maintenance: 5-15 mg/day. **Children:** Initially, 0.4-0.7 mg/kg/day in 3 divided doses 8 hr apart. Maintenance: One half the initial dose.

CONTRAINDICATIONS

Hypersensitivity to methimazole, breast-feeding

INTERACTIONS

Drug: Amiodarone, iodinated glycerol, iodine, potassium iodide: May decrease response to methimazole. **Digoxin:** May increase the blood concentration of digoxin as patient becomes euthyroid. **I^{131}:** May decrease thyroid uptake of I^{131}. **Oral anticoagulants:** May decrease the effects of oral anticoagulants. **Herbal:** None known. **Food:** None known.

DIAGNOSTIC TEST EFFECTS

May increase LDH, serum alkaline phosphatase, bilirubin, AST (SGOT), and ALT (SGPT) levels and prothrombin time. May decrease prothrombin level and WBC count.

SIDE-EFFECTS

Frequent (5%-4%): Fever, rash, pruritus. **Occasional (3%-1%):** Dizziness, loss of taste, nausea, vomiting, stomach pain, peripheral neuropathy or numbness in fingers, toes, face. **Rare (less than 1%):** Swollen lymph nodes or salivary glands

CRITICAL CARE CONSIDERATIONS

ADMINISTRATION/HANDLING

PO ALERT

- Store at room temperature in a light-resistant container.
- Administer methimazole with food if GI symptoms occur.

PRECAUTIONS

HEALTH-RELATED

- Use methimazole cautiously in patients taking methimazole with other agranulocytosis-inducing drugs and in those with impaired hepatic function.
- About 10% of patients with untreated hyperthyroidism have leukopenia.

AGE-RELATED

- **Children:** No age-related precautions have been noted.
- **Elderly:** Are more prone to experience adverse reactions. Use methimazole cautiously in patients over 40 yr.

PREGNANCY/LACTATION-RELATED

- Pregnancy category D. Use smallest possible dose to control maternal disease (propylthiouracil preferable, less likely to cross the placenta); excreted into breast milk.

MONITORING

- **Baseline assessment:** Obtain vital signs and weight.
- **Baseline lab work:** Thyroid function studies; biochemical panel including liver function studies, blood glucose, calcium and magnesium levels; CBC with WBC differential and platelet count; prothrombin time when beginning therapy and periodically thereafter. Elevated TSH level indicates methimazole dose should be reduced.
- **Bradycardia and weight gain:** Monitor heart rate and weight daily.
- **Hepatitis:** Monitor for anorexia, pruritis, right upper quadrant pain, and jaundice.
- **Rash:** Assess skin for rash, pruritus, and lymphadenopathy.
- **Bleeding and infection:** Note if invasive sites or gums are bleeding; check for hematuria; evaluate fever, sore throat, malaise, or areas causing discomfort.
- **Patient education:** Caution against exceeding the prescribed dosage. Explain how to space doses evenly around the clock. Teach how to count the resting pulse daily to monitor therapeutic drug effects. Urge restriction of iodine products and seafood. Instruct to report immediately illness or unusual bleeding or bruising to a health care provider. Instruct female patients to report promptly pregnancy or possible pregnancy to a health care provider.

SERIOUS ADVERSE REACTIONS

- **Bone marrow suppression:** Agranulocytosis as long as 4 mo after therapy, pancytopenia, leukopenia, thrombocytopenia, aplastic anemia, lupuslike syndrome.
- **Hypoprothrombinemia:** Low levels of prothrombin, which may lead to bleeding.

M

OVERDOSE/TOXICITY
- **Hepatotoxicity:** Fulminant hepatitis, hepatic necrosis, encephalopathy, death.
- **Insulin autoimmune syndrome:** Hypoglycemia that can result in hypoglycemic coma.
- **Nephrotoxicity:** Nephritis with elevated BUN and creatinine occurs rarely.
- **Management:** Discontinue methimazole immediately and treat symptoms using accepted protocols for supportive care.
- **GI decontamination:** No specific recommendations.

ANTIDOTE/DIALYSIS
- **Antidote:** No specific recommendations.
- **Dialysis:** Methimazole is not removed by hemodialysis or peritoneal dialysis. No data are available on removal using high-permeability hemodialysis.

methocarbamol

meth-oh-kar'-ba-mole

Classes
Chemical: carbamate derivative
Therapeutic: skeletal muscle relaxant

Pregnancy Category: C

Trade Names
Prescription: Carbacot, Robaxin

Combinations
Prescription: with aspirin (Robaxisal)

CLINICAL PHARMACOLOGY

Mechanism of Action

A carbamate derivative of guaifenesin that causes skeletal muscle relaxation by general CNS depression. **Therapeutic Effect:** Relieves muscle spasticity.

PHARMACOKINETICS

Rapidly and almost completely absorbed from the GI tract. Protein binding: 46%-50%. Metabolized in the liver by dealkylation and hydroxylation. Primarily excreted in urine as metabolites. **Half-life:** 1-2 hr.

AVAILABILITY

Injection: 100 mg/mL (Robaxin).
Tablets: 325 mg, 500 mg (Carbacot, Robaxin), 750 mg (Carbacot).

INDICATIONS AND DOSAGE

Musculoskeletal spasm

IM/IV

Adults, Children 16 yr and older: 1 g every 8 hr for no more than 3 consecutive days. May repeat course of therapy after a drug-free interval of 48 hr.

PO

Adults, Children 16 yr and older: 1.5 g 4 times/day for 2-3 days (up to 8 g/day may be given in severe conditions). Decrease to 4-4.5 g/day in 3-6 divided doses. **Elderly:** Initially 500 mg 4 times per day. May gradually increase dosage.

Tetanus spasm

IV

Adults: 1-3 g every 6 hr until oral dosing is possible. Injection should be used no more than 3 consecutive days. **Children:** 15 mg/kg/dose or 500 mg/m^2/dose every 6 hr as needed. Maximum: 1.8 g/m^2/day for 3 days only.

CONTRAINDICATIONS

Hypersensitivity to methocarbamol or any component of the formulation, renal impairment (injection formulation)

INTERACTIONS

Drug: CNS depressants, including alcohol: May potentiate effects when used with other CNS depressants, including alcohol. **Herbal: Gotu kola, kava kava, St. John's wort:** May increase CNS depression. **Food:** None known.

DIAGNOSTIC TEST EFFECTS

None known.

SIDE-EFFECTS

Frequent: Transient drowsiness, weakness, dizziness, lightheadedness, nausea, vomiting. **Occasional:** Headache, constipation, anorexia, hypotension, confusion, blurred vision, vertigo, facial flushing, rash. **Rare:** Paradoxic CNS excitement and restlessness, slurred speech, tremor, dry mouth, diarrhea, nocturia, impotence, bradycardia, hypotension, syncope

CRITICAL CARE CONSIDERATIONS

ADMINISTRATION/HANDLING

PO ALERT
- Give methocarbamol without regard to meals.
- Tablets may be crushed and mixed with food or liquid or given by nasogastric (NG) tube if needed.

IM ALERT
- Blood aspirated into the syringe will not mix with the medication. Maximum of 5

mL can be administered into each gluteal region.

IV ALERT

- **Storage:** Store at controlled room temperature.
- **IV push/direct injection:** May be administered undiluted as a direct intravenous bolus at a maximum rate of 3 mL/min. Solution should be hypertonic.
- **Dilution:** May dilute 1 g of methocarbamol to no more than 250 mL with IV solutions. Do not refrigerate after dilution.
- **Recumbent position:** Administer IV at no faster than 300 mg/min while in recumbent position. Adjust infusion for comfort. Maintain position for 15-30 min following infusion to avoid orthostatic hypotension.
- **Duration:** Do not use for more than 3 consecutive days.

PRECAUTIONS

HEALTH-RELATED

- Use oral formulation cautiously in patients with renal or hepatic impairment.
- Use injectable formulation cautiously in patients with a history of seizures or hepatic impairment.
- **Myasthenia gravis:** Use with caution in patients with myasthenia gravis receiving anticholinesterase agents (e.g., pyridostigmine [Neostigmine]) as effects of these agents are reduced by methocarbamol.

AGE-RELATED

- **Children:** Safety and efficacy of methocarbamol has not been established in children under 16 yr. Not recommended for children under 12 yr except in tetanus.
- **Elderly:** Are at increased risk of CNS toxicity (confusion, hallucinations, mental depression, and sedation); age-related renal impairment may require a decreased dosage. Men may experience more anticholinergic effects (dry mouth, urinary retention).

PREGNANCY/LACTATION-RELATED

- Pregnancy category C; compatible with breast-feeding.

MONITORING

- **Baseline assessment:** Assess duration, location, onset, and type of muscular spasm. Evaluate for immobility, stiffness, or swelling. Obtain history including allergies.
- **Baseline lab work:** Biochemical profile including renal (BUN and creatinine) and liver function (AST [SGOT], ALT [SGPT], alkaline phosphatase, bilirubin) studies; CBC with WBC differential. Monitor periodically throughout therapy.
- **Skin/limb assessment:** Monitor for pain at injection site, thrombophlebitis, or sloughing of tissue, indicative of extravasation.
- **Therapeutic response:** Evaluate for decreased intensity of skeletal muscle pain.
- **Patient education:** Explain the side effect of drowsiness usually diminishes with continued therapy. Warn to avoid tasks that require mental alertness or motor skills until response to the drug is known. Caution against abruptly discontinuing methocarbamol after long-term therapy. Urge avoidance of alcohol and CNS depressants.

SERIOUS ADVERSE REACTIONS

- Anaphylactoid reactions, leukopenia, and seizures (IV form) have been reported. Epinephrine, antihistamines, and steroids are used to manage anaphylaxis.

OVERDOSE/TOXICITY

- **Overdose:** Dysrhythmias, bradycardia, nausea, vomiting, drowsiness, and coma.
- **Management:** Maintain patent airway, support ventilation and BP.
- **GI decontamination:** No specific recommendations.

ANTIDOTE/DIALYSIS

- **Antidote:** No specific recommendations.
- **Dialysis:** No data are available on removal of methocarbamol by hemodialysis, peritoneal dialysis, or high-permeability hemodialysis.

M

methsuximide

See Anticonvulsants (p. 903)

methylcellulose

meth-ill-sell'-you-lose

Classes

Chemical: hydrophilic semisynthetic cellulose derivative

Therapeutic: laxative

Pregnancy Category: B

Trade Names

Over the Counter: Citrucel, Cologel

Do not confuse Citrucel with Citracal.

CLINICAL PHARMACOLOGY

Mechanism of Action

A bulk-forming laxative that dissolves and expands in water. **Therapeutic Effect:** Provides increased bulk and moisture content in stool, increasing peristalsis and bowel motility.

PHARMACOKINETICS

Route	Onset	Peak	Duration
PO	12-24 hr	N/A	N/A

Acts in small and large intestines. Full effect may not be evident for 2-3 days.

AVAILABILITY

Powder (Citrucel, Cologel).

INDICATIONS AND DOSAGE

Constipation

PO

Adults, Elderly: 1 tbsp (15 mL) in 8 oz water 1-3 times per day. **Children 6-12 yr:** 1 tsp (5 mL) in 8 oz water 1-3 times per day.

CONTRAINDICATIONS

Abdominal pain, dysphagia, nausea, partial bowel obstruction, symptoms of appendicitis, vomiting, hypersensitivity to methylcellulose

M

INTERACTIONS

Drug: Digoxin, oral anticoagulants, salicylates: May decrease the effects of digoxin, oral anticoagulants, and salicylates by decreasing absorption of these drugs. **Potassium-sparing diuretics, potassium supplements:** May interfere with the effects of potassium-sparing diuretics and potassium supplements. **Herbal:** None known. **Food:** None known.

DIAGNOSTIC TEST EFFECTS

May increase blood glucose level. May decrease serum potassium level.

SIDE-EFFECTS

Rare: Some degree of abdominal discomfort, nausea, mild cramps, griping, faintness

CRITICAL CARE CONSIDERATIONS

ADMINISTRATION/HANDLING

PO ALERT

- Drink 6-8 glasses of water per day to aid in stool softening.
- Methylcellulose should not be swallowed in dry form but should be mixed with at least 1 full glass (8 oz) of liquid.

PRECAUTIONS

HEALTH-RELATED

- Use methylcellulose with caution in patients with hypoactive bowel sounds, distended and painful abdomen because this may signal ileus or bowel obstruction.

AGE-RELATED

- **Children:** Safety and efficacy of methylcellulose have not been established in children under 6 yr. Methylcellulose use is not recommended in this age group.
- **Elderly:** No age-related precautions have been noted in the elderly.

PREGNANCY/LACTATION-RELATED

- Pregnancy category B. Bulk-forming laxatives are the laxative of choice during pregnancy; compatible with breast-feeding.

MONITORING

- **Baseline assessment:** Before methylcellulose administration, assess abdomen for signs of tenderness, rigidity, and the presence of bowel sounds. Try to determine when the last bowel movement occurred and find out the amount and consistency. Assess hydration status.
- **Baseline lab work:** Biochemical panel including electrolytes. Monitor serum electrolyte levels periodically in patients with excessive, frequent, or prolonged use of methylcellulose.
- **Ileus:** Assess bowel sounds for peristalsis. Assess pattern of daily bowel activity, stool consistency, and record time of evacuation.
- **Patient education:** Advise to institute measures to promote defecation, such as increasing fluid intake, exercising, and eating a high-fiber diet. Instruct to take each dose with a full glass of water. Warn that taking methylcellulose with an inadequate amount of fluid may cause choking or swelling in the throat. Encourage maintenance of adequate fluid intake.

SERIOUS ADVERSE REACTIONS

- Esophageal or bowel obstruction may occur if administered with less than 250 mL or 1 full glass of liquid.

OVERDOSE/TOXICITY

- Methylcellulose is not absorbed systemically. In large amounts, may cause bowel obstruction.
- **GI decontamination:** No specific recommendations.

ANTIDOTE/DIALYSIS

- **Antidote:** No specific recommendations.
- **Dialysis:** Methylcellulose is bulk forming inside the GI tract and is not absorbed systemically into the blood stream.

methylclothiazide

See Diuretics (p. 956)

methyldopa

See Antihypertensives, Miscellaneous (p. 931)

methylphenidate hydrochloride

meth-ill-fen'-i-date hye-droe-klor'-ide

DEA Schedule: II

Classes

Chemical: piperidine derivative of amphetamine

Therapeutic: cerebral stimulant

Pregnancy Category: C

Trade Names

Prescription: Concerta, Daytrana, Metadate CD, Metadate ER, Methylin, Methylin ER, Ritalin, Ritalin LA, Ritalin SR

Do not confuse Ritalin with Rifadin.

CLINICAL PHARMACOLOGY

Mechanism of Action

A CNS stimulant that blocks the reuptake of norepinephrine and *DOPamine into presynaptic neurons. **Therapeutic Effect:** Decreases motor restlessness and fatigue; increases motor activity, attention span, and mental alertness; produces mild euphoria.

PHARMACOKINETICS

Onset	Peak	Duration
Immediate release	2 hr	3-5 hr
Sustained release	4-7 hr	8 hr
Extended release	N/A	8-12 hr

Slowly and incompletely absorbed from the GI tract. Protein binding: 0%-33%. Metabolized in the liver. Eliminated in urine and in feces by biliary system. **Half-life:** 2-4 hr.

AVAILABILITY

Capsules (extended release): 10 mg (Metadate CD, Ritalin LA), 20 mg (Metadate CD, Ritalin LA), 30 mg (Metadate CD, Ritalin LA), 40 mg (Metadate CD, Ritalin LA), 50 mg (Metadate CD), 60 mg (Metadate CD).
Tablets (Ritalin): 5 mg, 10 mg, 20 mg.
Tablets (extended release): 10 mg (Metadate ER, Methylin ER), 18 mg (Concerta), 20 mg (Metadate ER, Methylin ER), 27 mg (Concerta), 36 mg (Concerta), 54 mg (Concerta), 72 mg (Concerta).
Tablets (sustained release [Ritalin SR]): 20 mg.
Tablets (chewable [Methylin]): 2.5 mg, 5 mg, 10 mg.
Oral solution (Methylin): 5 mg/5 mL, 10 mg/5 mL.
Topical patch (Daytrana): 10 mg/9 hr, 15 mg/9 hr, 20 mg/9 hr, 30 mg/9 hr.

INDICATIONS AND DOSAGE

Attention-deficit/hyperactivity disorder (ADHD)

PO (Immediate release)

Children 6 yr and older: Initially 2.5-5 mg before breakfast and lunch. May increase by 5-10 mg/day at weekly intervals. Maximum: 90 mg/day or 2 mg/kg/day.

PO (Concerta)

Children 6 yr and older: Initially 18 mg once per day; may increase by 18 mg/day at weekly intervals. Maximum: 72 mg/day (13-17 yr). Maximum: 54 mg/day (6-12 yr).

PO (Metadate CD)

Children 6 yr and older: Initially 20 mg/day. May increase by 10-20 mg/day at weekly intervals. Maximum: 60 mg/day.

PO (Ritalin LA)

Children 6 yr and older: Initially 20 mg/day. May increase by 10-20 mg/day at weekly intervals. Maximum: 60 mg/day.

PO (Metadate ER, Methylin ER, Ritalin SR)

Children 6 yr and older: May replace regular tablets after daily dose is titrated and 8-hr dosage corresponds to sustained-release or extended-release tablet size.

Topical patch (Daytrana)

Children: 10 mg once daily. Applied once per day and worn for 9 hr. Apply patch 2 hr before desired effect. Increase to next transdermal dose at weekly intervals.

Narcolepsy

PO

Adults, Elderly: 10 mg 2-3 times per day. Range: 10-60 mg/day.

M

OFF-LABEL USES

Treatment of disease-related fatigue, secondary mental depression

CONTRAINDICATIONS

Use within 14 days of MAOIs, hypersensitivity to methylphenidate, glaucoma

INTERACTIONS

Drug: MAOIs: May increase the effects of methylphenidate. **Other CNS stimulants:** May have an additive effect. **Herbal:** None known. **Food:** None known.

DIAGNOSTIC TEST EFFECTS

None known.

SIDE-EFFECTS

Frequent: Anxiety, insomnia, decreased appetite, nausea. **Occasional:** Dizziness, drowsiness, headache, nausea, abdominal pain, fever, rash, arthralgia, vomiting. **Rare:** Blurred vision, Tourette syndrome (marked by uncontrolled vocal outbursts, repetitive body movements, and tics), palpitations

CRITICAL CARE CONSIDERATIONS

M

ADMINISTRATION/HANDLING

PO ALERT

- Sustained- and extended-release tablets may be given in place of regular tablets once daily dose is titrated using regular tablets, and if titrated dosage corresponds to the sustained- or extended-release tablet strength.
- Give methylphenidate 30 to 45 min before meals (usually before breakfast and lunch). Give last dose before 6 PM to help prevent insomnia.
- Crush regular tablets as needed; do not crush or break extended-release capsules. May open Metadate CD capsule and sprinkle pellets on food.
- Ritalin LA has two distinct peaks of action approximately 4 hr apart.

PRECAUTIONS

HEALTH-RELATED

- Use methylphenidate cautiously in patients with hypertension, seizures, acute stress reaction, emotional instability, or a history of drug dependence.
- Methylphenidate should not be used for severe depression or to manage normal fatigue states. Clinical experience suggests administration of drug to psychotic patients may exacerbate thought and behavioral disorders. Drug may lower seizure threshold. BP and heart rate may increase in patients who may be compromised such as those with recent acute MI, preexisting hypertension, heart failure, or hyperthyroidism.

AGE-RELATED

- **Children:** Safety and efficacy of methylphenidate have not been established in children under 6 yr. Children are more prone to develop abdominal pain, anorexia, weight loss, and insomnia. Long-term methylphenidate use may inhibit growth.
- **Elderly:** No age-related precautions have been noted.

PREGNANCY/LACTATION-RELATED

- Pregnancy category C. Unknown if excreted in human breast milk.

MONITORING

- **Baseline assessment:** Obtain baseline height and weight; weigh patient regularly to detect delayed growth in children.
- **Baseline lab work:** CBC with WBC differential and platelet count before starting therapy and routinely during therapy.
- **Therapeutic effect:** Evaluate for improvement in attention span, ability to focus, and ability to sit quietly. Discontinue methylphenidate or reduce dosage if symptoms of ADHD return.
- **Patient education:** Instruct to take the last dose of methylphenidate before 6 PM to avoid insomnia. Caution against discontinuing the drug abruptly after prolonged use. Warn to avoid tasks that require mental alertness or motor skills until response to the drug is known. Instruct to report promptly fever, anxiety, chest discomfort, palpitations, rash, vomiting, or (for those with a seizure disorder) an increase in the number of seizures to a health care provider. Urge avoidance of caffeinated beverages during methylphenidate therapy. Suggest taking sips of water and chewing sugarless gum to relieve dry mouth.

SERIOUS ADVERSE REACTIONS

- **Growth delay:** Prolonged administration to children with ADHD may delay growth.
- **Visual disturbances:** Blurred vision and difficulty with accommodation.

- **Hypersensitivity reactions:** Rash, exfoliative dermatitis, fever, arthralgia, necrotizing vasculitis, and erythema multiforme.
- **Blood dyscrasias:** Leukopenia, anemia, and thrombocytopenic purpura.

OVERDOSE/TOXICITY

- **Overdose:** May produce tachycardia, palpitations, dysrhythmias, chest pain, frank psychotic episode, seizures, and coma.
- **Withdrawal:** Severe depression may result after withdrawal of methylphenidate following abusive use. Symptoms of original disorder may reemerge after stopping therapeutic use. Careful supervision is required.
- **GI decontamination:** No specific recommendations.

ANTIDOTE/DIALYSIS

- **Antidote:** No specific recommendations.
- **Dialysis:** Methylphenidate is unlikely to be removed using hemodialysis or peritoneal dialysis. No data are available on removal using high-permeability hemodialysis.

*methylPREDNISolone/ *methylPREDNISolone acetate/ *methylPREDNISolone sodium succinate

meth-ill-pred-niss'-oh-lone

Classes

Chemical: glucocorticoid, synthetic
Therapeutic: corticosteroid, systemic

Pregnancy Category: C

Trade Names

Prescription: Adlone-40, Adlone-80, A-Methapred, Depmedalone, Dep Medalone 80, Depoject-80, Depo-Medrol, Depopred, Med-Jec-40, Medralone 80, Medrol, Medrol Dosepak, Methacort 40, Methacort 80, Methylcotol, Methylcotolone, Methylpred DP, Solu-Medrol

Do not confuse *methylPREDNISolone with *medroxyPROGESTERone, or Medrol with Mebaral.

CLINICAL PHARMACOLOGY

Mechanism of Action

An adrenocortical steroid that suppresses migration of polymorphonuclear leukocytes and reverses increased capillary permeability. **Therapeutic Effect:** Decreases inflammation.

PHARMACOKINETICS

Route	Onset	Peak	Duration
PO	N/A	1-2 hr	30-36 hr
IM	N/A	4-8 days	1-4 week

Well absorbed after IM administration. Widely distributed. Metabolized in the liver. Excreted in urine. Removed by hemodialysis. **Half-life:** 3.5 hr.

AVAILABILITY

Tablets (Medrol, Medrol Dosepak, Methylpred DP): 2 mg, 4 mg, 8 mg, 16 mg, 32 mg.
Injection powder for reconstitution (A-Methapred, Solu-Medrol): 40 mg, 125 mg, 500 mg, 1 g.
Injection suspension: 20 mg/mL (Depo-Medrol), 40 mg/mL (Adlone-40, Depo-Medrol, Depopred, Depmedalone, Med-Jec-40, Methylcotol), 80 mg/mL (Adlone-80, Depmedalone, Dep Medalone 80, Depoject-80, Depopred, Depo-Medrol, Medralone 80, Methacort 80, Methylcotolone).

INDICATIONS AND DOSAGE

Antiinflammatory, immunosuppressive

IM (acetate)
Adults, Elderly: 10-80 mg every 1-2 wk.
IM (sodium succinate)
Adults, Elderly: 10-80 mg/day once daily.
IV
Adults, Elderly: 10-40 mg. May repeat as needed at 4- to 6-hr intervals. **Children:** 0.5-1.7 mg/kg/day or 5-25 mg/m^2/day in 2-4 divided doses.
PO
Adults, Elderly: 2-60 mg/day in 1-4 divided doses. **Children:** 0.5-1.7 mg/kg/day or 5-25 mg/m^2/day in 2-4 divided doses.

Status asthmaticus

IV (sodium succinate)
Adults, Elderly, Children: Initially, 2 mg/kg/dose, then 0.5-1 mg/kg/dose every 6 hr for up to 5 days.

Spinal cord injury

IV Bolus (sodium succinate)
Adults, Elderly: 30 mg/kg over 15 min. Maintenance dose: 5.4 mg/kg/h over 23 hr, to be given within 45 min of bolus dose.

Intraarticular, intralesional

IV (acetate)
Adults, Elderly: 20-60 mg, up to 80 mg every 1-5 wk or 20-80 mg (large joints) or 4-10 mg (small joints).

CONTRAINDICATIONS

Administration of live virus vaccines, systemic fungal infection, hypersensitivity to *methylPREDNISolone or related products

INTERACTIONS

Drug: Diuretics, insulin, oral hypoglycemics, potassium supplements: May decrease the effects of these drugs. **Hepatic enzyme inducers:** May decrease the effects of *methylPREDNISolone. **Live-virus vaccines:** May decrease antibody response to vaccine, increase vaccine side effects, and potentiate virus replication. **Herbal:** None known. **Food:** None known.

DIAGNOSTIC TEST EFFECTS

May increase blood cholesterol, glucose and serum lipid, amylase, and sodium levels. May decrease serum calcium, potassium, and thyroxine levels.

IV INCOMPATIBILITIES

Ciprofloxacin (Cipro), diltiazem (Cardizem), docetaxel (Taxotere), etoposide (VePesid), filgrastim (Neupogen), gemcitabine (Gemzar), paclitaxel (Taxol), potassium chloride, propofol (Diprivan), vinorelbine (Navelbine)

M

IV COMPATIBILITIES

*DOPamine (Intropin), heparin, midazolam (Versed), theophylline

SIDE-EFFECTS

Frequent: Insomnia, heartburn, anxiety, abdominal distention, diaphoresis, acne, mood swings, increased appetite, facial flushing, GI distress, delayed wound healing, increased susceptibility to infection, diarrhea, or constipation. **Occasional:** Headache, edema, tachycardia, change in skin color, frequent urination, depression. **Rare:** Psychosis, increased blood coagulability, hallucinations

CRITICAL CARE CONSIDERATIONS

ADMINISTRATION/HANDLING

PO ALERT

- Give *methylPREDNISolone with food or milk.
- Give single doses before 9 AM; give multiple doses at evenly spaced intervals. Individualize dosage based on the disease, patient, and response.

IV ALERT

- **Storage:** Store vials at room temperature.
- **Mix-o-Vial:** Follow package directions.
- **IV push/direct injection:** Add to D_5W or 0.9% NaCl. Give IV push over 2-3 min.
- **IV infusion:** Add to D_5W or 0.9% NaCl. Give IV piggyback over 10-20 min.
- ***MethylPREDNISolone acetate:** Do not give via IV line.

IM ALERT

- ***MethylPREDNISolone acetate:** Should not be further diluted.
- ***MethylPREDNISolone sodium succinate:** Reconstitute with bacteriostatic water for injection.
- **Administration:** Give deep IM injection into gluteus maximus.

PRECAUTIONS

HEALTH-RELATED

- Use *methylPREDNISolone cautiously in patients with cirrhosis, heart failure, diabetes mellitus, hypertension, hypothyroidism, thromboembolic disorders, or ulcerative colitis.
- **Hepatic enzyme inducers:** Patients receiving phenytoin, phenobarbital, rifampin (increase clearance of cortisone) may require an increased dose of *methylPREDNISolone.
- **Troleandomycin and ketoconazole:** Decrease clearance of cortisone; patients receiving these drugs may require decreased doses of *methylPREDNISolone.
- **Anticoagulants:** Effects on blood coagulation may increase or decrease when *methylPREDNISolone is administered with anticoagulants.
- **High dose aspirin** (cortisone increases clearance): Patients receiving chronic therapy may require higher doses of aspirin. Salicylate toxicity may occur if aspirin dose is not decreased when *methylPREDNISolone is decreased. Aspirin should be used cautiously with *methylPREDNISolone in patients with hypoprothrombinemia to avoid bleeding.

AGE-RELATED

- **Children:** Prolonged treatment or high dosages may decrease cortisol secretion and short-term growth rate in children.
- **Elderly:** Reduced muscle mass may indicate reduced dose is needed. Risk of osteoporosis and hypertension is increased. Avoid aluminum-based antacids to reduce risk of Alzheimer's disease.

PREGNANCY/LACTATION-RELATED

- Pregnancy category C; excreted in breast milk; could suppress infant's growth and interfere with endogenous corticosteroid production.

MONITORING

- **Baseline assessment:** Determine hypersensitivity to corticosteroids and if diabetes mellitus is present. Obtain vital signs, height, and weight. Antidiabetic drug regimen may need alteration to manage steroid-induced hyperglycemia.
- **Baseline lab work:** Biochemical panel including blood glucose and serum electrolyte levels. Determine serum digoxin level if patient is taking digoxin.
- **Adjusted drug doses:** If patients had drug dosages increased or decreased due to *methylPREDNISolone administration, when drug is withdrawn, ensure other medication doses are readjusted to avoid toxicity or ineffective levels of the other medications.
- **Hyperglycemia:** Determine if diabetes mellitus is present. Increase antidiabetic drug regimen if blood glucose becomes elevated.
- **Infection:** Be alert for infection caused by reduced immune response, including fever, sore throat, and vague symptoms.
- **Weight gain/BP elevation:** Monitor for salt and fluid retention-induced weight gain, edema, and increase in BP.
- **Hypokalemia:** Monitor ECG for dysrhythmias induced by increased potassium excretion such as premature ventricular beats, and ventricular and supraventricular tachycardias.
- **Electrolyte imbalance:** Monitor for hypocalcemia (muscle twitching, cramps, and positive Chvostek's or Trousseau's signs), or hypokalemia (ECG changes, nausea and vomiting, irritability, weakness and muscle cramps, numbness and tingling, especially in lower extremities).
- **Avoid adrenal insufficiency:** Wean cortisone slowly to discontinue both aggressive short-term and prolonged therapy.
- **GI bleeding:** Monitor for tarry or bloody stools, coffee-ground emesis or drainage from nasogastric (NG) tubes, hematemesis, or bloody NG tube drainage.
- **Sleep disturbance and emotional lability:** Assess sleep pattern and emotional status; drug may cause sleeplessness, euphoria, high energy, or labile emotional state. Inform patients that cortisone often causes mood swings.
- **Patient education:** When using *methylPREDNISolone outside the hospital, instruct to take it exactly as prescribed (not to change the dosage or schedule). Instruct to take oral *methylPREDNISolone with food or milk. Caution against abruptly discontinuing the drug because *methylPREDNISolone must be withdrawn gradually under medical supervision. Instruct to report promptly fever, muscle aches, sore throat, and sudden weight gain or swelling to a health care provider and to inform the dentist and other physicians about taking/having taken *methylPREDNISolone within the past 12 mo. Stress to maintain good personal hygiene and to avoid exposure to disease or trauma. Explain that severe stress, such as serious infection, surgery, or trauma, may require an increase in *methylPREDNISolone dosage. Stress that follow-up visits and laboratory tests are a necessary part of treatment and that children must be assessed for growth retardation.

SERIOUS ADVERSE REACTIONS

- **Long-term therapy:** May cause hypocalcemia, hypokalemia, muscle wasting (especially in arms and legs), osteoporosis, spontaneous fractures, amenorrhea, subcapsular cataracts, glaucoma, eye infections, peptic ulcer disease, and heart failure.
- **Abrupt withdrawal after long-term therapy:** May cause anorexia, nausea, fever, headache, sudden severe myalgia, rebound inflammation, fatigue, weakness, lethargy, dizziness, and orthostatic hypotension.

OVERDOSE/TOXICITY

- **Cushing's syndrome:** May be unavoidable and should resolve if medication dose can be reduced or discontinued. Syndrome reflects fluid retention, muscle wasting, possible hyperglycemia, vascular fragility which leads to bleeding and easy bruising, abnormal fat distribution, and the classic "moon face."
- **Severe hyperglycemia:** May occur if blood glucose is not monitored and managed appropriately. Thick blood viscosity secondary to associated dehydration may lead to thrombus formation and embolism.
- **Severe behavioral changes:** Extreme euphoria, personality changes, severe depression, frank psychosis (more likely in patients with mental health history).
- **Severe infection:** Patients who have underlying infection or acquire a significant infection may develop fatal septic shock.

M

- **Steroid-induced myopathy:** Generalized acute myopathy has been seen with high-dose steroids, more often in patients with neuromuscular degenerative diseases (myasthenia gravis) and those receiving neuromuscular blocking agents.
- **GI decontamination:** No specific recommendations.

ANTIDOTE/DIALYSIS

- **Antidote:** No specific recommendations.
- **Dialysis:** *MethylPREDNISolone is removed by hemodialysis and is likely removed by high-permeability hemodialysis. No data are available on removal using peritoneal dialysis.

metoclopramide hydrochloride

met-oh-kloe'-pra-mide hye-droe-klor'-ide

Classes

Chemical: para-aminobenzoic acid derivative

Therapeutic: antiemetic, gastrointestinal prokinetic agent

M

Pregnancy Category: B

Trade Names

Prescription: Apo-Metoclop ♣, Reglan

Do not confuse Reglan with Renagel.

CLINICAL PHARMACOLOGY

Mechanism of Action

A dopamine receptor antagonist that stimulates motility of the upper GI tract and decreases reflux into the esophagus. Also raises the threshold of activity in the chemoreceptor trigger zone. **Therapeutic Effect:** Accelerates intestinal transit and gastric emptying; relieves nausea and vomiting.

PHARMACOKINETICS

Route	Onset	Peak	Duration
PO	30-60 min	1-2 hr	2 hr
IV	1-3 min	N/A	N/A
IM	10-15 min	N/A	3 hr

Well absorbed from the GI tract. Metabolized in the liver. Protein binding: 30%. Primarily excreted in urine. Not removed by hemodialysis. **Half-life:** 4-6 hr.

AVAILABILITY

Syrup: 5 mg/5 mL.
Tablets: 5 mg, 10 mg.
Injection: 5 mg/mL.

INDICATIONS AND DOSAGE

Prevention of chemotherapy-induced nausea and vomiting

IV

Adults, Elderly, Children: 1-2 mg/kg 30 min before chemotherapy; repeat every 2 hr for 2 doses, then every 3 hr as needed for total of 5 doses/day.

Postoperative nausea, vomiting

IV

Elderly: 5 mg near end of surgery. **Adults:** 10 mg near end of surgery. **Children less than 14 yr:** 0.1-0.2 mg/kg/dose every 6-8 hr as needed.

Diabetic gastroparesis

PO, IV

Adults: 10 mg 30 min before meals and at bedtime for 2-8 wk.

PO

Elderly: Initially, 5 mg 30 min before meals and at bedtime. May increase to 10 mg.

IV

Elderly: 10 mg over 1-2 min.

Symptomatic gastroesophageal reflux

PO

Adults: 10-15 mg up to 4 times per day, or single doses up to 20 mg as needed. **Elderly:** Initially 5 mg 4 times per day. May increase to 10 mg. **Children:** 0.4-0.8 mg/kg/day in 4 divided doses.

To facilitate small bowel intubation (single dose)

IV

Adults, Elderly: 10 mg as a single dose. **Children 6-14 yr:** 2.5-5 mg as a single dose. **Children younger than 6 yr:** 0.1 mg/kg as a single dose.

Dosage in renal impairment

Dosage is modified based on creatinine clearance.

Creatinine Clearance	% of normal dose
50 mL/min	100%
10-50 mL/min	75%
Less than 10 mL/min	50%

OFF-LABEL USES

Prevention of aspiration pneumonia; treatment of drug-related postoperative nausea and vomiting, gastric stasis in preterm infants, persistent hiccups, slow gastric emptying, vascular headaches

CONTRAINDICATIONS

Concurrent use of medications likely to produce extrapyramidal reactions, GI hemorrhage, GI obstruction or perforation, history of seizure disorders, pheochromocytoma, hypersensitivity to metoclopramide

INTERACTIONS

Drug: Alcohol, other CNS suppressants: May increase CNS depressant effect. **Herbal:** None known. **Food:** None known.

DIAGNOSTIC TEST EFFECTS

May increase serum aldosterone and prolactin concentrations.

IV INCOMPATIBILITIES

Allopurinol (Aloprim), cefepime (Maxipime), *DOXOrubicin liposomal (Doxil), furosemide (Lasix), propofol (Diprivan)

IV COMPATIBILITIES

Dexamethasone, diltiazem (Cardizem), *diphenhydrAMINE (Benadryl), fentanyl (Sublimaze), heparin, hydromorphone (Dilaudid), morphine, potassium chloride, total parenteral nutrition (TPN)

SIDE-EFFECTS

Frequent (10%): Somnolence, restlessness, fatigue, lethargy. **Occasional (3%):** Dizziness, anxiety, headache, insomnia, breast tenderness, altered menstruation, constipation, rash, dry mouth, galactorrhea, gynecomastia. **Rare (less than 3%):** Hypotension or hypertension, tachycardia

CRITICAL CARE CONSIDERATIONS

ADMINISTRATION/HANDLING

PO ALERT

- Give metoclopramide 30 min before meals and at bedtime.
- Crush tablets as needed.
- Syrup comes in orange-colored, palatable, aromatic, sugar-free liquid.

IM ALERT

- **Storage:** Protect from light. Store at room temperature.
- Use only clear, colorless solution.

IV ALERT

- **Storage:** Store vials at room temperature. Protect from light. Use only clear, colorless solution.
- **Dilution:** Dilute doses greater than 10 mg in 50 mL D_5W, 0.9% NaCl, or lactated Ringer's solution.
- **Stability:** IV piggyback infusion is stable for 24 hr in normal light, 48 hr if protected from light after dilution.
- **Infusion:** Infuse over 15 min.
- **IV push/direct injection:** Give slow IV push of 10 mg over 1 to 2 min. Too-rapid IV injection may produce intense anxiety or restlessness, followed by drowsiness.
- Doses of 2 mg/kg or more, or prolonged therapy, may increase the incidence of side effects.

PRECAUTIONS

HEALTH-RELATED

- Use metoclopramide cautiously in patients with cirrhosis, heart failure, or renal impairment.
- **Postoperative nausea/vomiting:** Decision to use nasogastric tube versus metoclopramide in postoperative GI surgical patients should consider increased peristalsis from drug may place additional pressure on new gastric or bowel anastomosis sites.

AGE-RELATED

- **Children:** Children are more susceptible to dystonic reactions. Pharmacokinetics are highly variable in neonates and children. Safety profile is not fully established. Prolonged clearance in neonates may markedly elevate serum concentrations. May cause methemoglobinemia in premature and full-term neonates at doses greater than 0.5 mg/kg daily (24 hr).
- **Elderly:** More likely to have parkinsonian reactions and dyskinesias after long-term therapy.

PREGNANCY/LACTATION-RELATED

- Pregnancy category B. Has been used during pregnancy as an antiemetic and to decrease gastric emptying time. Excreted into milk; use during lactation a concern because of the potent CNS effects the drug is capable of producing.

MONITORING

- **Baseline assessment:** Assess vital signs and nutritional and hydration status.
- **Baseline lab work:** Biochemical panel including blood glucose level, BUN, and creatinine. For diabetic patients, hemoglobin $A1_C$ may help to assess compliance with glycemic control measures.
- **Dehydration:** Monitor patients taking metoclopramide as an antiemetic for dehydration (dry mucous membranes, longitudinal furrows in the tongue, and poor skin turgor).
- **Fluid retention:** Monitor for fluid retention in patients with heart failure, renal failure, or cirrhosis as the transient increase in aldosterone prompted by metoclopramide may induce volume overload.

M

- **Neurologic effects:** Monitor for anxiety, extrapyramidal symptoms, and restlessness during IV administration. Pretreatment with *diphenhydrAMINE may decrease extrapyramidal symptoms.
- **Diarrhea:** Assess pattern of daily bowel activity and stool consistency.
- **Hypersensitivity:** Assess for rash.
- **Gastroparesis:** Evaluate patients with gastroparesis for a therapeutic response including relief of bloating, nausea, and vomiting.
- **Patient education:** Warn to avoid tasks that require mental alertness or motor skills until response to the drug is known. Instruct to promptly report involuntary eye, facial, or limb movement to a health care provider. Urge avoidance of alcohol during metoclopramide therapy.

SERIOUS ADVERSE REACTIONS

- **Tardive dyskinesia:** Uncontrolled tongue, mouth, eye, facial, body/trunk, and extremity movements may occur with long-term use.
- **Extrapyramidal reactions:** Occur most commonly in children and young adults (18-30 yr) receiving large doses (2 mg/kg) during chemotherapy and are usually limited to akathisia (involuntary limb movement and facial grimacing).
- **Mental depression:** Mild to severe symptoms, including suicidal ideation, have occurred in patients without prior history of depression.
- **Methemoglobinemia:** Seen most often in premature and full-term neonates given metoclopramide. Methemoglobin does not transport oxygen; initially, generalized cyanosis is seen with a normal PO_2 and is unresponsive to oxygen, followed by dyspnea, tachypnea, tachycardia, mild hypertension, cyanosis, seizures, hypotension, ventricular dysrhythmias, headache, confusion, lactic acidosis. Methylene blue (1% solution) is the antidote given IV at 2 mg/kg initially in patients without glucose6-phosphate dehydrogenase (G6PD) deficiency. Methemoglobin appears chocolate brown in the blood.

OVERDOSE/TOXICITY

- **Neuroleptic malignant syndrome (NMS):** Hyperreflexia, muscle rigidity, altered mental status, autonomic nervous system irritability (labile BP, erratic heart rate, irregular pulse, tachycardia, dysrhythmias, diaphoresis), and fever.
- **Rhabdomyolysis:** May result if muscle rigidity and fever are not controlled. May lead to renal and respiratory failures, disseminated intravascular coagulation (DIC), and cardiovascular collapse.
- **Management:** Discontinue metoclopramide and other drugs nonessential to therapy (especially NMS-potentiating drugs including anticholinergics and lithium), aggressively manage symptoms. Maintain patent airway, manage dysrhythmias, reduce fever, support nutritional requirements, possible low-dose heparin to help reduce thromboembolism and manage organ failure per accepted standards.
- **GI decontamination:** No specific recommendations.

ANTIDOTE/DIALYSIS

- **Antidote:** Dantrolene may effectively manage muscle rigidity. dopamine agonists (e.g., bromocriptine, amantidine, carbidopa-levodopa, or levodopa alone) may be given to help manage neuroleptic-induced dopaminergic blockade.
- **Dialysis:** Metoclopramide is not removed using hemodialysis or peritoneal dialysis. No data are available on removal using high-permeability hemodialysis.

metolazone

me-tole'-a-zone

Classes

Chemical: quinazoline derivative

Therapeutic: antihypertensive; diuretic, thiazide-like

Pregnancy Category: B, D

Trade Names

Prescription: Mykrox (rapid acting), Zaroxolyn (slow acting)

Do not confuse metolazone with methazolamide, metoprolol, or miconazole or Zaroxolyn with Zarontin.

CLINICAL PHARMACOLOGY

Mechanism of Action

A thiazide-like diuretic and antihypertensive. As a diuretic, blocks reabsorption of sodium, potassium, and chloride at the distal convoluted tubule, increasing renal excretion of sodium and water. As an antihypertensive, reduces plasma and extracellular fluid volume and peripheral vascular resistance. Therapeutic Effect: Promotes diuresis and reduces BP.

PHARMACOKINETICS

Route	Onset	Peak	Duration
PO (diuretic)	1 hr	2 hr	12-24 hr

Incompletely absorbed from the GI tract. Protein binding: 95%. Primarily excreted unchanged in urine. Not removed by hemodialysis. Half-life: 6-20 hr.

AVAILABILITY

Tablets (prompt release [Mykrox]): 0.5 mg.
Tablets (extended release [Zaroxolyn]): 2.5 mg, 5 mg, 10 mg.

INDICATIONS AND DOSAGE

Edema

PO (Zaroxolyn)

Adults, Elderly: 2.5-20 mg/day. May increase to 20 mg/day in edema associated with renal disease or heart failure. **Children:** 0.2-0.4 mg/kg/day in 1-2 divided doses.

Hypertension

PO (Zaroxolyn)

Adults, Elderly: 2.5-5 mg/day.

PO (Mykrox)

Adults, Elderly: Initially, 0.5 mg/day. May increase up to 1 mg/day.

CONTRAINDICATIONS

Anuria; hepatic coma or precoma; history of hypersensitivity to metolazone, sulfonamides, or thiazide diuretics; renal decompensation

INTERACTIONS

Drug: **Cholestyramine, colestipol:** May decrease the absorption and effects of metolazone. **Digoxin:** May increase the risk of digoxin toxicity associated with metolazone-induced hypokalemia. **Lithium:** May increase the risk of lithium toxicity. Herbal: None known. Food: None known.

DIAGNOSTIC TEST EFFECTS

May increase blood glucose and serum cholesterol, LDL, bilirubin, calcium, creatinine, uric acid, and triglyceride levels. May decrease urinary calcium, and serum magnesium, potassium, and sodium levels.

SIDE-EFFECTS

Expected: Increase in urinary frequency and urine volume. **Frequent (10%-9%):** Dizziness, lightheadedness, headache. **Occasional (6%-4%):** Muscle cramps and spasm, fatigue, lethargy. **Rare (less than 2%):** Asthenia, palpitations, depression, nausea, vomiting, abdominal bloating, constipation, diarrhea, urticaria

CRITICAL CARE CONSIDERATIONS

ADMINISTRATION/HANDLING

PO ALERT

- Give metolazone with food or milk if GI upset occurs, preferably with breakfast to help prevent nocturia.
- Formulations bioequivalent to Zaroxolyn should not be interchanged with formulations bioequivalent to Mykrox because the formulations are not therapeutically equivalent. Mykrox is a more rapidly available and completely bioavailable metolazone formula than is Zaroxolyn.
- Mykrox should not be used for management of fluid retention related to heart failure or renal or hepatic disease because the correct dosage for these conditions and other edema states has not been established.

PRECAUTIONS

HEALTH-RELATED

- Use metolazone cautiously in patients with diabetes, elevated cholesterol and triglyceride levels, gout, hepatic impairment, hypokalemia, lupus erythematosus, or severe renal disease.

AGE-RELATED

- **Children:** Safety and efficacy of metolazone have not been established in children. Use is not recommended.
- **Elderly:** Age-related renal impairment may require cautious use. Elderly may be more sensitive to the drug's electrolyte and hypotensive effects.

PREGNANCY/LACTATION-RELATED

- Pregnancy category B (D if used in pregnancy-induced hypertension). Therapy for preexisting hypertension can be continued throughout pregnancy with minimal risk; initiating for simple edema

M

not recommended. Few unequivocal indications for diuretic therapy in pregnancy except for pulmonary edema or congestive heart failure. Excreted into breast milk in small amounts; considered compatible with breast-feeding.

MONITORING

- **Baseline assessment:** Monitor vital signs for hypotension before giving metolazone. Perform a baseline neurologic and mental status exam. Obtain baseline weight and temperature. Perform hemodynamic readings if pulmonary artery catheter is in place.
- **Baseline lab work:** Biochemical panel including sodium, potassium, magnesium, cholesterol, triglycerides, uric acid, BUN, and creatinine levels. Evaluate the patient for peripheral edema, and check mucous membranes and skin turgor to determine hydration status.
- **Neurologic changes:** Evaluate mental status and muscle strength, which may signal hypokalemia, hyponatremia, or other electrolyte imbalance.
- **Electrolyte disturbances:** Hypokalemia may result in altered mental status, muscle cramps, nausea and vomiting, tachycardia, ventricular dysrhythmias, tremor, and weakness. Hyponatremia may result in cold and clammy skin, confusion, and thirst.
- **Dysrhythmias:** Evaluate continuous ECG for tachycardias, ventricular dysrhythmias, and ST segment depression if patients become dehydrated or hypotensive.
- **Dehydration:** Begin monitoring fluid intake and output. Record amount of diuresis. Note pulmonary artery pressure decreases and right atrial pressure may approach 0-1 mmHg if dehydration is present.
- **Hypotension:** Continue monitoring for tachycardia, decreasing BP, markedly decreased CVP or right atrial pressure, and weight loss. Patients with coronary artery disease are at risk for acute MI if myocardial perfusion is severely decreased.
- **Patient education:** Advise to expect an increase in the frequency and volume of urination. Instruct about the need to change positions slowly and to pause momentarily before standing to reduce orthostatic hypotension. Encourage foods high in potassium such as apricots, bananas, raisins, orange juice, potatoes, legumes, meat, and whole grains (such as cereals).

SERIOUS ADVERSE REACTIONS

- **Cardiovascular:** Chest discomfort, angina, acute MI, orthostatic hypotension, lethal ventricular dysrhythmias including ventricular tachycardia, and ventricular fibrillation may result from hypokalemia or hypomagnesemia.
- **Dehydration/electrolyte imbalance:** Vigorous diuresis may prompt severe water and electrolyte depletion, resulting in hypokalemia and hyponatremia.
- **Hyperuricemia:** May prompt gout in patients who have no history of gout.
- **Gastrointestinal:** Pancreatitis, hepatitis, and cholestatic jaundice occur rarely.
- **Dermatologic:** Necrotizing angitis (cutaneous vasculitis) occurs rarely.
- **Neurologic:** Syncope, neuropathy, vertigo, and paresthesia occur rarely.
- **Hematologic:** Aplastic anemia, agranulocytosis, and leukopenia occur rarely.

OVERDOSE/TOXICITY

- **Overdose:** Lethargy and coma without changes in electrolytes or hydration.
- **Acute hypotensive episodes:** Seen following overly vigorous diuresis.
- **Hyperglycemia:** May occur during prolonged therapy.
- **Azotemia:** Oliguria, fluid retention, edema. May indicate renal insufficiency.
- **Systemic lupus erythematosus (SLE):** May exacerbate or activate SLE.
- **Management:** Discontinue metolazone. Provide IV hydration and electrolyte replacement. Manage dysrhythmias according to Advanced Cardiac Life Support (ACLS) guidelines, considering hypokalemia and hypomagnesemia may be present. Consider use of insulin infusion for hyperglycemia.
- **GI decontamination:** No specific recommendations.

ANTIDOTE/DIALYSIS

- **Antidote:** No specific recommendations.
- **Dialysis:** Metolazone is not removed by hemodialysis and is unlikely to be removed by peritoneal dialysis. No data are available on removal using high-permeability hemodialysis.

M

metoprolol tartrate

me-toe-proe'-lole tar-trayt

Classes

Chemical: β1-adrenergic blocker, cardioselective

Therapeutic: antianginal, antihypertensive

Pregnancy Category: C, D (2nd and 3rd trimester)

Trade Names

Prescription: Apo-Metoprolol ♣, Betaloc ♣, Lopressor, Nu-Metop ♣, PMS-Metoprolol ♣, Toprol XL

Combinations

Prescription: with hydrochlorothiazide (Lopressor Hct)

Do not confuse metoprolol with metaproterenol or metolazone.

CLINICAL PHARMACOLOGY

Mechanism of Action

An antianginal, antihypertensive, and MI adjunct that selectively blocks $beta_1$-adrenergic receptors; high dosages may block $beta_2$-adrenergic receptors. Decreases oxygen requirements. Large doses increase airway resistance. **Therapeutic Effect:** Slows sinus node heart rate, decreases cardiac output, and reduces BP. Also decreases myocardial ischemia severity.

PHARMACOKINETICS

Route	Onset	Peak	Duration
PO	10-15 min	N/A	6 hr
PO (extended release)	N/A	6-12 hr	24 hr
IV	Immediate	20 min	5-8 hr

Well absorbed from the GI tract. Protein binding: 12%. Widely distributed. Metabolized in the liver (undergoes significant first-pass metabolism). Primarily excreted in urine. Removed by hemodialysis. **Half-life:** 3-7 hr.

AVAILABILITY

Tablets (Lopressor): 25 mg, 50 mg, 100 mg.
Tablets (Extended Release [Toprol XL]): 25 mg, 50 mg, 100 mg, 200 mg.
Injection (Lopressor): 1 mg/mL.

INDICATIONS AND DOSAGE

Mild to moderate hypertension

PO

Adults: Initially, 100 mg/day as single or divided dose. Increase at weekly (or longer) intervals. Maintenance 100-450 mg/day. **Elderly:** Initially, 25 mg/day. Range: 25-300 mg/day.

PO (Extended Release)

Adults: 50-100 mg/day as single dose. May increase at least at weekly intervals until optimum BP attained. Maximum: 200 mg/day. **Elderly:** Initially, 25-50 mg/day as a single dose. May increase at 1-2 wk intervals.

Chronic, stable angina pectoris

PO

Adults: Initially, 100 mg/day as single or divided dose. Increase at weekly (or longer) intervals. Maintenance: 100-450 mg/day.

PO (Extended Release)

Adults: Initially, 100 mg/day as single dose. May increase at weekly intervals until optimum clinical response achieved. Maximum: 200 mg/day.

Congestive heart failure

PO (Extended Release)

Adults: Initially, 25 mg/day. May double dose every 2 wk. Maximum: 200 mg/day.

Early treatment of MI

IV

Adults: 5 mg every 2 min for 3 doses, followed by 50 mg orally every 6 hr for 48 hr. Begin oral dose 15 min after last IV dose. Or, in patients who do not tolerate full IV dose, give 25-50 mg orally every 6 hr, 15 min after last IV dose.

Late treatment and maintenance after MI

PO

Adults: 100 mg twice per day for at least 3 mo.

OFF-LABEL USES

To increase survival rate in diabetic patients with coronary artery disease (CAD); treatment or prevention of anxiety; cardiac dysrhythmias; hypertrophic cardiomyopathy; mitral valve prolapse syndrome; pheochromocytoma; tremors; thyrotoxicosis; vascular headache

CONTRAINDICATIONS

Cardiogenic shock, MI with a heart rate less than 45 beats/min or systolic BP less than 100 mmHg, overt heart failure, second- or third-degree heart block, sinus bradycardia

INTERACTIONS

Drug: Cimetidine: May increase metoprolol blood concentration. **Diuretics, other antihypertensives:** May increase hypotensive effect. **Insulin, oral hypoglycemics:** May mask symptoms of hypoglycemia and prolong hypoglycemic effect of these drugs. **NSAIDs:** May decrease antihypertensive effect. **Sympathomimetics, xanthines:** May

M

mutually inhibit effects. **Herbal:** None known. **Food:** None known.

DIAGNOSTIC TEST EFFECTS

May increase serum antinuclear antibody (ANA) titer and BUN, serum lipoprotein, serum LDH, serum alkaline phosphatase, serum bilirubin, serum creatinine, serum potassium, serum uric acid, AST (SGOT) and ALT (SGPT) levels, and serum triglyceride levels.

IV INCOMPATIBILITIES

Amphotericin B complex (Abelcet, AmBisome, Amphotec)

IV COMPATIBILITIES

Alteplase (Activase)

IV COMPATIBILITIES

Metoprolol is generally well tolerated, with transient and mild side effects. **Frequent:** Diminished sexual function, drowsiness, insomnia, unusual fatigue or weakness. **Occasional:** Anxiety, nervousness, diarrhea, constipation, nausea, vomiting, nasal congestion, abdominal discomfort, dizziness, difficulty breathing, cold hands or feet. **Rare:** Altered taste, dry eyes, nightmares, paresthesia, allergic reaction (rash, pruritus)

M

CRITICAL CARE CONSIDERATIONS

ADMINISTRATION/HANDLING

PO ALERT

- Absorption of metoprolol is enhanced if given after meals.
- Crush or break Lopressor tablets if necessary.
- Do not break or crush Toprol-XL.

IV ALERT

- **Storage:** Store at room temperature. After reconstitution, store parenteral form for up to 48 hr at room temperature.
- **Dilution:** Give undiluted or dilute in 10 to 50 mL 0.9% NaCl or D_5W.
- **IV push/direct IV:** Give IV push over 1 min. ECG must be monitored for heart block, bradycardia, and ST changes during direct IV injection.

PRECAUTIONS

HEALTH-RELATED

- Use metoprolol cautiously in patients with bronchospastic disease, diabetes mellitus, thyroid disease, impaired renal or hepatic function, inadequate cardiac function, or peripheral vascular disease.

AGE-RELATED

- **Children:** Safety and efficacy of metoprolol has not been established in children.
- **Elderly:** Use cautiously; elderly are at increased risk for age-related peripheral vascular disease, impaired renal function, and hypothermia; may exacerbate confusion or altered mental status.

PREGNANCY/LACTATION-RELATED

- Pregnancy category C; D if used in second or third trimester. Metoprolol crosses the placenta; may produce apnea, bradycardia, hypoglycemia, or hypothermia during childbirth; excreted in breast milk in small amounts.

MONITORING

- **Baseline assessment for heart rate:** Assess heart rate, BP, and ECG rhythm immediately before giving metoprolol. If heart rate is less than 45 beats/min, systolic BP is less than 100 mmHg, or the patient has second- or third-degree heart block, withhold the medication.
- **Baseline assessment for angina/myocardial infarction:** Record onset, quality (e.g., dull, sharp, or squeezing), radiation, location, intensity, and duration of anginal pain; document precipitating factors (e.g., emotional stress or exertion). Follow AHA/ACC guidelines including use of oxygen, aspirin, nitrates, and morphine, as appropriate based on patient assessment.
- **Baseline assessment for BP control:** Record baseline BP and monitor for effectiveness. If BP is extremely high, monitor for neurologic changes indicative of stroke or TIA.
- **Baseline lab work:** Biochemical profile including renal and hepatic function test results; CBC to rule out anemia if patients are being managed for angina. Cardiac enzymes including troponins and CKMB should be completed to assess for MI. Coagulation profile should be completed for MI patients.
- **Possible heart failure:** Monitor for distended neck veins, night cough, peripheral edema, hypotension, bradycardia, activity intolerance, and difficulty breathing.
- **Cardiac monitoring:** Observe ECG for dysrhythmias, including sinus bradycardia and heart block. If heart block progresses to significant first degree with PR interval more than 0.24 sec, second or third

degree, drug should be withheld. Monitor for ST segment changes for anginal/MI patients.

- **Fluid retention:** Monitor intake and output for oliguria and weight gain if patients are at risk for heart failure or cardiogenic shock secondary to MI.
- **Hypoglycemia:** Assess blood glucose before meals and at bedtime in diabetics. Metoprolol may mask tachycardia and diaphoresis associated with hypoglycemia.
- **Dizziness:** Assist with ambulation if dizziness occurs.
- **Patient education:** Warn not to abruptly discontinue metoprolol. Advise that compliance with therapy is essential to control angina and dysrhythmias. To reduce orthostatic effects, instruct to rise slowly from a lying to sitting position and pause momentarily before standing. If a dose is missed, the dose should not doubled, but rather the next dose should be taken when scheduled. Recommend avoidance of tasks requiring alertness or motor skills until response to the drug is known. Instruct to promptly report confusion, depression, dizziness, or rash to a health care provider. Warn not to take OTC cold and allergy medications, including stimulants, with prior physician approval. Discharge teaching should include the correct technique for monitoring BP and pulse before taking metoprolol. Urge restriction of alcohol and salt intake.

SERIOUS ADVERSE REACTIONS

- **Abrupt withdrawal:** May result in diaphoresis, tachydysrhythmias, ventricular dysrhythmias, palpitations, tremors, headache, angina, or myocardial infarction in patients with heart disease; thyroid storm in those with hyperthyroidism.
- **Respiratory:** Bronchospasms leading to severe respiratory distress in obstructive lung disease patients.
- **Cardiovascular:** Bradycardia, AV heart block, hypotension; heart failure in patients with cardiac disease, and peripheral ischemia in those with peripheral vascular disease.
- **Hypoglycemia:** May occur in patients with previously controlled diabetes.

OVERDOSE/TOXICITY

- **Overdose:** Profound bradycardia, heart block, bronchospasm or wheezing with respiratory distress, heart failure, hypoglycemia, and hypotension.
- **Management:** Upon withdrawing the medication following overdose, if patients experience acute angina, ST segment depression indicative of myocardial ischemia or ST segment elevation indicative of MI, patients must be provided with another therapy to promote myocardial perfusion immediately.
- **GI decontamination:** Activated charcoal is most effective versus whole bowel irrigation which has not been thoroughly tested in humans.

ANTIDOTE/DIALYSIS

- **Antidote:** Beta agonist high dose infusion such as *DOPamine, epinephrine, *DOBUTamine or isoproterenol (use cautiously to avoid extreme tachycardia) to counteract the effects of beta blockade including bradycardia, hypotension, and bronchospasms. Glucagon is often successful in increasing heart rate in beta blocker overdose. Phosphodiesterase inhibitors inamrinone and milrinone may be used to manage heart failure if other agents are ineffective. Other treatment options include glucose and insulin, cardiac pacing, crystalloid fluids, vasopressors such as norepinephrine for hypotension. Aerosolized bronchodilators (e.g., albuterol) may be effective in counteracting bronchospastic effects.
- **Dialysis:** Metoprolol is removed by hemodialysis, and is likely removed by high-permeability hemodialysis. It is not removed by peritoneal dialysis.

metronidazole

me-troe-nie-da-zole

Classes

Chemical: nitroimidazole derivative

Therapeutic: antibiotic, antihelmintic, antiprotozoal

Pregnancy Category: B

Trade Names

Prescription: Apo-Metronidazole ♣, Flagyl, Flagyl 375, Flagyl ER, Flagyl I.V. RTU, MetroCream, MetroGel, MetroGel-Vaginal, Metro IV, MetroLotion, Metronidazole Benzoate, Noritate, Novonidazole ♣, Protostat, Rozex, Vandazole

CLINICAL PHARMACOLOGY

Mechanism of Action

A nitroimidazole derivative that disrupts bacterial and protozoal DNA, inhibiting nucleic acid synthesis. **Therapeutic Effect:** Produces bactericidal, antiprotozoal, amebicidal, and trichomonacidal effects. Produces antiinflammatory and immunosuppressive effects when applied topically.

PHARMACOKINETICS

Well absorbed from the GI tract; minimally absorbed after topical application. Protein binding: less than 20%. Widely distributed; crosses blood-brain barrier. Metabolized in the liver to active metabolite. Primarily excreted in urine; partially eliminated in feces. Removed by hemodialysis. **Half-life:** 8 hr (increased in alcoholic hepatic disease and in neonates).

AVAILABILITY

Capsules (Flagyl 375): 375 mg.
Tablets (Flagyl, Protostat): 250 mg, 500 mg.
Tablets (extended release [Flagyl ER]): 750 mg.
Injection (infusion [Flagyl IV RTU]): 500 mg/100 mL.
Topical cream: 0.75% (MetroCream, Rozex), 1% (Noritate).
Topical gel (MetroGel): 0.75%, 1%.
Topical lotion (MetroLotion): 0.75%.
Vaginal gel (MetroGel-Vaginal, Vandazole): 0.75%.

INDICATIONS AND DOSAGE

Anaerobic infections

PO, IV

Adults, Elderly: 500 mg every 6-8 hr. Maximum: 4 g/day. **Children:** 7.5 mg/kg/dose every 6 hr. Maximum: 4 g/day.

Amebic dysentery

PO

Adults, Elderly: 750 mg 3 times per day for 5-10 days. **Children:** 35-50 mg/kg/day in 3 divided doses for 10 days. Maximum: 750 mg/dose.

Amebic liver abscess

PO

Adults, Elderly: 500-750 mg 3 times per day for 5-10 days. **Children:** 50 mg/kg/day in 3 divided doses. Maximum: 750 mg/dose.

Giardiasis

PO

Adults, Elderly: 250 mg 3 times per day for 5 days. **Children:** 15 mg/kg/day in 3 divided doses for 7-10 days. Maximum: 250 mg/dose.

Pseudomembranous colitis

PO

Adults, Elderly: 500-750 mg 3 times per day or 250-500 mg 4 times per day. **Children:** 7.5 mg/kg every 6 hr for 7-10 days.

Trichomoniasis

PO

Adults, Elderly: 250 mg 3 times per day or 375 mg twice per day or 500 mg twice per day or 2 g as a single dose. **Children:** 15-30 mg/kg/day in 3 divided doses for 7 days.

Bacterial vaginosis

PO

Adults (nonpregnant): 500 mg twice per day for 7 days or 750 mg (extended release) once daily for 7 days or 2 g as a single dose. **Adults (pregnant):** 250 mg 3 times per day for 7 days.

Intravaginal

Adults (pregnant, nonpregnant): 0.75% apply twice per day for 5 days. Centers for Disease Control does not recommend the use of topical agents during pregnancy.

Rosacea

Topical

Adults, Elderly: (1%): Apply to affected area once daily. **(0.75%)**: Apply to affected area twice per day.

OFF-LABEL USES

Treatment of bacterial vaginosis, grade III-IV decubitus ulcers with anaerobic infection, *Heliobacter pylori*–associated gastritis and duodenal ulcer, inflammatory bowel disease; topical treatment of acne rosacea

CONTRAINDICATIONS

Hypersensitivity to metronidazole or other nitroimidazole derivatives (also parabens with topical application)

INTERACTIONS

Drug: Alcohol: May cause a disulfiram-type reaction. **Disulfiram:** May increase the risk of toxicity. **Oral anticoagulants:** May increase the effects of these drugs. **Herbal:** None known. **Food:** None known.

DIAGNOSTIC TEST EFFECTS

May increase serum LDH, AST (SGOT), and ALT (SGPT) levels.

IV INCOMPATIBILITIES

Amphotericin B complex (Abelcet, AmBisome, Amphotec), filgrastim (Neupogen), total parenteral nutrition (TPN)

IV COMPATIBILITIES

Diltiazem (Cardizem), *DOPamine (Intropin), heparin, hydromorphone (Dilaudid), lorazepam (Ativan), magnesium sulfate, midazolam (Versed), morphine

SIDE-EFFECTS

Frequent: Systemic: Anorexia, nausea, dry mouth, metallic taste. **Vaginal:** Symptomatic cervicitis and vaginitis, abdominal cramps, uterine pain. **Occasional: Systemic:** Diarrhea or constipation, vomiting, dizziness, erythematous rash, urticaria, reddish brown urine. **Topical:** Transient erythema, mild dryness, burning, irritation, stinging, tearing when applied too close to eyes. **Vaginal:** Vaginal, perineal, or vulvar itching; vulvar swelling, vaginal discharge. **Rare:** Mild, transient leukopenia; thrombophlebitis with IV therapy

CRITICAL CARE CONSIDERATIONS

ADMINISTRATION/HANDLING

PO ALERT

- Give metronidazole without regard to food. Give with food if GI upset occurs.

IV ALERT

- **Storage:** Store ready-to-use infusion bags at room temperature. Discard diluted solutions after 24 hr. Do not refrigerate to avoid precipitate forming.
- **IV intermittent infusion:** Infuse over 30 to 60 min. Do not give as an IV bolus injection.

PRECAUTIONS

HEALTH-RELATED

- Use metronidazole cautiously in patients predisposed to edema, those taking corticosteroids, those with heart failure (drug contains 27-28 mEq sodium per gram), blood dyscrasias, CNS disorders, or severe hepatic dysfunction.

AGE-RELATED

- **Children:** Safety of metronidazole has not been established in infants and children. Safety and efficacy of topical administration in those under 21 yr have not been established.
- **Elderly:** Age-related hepatic impairment may require a dosage reduction.

PREGNANCY/LACTATION-RELATED

- Pregnancy category B. Use in pregnancy controversial; use in first trimester and single-dose therapy often avoided. Use with caution during breast-feeding; if single-dose therapy is used, discontinue breast-feeding for 12-24 hr to allow excretion of the drug.

MONITORING

- **Baseline assessment:** Determine history of hypersensitivity to metronidazole or other nitroimidazole derivatives (and parabens with topical form) before beginning therapy.
- **Baseline lab work:** CBC with WBC differential; biochemical profile including liver function tests. Obtain specimens for diagnostic tests and cultures before giving the first dose of metronidazole. Therapy may begin before the test results are known.
- **Diarrhea:** Assess pattern of daily bowel activity and stool consistency. Document the number and characteristics of stools in amebiasis patients.
- **Superinfection:** Assess for white patches on the mucous membranes in the mouth or tongue and for severe mouth or tongue soreness; assess for severe anal or genital pruritus or discharge.
- **Thrombophlebitis:** Monitor for redness and pain at IV insertion site. Rotate IV insertion site every 2-3 days, as possible.
- **Fluid retention:** Monitor intake and output; assess for oliguria and edema.
- **Neurologic effects:** Monitor for dizziness and paresthesia.
- **Hypersensitivity:** Assess for rash and urticaria.
- **Patient education:** Explain that urine may become reddish brown during metronidazole therapy. Urge avoidance of alcohol and alcohol-containing preparations (such as cough syrups and elixirs) while taking metronidazole to avoid toxic reactions. Warn to avoid tasks requiring mental alertness or motor skills until response to the drug is known. Instruct patients taking metronidazole for trichomoniasis to refrain from sexual intercourse until the full treatment is completed. Caution those using topical metronidazole to avoid drug contact with eyes. Explain cosmetics may be used after the drug is applied. Inform that metronidazole acts on papules, pustules, and erythema but has no effect on ocular problems (conjunctivitis, keratitis, blepharitis), rhinophyma (hypertrophy of nose), or telangiectasia. Urge rosacea patients to avoid alcohol; excessive sunlight; very hot or cold ambient temperatures; and hot, spicy foods.

M

SERIOUS ADVERSE REACTIONS
- Oral therapy may result in furry tongue, glossitis, cystitis, dysuria, pancreatitis, and flattening of T waves on ECG readings.

OVERDOSE/TOXICITY
- **Neurotoxicity:** Peripheral neuropathy, manifested as numbness and tingling in hands or feet, is usually reversible if treatment is stopped immediately after neurologic symptoms appear. Seizures occur occasionally.
- **GI decontamination:** No specific recommendations.

ANTIDOTE/DIALYSIS
- **Antidote:** No specific recommendations.
- **Dialysis:** Metronidazole is removed by hemodialysis and is likely removed by high-permeability hemodialysis. No data are available on removal by peritoneal dialysis.

mexiletine hydrochloride

mex'-i-leh-teen hye-droe-klor'-ide

Classes
Chemical: lidocaine derivative
Therapeutic: antidysrhythmic, class IB

Pregnancy Category: C

Trade Names
Prescription: Mexitil

CLINICAL PHARMACOLOGY
Mechanism of Action
An antidysrhythmic that shortens duration of action potential and decreases effective refractory period in the His-Purkinje system of the myocardium by blocking sodium transport across myocardial cell membranes. **Therapeutic Effect:** Suppresses ventricular dysrhythmias.

PHARMACOKINETICS
Well absorbed from the GI tract. Protein binding: 50%-70%. Metabolized in liver. Approximately 10% is excreted unchanged in urine. **Half-life:** 10-12 hr.

AVAILABILITY
Capsules: 150 mg, 200 mg, 250 mg.

INDICATIONS AND DOSAGE
Dysrhythmia
PO
Adults, Elderly: Initially, 200 mg every 8 hr. Adjust dosage by 50-100 mg at 2- to 3-day intervals. **Maximum:** 1200 mg/day.

OFF-LABEL USES
Treatment of diabetic neuropathy

CONTRAINDICATIONS
Cardiogenic shock, preexisting second- or third-degree AV block, right bundle-branch block without presence of pacemaker, hypersensitivity to mexiletine or related compounds

INTERACTIONS
Drug: **Antacids:** May reduce mexiletine absorption. **Phenobarbital, phenytoin, rifampin:** May decrease mexiletine blood concentration. **Herbal:** None known. **Food:** None known.

DIAGNOSTIC TEST EFFECTS
May increase liver enzymes, such as ALT (SGOT) and AST (SGPT). May decrease WBCs and thrombocytes.

SIDE-EFFECTS
Frequent (greater than 10%): GI distress, including nausea, vomiting, and heartburn; dizziness; lightheadedness; tremor. **Occasional (10%-1%):** Nervousness, change in sleep habits, headache, visual disturbances, paresthesia, diarrhea or constipation, palpitations, chest pain, rash, respiratory difficulty, edema

CRITICAL CARE CONSIDERATIONS

ADMINISTRATION/HANDLING
PO ALERT
- If 300 mg every 8 hr or less controls dysrhythmias, dose may be given every 12 hr.
- Swallow capsules whole; do not crush, open, or break capsules.
- **Transferring from lidocaine infusion:** The infusion should be stopped as soon as possible following the first dose of mexiletene.

PRECAUTIONS
HEALTH-RELATED
- Use mexiletine cautiously in patients with heart failure, impaired myocardial function, sick sinus syndrome, liver disease, leukopenia, or agranulocytosis.

AGE-RELATED
- **Children:** Safety and efficacy of mexiletine have not been established in children.
- **Elderly:** Age-related cardiac dysfunction may warrant a dosage adjustment.

PREGNANCY/LACTATION-RELATED

- Pregnancy category C; limited data do not suggest significant risk to the fetus; compatible with breast-feeding.

MONITORING

- **Baseline assessment:** Discern the cardiovascular and medication history, especially use of other antidysrhythmics.
- **Baseline lab work:** CBC with WBC differential, biochemical profile including potassium, magnesium, calcium, CPK and renal function studies. Beta natriuretic peptide to assess for heart failure.
- **Baseline diagnostic tests:** Baseline 12-lead ECG to identify dysrhythmias and to assess for myocardial ischemia (ST depression).
- **Dysrhythmias:** Monitor ECG continuously for heart block and bradycardia.
- **Heart failure:** Monitor for hypotension, difficulty breathing, chest discomfort or heaviness, and activity intolerance.
- **CNS effects:** Monitor for dizziness, light headedness, tremors, nervousness, and coordination difficulties.
- **GI effects:** Monitor for nausea, vomiting, and heartburn.
- **Liver dysfunction:** Monitor for dark urine, pale stools, liver enzyme elevation, right upper quadrant pain, edema, and jaundice.
- **Therapeutic serum level:** 0.5 to 2 mcg/mL.
- **Patient education:** Instruct to report promptly dark urine, cough, generalized fatigue, activity intolerance, shortness of breath, nausea, pale stools, severe or persistent abdominal pain, unexplained sore throat or fever, vomiting, or yellowing of the eyes or skin to a health care provider. Caution against using nasal decongestants and OTC cold preparations without discussing with a health care provider prior to taking the medication.

SERIOUS ADVERSE REACTIONS

- **Heart failure:** May occur and existing heart failure may worsen. Heart failure may be preceded by heart block and bradycardia.

OVERDOSE/TOXICITY

- **Proarrhythmia:** Mexiletine has the ability to worsen existing dysrhythmias or produce new ones including lethal ventricular dysrhythmias.
- **Bone marrow suppression:** Agranulocytosis and leukopenia may occur in patients receiving other medications which create blood dyscrasias. Patients may manifest an infection signaling immune dysfunction.
- **Hepatotoxicity:** AST (SGOT) elevation up to 3 times normal, rare hepatic necrosis.
- **CNS toxicity:** Tremors, extreme nervousness or panic, rare seizures. CNS stimulation may be managed with benzodiazepines (diazepam [Valium] or lorazepam [Ativan]), short-acting barbiturates (thiopental [Pentothal]), or, if anesthetized, neuromuscular blocking agents (succinylcholine, vecuronium).
- **Management:** Discontinue mexiletine immediately. Manage dysrhythmias using Advanced Cardiac Life Support (ACLS) guidelines. Provide supportive care for conditions present.
- **GI decontamination:** No specific recommendations.

ANTIDOTE/DIALYSIS

- **Antidote:** No specific recommendations.
- **Dialysis:** Mexiletine is removed by hemodialysis and is likely removed by high-permeability hemodialysis. It is not removed by peritoneal dialysis.

micafungin

See Antifungals (p. 922)

miconazole

mye-con'-a-zole

Classes

Chemical: imidazole derivative
Therapeutic: antifungal

Pregnancy Category: C, B

Trade Names

Prescription: Monistat-Derm
Over the Counter: DiabetAid, Femizol-M, Fungoid, Lotrimin AF, Micatin Athlete's Foot, Monistat 3, Monistat 7, Neosporin AF, Tetterine, Zeasorb-AF

Do not confuse miconazole with metolazone.

CLINICAL PHARMACOLOGY

Mechanism of Action

An imidazole derivative that inhibits synthesis of ergosterol (vital component of fungal cell formation), damaging cell membrane. **Therapeutic Effect:** Fungistatic; may be fungicidal, depending on concentration.

PHARMACOKINETICS

Parenteral: Widely distributed in tissues. Metabolized in liver. Primarily excreted in urine. **Half-life:** 24 hr. **Topical:** No systemic absorption following application to intact skin. **Intravaginally:** Small amount absorbed systemically.

AVAILABILITY

Injection: 10 mg/mL.
Effervescent tablet: 2% topical fungal foot bath (DiabetAid).
Vaginal suppository: 100 mg (Monistat 7), 200 mg (Monistat 3).
Topical cream: 2% (Micatin, Monistat-Derm, Neosporin AF).
Vaginal cream: 2% (Femizol-M, Monistat 3 [4%], Monistat 7 [2%]).
Topical powder: 2% (Micatin, Lotrimin AF, Zeasorb-AF [2%]).
Topical lotion, powder: 2% (Zeasorb-AF).
Topical spray: 2% (Lotrimin AF, Micatin Athlete's Foot [2%], Neosporin AF [2%]).
Topical ointment: 2% (Tetterine).
Topical tincture: 2% (Fungoid).

M

INDICATIONS AND DOSAGE

Vulvovaginal candidiasis

Intravaginally

Adults, Elderly: One 200-mg suppository at bedtime for 3 days (Monistat 3); one 100-mg suppository or one applicator full at bedtime for 7 days (Monistat 7). Insert 2% vaginal cream (one applicator full) at bedtime for 7 days. Insert 4% vaginal cream (one applicator full) at bedtime for 3 days. Insert vaginal suppository 100 mg once daily for 7 days; 200 mg once daily for 3 days; 1200 mg once daily for 1 day.

Topical fungal infections

Topical, tinea corporis

Adults, Elderly, Children 2 yr and older: Apply twice daily for 4 wk.

Topical, tinea pedis

Adults, Elderly, Children 2 yr and older: Apply twice daily for 4 wk.

Effervescent tablet, tinea pedis

Adults, Elderly, Children 2 yr and older: Dissolve 1 tablet in 1 gallon water and soak feet for 15-30 min, then pat dry.

Topical, tinea cruris

Adults, Elderly, Children 2 yr and older: Apply twice daily for 2 wk.

CONTRAINDICATIONS

Children younger than 1 yr, hypersensitivity to miconazole or any component of the formulation. **Topically:** Children younger than 2 yr

INTERACTIONS

Drug: Oral anticoagulants, oral hypoglycemics: May increase effects of these drugs. **Isoniazid, rifampin:** May decrease concentrations. **Herbal:** None known. **Food:** None known.

DIAGNOSTIC TEST EFFECTS

None known.

IV INCOMPATIBILITIES

Do not administer other medications via Y-site.

SIDE-EFFECTS

Frequent: Phlebitis, fever, chills, rash, itching, nausea, vomiting. **Occasional:** Dizziness, drowsiness, headache, flushed face, abdominal pain, constipation, diarrhea, decreased appetite. **Topical:** Itching, burning, stinging, erythema, urticaria. **Vaginal:** Vulvovaginal burning, itching, irritation, headache, skin rash

CRITICAL CARE CONSIDERATIONS

ADMINISTRATION/HANDLING

INTRAVAGINAL ALERT

- Insert high in vagina.

TOPICAL ALERT

- **Preparation:** Wash and dry area before applying medication.
- **Application:** Apply a thin layer on affected area. Avoid contact with eyes.

PRECAUTIONS

HEALTH-RELATED

- Use cautiously in patients with liver impairment.
- Soft gel vaginal inserts and external vulvar cream contain a base that may interact with certain latex products. Condoms and diaphragms should not be relied on to prevent sexually transmitted diseases or pregnancy until 3 days after the last use of the vaginal inserts or vulvar cream.

AGE-RELATED

- **Children:** Use in children under 2 yr has not been studied extensively. Safety and

efficacy of soft gel vaginal inserts and external vulvar cream in premenarchal females has not been studied.
- **Elderly:** No age-related precautions have been noted.

PREGNANCY/LACTATION-RELATED

- Pregnancy category C (topical: category B); unknown if excreted into breast milk.

MONITORING

- **Baseline assessment:** Antiemetics and antihistamines should be given before infusion to reduce nausea, vomiting.
- **Baseline lab work:** Confirm that cultures or histologic tests were done. CBC with WBC differential and platelet count. Biochemical profile including liver function studies. Monitor periodically throughout therapy.
- **IV therapy adverse reactions:** Assess for phlebitis, pruritus, nausea, vomiting, fever, chills, and rash.
- **Topical/vaginal:** Assess for burning, itching, irritation.
- **Patient education:** Instruct to continue full length of treatment. Prolonged therapy (weeks or months) may be necessary for some conditions. Advise those using a vaginal preparation that the base interacts with certain latex products such as contraceptive diaphragms or condoms and may render them ineffective. Explain douching and sexual intercourse may remove medication, reducing effectiveness of treatment. Instruct those using the topical formulation to rub well into affected areas. Avoid getting in eyes. Keep areas clean, dry; wear light clothing for ventilation. Separate personal items in contact with affected areas.

SERIOUS ADVERSE REACTIONS

- None noted.

OVERDOSE/TOXICITY

- **Bone marrow suppression:** Anemia and thrombocytopenia.
- **Hepatotoxicity:** Elevated liver enzymes, right upper quadrant pain, jaundice, edema.
- **GI decontamination:** No specific recommendations.

ANTIDOTE/DIALYSIS

- **Antidote:** No specific recommendations.
- **Dialysis:** Miconazole is not removed by hemodialysis or peritoneal dialysis. No data are available on removal using high-permeability hemodialysis.

midazolam hydrochloride ⚑

mid'-ay-zoe-lam hye-droe-klor'-ide

DEA Schedule: IV

Classes

Chemical: benzodiazepine
Therapeutic: sedative/hypnotic

Pregnancy Category: D

Trade Names

Prescription: Apo-Midazolam ♣, Versed

Do not confuse Versed with VePesid.

CLINICAL PHARMACOLOGY

Mechanism of Action

A benzodiazepine that enhances the action of gamma-aminobutyric acid, one of the major inhibitory neurotransmitters in the brain. **Therapeutic Effect:** Produces anxiolytic, hypnotic, anticonvulsant, muscle relaxant, and amnestic effects.

PHARMACOKINETICS

Route	Onset	Peak	Duration
PO	10-20 min	20-50 min	N/A
IV	1-5 min	5-7 min	20-30 min
IM	5-15 min	30-60 min	1.5 hr

Well absorbed after IM administration. Protein binding: 97%. Metabolized in the liver to active metabolite. Primarily excreted in urine. Not removed by hemodialysis. **Half-life:** 1-5 hr.

AVAILABILITY

Syrup: 2 mg/mL.
Injection: 1 mg/mL, 5 mg/mL.
Injection (preservative-free): 1 mg/mL, 5 mg/mL.

INDICATIONS AND DOSAGE

Preoperative sedation

PO

Children: 0.25-0.5 mg/kg. Maximum: 20 mg. Administer 3-40 min before procedure. Children under 6 yr may require up to 1 mg/kg.

IV

Adults, Elderly: 0.02-0.04 mg/kg. **Children 6-12 yr:** 0.025-0.05 mg/kg. Maximum: 10 mg. **Children 6 mo-5 yr:** 0.05-0.1 mg/kg. Maximum: 6 mg.

IM

Adults, Elderly: 0.07-0.08 mg/kg 30-60 min before surgery. **Children:** 0.1-0.15

mg/kg 30-60 min before surgery. Maximum: 10 mg.

Conscious sedation for diagnostic, therapeutic, and endoscopic procedures

IV

Adults, Elderly: 0.5-2 mg over 2 min. May repeat every 2-3 min. Maximum total dose: 2.5-5 mg. **Children 6-12 yr:** 0.025-0.05 mg/kg. Total dose of 0.4 mg/kg may be necessary. Maximum total dose: 10 mg. **Children 6 mo-5 yr:** 0.05-0.1 mg/kg. Total dose of 0.6 mg/kg may be necessary. Maximum total dose: 6 mg.

Conscious sedation during mechanical ventilation

IV

Adults, Elderly: Initially, 0.02-0.08 mg/kg. May repeat at 5- to 15-min intervals or continuous infusion rate of 0.04-0.2 mg/kg/hr and titrated to desired effect. **Children:** Initially, 1-2 mg/kg followed by a continuous infusion of 0.06-0.12 mg/kg/hr (0.05-0.2 mg/kg) titrated to desired effect.

Status epilepticus

IV

Children older than 2 mo: Loading dose of 0.15 mg/kg followed by continuous infusion of 1 mcg/kg/min. Titrate every 5 min until seizure activity is controlled. Range: 1-18 mcg/kg/min.

M

OFF-LABEL USES

Anxiety, status epilepticus

CONTRAINDICATIONS

Acute alcohol intoxication, acute angle-closure glaucoma, pregnancy, allergies to cherries, coma, shock, hypersensitivity to midazolam

INTERACTIONS

Drug: **Alcohol, other CNS depressants:** May increase CNS and respiratory depression and hypotensive effects of midazolam. **Hypotension-producing medications:** May increase hypotensive effects of midazolam. **Ketoconazole:** May increase midazolam concentration. **Herbal:** **Kava kava, valerian:** May increase CNS depression. **Food:** **Grapefruit, grapefruit juice:** Increases the oral absorption and systemic availability of midazolam.

DIAGNOSTIC TEST EFFECTS

None known.

IV INCOMPATIBILITIES

Albumin, ampicillin and sulbactam (Unasyn), amphotericin B complex (Abelcet, AmBisome, Amphotec), ampicillin (Polycillin), bumetanide (Bumex), co-trimoxazole (Bactrim), dexamethasone (Decadron), fosphenytoin (Cerebyx), furosemide (Lasix), hydrocortisone (Solu-Cortef), methotrexate, nafcillin (Nafcil), sodium bicarbonate, sodium pentothal (Thiopental)

IV COMPATIBILITIES

Amiodarone (Cordarone), atropine, calcium gluconate, diltiazem (Cardizem), *diphenhydrAMINE (Benadryl), *DOBUTamine (Dobutrex), *DOPamine (Intropin), etomidate (Amidate), fentanyl (Sublimaze), glycopyrrolate (Robinul), heparin, hydromorphone (Dilaudid), *hydrOXYzine (Vistaril), insulin, lorazepam (Ativan), milrinone (Primacor), morphine, nitroglycerin, norepinephrine (Levophed), potassium chloride, propofol (Diprivan)

SIDE-EFFECTS

Frequent (10%-4%): Decreased respiratory rate, tenderness at IM or IV injection site, pain during injection, oxygen desaturation, hiccups. **Occasional (3%-2%):** Hypotension, paradoxic CNS reaction. **Rare (less than 2%):** Nausea, vomiting, headache, coughing

CRITICAL CARE CONSIDERATIONS

ADMINISTRATION/HANDLING

IV ALERT

- **Storage:** Store vials at room temperature.
- **Preparation:** Ensure that resuscitative supplies including endotracheal tubes, suction equipment, reversal agents (antidote), and oxygen are readily available.
- **IV push/direct injection:** Midazolam may be given undiluted. Administer by slow IV injection in incremental doses. Give each incremental dose over 2 min or more and wait at least 2 min between doses.
- **IV infusion dilution:** May be diluted with D_5W or normal saline for IV continuous infusion. Maximum concentration following dilution should not exceed 0.5 mg/mL.
- **IV continuous infusion:** Reduce IV rate in patients older than 60 yr, debilitated patients, those with chronic diseases or impaired pulmonary function. A too-rapid IV rate, excessive doses, or a single large dose increases the risk of respiratory depression or arrest.
- **Dosage:** Individualized based on patient age, underlying disease, medications, and on the desired effect.

IM ALERT

- **Administration:** Inject drug deep into a large muscle mass, such as the gluteus maximus. Do not use for intrathecal or epidural administration; contains benzyl alcohol. Drug is for IV or IM use only.

PO ALERT

- Syrup should be stored at controlled room temperature (15-30°C or 59-86°F.) Disposal of schedule IV controlled substances must be consistent with state and federal regulations.
- Syrup is clear, red to purplish red, cherry flavored.

PRECAUTIONS

HEALTH-RELATED

- Use midazolam cautiously in patients with acute illness; heart failure; pulmonary, renal, or hepatic impairment; severe fluid or electrolyte imbalance; and treated angle-closure glaucoma.
- **Cytochrome P450 metabolism:** Midazolam should be used with caution when given with other medications that inhibit the cytochrome P4503A4 enzyme system including cimetidine, erythromycin, diltiazem, verapamil, ketoconazole, and itraconazole.

AGE-RELATED

- **Children:** Neonates are more likely to experience respiratory depression. Clearance is decreased and half-life is increased in critically ill neonates. Elimination rate is faster in infants and children. Midazolam syrup has not been studied in children under 6 mo.
- **Elderly:** Age-related renal impairment may require dosage adjustment. Clearance is reduced and time for recovery may be prolonged. May have prolonged respiratory depression.

PREGNANCY/LACTATION-RELATED

- Pregnancy category D; excreted in breast milk, use with caution in nursing mothers.

MONITORING

- **Baseline assessment:** Obtain presedation history including medical conditions and medications used. Check for airway abnormalities. Take vital signs before administering midazolam and implement continuous pulse oximetry.
- **Baseline lab work:** Biochemical panel including renal and liver function studies.
- **Paradoxic reactions:** Assess for paradoxic CNS reactions (increased agitation), particularly early in therapy.
- **Sedation management:** Use standardized sedation and pain management scoring throughout therapy. A designated professional should monitor level of sedation and respiratory function throughout deep sedation.
- **Pain management:** Assess for pain in patients who are unable to communicate well. Patients in pain are sometimes given large doses of sedatives to control restlessness that is due to pain. Reduced rate of midazolam infusion may be needed if opioid analgesia is added.
- **Respiratory status:** Assess for patent airway, respiratory rate and oxygen saturation (pulse oximetry) continuously during parenteral administration to detect apnea and respiratory depression. Critically ill patients and others who are intubated and mechanically ventilated are better protected from respiratory compromise.
- **Level of sedation:** Monitor level of sedation every 3 to 5 min, and assess vital signs during the recovery period.
- **Patient education:** Inform before the procedure that midazolam produces an amnesic effect. Patients should not drive or perform tasks requiring full mental alertness for at least 24 hr following discontinuation of the drug. Encourage avoidance of use of alcohol or other CNS depressants (antihistamines, barbiturates) before receiving midazolam. Drug should not be used outside of a facility that can provide continuous monitoring of respiratory and cardiac function by licensed health or dental care professionals. Female patients should report if they are pregnant or suspect pregnancy before receiving midazolam; the health care provider may reconsider using the drug.

SERIOUS ADVERSE REACTIONS

- **Abrupt or too-rapid withdrawal:** May result in pronounced restlessness, irritability, insomnia, hand tremor, abdominal or muscle cramps, diaphoresis, vomiting, and seizures.
- **Paradoxic reactions:** Some patients are intolerant of benzodiazepines and respond to the drug with cerebral hypoxia, agitation, involuntary movements, hyperactivity, and combativeness.
- **Respiratory depression:** A too-rapid IV rate, excessive doses, or a single large dose increases the risk of respiratory

depression, apnea, hypoxia, and cardiac arrest.

OVERDOSE/TOXICITY

- **Symptoms:** Somnolence, confusion, diminished reflexes, hypotension, and coma.
- **Management:** Ensure patent airway with endotracheal intubation if necessary, along with mechanical ventilation. Support blood pressure with fluids and vasopressors if needed. Administer benzodiazepine antidote flumazenil. Forced diuresis and osmotic diuretics (e.g., mannitol) may facilitate elimination.
- **GI decontamination:** No specific recommendations.

ANTIDOTE/DIALYSIS

- **Antidote:** Cautiously use flumazenil (Romazicon) 0.2 mg (2 mL) over 30 sec; may repeat after 30 sec with 0.3 mg (3 mL) over 30 sec. Further doses may be given up to 0.5 mg (5 mL) up to a total of 3 mg (30 mL). Flumazenil reverses CNS depressive effects. Naloxone (Narcan) should be considered in addition to flumazenil if patients have significant respiratory depression.
- **Dialysis:** Midazolam is not removed by hemodialysis and is unlikely to be removed by peritoneal dialysis. No data are available on removal using high-permeability hemodialysis.

M

midodrine hydrochloride

mye'-doe-drene hye-droe-klor'-ide

Classes

Chemical: catecholamine, synthetic
Therapeutic: vasopressor, α-adrenergic sympathomimetic amine

Pregnancy Category: C

Trade Names

Prescription: Amatine ♣, ProAmatine

Do not confuse Amatine or ProAmatine with amantadine or protamine.

CLINICAL PHARMACOLOGY

Mechanism of Action

A vasopressor that forms the active metabolite desglymidodrine, an alpha$_1$-agonist, activating alpha receptors of the arteriolar and venous vasculature. **Therapeutic Effect:** Increases vascular tone and BP.

PHARMACOKINETICS

Rapid absorption from the GI tract following PO administration. Protein binding: Minimal. Undergoes enzymatic hydrolysis (deglycination) in the systemic circulation. Excreted in urine. **Half-life:** 3-4 hr (active metabolite).

AVAILABILITY

Tablets: 2.5 mg, 5 mg, 10 mg.

INDICATIONS AND DOSAGE

Orthostatic hypotension

PO

Adults, Elderly: 10 mg 3 times per day. Give during the day when patient is upright, such as upon arising, midday, and late afternoon. Do not give later than 6 PM

Dosage in renal impairment

Adults, Elderly: 2.5 mg 3 times per day; increase gradually, as tolerated.

OFF-LABEL USES

Infection-related hypotension, intradialytic hypotension, psychotropic agent-induced hypotension, urinary incontinence

CONTRAINDICATIONS

Acute renal function impairment, persistent hypertension, pheochromocytoma, severe cardiac disease, thyrotoxicosis, urine retention, hypersensitivity to midodrine

INTERACTIONS

Drug: Digoxin: May have additive bradycardia effects. **Sodium-retaining steroids (such as fludrocortisone):** May increase sodium retention and intraocular pressure. **Vasoconstrictors:** May have an additive vasoconstricting effect. **Herbal:** None known. **Food:** None known.

DIAGNOSTIC TEST EFFECTS

None known.

SIDE-EFFECTS

Frequent (20%-7%): Paresthesia, piloerection, pruritus, dysuria, supine hypertension. **Occasional (less than 7%-1%):** Pain, rash, chills, headache, facial flushing, confusion, dry mouth, anxiety

CRITICAL CARE CONSIDERATIONS

ADMINISTRATION/HANDLING

PO ALERT

- Store at controlled room temperature.
- Give midodrine without regard to meals.

- Give midodrine when patients are upright (not lying down) upon arising, midday, or late afternoon (not past 6 PM).

PRECAUTIONS

HEALTH-RELATED

- Use midodrine cautiously in patients with a history of vision problems and renal or hepatic impairment.

AGE-RELATED

- **Children:** Safety and efficacy of midodrine have not been established in children.
- **Elderly:** Age-related organ impairment may prompt a dosage adjustment.

PREGNANCY/LACTATION-RELATED

- Pregnancy category C; unknown if excreted in breast milk.

MONITORING

- **Baseline assessment:** Assess for hypersensitivity to midodrine; determine medical and medication history including acute renal function impairment, severe hypertension, and cardiac disease. Note current medications, especially digoxin, sodium-retaining steroids, and vasoconstrictors.
- **Baseline lab work:** Biochemical profile including liver and renal function studies.
- **Therapeutic effect:** Observe for resolution of orthostatic hypotension.
- **Patient education:** Instruct not to take the last dose of the day after the evening meal or less than 4 hr before bedtime. Caution not to take the medication while lying down. Advise cautious use of OTC medications, such as cough, cold, and diet preparations, because they may affect further increase in BP.

SERIOUS ADVERSE REACTIONS

- **Cardiac effects:** Bradycardia, hypertension.
- **Renal:** Sodium retention leading to hypervolemia with possible hypernatremia.

OVERDOSE/TOXICITY

- **CNS effects:** Hyperpyrexia, altered mental status, possible seizures, and stroke.
- **Cardiovascular:** Tachycardia, ventricular dysrhythmias, hypertension followed by hypotension in the premorbid state.
- **Anticholinergic effects:** Urinary retention, hypoactive bowel sounds.
- **GI decontamination:** No specific recommendations.

ANTIDOTE/DIALYSIS

- **Antidote:** No specific recommendations.
- **Dialysis:** Midodrine is removed by high-permeability hemodialysis. No data are available on removal by hemodialysis or peritoneal dialysis.

miglitol

See Antidiabetics (p. 911)

miglustat

mig'-loo-stat

Classes

Chemical: N-alkylated imino sugar, synthetic D-glucose analog
Therapeutic: metabolic agent

Pregnancy Category: X

Trade Names

Prescription: Zavesca

CLINICAL PHARMACOLOGY

Mechanism of Action

A Gaucher disease agent that inhibits the enzyme glucosylceramide synthase, reducing the rate of synthesis of most glycosphingolipids. Allows the residual activity of the deficient enzyme, glucocerebrosidase, to be more effective in degrading lysosomal storage within tissues. **Therapeutic Effect:** Minimizes conditions associated with Gaucher's disease, such as anemia and bone disease.

PHARMACOKINETICS

The average bioavailability is 97%. Not protein bound. Crosses blood-brain barrier. Not metabolized. Excreted in urine. **Half-life:** 6-7 hr.

AVAILABILITY

Capsules: 100 mg.

INDICATIONS AND DOSAGE

Gaucher's disease

PO

Adults, Elderly: One 100-mg capsule 3 times per day at regular intervals.

Dosage in renal impairment

For patients with creatinine clearance of 50-75 mL/min, dosage is reduced to 100 mg twice per day. For patients with creatinine clearance of 30-49 mL/min, dosage is 100 mg once per day. Drug is not recommended

M

if creatinine clearance is less than 30 mL/min.

CONTRAINDICATIONS

Women who are or may become pregnant, hypersensitivity to miglustat

INTERACTIONS

Drug: Imiglucerase: May decrease the effects of imiglucerase. **Herbal:** None known. **Food:** None known.

DIAGNOSTIC TEST EFFECTS

None known.

SIDE-EFFECTS

Expected (89%-65%): Diarrhea, weight loss. **Frequent (39%-11%):** Hand tremor, flatulence, headache, abdominal pain, nausea. **Occasional (7%-4%):** Paresthesia, anorexia, dyspepsia, leg cramps, vomiting

CRITICAL CARE CONSIDERATIONS

ADMINISTRATION/HANDLING

PO ALERT

- Give miglustat without regard to food.
- Swallow capsules whole; do not open, crush, or break capsules.

PRECAUTIONS

HEALTH-RELATED

- Use miglustat cautiously in patients with impaired fertility or renal function.

AGE-RELATED

- **Children:** Safety and efficacy of miglustat have not been established in children.
- **Elderly:** Age-related renal impairment may prompt a dosage adjustment.

PREGNANCY/LACTATION-RELATED

- Pregnancy category X; use cautiously in breast-feeding women.

MONITORING

- **Baseline assessment:** Perform a baseline neurologic evaluation with follow-up evaluations every 6 mo throughout treatment.
- **Baseline lab work:** Biochemical profile including renal function studies.
- **Hydration:** Provide or encourage patients to maintain adequate fluid intake.
- **Diarrhea:** Assess bowel sounds for peristalsis, pattern of daily bowel activity, and stool consistency.
- **Weight loss:** Weigh patients weekly and provide adequate nutrition.
- **Hand tremors:** Observe for hand tremor.
- **Patient education:** Instruct to avoid high-carbohydrate foods during miglustat treatment if diarrhea occurs. Stress the need to use reliable contraceptive methods during miglustat treatment and for 3 mo afterward. Remind to report intention of getting pregnant to a health care provider and plan to stop miglustat therapy before trying to conceive.

SERIOUS ADVERSE REACTIONS

- Thrombocytopenia occurs in 7% of patients.

OVERDOSE/TOXICITY

- Overdose produces dizziness and neutropenia.
- **GI decontamination:** No specific recommendations.

ANTIDOTE/DIALYSIS

- **Antidote:** No specific recommendations.
- **Dialysis:** No data are available on removal using hemodialysis, high-permeability hemodialysis, or peritoneal dialysis.

milrinone lactate 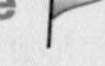

mill'-re-none lak'-tate

Classes

Chemical: bipyridine derivative
Therapeutic: cardiac inotropic agent

Pregnancy Category: C

Trade Names

Prescription: Primacor, Primacor IV

CLINICAL PHARMACOLOGY

Mechanism of Action

A cardiac inotropic agent that inhibits phosphodiesterase, which increases cyclic adenosine monophosphate and potentiates the delivery of calcium to myocardial contractile systems. **Therapeutic Effect:** Relaxes vascular muscle, causing vasodilation. Increases cardiac output; decreases pulmonary capillary wedge pressure and vascular resistance.

PHARMACOKINETICS

Route	Onset	Peak	Duration
IV	5-15 min	N/A	3-5 hr

Protein binding: 70%. Primarily excreted unchanged in urine. **Half-life:** 2.4 hr.

AVAILABILITY

Injection (Primacor, Primacor IV): 1 mg/mL, 10-mL single-dose vial, 20-mL single-dose vial, 50-mL single-dose vial, 5-mL sterile cartridge unit.
Injection (Premix [Primacor]): 200 mcg/mL.

INDICATIONS AND DOSAGE

Short-term management of heart failure

IV

Adults: Initially, 50 mcg/kg over 10 min. Continue with maintenance infusion rate of 0.375-0.75 mcg/kg/min based on hemodynamic and clinical response. Total daily dosage: 0.59-1.13 mg/kg.

Dosage in renal impairment

For patients with severe renal impairment (creatinine clearance 5 mL/min/1.73 m^2-50 mL/min/1.73 m^2), reduce dosage to 0.2-0.43 mcg/kg/min.

CONTRAINDICATIONS

Hypersensitivity to milrinone or inamrinone

INTERACTIONS

Drug: **Other cardiac glycosides:** Produces additive inotropic effects. **Herbal:** None known. **Food:** None known.

DIAGNOSTIC TEST EFFECTS

None known.

IV INCOMPATIBILITIES

Furosemide (Lasix)

IV COMPATIBILITIES

Calcium gluconate, digoxin (Lanoxin), diltiazem (Cardizem), *DOBUTamine (Dobutrex), *DOPamine (Intropin), heparin, lidocaine, magnesium, midazolam (Versed), nitroglycerin, potassium, propofol (Diprivan)

SIDE-EFFECTS

Frequent (4%-12%): Ventricular dysrhythmias, ventricular ectopy, supraventricular dysrhythmias. **Occasional (3%-1%):** Headache, hypotension, nonsustained and sustained ventricular tachycardia, ventricular fibrillation. **Rare (less than 1%):** Angina, chest pain, anaphylaxis, atrial fibrillation, liver dysfunction

CRITICAL CARE CONSIDERATIONS

ADMINISTRATION/HANDLING

IV ALERT

- **Storage:** Store at room temperature.
- **Loading dose IV injection:** Administer milrinone undiluted slowly over 10 min.

MILRINONE LOADING DOSE (1 mg/mL)

WEIGHT (Kg)	20	30	40	50	60	70	80	90	100
mL given	1	1.5	2	2.5	3	3.5	4	4.5	5

- **IV infusion:** Dilute 20-mg (20-mL) vial with 80 or 180 mL diluent (0.9% NaCl, D_5W) or 10-mg (10-mL) vial with 40 or 90 mL diluent to provide concentration of 200 or 100 mcg/mL, respectively. Maximum concentration: 100 mg/250 mL.

MILRINONE MAINTENANCE DOSE INFUSION RATE (100 mcg/mL) in mL/hr

DOSE (mcg/kg/min)	WEIGHT (kg)								
	20	30	40	50	60	70	80	90	100
0.375	4.5	6.8	9	11.3	13.5	15.8	18	20.3	22.5
0.4	4.8	7.2	9.6	12	14.4	16.8	19.2	21.6	24
0.5	6	9	12	15	18	21	24	27	30
0.6	7.2	10.8	14.4	18	21.6	25.2	28.8	32.4	36
0.7	8.4	12.6	16.8	21	25.2	29.4	33.6	37.8	42
0.75	9	13.5	18	22.5	27	31.5	36	40.5	45

PRECAUTIONS

HEALTH-RELATED

- Use milrinone cautiously in patients with atrial fibrillation or flutter, history of ventricular dysrhythmias, impaired renal function, or severe obstructive aortic or pulmonic valvular disease.

AGE-RELATED

- **Children:** Safety and efficacy of milrinone have not been established in children.
- **Elderly:** Age-related renal impairment may require dosage adjustment.

PREGNANCY/LACTATION-RELATED

- Pregnancy category C; use caution with breast-feeding mothers until more is known about excretion in breast milk.

MONITORING

- **Baseline assessment:** Assess heart rate, heart rhythm, and BP before starting treatment and throughout therapy. Assess breath sounds for crackles and rhonchi; check for dependent edema.
- **Baseline lab work:** Biochemical profile including potassium level, liver and renal function studies, cholesterol, triglyerides, CPK, and LDH. Obtain beta natriuretic peptide to assess for heart failure.

M

- **Diagnostic tests:** Echocardiogram to assess cardiac wall motion and ejection fraction.
- **Ongoing monitoring:** Monitor for hypotension, use continuous cardiac monitoring for dysrhythmias, possible pulmonary artery catheter for cardiac output, heart rate; assess for elevated BUN, creatinine, and serum potassium levels. If hypotension or dysrhythmias are noted, reduce or temporarily discontinue infusion until condition stabilizes.
- **Heart failure:** Assess for heart failure including elevated pulmonary capillary wedge pressure, elevated pulmonary artery systolic and diastolic pressures, and possibly elevated central venous pressure. Observe for shortness of breath, activity intolerance, edema, chest discomfort.
- **Patient education:** Instruct to report immediately palpitations or chest pain to a health care provider. Explain that milrinone is not a cure for heart failure but will help relieve symptoms.

SERIOUS ADVERSE REACTIONS

- Supraventricular and ventricular dysrhythmias (12%), nonsustained ventricular tachycardia (3%), and sustained ventricular tachycardia (1%) may occur.

M

OVERDOSE/TOXICITY

- **Hepatotoxicity:** Elevated liver enzymes.
- **Hypotension:** Low BP secondary to vasodilation.
- **Management:** Drug dose should be decreased, fluid resuscitation initiated if tolerated; otherwise, vasopressors to correct hypotension.
- **GI decontamination:** No specific recommendations.

ANTIDOTE/DIALYSIS

- **Antidote:** No specific recommendations.
- **Dialysis:** No data are available on removal of milrinone by hemodialysis, high-permeability hemodialysis, or peritoneal dialysis.

minocycline hydrochloride

mi-noe-sye'-kleen hye-droe-klor'-ide

Classes

Chemical: tetracycline derivative
Therapeutic: antibiotic

Pregnancy Category: D

Trade Names

Prescription: Arestin, Dynacin, Minocin, Myrac, Solodyn, Vectrin

Do not confuse Dynacin with Dynabac or Minocin with Mithracin or niacin.

CLINICAL PHARMACOLOGY

Mechanism of Action

A tetracycline antibiotic that inhibits bacterial protein synthesis by binding to ribosomes. **Therapeutic Effect:** Bacteriostatic.

PHARMACOKINETICS

Protein binding: 76%. Partial elimination in feces; minimal excretion in urine. Not removed by hemodialysis. **Half-life:** 11-12 hr (oral capsule).

AVAILABILITY

Capsules (Dynacin, Minocin, Vectrin): 50 mg, 75 mg, 100 mg.
Capsules (pellet-filled [Minocin]): 50 mg, 100 mg.
Tablets (Minocin, Myrac): 50 mg, 75 mg, 100 mg.
Extended-release tablets (Solodyn): 45 mg, 90 mg, 135 mg.
Powder for injection (Minocin, Myrac): 100 mg.

INDICATIONS AND DOSAGE

Mild, moderate, or severe prostate, urinary tract, and CNS infections (excluding meningitis); uncomplicated gonorrhea; inflammatory acne; brucellosis; skin granulomas; cholera; trachoma; nocardiasis; yaws; and syphilis when penicillins are contraindicated

PO

Adults, Elderly: Initially, 100-200 mg, then 100 mg every 12 hr or 50 mg every 6 hr. Maximum: 400 mg/day. **Adults, Elderly, Children over 12 yr:** Soldyn (acne) 45 mg once daily (45-59 kg), 90 mg once daily (60-90 kg), 135 mg once daily (91-136 kg) for 12 wk.

IV

Adults, Elderly: Initially, 200 mg, then 100 mg every 12 hr up to 400 mg/day.

PO, IV

Children older than 8 yr: Initially, 4 mg/kg, then 2 mg/kg every 12 hr.

OFF-LABEL USES

Treatment of atypical mycobacterial infections, rheumatoid arthritis, scleroderma

CONTRAINDICATIONS

Children younger than 8 yr, children younger than 12 yr for Solodyn, hypersensitivity to minocycline or other tetracyclines, last half of pregnancy

INTERACTIONS

Drug: **Carbamazepine, phenytoin:** May decrease minocycline blood concentration. **Cholestyramine, colestipol:** May decrease minocycline absorption. **Ergot:** May increase the risk of ergotism. **Oral contraceptives:** May decrease the effects of oral contraceptives. **Herbal:** **St. John's wort:** May increase the risk of photosensitivity. **Food:** None known.

DIAGNOSTIC TEST EFFECTS

May increase serum alkaline phosphatase, amylase, bilirubin, AST (SGOT), and ALT (SGPT) levels.

IV INCOMPATIBILITIES

Piperacillin and tazobactam (Zosyn)

IV COMPATIBILITIES

Heparin, magnesium, potassium

SIDE-EFFECTS

Frequent: Dizziness, lightheadedness, diarrhea, nausea, vomiting, abdominal cramps, possibly severe photosensitivity, drowsiness, vertigo. **Occasional:** Altered pigmentation of skin or mucous membranes, rectal or genital pruritus, stomatitis

CRITICAL CARE CONSIDERATIONS

ADMINISTRATION/HANDLING

PO ALERT

- Store the oral drug at room temperature.
- Give capsules and tablets with a full glass of water.
- Space drug doses evenly around the clock.

IV ALERT

- **Storage:** IV solution may be stored for up to 24 hr at room temperature. Discard the solution if a precipitate forms.
- **Intermittent IV reconstitution:** Reconstitute each 100-mg vial with 5 to 10 mL of sterile water for injection to provide a concentration of 20 or 10 mg/mL, respectively.
- **Further dilution:** Further dilute with 500 to 1000 mL D_5W or 0.9% NaCl.
- **IV intermittent (piggyback) infusion:** Administer immediately after reconstitution. Infuse over 6 hr.

PRECAUTIONS

HEALTH-RELATED

- Use minocycline cautiously in patients with renal impairment and in those who are unable to avoid sun or ultraviolet exposure; exposure may produce a severe photosensitivity reaction.

AGE-RELATED

- **Children:** Minocycline use during infancy through 8 yr may result in permanent discoloration of the teeth.
- **Elderly:** Age-related renal impairment may prompt a need for decreased dosage.

PREGNANCY/LACTATION-RELATED

- Pregnancy category D. Not recommended in last half of pregnancy secondary to adverse effects on fetal teeth. Not recommended during breast-feeding.

MONITORING

- **Baseline assessment:** Determine history of allergies, especially to tetracyclines or sulfites, before beginning drug therapy.
- **Baseline lab work:** Biochemical panel including renal (BUN, creatinine) and liver function (AST [SGOT], AST [SGPT], alkaline phosphatase) studies; amylase and lipase to evaluate for pancreatitis; obtain appropriate cultures to diagnose suspected infection before beginning treatment.
- **Neurologic side effects:** Check BP and mental status because of the potential for benign intracranial hypertension. Assess ability to ambulate; minocycline may cause dizziness, drowsiness, or vertigo.
- **Diarrhea:** Assess pattern of daily bowel activity and stool consistency.
- **GI side effects:** Monitor for anorexia, nausea, vomiting, dysphagia, and glossitis.
- **Hypersensitivity:** Examine skin for rash; note any itching.
- **Superinfection:** Be alert for anal or genital pruritus, diarrhea, furry or white-coated tongue, and stomatitis.
- **Patient education:** Instruct to drink a full glass of water with minocycline capsules or tablets. Dosing immediately before lying down may increase nausea. Advise spacing drug doses evenly around the clock and to continue taking minocycline for the full course of treatment. Warn to avoid tasks that require mental alertness or motor skills until response to the drug is known. Instruct to report diarrhea, rash, or other new symptoms to a health care provider. Encourage avoidance of overexposure to the sun or

ultraviolet light to prevent a photosensitivity reaction.

SERIOUS ADVERSE REACTIONS

- **Superinfection:** Fungal infections are seen most often.
- **Hypersensitivity reaction:** Rash, urticaria, angioneurotic edema, pericarditis, exacerbation of systemic lupus erythematosus, and rarely pulmonary infiltrates and anaphylaxis.
- **Benign intracranial hypertension:** Headache and blurred vision may occur in adults and children; may rarely cause bulging fontanelles in infants.

OVERDOSE/TOXICITY

- **Hepatotoxicity:** Elevated liver enzymes (AST [SGOT], AST [SGPT], alkaline phosphatase, bilirubin) with right upper quadrant pain, edema, and jaundice; seen more often in patients with renal impairment; drug accumulates because of a lack of normal elimination.
- **Nephrotoxicity:** Elevated BUN and creatinine, decreased creatinine clearance, oliguria, nausea, and vomiting.
- **Pancreatitis:** Elevated amylase and lipase with abdominal pain.
- **Blood dyscrasias:** Hemolytic anemia, thrombocytopenia, neutropenia, eosinophilia.
- **Management:** Discontinue drug and symptoms should resolve. If not, supportive care is required for each problem based on current standard of care.
- **GI decontamination:** No specific recommendations.

ANTIDOTE/DIALYSIS

- **Antidote:** No specific recommendations.
- **Dialysis:** Minocycline is not removed by hemodialysis or peritoneal dialysis. No data are available on removal using high-permeability hemodialysis.

minoxidil

See Antihypertensives, Miscellaneous (p. 931)

mirtazapine

mir-taz'-a-peen

Classes

Chemical: tetracyclic piperazino-azepine derivative
Therapeutic: antidepressant

Pregnancy Category: C

Trade Names

Prescription: Remeron, Remeron Soltab

Do not confuse Remeron with Premarin.

CLINICAL PHARMACOLOGY

Mechanism of Action

A tetracyclic compound that acts as an antagonist at presynaptic $alpha_2$-adrenergic receptors, increasing both norepinephrine and serotonin neurotransmission. Has low anticholinergic activity. **Therapeutic Effect:** Relieves depression and produces sedative effects.

PHARMACOKINETICS

Rapidly and completely absorbed after PO administration; absorption not affected by food. Protein binding: 85%. Metabolized in the liver. Primarily excreted in urine. **Half-life:** 20-40 hr (longer in males [37 hr] than females [26 hr]).

AVAILABILITY

Tablets: 7.5 mg, 15 mg, 30 mg, 45 mg.
Tablets (disintegrating): 15 mg, 30 mg, 45 mg.

INDICATIONS AND DOSAGE

Depression

PO

Adults: Initially, 15 mg at bedtime. May increase by 15 mg/day every 1-2 wk. Maximum: 45 mg/day. **Elderly:** Initially, 7.5 mg at bedtime. May increase by 7.5-15 mg/day every 1-2 wk. Maximum: 45 mg/day.

CONTRAINDICATIONS

Use within 14 days of MAOIs, hypersensitivity to mirtazapine

INTERACTIONS

Drug: **Alcohol, diazepam:** May increase impairment of cognition and motor skills. **Clonidine:** May decrease the effect of clonidine; may increase BP significantly if clonidine is abruptly discontinued. **MAOIs:** May increase the risk of neuroleptic malignant syndrome, hypertensive crisis, and severe seizures. **Linezolid:** Avoid if possible if MAOIs are being used. **Tramadol:** May increase the risk of serotonin syndrome. **Herbal:** None known. **Food:** None known.

DIAGNOSTIC TEST EFFECTS

May increase serum cholesterol, triglyceride, AST (SGOT), and ALT (SGPT) levels.

SIDE-EFFECTS

Frequent: Somnolence (54%), dry mouth (25%), increased appetite (17%), constipation (13%), weight gain (12%). **Occasional:** Asthenia (8%), dizziness (7%), flulike symptoms (5%), abnormal dreams (4%). **Rare:** Abdominal discomfort, vasodilation, paresthesia, acne, dry skin, thirst, arthralgia

CRITICAL CARE CONSIDERATIONS

ADMINISTRATION/HANDLING

PO ALERT

- Give mirtazapine without regard to food.
- Scored tablets may be crushed or broken if needed.

PRECAUTIONS

HEALTH-RELATED

- **MAOIs:** Make sure at least 14 days elapse between the use of MAOIs and mirtazapine.
- Use mirtazapine cautiously in patients with cardiovascular disorders, GI disorders, angle-closure glaucoma, benign prostatic hyperplasia, hepatic or renal impairment, or urine retention.

AGE-RELATED

- **Children:** Safety and efficacy of mirtazapine have not been established in children.
- **Elderly:** Age-related renal impairment may require cautious use.

PREGNANCY/LACTATION-RELATED

- Pregnancy category C; not recommended for use in breast-feeding women.

MONITORING

- **Baseline assessment:** Assess appearance, behavior, level of interest, mood, and sleep pattern.
- **Baseline lab work:** CBC with WBC differential; biochemical panel including renal (BUN and creatinine) and liver function tests (alkaline phosphatase, bilirubin, AST [SGOT], and ALT [SGPT]) levels before and periodically in patients on long-term therapy.
- **Baseline diagnostic tests:** 12-lead ECG to assess for dysrhythmias.
- **Suicide precautions:** Closely supervise suicidal patients during early therapy. As depression lessens, energy level improves, increasing the suicide potential.
- **Cardiac effects:** Continuously monitor ECG in patients at high risk for dysrhythmias and hypotension.
- **Neurologic effects:** Monitor for tremors and seizures.
- **Therapeutic effects:** Assess for improvement in appearance, behavior, level of interest, mood, and sleep pattern.
- **Patient education:** Instruct to take mirtazapine as a single bedtime dose. Urge avoidance of alcohol as well as other sedating medications during therapy. Warn to avoid tasks that require mental alertness or motor skills until response to the drug is known.

SERIOUS ADVERSE REACTIONS

- **Seizures:** Mirtazapine poses a higher risk of seizures than tricyclic antidepressants, especially in those with no previous history of seizures.
- **Withdrawal:** Abrupt discontinuation after prolonged therapy may produce headache, malaise, nausea, vomiting, and vivid dreams.
- **Use within 14 days of MAOIs:** Nausea; vomiting; agitation; flushing; diaphoresis; dizziness; tremor; myoclonus; hyperthermia with rapid fluctuations in vital signs resulting in seizures, coma, and death.

OVERDOSE/TOXICITY

- **Bone marrow suppression:** Agranulocytosis and neutropenia occur rarely.
- **Overdose:** Hypotension, altered mental status, tremors, dizziness, tachycardia, palpitations, seizures, and dysrhythmias.
- **Management:** Maintain patent airway, support ventilation, support BP with IV fluids and vasopressors if needed, benzodiazepines for seizures.
- **GI decontamination:** No specific recommendations.

ANTIDOTE/DIALYSIS

- **Antidote:** No specific recommendations.
- **Dialysis:** Mirtazapine is unlikely to be removed by hemodialysis or peritoneal dialysis. No data are available on removal using high-permeability hemodialysis.

modafinil

moe-daf′-ih-nil

Classes

Chemical: benzhydrylsulfinylacetamide compound

Therapeutic: central nervous system stimulant

M

Pregnancy Category: C

Trade Names
Prescription: Alertec ♣, Provigil, Sparlon

Do not confuse modafinil with moexipril.

CLINICAL PHARMACOLOGY
Mechanism of Action
An $alpha_1$-agonist that may bind to dopamine reuptake carrier sites, increasing alpha activity and decreasing delta, theta, and beta brain wave activity. **Therapeutic Effect:** Reduces the number of sleep episodes and total daytime sleep.

PHARMACOKINETICS
Well absorbed. Protein binding: 60%. Widely distributed. Metabolized in the liver. Excreted by the kidneys. Unknown if removed by hemodialysis. **Half-life:** 8-10 hr.

AVAILABILITY
Tablets: 85 mg (Sparlon), 100 mg (Provigil), 170 mg (Sparlon), 200 mg (Provigil), 255 mg (Sparlon), 340 mg (Sparlon), 425 mg (Sparlon).

INDICATIONS AND DOSAGE
Narcolepsy, other sleep disorders
PO
Adults, Elderly: 200 mg/day taken at 1 hr before work shift. Sparlon: 85-425 mg once per day.
Attention-deficit/hyperactivity disorder (ADHD)
PO
Adults, Elderly: 100-300 mg daily. **Children:** 50-100 mg daily.

OFF-LABEL USES
Treatment of ADHD, brain injury–related underarousal, depression, endozepine stupor, multiple sclerosis–related fatigue, Parkinson-related fatigue, seasonal affective disorder

CONTRAINDICATIONS
Hypersensitivity to modafinil

INTERACTIONS
Drug: *CycloSPORINE, oral contraceptives, theophylline: May decrease plasma concentrations of these drugs. **Diazepam, phenytoin, propranolol, tricyclic antidepressants, warfarin:** May increase plasma concentrations of these drugs. **Other CNS stimulants:** May increase CNS stimulation.
Herbal: None known. **Food:** None known.

DIAGNOSTIC TEST EFFECTS
None known.

SIDE-EFFECTS
Frequent: Anxiety, insomnia, nausea.
Occasional: Anorexia, diarrhea, dizziness, dry mouth or skin, muscle stiffness, polydipsia, rhinitis, paresthesia, tremor, headache, vomiting

CRITICAL CARE CONSIDERATIONS

ADMINISTRATION/HANDLING
PO ALERT
- Give modafinil without regard to food.

PRECAUTIONS
HEALTH-RELATED
- Use modafinil cautiously in patients with hepatic or renal impairment, or a history of clinically significant mitral valve prolapse, left ventricular hypertrophy, or seizures.
- **Steroidal/hormonal contraceptives:** Effectiveness of hormonal contraceptives may be reduced while on modafinil therapy and up to 1 mo following discontinuation.
- **Cytochrome P450 enzyme drug interactions:** Modafinil has several actions among the cytochrome P450 enzyme pathways; may prompt drug interactions when given concomitantly with cytochrome P450 enzyme inhibitors. Drugs affected may include ketoconazole, itraconazole, carbamazepine, phenobarbital, rifampin, *cycloSPORINE, theophylline, warfarin, phenytoin, diazepam, propranolol, and tricyclic antidepressants.

AGE-RELATED
- **Children:** Safety and efficacy of modafinil have not been established in children under 16 yr.
- **Elderly:** Safety and efficacy have not been established. Age-related hepatic or renal impairment may require decreased dosage.

PREGNANCY/LACTATION-RELATED
- Pregnancy category C; no mutagenic or clastogenic potential in several *in vitro* assays; *in vivo* mouse bone marrow micronucleus assays were also negative for mutagenicity; not fully evaluated; breast milk excretion unknown

MONITORING
- **Baseline assessment:** Obtain history of narcolepsy or other sleep disorders, including

the duration, pattern, frequency, and severity of sleep episodes and the environmental situations in which they occurred. Ask patients if they have experienced a sudden loss of muscle tone (cataplexy) precipitated by strong emotional responses before a sleep episode.

- **Baseline lab work:** Biochemical profile including renal (BUN, creatinine) and liver function tests (AST [SGOT], ALT [SGPT], alkaline phosphatase, bilirubin), CPK and LDH.
- **Baseline diagnostic tests:** Echocardiogram for patients with mitral valve prolapse or left ventricular hypertrophy if not recently done.
- **Sleep pattern:** Monitor sleep pattern including restlessness during sleep and the duration of insomnia at night.
- **Neurologic/behavioral effects:** Assess for anxiety and dizziness. Institute safety precautions as needed.
- **Patient education:** Instruct not to increase the drug dose without prior approval from a health care provider. Warn to avoid tasks that require mental alertness or motor skills until response to the drug is known. Advise to use a nonhormonal contraceptive method during modafinil therapy and for 1 mo afterward. Modafinil decreases the effectiveness of hormonal contraceptives. Sipping water and chewing sugarless gum may relieve dry mouth.

SERIOUS ADVERSE REACTIONS

- **Insomnia:** Occasionally occurs.
- **Cardiac effects:** Hypertension; ST-T wave changes may occur in patients with cardiac disease.
- **Behavioral effects:** Agitation, excitation; rare delusions and hallucinations.

OVERDOSE/TOXICITY

- **Overdose:** Fever, altered mental status, seizures, hypertension, tachycardia, dysrhythmias.
- **Management:** Discontinue modafinil. Provide symptom-specific, supportive care.
- **GI decontamination:** No specific recommendations.

ANTIDOTE/DIALYSIS

- **Antidote:** No specific recommendations.
- **Dialysis:** No data are available on removal of modafinil by hemodialysis, high-permeability hemodialysis, or peritoneal dialysis.

moexipril hydrochloride

See ACE Inhibitors (p. 883)

molindone

See Antipsychotics (p. 934)

mometasone furoate monohydrate

See Bronchodilators (p. 947)

montelukast

See Bronchodilators (p. 947)

moricizine hydrochloride

See Antidysrhythmics (p. 919)

M

morphine sulfate 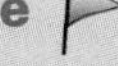

mor'-feen sul'-fate

DEA Schedule: II

Classes

Chemical: natural opium alkaloid, phenanthrene derivative

Therapeutic: narcotic analgesic

Pregnancy Category: C, D

Trade Names

Prescription: Astramorph PF, Avinza, Depo-Dur, Duramorph PF, Infumorph, Kadian, M-Eslon, MS Contin, MSIR, MS/S, Oramorph SR, Rapi-Ject, RMS, Roxanol, Roxanol-T, Statex ♣

Do not confuse morphine with hydromorphone, or Roxanol with Roxicet.

CLINICAL PHARMACOLOGY

Mechanism of Action

An opioid agonist that binds with opioid receptors in the CNS. **Therapeutic Effect:** Alters the perception of and emotional response to pain; produces generalized CNS depression.

PHARMACOKINETICS

Route	Onset	Peak	Duration
Oral solution	N/A	1 hr	3-5 hr
Tablets	30 min	1 hr	3-5 hr
Tablets (ER)	N/A	3-4 hr	8-12 hr
IV	Rapid	0.3 hr	3-5 hr
IM	5-30 min	0.5-1 hr	3-5 hr
Epidural	15-60 min	1 hr	12-24 hr
Subcutaneous	15-30 min	1.1-5 hr	3-5 hr
Rectal	20-60 min	0.5-1 hr	3-7 hr

Variably absorbed from the GI tract. Readily absorbed after IM or subcutaneous administration. Protein binding: 30%-35%. Widely distributed. Metabolized in the liver. Primarily excreted in urine. **Half-life:** 2-4 hr (increased in patients with hepatic disease).

AVAILABILITY

Capsules (extended release): 20 mg (Kadian), 30 mg (Avinza, Kadian), 50 mg (Kadian), 60 mg (Avinza, Kadian), 90 mg (Avinza), 100 mg (Kadian), 120 mg (Avinza).
Capsules (MSIR): 15 mg, 30 mg.
Solution for injection: 0.5 mg/mL, 1 mg/mL, 2 mg/mL, 4 mg/mL, 5 mg/mL, 8 mg/mL, 10 mg/mL, 15 mg/mL, 25 mg/mL, 50 mg/mL.
Solution for injection: 5% dextrose-20 mg morphine/100 mL, 5% dextrose-100 mg morphine/100 mL.
Solution for injection (preservative free): 0.5 mg/mL (Astramorph PF, Duramorph PF), 1 mg/mL (Astramorph PF, Duramorph PF), 10 mg/mL (Infumorph), 25 mg/mL (Infumorph), 50 mg/mL.
Epidural and intrathecal via infusion device (Infumorph): 10 mg/mL, 25 mg/mL.
Oral solution: 10 mg/5 mL (MSIR), 20 mg/5 mL (MSIR, Roxanol), 100 mg/5 mL (Roxanol).
Suppositories (RMS): 5 mg, 10 mg, 20 mg, 30 mg.
Tablets (MSIR): 15 mg, 30 mg.
Tablets (extended release): 15 mg (MS Contin, Oramorph SR), 30 mg (MS Contin, Oramorph SR), 60 mg (MS Contin, Oramorph SR), 100 mg (MS Contin, Oramorph SR), 200 mg (MS Contin).
Liposomal injection (DepoDur): 10 mg/mL, 15 mg/1.5 mL, 20 mg/2 mL.

INDICATIONS AND DOSAGE

Alert: Dosage should be titrated to desired effect.

Analgesia

PO (prompt release)

Adults, Elderly: 10-30 mg every 3-4 hr as needed. **Children over 6 mo, less than 50 kg:** 0.15-0.3 mg/kg every 3-4 hr as needed. **Alert:** For the Avinza dosage below, be aware that this drug is to be administered once per day only. **Alert:** For the Kadian dosage information that follows, be aware that this drug is to be administered every 12 hr or once per day only. **Alert:** Be aware that pediatric dosages of extended-release preparations Kadian and Avinza have not been established. **Alert:** For the MS Contin and Oramorph SR dosage information below, be aware that the daily dosage is divided and given every 8 hr or every 12 hr.

PO (Extended Release [Avinza])

Adults, Elderly: Dosage requirement should be established using prompt-release formulations and is based on total daily dose. Avinza is given once per day only.

PO (Extended Release [Kadian])

Adults, Elderly: Dosage requirement should be established using prompt-release formulations and is based on total daily dose. Dose is given once per day or divided and given every 12 hr.

PO (Extended Release [MS Contin, Oramorph SR])

Adults, Elderly: Dosage requirement should be established using prompt-release formulations and is based on total daily dose. Daily dose is divided and given every 8 hr or every 12 hr. **Children:** 0.3-0.6 mg/kg/dose every 12 hr.

IV

Adults, Elderly: 2.5-5 mg every 3-4 hr as needed. Note: Repeated doses (e.g., 1-2 mg) may be given more frequently (e.g., every hr) if needed. **Children:** 0.05-0.1 mg/kg every 2-4 hr as needed. Maximum: 15 mg/dose.

IV Continuous Infusion

Adults, Elderly: 0.8-10 mg/hr. Range: Up to 80 mg/hr. **Children:** 0.01 mg/kg/hr to 0.03 mg/kg/hr.

IM

Adults, Elderly: 5-10 mg every 3-4 hr as needed. **Children:** 0.1-0.2 mg/kg every 2-4 hr as needed. Maximum: 15 mg/dose.

Epidural

Adults, Elderly: Initially, 3-5 mg bolus, infusion rate: 0.1-0.2 mg/h. Maximum: 10 mg/24 hr.

Intrathecal

Adults, Elderly: One-tenth of the epidural dose: 0.2-0.25 mg/dose.

Patient-controlled analgesia

IV

Adults, Elderly: Loading dose: 5-10 mg. Intermittent bolus: 0.5-3 mg. Lockout interval: 5-12 min. Continuous infusion: 1-10 mg/hr. 4-hr limit: 20-30 mg.

CONTRAINDICATIONS

Acute or severe asthma, GI obstruction, paralytic ileus, severe hepatic or renal impairment, severe respiratory depression, hypersensitivity to morphine

INTERACTIONS

Drug: **Alcohol, other CNS depressants:** May increase CNS or respiratory depression and hypotension. **MAOIs:** May produce a severe, sometimes fatal reaction; expect to administer one quarter of usual morphine dose. **Herbal:** None known. **Food:** None known.

DIAGNOSTIC TEST EFFECTS

May increase serum amylase and lipase levels.

IV INCOMPATIBILITIES

Amphotericin B complex (Abelcet, AmBisome, Amphotec), cefepime (Maxipime), *DOXOrubicin liposomal (Doxil), thiopental

IV COMPATIBILITIES

Amiodarone (Cordarone), atropine, bumetanide (Bumex), bupivacaine (Marcaine, Sensorcaine), diltiazem (Cardizem), *diphenhydrAMINE (Benadryl), *DOBUTamine (Dobutrex), *DOPamine (Intropin), glycopyrrolate (Robinul), heparin, *hydrOXYzine (Vistaril), lidocaine, lorazepam (Ativan), magnesium, midazolam (Versed), milrinone (Primacor), nitroglycerin, potassium, propofol (Diprivan), total parenteral nutrition (TPN)

SIDE-EFFECTS

Frequent: Sedation, decreased BP (including orthostatic hypotension), diaphoresis, facial flushing, constipation, dizziness, somnolence, nausea, vomiting. **Occasional:** Allergic reaction (rash, pruritus), dyspnea, confusion, palpitations, tremors, urine retention, abdominal cramps, vision changes, dry mouth, headache, decreased appetite, pain or burning at injection site. **Rare:** Paralytic ileus

CRITICAL CARE CONSIDERATIONS

ADMINISTRATION/HANDLING

PO ALERT

- Mix the liquid form with fruit juice to improve the taste.
- Do not crush, open, or break extended-release capsules.
- Kadian (extended-release capsules) may be mixed with soft food such as applesauce just before administration.

IV ALERT

- **Storage:** Store vials at room temperature.
- **Preparation:** Place patients in the recumbent position before giving parenteral morphine.
- **IV push/direct injection:** Morphine may be given undiluted as IV push; or 2.5 to 15.0 mg morphine may be diluted in 4 to 5 mL sterile water for injection.
- **IV administration:** Administer IV morphine very slowly because rapid IV administration increases the risk of a severe anaphylactic reaction (apnea, cardiac arrest, and circulatory collapse).
- **Continuous IV infusion:** Dilute to a concentration of 0.1 to 1.0 mg/mL in D_5W and administer through a controlled infusion device.

IM, SUBCUTANEOUS ALERT

- **Administration:** Inject the drug slowly; rotate injection sites.
- **Circulatory impaired patients:** Patients with circulatory impairment are at increased risk for overdose because of delayed absorption of repeated injections.

RECTAL ALERT

- **Preparation:** If the suppository is too soft, refrigerate it for 30 min or run cold water over the foil wrapper.
- **Administration:** Moisten the suppository with cold water before inserting well into the rectum.

PRECAUTIONS

HEALTH-RELATED

- Use morphine extremely cautiously in patients with chronic obstructive pulmonary disease, cor pulmonale, head injury, hypoxia, hypercapnia, increased intracranial pressure, preexisting respiratory depression, or severe hypotension.
- Use morphine cautiously in debilitated patients and in those with Addison's disease, alcoholism, biliary tract disease, CNS depression, hypothyroidism, pancreatitis, benign prostatic hyperplasia, seizure disorders, toxic psychosis, or urethral stricture.
- **Reduce morphine dosage:** For debilitated and elderly patients and those using CNS depressants concurrently. Titrate dosage to desired effect.
- **Side effects:** Morphine's side effects are dependent on the dosage, route of

M

administration, patient position, and level of pain. Ambulatory patients with mild to moderate pain may experience dizziness, nausea, and vomiting more than those in severe pain who are recumbent in the supine position.

AGE-RELATED

- **Children:** Children are more prone to experience paradoxic excitement. Children under 2 yr are more susceptible to the drug's respiratory depressant effects.
- **Elderly:** Age-related renal impairment may increase the risk of urine retention in the elderly. Elderly are more prone to experience paradoxic excitement and the drug's respiratory depressant effects.

PREGNANCY/LACTATION-RELATED

- Pregnancy category C (D if used for prolonged periods or at high dosages at term); trace amounts enter breast milk; compatible with breast-feeding.

MONITORING

- **Baseline assessment:** Assess the duration, location, onset, and type of pain. Obtain vital signs before administering morphine. If cough is being treated, assess the frequency, severity, and type of cough. If not receiving comfort care, withhold the drug if the respiratory rate is less than 9 breaths/min or less than 16 breaths/min in a child.
- **Persistent pain:** The drug's effect is reduced if the full pain response recurs before the next dose. Instruct to report when pain begins to return. It is inappropriate to tell patients in pain it is not yet time for medication. Medication should be provided at the proper frequency and dosage to keep patients comfortable.
- **Autonomic nervous system depression:** Monitor vital signs for bradycardia, hypotension, and bradypnea. If respiratory rate is consistently below 10 breaths/min or very shallow, pulse rate is consistently below 50 beats/min, and BP is consistently below 85 mmHg systolic, with difficulty awakening patients or keeping patients awake, consider reducing medication dose or frequency of administration unless patients are receiving end-of-life comfort care.
- **Ventilation/oxygenation:** Monitor pulse oximetry (SpO_2) continuously on patients receiving high doses or continuous IV or epidural medication infusions. Use reading to augment assessment of ventilation and oxygenation, rather than *in place of* the assessment. Low readings may be corrected using supplemental oxygen and/or noninvasive positive pressure ventilation (bilevel positive airway pressure [BiPAP] or continuous positive airway pressure [CPAP]) on nonintubated/mechanically ventilated patients if drug dosage reduction results in patient experiencing severe pain.
- **Pulmonary hygiene:** Initiate deep-breathing and coughing exercises, particularly in patients with impaired respiratory function.
- **Persistent coughing:** For patients being treated for a cough, auscultate the lungs for adventitious breath sounds, and increase fluid intake and environmental humidity to decrease the viscosity of lung secretions.
- **Constipation:** Assess pattern of daily bowel activity and stool consistency, especially with long-term use.
- **Therapeutic response:** Assess for clinical improvement and record the onset of pain or cough relief. The effect of morphine is reduced if a full pain response recurs before the next dose.
- **Tolerance and dependence:** Monitor usage pattern for development of tolerance and assess for physical dependence.
- **Patient education:** Instruct to alert a health care provider when pain starts to return; morphine is less effective if a full pain response recurs before the next dose. Explain that drug dependence and tolerance may occur with prolonged use of high dosages. Urge avoidance of alcohol during hydromorphone therapy. Warn to avoid tasks that require mental alertness and motor skills until response to the drug is known. Instruct to change positions slowly to avoid orthostatic hypotension. Inform that injection of morphine may cause discomfort.

SERIOUS ADVERSE REACTIONS

- **Tolerance:** Drug tolerance is common when managing chronic pain patients and requires increasing doses of medication or combinations of medications to provide pain relief.
- **Dependence:** Addiction to narcotics occurs infrequently compared with drug tolerance, but chronic pain patients are often viewed as addicted when tolerance has occurred. Patients with cancer pain or other severe pain may require extraordinary doses to attain pain relief due to drug tolerance or low pain tolerance,

rather than addiction. Do not withhold medication from patients based on dosage norms when dealing with patients in severe, persistent pain.

- **Cumulative effect:** Morphine may have a prolonged duration of action and cumulative effect in patients with hepatic or renal impairment.

OVERDOSE/TOXICITY

- **Overdose:** Respiratory depression, difficulty awakening, disorientation, skeletal muscle flaccidity, cold or clammy skin, cyanosis, and extreme somnolence progressing to seizures, stupor, coma, and death.
- **Death from "double effect":** Terminally ill patients sometimes require dosage of medication for pain relief that may be lethal. If patients will not be resuscitated and have been informed of the potential complications of high-dose narcotic administration, if death ensues, the ethics principle of double effect makes it permissible for health care providers to administer potentially lethal doses of medication as long as the intent is pain relief rather than euthanasia.
- **Management:** Initiate Advanced Cardiac Life Support (ACLS) guidelines for respiratory depression and management of bradycardia and hypotension, if present.
- **GI decontamination:** No specific recommendations.

ANTIDOTE/DIALYSIS

- **Antidote:** Naloxone 0.4-2 mg IV, subcutaneous, or IM; may repeat if ineffective; well absorbed IM and subcutaneous in noncirculatory impaired patients. Use with caution in patients with cardiovascular disease to avoid compromise if opiates rapidly displace from receptors. Hypertension, tachypnea, and return of extreme pain may immediately occur, causing extreme increases in myocardial oxygen consumption.
- **Dialysis:** Morphine is not removed by high-permeability hemodialysis or peritoneal dialysis. No data are available on removal by conventional hemodialysis.

moxifloxacin hydrochloride

See Antibiotics (p. 892)

muromonab-CD3

myoo-roe-moe'-nab

Classes

Chemical: monoclonal antibody
Therapeutic: immunosuppressant

Pregnancy Category: C

Trade Names

Prescription: Orthoclone OKT3

CLINICAL PHARMACOLOGY

Mechanism of Action

A monoclonal antibody derived from purified IgG_2 that reacts with a T-3 (CD3) antigen of human T-cell membranes, blocking the production and function of T cells, which play a major role in acute organ rejection. Therapeutic Effect: Reverses organ rejection.

PHARMACOKINETICS

Primarily eliminated by binding to T lymphocytes. Half-life: approximately 18 hr.

AVAILABILITY

Injection: 1 mg/mL.

INDICATIONS AND DOSAGE

Treatment of acute renal allograft rejection

IV

Adults, Elderly, Children 12 yr and older: 5 mg/day for 10-14 days, beginning as soon as acute renal rejection is diagnosed. **Children more than 30 kg:** 5 mg IV once daily for 10-14 days, beginning as soon as acute renal rejection is diagnosed. **Children less than 30 kg:** 2.5 mg IV once daily for 10-14 days, beginning as soon as acute renal rejection is diagnosed.

CONTRAINDICATIONS

History of hypersensitivity to muromonab-CD3 or any murine-derived product (antibody titers more than 1:1000), fluid overload (as evidenced by chest x-ray or weight gain of more than 3%) in the week before initial treatment, pregnancy, history of seizures, uncontrolled hypertension

INTERACTIONS

Drug: **Live-virus vaccines:** May potentiate virus replication, increase the vaccine's side effects, and decrease the patient's response to the vaccine. **Other immunosuppressants:** May increase the risk of infection or lymphoproliferative disorders. Herbal:

M

Echinacea: May decrease the effects of muromonab-CD3. **Food:** None known.

DIAGNOSTIC TEST EFFECTS

None known.

IV INCOMPATIBILITIES

Do not mix muromonab with any other medications.

SIDE-EFFECTS

Frequent: Fever, chills, dyspnea, malaise frequently occur 30 min to 6 hr after first dose (this reaction markedly diminishes after the second day of treatment), nausea (32%), vomiting (25%), diarrhea (37%), hypotension (25%), hypertension (19%), rash (14%), headache (28%), tremor (14%).

CRITICAL CARE CONSIDERATIONS

ADMINISTRATION/HANDLING

IV ALERT

- **Preparation:** Resuscitative drugs and equipment should be immediately available.
- **Storage:** Refrigerate ampules. Do not use if drug has been left out of the refrigerator for longer than 4 hr. Solution may develop fine translucent particles, which will not affect potency; use of filter will clear particles.
- **Prior to use:** Do not shake ampules before using. Draw solution into the syringe through a 0.22-micron, low protein binding filter. Discard the filter; use a needle for IV administration.
- **IV push and direct injection:** Administer by IV push over less than 1 min.
- **Following injection:** Give 1 mg/kg methylprednisolone 1-4 hr before and 100 mg hydrocortisone 30 min after the first dose of muromonab, to decrease the risk and severity of cytokine release syndrome.

PRECAUTIONS

HEALTH-RELATED

- Use muromonab-CD3 cautiously in patients with impaired cardiac, hepatic, or renal function.
- **Experienced users only:** Only physicians experienced in immunosuppressive therapy and management of solid organ transplant patients should use muromonab-CD3. There is increased likelihood of greater morbidity and mortality when drug is used outside a facility staffed for close, expert monitoring by health care professionals familiar with the drug and transplant patients.

AGE-RELATED

- **Children:** Safety and efficacy of muromonab have not been established in children over 2 yr, but drug has been used; may be more likely to develop cerebral edema with or without herniation.
- **Elderly:** No adequate and well-controlled studies are available.

PREGNANCY/LACTATION-RELATED

- Pregnancy category C; safety for use in pregnancy and effect on fertility of both men and women has not been established. Breastfeeding should be discontinued.

MONITORING

- **Baseline assessment:** Check for fluid overload before beginning muromonab treatment to decrease the risk of pulmonary edema.
- **Baseline lab work:** Monitor immunologic test results (including plasma drug levels and quantitative T-lymphocyte surface phenotyping); obtain biochemical profile including liver and renal function test results, and CBC with WBC differential before and during therapy.
- **Baseline diagnostic tests:** Obtain chest x-ray within 24 hr of beginning muromonab therapy to ensure lungs are free of fluid.
- **Fever:** Give antipyretics to patients with a fever above 100°F.
- **Fluid overload:** Obtain chest x-rays and auscultate breath sounds to detect rales indicative of fluid overload. Assess for weight gain of more than 3% over pretherapy weight. Monitor intake and output.
- **Seizures:** Initiate seizure precautions and monitor for encephalopathy.
- **Cytokine release syndrome versus hypersensitivity reaction:** Monitor for reaction 30-60 min after administration of a dose. May range from flulike symptoms to shock. Patients experiencing a hypersensitivity reaction are more likely to begin symptoms within 10 min of the start of the infusion.
- **Thrombosis:** Drug can induce thrombus formation in any vascular bed of the body. Monitor for unexplained system failure, including heart attack, stroke, acute renal failure, bowel infarction, etc.
- **Patient education:** Warn to expect a first-dose reaction, including chest tightness, chills, fever, diarrhea, nausea, vomiting,

and wheezing. Urge avoidance of receiving immunizations and coming in contact with crowds and people with known infections during muromonab therapy.

SERIOUS ADVERSE REACTIONS

- **Cytokine release syndrome:** A common reaction; symptoms include mild flulike symptoms to a life-threatening, shock-like reaction with high fever, rigors/chills, headache, tremors, diarrhea, nausea, vomiting.
- **Fatal hypersensitivity reactions:** Occur occasionally. Pretreat with antipyretics and antihistamines to try to avoid reactions.
- **Infection due to immunosuppression:** Generally occurs within 45 days after initial treatment. Cytomegalovirus occurs in 19% of patients, and herpes simplex occurs in 27% of patients. Epstein-Barr virus is possible. A severe life-threatening infection occurs in fewer than 5% of patients.
- **Severe pulmonary edema:** Occurs in fewer than 2% of patients.
- **Thrombosis:** Arterial, venous, and capillary thromboses of allografts and other vascular beds (brain, heart, lungs, kidney, small and large bowel, etc.) are possible.

OVERDOSE/TOXICITY

- **Neurotoxicity:** Seizures, encephalopathy, aseptic meningitis syndrome.
- **Neoplasia:** Lymphoproliferative disorders, squamous cell carcinoma of the lip, skin, and sarcomas.
- **Management:** Manage according to current guidelines for the disorder.
- **GI decontamination:** No specific recommendations.

ANTIDOTE/DIALYSIS

- **Antidote:** No specific antidote.
- **Dialysis:** Muromonab-CD3 is unlikely to be removed by hemodialysis or peritoneal dialysis. No data are available on removal using high-permeability hemodialysis.

mycophenolate mofetil

mye-koe-fen'-oh-late moe-fet'-ill

Classes

Chemical: mycophenolic acid derivative
Therapeutic: immunosuppressant

Pregnancy Category: C

Trade Names

Prescription: CellCept, Myfortic

CLINICAL PHARMACOLOGY

Mechanism of Action

An immunologic agent that suppresses the immunologically mediated inflammatory response by inhibiting inosine monophosphate dehydrogenase, an enzyme that deprives lymphocytes of nucleotides necessary for DNA and RNA synthesis, thus inhibiting the proliferation of T and B lymphocytes. **Therapeutic Effect:** Prevents transplant rejection.

PHARMACOKINETICS

Rapidly and extensively absorbed after PO administration (food decreases drug plasma concentration but does not affect absorption). Protein binding: 97%. Completely hydrolyzed to active metabolite mycophenolic acid. Primarily excreted in urine. Not removed by hemodialysis. **Half-life:** 16-18 hr; delayed-release tablet: 8-16 hr.

AVAILABILITY

Capsules (CellCept): 250 mg.
Oral Suspension (CellCept): 200 mg/mL.
Tablets (CellCept): 500 mg.
Tablets (delayed release [Myfortic]): 180 mg, 360 mg.
Injection (CellCept): 500 mg.

INDICATIONS AND DOSAGE

Prevention of renal transplant rejection

PO, IV (CellCept)

Adults, Elderly: 1 g twice per day.

PO (Myfortic)

Adults, Elderly: 720 mg twice per day.
Children 5-16 yr: 400 mg/m^2 twice per day. Maximum: 720 mg twice per day.

Prevention of heart transplant rejection

PO, IV (CellCept)

Adults, Elderly: 1.5 g twice per day.

Prevention of liver transplant rejection

PO (CellCept)

Adults, Elderly: 1.5 g twice per day.

IV (CellCept)

Adults, Elderly: 1 g twice per day.

Usual pediatric dosage

PO (CellCept)

Children 3 mo and older: Oral suspension: 600 mg/m^2/dose twice per day. Capsule: 750 mg twice per day (body surface area [BSA] 1.25-1.5 m^2). Capsule/tablet: 1000 mg twice per day (BSA greater than 1.5 m^2). Maximum: 2 g/day.

OFF-LABEL USES

Treatment of liver transplantation rejection, mild heart transplant rejection, moderate to severe psoriasis

M

CONTRAINDICATIONS

Hypersensitivity to mycophenolate, mycophenolic acid, or polysorbate 80 (IV formulation)

INTERACTIONS

Drug: **Acyclovir, ganciclovir:** May increase plasma concentrations of both drugs in patients with renal impairment. **Antacids (aluminum- and magnesium-containing), cholestyramine:** May decrease the absorption of mycophenolate. **Live-virus vaccines:** May potentiate virus replication, increase vaccine side effects and decrease antibody response to the vaccine. **Other immunosuppressants:** May increase the risk of infection or lymphomas. **Probenecid:** May increase mycophenolate plasma concentration. Herbal: **Echinacea:** May decrease the effects of mycophenolate. Food: **All foods:** May decrease mycophenolate plasma concentration.

DIAGNOSTIC TEST EFFECTS

May increase serum cholesterol, alkaline phosphatase, creatinine, AST (SGOT), and ALT (SGPT) levels. May increase or decrease blood glucose as well as serum lipid, calcium, potassium, phosphate, and uric acid levels.

IV INCOMPATIBILITIES

Mycophenolate is compatible only with D_5W. Do not infuse it concurrently with other drugs or IV solutions.

SIDE-EFFECTS

Frequent (37%-20%): Urinary tract infection, hypertension, peripheral edema, diarrhea, constipation, fever, headache, nausea. Occasional (18%-10%): Dyspepsia; dyspnea; cough; hematuria; asthenia; vomiting; edema; tremors; abdominal, chest, or back pain; oral candidiasis; acne. Rare (9%-6%): Insomnia, respiratory tract infection, rash, dizziness

CRITICAL CARE CONSIDERATIONS

ADMINISTRATION/HANDLING

PO ALERT

- Store reconstituted suspension in the refrigerator or at room temperature. Remains stable for 60 days after reconstitution.
- Give mycophenolate on an empty stomach.
- Swallow capsules whole; do not open or crush capsules.
- Suspension can be administered orally or by nasogastric tube (minimum size: 8 French).
- **Avoid skin/eye contact:** Avoid inhaling the powder in capsules and keep the powder away from skin and mucous membranes. If contact occurs, wash thoroughly with soap and water and rinse the eyes profusely with plain water.

IV ALERT

- **Storage:** Store vials at room temperature.
- **Reconstitution:** Reconstitute 500-mg vial with 14 mL D_5W. Gently agitate vial.
- **Further dilution:** For a 1-g dose, further dilute with 140 mL D_5W; for a 1.5-g dose, further dilute with 210 mL D_5W to provide a concentration of 6 mg/mL.
- **IV intermittent infusion:** Infuse the drug over at least 2 hr.

PRECAUTIONS

HEALTH-RELATED

- Use mycophenolate cautiously in female patients of child-bearing age and in patients with active serious digestive disease, neutropenia, or renal impairment.
- **Experienced users only:** Only physicians experienced in immunosuppressive therapy and management of solid organ transplant patients should use mycophenolate. There is increased likelihood of greater morbidity and mortality when drug is used outside a facility staffed for close, expert monitoring by health care professionals familiar with the drug and transplant patients.

AGE-RELATED

- **Children:** Safety and efficacy of mycophenolate have not been established in children.
- **Elderly:** Age-related renal impairment may require a dosage adjustment.

PREGNANCY/LACTATION-RELATED

- Pregnancy category C; mycophenolic acid is excreted in breast milk; not recommended during breast-feeding.

MONITORING

- **Baseline assessment:** Assess medical history, especially for renal function, active digestive disease, and medication use, including other immunosuppressants.
- **Baseline lab work:** Perform a pregnancy test in female patients of child-bearing age within 1 wk before beginning mycophenolate therapy. Biochemical profile including renal, liver, and cardiac function

tests, along with cholesterol and triglyceride screening. Obtain CBC with WBC differential weekly during the first mo of therapy, twice monthly during the second and third mo, then monthly for the first yr.

- **Thrombosis:** Mycophenolate can induce thrombus formation in any vascular bed of the body. Monitor for unexplained system failure, including heart attack, stroke, acute renal failure, bowel infarction, etc.
- **GI bleeding:** Monitor for coffee ground nasogastric secretions, black tarry stools, hematemesis, bloody stools.
- **Sepsis/infection:** Monitor for fever, malaise, abnormal lab values related to organ function.
- **Reduced dosage:** Reduce the dosage or discontinue mycophenolate if patients experience a rapid fall in WBC count. Assess for delayed myelosuppression.
- **Patient education:** Instruct female patients of child-bearing age to use effective contraception before, during, and for 6 wk after discontinuing mycophenolate therapy, even if there is a history of infertility. Advise use of two forms of contraception concurrently unless patients will remain abstinent. Instruct to report promptly abdominal pain, fever, sore throat, or unusual bleeding or bruising to a health care provider. Stress the need for regular laboratory tests during mycophenolate therapy. Inform patients that malignancies may occur. Be prepared to answer questions and provide additional information.

SERIOUS ADVERSE REACTIONS

- **Sepsis and infection:** Occur occasionally.
- **GI bleeding:** Occurs rarely.

OVERDOSE/TOXICITY

- **Blood dyscrasias:** Significant anemia, leukopenia, thrombocytopenia, neutropenia, and leukocytosis may occur, particularly in those undergoing renal transplant rejection.
- **Neoplasia:** Patients have an increased risk of developing neoplasms.
- **GI decontamination:** No specific recommendations.

ANTIDOTE/DIALYSIS

- **Antidote:** Mycophenolic acid (MPA) may be removed by bile and acid sequestrants (e.g., cholestyramine [Questran]).
- **Dialysis:** Mycophenolate is not removed by hemodialysis or peritoneal dialysis. No data are available on removal using high-permeability hemodialysis. At high concentrations, small amounts of the inactive metabolite mycophenolic acid glucuronide (MPAG) are removed by hemodialysis.

M

nabumetone

See NSAIDs and Cox-2 Inhibitors (p. 976)

nadolol

nay-doe'-lole

Classes

Chemical: β-adrenergic blocker, nonselective

Therapeutic: antianginal, antiglaucoma agent, antihypertensive

Pregnancy Category: C, D (2nd and 3rd trimesters)

Trade Names

Prescription: Corgard

Combinations

Prescription: With bendroflumethiazide (Corzide)

CLINICAL PHARMACOLOGY

Mechanism of Action

A nonselective beta-blocker that blocks $beta_1$- and $beta_2$-adrenergic receptors. Large doses increase airway resistance. **Therapeutic Effect:** Slows sinus heart rate, decreases cardiac output and BP. Decreases myocardial ischemia severity by decreasing oxygen requirements.

PHARMACOKINETICS

Variable absorption after PO administration. Protein binding: 28%-30%. Not metabolized. Excreted unchanged in feces. **Half-life:** 20-24 hr.

AVAILABILITY

Tablets: 20 mg, 40 mg, 80 mg, 120 mg, 160 mg.

INDICATIONS AND DOSAGE

Mild to moderate hypertension, angina

PO

Adults: Initially, 40 mg/day. May increase by 40-80 mg at 3- to 7-day intervals. Maximum: 240-360 mg/day. **Elderly:** Initially, 20 mg/day. May increase gradually. Range: 20-240 mg/day.

Dosage in renal impairment

Dosage is modified based on creatinine clearance.

Creatinine Clearance	Dosage Interval Increase
31-50 mL/min/1.73 m^2	Every 24-36 hr
10-30 mL/min/1.73 m^2	Every 24-48 hr
Less than 10 mL/min/1.73 m^2	Every 40-60 hr

OFF-LABEL USES

Treatment of dysrhythmias, hypertrophic cardiomyopathy, MI, mitral valve prolapse syndrome, neuroleptic-induced akathisia, pheochromocytoma, tremors, thyrotoxicosis, vascular headaches

CONTRAINDICATIONS

Bronchial asthma, cardiogenic shock, heart failure secondary to tachyarrhythmias, chronic obstructive pulmonary disease (COPD), second- or third-degree heart block, sinus bradycardia, uncontrolled cardiac failure, hypersensitivity to nadolol

INTERACTIONS

Drug: **Clonidine:** If clonidine is withdrawn, remove nadolol first to prevent rebound hypertension due to unopposed alpha-adrenergic effects. Consider labetalol or alpha-blockers to prevent rebound hypertension when clonidine is removed. **Diuretics, other antihypertensives:** May increase hypotensive effect. **Insulin, oral hypoglycemics:** May mask symptoms of hypoglycemia and prolong the hypoglycemic effect of insulin and oral hypoglycemics. **Lidocaine:** May increase lidocaine levels by 20%-30%. **NSAIDs:** May decrease antihypertensive effect. **Sympathomimetics, xanthines:** May mutually inhibit effects. **Herbal:** None known. **Food:** None known.

DIAGNOSTIC TEST EFFECTS

May increase serum antinuclear antibody (ANA) titer and BUN, serum LDH, serum lipoprotein, serum alkaline phosphatase, serum bilirubin, serum creatinine, serum potassium, serum uric acid, AST (SGOT), ALT (SGPT), and serum triglyceride levels.

SIDE-EFFECTS

Frequent: Nadolol is generally well tolerated, with transient and mild side effects. Diminished sexual ability, drowsiness, unusual fatigue or weakness. **Occasional:** Bradycardia (2%), difficulty breathing, depression, cold hands or feet, diarrhea, constipation, anxiety, nasal congestion, nausea, vomiting. **Rare:** Altered taste, dry eyes, itching

CRITICAL CARE CONSIDERATIONS

ADMINISTRATION/HANDLING

PO ALERT

- Give nadolol without regard to meals.
- Tablets may be crushed.

PRECAUTIONS

HEALTH-RELATED

- Use nadolol cautiously in patients with diabetes mellitus, hyperthyroidism, peripheral vascular disease, impaired hepatic or renal function, or inadequate cardiac function.

AGE-RELATED

- **Children:** Safety and efficacy of nadolol have not been established in children.
- **Elderly:** Age-related organ impairment may prompt a dosage reduction.

PREGNANCY/LACTATION-RELATED

- Pregnancy category C (D if used in second or third trimester). A similar drug, atenolol, is frequently used in the third trimester for treatment of hypertension (many studies of efficacy and safety of atenolol in pregnancy-induced hypertension). Long-term use has been associated with intrauterine growth retardation; mean milk: plasma ratio, 0.80 in one study. Quantity of drug ingested by breast-feeding infant unlikely to be therapeutically significant.

MONITORING

- **Baseline assessment for hypertension:** Assess heart rate and BP immediately before giving nadolol. For heart rate less than 60 beats/min or systolic BP less than 90 mmHg, withhold medication.
- **Baseline assessment for chest discomfort:** Record the onset, type (sharp, dull, or squeezing), radiation, location, intensity, and duration of anginal pain and its precipitating factors, such as exertion and emotional stress.
- **Baseline lab work:** Biochemical profile including hepatic and renal function tests. Thyroid studies if history of heart disease is present. Beta natriuretic peptide (BNP) level for history of heart failure.
- **Heart failure:** Monitor for hypotension, activity intolerance, distended neck veins, dyspnea (on exertion or at rest), night cough, and peripheral edema.
- **Fluid retention:** Monitor intake and output; note weight gain. An increase in weight or a decrease in urine output may indicate heart failure.
- **Dysrhythmias:** Continuous cardiac monitoring for bradycardia and heart block.
- **Raynaud's disease:** Assess hands and feet for coldness, numbness, and tingling.
- **Hypoglycemia:** Assess blood glucose at least before meals and at bedtime in diabetics because atenolol may mask sympathetic nervous system effects (e.g., tachycardia and diaphoresis) associated with hypoglycemia.
- **Diarrhea:** Assess pattern of daily bowel activity and stool consistency.
- **Patient education:** Caution against abruptly discontinuing nadolol, which may precipitate angina. Instruct to report promptly confusion, depression, difficulty breathing, dizziness, fever, night cough, rash, slow pulse, sore throat, swelling of arms and legs, or unusual bleeding or bruising to a health care provider. Advise avoidance of tasks requiring mental alertness or motor skills until response to the drug is known.

SERIOUS ADVERSE REACTIONS

- **Abrupt withdrawal:** May result in diaphoresis, palpitations, headache, tremulousness, exacerbation of angina, MI, and ventricular dysrhythmias.
- **Cardiovascular disease:** May precipitate heart failure and MI and peripheral ischemia in those with existing peripheral vascular disease.
- **Thyroid disease:** May cause thyroid storm in those with thyrotoxicosis.
- **Diabetes:** Hypoglycemia may occur in patients with previously controlled diabetes.

OVERDOSE/TOXICITY

- **Overdose:** Profound bradycardia, heart block, bronchospasm or wheezing with respiratory distress, heart failure, hypoglycemia, and hypotension.
- **Management:** Upon withdrawing nadolol following overdose, if patients experience acute angina, ST segment depression indicative of myocardial ischemia, or ST segment elevation indicative of MI, immediately provide another therapy to promote myocardial perfusion.
- **GI decontamination:** Activated charcoal is more effective than whole bowel irrigation, which has not been thoroughly tested in humans.

ANTIDOTE/DIALYSIS

- **Antidote:** Beta-agonist high-dose infusion such as *DOPamine, epinephrine, *DOBUTamine or isoproterenol (use cautiously to avoid extreme tachycardia) to counteract the effects of beta blockade including bradycardia, hypotension, and bronchospasms. Glucagon is often successful in increasing heart rate in beta-blocker overdose. Phosphodiesterase inhibitors inamrinone and milrinone may be used to manage heart failure if other agents are ineffective. Other treatment options include glucose and insulin, cardiac pacing, crystalloid fluids, vasopressors such as norepinephrine for hypotension. Aerosolized bronchodilators (e.g., albuterol) may be effective in counteracting bronchospastic effects.

- **Dialysis:** Nadolol is removed by hemodialysis and is likely removed by high-permeability hemodialysis. No data are available on removal using peritoneal dialysis.

nafcillin

See Antibiotics (p. 892)

nalbuphine hydrochloride

nal'-byoo-feen

Classes

Chemical: opiate derivative, phenanthrene derivative

Therapeutic: narcotic agonist-antagonist analgesic

Pregnancy Category: B, D

Trade Names

Prescription: Nubain

Do not confuse Nubain with Navane.

CLINICAL PHARMACOLOGY

Mechanism of Action

A narcotic agonist-antagonist that binds with opioid receptors in the CNS. May displace opioid agonists and competitively inhibit their action; may precipitate withdrawal symptoms. **Therapeutic Effect:** Alters the perception of and emotional response to pain.

PHARMACOKINETICS

Route	Onset	Peak	Duration
IV	2-3 min	30 min	3-6 hr
IM	Less than 15 min	60 min	3-6 hr
Subcutaneous	Less than 15 min	N/A	3-6 hr

Well absorbed after IM or subcutaneous administration. Protein binding: 50%. Metabolized in the liver. Primarily eliminated in feces by biliary secretion. **Half-life:** 5 hr.

AVAILABILITY

Injection: 10 mg/mL, 20 mg/mL.

INDICATIONS AND DOSAGE

Analgesia

IV, IM, Subcutaneous

Adults, Elderly: 10 mg every 3-6 hr as needed. Do not exceed maximum single dose of 20 mg or daily dose of 160 mg. For patients receiving long-term narcotic analgesics of similar duration of action, give 25% of usual dose. **Children.** 0.1-0.15 mg/kg every 3-6 hr as needed.

Supplement to anesthesia

IV

Adults, Elderly: Induction: 0.3-3 mg/kg over 10-15 min. Maintenance: 0.25-0.5 mg/kg as needed.

CONTRAINDICATIONS

Respiratory rate less than 12 breaths/min, hypersensitivity to nalbuphine

INTERACTIONS

Drug: Alcohol, other CNS depressants: May increase CNS or respiratory depression and hypotension. **Buprenorphine:** May decrease the effects of nalbuphine. **MAOIs:** May produce a severe, possibly fatal reaction; plan to administer 25% of the usual nalbuphine dose. **Herbal:** None known. **Food:** None known.

DIAGNOSTIC TEST EFFECTS

May increase serum amylase and lipase levels.

IV INCOMPATIBILITIES

Amphotericin B complex (Abelcet, AmBisome, Amphotec), cefepime (Maxipime), docetaxel (Taxotere), methotrexate, nafcillin (Nafcil), piperacillin and tazobactam (Zosyn), sargramostim (Leukine, Prokine), sodium bicarbonate

IV COMPATIBILITIES

*DiphenhydrAMINE (Benadryl), droperidol (Inapsine), glycopyrrolate (Robinul), *hydrOXYzine (Vistaril), ketorolac (Toradol), lidocaine, midazolam (Versed), propofol (Diprivan)

SIDE-EFFECTS

Frequent (35%): Sedation. **Occasional (9%-3%):** Diaphoresis, cold and clammy skin, nausea, vomiting, dizziness, vertigo, dry mouth, headache. **Rare (less than 1%):** Restlessness, emotional lability, paresthesia, flushing, paradoxic reaction

CRITICAL CARE CONSIDERATIONS

ADMINISTRATION/HANDLING

IV ALERT

- **Storage:** Store vials at room temperature; avoid freezing and prolonged exposure to sunlight.
- **IV push/direct injection:** Nalbuphine may be given undiluted: administer each 10 mg over 3-5 min.
- **Dosage:** Nalbuphine dosage is based on physical condition, severity of pain, and concurrent use of other drugs.

IM ALERT

- Rotate IM injection sites.

PRECAUTIONS

HEALTH-RELATED

- Use nalbuphine cautiously in pregnant patients; opioid-dependent patients; patients with head trauma, increased intracranial pressure, hepatic or renal impairment, recent MI, or respiratory depression; and those preparing for biliary tract surgery.
- **Supplement to anesthesia:** Nalbuphine should be administered as a supplement to general anesthesia only by people trained in administration of IV anesthetics and management of possible respiratory compromise.

AGE-RELATED

- **Children:** May experience paradoxic excitement; those under 2 yr are more likely to develop respiratory depression.
- **Elderly:** Age-related renal impairment may increase the risk of urine retention; elderly are more likely to develop respiratory depression.

PREGNANCY/LACTATION-RELATED

- Pregnancy category B (D if used for prolonged periods or at high dosages at term); not recommended for use with breast-feeding.

MONITORING

- **Baseline assessment:** Assess the duration, location, onset, and type of pain. Obtain vital signs before giving nalbuphine. Withhold drug if respiratory rate is less than 12 breaths/min in adults or less than 20 breaths/min in children.
- **Baseline lab work:** Biochemical profile including renal and liver function studies.
- **Evenly spaced dosing:** Evenly spaced dosing may help prevent reoccurrence of severe pain. The analgesic effect is reduced if a full pain response recurs before the next dose.
- **Low abuse potential:** Nalbuphine has a low abuse potential.
- **Increased intracranial pressure (ICP):** Monitor for deterioration in level of consciousness and neurological assessment findings. Vasodilation from retention of carbon dioxide secondary to the drug's respiratory depressant effects may be exaggerated in head-injury patients, those with brain tumors/intracranial lesions or preexisting increased ICP.
- **Other CNS depressants:** May have an additive effect when used with opioid analgesics, sedatives, hypnotics, general anesthetics, phenothiazines, and other tranquilizers.
- **Nausea/vomiting:** Monitor tolerance of food and tube feedings.
- **Respiratory depression:** Initiate deep-breathing and coughing exercises, particularly in patients with impaired pulmonary function.
- **Therapeutic effects:** Assess for relief of pain. Dosage should be modified if pain relief is inadequate, or other agents should be added to control pain.
- **Patient education:** Instruct to report pain as soon as it occurs and not to wait until the pain is unbearable because nalbuphine is more effective when given at the onset of pain. Inform that nalbuphine may be habit-forming. Urge to avoid alcohol and CNS depressants during nalbuphine therapy. Warn to avoid tasks that require mental alertness or motor skills until response to the drug is known. Inform that nalbuphine may cause dry mouth.

SERIOUS ADVERSE REACTIONS

- **Abrupt withdrawal after prolonged use:** May produce symptoms of narcotic withdrawal such as abdominal cramping, rhinorrhea, lacrimation, anxiety, fever, and piloerection (goose bumps).
- **Tolerance and dependence:** May result from repeated use.
- **Hypersensitivity:** Anaphalaxis, shock, respiratory distress, respiratory arrest, bradycardia, cardiac arrest, hypotension, and laryngeal edema have been reported.

OVERDOSE/TOXICITY

- **Overdose:** Severe respiratory depression, skeletal muscle flaccidity, cyanosis, and extreme somnolence progressing to seizures, stupor, and coma.

- **Management:** Maintain patent airway, support ventilation; administer IV fluids and then vasopressors if needed to control hypotension. Endotracheal intubation and mechanical ventilation may be required.
- **GI decontamination:** No specific recommendations.

ANTIDOTE/DIALYSIS

- **Antidote:** Naloxone will reverse respiratory depression, somnolence, and other symptoms of overdose.
- **Dialysis:** No data are available on removal of nalbuphine by hemodialysis, high-permeability hemodialysis, or peritoneal dialysis.

nalidixic acid

See Antibiotics (p. 892)

nalmefene hydrochloride

See Antidotes (p. 918)

naloxone hydrochloride

nal-oks'-one hye-droe-klor'-ide

N

Classes

Chemical: thebaine derivative
Therapeutic: antidote, opiate

Pregnancy Category: C

Trade Names

Prescription: Narcan

Combinations

Prescription: with pentazocine (Talwin NX); with buprenorphine (Suboxone)

Do not confuse naltrexone or Narcan with Norcuron.

CLINICAL PHARMACOLOGY

Mechanism of Action

A narcotic antagonist that displaces opioids at opioid-occupied receptor sites in the CNS. **Therapeutic Effect:** Reverses opioid-induced sleep or sedation, increases respiratory rate, raises BP to normal range.

PHARMACOKINETICS

Route	Onset	Peak	Duration
IV	1-2 min	N/A	20-60 min
IM	2-5 min	N/A	20-60 min
Subcutaneous	2-5 min	N/A	20-60 min

Well absorbed after IM or subcutaneous administration. Metabolized in the liver. Primarily excreted in urine. **Half-life:** 60-90 min.

AVAILABILITY

Injection: 0.02 mg/mL, 0.4 mg/mL, 1 mg/mL.

INDICATIONS AND DOSAGE

Opioid toxicity

IV, IM, Subcutaneous

Adults, Elderly: 0.4-2 mg every 2-3 min as needed. May repeat every 20-60 min. **Children 5 yr and older and weighing 20 kg and more:** 2 mg/dose; if no response, may repeat every 2-3 min. May need to repeat dose every 20-60 min. **Children younger than 5 yr and weighing less than 20 kg:** 0.1 mg/kg; if no response, repeat every 2-3 min. May need to repeat dose every 20-60 min.

Postanesthesia narcotic reversal

IV

Adults, Elderly: 0.1-0.2 mg. May repeat every 2-3 min as needed. **Children:** 0.01 mg/kg; may repeat every 2-3 min.

Neonatal opioid-induced depression

IV

Neonates: 0.01 mg/kg. May repeat every 2-3 min as needed. May need to repeat dose every 1-2 hr.

OFF-LABEL USES

Treatment of ethanol ingestion, *Pneumocystitis carinii* pneumonia (PCP)

CONTRAINDICATIONS

Respiratory depression due to nonopioid drugs, hypersensitivity to naloxone

INTERACTIONS

Drug: Butorphanol, nalbuphine, opioid agonist analgesics, pentazocine: Reverses the analgesic and adverse effects of these drugs and may precipitate withdrawal symptoms. **Herbal:** None known. **Food:** None known.

DIAGNOSTIC TEST EFFECTS

None known.

IV INCOMPATIBILITIES

Amphotericin B complex (Abelcet, AmBisome, Amphotec)

IV COMPATIBILITIES

Heparin, ondansetron (Zofran), propofol (Diprivan), linezolid (Zyvox)

SIDE-EFFECTS

None known; little or no pharmacologic effect in absence of narcotics.

CRITICAL CARE CONSIDERATIONS

ADMINISTRATION/HANDLING

IV ALERT

- **Storage:** Store parenteral form at room temperature: protect from light.
- **Stability:** Reconstituted solution remains stable in D_5W or 0.9% NaCl at 4 mcg/mL for 24 hr. Discard any unused solution.
- **IV injection:** Naloxone may be administered undiluted; may also dilute 1 mg/mL with 50 mL sterile water for injection to provide a concentration of 0.02 mg/mL. Give each 0.4 mg as IV push over 15 sec.
- **Continuous IV infusion:** Dilute each 2 mg of naloxone with 500 mL D_5W or 0.9% NaCl to provide a concentration of 0.004 mg/mL.
- **Adult versus neonatal vials:** Use the 0.4-mg/mL and 1-mg/mL vials for adults and the 0.02-mg/mL concentration for neonates.
- **Pediatric dosage:** The American Academy of Pediatrics recommends an initial dose of 0.1 mg/kg for infants and children under 5 yr and weighing less than 20 kg, and an initial dose of 2 mg for children 5 yr and older and weighing more than 20 kg.
- **Neonatal opiate depression:** Administration into umbilical vein is preferred using 0.01 to 0.1 mg/kg initially, based on estimated degree of overdose and respiratory depression. May repeat every 2-3 min to attain response.

IM ALERT

- Inject naloxone in a large muscle mass if IV route is not available.

SUBCUTANEOUS ALERT

- Inject naloxone into subcutaneous tissue in a well-perfused area if IV route is not available.

PRECAUTIONS

HEALTH-RELATED

- Use naloxone cautiously in patients with chronic cardiovascular or pulmonary disease, postoperative patients (to avoid cardiovascular complications), and patients suspected of being opioid dependent.

AGE-RELATED

- **Children:** No age-related precautions have been noted. Extreme caution should be used when administering naloxone to a newborn of a narcotic-addicted mother; drug may prompt acute abstinence syndrome.
- **Elderly:** No age-related precautions have been noted.

PREGNANCY/LACTATION-RELATED

- Pregnancy category C; excretion into breast milk unknown, use caution in nursing mothers.

MONITORING

- **Baseline assessment:** Assess to determine prior history of cardiac or pulmonary disease; determine probability of prior opioid dependence. Establish and maintain airway. Obtain weight of pediatric patients to calculate drug dosage.
- **Baseline lab work:** Perform drug screening as possible to determine opioid dependence and to assess for other medications the patient may have ingested if being managed for drug overdose.
- **Challenge test for suspected opioid dependency:** Administer 0.2 mg naloxone IV and observe for withdrawal symptoms (abdominal cramps, diaphoresis, nausea, rhinorrhea, and vomiting) for 30 seconds. If no withdrawal symptoms occur, administer naloxone 0.6 mg IV and observe for an additional 20 min.
- **Dysrhythmias:** Continuous cardiac monitoring should be used for patients with history of cardiac and pulmonary disease. Lethal dysrhythmias including ventricular fibrillation have been reported.
- **Response and reoccurrence of symptoms:** Monitor vital signs, especially respiratory rate, depth, and rhythm, during and frequently after administration. Continue to monitor after a satisfactory response has been achieved. If the duration of action of the opioid exceeds that of naloxone, respiratory depression may recur.
- **Exacerbation of pain:** Assess for increased pain with reversal of the opioid.
- **Patient education:** Instruct to report pain or increased sedation after receiving naloxone.

SERIOUS ADVERSE REACTIONS

- **Too-rapid reversal of narcotic-induced respiratory depression:** May result in nausea, vomiting, diaphoresis, tremors, increased BP, and tachycardia.
- **Excessive dosage in postoperative patients:** Significant excitement, tremors, and reversal of analgesia.

- **Patients with cardiovascular disease:** Hypotension or hypertension, ventricular tachycardia and fibrillation, and pulmonary edema.
- **Opioid withdrawal:** Stuffy or runny nose, tearing, yawning, diaphoresis, tremor, vomiting, piloerection, feeling of temperature change, bone pain, arthralgia, myalgia, abdominal cramps, and feeling of skin crawling.

OVERDOSE/TOXICITY

- **Overdose:** Nausea, vomiting, excitement, tremors, increased BP, tachycardia, hypotension or hypertension, ventricular tachycardia and fibrillation, and pulmonary edema. Increased crying may be noted in the newborn.
- **Management:** Maintain patent airway and protect from aspiration. Treat dysrhythmias and resuscitate for other symptoms according to Advanced Cardiac Life Support (ACLS) guidelines.
- **GI decontamination:** No specific recommendations.

ANTIDOTE/DIALYSIS

- **Antidote:** No specific recommendations.
- **Dialysis:** No data are available on removal of naloxone by hemodialysis, high-permeability hemodialysis, or peritoneal dialysis.

N

naltrexone hydrochloride

nal-trex'-one hye-droe-klor'-ide

Classes

Chemical: thebaine derivative

Therapeutic: alcohol deterrent, antidote, opiate

Pregnancy Category: C

Trade Names

Prescription: Depade, ReVia, Vivitrol

CLINICAL PHARMACOLOGY

Mechanism of Action

A narcotic antagonist that displaces opioids at opioid-occupied receptor sites in the CNS. **Therapeutic Effect:** Blocks physical effects of opioid analgesics; decreases craving for alcohol and relapse rate in alcoholism.

PHARMACOKINETICS

Well absorbed following oral administration. Metabolized in liver; undergoes first-pass metabolism. Excreted primarily in urine; partial elimination in feces. **Half-life:** 4 hr.

AVAILABILITY

Injection: 380 mg (Vivitrol [extended release]).

Tablets: 50 mg (ReVia); 25 mg, 50 mg, 100 mg (Depade)

INDICATIONS AND DOSAGE

Naloxone challenge test to determine whether patient is opioid dependent

IV

Alert: Perform the naloxone challenge test if there is any question that the patient is opioid dependent. Do not administer naltrexone until the naloxone challenge test is negative. **Adults, Elderly:** Draw 2 mL (0.8 mg) of naloxone into syringe. Inject 0.5 mL (0.2 mg); while needle is still in vein, observe patient for 30 sec for withdrawal signs or symptoms. If no evidence of withdrawal, inject remaining 1.5 mL (0.6 mg); observe patient for additional 20 min for withdrawal signs or symptoms.

Subcutaneous

Adults, Elderly: Inject 2 mL (0.8 mg) of naloxone; observe patient for 45 min for withdrawal signs or symptoms.

Treatment of opioid dependence in patients who have been opioid free for at least 7-10 days

PO

Adults, Elderly: Initially, 25 mg. Observe patient for 1 hr. If no withdrawal signs or symptoms appear, give another 25 mg. May be given as 100 mg every other day or 150 mg every 3 days.

Adjunctive treatment of alcohol dependence

PO

Adults, Elderly: 25 mg initially. Observe for withdrawal symptoms for 1 hr. If asymptomatic, repeat 25 mg dose once. Maintenance: 50 mg daily or 100-150 mg given 3 times per wk.

IM

Adults, Elderly: 380 mg once per mo. Inject into gluteal muscle, alternate buttocks monthly.

OFF-LABEL USES

Treatment of eating disorders, postconcussional syndrome unresponsive to other treatments

CONTRAINDICATIONS

Acute hepatitis, acute opioid withdrawal, failed naloxone challenge test, hepatic failure, history of hypersensitivity to naltrexone, opioid dependence, positive urine screen for opioids

INTERACTIONS

Drug: **Opioid-containing products (including analgesics, antidiarrheals, and antitussives):** Blocks the therapeutic effects of these drugs. **Thioridazine:** May produce lethargy and somnolence. **Herbal:** None known. **Food:** None known.

DIAGNOSTIC TEST EFFECTS

May increase AST (SGOT) and ALT (SGPT) levels.

SIDE-EFFECTS

Frequent (more than 10%): Nausea, headache, injection site reaction, abdominal cramps, vomiting, arthalgia, myalgia, dizziness. **Occasional (10%-5%):** Fatigue, insomnia, anxiety, nervousness. **Rare (4%-2%):** Narcotic addiction, alcoholism, irritability, increased energy, anorexia, constipation, rash, chills, increased thrist.

CRITICAL CARE CONSIDERATIONS

ADMINISTRATION/HANDLING

PO ALERT

- Give naltrexone with antacids, after meals, or with food to avoid adverse GI effects.

IM ALERT

- Administer into upper outer quadrant of gluteal muscle. Alternate buttocks.

PRECAUTIONS

HEALTH-RELATED

- **Hepatic disease:** Use naltrexone cautiously in patients with active hepatic disease. The margin of safety between the recognized safe dose and the dose causing hepatic injury may be less than fivefold.
- **When reversal of naltrexone blockade/pain control is required:** If possible, regional analgesia, conscious sedation using benzodiazepines, use of nonopioid analgesics or general anesthesia should be used. If opioids are needed, larger than usual doses may be required and respiratory depression may be significant and prolonged. Rapid-acting opioid analgesics are preferred. Close monitoring for complications is necessary until patient is fully stabilized.

AGE-RELATED

- **Children:** Safety and efficacy of naltrexone have not been established in children under 18 yr.
- **Elderly:** No age-related precautions have been noted.

PREGNANCY/LACTATION-RELATED

- Pregnancy category C; excretion in breast milk is unknown; use with caution in nursing mothers.

MONITORING

- **Baseline assessment:** Establish the medication history, especially opioid use, and other medical conditions including hepatitis or other hepatic disease.
- **Baseline lab work:** Biochemical profile including renal function (BUN/creatinine), liver function (serum bilirubin, AST [SGOT], and ALT [SGPT]) testing. Creatinine clearance may be done to further evaluate for renal failure.
- **Suicide:** Evaluate for suicidal behaviors. Risk of suicide is known to be higher in patients with substance abuse, with and without depression.
- **Patient education:** Instruct to take naltrexone tablets with antacids, after meals, or with food to avoid GI upset. Inform that any opioid-containing drugs used during naltrexone therapy will have no effect. Stress that any attempt to overcome naltrexone's prolonged 24- to 72-hr blockade of opioid effects by taking large amounts of opioids (including methadone and levo-alpha acetyl methadol) may result in coma, serious injury, or death. Inform about the high risk of hepatic injury using the drug. Instruct to report promptly abdominal pain that lasts longer than 3 days, dark urine, white stools, or yellowing of the whites of the eyes to a health care provider. Refer patients to an alcohol or drug rehab center.

SERIOUS ADVERSE REACTIONS

- **Opioid withdrawal:** Stuffy or runny nose, tearing, yawning, diaphoresis, tremor, vomiting, piloerection, feeling of temperature change, bone pain, arthralgia, myalgia, abdominal cramps, and feeling of skin crawling. Death has been reported in patients undergoing ultrarapid opiate detoxification programs.

OVERDOSE/TOXICITY

- **Hepatotoxicity:** Elevated AST (SGOT), ALT (SGPT), bilirubin, alkaline phosphatase, right upper quadrant pain, nausea, fluid retention, edema.

N

- **Accidental ingestion:** Produces withdrawal symptoms in opioid-dependent people within 5 min of ingestion that may last for up to 48 hr. Symptoms include confusion, visual hallucinations, somnolence, and significant vomiting and diarrhea.
- **GI decontamination:** No specific recommendations.

ANTIDOTE/DIALYSIS

- **Antidote:** No specific recommendations.
- **Dialysis:** No data are available on removal of naltrexone by hemodialysis, high-permeability hemodialysis, or peritoneal dialysis.

naproxen/naproxen sodium

na-prox'-en soe'-dee-um

Classes

Chemical: propionic acid derivative
Therapeutic: NSAID, antipyretic, nonnarcotic analgesic

Pregnancy Category: B, D (3rd trimester)

Trade Names

Prescription: (naproxen) EC-Naprosyn, Naprelan, Naprelan 375, Naprelan 500, Naprosyn, Naxen ♣; (naproxen sodium) Aflaxen, Aleve, Anaprox, Anaprox DS, Apo-Naproxen ♣, Novo-naprox ♣, Pamprin

Combinations

Prescription: with lansoprazole (NapraPAC)

Do not confuse Aleve with Allese, or Anaprox with Anaspaz.

CLINICAL PHARMACOLOGY

Mechanism of Action

An NSAID that produces analgesic and antiinflammatory effects by inhibiting prostaglandin synthesis. **Therapeutic Effect:** Reduces the inflammatory response and intensity of pain.

PHARMACOKINETICS

Route	Onset	Peak	Duration
PO (analgesic)	Less than 1 hr	N/A	7 hr or less
PO (antiinflammatory)	14 days	2-4 wk	Less than 12 hr

Completely absorbed from the GI tract. Protein binding: 99%. Metabolized in the liver. Primarily excreted in urine. Not removed by hemodialysis. **Half-life:** 13 hr.

AVAILABILITY

Gelcaps (Aleve): 220 mg naproxen sodium (equivalent to 200 mg naproxen).
Oral Suspension (Naprosyn): 125 mg/5 mL naproxen.
Tablets: 220 mg naproxen (Aleve), 250 mg (Naprosyn), 275 mg naproxen sodium (equivalent to 250 mg naproxen) (Anaprox), 550 mg naproxen sodium (equivalent to 500 mg naproxen) (Aflaxen, Anaprox DS).
Tablets (controlled release): 375 mg naproxen (EC-Naprosyn), 421 mg naproxen (Naprelan), 500 mg naproxen (EC-Naprosyn), 550 mg naproxen sodium (equivalent to 500 mg naproxen) (Naprelan).

INDICATIONS AND DOSAGE

Rheumatoid arthritis, osteoarthritis, ankylosing spondylitis

PO

Adults, Elderly: 250-500 mg naproxen (275-550 mg naproxen sodium) twice per day or 250 mg naproxen (275 mg naproxen sodium) in morning and 500 mg naproxen (550 mg naproxen sodium) in evening. Naprelan: 750-1000 mg once per day.

Acute gouty arthritis

PO

Adults, Elderly: Initially 750 mg naproxen (825 mg naproxen sodium), then 250 mg naproxen (275 mg naproxen sodium) every 8 hr until attack subsides. Naprelan: Initially 1000-1500 mg, then 1000 mg once per day until attack subsides.

Mild to moderate pain, dysmenorrhea, bursitis, tendinitis

PO

Adults, Elderly: Initially, 500 mg naproxen (550 mg naproxen sodium), then 250 mg naproxen (275 mg naproxen sodium) every 6-8 hr as needed. Maximum: 1.25 g/day naproxen (1.375 g/day naproxen sodium). Naprelan: 1000 mg once per day.

Juvenile rheumatoid arthritis

PO (naproxen only)

Children less than 2 yr: 10-15 mg/kg/day in 2 divided doses. Maximum: 1000 mg/day.

OTC uses

PO

Adults 65 yr and younger, Children 12 yr and older: 220 mg (200 mg naproxen sodium) every 8-12 hr. May take 440 mg (200 mg naproxen sodium) as initial dose.
Adults older than 65 yr: 220 mg (200 mg naproxen sodium) every 12 hr.

OFF-LABEL USES
Treatment of vascular headaches

CONTRAINDICATIONS
Hypersensitivity to aspirin, naproxen, or other NSAIDs

INTERACTIONS
Drug: Antihypertensives, diuretics: May decrease the effects of these drugs. **Aspirin, other salicylates:** May increase the risk of GI side effects such as bleeding. **Bone marrow depressants:** May increase the risk of hematologic reactions. **Heparin, oral anticoagulants, thrombolytics:** May increase the effects of these drugs. **Lithium:** May increase the blood concentration and risk of toxicity of lithium. **Methotrexate:** May increase the risk of methotrexate toxicity. **Probenecid:** May increase the naproxen blood concentration. **Herbal: Feverfew:** May decrease the effects of feverfew. **Ginkgo biloba:** May increase the risk of bleeding. **Food:** None known.

DIAGNOSTIC TEST EFFECTS
May prolong bleeding time and alter blood glucose level. May increase serum hepatic function test results. May decrease serum sodium and uric acid levels.

SIDE-EFFECTS
Frequent (9%-4%): Nausea, constipation, abdominal cramps or pain, heartburn, dizziness, headache, somnolence. **Occasional (3%-1%):** Stomatitis, diarrhea, indigestion. **Rare (less than 1%):** Vomiting, confusion

CRITICAL CARE CONSIDERATIONS

ADMINISTRATION/HANDLING

PO ALERT
- **Naproxen versus naproxen sodium:** Each 275- or 550-mg tablet of naproxen sodium equals 250 or 500 mg of naproxen, respectively.
- Swallow enteric-coated tablets whole.
- Scored tablets may be broken or crushed.
- Give naproxen with food, milk, or antacids if GI distress is experienced.

PRECAUTIONS

HEALTH-RELATED
- Use naproxen cautiously in patients with cardiac disease, GI disease, impaired hepatic or renal function, and in patients using anticoagulants concurrently.

AGE-RELATED
- **Children:** Safety and efficacy of naproxen have not been established in children under 2 yr. Children over 2 yr are at an increased risk for developing a rash during naproxen therapy.
- **Elderly:** GI bleeding or ulceration is more likely to cause serious complications and age-related renal impairment may increase the risk of hepatotoxicity and renal toxicity; a reduced dosage is recommended.

PREGNANCY/LACTATION-RELATED
- Pregnancy category B (category D if used in third trimester or near delivery). Could cause constriction of the ductus arteriosus in utero, persistent pulmonary hypertension of the newborn, or prolonged labor. Passes into breast milk in small quantities; compatible with breast-feeding.

MONITORING
- **Baseline assessment:** Assess the duration, location, onset, and type of inflammation or pain. Inspect arthritic affected joints for deformity, immobility, and skin condition.
- **Baseline and ongoing lab work:** CBC with WBC differential, biochemical profile including renal function studies (BUN and creatinine) and liver function studies (serum alkaline phosphatase, bilirubin, AST [SGOT], and ALT [SGPT] levels).
- **Side effects:** Monitor for dyspepsia, headache, and a change in daily bowel activity and stool consistency.
- **Therapeutic response:** Evaluate for pain relief, improved grip strength, increased joint mobility, and decreased joint pain, tenderness, stiffness, and swelling.
- **Patient education:** Instruct to swallow enteric-coated tablets whole and not to crush or chew. Advise taking ibuprofen with food or milk if experiencing GI upset. Warn to avoid alcohol and aspirin during ibuprofen therapy because these substances increase the risk of GI bleeding. Instruct to report persistent headache, black stools, changes in vision, pruritus, rash, or weight gain. Advise female patients to discuss if planning a pregnancy with a health care provider before becoming pregnant.

SERIOUS ADVERSE REACTIONS
- **Long-term or high-dose use:** Peptic ulcer disease, GI bleeding, gastritis, severe hepatic reactions (cholestasis, jaundice), nephrotoxicity (dysuria, hematuria, proteinuria, nephrotic syndrome).

N

- **Severe hypersensitivity reaction:** Fever, chills, bronchospasm; most often seen in patients with systemic lupus erythematosus or other collagen diseases.

OVERDOSE/TOXICITY

- **Overdose:** Hypotonia, muscle fasciculations, twitching, bone marrow suppression, metabolic acidosis, nausea, vomiting, diarrhea, GI bleeding, abdominal pain, volume depletion with secondary hypotension, tachycardia, pulmonary edema and acute respiratory distress syndrome, acute psychosis, seizures, CNS depression following agitation.
- **Nephrotoxicity:** Elevated BUN, creatinine, dysuria, hematuria, proteinuria, oliguria or anuria, possible hyperkalemia, and nephrotic syndrome.
- **GI decontamination:** No specific recommendations.

ANTIDOTE/DIALYSIS

- **Antidote:** No specific antidote. Treatment should be supportive and directed at symptoms.
- **Dialysis:** Naproxen is not removed by hemodialysis and is unlikely to be removed by peritoneal dialysis. No data are available on removal using high-permeability hemodialysis.

N

naratriptan hydrochloride

See Triptans (p. 984)

nateglinide

See Antidiabetics (p. 911)

nedocromil sodium

See Bronchodilators (p. 947)

nefazodone hydrochloride

See Antidepressants (p. 906)

nelfinavir mesylate

See HIV Medications (p. 961)

neomycin sulfate

nee-oh-mye'-sin sul'-fayt

Classes

Chemical: aminoglycoside
Therapeutic: antibiotic

Pregnancy Category: D

Trade Names

Prescription: Myciguent, Neo-Fradin, Neo-Rx, Neo-Tab

Combinations

Prescription: with polymyxin B (Neosporin G.U. irrigant)
Over the Counter: with polymyxin B, bacitracin (Neosporin, Mycitracin)

CLINICAL PHARMACOLOGY

Mechanism of Action

An aminoglycoside antibiotic that binds to bacterial microorganisms. **Therapeutic Effect:** Interferes with bacterial protein synthesis.

PHARMACOKINETICS

Poorly absorbed (less than 3%) from the GI tract following PO administration. Protein binding: Low. Primarily eliminated unchanged in the feces; minimal excretion in urine. Removed by hemodialysis. **Half-life:** 3 hr.

AVAILABILITY

Tablets (Neo-Tab): 500 mg.
Ointment (Myciguent): 0.5%, 0.35%.
Cream (Myciguent): 0.5%, 0.35%.
Oral solution (Neo-Fradin): 125 mg/5 mL.
Powder for compounding (Neo-Rx): 100%.

INDICATIONS AND DOSAGE

Preoperative bowel antisepsis

PO

Adults, Elderly: 1 g/hr for 4 doses; then 1 g every 4 hr for 5 doses or 1 g at 1 PM, 2 PM, and 10 PM (with erythromycin) on day before surgery. **Children:** 90 mg/kg/day in divided doses every 4 hr for 2 days or 25 mg/kg at 1 PM, 2 PM, and 10 PM on day before surgery.

Hepatic encephalopathy

PO

Adults, Elderly: 4-12 g/day in divided doses every 4-6 hr for 5-6 days. **Children:** 2.5-7 g/m^2/day in divided doses every 4-6 hr for 5-6 days, or 50-100 mg/kg/day in divided doses every 6-8 hr. Maximum: 12 g/day.

Minor skin infections
Topical
Adults, Elderly, Children: Usual dosage, apply to affected area 1-3 times per day.

CONTRAINDICATIONS

Hypersensitivity to neomycin, other aminoglycosides (cross-sensitivity), or their components

INTERACTIONS

Drug: **Nephrotoxic medications, other aminoglycosides, ototoxic medications:** May increase nephrotoxicity and ototoxicity if significant systemic absorption occurs. **Herbal:** None known. **Food:** None known.

DIAGNOSTIC TEST EFFECTS

None known.

SIDE-EFFECTS

Frequent: **Systemic:** Nausea, vomiting, diarrhea, irritation of mouth or rectal area. **Topical:** Itching, redness, swelling, rash. **Rare:** **Systemic:** Malabsorption syndrome, neuromuscular blockade (difficulty breathing, drowsiness, weakness)

CRITICAL CARE CONSIDERATIONS

ADMINISTRATION/HANDLING

PO ALERT

- Store capsules at room temperature.
- Neomycin may be taken without regard to food.
- Give neomycin with 8 oz of water.
- After reconstitution, oral solution is stable for 2 wk at room temperature. Do not refrigerate oral solution to avoid thickening.

TOPICAL ALERT

- Do not apply topical preparations to abraded areas or near the eyes.

PRECAUTIONS

HEALTH-RELATED

- Use neomycin cautiously in elderly patients, infants, and other patients with renal insufficiency or immaturity as well as those with neuromuscular disorders, hearing loss, or vertigo.

AGE-RELATED

- **Children:** Safety and efficacy of neomycin have not been established in children under 1 yr.
- **Elderly:** Age-related organ impairment may prompt a dosage adjustment.

PREGNANCY/LACTATION-RELATED

- Pregnancy category D. Ototoxicity has not been reported as an effect of in-utero exposure. Eighth cranial nerve toxicity in the fetus is well known following exposure to other aminoglycosides and could potentially occur with neomycin.

MONITORING

- **Baseline assessment:** Evaluate for and correct dehydration before beginning neomycin therapy. Establish baseline hearing acuity before beginning therapy.
- **Baseline lab work:** CBC with WBC differential to evaluate infection; biochemical panel with BUN and creatinine to evaluate renal function and to assess hydration. Obtain culture of infected area before drug administration (wound, blood, sputum, urine).
- **Neuromuscular blockade:** Avoid concurrent use if possible to avoid potentiating neuromuscular blockade, causing severe respiratory depression.
- **Toxicity:** Assess for hearing loss, dizziness, ringing in the ears (ototoxicity) and headache, dizziness, lethargy, tremor, and visual disturbances (neurotoxicity).
- **Hypersensitivity reaction:** With topical application symptoms may include rash, redness, or itching.
- **Superinfection:** Assess the mouth for white patches on the mucous membranes or tongue or for severe mouth or tongue soreness; assess for severe anal or genital pruritus or discharge (even with topical neomycin).
- **Possible *Clostridium difficile* colitis:** Assess pattern of daily bowel activity and stool consistency. Although mild GI effects may be tolerable, severe symptoms including abdominal pain or cramping and moderate to severe diarrhea may indicate the onset of antibiotic-associated colitis.
- **Hand washing:** If *C. difficile* (antibiotic-associated) colitis develops, wash hands with antibacterial soap. Alcohol-based foam is ineffective against *C. difficile* spores.
- **Skin:** Assess skin for dryness, irritation, and rash with topical application.
- **Eye irritation:** If topical neomycin accidentally comes in contact with the eyes, they should be rinsed with copious amounts of cool tap water.
- **Nephrotoxicity:** Monitor for fluid retention (edema, positive fluid balance) and renal function test results to assess for toxicity.

N

- **Patient education:** Advise on taking neomycin for the full course of treatment and to space doses evenly around the clock. Instruct to report promptly dizziness, impaired hearing, or ringing in the ears to a health care provider. Instruct patients using topical neomycin to clean the affected area gently before applying the drug and report if itching or redness occurs to the prescriber.

SERIOUS ADVERSE REACTIONS

- **Hypersensitivity:** Severe respiratory depression and anaphylaxis occur rarely.
- **Superinfection:** Particularly fungal infections, may occur.

OVERDOSE/TOXICITY

- **Nephrotoxicity:** Increased BUN and serum creatinine levels; decreased creatinine clearance. May be reversible if neomycin is stopped at the first sign of nephrotoxic symptoms.
- **Ototoxicity:** Tinnitus, dizziness, and impaired hearing.
- **Neurotoxicity:** Headache, dizziness, lethargy, tremor, and visual disturbances.
- **GI decontamination:** No specific recommendations.

ANTIDOTE/DIALYSIS

- **Antidote:** No specific recommendations.
- **Dialysis:** Neomycin is removed by hemodialysis and peritoneal dialysis and is likely to be removed by high-permeability hemodialysis.

neostigmine bromide

nee-oh-stig'-meen broe'-mide

Classes

Chemical: cholinesterase inhibitor, quaternary ammonium derivative
Therapeutic: cholinergic

Pregnancy Category: C

Trade Names

Prescription: Prostigmin, Prostigmin Bromide

Do not confuse neostigmine with physostigmine.

CLINICAL PHARMACOLOGY

Mechanism of Action

A cholinergic that prevents destruction of acetylcholine by inhibiting the enzyme acetylcholinesterase, thus enhancing impulse transmission across the myoneural junction. **Therapeutic Effect:** Improves intestinal and skeletal muscle tone; stimulates salivary and sweat gland secretions.

PHARMACOKINETICS

Poorly absorbed from the GI tract following oral administration. Partially eliminated in urine. **Half-life:** 0.5-2 hr. Onset: IV is 1-20 min, IM 20-30 min. Duration: IV is 1-2 hr, IM 2.5-4 hr.

AVAILABILITY

Tablets (Prostigmin Bromide): 15 mg.
Injection (Prostigmin): 0.25 mg/mL, 0.5 mg/mL, 1 mg/mL.

INDICATIONS AND DOSAGE

Myasthenia gravis

PO

Adults, Elderly: Initially, 15-30 mg every 3-4 hr. Increase as necessary. Maintenance: 150 mg/day (range of 15-375 mg). **Children:** 2 mg/kg/day divided every 3-4 hr.

IV, IM, Subcutaneous

Adults: 0.5-2.5 mg as needed every 1-3 hr. Maximum: 10 mg in 24 hr. **Children:** 0.01-0.04 mg/kg every 2-4 hr.

Diagnosis of myasthenia gravis

IM

Adults, Elderly: 0.02 mg/kg. If cholinergic reaction occurs, discontinue tests and administer 0.4-0.6 mg or more atropine sulfate IV. **Children:** 0.025-0.04 mg/kg preceded by atropine sulfate 0.01 mg/kg subcutaneously.

Prevention of postoperative urinary retention

IM, Subcutaneous

Adults, Elderly: 0.25 mg every 4-6 hr for 2-3 days.

Postoperative abdominal distention and urine retention

IM, Subcutaneous

Adults, Elderly: 0.5-1 mg. Catheterize patient if voiding does not occur within 1 hr. After voiding, administer 0.5 mg every 3 hr for 5 injections.

Reversal of neuromuscular blockade

IV

Adults, Elderly: 0.5-2.5 mg given slowly. **Children:** 0.025-0.08 mg/kg/dose. **Infants:** 0.025-0.1 mg/kg/dose.

CONTRAINDICATIONS

GI or GU obstruction, history of hypersensitivity reaction to neostigmine or bromides, peritonitis

INTERACTIONS

Drug: Anticholinergics: Reverse or prevent the effects of neostigmine. **Cholinesterase**

inhibitors: May increase the risk of toxicity. **Neuromuscular blockers:** Antagonizes the effects of these drugs. **Procainamide, quinidine:** May antagonize the action of neostigmine. **Herbal:** None known. **Food:** None known.

DIAGNOSTIC TEST EFFECTS

None known.

IV INCOMPATIBILITIES

None known.

IV COMPATIBILITIES

Glycopyrrolate (Robinul), heparin, ondansetron (Zofran), potassium chloride, thiopental (Pentothal)

SIDE-EFFECTS

Frequent: Muscarinic effects (diarrhea, diaphoresis, increased salivation, nausea, vomiting, abdominal cramps or pain). **Occasional:** Muscarinic effects (urinary urgency or frequency, increased bronchial secretions, miosis, lacrimation)

CRITICAL CARE CONSIDERATIONS

ADMINISTRATION/HANDLING

IV ALERT

- **Storage:** Store below 40°C. Protect from light.
- **Tensilon (edrophonium) testing:** Discontinue all anticholinesterase therapy at least 8 hr before diagnostic testing for myasthenia gravis.
- **Premedicate with atropine:** Give 0.01 mg/kg atropine sulfate IV simultaneously with neostigmine or IM 30 min before administering neostigmine to prevent adverse effects.
- **Neostigmine overdose:** Atropine may mask the symptoms of neostigmine overdose. Glycopyrrolate 0.2 mg for every 1 mg neostigmine may be given instead of atropine.
- **Increased weakness and fatigue:** Larger doses may be needed to manage myasthenia gravis when patients are most tired.

PRECAUTIONS

HEALTH-RELATED

- Use neostigmine cautiously in patients with dysrhythmias, asthma, bradycardia, epilepsy, hyperthyroidism, peptic ulcer disease, or recent coronary occlusion.

AGE-RELATED

- **Children:** No age-related precautions have been noted. Differentiate cholinergic crisis from myasthenic crisis in neonates with edrophonium test.
- **Elderly:** Length of reversal of neuromuscular blockade is prolonged.

PREGNANCY/LACTATION-RELATED

- Pregnancy category C. Transient muscle weakness occurred in 20% of infants born to mothers using neostigmine and similar drugs. Ionized at physiologic pH; would not be expected to be excreted in breast milk

MONITORING

- **Baseline assessment:** Before beginning therapy, assess for reduced GI motility or megacolon because these patients should not receive large doses.
- **Muscle relaxant antagonist effects:** Monitor muscle strength and vital signs when reversing nondepolarizing drug induced (doxacurium [Neuromax], mivacurium [Mivachron], tubocurarine [Curare]) neuromuscular blockade. Heart rate should be at least 80 beats/min when drug is given. A peripheral nerve stimulator may be used to monitor effectiveness.
- **Therapeutic response for myasthenia gravis:** Monitor for decreased fatigue, improved chewing and swallowing, and increased muscle strength.
- **Urinary retention or urgency:** Monitor fluid intake and output. Palpate bladder for distention and note urinary urgency or incontinence. Too much neostigmine may create cholinergic crisis (frequency), and inadequate dosing may prompt urinary retention.
- **Narcotic analgesics:** Monitor vital signs and neurologic status closely in patients receiving narcotics (e.g., morphine, meperidine, codeine, hydromorphone) to avoid respiratory depression, bradycardia, and hypotension.
- **Patient education:** Instruct to report promptly diarrhea, difficulty breathing, increased salivation, irregular heartbeat, muscle weakness, nausea and vomiting, severe abdominal pain, or increased sweating to a health care provider. When at home, urge to keep a log of their energy level and muscle strength to help guide drug dosing.

SERIOUS ADVERSE REACTIONS

- **Impending cholinergic crisis:** Bradycardia, hypotension, urinary frequency,

N

muscle fasiculations, which may indicate cholinergic crisis.

- **Hypersensitivity:** Difficulty breathing, angioedema, urticaria. Manage with epinephrine.

OVERDOSE/TOXICITY

- **Cholinergic crisis:** Abdominal discomfort or cramps, nausea, vomiting, diarrhea, possible shock, flushing, facial warmth, excessive salivation, diaphoresis, urinary incontinence or urgency, lacrimation, pallor, bradycardia or tachycardia, hypotension, bronchospasm, blurred vision, miosis, and fasciculation (involuntary muscular contractions visible under the skin).
- **Management:** Endotracheal intubation, support of ventilation, possible mechanical ventilation, management of hypotension with IV fluids and vasopressors if IV fluids are ineffective, management of heart rate using Advanced Cardiac Life Support (ACLS) guidelines. Atropine, often given before neostigmine, may mask the symptoms of overdose.
- **GI decontamination:** No specific recommendations.

ANTIDOTE/DIALYSIS

- **Antidote:** Atropine sulfate 0.6 mg given IV should reverse side effects; may repeat every 3-10 min. Pralidoxime chloride (PAM) 2 g IV may be required to reactivate cholinesterase and reverse paralysis.
- **Dialysis:** No data are available on removal of neostigmine by hemodialysis, peritoneal dialysis, or high-permeability hemodialysis.

nesiritide ⚑

ni-sir'-i-tide

Classes

Chemical: recombinant human peptide
Therapeutic: vasodilator

Pregnancy Category: C

Trade Names

Prescription: Natrecor

CLINICAL PHARMACOLOGY

Mechanism of Action

A brain natriuretic peptide that facilitates cardiovascular homeostasis and fluid status through counterregulation of the renin-angiotensin-aldosterone system, stimulating cyclic guanosine monophosphate, thereby leading to smooth-muscle-cell relaxation. **Therapeutic Effect:** Promotes vasodilation, natriuresis, and diuresis, correcting heart failure.

PHARMACOKINETICS

Route	Onset	Peak	Duration
IV	15-30 min	1-2 hr	4 hr

Excreted primarily in the heart by the left ventricle. Metabolized by the natriuretic neutral endopeptidase enzymes on the vascular luminal surface. **Half-life:** 18-23 min.

AVAILABILITY

Injection powder for reconstitution: 1.5-mg/5-mL vial.

INDICATIONS AND DOSAGE

Treatment of acutely decompensated heart failure in patients with dyspnea at rest or with minimal activity

IV bolus

Adults, Elderly: 2 mcg/kg followed by a continuous IV infusion of 0.01 mcg/kg/min. At intervals of 3 hr or longer, may be increased by 0.005 mcg/kg/min (preceded by a bolus of 1 mcg/kg), up to a maximum of 0.03 mcg/kg/min.

CONTRAINDICATIONS

Cardiogenic shock, systolic BP less than 90 mmHg, hypersensitivity to nesiritide

INTERACTIONS

Drug: ACE inhibitors, IV nitroglycerin, milrinone, nitroprusside: May increase risk of hypotension. **Arsenic trioxide:** May increase the risk of QT prolongation. **Herbal:** None known. **Food:** None known.

DIAGNOSTIC TEST EFFECTS

None known.

IV INCOMPATIBILITIES

Sodium metabisulfite, bumetanide (Bumex), enalapril (Vasotec), ethacrynic acid (Edecrin), furosemide (Lasix), heparin, *hydrALAZINE (Apresoline), insulin

SIDE-EFFECTS

Frequent (11%): Hypotension. **Occasional (8%-2%):** Headache, nausea, bradycardia. **Rare (1% or less):** Confusion, paresthesia, somnolence, tremor

CRITICAL CARE CONSIDERATIONS

ADMINISTRATION/HANDLING

IV ALERT

- **Storage/stability:** Store vial at room temperature. Once reconstituted, store at room temperature or refrigerate; use within 24 hr.
- **Reconstitution/dilution:** Reconstitute one 1.5-mg vial with 5 mL D_5W, 0.9% NaCl, 0.2% NaCl, or any combination thereof. Swirl or rock gently and add to 250-mL bag D_5W, 0.9% NaCl, 0.2% NaCl, or any combination thereof, yielding a solution of 6 mcg/mL.
- **IV bolus:** Give initially as an IV bolus over approximately 60 sec, followed by continuous IV infusion.
- **Dedicated IV line:** Do not mix with other injections or infusions. Do not give IM.

NESIRITIDE BOLUS AND INFUSION TABLE (6 mcg/mL CONCENTRATION)

Weight (kg)	Bolus Volume (mL) 2 mcg/kg	IV Infusion Rate (mL/hr) 0.01 mcg/kg/min
50	16.7	5
60	20	6
70	23.3	7
80	26.7	8
90	30	9
100	33.3	10

PRECAUTIONS

HEALTH-RELATED

- Use nesiritide cautiously in patients with AV conduction defects, atrial fibrillation, ventricular dysrhythmias, constrictive pericarditis, hypotension, hepatic impairment, pericardial tamponade, renal impairment, restrictive or obstructive cardiomyopathy, significant valvular stenosis, and suspected low cardiac filling pressures.
- Safety and efficacy for use longer than 48 hr has not been established.

AGE-RELATED

- **Children:** Safety and efficacy of nesiritide have not been established in children.
- **Elderly:** No age-related precautions have been noted; elderly may be more sensitive to effects.

PREGNANCY/LACTATION-RELATED

- Pregnancy category C (neither animal or human studies have been done); breast milk data unavailable.

MONITORING

- **Baseline assessment:** Obtain BP immediately before each nesiritide dose, in addition to regular monitoring. Place patients in the supine position with legs elevated when hypotensive. Assess prior strategies used to manage heart failure, including dosage, frequency, and duration of management with diuretics.
- **Baseline lab work:** Biochemical profile to screen for electrolyte imbalance (hypokalemia) if diuretics have been used and renal function (BUN, creatinine levels). Digoxin level if digoxin is currently being used. Beta natriuretic peptide (BNP) level to assess for degree of heart failure.
- **Baseline diagnostic testing:** 12-lead ECG to assess for myocardial ischemia; if heart failure is worsening, echocardiogram to assess ejection fraction, ventricular wall motion, and status of heart valves.
- **Fluid retention:** Maintain accurate intake and output records; assess urine output frequently. Administer diuretics as appropriate to manage fluid retention.
- **Acute renal failure:** Biochemical profile monitoring for increased BUN and creatinine; monitor for oliguria and increased edema. Nesiritide may induce azotemia in patients with severe heart failure whose renal function is dependent on the renin-angiotensin-aldosterone system. Need for first time dialysis has presented in patients receiving nesiritide.
- **Hemodynamic monitoring:** Monitoring of pulmonary artery pressures and cardiac index are helpful but not mandatory. Decreasing pulmonary artery pressures and increased cardiac index are indicative drug is effective in managing heart failure.
- **Hypotension and heart rate changes:** Frequently monitor blood hypotension and heart rate for tachycardia and bradycardia.
- **Dysrhythmias:** Use continuous cardiac monitoring to assess for ventricular dysrhythmias, atrial fibrillation, tachycardias, and bradycardia.
- **Treatment parameters:** Establish parameters with all health care providers for adjusting the rate or stopping the infusion.
- **Patient education:** Explain that nesiritide is not a cure for heart failure but will help relieve symptoms. Instruct to report chest pain or palpitations immediately to a health care provider.

N

SERIOUS ADVERSE REACTIONS

- Ventricular dysrhythmias, including ventricular tachycardia, atrial fibrillation, AV node conduction abnormalities, and angina pectoris occur rarely.
- **Hypersensitivity:** Urticaria, injection site reaction, possible anaphylaxis because drug is a protein substance.

OVERDOSE/TOXICITY

- **Overdose:** Hypotension, respiratory distress, ventricular dysrhythmias, and chest discomfort. Symptoms may last for several hr.
- **Management:** Discontinue nesiritide. Maintain patent airway, administer oxygen and support ventilation. Careful IV fluid administration may be used to manage BP, ensuring patient does not experience fluid overload. Elevate legs to increase venous return. Vasopressors and positive inotropic agents are difficult to manage in heart failure patients, as drugs may increase myocardial workload and oxygen demand. When stabilized, nesiritide may be restarted; bolus should not be given when restarting and infusion rate should be reduced by at least 30% from last dose.
- **GI decontamination:** No specific recommendations.

ANTIDOTE/DIALYSIS

- **Antidote:** No specific recommendations.
- **Dialysis:** Nesiritide is unlikely to be removed by hemodialysis, peritoneal dialysis, or high permeability hemodialysis.

N

netilmicin

See Antibiotics (p. 892)

nevirapine

See HIV Medications (p. 961)

niacin, nicotinic acid

nye'-a-sin nik-oh-tin'-ik as'-id

Classes

Chemical: vitamin B complex
Therapeutic: antilipemic, vitamin

Pregnancy Category: C, A

Trade Names

Prescription: Niacor, Niaspan ER, Nicotinex
Over the Counter: Slo-Niacin

Combinations

Prescription: with lovastatin (Advicor)

Do not confuse niacin, Niacor, or Niaspan with minocin or Nitro-Bid.

CLINICAL PHARMACOLOGY

Mechanism of Action

An antihyperlipidemic, water-soluble vitamin that is a component of two coenzymes needed for tissue respiration, lipid metabolism, and glycogenolysis. Inhibits synthesis of very low-density lipoproteins. **Therapeutic Effect:** Reduces total, LDL, and VLDL cholesterol levels and triglyceride levels; increases HDL cholesterol concentration.

PHARMACOKINETICS

Readily absorbed from the GI tract. Widely distributed. Metabolized in the liver. Primarily excreted in urine. **Half-life:** 45 min.

AVAILABILITY

Capsules (timed release): 125 mg, 250 mg, 400 mg, 500 mg.
Tablets (Niacor): 50 mg, 100 mg, 250 mg, 500 mg.
Tablets (timed release [Slo-Niacin]): 250 mg, 500 mg, 750 mg.
Tablets (timed release [Niaspan]): 500 mg, 750 mg, 1000 mg.
Elixir (Nicotinex): 50 mg/5 mL.

INDICATIONS AND DOSAGE

Hyperlipidemia

PO (Immediate-Release)

Adults, Elderly: Initially, 50-100 mg twice per day for 7 days. Increase gradually by doubling dose every wk up to 1-1.5 g/day in 2-3 doses. Maximum: 4.5 g/day. **Children:** Initially 100-250 mg/day (maximum: 10 mg/kg/day) in 3 divided doses. May increase by 100 mg/wk or 250 mg every 2-3 wk. Maximum: 2250 mg/day.

PO (Timed-Release)

Adults, Elderly: Initially 500 mg/day in 2 divided doses for 1 wk; then increase to 500 mg twice per day. Maintenance: 2 g/day.

Nutritional supplement

PO

Adults, Elderly: 10-20 mg/day. Maximum: 100 mg/day.

Pellegra

PO

Adults, Elderly: 50-100 mg 3-4 times per day. Maximum: 500 mg/day. **Children:** 50-100 mg 3 times per day.

CONTRAINDICATIONS

Active peptic ulcer disease; arterial hemorrhaging; hepatic dysfunction; hypersensitivity to niacin, nicotinic acid, or tartrazine (frequently seen in patients sensitive to aspirin); severe hypotension

INTERACTIONS

Drug: Alcohol: May increase risk of niacin side effects, such as flushing. **Lovastatin, pravastatin, simvastatin:** May increase the risk of acute renal failure and rhabdomyolysis. **Herbal:** None known. **Food:** None known.

DIAGNOSTIC TEST EFFECTS

May increase serum uric acid level.

SIDE-EFFECTS

Frequent: Flushing (especially of the face and neck) occurring within 20 min of drug administration and lasting for 30-60 min, GI upset, pruritus. **Occasional:** Dizziness, hypotension, headache, blurred vision, burning or tingling of skin, flatulence, nausea, vomiting, diarrhea. **Rare:** Hyperglycemia, glycosuria, rash, hyperpigmentation, dry skin

CRITICAL CARE CONSIDERATIONS

ADMINISTRATION/HANDLING

PO ALERT

- Give niacin without regard to meals.
- Administer niacin at bedtime.

PRECAUTIONS

HEALTH-RELATED

- Use niacin cautiously in patients with diabetes mellitus, gallbladder disease, gout, or a history of hepatic disease or jaundice.

AGE-RELATED

- **Children:** Niacin use is not recommended in children under 2 yr. Safety and efficacy have not been established.
- **Elderly:** No age-related precautions have been noted.

PREGNANCY/LACTATION-RELATED

- Pregnancy category A (category C if used in doses greater than recommended daily allowance [RDA]); actively excreted in human breast milk; RDA during lactation is 18-20 mg

MONITORING

- **Baseline assessment:** Determine history of hypersensitivity to aspirin, niacin, nicotinic acid, or tartrazine before beginning drug therapy; determine history of liver disease or gout.
- **Baseline and ongoing lab work:** Biochemical profile including blood glucose and potassium levels, uric acid, cholesterol, triglyceride levels and liver function tests (serum alkaline phosphatase, bilirubin, uric acid level, AST [SGOT], and ALT [SGPT] levels).
- **Diarrhea:** Assess pattern of daily bowel activity, degree of GI discomfort and stool consistency.
- **Hyperglycemia:** Monitor point of care blood glucose before meals and at bedtime in patients with hyperglycemia (blood glucose more than 140 mg/dL) on a biochemical profile.
- **Urticaria:** Assess the skin for dryness.
- **Side effects:** Monitor for flushing, blurred vision, dizziness, and headache.
- **Patient education:** Advise taking niacin at bedtime and to avoid alcohol consumption to reduce severity of flushing. Inform that itching, flushing of the skin, sensation of warmth, and tingling may occur. Instruct to report promptly dark urine, dizziness, loss of appetite, nausea, vomiting, weakness, or yellowing of the skin to a health care provider. Suggest avoidance of sudden changes in posture to help prevent bouts of dizziness.

SERIOUS ADVERSE REACTIONS

- **Dysrthythmias:** Atrial fibrillation, tachycardia, ventricular dysrhythmias occur rarely.
- **Hyperglycemia:** Tight glycemic control should be practiced to avoid increased morbidity and mortality in critically ill patients.
- **GI effects:** Severe nausea/vomiting, peptic ulcer disease.
- **Gout:** May result from elevated uric acid level.

OVERDOSE/TOXICITY

- **Hepatotoxicity:** Elevated liver enzymes, right upper quadrant pain, fluid retention, edema, weight gain, jaundice, abdominal distention, dark urine, nausea.
- **Ocular:** Toxic amblyopia, cystic macular edema.
- **Rhabdomyolysis:** Dark/tea-colored urine (myoglobinuria); metabolic acidosis; elevated CPK, AST (SGOT) and ALT (SGPT); hyperkalemia; hypocalcemia; muscle pain; dehydration; weakness; acute renal failure prompting hyperphosphatemia; rare septic syndrome with disseminated

intravascular coagulation (DIC). Seen when niacin is used with hydromethyl-glutyrl-CoA reductase inhibitors (lovastatin, simvastatin, pravastatin) to lower cholesterol.
- **GI decontamination:** No specific recommendations.

ANTIDOTE/DIALYSIS
- **Antidote:** No specific recommendations.
- **Dialysis:** No data are available on removal of niacin by hemodialysis, high-permeability hemodialysis, or peritoneal dialysis.

*niCARdipine hydrochloride

nye-kar'-de-peen hye-droe-klor'-ide

Classes
Chemical: dihydropyridine
Therapeutic: antianginal, antihypertensive, calcium channel blocker

Pregnancy Category: C

Trade Names
Prescription: Cardene, Cardene IV, Cardene SR

Do not confuse *niCARdipine with *NIFEdipine, Cardene with codeine, or Cardene SR with Cardizem SR or codeine.

N

CLINICAL PHARMACOLOGY
Mechanism of Action
An antianginal and antihypertensive agent that inhibits calcium ion movement across cell membranes, depressing contraction of cardiac and vascular smooth muscle. **Therapeutic Effect:** Increases heart rate and cardiac output. Decreases systemic vascular resistance and BP.

PHARMACOKINETICS

Route	Onset	Peak	Duration
PO	0.5-2 hr	1-2 hr	8 hr
IV	10 min	N/A	3 hr

Rapidly, completely absorbed from the GI tract. Protein binding: 95%. Undergoes first-pass metabolism in the liver. Primarily excreted in urine. Not removed by hemodialysis. **Half-life:** 2-4 hr.

AVAILABILITY
Capsules (Cardene): 20 mg, 30 mg.
Capsules (sustained release [Cardene SR]): 30 mg, 45 mg, 60 mg.
Injection (Cardene IV): 2.5 mg/mL.

INDICATIONS AND DOSAGE
Chronic stable (effort-associated) angina
PO
Adults, Elderly: Initially, 20 mg 3 times per day. Range: 20-40 mg 3 times per day. Increase dose at 3-day intervals.

Essential hypertension
PO
Adults, Elderly: Initially, 20 mg 3 times per day. Range: 20-40 mg 3 times per day.
PO (Sustained Release)
Adults, Elderly: Initially, 30 mg twice per day. Range: 30-60 mg twice per day.

Short-term treatment of hypertension when oral therapy is not feasible or desirable (substitute for oral *niCARdipine)
IV
Adults, Elderly: 0.5 mg/hr (for patient receiving 20 mg PO every 8 hr); 1.2 mg/hr (for patient receiving 30 mg PO every 8 hr); 2.2 mg/hr (for patient receiving 40 mg PO every 8 hr).

Patients not already receiving *niCARdipine
IV
Adults, Elderly (gradual BP decrease): Initially, 5 mg/hr. May increase by 2.5 mg/hr every 15 min. After BP goal is achieved, decrease rate to 3 mg/hr. **Adults, Elderly (rapid BP decrease):** Initially, 5 mg/hr. May increase by 2.5 mg/hr every 5 min. Maximum: 15 mg/hr until desired BP attained. After BP goal achieved, decrease rate to 3 mg/hr.

Changing from IV to oral antihypertensive therapy
Adults, Elderly: Begin antihypertensives other than *niCARdipine when IV has been discontinued; for *niCARdipine, give first dose 1 hr before discontinuing IV.

Dosage in hepatic impairment
Adults, Elderly: Initially 20 mg twice per day, then titrate.

Dosage in renal impairment
Adults, Elderly: Initially 20 mg every 8 hr (30 mg twice per day [sustained-release capsules]), then titrate.

OFF-LABEL USES
Treatment of associated neurologic deficits, Raynaud's phenomenon, subarachnoid hemorrhage, vasospastic angina

CONTRAINDICATIONS
Atrial fibrillation or flutter associated with accessory conduction pathways, advanced aortic stenosis, cardiogenic shock, heart failure, second- or third-degree heart block, severe hypotension, sinus bradycardia, ventricular tachycardia, within several hr of

IV beta-blocker therapy, hypersensitivity to *niCARdipine

INTERACTIONS

Drug: Beta-blockers: May have additive effect. **Digoxin:** May increase *niCARdipine blood concentration. **Hypokalemia-producing agents (such as furosemide and certain other diuretics):** May increase risk of dysrhythmias. **Procainamide, quinidine:** May increase risk of QT-interval prolongation. **Herbal:** None known. **Food: Grapefruit, grapefruit juice:** May alter absorption of *niCARdipine.

DIAGNOSTIC TEST EFFECTS

None known.

IV INCOMPATIBILITIES

Furosemide (Lasix), heparin, thiopental (Pentothal)

IV COMPATIBILITIES

Diltiazem (Cardizem), *DOBUTamine (Dobutrex), *DOPamine (Intropin), epinephrine, hydromorphone (Dilaudid), labetalol (Trandate), lorazepam (Ativan), midazolam (Versed), milrinone (Primacor), morphine, nitroglycerin, norepinephrine (Levophed)

SIDE-EFFECTS

Frequent (10%-7%): Headache, facial flushing, peripheral edema, lightheadedness, dizziness. **Occasional (6%-3%):** Asthenia (loss of strength, energy), palpitations, angina, tachycardia. **Rare (less than 2%):** Nausea, abdominal cramps, dyspepsia, dry mouth, rash

CRITICAL CARE CONSIDERATIONS

ADMINISTRATION/HANDLING

PO ALERT

- Do not crush, open, or break sustained-release capsules.
- Give *niCARdipine without regard to food.
- Concurrent administration of sublingual nitroglycerin therapy may be used for relief of anginal pain.

IV ALERT

- **Storage:** Store at room temperature. Store diluted IV solution for up to 24 hr at room temperature.
- **Dilution:** Dilute each 25-mg ampule with 250 mL D_5W, 0.9% NaCl, 0.45% NaCl, or any combination thereof to provide a concentration of 1 mg/10 mL. Maximum concentration is 4 mg/10 mL.
- **IV infusion:** Give by slow IV infusion.
- **Rotate peripheral IV site:** Change IV site every 12 hr if *niCARdipine is administered by a peripheral rather than a central venous catheter line.

PRECAUTIONS

HEALTH-RELATED

- Use *niCARdipine cautiously in patients with cardiomyopathy, edema, hepatic or renal impairment, severe left ventricular dysfunction, or sick sinus syndrome and in those concurrently receiving beta-blockers or digoxin.
- **Aortic stenosis:** *NiCARdipine is not recommended for use in reducing diastolic BP of patients with advanced aortic stenosis, as reduced diastolic BP may prompt instability.

AGE-RELATED

- **Children:** Safety and efficacy of *niCARdipine have not been established in children.
- **Elderly:** Age-related renal impairment may require cautious use because half-life may be prolonged; drug-induced tinnitus may ensue.

PREGNANCY/LACTATION-RELATED

- Pregnancy category C; significant excretion into rat maternal milk.

MONITORING

- **Baseline assessment for stroke:** Assess for hypertension and use *niCARdipine according to current acute stroke management guidelines. Monitor neurologic changes associated with use of *niCARdipine when used to control hypertension associated with strokes.
- **Baseline assessment for angina:** Record the onset, type (sharp, dull, or squeezing), radiation, location, intensity, and duration of anginal pain and its precipitating factors, such as exertion and emotional stress.
- **Baseline lab work:** Biochemical profile to rule out electrolyte imbalance associated with other medications and to assess liver function; CBC to assess for anemia in angina patients.
- **Baseline diagnostic tests:** 12-lead ECG to assess myocardial ischemia in angina patients.
- **Dysrhythmias:** Assess continuously monitored ECG for tachycardia, ST depression

N

(myocardial ischemia), and ST elevation (acute MI).

- **Hypertension management:** Monitor BP during and following the IV infusion.
- **Edema:** Assess for peripheral edema behind the medial malleolus and on the sacrum.
- **Skin side effects:** Examine skin for dermatitis, facial flushing, and rash.
- **Neurologic/neuromuscular effects:** Evaluate for asthenia and headache. If acute stroke occurs, monitor for changes in neurologic status every 15 min while evaluating other diagnostic tests (CT brain scan). Assess for appropriateness of patients receiving thrombolysis with rTPA (alteplase).
- **Patient education:** Instruct to take *niCARdipine's sustained-release form with food and not to crush or open capsules. Urge avoidance of alcohol and limiting caffeine while taking *niCARdipine. Instruct to report promptly anginal pain not relieved by the medication, constipation, dizziness, irregular heartbeat, nausea, shortness of breath, or swelling, or symptoms of hypotension such as lightheadedness to a health care provider.

SERIOUS ADVERSE REACTIONS

- **Cardiac effects:** Angina, hypotension, palpitations, tachycardia, premature ventricular contractions.

OVERDOSE/TOXICITY

- **Overdose:** Confusion, slurred speech, headache, somnolence, marked hypotension, progressive AV heart block, and bradycardia.
- **Management:** Maintain patent airway, administer oxygen, support ventilation; administer IV fluids and if ineffective in increasing blood pressure, administer vasopressors (norepinephrine, high-dose *DOPamine). Catecholamine infusion (*DOPamine, epinephrine) to increase heart rate. IV calcium may facilitate more rapid stabilization.
- **GI decontamination:** No specific recommendations.

ANTIDOTE/DIALYSIS

- **Antidote:** IV calcium gluconate may be effective in reversing calcium channel blockade.
- **Dialysis:** *NiCARdipine is not removed by hemodialysis and is unlikely to be removed by peritoneal dialysis. No data are available on removal by high-permeability hemodialysis.

nicotine

nik'-oh-teen

Classes

Chemical: pyridine alkaloid
Therapeutic: smoking deterrent

Pregnancy Category: D

Trade Names

Prescription: Commit, NicoDerm CQ, NicoDerm CQ Clear, Nicorette, Nicotrol, Nictrol Inhaler, Nicotrol NS

Do not confuse Nicoderm with Nitroderm.

CLINICAL PHARMACOLOGY

Mechanism of Action

A cholinergic-receptor agonist that binds to acetylcholine receptors, producing both stimulating and depressant effects on the peripheral and central nervous systems. **Therapeutic Effect:** Provides a source of nicotine during nicotine withdrawal and reduces withdrawal symptoms.

PHARMACOKINETICS

Absorbed slowly after transdermal administration. Protein binding: 5%. Metabolized in the liver. Excreted primarily in urine. **Half-life:** 4 hr.

AVAILABILITY

Chewing gum (Nicorette): 2 mg, 4 mg.
Lozenge (Commit): 2 mg, 4 mg.
Transdermal patch (NicoDerm CQ, Nicotrol): 5 mg/16 hr, 7 mg/24 hr, 10 mg/16 hr, 14 mg/24 hr, 21 mg/24 hr.
Nasal spray (Nicotrol NS): 0.5 mg/spray.
Inhalation (Nicotrol Inhaler): 10 mg cartridge.

INDICATIONS AND DOSAGE

Smoking cessation aid to relieve nicotine withdrawal symptoms

PO (Chewing gum)

Adults, Elderly: Usually, 10-12 pieces/day. Maximum: 30 pieces/day.

PO (Lozenge)

Alert: For those who smoke the first cigarette within 30 min of waking, administer the 4 mg-lozenge; otherwise administer the 2-mg lozenge. **Adults, Elderly:** 1 4-mg or 2-mg lozenge every 1-2 hr for the first 6 wk; 1 lozenge every 2-4 hr for wk 7-9; and 1 lozenge every 4-8 hr for wk 10-12. Maximum: 1 lozenge at a time, 5 lozenges/6 hr, 20 lozenges/day.

Transdermal

Adults, Elderly who smoke 10 cigarettes or more per day: Follow the guidelines below. **Step 1:** 21 mg/day for 4-6 wk. **Step 2:** 14 mg/day for 2 wk. **Step 3:** 7 mg/day for 2 wk. **Adults, Elderly who smoke fewer than 10 cigarettes per day:** Follow the guidelines below. **Step 1:** 14 mg/day for 6 wk. **Step 2:** 7 mg/day for 2 wk. **Patients weighing less than 100 lb, patients with a history of cardiovascular disease:** Initially, 14 mg/day for 4-6 wk, then 7 mg/day for 2-4 wk.

Transdermal (Nicotrol)

Adults, Elderly: One patch per day for 6 wk.

Nasal

Adults, Elderly: 1-2 doses/hr (1 dose = 2 sprays [1 in each nostril] = 1 mg). Maximum: 5 doses (5 mg)/hr; 40 doses (40 mg)/day.

Inhaler (Nicotrol)

Adults, Elderly: Puff on nicotine cartridge mouthpiece for about 20 min as needed.

CONTRAINDICATIONS

Immediate post-MI period, life-threatening dysrhythmias, severe or worsening angina, hypersensitivity to nicotine

INTERACTIONS

Drug: Beta-adrenergic blockers, bronchodilators (such as theophylline), insulin, propoxyphene: May increase the effects of these drugs. **Herbal:** None known. **Food:** None known.

DIAGNOSTIC TEST EFFECTS

None known.

SIDE-EFFECTS

Frequent: All forms: Hiccups, nausea. **Gum:** Mouth or throat soreness, nausea. **Transdermal:** Erythema, pruritus, or burning at application site. **Occasional: All forms:** Eructation, GI upset, dry mouth, insomnia, diaphoresis, irritability. **Gum:** Hoarseness. **Inhaler:** Mouth or throat irritation, cough. **Rare: All forms:** Dizziness, myalgia, arthralgia

CRITICAL CARE CONSIDERATIONS

ADMINISTRATION/HANDLING

PO ALERT (GUM)

- Chew 1 piece slowly and intermittently for 30 min when the urge to smoke begins, then continue chewing until the distinctive, peppery nicotine taste or slight tingling in mouth occurs. When the tingling or taste is almost gone (approximately 1 min), continue chewing slowly to allow constant, slow buccal absorption. Do not chew too rapidly to avoid excessive release of nicotine, resulting in adverse effects such as nausea and throat irritation. Discard gum when finished; do not swallow gum.

TRANSDERMAL ALERT

- **Cimetidine:** Decrease dosage for patients taking more than 600 mg cimetidine (Tagamet) daily.
- **Dose response:** Individualize nicotine dosage based on patient response.
- **Smoking cessation:** Ideally, nicotine is administered when patients plan to stop smoking; appropriate critically ill patients may benefit from the drug regardless of plans for smoking cessation to help control agitation and anxiety.
- **Application:** Apply patch as soon as it has been removed from the protective pouch to prevent evaporation and loss of nicotine. Use only an intact pouch. Do not cut the patch. Apply only once daily to a hairless, clean, dry area on the upper body or outer arm. Wash hands with water alone after applying the patch because soap may increase nicotine absorption.
- **Rotate application sites:** Do not use the same site for 7 days or the same patch for longer than 24 hr.
- **Discard used patches:** Fold the patch in half with the sticky sides together, place it in the pouch of the new patch, and discard it in a receptacle that is not accessible to children or pets.

INHALER ALERT

- **Preparation:** Insert the cartridge into the mouthpiece.
- **Administration:** Puff vigorously for 20 min.

PRECAUTIONS

HEALTH-RELATED

- Use nicotine cautiously in patients with eczematous dermatitis, esophagitis, hyperthyroidism, insulin-dependent diabetes mellitus, oral or pharyngeal inflammation, peptic ulcer disease, pheochromocytoma, or severe renal impairment.

AGE-RELATED

- **Children:** Nicotine use is not recommended for children.
- **Elderly:** An age-related decrease in cardiac function may require cautious use.

N

PREGNANCY/LACTATION-RELATED

- Pregnancy category D. Use of nicotine gum during last trimester has been associated with decreased fetal breathing movements. Passes freely into breast milk; however, lower concentrations in milk can be expected with transdermal systems than cigarette smoking when used as directed.

MONITORING

- **Baseline assessment:** Obtain baseline vital signs, including BP and heart rate. Assess smoking habits in relation to sleep patterns. Screen and evaluate patients with Buerger's disease, coronary artery disease (including angina pectoris and history of MI), Prinzmetal's variant angina, and serious cardiac dysrhythmias.
- **Baseline lab work:** CBC to assess for anemia and biochemical profile to assess for renal insufficiency.
- **Baseline diagnostic testing:** 12-lead ECG.
- **Transdermal system:** Monitor application site for burning, erythema, and pruritus.
- **Cardiac monitoring:** Monitor for dysrhythmias (tachycardia, premature ventricular beats) following nicotine administration.
- **Withdrawal:** Assess for irritability, anxiety, and agitation, which may indicate need for a higher dose. All patients who were smoking before hospitalization should be considered for use of the transdermal system to avoid nicotine withdrawal during smoking abstinence, regardless of whether they plan smoking cessation post-hospitalization.
- **Substance abuse:** If being managed for other substance abuse, other medications used for withdrawal may also assist in managing smoking cessation symptoms. When other medications are weaned, signs of nicotine withdrawal may then be exhibited.
- **Patient education:** Instruct patients using nicotine gum to chew slowly to avoid jaw ache, nausea, and throat irritation, and to maximize therapeutic benefits; patients should not swallow the gum. Teach how to apply and discard nicotine patches properly. Instruct not to cut patches. Instruct to promptly report itching or a persistent rash during treatment with the transdermal patch to a health care provider. Urge not to smoke while wearing nicotine transdermal patches; this results in very large doses of nicotine, which may promote undesirable elevation of BP and heart rate and may prompt nausea and chest discomfort.

SERIOUS ADVERSE REACTIONS

- **Cardiovascular effects:** Tachycardia, ventricular dysrhythmias, hypertension or hypotension, chest discomfort, dyspnea.
- **GI effects:** Severe nausea, vomiting, heartburn.

OVERDOSE/TOXICITY

- **Overdose:** Palpitations, tachydysrhythmias, seizures, depression, confusion, diaphoresis, hypotension, rapid or weak pulse, and dyspnea. Lethal dose for adults is 40-60 mg. Death results from respiratory paralysis.
- **Management:** Maintain patent airway and support breathing. May require endotracheal intubation and mechanical ventilation. Support BP with IV fluids, then vasopressors if needed. Manage heart rate according to Advanced Cardiac Life Support (ACLS) guidelines.
- **GI decontamination:** No specific recommendations.

ANTIDOTE/DIALYSIS

- **Antidote:** No specific recommendations.
- **Dialysis:** No data are available on removal of nicotine using hemodialysis, high-permeability hemodialysis, or peritoneal dialysis.

N

*NIFEdipine

nye-fed'-i-peen

Classes

Chemical: dihydropyridine

Therapeutic: antianginal, antihypertensive, calcium channel blocker

Pregnancy Category: C

Trade Names

Prescription: Adalat CC, Adalat FT ♣, Adalat PA ♣, Apo-Nifed ♣, Nifedical XL, Novo Nifedin ♣, Procardia, Procardia XL

Do not confuse *NIFEdipine with *niCARdipine or nimodipine.

CLINICAL PHARMACOLOGY

Mechanism of Action

An antianginal and antihypertensive agent that inhibits calcium ion movement across cell membranes, depressing contraction of cardiac and vascular smooth muscle. **Therapeutic Effect:** Increases heart rate and cardiac output. Decreases systemic vascular resistance and BP.

PHARMACOKINETICS

Route	Onset	Peak	Duration
Sublingual	1-5 min	20-30 min	N/A
PO	20-30 min	N/A	4-8 hr
PO (extended release)	2 hr	N/A	24 hr

Rapidly, completely absorbed from the GI tract. Protein binding: 92%-98%. Undergoes first-pass metabolism in the liver. Primarily excreted in urine. Not removed by hemodialysis. **Half-life:** 2-5 hr.

AVAILABILITY

Capsules (Procardia): 10 mg.
Tablets (extended release): 30 mg (Adalat CC, Nifedical XL, Procardia XL), 60 mg (Adalat CC, Nifedical XL, Procardia XL), 90 mg (Adalat CC, Procardia XL).

INDICATIONS AND DOSAGE

Prinzmetal's variant angina, chronic stable (effort-associated) angina
PO
Adults, Elderly: Initially, 10 mg 3 times per day. Increase at 7- to 14-day intervals. Maintenance: 10 mg 3 times per day up to 30 mg 4 times per day.
PO (Extended Release)
Adults, Elderly: Initially, 30-60 mg/day. Maintenance: Up to 120 mg/day.
Essential hypertension
PO (Extended Release)
Adults, Elderly: Initially, 30-60 mg/day. Maintenance: Up to 120 mg/day.

OFF-LABEL USES

Treatment of Raynaud's phenomenon

CONTRAINDICATIONS

Advanced aortic stenosis, acute MI, severe hypotension, hypersensitivity to *NIFEdipine, immediate release preparation for treatment of urgent or emergent hypertension

INTERACTIONS

Drug: Beta-blockers: May have additive effect. **Digoxin:** May increase digoxin blood concentration. **Hypokalemia-producing agents (such as furosemide and certain other diuretics):** May increase risk of dysrhythmias. **Herbal:** None known. **Food: Grapefruit, grapefruit juice:** May increase *NIFEdipine plasma concentration.

DIAGNOSTIC TEST EFFECTS

May cause positive antinuclear antibodies and direct Coombs' test.

SIDE-EFFECTS

Frequent (30%-11%): Peripheral edema, headache, flushed skin, dizziness. **Occasional (12%-6%):** Nausea, shakiness, muscle cramps and pain, somnolence, palpitations, nasal congestion, cough, dyspnea, wheezing. **Rare (5%-3%):** Hypotension, rash, pruritus, urticaria, constipation, abdominal discomfort, flatulence, sexual difficulties

CRITICAL CARE CONSIDERATIONS

ADMINISTRATION/HANDLING

PO ALERT

- Do not crush or break extended-release tablets.
- Give *NIFEdipine without regard to meals.
- Grapefruit juice may alter absorption (cytochrome P450 enzyme inhibitor).

SUBLINGUAL ALERT

- **Angina:** May give 10-20 mg of *NIFEdipine sublingually as needed for acute attack of angina if nitrates are ineffective or unavailable.
- Capsules must be punctured with a sterile pin or needle and squeezed to express liquid under the tongue.

PRECAUTIONS

HEALTH-RELATED

- Use *NIFEdipine cautiously in patients with impaired hepatic or renal function.
- **Cytochrome P450 enzyme metabolism:** *NIFEdipine's first-pass metabolism may be mediated by the cytochrome P450 enzyme system. Drugs that inhibit the enzyme pathway (cimetidine, ranitidine) used concomitantly may alter the effects of *NIFEdipine, or *NIFEdipine may alter levels of other cytochrome P450 enzyme inhibitors.

AGE-RELATED

- **Children:** Safety and efficacy of *NIFEdipine have not been established in children.
- **Elderly:** Age-related renal impairment may require cautious use.

PREGNANCY/LACTATION-RELATED

- Pregnancy category C; an insignificant amount is excreted into breast milk.

N

MONITORING

- **Baseline assessment:** Record onset, type (sharp, dull, or squeezing), radiation, location, intensity, and duration of anginal pain and precipitating factors (exertion and emotional stress). Assess for hypotension immediately before *NIFEdipine administration. Concurrent sublingual nitroglycerin therapy may be used for relief of anginal pain.
- **Lab work:** CBC to assess for anemia; biochemical profile including renal (BUN, creatinine) and hepatic function (AST [SGOT], ALT [SGPT], alkaline phosphatase) tests.
- **Diagnostic tests:** 12-lead ECG to assess for myocardial ischemia. Monitor liver function weekly throughout therapy.
- **Dizziness:** Assist patients with ambulation if dizziness or lightheadedness occurs.
- **Edema:** Assess for peripheral edema behind the medial malleolus in ambulatory patients or the sacral area in bedridden patients.
- **Flushing:** Examine skin for redness or flushing following use.
- **Dysrhythmias:** Monitor ECG continuously for bradycardia, heart block, ST depression or elevation in critically ill patients.
- **Patient education:** Instruct to rise slowly from a lying to a sitting position and to pause momentarily before standing to reduce drug's hypotensive effect. Instruct to report promptly irregular heartbeat, prolonged dizziness, nausea, or shortness of breath to a health care provider. Urge avoidance of alcohol, grapefruit, and grapefruit juice.

SERIOUS ADVERSE REACTIONS

- *NIFEdipine may precipitate heart failure and MI in patients with cardiac disease and peripheral ischemia.
- Severe peripheral edema with weight gain, headache, and flushing.
- Nausea, somnolence, confusion, and slurred speech.
- **Acute liver injury:** Liver failure has been reported in rare cases.

OVERDOSE/TOXICITY

- **Overdose:** Hypotension, bradycardia, heart block, dysrhythmias, altered mental status most commonly. Less commonly, tachycardia, respiratory arrest, seizures, gastroenteritis, hyperglycemia, noncardiogenic pulmonary edema (acute respiratory distress syndrome), lactic acidosis, and cardiac arrest.
- **Management:** Maintain patent airway, ventilation, oxygenation and support of BP with fluids, and then vasopressors and/or inotropes if needed. Continuous cardiac monitoring should be initiated. A pulmonary artery catheter may be needed to differentiate the cause of hypotension between decreased cardiac output and decreased systemic vascular resistance. Effects of overdose are fully reversible if resuscitative efforts can be sustained for several hr. Initial drug for bradycardia is atropine. Calcium, glucagon, catecholamine infusions, insulin-glucose, inamrinone (Inocor), cardiac pacing, and ventricular assist devices have been used to help support severely unstable patients. Differential diagnosis of the cause of hypotension is important in selection of the appropriate catecholamine (low cardiac output may respond to a strong beta agonist, while vasodilation may respond to a strong alpha agonist).
- **GI decontamination:** Single-dose activated charcoal, ideally administered within 1-2 hr of ingestion.

ANTIDOTE/DIALYSIS

- **Antidote:** Calcium chloride (10% CaCl) is the preferred calcium salt because it has 3 times the molar calcium concentration (270 mg) as calcium gluconate (90 mg). CaCl 10% (10 mL) given over 2-3 min until adequate clinical response is obtained, QT narrowing occurs, or ionized calcium at least doubles; may be helpful in reversing effects of calcium channel blockade. If patient stabilizes, an infusion of 10% CaCl at 10 mL/hr can be initiated. Doses of 30 g of calcium over 12 hr have resulted in only a transient rise in serum calcium concentrations, without clinical symptoms of hypercalcemia. *Pediatric dose is 0.2 mL/kg of 10% CaCl or 1 mL/kg of calcium gluconate.*
- **Dialysis:** *NIFEdipine is not removed by hemodialysis or peritoneal dialysis. No data are available on removal using high-permeability hemodialysis.

nimodipine

nye-moe'-di-peen

Classes

Chemical: dihydropyridine

Therapeutic: calcium channel blocker, cerebral vasodilator

Pregnancy Category: C

Trade Names

Prescription: Nimotop

Do not confuse nimodipine with *NIFEdipine.

CLINICAL PHARMACOLOGY

Mechanism of Action

A cerebral vasospasm agent that inhibits movement of calcium ions across vascular smooth-muscle cell membranes. **Therapeutic Effect:** Produces favorable effect on severity of neurologic deficits due to cerebral vasospasm. Exerts greatest effect on cerebral arteries; may prevent cerebral spasm.

PHARMACOKINETICS

Rapidly absorbed from the GI tract. Protein binding: 95%. Metabolized in the liver. Excreted in urine; eliminated in feces. Not removed by hemodialysis. **Half-life:** terminal, 3 hr.

AVAILABILITY

Capsules: 30 mg.

INDICATIONS AND DOSAGE

Improvement of neurologic deficits after subarachnoid hemorrhage from ruptured congenital aneurysms

PO

Adults, Elderly: 60 mg every 4 hr for 21 days. Begin within 96 hr of subarachnoid hemorrhage.

OFF-LABEL USES

Treatment of chronic and classic migraine, chronic cluster headaches

CONTRAINDICATIONS

Atrial fibrillation or flutter, cardiogenic shock, heart failure, heart block, sinus bradycardia, ventricular tachycardia, within several hr of IV beta-blocker therapy, hypersensitivity to nimodipine

INTERACTIONS

Drug: Beta-blockers: May prolong SA and AV conduction, which may lead to severe hypotension, bradycardia, and cardiac failure. **Erythromycin, itraconazole, ketoconazole, protease inhibitors:** May inhibit the metabolism of nimodipine. **Rifabutin, rifampin:** May increase the metabolism of nimodipine. **Herbal: Garlic:** May increase antihypertensive effect. **Ginseng, yohimbe:** May worsen hypertension. **Food: Grapefruit juice:** May increase nimodipine blood concentration and risk of toxicity.

DIAGNOSTIC TEST EFFECTS

None known.

SIDE-EFFECTS

Occasional (6%-2%): Hypotension, peripheral edema, diarrhea, headache. **Rare (less than 2%):** Allergic reaction (rash, hives), tachycardia, flushing of skin

CRITICAL CARE CONSIDERATIONS

ADMINISTRATION/HANDLING

PO ALERT

- **Nasogastric administration:** If patients are unable to swallow, place a hole in both ends of a capsule with an 18-gauge needle to extract contents into a syringe. Empty contents of syringe into a nasogastric tube; flush tube with 30 mL normal saline.

PRECAUTIONS

HEALTH-RELATED

- Use nimodipine cautiously in patients with impaired hepatic or renal function.
- **Cytochrome P450 enzyme metabolism:** Drugs that inhibit the enzyme pathway (erythromycin, itraconazole, ketoconazole, protease inhibitors, rifabutin, rifampin) used concomitantly may alter the effects of nimodipine, or nimodipine may alter levels of other cytochrome P450 enzyme inhibitors.

AGE-RELATED

- **Children:** Safety and efficacy of nimodipine have not been established in children.
- **Elderly:** Age-related renal impairment may require cautious use; elderly may also experience greater hypotensive response and constipation.

PREGNANCY/LACTATION-RELATED

- Pregnancy category C; unknown if distributed in breast milk.

MONITORING

- **Baseline assessment:** Assess LOC and neurologic response, initially and throughout nimodipine therapy. Assess for bradycardia

N

and hypotension before giving nimodipine. If heart rate is less than 60 beats/min or systolic BP is less than 90 mmHg, withhold the medication.

- **Lab work:** CBC to assess for anemia; biochemical profile including renal (BUN, creatinine) and hepatic function (AST [SGOT], ALT [SGPT], alkaline phosphatase) tests.
- **Diagnostic tests:** CT brain scan to assess for stroke. Monitor liver function weekly throughout therapy.
- **Dizziness:** Assist with ambulation if dizziness or lightheadedness occurs.
- **Edema:** Assess for peripheral edema behind the medial malleolus in ambulatory patients or sacral area in bedridden patients.
- **Neurologic monitoring:** Assess neurologic status based on patient instability. Drug should improve cerebral perfusion, but overt signs of improvement may not be apparent.
- **Patient education:** Warn not to crush or chew capsules. Instruct to report constipation, dizziness, irregular heartbeat, nausea, shortness of breath, or swelling promptly to a health care provider.

SERIOUS ADVERSE REACTIONS

- Nimodipine may precipitate heart failure and MI in patients with cardiac disease and peripheral ischemia.
- Peripheral edema with weight gain, headache, and flushing.
- Nausea, somnolence, confusion, and slurred speech.
- **Acute liver injury:** Liver failure has been reported in rare cases.

OVERDOSE/TOXICITY

- **Overdose:** Hypotension, bradycardia, heart block, dysrhythmias, altered mental status most commonly. Less commonly, tachycardia, respiratory arrest, seizures, gastroenteritis, hyperglycemia, noncardiogenic pulmonary edema (acute respiratory distress syndrome), lactic acidosis, and cardiac arrest.
- **Management:** Maintain patent airway, ventilation, oxygenation and support of BP with fluids, and then vasopressors and/or inotropes if needed. Continuous cardiac monitoring should be initiated. A pulmonary artery catheter may be needed to differentiate the cause of hypotension between decreased cardiac output and decreased systemic vascular resistance. Effects of overdose are fully reversible if resuscitative efforts can be sustained for several hr. Initial drug for bradycardia is atropine. Calcium, glucagon, catecholamine infusions, insulin-glucose, inamrinone (Inocor), cardiac pacing, and ventricular assist devices have been used to help support severely unstable patients. Differential diagnosis of the cause of hypotension is important in selection of the appropriate catecholamine (low cardiac output may respond to a strong beta agonist, while vasodilation may respond to a strong alpha agonist).
- **GI decontamination:** Single-dose activated charcoal, ideally administered within 1-2 hr of ingestion.

ANTIDOTE/DIALYSIS

- **Antidote:** Calcium chloride (10% CaCl) is the preferred calcium salt because it has 3 times the molar calcium concentration (270 mg) as calcium gluconate (90 mg). CaCl 10% (10 mL) given over 2-3 min until adequate clinical response is obtained, QT narrowing occurs, or ionized calcium at least doubles; may be helpful in reversing effects of calcium channel blockade. If patient stabilizes, an infusion of 10% CaCl at 10 mL/hr can be initiated. Doses of 30 g of calcium over 12 hr have resulted in only a transient rise in serum calcium concentrations without clinical symptoms of hypercalcemia. *Pediatric dose is 0.2 mL/kg of 10% CaCl or 1 mL/kg of calcium gluconate.*
- **Dialysis:** Nimodipine is not removed by hemodialysis or peritoneal dialysis. No data are available on removal by high-permeability hemodialysis.

nitazoxanide

nye-ta-zox'-ah-nide

Classes

Chemical: benzamide derivative
Therapeutic: antiprotozoal

Pregnancy Category: B

Trade Names

Prescription: Alinia

CLINICAL PHARMACOLOGY

Mechanism of Action

An antiparasitic that interferes with the body's reaction to pyruvate ferredoxin oxidoreductase, an enzyme essential for anaerobic energy metabolism. **Therapeutic**

Effect: Produces antiprotozoal activity, reducing or terminating diarrheal episodes.

PHARMACOKINETICS

Rapidly hydrolyzed to an active metabolite. Protein binding: 99%. Excreted in the urine, bile, and feces. **Half-life:** 2-4 hr.

AVAILABILITY

Powder for oral suspension: 100 mg/5 mL.
Tablets: 500 mg.

INDICATIONS AND DOSAGE

Diarrhea caused by *Cryptosporidium parvum*

PO

Children 4-11 yr: 200 mg every 12 hr for 3 days. **Children 12-47 mo:** 100 mg every 12 hr for 3 days.

Diarrhea caused by *Giardia lamblia*

PO

Adults, Elderly, Children 12 yr and older: 500 mg every 12 hr for 3 days. **Children 4-11 yr:** 200 mg every 12 hr for 3 days. **Children 12-47 mo:** 100 mg every 12 hr for 3 days.

CONTRAINDICATIONS

History of sensitivity to aspirin and salicylates or nitazoxanide

INTERACTIONS

Drug: None known. **Herbal:** None known. **Food:** None known.

DIAGNOSTIC TEST EFFECTS

May increase serum creatinine and ALT (SGOT) levels.

SIDE-EFFECTS

Occasional (8%): Abdominal pain. **Rare (2%-1%):** Diarrhea, vomiting, headache

CRITICAL CARE CONSIDERATIONS

ADMINISTRATION/HANDLING

PO ALERT

- **Storage:** Store unreconstituted powder at room temperature.
- **Reconstitution:** Reconstitute oral suspension with 48 mL water to provide a concentration of 100 mg/5 mL. Shake vigorously to suspend powder.
- **Stability:** Reconstituted solution is stable for 7 days at room temperature.
- Give nitazoxanide with food.

PRECAUTIONS

HEALTH-RELATED

- Use nitazoxanide cautiously in patients with biliary or hepatic disease, GI disorders, or renal impairment.

AGE-RELATED

- **Children:** Safety and efficacy of nitazoxanide have not been established in children under 1 yr or over 11 yr.
- **Elderly:** Nitazoxanide is not indicated for use in the elderly.

PREGNANCY/LACTATION-RELATED

- Pregnancy category B; excretion into breast milk unknown; use caution in nursing mothers.

MONITORING

- **Baseline assessment:** Assess for dehydration (hypotension, weight loss, poor skin turgor, hemoconcentration) secondary to diarrhea.
- **Baseline lab work:** CBC with WBC differential and biochemical panel including blood glucose and electrolyte levels, renal (BUN, creatinine) and liver (AST [SGOT], ALT [SGPT], alkaline phosphatase, bilirubin) function tests. Stool cultures to identify *C. parvum* or *G. lamblia.*
- **Hyperglycemia:** Evaluate blood glucose level, especially in diabetic patients.
- **Fluid and electrolyte imbalance:** Assess electrolyte levels for abnormalities daily in critically ill patients. Weigh daily.
- **Hydration:** Provide IV hydration and encourage patients to try to maintain adequate fluid intake.
- **Abdominal pain:** Monitor and manage pain. Assess for peristalsis.
- **Diarrhea:** Assess pattern of daily bowel activity and stool consistency.
- **Patient education:** Tell parents of children with diabetes mellitus that the oral suspension of nitazoxanide contains 1.48 g of sucrose per 5 mL. Explain that nitazoxanide therapy should significantly help resolve diarrhea. Instruct patients and parents to make sure the drug is taken with food.

SERIOUS ADVERSE REACTIONS

- Nitazoxanide is highly protein bound and may compete for binding sites with other highly bound drugs.

OVERDOSE/TOXICITY

- Abdominal pain, vomiting, headache.
- **GI decontamination:** No specific recommendations.

N

ANTIDOTE/DIALYSIS

- **Antidote:** No specific recommendations.
- **Dialysis:** Nitazoxanide is unlikely to be removed by hemodialysis, high-permeability hemodialysis, or peritoneal dialysis.

nitroglycerin

nye-troe-gli'-ser-in

Classes

Chemical: nitrate, organic
Therapeutic: antianginal, vasodilator

Pregnancy Category: C

Trade Names

Prescription: Minitran, Nitrek, Nitro-Bid, Nitro-Bid IV, Nitrocot, Nitro-Dur, Nitrogard, Nitroglyn E-R, Nitrol ♣, Nitrol Appli-Kit, Nitrolingual, Nitrong, Nitro-Quick, Nitrostat, Nitro-Tab, Nitro TD Patch-A, Nitro-Time, Transderm-Nitro ♣, Tridil

Do not confuse nitroglycerin with nitroprusside; Nitro-Bid with Nicobid; Nitro-Dur with Nicoderm; Nitrostat with Hyperstat, Nilstat, or Nystatin; or Nitrong-SR with Nizoral.

N

CLINICAL PHARMACOLOGY

Mechanism of Action

A nitrate that decreases myocardial oxygen demand. Reduces left ventricular preload and afterload. **Therapeutic Effect:** Dilates coronary arteries and improves collateral blood flow to ischemic areas within myocardium. IV form produces peripheral vasodilation.

PHARMACOKINETICS

Route	Onset	Peak	Duration
Sublingual	1-3 min	4-8 min	30-60 min
Translingual spray	2 min	4-10 min	30-60 min
Buccal tablet	2-5 min	4-10 min	2 hr
PO (extended release)	20-45 min	45-120 min	4-8 hr
Topical	15-60 min	30-120 min	2-12 hr
Transdermal patch	40-60 min	60-180 min	18-24 hr
IV	1-2 min	Immediate	3-5 min

Well absorbed after PO, sublingual, and topical administration. Undergoes extensive first-pass metabolism. Metabolized in the liver and by enzymes in the bloodstream. Primarily excreted in urine. Not removed by hemodialysis. **Half-life:** 1-4 min.

AVAILABILITY

Capsules (extended release [NitroBid, Nitrocot, Nitroglyn E-R, Nitro-Time]): 2.5 mg, 6.5 mg, 9 mg.
Tablets (extended release, oral transmucosal): 1 mg (Nitrogard), 2.6 mg (Nitrong), 3 mg (Nitrogard), 6.5 mg (Nitrong).
Tablets (sublingual [NitroQuick, Nitrostat, Nitro-Tab]): 0.3 mg, 0.4 mg, 0.6 mg.
Spray (translingual [Nitrolingual]): 0.4 mg/spray.
Infusion solution: 0.1 mg/mL, 0.2 mg/mL, 0.4 mg/mL.
Intravenous solution (Nitro-Bid IV, Tridil): 5 mg/mL.
Intravenous solution: 5% dextrose-10 mg nitroglycerin/100 mL, 5% dextrose-20 mg nitroglycerin/100 mL, 5% dextrose-40 mg nitroglycerin/100 mL.
Topical ointment (Nitro-Bid, Nitrol, Nitrol Appli-Kit): 2%.
Transdermal patch (Minitran): 0.1 mg/hr (Minitran, Nitro-Dur), 0.2 mg/hr (Minitran, Nitrek, Nitro-Dur), 0.3 mg/hr (Minitran, Nitro-Dur), 0.4 mg/hr (Minitran, Nitrek, Nitro-Dur), 0.6 mg/hr (Nitrek, Nitro-Dur), 0.8 mg/hr (Nitro-Dur).

INDICATIONS AND DOSAGE

Acute relief of angina pectoris, acute prophylaxis

Lingual Spray

Adults, Elderly: 1 spray onto or under tongue every 3-5 min until relief is noted (no more than 3 sprays in 15-min period).

Sublingual

Adults, Elderly: 0.4 mg every 5 min until relief is noted (no more than 3 doses in 15-min period). Use prophylactically 5-10 min before activities that may cause an acute attack.

Long-term prophylaxis of angina

PO (Extended Release)

Adults, Elderly: 2.5-9 mg 2-4 times per day. Maximum: 26 mg 4 times per day.

Topical

Adults, Elderly: Initially half inch every 8 hr. Increase by half inch with each application. Range: 1-2 inches every 8 hr up to 4-5 inches every 4 hr.

Transdermal Patch

Adults, Elderly: Initially, 0.2-0.4 mg/hr. Maintenance: 0.4-0.8 mg/hr. Consider patch on for 12-14 hr, patch off for 10-12 hr (prevents tolerance).

Heart failure associated with acute MI

IV

Adults, Elderly: Initially, 5 mcg/min via infusion pump. Increase in 5-mcg/min increments at 3- to 5-min intervals until BP response is noted or until dosage reaches 20 mcg/min; then increase as needed by 10 mcg/min. Dosage may be further titrated according to clinical, therapeutic response up to 200 mcg/min. **Children:** Initially 0.25-0.5 mcg/kg/min; titrate by 0.5-1 mcg/kg/min up to 20 mcg/kg/min.

CONTRAINDICATIONS

Allergy to adhesives (transdermal), closed-angle glaucoma, constrictive pericarditis (IV), early MI (sublingual), GI hypermotility or malabsorption (extended release), head trauma, hypotension (IV), inadequate cerebral circulation (IV), increased intracranial pressure (ICP), nitrates, orthostatic hypotension, pericardial tamponade (IV), severe anemia, uncorrected hypovolemia (IV), hypersensitivity to nitroglycerin

INTERACTIONS

Drug: Alcohol, other antihypertensives, vasodilators: May increase risk of orthostatic hypotension. **Sildenafil, tadalafil, vardenafil:** Concurrent use of these drugs produces significant hypotension. **Cisatracurium, atracurium, vecuronium, pancuronium:** Nitroglycerin may increase effects of neuromuscular blockade. **Herbal:** None known. **Food:** None known.

DIAGNOSTIC TEST EFFECTS

May increase blood methemoglobin, urine catecholamine, and urine vanillylmandelic acid concentrations (VMA).

IV INCOMPATIBILITIES

Alteplase (Activase)

IV COMPATIBILITIES

Amiodarone (Cordarone), diltiazem (Cardizem), *DOBUTamine (Dobutrex), *DOPamine (Intropin), epinephrine, famotidine (Pepcid), fentanyl (Sublimaze), furosemide (Lasix), heparin, hydromorphone (Dilaudid), insulin, labetalol (Trandate), lidocaine, lorazepam (Ativan), midazolam (Versed), milrinone (Primacor), morphine, *niCARdipine (Cardene), nitroprusside (Nipride), norepinephrine (Levophed), propofol (Diprivan)

SIDE-EFFECTS

Frequent: Headache (possibly severe; occurs mostly in early therapy, diminishes rapidly in intensity, and usually disappears during continued treatment), transient flushing of face and neck, dizziness (especially if patient is standing immobile or is in a warm environment), weakness, orthostatic hypotension. **Sublingual:** Burning, tingling sensation at oral point of dissolution. **Ointment:** Erythema, pruritus. **Occasional:** GI upset. **Transdermal:** Contact dermatitis

CRITICAL CARE CONSIDERATIONS

ADMINISTRATION/HANDLING

PO ALERT

- Swallow extended-release capsules whole. Capsules should not be chewed or crushed.
- Do not shake aerosol canister before lingual spraying.

SUBLINGUAL ALERT

- Dissolve the sublingual form under the tongue and avoid swallowing. Administer while seated or lying down.
- To lessen the burning sensation under the tongue, place the tablet in the buccal pouch.
- **Storage:** Keep sublingual tablets in their original container.

TOPICAL ALERT

- **Application:** Use the applicator or dose measuring papers to spread a thin layer on clean, dry, hairless skin of the upper arm or body and not below the knee or elbow. Do not use fingers; do not rub or massage into skin.

TRANSDERMAL ALERT

- **Application:** Apply patch on clean, dry, hairless skin of the upper arm or body and not below the knee or elbow.

IV ALERT

- **Storage:** Store at room temperature. The IV form is available in ready-to-use injectable containers.
- **Dilution:** Dilute vials in 250 or 500 mL D_5W or 0.9% NaCl to a maximum concentration of 250 mg/250 mL.
- **Infusion:** Use microdrop or infusion pump. Nitroglycerin manufacturer may recommend special IV tubing to help reduce its adsorption into polyvinyl chloride (PVC) tubing.

N

NITROGLYCERIN INFUSION TABLE

NITROGLYCERIN 50 mg/250 mL [0.2 mg/mL]		NITROGLYCERIN 100 mg/250 mL [0.4 mg/mL]	
Dose (mcg/min)	Rate (mL/hr)	Dose (mcg/min)	Rate (mL/hr)
10	3	10	1.5
15	4.5	15	2.3
20	6	20	3
25	7.5	25	3.8
30	9	30	4.5
35	10.5	35	5.3
40	12	40	6
45	13.5	45	6.8
50	15	50	7.5
55	16.5	55	8.3
60	18	60	9
65	19.5	65	9.8
70	21	70	10.6
75	22.5	75	11.3
80	24	80	12
85	25.5	85	12.8
90	27	90	13.5
95	28.5	95	14.3
100	30	100	15

PRECAUTIONS

N

HEALTH-RELATED

- Use nitroglycerin cautiously in patients with acute MI, blood volume depletion from diuretic therapy, glaucoma (contraindicated in closed-angle glaucoma), hepatic or renal disease, or systolic BP less than 90 mmHg.
- **Erectile dysfunction:** To avoid irreversible hypotension, do not give nitrates within 24 hr of the patient taking Cialis, Levitra, or Viagra.
- **Defibrillation:** The defibrillator must not be discharged through a paddle electrode overlying a nitroglycerin system because this may cause burns or damage the paddle via arcing.
- **Neuromuscular blockade:** Nitroglycerin potentiates nondepolarizing neuromuscular blocking agents; dosage may need to be reduced.

AGE-RELATED

- **Children:** Safety and efficacy of nitroglycerin have not been established in children.
- **Elderly:** More susceptible to the hypotensive effects of nitroglycerin; age-related renal impairment may require cautious use. Lower initial doses may be indicated.

PREGNANCY/LACTATION-RELATED

- Pregnancy category C; use of sublingual form for angina during pregnancy without fetal harm has been reported.

MONITORING

- **Baseline assessment:** Assess for hypovolemia before administration. Record onset, type (sharp, dull, or squeezing), radiation, location, intensity, and duration of anginal pain and precipitating factors (exertion and emotional stress). Assess for hypotension immediately before nitroglycerin administration. Concurrent sublingual *NIFEdipine therapy may be used for relief of anginal pain.
- **Lab work:** CBC to assess for anemia; biochemical profile including renal (BUN, creatinine) and hepatic function (AST [SGOT], ALT [SGPT], alkaline phosphatase) tests.
- **Diagnostic tests:** 12-lead ECG to assess for myocardial ischemia. Monitor the liver function weekly throughout therapy.
- **Acute MI:** Use of alteplase (Activase, r-TPA) with nitroglycerin reduces the thrombolytic effect of alteplase.
- **Hypovolemia:** Correct hypovolemia with careful administration of IV fluids. If history of heart failure is present, volume infusion may be done while monitoring central venous pressure increases or pulmonary capillary wedge pressure increases if a pulmonary artery catheter is in place.
- **Postoperative hypertension:** Nitroglycerin may be used to lower BP following a surgical procedure; if BP is not effectively controlled, consider using a drug with stronger systemic arterial dilating effects.
- **Hemodynamic monitoring:** Observe for decreased pulmonary capillary wedge pressure, which may precede systemic hypotension or shock. If tachycardia is present, note at what heart rate the tachycardia no longer increases cardiac output.
- **Dysrhythmias:** Monitor ECG continuously for dysrhythmias and ST depression or elevation in critically ill patients. Tachycardia must be controlled to preserve diastolic filling time to avoid hypotension secondary to decreased cardiac output.
- **Dizziness:** Assist patients with ambulation if dizziness or lightheadedness occurs.
- **Edema:** Assess for pedal or ankle edema in ambulatory patients or sacral area in bedridden patients, which may indicate heart or renal failure.

- **Flushing:** Examine for redness or flushing of face and neck following or during use.
- **Defibrillation:** Remove the transdermal patch before cardioversion or defibrillation because the electrical current may cause arcing, which can burn patients and damage the paddles.
- **Patient education:** Instruct to take sublingual tablets at the first sign of angina because if anginal pain is not relieved within 5 min of the first dose, a second tablet should be dissolved under the tongue. If the second dose does not relieve anginal pain within 5 min, a third tablet should be dissolved under the tongue. Warn that if anginal pain continues with no relief from the third tablet, patients should immediately seek emergency medical help. Instruct to expel any remaining intrabuccal, buccal, lingual, or sublingual tablets after the anginal pain is completely relieved. Teach to take oral nitroglycerin on an empty stomach if tolerated. If headache occurs, advise taking the medication with food. Remind to dissolve sublingual nitroglycerin tablets under the tongue and not to swallow tablets. Teach patients using nitroglycerin lingual aerosol to spray it on or under the tongue only when lying down. Explain that inhaling or swallowing the lingual aerosol should be avoided. Teach to place transmucosal tablets under the upper lip or buccal pouch, which is between the cheek and gum. Advise against chewing or swallowing transmucosal tablets. Caution against changing brands of nitroglycerin. Instruct about rising slowly from a lying to a sitting position and pausing momentarily before standing to avoid hypotension. Recommend that patients avoid alcohol during nitroglycerin therapy; alcohol causes further lowering of BP. Warn that alcohol ingested soon after taking nitroglycerin can cause acute hypotension (dizziness, pallor, fainting). Drug container should be kept away from heat and moisture.

SERIOUS ADVERSE REACTIONS

- **Methemoglobinemia:** Cyanosis, respiratory distress, falsely elevated or falsely low O_2 saturation using pulse oximetry in the presence of normal PO_2; if cooximeter is used for arterial blood gas (ABG) analysis, the cooximeter O_2 saturation will be lower than older or less precise ABG analyzers; chocolate brown or abnormally dark arterial blood sample; manage with methylene blue 1-2 mg/kg and high-flow oxygen.
- Nitroglycerin should be discontinued if blurred vision or dry mouth occurs.
- Severe orthostatic hypotension may occur manifested by fainting, pulselessness, cold or clammy skin, and diaphoresis.
- Tolerance may occur with repeated, prolonged therapy; minor tolerance may occur with intermittent use of sublingual tablets.
- High doses of nitroglycerin tend to produce severe headache.

OVERDOSE/TOXICITY

- **Overdose:** Severe hypotension, shock, tachycardia, reflex paradoxic bradycardia, heart block, dyspnea, flushing, bloody diarrhea, visual disturbances, constrictive pericarditis, cardiac tamponade, death.
- **Management:** Temporarily discontinue nitroglycerin. Lower head of bed, elevate legs, administer IV fluids and if needed, alpha-adrenergic vasopressors (methoxamine [Vasoxyl], phenylephrine [Neosynephrine]) to increase BP. Epinephrine and related drugs (*DOPamine) are contraindicated. Resuscitate according to Advanced Cardiac Life Support (ACLS) guidelines.
- **GI decontamination:** No specific recommendations.

ANTIDOTE/DIALYSIS

- **Antidote:** No specific recommendations.
- **Dialysis:** Nitroglycerin is not removed by hemodialysis or peritoneal dialysis. No data are available on removal by high-permeability hemodialysis.

nitroprusside sodium 

nye-troe-pruss'-ide soe'-dee-um

Classes

Chemical: cyanonitrosylferrate derivative
Therapeutic: antihypertensive

Pregnancy Category: C

Trade Names

Prescription: Nipride 🍁, Nitropress

Do not confuse nitroprusside with nitroglycerin or Nitrostat.

CLINICAL PHARMACOLOGY

Mechanism of Action

A potent vasodilator used to treat emergent hypertensive conditions; acts directly on arterial and venous smooth muscle. Decreases peripheral vascular resistance, preload and afterload; improves cardiac output. **Therapeutic Effect:** Dilates coronary arteries, decreases oxygen consumption, and relieves persistent chest pain.

PHARMACOKINETICS

Route	Onset	Peak	Duration
IV	1-2 min	Dependent on infusion rate	1-10 min

Reacts with Hgb in erythrocytes, producing cyanmethemoglobin and cyanide ions. Primarily excreted in urine. **Half-life:** less than 10 min.

AVAILABILITY

Injection: 25 mg/mL.
Powder for injection: 50 mg.

INDICATIONS AND DOSAGE

Immediate reduction of BP in hypertensive crisis; to produce controlled hypotension in surgical procedures to reduce bleeding; treatment of acute heart failure

IV Infusion

Adults, Elderly: Initially, 0.3-0.5 mcg/kg/min. May increase by 0.5 mcg/kg/min to desired hemodynamic effect or appearance of headache or nausea. Usual dose: 3 mcg/kg/min. Maximum: 10 mcg/kg/min.

N

OFF-LABEL USES

Control of paroxysmal hypertension before and during surgery for pheochromocytoma, peripheral vasospasm caused by ergot alkaloid overdose, treatment adjunct for MI, valvular regurgitation

CONTRAINDICATIONS

Compensatory hypertension (atrioventricular [AV] shunt or coarctation of aorta), congenital (Leber's) optic atrophy, inadequate cerebral circulation, moribund patients, tobacco amblyopia, hypersensitivity to nitroprusside

INTERACTIONS

Drug: ***DOBUTamine:** May increase cardiac output and decrease pulmonary wedge pressure. **Hypotension-producing medications:** May increase hypotensive effect. **Herbal:** None known. **Food:** None known.

DIAGNOSTIC TEST EFFECTS

None known.

IV INCOMPATIBILITIES

Cisatracurium (Nimbex), levofloxacin (Levaquin), haloperidol (Haldol)

IV COMPATIBILITIES

Diltiazem (Cardizem), *DOBUTamine (Dobutrex), *DOPamine (Intropin), enalapril (Vasotec), heparin, insulin, labetalol (Normodyne, Trandate), lidocaine, midazolam (Versed), milrinone (Primacor), nitroglycerin, propofol (Diprivan)

SIDE-EFFECTS

Occasional: Flushing of skin, increased intracranial pressure, rash, pain or redness at injection site

CRITICAL CARE CONSIDERATIONS

ADMINISTRATION/HANDLING

IV ALERT

- **Storage:** Protect solution from light. Inspect solution, which normally appears as very faint brown. A color change from brown to blue, green, or dark red indicates drug deterioration.
- **Stability:** Use only freshly prepared solution. Once the solution has been prepared, it must be used within 24 hr. Discard unused portion.
- **Reconstitution:** Reconstitute 50-mg vial with 2-3 mL D_5W or sterile water for injection without preservative.
- **Further dilution:** Further dilute with 250 to 1000 mL D_5W to provide a concentration of 200 mcg/mL to 50 mcg/mL, respectively, up to a maximum concentration of 200 mg/250 mL.
- **Light sensitive:** Wrap infusion bottle in aluminum foil immediately after mixing.
- **IV infusion:** Give by IV infusion using infusion rate chart from manufacturer or facility protocol. Administer using IV infusion pump.

NITROPRUSSIDE INFUSION TABLE 50 mg/250 mL D_5W [0.2 mg/mL]

	DESIRED DOSES (mcg/kg/min)				
	1	2	5	7.5	9.5
Weight	Infusion Rate in mL/hr				
40	12	24	60	90	120
50	15	30	75	112.5	150
60	18	36	90	135	180
70	21	42	105	157.5	210
80	24	48	120	180	240
90	27	54	135	202.5	270
100	30	60	150	225	300

PRECAUTIONS

HEALTH-RELATED

- Use nitroprusside cautiously in patients with hyponatremia, hypothyroidism, or severe hepatic or renal impairment.

AGE-RELATED

- **Children:** Safety and efficacy of nitroprusside have not been established in children.
- **Elderly:** More sensitive to hypotensive effects; age-related renal impairment may require cautious use.

PREGNANCY/LACTATION-RELATED

- Pregnancy category C; excretion into breast milk is unknown; use caution in nursing mothers.

MONITORING

- **Baseline assessment:** Obtain baseline vital signs. Determine desired BP level. BP is normally maintained at about 30%-40% below pretreatment levels.
- **Baseline lab work:** Biochemical profile including renal (BUN, creatinine) and liver (AST [SGOT], ALT [SGPT], alkaline phosphatase, bilirubin) function tests.
- **Baseline diagnostic tests:** 12-lead ECG to assess for myocardial ischemia and prior myocardial infarctions.
- **Hypotension:** Monitor BP continuously or frequently. Consider use of an arterial line for BP monitoring.
- **Hemodynamic monitoring:** Observe for decreased pulmonary capillary wedge pressure, which may precede systemic hypotension or shock. If tachycardia is present, note at what heart rate the tachycardia no longer increases cardiac output.
- **Dysrhythmias:** Monitor ECG continuously for dysrhythmias or ST depression or elevation in critically ill patients. Tachycardia must be controlled to preserve diastolic filling time to avoid hypotension secondary to decreased cardiac output.
- **Hypovolemia:** Correct hypovolemia with careful administration of IV fluids. If history of heart failure is present, volume infusion may be done while monitoring central venous pressure increases or pulmonary capillary wedge pressure increases if pulmonary artery catheter is in place.
- **Extravasation:** Examine IV site for redness, sloughing, and severe pain.
- **Fluid and electrolyte balance:** Monitor acid-base balance with arterial blood gas analysis, electrolyte levels.
- **Acid-base imbalance:** Assess for signs of metabolic acidosis, including disorientation, headache, hyperventilation, nausea, vomiting, and weakness.
- **Therapeutic response:** Discontinue nitroprusside if the therapeutic response is not achieved within 10 min after IV infusion at 10 mcg/kg/min is initiated.
- **Discontinued infusion:** Monitor BP for potential rebound hypertension after the infusion has been discontinued.
- **Patient education:** Instruct to immediately report dizziness, headache, nausea, palpitations and pain, redness, or swelling at the IV insertion site.

SERIOUS ADVERSE REACTIONS

- **Hypotension:** Too-rapid IV infusion rate reduces BP too quickly.
- **Methemoglobinemia:** Cyanosis, respiratory distress, falsely elevated or falsely low O_2 saturation using pulse oximetry in the presence of normal PO_2; If cooximeter is used for arterial blood gas (ABG) analysis, the cooximeter O_2 saturation will be lower than older or less precise ABG analyzers; chocolate brown or abnormally dark arterial blood sample; manage with methylene blue 1-2 mg/kg and high-flow oxygen.

N

OVERDOSE/TOXICITY

- **Overdose:** Thiocyanate toxicity with hypotension, abdominal pain, ileus, increased intracranial pressure, air hunger, bright red venous blood, confusion, metabolic acidosis, and tolerance to therapeutic effect.
- **Thiocyanate (cyanide) toxicity:** May occur with doses less than the average therapeutic dose; will occur as maximum dose of 10 mcg/kg/min is approached. Nausea, vomiting, diaphoresis, apprehension, headache, restlessness, muscle twitching, dizziness, palpitations, retrosternal pain, and abdominal pain may occur. Symptoms disappear rapidly if rate of administration is slowed or drug is temporarily discontinued.
- **Management:** Stop the infusion and monitor BP, which will return to pretreatment level in 10 min. Persistent hypotension following discontinuation of the drug is due to another source. Prepare to administer sodium thiosulfate/nitrite antidote. Position patients supine, flat with legs elevated. Maintain patent airway and support ventilation. Manage hypotension

with IV fluids as tolerated; use with caution in heart failure patients.
- **GI decontamination:** No specific recommendations.

ANTIDOTE/DIALYSIS
- **Antidote:** Sodium nitrite/sodium thiosulfate IV infusion, preceded by amyl nitrite inhalations for 15-30 sec each min until sodium nitrite infusion is ready.
- **Dialysis:** Nitroprusside is removed by hemodialysis, peritoneal dialysis, and is likely removed by high-permeability hemodialysis.

nizatidine

See Acid Secretion Inhibitors (p. 884)

norepinephrine bitartrate

nor-ep-i-nef′-rin bi-tar′-trate

Classes
Chemical: catecholamine, synthetic
Therapeutic: vasopressor, α- and β-adrenergic sympathomimetic

Pregnancy Category: C

Trade Names
Prescription: Levophed

Do not confuse Levophed with Levid, or norepinephrine with epinephrine.

CLINICAL PHARMACOLOGY
Mechanism of Action
A sympathomimetic that stimulates $beta_1$-adrenergic receptors and alpha-adrenergic receptors, increasing peripheral resistance. Enhances contractile myocardial force and increases cardiac output. Constricts resistance and capacitance vessels. **Therapeutic Effect:** Increases systemic BP and coronary blood flow.

PHARMACOKINETICS

Route	Onset	Peak	Duration
IV	Rapid	1-2 min	N/A

Localized in sympathetic tissue. Metabolized in the liver. Primarily excreted in urine.

AVAILABILITY
Injection: 1-mg/mL ampules.

INDICATIONS AND DOSAGE
Acute hypotension unresponsive to fluid volume replacement
IV
Adults, Elderly: Initially, administer at 0.5-1 mcg/min. Adjust rate of flow to establish and maintain desired BP (40 mmHg below preexisting systolic pressure). Average maintenance dose: 8-30 mcg/min. **Children:** Initially, 0.05-0.1 mcg/kg/min; titrate to desired effect. Maximum: 1-2 mcg/kg/min. Range: 0.5-3 mcg/min.

CONTRAINDICATIONS
Hypovolemic states (unless as an emergency measure), mesenteric or peripheral vascular thrombosis, profound hypoxia, hypersensitivity to norepinephrine or any component of the product

INTERACTIONS
Drug: Beta-blockers: May have mutually inhibitory effects. **Digoxin:** May increase risk of dysrhythmias. **Ergonovine, oxytocin:** May increase vasoconstriction. **MAOIs:** May cause prolonged hypertension. **Maprotiline, tricyclic antidepressants:** May increase cardiovascular effects. **Methyldopa:** May decrease the effects of methyldopa. **Herbal:** None known. **Food:** None known.

DIAGNOSTIC TEST EFFECTS
None known.

IV INCOMPATIBILITIES
Regular insulin

IV COMPATIBILITIES
Amiodarone (Cordarone), calcium gluconate, diltiazem (Cardizem), *DOBUTamine (Dobutrex), *DOPamine (Intropin), epinephrine, esmolol (Brevibloc), fentanyl (Sublimaze), furosemide (Lasix), haloperidol (Haldol), heparin, hydromorphone (Dilaudid), labetalol (Trandate), lorazepam (Ativan), magnesium, midazolam (Versed), milrinone (Primacor), morphine, *niCARdipine (Cardene), nitroglycerin, potassium chloride, propofol (Diprivan)

SIDE-EFFECTS
Norepinephrine produces less pronounced and less frequent side effects than epinephrine. **Occasional (5%-3%):** Anxiety, bradycardia, palpitations. **Rare (2%-1%):** Nausea, anginal pain, shortness of breath, fever

CRITICAL CARE CONSIDERATIONS

ADMINISTRATION/HANDLING

IV ALERT

- **Storage:** Store ampules at room temperature. Do not use if solution is brown or contains precipitate.
- **Preparation:** Restore blood and fluid volume (correct hypovolemia) before administering norepinephrine.
- **Dilution:** Add 4 mL (4 mg) to 250 mL of D_5W for a 16 mcg/mL solution.
- **Maximum concentration:** 128 mcg/mL
- **Administration:** Administer infusion through a central venous catheter, as possible, to avoid extravasation. Closely monitor the infusion rate with a microdrip or infusion pump.
- **Possible hypertension:** Monitor BP every 2 min during the infusion until desired therapeutic response is achieved, then every 5 min during the remainder of the infusion. Never leave patients unattended during the infusion.
- **Possible headache:** Manage complaint of headache.
- **BP management:** Plan to maintain BP at 80-100 mmHg in previously normotensive patients, and 30-40 mmHg below preexisting BP in previously hypertensive patients. Reduce the infusion gradually. Avoid abrupt withdrawal.
- **Possible extravasation:** Check the peripherally inserted catheter IV site frequently for signs of extravasation, including blanching, coldness, hardness, and pallor to the extremity.

NOREPINEPHRINE DOSAGE/RATE INFUSION TABLE

4 mg/250 mL (16 mcg/mL)		8 mg/250 mL (32 mcg/mL)	
Dosage (mcg/min)	Rate (mL/hr)	Dosage (mcg/min)	Rate (mL/hr)
1	3.8	1	1.9
2	7.5	2	3.8
5	18.8	5	9.4
10	37.5	10	18.8
15	56.3	15	28.1
20	75	20	37.5
30	112.5	30	56.3

PRECAUTIONS

HEALTH-RELATED

- Use norepinephrine cautiously in patients with hypertension, hypothyroidism, or severe cardiac disease.
- Use cautiously in patients on concurrent MAOI therapy.

AGE-RELATED

- **Children:** No age-related precautions have been noted in children.
- **Elderly:** Age-related renal impairment may prompt lower dosing.

PREGNANCY/LACTATION-RELATED

- Pregnancy category C; use caution with breast-feeding mothers.

MONITORING

- **Baseline assessment:** Assess vital signs and for hypotension continuously. Assess for hypovolemia and correct before starting norepinephrine.
- **Baseline lab work:** Biochemical profile with renal (BUN, creatinine) and liver (AST [SGOT], ALT [SGPT], alkaline phosphatase) function tests.
- **Diagnostic tests:** 12-lead ECG to assess for myocardial ischemia.
- **Dysrhythmias:** Continuous cardiac monitoring to assess for tachycardia, ventricular and other dysrhythmias.
- **Hemodynamic monitoring:** Norepinephrine increases systemic vascular resistance (SVR), and increases venous return (CVP) but must not be given to hypovolemic patients. Pulmonary catheter pressure monitoring is helpful to assess progress in severely hypotensive patients and for differential diagnosis of shock state.
- **Peripheral ischemia:** Assess peripheral pulses, capillary refill, monitor urine output and auscultate bowel sounds to ensure areas outside the central circulation are being perfused effectively.
- **Oliguria:** Monitor intake and output hourly. In patients with a urine output of less than 0.5 mL/kg/hr, decrease or stop the infusion unless the systolic BP falls below 80 mmHg. Consider whether additional inotropic agents may help to increase renal perfusion.
- **Extravasation:** Assess skin at IV insertion site for extravasation. If extravasation occurs, infiltrate the affected area with 10-15 mL sterile saline containing 5-10 mg

phentolamine. Phentolamine does not alter the pressor effects of norepinephrine. Monitor the IV flow rate diligently.
- **Patient education:** Instruct to report immediately burning, pain, or coolness at the IV site to a health care provider.

SERIOUS ADVERSE REACTIONS
- **Extravasation:** May produce tissue necrosis and sloughing. Blanching along the vein may be an early indicator that extravasation is present.
- **Hypovolemia:** Prolonged therapy may result in plasma volume depletion. Hypotension may recur if plasma volume is not restored.

OVERDOSE/TOXICITY
- **Overdose:** Severe hypertension with violent headache (which may be the first clinical sign of overdose), dysrhythmias, photophobia, retrosternal or pharyngeal pain, pallor, excessive sweating, and vomiting.
- **Management:** Decrease dosage or stop infusion, as tolerated.
- **Severe, uncontrolled hypertension:** Discontinue norepinephrine. Patients may require an adrenergic-blocking drug (phentolamine [Regitine] or phenoxybenzamine [Dibenzyline]) to correct hypertensive event.
- **GI decontamination:** No specific recommendations.

ANTIDOTE/DIALYSIS
- **Antidote:** Phentolamine (Regitine 10-15 mL) injected throughout the affected tissue with a fine needle may be used to help prevent sloughing of tissue around IV site if extravasation occurred. May also be effective if a persistent episode of uncontrolled hypertension occurs.
- **Dialysis:** No data are available on removal of norepinephrine by hemodialysis, high-permeability hemodialysis, or peritoneal dialysis.

norfloxacin

See Antibiotics (p. 892)

nortriptyline hydrochloride

noor-trip'-ti-leen hye-droe-klor'-ide

Classes
Chemical: dibenzocycloheptene derivative, secondary amine
Therapeutic: antidepressant, tricyclic

Pregnancy Category: D

Trade Names
Prescription: Aventyl, Norventyl ♣, Pamelor

Do not confuse nortriptyline with amitriptyline, or Aventyl with Ambenyl or Bentyl.

CLINICAL PHARMACOLOGY
Mechanism of Action
A tricyclic antidepressant (TCA) that blocks reuptake of the neurotransmitters norepinephrine and serotonin at neuronal presynaptic membranes, increasing their availability at postsynaptic receptor sites. **Therapeutic Effect:** Relieves depression.

PHARMACOKINETICS
Well absorbed from the GI tract. Protein binding: 90%-95%. Metabolized in the liver. Primarily excreted in urine. **Half-life:** 28-30 hr.

AVAILABILITY
Capsules (Aventyl): 10 mg, 25 mg.
Capsules (Pamelor): 10 mg, 25 mg, 50 mg, 75 mg.
Oral solution (Aventyl, Pamelor): 10 mg/5 mL.

INDICATIONS AND DOSAGE
Depression
PO

Adults: 75-100 mg/day in 1-4 divided doses until therapeutic response is achieved. Reduce dosage gradually to effective maintenance level. **Elderly:** Initially, 10-25 mg at bedtime. May increase by 25 mg every 3-7 days. Maximum: 150 mg/day. **Children 12 yr and older:** 30-50 mg/day in 3-4 divided doses. Maximum: 150 mg/day. **Children 6-11 yr:** 10-20 mg/day in 3-4 divided doses.

Enuresis
PO

Children 12 yr and older: 25-35 mg/day. **Children 8-11 yr:** 10-20 mg/day. **Children 6-7 yr:** 10 mg/day.

OFF-LABEL USES

Treatment of neurogenic pain, panic disorder; prevention of migraine headache

CONTRAINDICATIONS

Acute recovery period after MI, angle-closure glaucoma, use within 14 days of MAOIs, hypersensitivity to nortriptyline

INTERACTIONS

Drug: Alcohol, other CNS depressants: May increase CNS and respiratory depression and the hypotensive effects of nortriptyline. **Antithyroid agents:** May increase the risk of agranulocytosis. **Cimetidine:** May increase the blood concentration and risk of toxicity of nortriptyline. **Clonidine, guanadrel:** May decrease the effects of these drugs. **MAOIs:** May increase the risk of neuroleptic malignant syndrome, seizures, hyperpyrexia, and hypertensive crisis. **Phenothiazines:** May increase the anticholinergic and sedative effects of nortriptyline. **Sympathomimetics:** May increase the risk of cardiac effects. **Herbal:** None known. **Food:** None known.

DIAGNOSTIC TEST EFFECTS

May alter blood glucose level and ECG readings. Therapeutic peak serum level is 6-10 mcg/mL; therapeutic trough serum level is 0.5-2 mcg/mL. Toxic peak serum level is greater than 12 mcg/mL; toxic trough serum level is greater than 2 mcg/mL.

SIDE-EFFECTS

Frequent: Somnolence, fatigue, dry mouth, blurred vision, constipation, delayed micturition, orthostatic hypotension, diaphoresis, impaired concentration, increased appetite, urine retention. **Occasional:** GI disturbances (nausea, GI distress, metallic taste), photosensitivity. **Rare:** Paradoxic reactions (agitation, restlessness, nightmares, insomnia), extrapyramidal symptoms (particularly fine hand tremor)

CRITICAL CARE CONSIDERATIONS

ADMINISTRATION/HANDLING

PO ALERT

- Give nortriptyline with food or milk if GI distress occurs.
- Make sure at least 14 days elapse between the use of MAOIs and nortriptyline.

PRECAUTIONS

HEALTH-RELATED

- Use nortriptyline cautiously in patients with cardiac disease, diabetes mellitus, glaucoma, hiatal hernia, history of seizures, history of urinary obstruction or urine retention, hyperthyroidism, increased intraocular pressure, prostatic hypertrophy, hepatic or renal disease, or schizophrenia.

AGE-RELATED

- **Children:** Safety and efficacy of nortriptyline have not been established in children.
- **Elderly:** Age-related organ impairment may warrant a dosage reduction.

PREGNANCY/LACTATION-RELATED

- Pregnancy category D; effect on nursing infant unknown but may be of concern, especially after prolonged exposure.

MONITORING

- **Baseline assessment:** Observe and document appearance, behavior, interest in the environment, mood, and sleep pattern.
- **Lab work:** CBC with WBC differential and biochemical profile with blood glucose, hepatic and renal function tests before and periodically during long-term therapy.
- **Baseline diagnostic tests:** Perform a baseline 12-lead ECG if risk for dysrhythmias is present.
- **Suicidal patients:** Closely supervise patients at risk for suicide during early therapy. As depression lessens, energy level improves, increasing the likelihood of suicide attempts.
- **Therapeutic response:** Assess appearance, behavior, level of interest, mood, and sleep pattern to determine the drug's therapeutic effect. Inform that the drug's full therapeutic effect may be noted in 2-4 wk.
- **Side effects:** Monitor BP and pulse rate to detect dysrhythmias and hypotension.
- **Constipation:** Assess pattern of daily bowel activity and stool consistency. Encourage eating high-fiber foods and drinking plenty of fluids to help prevent constipation.
- **Hypotension:** Monitor for low BP; tachycardia may indicate that hypotension could ensue if volume status is not corrected or heart rate is not maintained.
- **Dysrhythmias:** Continuous ECG monitoring to detect dysrhythmias.

N

- **Urinary retention:** Palpate bladder for signs of urine retention, and monitor urine output.
- **Serum levels:** Monitor drug serum drug levels. Therapeutic peak level is 6-10 mcg/mL; trough level is 0.5-2 mcg/mL. Toxic peak level is greater than 12 mcg/mL; trough level is greater than 2 mcg/mL
- **Patient education:** Warn to avoid tasks that require alertness or motor skills until response to the drug is known. Caution against abruptly discontinuing nortriptyline. Inform that nortriptyline's therapeutic effect may be noted in 2 wk or longer. Instruct patients to change positions slowly to avoid dizziness. Inform that tolerance will develop to the drug's anticholinergic, hypotensive, and sedative effects during early therapy. Advise patients to notify the physician if they experience visual disturbances. Encourage use of sunscreens and protective clothing to avoid sunburn from photosensitivity. Suggest sips of tepid water or chew sugarless gum to relieve dry mouth.

SERIOUS ADVERSE REACTIONS

- **Abrupt withdrawal:** Abrupt discontinuation after prolonged therapy may produce headache, malaise, nausea, vomiting, and vivid dreams.
- Blood dyscrasias and cholestatic jaundice occur rarely.

OVERDOSE/TOXICITY

- **Cardiac:** Dysrhythmias, fatigue, dyspnea.
- **Dysrhythmias/ECG changes:** Sinus tachycardia, prolonged PR interval, prolonged QT interval, widened QRS complex greater than 100 msec, right axis deviation (positive deflection) of terminal QRS complex in lead AVR greater than 3 mm.
- **Neurologic:** Seizures, severe somnolence, hallucinations, agitation, weakness, fever.
- **Antimuscarinic effects:** Dilated pupils, blurred vision, tachycardia, hyperthermia, hypertension, decreased oral and bronchial secretions, dry skin, ileus, urinary retention, increased muscle tone, tremor.
- **Toxicity:** Symptoms occur within the first 2 hr of ingestion or not at all. Should be screened by the ECG and serum and/or urine TCA levels.
- **Management:** Ventilator driven hyperventilation with intravenous saline to raise the pH to 7.50-7.55 to induce respiratory alkalosis. Sodium bicarbonate intravenous infusion with initial bolus of 1-2 mEq/kg until clinical improvement is noted or blood pH is 7.50-7.55 (induced metabolic alkalosis). Higher blood pH may be deleterious to the patient. IV potassium supplementation may be needed to correct hypokalemia which results from use of bicarbonate infusion. IV fluid infusion is used to manage hypotension. Vasopressors are used only when patients do not respond to fluid therapy. Seizures may respond spontaneously; if persistent, benzodiazepines (lorazepam, diazepam) may be used; phenobarbital or propofol may be used if other medications fail.
- **GI decontamination:** Activated charcoal binds TCAs effectively and if used should be given in one dose within the first few hr of ingestion. The risks of using ipecac to induce vomiting outweigh the benefits. Adding gastric lavage to activated charcoal may enhance removal effects if done within the first hr of ingestion.

ANTIDOTE/DIALYSIS

- **Antidote:** No specific recommendations.
- **Dialysis:** Nortriptyline is not removed by hemodialysis or peritoneal dialysis. No data are available on removal by high-permeability hemodialysis.

N

nystatin

nye-stat'-in

Classes

Chemical: amphoteric polyene macrolide
Therapeutic: antifungal

Pregnancy Category: C

Trade Names

Prescription: Bio-Statin, Mycostatin, Mycostatin Pastilles, Mycostatin Topical, Nyaderm, Nystat-Rx, Nystex, Nystop, Pedi-Dri

Combinations

Prescription: *Topical:* with triamcinolone (Mycolog-II, Mycomer, Mycasone, Myco Biotic II, Tri-Statin II, Mytrex, Myco-Triacet II, Mycogen II)

Do not confuse nystatin or Mycostatin with Nitrostat.

CLINICAL PHARMACOLOGY

Mechanism of Action

A fungistatic antifungal that binds to sterols in the fungal cell membrane. **Therapeutic Effect:** Increases fungal cell-membrane permeability, allowing loss of potassium and other cellular components.

PHARMACOKINETICS

PO: Poorly absorbed from the GI tract. Eliminated unchanged in feces. **Topical:** Not absorbed systemically from intact skin.

AVAILABILITY

Oral suspension (Mycostatin): 100,000 units/mL.
Tablets (Mycostatin): 500,000 units.
Capsules (Bio-Statin): 500,000 units, 1 million units.
Oral lozenge (Mycostatin Pastilles): 200,000 units.
Vaginal tablets: 100,000 units.
Cream (Mycostatin Topical): 100,000 units/g.
Ointment: 100,000 units/g.
Topical powder (Mycostatin Topical, Nystop, Pedi-Dri): 100,000 units/g.
Powder (compounding): 50 million units (Nystat-Rx), 150 million units (Bio-Statin, Nystat-Rx), 500 million units (Nystat-Rx), 1 billion units, 2 billion units (Bio-Statin, Nystat-Rx).

INDICATIONS AND DOSAGE

Intestinal infections

PO

Adults, Elderly: 500,000-1 million units every 8 hr.

Oral candidiasis

PO

Adults, Elderly, Children: 400,000-600,000 units 4 times per day. **Infants:** 200,000 units 4 times per day.

Vaginal infections

Vaginal

Adults, Elderly, Adolescents: 1 tablet/day at bedtime for 14 days.

Cutaneous candidal infections

Topical

Adults, Elderly, Children: Apply 2-4 times per day.

OFF-LABEL USES

Prophylaxis and treatment of oropharyngeal candidiasis, tinea barbae, tinea capitis

CONTRAINDICATIONS

Hypersensitivity to nystatin

INTERACTIONS

Drug: None known. **Herbal:** None known. **Food:** None known.

DIAGNOSTIC TEST EFFECTS

None known.

SIDE-EFFECTS

Occasional: **PO:** None known. **Topical:** Skin irritation. **Vaginal:** Vaginal irritation

CRITICAL CARE CONSIDERATIONS

ADMINISTRATION/HANDLING

PO ALERT

- Dissolve lozenges (troches) slowly and completely in the mouth to ensure an optimal therapeutic effect. Do not chew or swallow whole.
- Shake the oral suspension well before administration. Swish the oral suspension in the mouth for as long as possible before swallowing.

TOPICAL ALERT

- Use sparingly; apply nystatin cream or powder sparingly on erythematous areas.

PRECAUTIONS

HEALTH-RELATED

- None known.

AGE-RELATED

- **Children:** Lozenges (troches) are not recommended for use in children under 5 yr. No age-related precautions have been noted for use of oral suspension or topical forms in children.
- **Elderly:** No age-related precautions have been noted.

PREGNANCY/LACTATION-RELATED

- Pregnancy category C; due to poor bioavailability, serum and breast milk levels do not occur.

MONITORING

- **Baseline assessment:** Assess history of infection.
- **Baseline lab work:** Biochemical profile including BUN and creatinine. Confirm that cultures or histologic tests were done to ensure an accurate diagnosis before giving nystatin.
- **Adverse effects:** Assess for increased irritation with topical application or increased vaginal discharge with vaginal application.
- **Patient education:** Advise not to miss a dose and to complete the full course of treatment. Instruct to swish the oral suspension in the mouth for as long as possible before swallowing. Advise inserting the vaginal form high into the vagina

N

and to continue using the drug during menstruation. Douching is unnecessary during therapy. Sexual intercourse may increase vaginal irritation. Caution not to let the topical form come in contact with the eyes. Explain that nystatin cream or powder should be used sparingly on erythematous areas. Teach rubbing the topical form well into affected areas, to keep affected areas clean and dry, and to wear light clothing for ventilation. Encourage to separate personal items that come in contact with affected areas. Instruct to report promptly diarrhea, nausea, vomitting, or abdominal pain to a health care provider.

SERIOUS ADVERSE REACTIONS

- **Hypersensitivity:** Redness, irritation increasing or ensuing following use. If swallowed, urticaria, itching may be present.

OVERDOSE/TOXICITY

- **High dosages of oral form:** May produce nausea, vomiting, diarrhea, and GI distress.
- **GI decontamination:** No specific recommendations.

ANTIDOTE/DIALYSIS

- **Antidote:** No specific recommendations.
- **Dialysis:** Nystatin is unlikely to be removed by hemodialysis, high-permeability hemodialysis, or peritoneal dialysis.

octreotide acetate

ok-tree'-oh-tide ass'-eh-tate

Classes

Chemical: somatostatin analog
Therapeutic: acromegaly agent, antidiarrheal

Pregnancy Category: B

Trade Names

Prescription: Sandostatin, Sandostatin LAR Depot

Do not confuse octreotide with OctreoScan, or Sandostatin with Sandimmune or Sandoglobulin.

CLINICAL PHARMACOLOGY

Mechanism of Action

An antidiarrheal and growth hormone suppressant that suppresses the secretion of serotonin and gastroenteropancreatic peptides and enhances fluid and electrolyte absorption from the GI tract. **Therapeutic Effect:** Prolongs intestinal transit time.

PHARMACOKINETICS

Route	Onset	Peak	Duration
Subcutaneous	N/A	15-30 min	6-12 hr

Rapidly and completely absorbed from injection site. Excreted in urine. Removed by hemodialysis. **Half-life:** 1.5 hr.

AVAILABILITY

Injection (Sandostatin): 0.05 mg/mL, 0.1 mg/mL, 0.2 mg/mL, 0.5 mg/mL, 1 mg/mL.
Suspension for injection (Sandostatin LAR Depot): 10-mg, 20-mg, 30-mg vials.

INDICATIONS AND DOSAGE

Diarrhea

IV (Sandostatin)

Adults, Elderly: Initially 50-100 mcg every 8 hr. May increase by 100 mcg/dose every 48 hr. Maximum: 500 mcg every 8 hr.

Subcutaneous (Sandostatin)

Adults, Elderly: 50 mcg 1-2 times per day.

IV, Subcutaneous (Sandostatin)

Children: 1-10 mcg/kg every 12 hr.

Carcinoid tumors

IV, Subcutaneous (Sandostatin)

Adults, Elderly: 100-600 mcg/day in 2-4 divided doses.

IM (Sandostatin LAR Depot)

Adults, Elderly: 20 mg every 4 wk.

Vipomas

IV, Subcutaneous (Sandostatin)

Adults, Elderly: 200-300 mcg/day in 2-4 divided doses. Range: 150-750 mg/day.

IM (Sandostatin LAR Depot)

Adults, Elderly: 20 mg every 4 wk.

Esophageal varices

IV (Sandostatin)

Adults, Elderly: Bolus of 25-50 mcg followed by IV infusion of 25-50 mcg/hr for 48 hr.

Acromegaly

IV, Subcutaneous (Sandostatin)

Adults, Elderly: 50 mcg 3 times per day. Increase as needed. Maximum: 500 mcg 3 times per day.

IM (Sandostatin LAR Depot)

Adults, Elderly: 20 mg every 4 wk for 3 mo. Maximum: 40 mg every 4 wk.

OFF-LABEL USES

Control of bleeding esophageal varices, treatment of AIDS-associated secretory diarrhea, chemotherapy-induced diarrhea, insulinomas, small-bowel fistulas, control of bleeding esophageal varices

CONTRAINDICATIONS

Hypersensitivity to octreotide

INTERACTIONS

Drug: ***CycloSPORINE:** May decrease the effectiveness of *cycloSPORINE. **Glucagon, growth hormone, insulin, oral antidiabetics:** May alter glucose concentrations.
Herbal: None known. **Food:** None known.

DIAGNOSTIC TEST EFFECTS

May decrease serum thyroxine (T_4) concentration.

SIDE-EFFECTS

Frequent (10%-6%, 58%-30% in acromegaly patients): Diarrhea, nausea, abdominal discomfort, headache, injection site pain.
Occasional (5%-1%): Vomiting, flatulence, constipation, alopecia, facial flushing, pruritus, dizziness, fatigue, dysrhythmias, ecchymosis, blurred vision. **Rare (less than 1%):** Depression, diminished libido, vertigo, palpitations, dyspnea

CRITICAL CARE CONSIDERATIONS

ADMINISTRATION/HANDLING

SUBCUTANEOUS ALERT

- **Storage:** Store in refrigerator before use. May store at room temperature the day

O

of use. Do not use solution if it becomes discolored or contains particulates.

- **Administration:** Octreotide (Sandostatin) is usually given subcutaneously. May be given undiluted.
- **Rotate sites:** Avoid multiple injections at the same site within a short period.
- Multidose vials must be discarded after using for 14 days.

IM ALERT

- **Sandostatin LAR:** Sandostatin LAR (octreotide) may be given only IM. Give the drug immediately after mixing.
- **Administration:** Inject octreotide deep IM in a large muscle mass at 4-wk intervals. Avoid deltoid injections.

IV ALERT

- **Route:** Octreotide (Sandostatin) is given least often IV; route is helpful in dose finding. Convert patients to IM (Sandostatin LAR) or subcutaneous as soon as possible.
- **Dosing:** Begin with smallest dose and increase gradually.
- **IV direct injection (IV push):** Give over 3 min. May be given undiluted.
- **Life-threatening hypoglycemia:** 100 mcg IV push is used as a lifesaving antihypoglycemic agent for patients with hypoglycemic crisis secondary to an insulinoma.
- **Dilution:** May dilute with 50-200 mL of D_5W or normal saline. May be further diluted in a fluid volume suitable for continuous IV infusion.
- **IV intermittent infusion (piggyback):** Infuse over 15-30 min.
- **Continuous IV infusion:** Infusion rate is calculated based on required dose and concentration of drug in the infusion. Dosing is individualized for patient's disease process and overall tolerance to the drug/fluid volume.

PRECAUTIONS

HEALTH-RELATED

- Use octreotide cautiously in patients with insulin-dependent diabetes or renal failure; patients with gallbladder disease may have worsened symptoms.
- **Carcinoid crisis during anesthesia:** Octreotide (Sandostatin) may be used before or during induction to help abate crisis in patients with carcinoid tumors undergoing surgery; patients must be closely monitored for hypoglycemia and hyperglycemia during induction.
- ***CycloSPORINE:** May inhibit action of *cycloSPORINE resulting in acute rejection of transplanted organs.

AGE-RELATED

- **Children:** Dosage is not firmly established but seems well tolerated in infants and young children when given 1-10 mcg/kg/day for most conditions. Nesidioblastosis (pancreatic tumors) require IV continuous dosage 1 mcg/kg/hr until vasoactive intestinal peptide levels (VIP) decrease. When fluid absorption normalizes, children can be converted to subcutaneous injection.
- **Elderly:** Age-related renal function and increased sensitivity to side effects warrant a dosage reduction; half-life is extended and clearance is reduced.

PREGNANCY/LACTATION-RELATED

- Pregnancy category B; breast milk excretion unknown.

MONITORING

- **Baseline assessment:** Vital signs and weight should be measured. Assess for dehydration due to diarrhea, bony changes associated with acromegaly, history of cancer with carcinoid tumors including insulinoma. Blood glucose monitoring must be done judiciously; octreotide helps regulate blood glucose levels.
- **Lab work:** Biochemical profile including blood glucose level, hepatic (AST [SGOT], ALT [SGPT], alkaline phosphatase) and renal function studies (BUN, creatinine), thyroid stimulating hormone levels and thyroid hormones. For carcinoid tumors, 5-HIAA, plasma serotonin and plasma substance P; for vipoma, plasma vasoactive intestinal peptide (VIP); for acromegaly, IGF-1 and growth hormone levels. Periodic fecal fat and carotene studies should be done.
- **Dysrhythmias:** Monitor ECG continuously for sinus bradycardia. Assess for hypotension with slowing heart rate.
- **Fluid and electrolyte imbalance:** Monitor lab work and for symptoms of common electrolyte imbalances.
- **Blood glucose changes:** Monitor blood glucose at bedside before meals, at bedtime, and at 3 AM. Hyperglycemia and hypoglycemia are possible.
- **Weight gain:** Weigh patients every 2-3 days; weight gain of more than 5 lb per wk may indicate fluid retention. Be alert for decreased urine output and peripheral

edema, especially of the ankles, which may signal renal insufficiency.

- **Hypothyroidism:** Monitor acromegalic patients for symptoms of hypothyroidism including lack of energy, activity intolerance, sense of coldness, and weight gain.
- **Diarrhea:** Assess pattern of daily bowel activity and stool consistency. May be associated with abdominal pain and flatulence.
- **Cholelithiasis:** Monitor for chest pressure, right shoulder pain, dyspepsia, bloating, abdominal discomfort, fatty stools, fatty food intolerance.
- **Acute rejection:** Monitor for acute organ rejection in transplanted patients.
- **Patient education:** Instruct to report promptly any unusual symptoms, such as palpitations or unusual bleeding, to a health care provider. Advise to weigh themselves daily; weight gain of more than 5 lb per wk should be promptly reported to a health care provider. Teach symptoms of gallbladder disease and instruct to report symptoms promptly to a health care provider.

SERIOUS ADVERSE REACTIONS

- **Acute rejection:** May cause acute rejection of transplanted organs if *cycloSPORINE dosage is not increased.
- **GI effects:** Cholelithiasis, pancreatitis, GI bleeding, hepatitis.
- **Hypothyroidism:** With prolonged high dosages with acromegalic patients.
- **Neurologic:** Paresthesias, decreased sensation, paresis; seizures occur rarely.
- **Hypersensitivity:** Reactions from urticaria and injection site reactions to anaphylaxis (rare) have been reported.

OVERDOSE/TOXICITY

- **Overdose:** Hyperglycemia or hypoglycemia, renal insufficiency or renal failure, hepatitis, weakness, rigors, edema, dyspepsia, palpitations, aphasia, hot flashes, bradycardia.
- **Management:** Discontinue octreotide temporarily and monitor patients. Symptom-specific management should be effective in stabilizing patients. Resuscitate as needed according to Advanced Cardiac Life Support (ACLS) guidelines. Manage hypoglycemia with dextrose 50% (D50) IV push. Beta-blockers and calcium channel blockers may have altered effects, including promoting hyperglycemia. Manage hyperglycemia with continuous insulin infusion.
- **GI decontamination:** No specific recommendations.

ANTIDOTE/DIALYSIS

- **Antidote:** No specific recommendations.
- **Dialysis:** Octreotide is removed by hemodialysis and is likely removed by high-permeability hemodialysis. No data are available on removal by peritoneal dialysis.

ofloxacin

See Antibiotics (p. 892)

olanzapine

oh-lan'-zah-peen

Classes

Chemical: thienbenzodiazepine derivative
Therapeutic: antipsychotic

Pregnancy Category: C

Trade Names

Prescription: Zyprexa, Zyprexa Intramuscular, Zyprexa Zydis

Combinations

Prescription: with fluoxetine (Symbyax)

Do not confuse olanzapine with olsalazine, or Zyprexa with Zyrtec.

O

CLINICAL PHARMACOLOGY

Mechanism of Action

A thienobenzodiazepine derivative that antagonizes alpha$_1$-adrenergic, dopamine, histamine, muscarinic, and serotonin receptors. Produces anticholinergic, histaminic, and CNS depressant effects. **Therapeutic Effect:** Diminishes manifestations of psychotic symptoms.

PHARMACOKINETICS

Well absorbed after PO administration. Protein binding: 93%. Extensively distributed throughout the body. Undergoes extensive first-pass metabolism in the liver. Excreted primarily in urine and, to a lesser extent, in feces. Not removed by dialysis. **Half-life:** 21-54 hr.

AVAILABILITY

Tablets (Zyprexa): 2.5 mg, 5 mg, 7.5 mg, 10 mg, 15 mg, 20 mg.
Tablets (orally disintegrating [Zyprexa Zydis]): 5 mg, 10 mg, 15 mg, 20 mg.
Injection (Zyprexa Intramuscular): 10 mg.

INDICATIONS AND DOSAGE

Schizophrenia

PO

Adults: Initially, 5-10 mg once daily. May increase by 10 mg/day at 5- to 7-day intervals. If further adjustments are indicated, may increase by 5-10 mg/day at 7 day intervals. Range: 10-30 mg/day. **Elderly:** Initially, 2.5 mg/day. May increase as indicated. Range: 2.5-10 mg/day. **Children:** Initially, 2.5 mg/day. Titrate as necessary up to 20 mg/day.

Bipolar mania

PO

Adults: Initially, 10-15 mg/day. May increase by 5 mg/day at intervals of at least 24 hr. Maximum: 20 mg/day. **Children:** Initially 2.5 mg/day. Titrate as necessary up to 20 mg/day.

Dosage for elderly or debilitated patients and those predisposed to hypotensive reactions

The initial dosage for these patients is 2.5-5 mg/day.

Control agitation in schizophrenic or bipolar patients

IM

Adults, Elderly: 2.5-10 mg. May repeat 2 hr after first dose and 4 hr after second dose. Maximum: 30 mg/day.

OFF-LABEL USES

Treatment of anorexia, apathy, borderline personality disorder, Huntington's disease; maintenance of long-term treatment response in schizophrenic patients; nausea; vomiting

CONTRAINDICATIONS

Hypersensitivity to olanzapine

INTERACTIONS

Drug: Alcohol, other CNS depressants: May increase CNS depressant effects. **Antihypertensives:** May increase the hypotensive effects of these drugs. **Carbamazepine:** Increases olanzapine clearance. **Ciprofloxacin, fluvoxamine:** May increase the olanzapine blood concentration. **Dopamine agonists, levodopa:** May antagonize the effects of these drugs. **Imipramine, theophylline:** May inhibit the metabolism of these drugs. **Herbal:** None known. **Food:** None known.

DIAGNOSTIC TEST EFFECTS

May significantly increase serum GGT, prolactin, AST (SGOT), and ALT (SGPT) levels.

SIDE-EFFECTS

Frequent: Somnolence (26%), agitation (23%), insomnia (20%), headache (17%), nervousness (16%), hostility (15%), dizziness (11%), rhinitis (10%). **Occasional:** Anxiety, constipation (9%); nonaggressive atypical behavior (8%); dry mouth (7%); weight gain (6%); orthostatic hypotension, fever, arthralgia, restlessness, cough, pharyngitis, visual changes (dim vision) (5%). **Rare:** Tachycardia; back, chest, abdominal, or extremity pain; tremor

CRITICAL CARE CONSIDERATIONS

ADMINISTRATION/HANDLING

PO ALERT

- Give olanzapine without regard to food.

PRECAUTIONS

HEALTH-RELATED

- Use olanzapine cautiously in patients with a hypersensitivity to clozapine, hepatic impairment, cerebrovascular disease, cardiovascular disease (such as conduction abnormalities, heart failure, or history of MI or ischemia), history of seizures or conditions that lower the seizure threshold (such as Alzheimer's disease), and conditions predisposing patients to hypotension (such as dehydration, hypovolemia, and use of antihypertensives).
- Use the drug cautiously in elderly patients, patients at risk for aspiration pneumonia, patients concurrently taking hepatotoxic drugs, and those who should avoid anticholinergics (such as patients with benign prostatic hyperplasia).
- Use caution with each dosage increase.
- **Cytochrome P450:** Olanzapine is metabolized by CYP450 enzymes; significant alterations in drug actions are not likely to occur when other CYP450 enzyme-inhibiting medications are used.

AGE-RELATED

- **Children:** Safety and efficacy of olanzapine have not been established in children.
- **Elderly:** May be more susceptible to orthostatic hypotension, urinary retention, and constipation.

PREGNANCY/LACTATION-RELATED

- Pregnancy category C; excretion into human breast milk unknown; excreted in the milk of treated rats.

MONITORING

- **Baseline assessment:** Assess appearance, behavior, emotional status, response to

O

environment, speech pattern, and thought content.

- **Baseline lab work:** CBC with WBC differential; biochemical profile with liver function tests (AST [SGOT], ALT [SGPT], alkaline phosphatase, bilirubin).
- **ECG:** Monitor for hypertension or hypotension which may indicate the onset of an adverse drug reaction.
- **Neurologic changes:** Observe for involuntary movements, tremors, drowsiness, restlessness, agitation, confusion, fatigue, visual disturbances, sweating, excessive salivation.
- **Suicidal patients:** Closely supervise suicidal patients during early therapy. As depression lessens, energy level improves, which increases the suicide potential.
- **Therapeutic response:** Assess for increased interest in surroundings and ability to concentrate, improvement in self-care, and relaxed facial expression.
- **Dosing:** Do not abruptly discontinue olanzapine to avoid reoccurrence of psychotic symptoms.
- **Anticholinergic effects:** Monitor for urinary retention, constipation, and dry mouth.
- **Somnolence:** Assess sleep pattern for difficulty awakening or staying awake.
- **Tardive dyskinesia:** Monitor for extrapyramidal symptoms.
- **Patient education:** Instruct to take olanzapine as ordered. Caution against abruptly discontinuing the drug or increasing the dosage. Inform that drowsiness generally subsides with continued therapy. Warn to avoid tasks requiring mental alertness or motor skills until response to the drug is known. Instruct female patients to report if they become pregnant or intend to become pregnant during olanzapine therapy. Advise to keep well hydrated, particularly during exercise, exposure to extreme heat, and concurrent use of medications that cause dry mouth or other drying effects. Suggest taking sips of water and chewing sugarless gum to help relieve dry mouth. Instruct to maintain a healthy diet and exercise program to prevent weight gain.

SERIOUS ADVERSE REACTIONS

- **Seizures:** Occur in less than 1% of patients.
- **Neurologic:** Extrapyramidal symptoms, akathisia, tardive dyskinesia, and neuroleptic malignant syndrome occur rarely and are dose dependent.
- **Tardive dyskinesia:** Has infrequently occurred in several patients after a brief period of treatment at low doses. Seen more commonly after a prolonged course of therapy and/or when using higher doses.

OVERDOSE/TOXICITY

- **Overdose:** 300 mg of olanzapine produces drowsiness and slurred speech.
- **Symptoms:** CNS depression (sedation, coma, delirium), hypersalivation, seizures, aganulocytosis, respiratory depression, respiratory arrest, fatal myocarditis, dysrhythmias, orthostatic hypotension, cardiac arrest.
- **Neuroleptic malignant syndrome (NMS):** High fever, muscle rigidity, altered mental status, irregular pulse, labile blood pressure, tachycardia, diaphoresis, and cardiac dysrhythmias.
- **Management of NMS:** Discontinue olanzapine immediately; aggressive management of BP, heart rate, and dysrhythmias according to accepted Advanced Cardiac Life Support (ACLS) guidelines; manage other associated medical problems per accepted guidelines. When reintroducing olanzapine, monitor carefully, as repeat episodes of NMS may occur.
- **GI decontamination:** No specific recommendations.

ANTIDOTE/DIALYSIS

- **Antidote:** Benztropine and/or diazepam or lorazepam may help resolve acute dystonic reactions.
- **Dialysis:** Olanzapine is not removed by hemodialysis or peritoneal dialysis. No data are available on removal by high-permeability hemodialysis.

olmesartan medoxomil

See Angiotensin II Receptor Antagonists (p. 889)

olsalazine sodium

ole-sal'-a-zeen soe'-dee-um

Classes

Chemical: salicylate derivative
Therapeutic: gastrointestinal antiinflammatory

Pregnancy Category: C

O

Trade Names
Prescription: Dipentum

Do not confuse olsalazine with olanzapine.

CLINICAL PHARMACOLOGY

Mechanism of Action

A salicylic acid derivative that is converted to mesalamine in the colon by bacterial action. Blocks prostaglandin production in bowel mucosa. **Therapeutic Effect:** Reduces colonic inflammation in inflammatory bowel disease.

PHARMACOKINETICS

Small amount absorbed. Protein binding: 99%. Metabolized by bacteria in the colon. Minimal elimination in urine and feces. **Half-life:** 1 hr.

AVAILABILITY

Capsules: 250 mg.

INDICATIONS AND DOSAGE

Maintenance of controlled ulcerative colitis

PO

Adults, Elderly: 1 g/day in 2 divided doses, preferably every 12 hr.

OFF-LABEL USES

Treatment of inflammatory bowel disease

CONTRAINDICATIONS

History of hypersensitivity to olsalazine or other salicylates, hypersensitivity to sulfites

O

INTERACTIONS

Drug: Warfarin: May increase prothrombin time. **Herbal:** None known. **Food:** None known.

DIAGNOSTIC TEST EFFECTS

May increase AST (SGOT) and ALT (SGPT) levels.

SIDE-EFFECTS

Frequent (10%-5%): Headache, diarrhea, abdominal pain or cramps, nausea. **Occasional (5%-1%):** Depression, fatigue, dyspepsia, upper respiratory tract infection, decreased appetite, rash, itching, arthralgia. **Rare (1%):** Dizziness, vomiting, stomatitis

CRITICAL CARE CONSIDERATIONS

ADMINISTRATION/HANDLING

PO ALERT

- Give olsalazine with food in evenly divided doses.

PRECAUTIONS

HEALTH-RELATED

- Use olsalazine cautiously in patients with preexisting renal disease.

AGE-RELATED

- **Children:** Safety and efficacy of olsalazine have not been established in children.
- **Elderly:** Dosage reduction may be necessary; elderly may be more susceptible to adverse effects.

PREGNANCY/LACTATION-RELATED

- Pregnancy category C; olsalazine has produced adverse effects in a nursing infant and should be used with caution during breast-feeding. Observe nursing infant closely for changes in stool consistency.

MONITORING

- **Baseline assessment:** Before administering olsalazine, determine if allergy to sulfa-based products is present.
- **Baseline lab work:** Biochemical profile including liver function tests (alkaline phosphatase, AST [SGOT], and ALT [SGPT] levels).
- **Diarrhea and constipation:** Assess bowel sounds for peristalsis; note pattern of daily bowel activity and stool consistency. Evaluate for abdominal discomfort. Discontinue olsalazine if cramping, diarrhea, fever, and rash are experienced.
- **Dysrhythmias:** In critically ill patients, continuously monitor for tachycardia, heart block, and other abnormal cardiac rhythms. Chest discomfort may be associated with dysrhythmias.
- **Neurologic effects:** Monitor for headache, fatigue, lethargy, depression; paresthesia, tremors, and insomnia have been reported.
- **Hypersensitivity:** Assess skin for hives and rash.
- **Patient education:** Instruct to report promptly persistent or increasing cramping, diarrhea, fever, pruritus, and rash to a health care provider. Encourage adequate fluid intake.

SERIOUS ADVERSE REACTIONS

- **Sulfite sensitivity:** May occur in susceptible patients manifested by cramping, headache, diarrhea, fever, rash, hives, itching, and wheezing. Discontinue olsalazine immediately.
- **Bowel effects:** Excessive diarrhea associated with extreme fatigue is noted rarely. Debilitated patients and infants may develop impaction.
- **Cardiopulmonary effects:** Pericarditis, palpitations, hypertension, orthostatic

hypotension, chest discomfort, heart block, tachycardia, shortness of breath, and bronchospasms.

OVERDOSE/TOXICITY

- **Hepatotoxicity:** Elevated AST (SGOT), AST (SGPT), GGT, LDH, alkaline phosphatase, bilirubin, jaundice, cirrhosis, possible hepatocellular damage/necrosis, and liver failure.
- **GI decontamination:** No specific recommendations.

ANTIDOTE/DIALYSIS

- **Antidote:** No specific recommendations.
- **Dialysis:** Olsalazine is unlikely to be removed by hemodialysis or peritoneal dialysis. No data are available on removal by high-permeability hemodialysis.

omalizumab

See Bronchodilators (p. 947)

omeprazole

See Acid Secretion Inhibitors (p. 884)

ondansetron hydrochloride

on-dan'-seh-tron hye-droe-klor'-ide

Classes

Chemical: carbazole derivative
Therapeutic: antiemetic

Pregnancy Category: B

Trade Names

Prescription: Zofran, Zofran ODT

Do not confuse Zofran with Zantac or Zosyn.

CLINICAL PHARMACOLOGY

Mechanism of Action

An antiemetic that blocks serotonin, both peripherally on vagal nerve terminals and centrally in the chemoreceptor trigger zone. **Ther apeutic Effect:** Prevents nausea and vomiting.

PHARMACOKINETICS

Readily absorbed from the GI tract. Protein binding: 70%-76%. Metabolized in the liver. Primarily excreted in urine. Unknown if removed by hemodialysis. **Half-life:** 4 hr; in moderate to severe hepatic impairment, 12-20 hr.

AVAILABILITY

Oral solution (Zofran): 4 mg/5 mL.
Tablets (Zofran): 4 mg, 8 mg, 24 mg.
Tablets (orally disintegrating [Zofran ODT]): 4 mg, 8 mg.
Injection (Zofran): 2 mg/mL.
Injection (Premix): 32 mg/50 mL.

INDICATIONS AND DOSAGE

Chemotherapy-induced emesis

IV

Adults, Elderly: 0.15 mg/kg 3 times per day beginning 30 min before chemotherapy or 0.45 mg/kg once daily or 8-10 mg 1-2 times/day or 24-32 mg once daily. **Children 6 mo-18 yr:** 0.15 mg/kg 3 times per day beginning 30 min before chemotherapy and again 4 and 8 hr after first dose or 0.45 mg/kg as a single dose.

PO

Adults, Elderly: highly emetogenic—24 mg 30 min before start of chemotherapy; moderately emetogenic—8 mg every 12 hr beginning 30 min before chemotherapy and continuing for 1-2 days after completion of chemotherapy. **Children 4-11 yr:** 4 mg 30 min before start of chemotherapy. Repeat 4 hr and 8 hr after initial dose, then 4 mg every 8 hr for 1-2 days.

Prevention of postoperative nausea and vomiting

IV, IM

Adults, Elderly: 4 mg as a single dose **Children 2-12 yr, weighing more than 40 kg:** 4 mg. **Children 2-12 yr, weighing 40 kg and less:** 0.1 mg/kg.

PO

Adults, Elderly: 16 mg 1 hr before induction of anesthesia.

Prevention of radiation-induced nausea and vomiting

PO

Adults, Elderly: Total body irradiation—8 mg 1-2 hr daily before each fraction of radiotherapy; single high-dose radiotherapy to abdomen—8 mg 1-2 hr before irradiation, then 8 mg every 8 hr after first dose for 1-2 days after completion of radiotherapy; daily fractionated radiotherapy to abdomen—8 mg 1-2 hr before irradiation, then 8 mg 8 hr after first dose for each day of radiotherapy.

OFF-LABEL USES

Treatment of postoperative nausea and vomiting

CONTRAINDICATIONS

Hypersensitivity to ondansetron

O

INTERACTIONS

Drug: **Apomorphine:** May cause profound hypotension and alter consciousness. **Herbal:** None known. **Food:** None known.

DIAGNOSTIC TEST EFFECTS

May transiently increase serum bilirubin, AST (SGOT), and ALT (SGPT) levels.

IV INCOMPATIBILITIES

Acyclovir (Zovirax), allopurinol (Aloprim), aminophylline, amphotericin B (Fungizone), amphotericin B complex (Abelcet, AmBisome, Amphotec), ampicillin (Polycillin), ampicillin and sulbactam (Unasyn), cefepime (Maxipime), cefoperazone (Cefobid), 5-fluorouracil, lorazepam (Ativan), meropenem (Merrem IV), *methylPREDNISolone (Solu-Medrol)

IV COMPATIBILITIES

Carboplatin (Paraplatin), cisplatin (Platinol), cyclophosphamide (Cytoxan), cytarabine (Cytosar), dacarbazine (DTIC-Dome), daunorubicin (Cerubidine), dexamethasone (Decadron), *diphenhydrAMINE (Benadryl), docetaxel (Taxotere), *DOPamine (Intropin), etoposide (VePesid), gemcitabine (Gemzar), heparin, hydromorphone (Dilaudid), ifosfamide (Ifex), magnesium, mannitol, mesna (Mesnex), methotrexate, metoclopramide (Reglan), mitomycin (Mutamycin), mitoxantrone (Novantrone), morphine, paclitaxel (Taxol), potassium chloride, teniposide (Vumon), topotecan (Hycamtin), *vinBLAStine (Velban), *vinCRIStine (Oncovin), vinorelbine (Navelbine)

SIDE-EFFECTS

Frequent (13%-5%): Anxiety, dizziness, somnolence, headache, fatigue, constipation, diarrhea, hypoxia, urine retention. **Occasional (4%-2%):** Abdominal pain, xerostomia, fever, feeling of cold, redness and pain at injection site, paresthesia, asthenia. **Rare (1%):** Hypersensitivity reaction (including rash and pruritus), blurred vision

CRITICAL CARE CONSIDERATIONS

ADMINISTRATION/HANDLING

PO ALERT

- Give all oral doses 30 min before chemotherapy and repeat at 8-hr intervals.
- Give ondansetron without regard to food.

IV ALERT

- **Storage:** Store vials at room temperature. Protect from light.
- **IV push/direct injection:** Ondansetron 4 mg may be given undiluted as an IV push over 2 to 5 min.
- **IV intermittent (piggyback) infusion:** Dilute with 50 mL D_5W or 0.9% NaCl before administration, and infuse over 15 min.
- **Stability:** Solution is stable for 48 hr after dilution.

IM ALERT

- **Administration:** Inject into a large muscle mass.

PRECAUTIONS

HEALTH-RELATED

- Use caution in patients with cardiac dysrhythmias, including tachycardia, cardiomyopathy, coronary artery disease, and cardiac decompensation.
- Ondansetron may not be used instead of gastric suction; it does not stimulate gastric or intestinal peristalsis.

AGE-RELATED

- **Children:** Safety and efficacy of ondansetron have not been established in children. For postoperative nausea management in children 2-12 yr, give before anesthesia induction or immediately after surgery. Safety for use in children under 2 yr has not been established.
- **Elderly:** No age-related precautions have been noted.

PREGNANCY/LACTATION-RELATED

- Pregnancy category B. Has been used in the treatment of hyperemesis gravidarum. Use caution if required during breastfeeding.

MONITORING

- **Baseline assessment:** Assess for dehydration (dry mucous membranes, furrows in the tongue and poor skin turgor) in patients experiencing severe vomiting.
- **Baseline lab work:** Biochemical profile including liver function studies (serum bilirubin, AST [SGOT] and ALT [SGPT]).
- **Constipation or diarrhea:** Assess pattern of daily bowel activity and stool consistency, and auscultate bowel sounds for peristalsis. Constipation is common.

- **Neurologic effects:** Monitor for dizziness, somnolence, and visual disturbances.
- **Therapeutic effect:** Has relieved nausea effectively in patients receiving cyclophosphamide (Cytoxan), *DOXOrubicin (Adriamycin), etoposide (VePesid), fluorouracil (Adrucil), ifosfamide (Ifex), methotrexate (Folex), mitoxantone (Novantrone), and *vinCRIStine (Oncovin). May be effective when used in combination with dexamethasone when managing cisplatin-induced nausea and vomiting.
- **Patient education:** Inform that nausea and vomiting should be relieved shortly after drug administration. Instruct to report promptly to a health care provider if vomiting persists. Inform that ondansetron may cause dizziness or drowsiness; urge avoidance of alcohol and barbiturates while taking ondansetron. Teach other methods of reducing nausea and vomiting (lying quietly and avoiding strong odors). Warn to avoid performing tasks that require mental alertness or motor skills until response to the drug is known.

SERIOUS ADVERSE REACTIONS

- **Cardiovascular:** Dysrhythmias (including supraventricular and ventricular tachycardia, atrial fibrillation, second- and third-degree heart block), ST depression, chest pain, and syncope.
- **Neurologic:** Oculogyric crisis; either alone or as part of other dystonia, transient blurred vision; rare cases of grand mal seizures and one case of blindness.
- **Hypersensitivity:** Rash, rare anaphylaxis, angioedema, bronchospasm, laryngospasm, dyspnea, and stridor.

OVERDOSE/TOXICITY

- **Overdose:** Possible CNS stimulant and depressant effects.
- **Hepatotoxicity:** Elevated liver enzymes; liver failure, and death have been reported in patients with cancer receiving other medications including chemotherapy and antibiotics.
- **GI decontamination:** No specific recommendations.

ANTIDOTE/DIALYSIS

- **Antidote:** No specific recommendations.
- **Dialysis:** Ondansetron is unlikely to be removed by hemodialysis or peritoneal dialysis. No data are available on removal by high-permeability hemodialysis.

oprelvekin (interleukin-11, IL-11)

oh-prel'-ve-kin

Classes

Chemical: synthetic hematopoietic, recombinant interleukin eleven

Therapeutic: thrombocytogenic, thrombopoietic growth factor

Pregnancy Category: C

Trade Names

Prescription: Neumega

Do not confuse Neumega with Neupogen.

CLINICAL PHARMACOLOGY

Mechanism of Action

A hematopoietic that stimulates production of blood platelets, essential to the blood-clotting process. **Therapeutic Effect:** Increases platelet production.

PHARMACOKINETICS

Renal elimination. **Half-life:** 5-8 hr.

AVAILABILITY

Injection: 5 mg.

INDICATIONS AND DOSAGE

Prevention of thrombocytopenia (following chemotherapy)

Subcutaneous

Adults: 50 mcg/kg once per day for 10-21 days until postnadir platelet count increases to more than 50,000. **Children:** 75-100 mcg/kg once per day. Continue for 10-21 days or until platelet count reaches 50,000 cells/mcL after its nadir.

CONTRAINDICATIONS

Hypersensitivity to oprelvekin or any component of the product

INTERACTIONS

Drug: None known. **Herbal:** None known. **Food:** None known.

DIAGNOSTIC TEST EFFECTS

May decrease Hgb and Hct, usually within 3-5 days of initiation of therapy; reverses about 1 wk after discontinuance of therapy.

SIDE-EFFECTS

Frequent: Nausea or vomiting (77%); fluid retention (59%); neutropenic fever (48%); diarrhea (43%); rhinitis (42%); headache (41%); dizziness (38%); fever (36%); insomnia (33%); cough (29%); rash, pharyngitis (25%); tachycardia (20%); vasodilation (19%)

O

CRITICAL CARE CONSIDERATIONS

ADMINISTRATION/HANDLING

SUBCUTANEOUS ALERT

- **Dosage timing:** Begin oprelvekin administration 6-24 hr following completion of chemotherapy dose.
- **Storage/stability:** Store in refrigerator. Once reconstituted, use within 3 hr.
- **Reconstitution:** Inject 1 mL sterile water along inside surface of vial for concentration of 5 mg/mL oprelvekin; gently swirl contents; avoid agitation.
- **Administration:** Give single injection in the abdomen, thigh, hip, or upper arm. Discard unused portion.

PRECAUTIONS

HEALTH-RELATED

- Use oprelvekin cautiously in patients with heart disease susceptible to developing heart failure, those with heart failure, and those with atrial dysrhythmias.

AGE-RELATED

- **Children:** Safety and efficacy of oprelvekin have not been established in children.
- **Elderly:** No age-related precautions have been noted.

PREGNANCY/LACTATION-RELATED

- Pregnancy category C; use with caution in breast-feeding women.

MONITORING

- **Baseline assessment:** Assess for ecchymosis and bleeding. Perform vital signs before injection. Assess for heart disease.
- **Baseline and ongoing lab work:** CBC with platelet count before chemotherapy and at regular intervals thereafter. Biochemical profile including potassium. Monitor platelet count periodically to assess therapeutic response. Continue drug dosing until postnadir platelet count is greater than 50,000 cells/mcL.
- **Baseline diagnostic tests:** 12-lead ECG with rhythm strip to assess for dysrhythmias.
- **Fluid retention:** Assess for dyspnea on exertion and peripheral edema, which generally occurs during the first wk of therapy and continues for the duration of treatment. Closely monitor fluid and electrolyte status, particularly if receiving diuretic therapy.
- **Hypokalemia:** Monitor continuous ECG for atrial and ventricular dysrhythmias, ST segment depression, flattened T wave, presence of U waves, PR and QT interval prolongation; may have muscle weakness and cramps or nausea and vomiting.
- **Chemotherapy:** Discontinue oprelvekin more than 2 days before starting next round of chemotherapy.
- **Patient education:** Explain that follow-up blood tests will be performed to assess the results of therapy. Instruct on using an electric razor and soft toothbrush to prevent bleeding until platelet count is within normal range. Remind to promptly report palpitations or dyspnea to a health care provider.

SERIOUS ADVERSE REACTIONS

- **Transient atrial fibrillation or flutter:** Occurs in 10% of patients and may be caused by increased plasma volume; oprelvekin is not directly arrhythmogenic. Dysrhythmias usually are brief in duration and spontaneously convert to normal sinus rhythm.
- **Papilledema:** May occur in children.
- **Hypersensitivity:** Rash, angioedema, exfoliative dermatitis (rare).

OVERDOSE/TOXICITY

- **Cardiac:** Ventricular dysrhythmias, heart failure, rare cardiac arrest.
- **Management:** Potassium replacement, diuretic therapy for heart failure. Resuscitate according to Advanced Cardiac Life Support (ACLS) guidelines.
- **GI decontamination:** No specific recommendations.

ANTIDOTE/DIALYSIS

- **Antidote:** No specific recommendations.
- **Dialysis:** No data are available on removal of oprelvekin by hemodialysis, high-permeability hemodialysis, or peritoneal dialysis.

orlistat

or'-li-stat

Classes

Chemical: lipase inhibitor
Therapeutic: weight loss

Pregnancy Category: B

Trade Names

Prescription: Xenical

Do not confuse Xenical with Xeloda.

O

CLINICAL PHARMACOLOGY

Mechanism of Action

A gastric and pancreatic lipase inhibitor that inhibits absorption of dietary fats by inactivating gastric and pancreatic enzymes. **Therapeutic Effect:** Resulting caloric deficit may positively affect weight control.

PHARMACOKINETICS

Minimal absorption after administration. Protein binding: 99%. Primarily eliminated unchanged in feces. Unlikely to be removed by hemodialysis. **Half-life:** 1–2 hr.

AVAILABILITY

Capsules: 120 mg.

INDICATIONS AND DOSAGE

Weight reduction

PO

Adults, Elderly, Children 12-16 yr: 120 mg 3 times per day with each main meal containing fat (omit if meal is occasionally missed or contains no fat).

OFF-LABEL USES

Type 2 diabetes

CONTRAINDICATIONS

Cholestasis, chronic malabsorption syndrome, hypersensitivity to orlistat

INTERACTIONS

Drug: ***CycloSPORINE:** May decrease *cycloSPORINE levels. **Warfarin:** May increase anticoagulant effects of warfarin secondary to decreased vitamin K absorption. Prothrombin time and INR should be closely monitored. **Herbal:** None known. **Food:** Decreased absorption of fat soluble vitamins (A, D, E, K).

DIAGNOSTIC TEST EFFECTS

Decreases blood glucose, total serum cholesterol, and serum LDL levels. Decreases absorption and levels of vitamins A and E.

SIDE-EFFECTS

Frequent (30%-20%): Headache, abdominal discomfort, flatulence, fecal urgency, fatty or oily stool. **Occasional (14%-5%):** Back pain, menstrual irregularity, nausea, fatigue, diarrhea, dizziness. **Rare (less than 4%):** Anxiety, rash, myalgia, dry skin, vomiting

CRITICAL CARE CONSIDERATIONS

ADMINISTRATION/HANDLING

PO ALERT

- Give orlistat without regard to food.
- Store at controlled room temperature with bottle tightly closed.
- **Side effects:** Orlistat's side effects tend to be mild and transient in nature, gradually diminishing during treatment.

PRECAUTIONS

HEALTH-RELATED

- Organic causes of obesity (e.g., hypothyroidism) should be ruled out before prescribing orlistat.
- Patients must adhere to strict dietary guidelines to avoid gastrointestinal adverse effects; fat soluble vitamins should be included in nutritional supplements, as orlistat may reduce absorption of some fat soluble vitamins (A, D, E, possibly K) and beta carotene.

AGE-RELATED

- **Children:** Safety and efficacy of orlistat have not been established in children.
- **Elderly:** No age-related precautions have been noted.

PREGNANCY/LACTATION-RELATED

- Pregnancy category B; unknown if excreted in breast milk.

MONITORING

- **Baseline assessment:** Obtain an accurate assessment of height and weight to help determine weight loss goals. Measure vital signs noting hypertension. Consult a registered dietitian to review current diet and to make dietary recommendations. If patients meet criteria for metabolic syndrome, consider consulting with an endocrinologist.
- **Baseline lab work:** Biochemical profile with blood glucose levels and lipid profile (LDL, cholesterol), coagulation profile, CBC when beginning therapy and ongoing.
- **Diagnostic tests:** For patients with metabolic syndrome, a 12-lead ECG to assess for myocardial ischemia and chest x-ray to assess heart size.

O

- **GI side effects:** Flatulence with oily rectal discharge, fatty stools, and fecal incontinence are commonly seen with use of orlistat.
- **Patient education:** Instruct to maintain a nutritionally balanced, reduced-calorie diet. Teach to distribute daily intake of carbohydrates, fats, and protein over three main meals. Tell that some of the unpleasant side effects, such as flatulence and fecal urgency, should diminish with time.

SERIOUS ADVERSE REACTIONS
- **Hypersensitivity:** Pruritis, rash, urticaria, angioedema, anaphylaxis (rare).
- **Misuse:** Anorexic and bulimic patients may abuse orlistat to lose weight.

OVERDOSE/TOXICITY
- **GI side effects:** Extreme GI side effects, possible fatty diarrhea if uncontrolled can lead to fluid/electrolyte and acid/base imbalance.
- **GI decontamination:** No specific recommendations.

ANTIDOTE/DIALYSIS
- **Antidote:** No specific recommendations.
- **Dialysis:** Orlistat is unlikely to be removed by hemodialysis, high-permeability hemodialysis, or peritoneal dialysis.

O

oseltamivir phosphate

See Antivirals (p. 937)

oxacillin sodium

ox-a-sill'-in soe'-dee-um

Classes
Chemical: penicillin derivative, penicillinase-resistant
Therapeutic: antibiotic

Pregnancy Category: B

Trade Names
Prescription: Bactocill

CLINICAL PHARMACOLOGY
Mechanism of Action
A penicillin that binds to bacterial membranes. **Therapeutic Effect:** Bactericidal.

PHARMACOKINETICS
Rapid and incomplete absorption following PO administration. Protein binding: 94%. Rapidly excreted as unchanged drug in urine. **Half-life:** 30 min.

AVAILABILITY
Capsules: 250 mg, 500 mg.
Powder for reconstitution (Oral): 250 mg/5 mL.
Powder for injection: 500-mg vials, 1-g vials, 2-g vials, 4-g vials, 10-g vials.
Intravenous solution: 1 g/50 mL, 2 g/50 mL.

INDICATIONS AND DOSAGE
Upper respiratory tract, skin, and skin structure infections
IV, IM
Adults, Elderly, Children weighing 40 kg or more: 250-500 mg every 4-6 hr. **Children weighing less than 40 kg:** 50 mg/kg/day in divided doses every 6 hr. Maximum: 12 g/day.
Lower respiratory tract and other serious infections
IV, IM
Adults, Elderly, Children weighing 40 kg or more: 2 g every 4 hr. Maximum: 12 g/day. **Children weighing less than 40 kg:** 100 mg/kg/day in divided doses every 4-6 hr. Maximum 12 g/day.
Mild to moderate infections
PO
Adults, Elderly, Children weighing 40 kg and more: 500-1000 mg every 4-6 hr. **Children weighing less than 40 kg:** 50 mg/kg/day in divided doses every 6 hr. Maximum: 4 g/day.
Severe infections
PO
Adults, Elderly, Children weighing 40 kg and more: 500-1000 mg every 4-6 hr. **Children weighing less than 40 kg:** 100 mg/kg/day in divided doses every 4-6 hr.
Endocarditis
IV
Adults, Elderly, Children weighing 40 kg and more: 2 g every 4 hr for 4-6 wks. Maximum: 18 g/day.
IM/IV
Neonates 0-4 wk or weighing less than 1200 g: 50 mg/kg/day divided every 12 hr. **Neonates postnatal less than 7 days:** Weighing 1200-2000 g, 50-100 mg/kg/day divided every 12 hr. Weighing more than 2000 g, 75-150 mg/kg/day divided every 8 hr. **Neonates postnatal more than 7 days:** Weighing 1200-2000 g, 75-150 mg/kg/day divided every 8 hr. Weighing more than 2000 g, 100-200 mg/kg/day divided every 6 hr.

CONTRAINDICATIONS
Hypersensitivity to oxacillin or any penicillin

INTERACTIONS

Drug: Probenecid: May increase oxacillin blood concentration and risk of toxicity. **Herbal:** None known. **Food:** None known.

DIAGNOSTIC TEST EFFECTS

May increase AST (SGOT) levels. May cause a positive Coombs' test.

SIDE-EFFECTS

Frequent: Mild hypersensitivity reaction (fever, rash, pruritus), GI effects (nausea, vomiting, diarrhea). **Occasional:** Phlebitis, thrombophlebitis (more common in elderly), hepatotoxicity (with high IV dosage)

CRITICAL CARE CONSIDERATIONS

ADMINISTRATION/HANDLING

PO ALERT

- Oral solutions should be prepared at the time of dispensing.

IV ALERT

- **Storage:** Store vials at room temperature.
- **Reconstitution:** Add 10 mL sterile water for injection to each 1-g vial to provide a concentration of 100 mg/mL.
- **IV (push) direct injection:** Administer IV push over 10 min and IV piggyback over 30 min.
- **Stability:** Once reconstituted, the solution remains stable for 3 days at room temperature or 7 days refrigerated. When further diluted with D_5W or 0.9% NaCl, the solution is stable for 24 hr.
- **Further dilution for piggyback administration:** Dilute with 50-100 mg D_5W or 0.9% NaCl.

PRECAUTIONS

HEALTH-RELATED

- Use oxacillin cautiously in patients with impaired renal function or a history of allergies, especially to cephalosporins (not absolute).

AGE-RELATED

- **Children:** Elimination rate is significantly reduced in neonates; limited experience with premature infants and neonates.
- **Elderly:** Age-related organ impairment may prompt a dosage adjustment; may be more sensitive to side effects.

PREGNANCY/LACTATION-RELATED

- Pregnancy category B; potential exists for modification of bowel flora in nursing infant, allergy or sensitization, and interference with interpretation of culture results if fever workup required.

MONITORING

- **Baseline assessment:** Determine history of allergies, especially to cephalosporins or penicillin, before starting oxacillin therapy.
- **Baseline lab work:** CBC with WBC differential; biochemical profile including liver (AST [SGOT], ALT [SGPT], alkaline phosphatase, bilirubin) and renal (BUN, creatinine) function studies. Test patients with syphilis for HIV.
- **Fluid retention:** Oxacillin has a high content of sodium; may worsen heart failure and prompt hypokalemia. Monitor intake and output, liver and renal function test results, and urinalysis.
- **Dysrhythmias:** Continously monitor ECG in critically ill patients for ventricular dysrhythmias, sinus tachycardia, and ST-T wave changes indicative of hypokalemia.
- **Allergy/reaction:** Withhold oxacillin if rash or diarrhea occurs. Although rash is a common side effect of oxacillin, it may also indicate hypersensitivity.
- **Colitis:** Severe diarrhea with abdominal pain, blood or mucus in stools, and fever may indicate antibiotic-associated colitis.
- **Nausea/vomiting:** Manage with standard measures. Provide IV hydration if severe symptoms occur. Consider use of another antibiotic.
- **Superinfection:** Be alert for signs and symptoms of superinfection, including anal or genital pruritus, black hairy tongue, diarrhea, increased fever, sore throat, ulceration or changes of oral mucosa, and vomiting.
- **Evenly space dosing:** Administer doses evenly around the clock.
- **Phlebitis:** Evaluate IV insertion site frequently for signs of phlebitis, such as heat, pain, and red streaking over the vein.
- **Patient education:** Warn to report immediately burning or pain at the IV site. Instruct to report immediately signs of an allergic reaction such as shortness of breath, chest tightness, or hives. Encourage good oral hygiene.

SERIOUS ADVERSE REACTIONS

- **Colitis:** Antibiotic-associated colitis, pseudomembranous colitis, or *Clostridium difficile* colitis, and other superinfections may result from altered bacterial balance.

- **Hypersensitivity:** Mild to severe reactions may occur in penicillin-sensitive patients.
- **Hematologic:** Anemia, hemolytic anemia, thrombocytopenia, leukopenia, agranulocytosis, eosinophilia, and thrombocytopenic purpura.
- **Central nervous system:** Agitation, anxiety, seizures, behavioral changes, dizziness.
- **Management:** Discontinue oxacillin, treat allergic reactions with IV *diphenhydrAMINE, epinephrine, and corticosteroids. Resuscitate according to Advanced Cardiac Life Support (ACLS) guidelines if needed.

OVERDOSE/TOXICITY

- **Gastrointestinal:** Nausea, vomiting, diarrhea. Severe diarrhea with abdominal pain, blood or mucus in stool, and fever may indicate antibiotic-associated colitis.
- **Hepatotoxicity:** Elevated liver enzymes (AST [SGOT], ALT [SGPT]), confusion, fever, nausea, vomiting, altered behavior, right upper quadrant pain, edema.
- **Nephrotoxicity:** Elevated BUN, creatinine, nausea, oliguria, back pain, edema, renal tubular damage, interstitial nephritis.
- **GI decontamination:** No specific recommendations.

ANTIDOTE/DIALYSIS

- **Antidote:** No specific recommendations.
- **Dialysis:** Oxacillin is not removed by hemodialysis or peritoneal dialysis. No data are available on removal by high-permeability hemodialysis.

O

oxaprozin

See NSAIDs and Cox-2 Inhibitors (p. 976)

oxazepam

See Antianxiety Agents (p. 890)

oxcarbazepine

ox-car-baz'-e-peen

Classes

Chemical: dibenzazepine derivative
Therapeutic: anticonvulsant

Pregnancy Category: C

Trade Names

Prescription: Trileptal

CLINICAL PHARMACOLOGY

Mechanism of Action

An anticonvulsant that blocks sodium channels, resulting in stabilization of hyperexcited neural membranes, inhibition of repetitive neuronal firing, and diminishing synaptic impulses. **Therapeutic Effect:** Prevents seizures.

PHARMACOKINETICS

Completely absorbed from GI tract and extensively metabolized in the liver to active metabolite. Protein binding: 40%. Primarily excreted in urine. **Half-life:** 2 hr; metabolite, 6-10 hr.

AVAILABILITY

Oral suspension: 300 mg/5 mL.
Tablets: 150 mg, 300 mg, 600 mg.

INDICATIONS AND DOSAGE

Adjunctive treatment of seizures

PO

Adults, Elderly: Initially, 600 mg/day in 2 divided doses. May increase by up to 600 mg/day at weekly intervals. Maximum: 2400 mg/day. **Children 4-16 yr:** 8-10 mg/kg. Maximum: 600 mg/day. Maintenance (based on weight): 1800 mg/day for children weighing more than 39 kg; 1200 mg/day for children weighing 29.1-39 kg; and 900 mg/day for children weighing 20-29 kg.

Conversion to monotherapy

PO

Adults, Elderly: 600 mg/day in 2 divided doses (while decreasing concomitant anticonvulsant over 3-6 wk). May increase by 600 mg/day at weekly intervals up to 2400 mg/day. **Children:** Initially 8-10 mg/kg/day in 2 divided doses. Increase at 3-day intervals by 5 mg/kg/day to achieve maintenance dose by weight; (70 kg)—1500-2100 mg/day; (60-69 kg)—1200-2100 mg/day; (50-59 kg)—1200-1800 mg/day; (41-49 kg)—1200-1500 mg/day; (35-40 kg)—900-1500 mg/day; (25-34 kg)—900-1200 mg/day—(20-24 kg)—600-900 mg/day.

Initiation of monotherapy

PO

Adults, Elderly: 600 mg/day in 2 divided doses. May increase by 300 mg/day every 3 days up to 1200 mg/day. **Children:** Initially, 8-10 mg/kg/day in 2 divided doses. Increase at 3-day intervals by 5 mg/kg/day to achieve maintenance dose by weight; (70 kg)—1500-2100 mg/day; (60-69 kg)—1200-2100 mg/day; (50-59 kg)—1200-1800 mg/day; (41-49 kg)—1200-1500 mg/day; (35-40 kg)—900-1500 mg/day; (25-34 kg)—900-1200 mg/day; (20-24 kg)—600-900 mg/day.

Dosage in renal impairment

For patients with creatinine clearance less than 30 mL/min, give 50% of normal starting dose, then titrate slowly to desired dose.

OFF-LABEL USES

Atypical panic disorder, bipolar disorders, neuralgia/neuropathy

CONTRAINDICATIONS

Hypersensitivity to oxcarbazepine

INTERACTIONS

Drug: **Carbamazepine:** May decrease the blood concentration and effects of oxcarbazepine up to 40%. **Felodipine, oral contraceptives:** May decrease the effectiveness of these drugs. **Phenobarbital, phenytoin:** May increase the blood concentration and risk of toxicity of these drugs. Phenobarbital levels may increase 14% (average), and oxcarbazepine levels decrease by 25% with phenobarbital. **Valproic acid:** May decrease oxcarbazepine levels by 18% (average). **Herbal:** None known. **Food:** None known.

DIAGNOSTIC TEST EFFECTS

May increase GGT level and other hepatic function test results. May increase or decrease blood glucose level. May decrease serum calcium, potassium, and sodium levels.

SIDE-EFFECTS

Frequent: Dizziness (22%-49%), nausea (15%-29%), headache (13%-32%), vomiting (8%-36%), diplopia (14%-40%), nystagmus (8%-26%). **Occasional (7%-5%):** Vomiting, diarrhea, ataxia, nervousness, heartburn, indigestion, epigastric pain, constipation. **Rare (4%):** Tremor, rash, back pain, epistaxis, sinusitis, diplopia

CRITICAL CARE CONSIDERATIONS

ADMINISTRATION/HANDLING

PO ALERT

- Plan to give all doses in a twice-daily regimen.
- Give oxcarbazepine without regard to food.
- Do not administer oxcarbazepine with grapefruit juice because it may increase drug concentration in the blood.
- If patients must change to another anticonvulsant, plan to decrease the oxcarbazepine dose gradually as therapy begins with a low dose of the replacement drug.
- When transferring from tablets to suspension, divide the total daily tablet dose into smaller, more frequent doses of suspension.
- Shake the oral suspension well. Do not administer simultaneously with any other liquid medicine.

PRECAUTIONS

HEALTH-RELATED

- Use oxcarbazepine cautiously in patients with renal impairment or a hypersensitivity to carbamazepine.
- **Cytochrome P450 enzyme metabolism:** Oxcarbazepine can inhibit CYP2C19 and induce CYP3A4/5, which may have significant effects on other medications metabolized by these enzyme pathways. Other CYP450-inducing antiepileptic drugs may affect oxcarbazepine levels.

AGE-RELATED

- **Children:** No age-related precautions have been noted in children over 4 yr.
- **Elderly:** Age-related renal impairment may require dosage adjustment. Elderly are more susceptible to agitation, AV block, bradycardia, confusion, and syndrome of inappropriate antidiuretic hormone secretion (SIADH).

PREGNANCY/LACTATION-RELATED

- Pregnancy category C. Increased incidence of fetal structural abnormalities and other manifestations of developmental toxicity have been observed in the offspring of animals. No adequate and well-controlled data in humans. Oxcarbazepine and monohydroxy derivation (MHD), an active metabolite, both excreted in human breast milk; milk:plasma ratio: 0.5 (both).

MONITORING

- **Baseline assessment:** Assess LOC and review the history of the seizure disorder, including the duration, frequency, intensity, onset, type of seizures, and the drug history, especially the use of other anticonvulsants.
- **Baseline lab work:** Biochemical panel including serum sodium level, glucose, calcium, potassium, and liver enzymes.
- **Seizure precautions:** Have airway management equipment at the bedside. Do not force anything into the mouth when seizing. Provide a quiet, dark environment and institute safety precautions. Observe seizure patients frequently for recurrence of seizure activity.
- **Neurologic effects:** Assist with ambulation during experiences of ataxia or

dizziness. Assess for headache and visual abnormalities.

- **Hyponatremia:** Monitor serum sodium levels. Assess for confusion, headache, lethargy, malaise, and nausea. With SIADH, note weight gain, headache, lassitude, and muscle spasms.
- **Dysrhythmias:** Monitor for bradycardia and heart block.
- **Therapeutic effect:** Assess for decrease in the frequency or intensity of seizures.
- **Toxicity:** Assess for early toxic signs of toxicity such as ecchymosis, fever, joint pain, mouth ulcerations, sore throat, and unusual bleeding from any site.
- **Patient education:** Caution against discontinuing oxcarbazepine abruptly to avoid increasing seizure frequency. Instruct to report promptly dizziness, headache, nausea, and rash to a health care provider; explain that periodic blood tests may be necessary. Advise to always carry an identification card or wear an identification bracelet that displays the seizure disorder and anticonvulsant therapy.

SERIOUS ADVERSE REACTIONS

- **Hyponatremia:** Neurologic symptoms (irritability, apprehension, nervousness, confusion) occur when sodium decreases to 120-125 mEq/L. Tremors, seizures, coma may occur when sodium is less than 115 mEq/L.
- **Status epilepticus:** Abrupt withdrawal may precipitate status epilepticus.
- **Blood dyscrasias:** Aplastic anemia, agranulocytosis, thrombocytopenia, leukopenia, leukocytosis, and eosinophilia (rare).
- **Cardiovascular:** Heart block, heart failure, hypotension or hypertension, and dysrhythmias secondary to fluid and electrolyte imbalance (rare).
- **Dermatologic effects:** Rash, urticaria, pruritus, Stevens–Johnson syndrome, toxic epidermal necrolysis, and photosensitivity (rare).

OVERDOSE/TOXICITY

- **Symptoms:** Encephalopathy, coma, respiratory failure, seizures, tachycardia, cardiac conduction disturbance (prolonged QRS complex), and hypotension.
- **Supportive care:** Endotracheal intubation, mechanical ventilation, fluid volume resuscitation done carefully to avoid development of pulmonary edema, possible use of hypertonic sodium bicarbonate or saline therapy, intravenous vasopressor infusions, and seizure control with benzodiazepines and barbiturates.
- **GI decontamination:** No specific recommendations, but if patients are seen within 3 hr of overdose, activated charcoal and gastric lavage are both recommended.

ANTIDOTE/DIALYSIS

- **Antidote:** No specific recommendations.
- **Dialysis:** No data are available on removal of oxcarbazepine by hemodialysis, high-permeability hemodialysis, or peritoneal dialysis.

O

oxybutynin

ox-i-byoo'-ti-nin

Classes

Chemical: tertiary amine

Therapeutic: antispasmodic, gastrointestinal, genitourinary muscle relaxant

Pregnancy Category: B

Trade Names

Prescription: Ditropan, Ditropan XL, Oxytrol, Urotrol

Do not confuse oxybutynin with Oxycontin, or Ditropan with diazepam.

CLINICAL PHARMACOLOGY

Mechanism of Action

An anticholinergic that exerts antispasmodic (papaverine-like) and antimuscarinic (atropine-like) action on the detrusor smooth muscle of the bladder. **Therapeutic Effect:** Increases bladder capacity and delays desire to void.

PHARMACOKINETICS

Route	Onset	Peak	Duration
PO	0.5-1 hr	3-6 hr	6-10 hr

Rapidly absorbed from the GI tract. Metabolized in the liver. Primarily excreted in urine. Unknown if removed by hemodialysis. **Half-life:** 2-3 hr.

AVAILABILITY

Syrup (Ditropan): 5 mg/5 mL .
Tablets (Ditropan, Urotrol): 5 mg.
Tablets (extended release [Ditropan XL]): 5 mg, 10 mg, 15 mg.
Transdermal (Oxytrol): 3.9 mg.

INDICATIONS AND DOSAGE

Neurogenic bladder

PO

Adults: 5 mg 2-3 times per day. Maximum: 20 mg/day. **Elderly:** 2.5-5 mg twice per day. May increase by 2.5 mg/day every 1-2 days. **Children 5 yr and older:** 5 mg twice per day. Maximum: 15 mg/day. **Children 1-4 yr:** 0.2 mg/kg/dose 2-4 times per day.

PO (Extended Release)

Adults, Elderly: 5-10 mg/day up to 30 mg/day. **Children 6 yr and older:** Initially, 5 mg once daily. May increase in 5-10 mg increments. Maximum: 20 mg/day.

Transdermal

Adults: 3.9 mg applied twice per wk. Apply every 3-4 days.

CONTRAINDICATIONS

GI or GU obstruction, untreated glaucoma, myasthenia gravis, toxic megacolon, ulcerative colitis, hypersensitivity to oxybutynin

INTERACTIONS

Drug: Medications with anticholinergic effects (such as antihistamines): May increase the anticholinergic effects of oxybutynin. **Herbal:** None known. **Food:** May decrease absorption of immediate-release tablets and solution.

DIAGNOSTIC TEST EFFECTS

None known.

SIDE-EFFECTS

Frequent: Constipation (13%), dry mouth (60%-70%), somnolence (12%-13%), dizziness (6%-16%). **Occasional:** Decreased lacrimation, perspiration, and salivation; impotence; urinary hesitancy and retention; suppressed lactation; blurred vision; mydriasis; nausea or vomiting; insomnia

CRITICAL CARE CONSIDERATIONS

ADMINISTRATION/HANDLING

PO ALERT

- Give extended-release oxybutynin without regard to food. Immediate-release tablets and solution should be given on an empty stomach with water.
- Swallow extended release tablets whole; do not chew or crush.

TRANSDERMAL ALERT

- **Application:** Apply patch to dry, intact skin on the abdomen, hip, or buttock.
- **Rotate sites:** Use a new application site for each new patch; avoid reapplication to the same site within 7 days.

PRECAUTIONS

HEALTH-RELATED

- Use oxybutynin cautiously in patients with cardiovascular disease, hypertension, hyperthyroidism, hepatic or renal impairment, neuropathy, benign prostatic hyperplasia, or reflux esophagitis.

AGE-RELATED

- **Children:** No age-related precautions are noted in children over 5 yr.
- **Elderly:** May be more sensitive to the drug's anticholinergic effects, such as dry mouth and urine retention.

PREGNANCY/LACTATION-RELATED

- Pregnancy category B; may suppress lactation.

MONITORING

- **Baseline assessment:** Assess urinary symptoms (dysuria; urinary frequency, urgency, or incontinence).
- **Baseline lab work:** CBC with WBC count; urine culture and sensitivity to identify urinary tract infection; biochemical panel with BUN and creatinine.
- **Therapeutic response:** Monitor for relief in problems related to voiding.
- **Urinary retention:** Monitor intake and output and palpate the bladder for fullness indicative of retention.
- **Constipation:** Assess pattern of daily bowel activity and stool consistency.
- **Patient education:** Inform that oxybutynin may cause drowsiness and dry mouth. Urge avoidance of alcohol and performing tasks that require mental alertness or motor skills until response to the drug is known. Avoid prolonged exposure to hot environments; heat prostration may result because oxybutynin inhibits sweating.

SERIOUS ADVERSE REACTIONS

- Palpitations, edema, insomnia, tachycardia, hallucinations, urinary retention, impotence.

OVERDOSE/TOXICITY

- **Anticholinergic syndrome:** CNS excitation (including nervousness, restlessness, hallucinations, agitation, irritability), dry mouth and skin, decreased bowel sounds, myoclonus, cardiogenic shock, hyperthermia, hypertension, confusion, tachycardia, facial flushing, respiratory depression, cardiac arrest, extrapyramidal reactions, muscle rigidity, and seizures. Rhabdomyolysis may occur due to fever, muscle rigidity, and agitation. Manage rhabdomyolysis

O

with IV hydration, mannitol, and sodium bicarbonate infusion to alkaline urine and help prevent precipitation of myoglobin in the urine.
- **Management:** Supportive care is usually sufficient to manage patients with careful monitoring so that patients do not injure themselves; control of agitation, seizures, and fever is imperative; if haloperidol is used, QT interval should be monitored for prolongation.
- **GI decontamination:** No specific recommendations.

ANTIDOTE/DIALYSIS
- **Antidote:** Agitation and seizures may be reversed by an anticholinesterase (physostigmine) or sedation with benzodiazepines. Muscle rigidity may be managed with dantrolene.
- **Dialysis:** No data are available on removal of oxybutinin by hemodialysis, high-permeability hemodialysis, or peritoneal dialysis.

oxycodone hydrochloride

ox-i-koe'-done hye-droe-klor'-ide

O

DEA Schedule: II

Classes
Chemical: opiate derivative, phenanthrene derivative
Therapeutic: narcotic analgesic

Pregnancy Category: B, D

Trade Names
Prescription: M-Oxy, OxyContin, Oxydose, OxyFast, OxyIR, Percolone, Roxicodone, Roxicodone Intensol

Combinations
Prescription: with aspirin (Percodan, Endodan, Roxiprin); with acetaminophen (Percocet, Endocet, Tylox, Roxicet, Roxilox)

Do not confuse oxycodone with oxybutynin.

CLINICAL PHARMACOLOGY
Mechanism of Action
An opioid analgesic that binds with opioid receptors in the CNS. Therapeutic Effect: Alters the perception of and emotional response to pain.

PHARMACOKINETICS

Route	Onset	Peak	Duration
PO, immediate release	10-15 min	30-60 min	4-5 hr
PO, controlled release	30 min	60 min	12 hr

Moderately absorbed from the GI tract. Protein binding: 38%-45%. Widely distributed. Metabolized in the liver. Excreted in urine. Unknown if removed by hemodialysis. Half-life: 3 hr (4.5 hr controlled-release).

AVAILABILITY
Capsules (immediate release [OxyIR]): 5 mg.
Oral concentrate (Oxydose, OxyFast, Roxicodone Intensol): 20 mg/mL.
Oral solution (Roxicodone): 5 mg/5 mL.
Tablets (M-Oxy, Percolone, Roxicodone): 5 mg, 15 mg, 30 mg.
Tablets (extended release [OxyContin]): 10 mg, 20 mg, 40 mg, 80 mg, 160 mg.

INDICATIONS AND DOSAGE
Analgesia
PO (Controlled Release)
Adults, Elderly: Initially, 10 mg every 12 hr. May increase every 1-2 days by 25%-50%. Usual: 40 mg/day (100 mg/day for cancer pain).
PO (Immediate Release)
Adults, Elderly: Initially, 5 mg every 6 hr as needed. May increase up to 30 mg every 4 hr. Usual: 10-30 mg every 4 hr as needed.
Children: 0.05-0.15 mg/kg/dose every 4-6 hr.

CONTRAINDICATIONS
Acute bronchial asthma or hypercapnia, paralytic ileus, respiratory depression, hypersensitivity to oxycodone

INTERACTIONS
Drug: **Alcohol, other CNS depressants:** May increase CNS or respiratory depression and hypotension. **MAOIs:** May produce a severe, sometimes fatal reaction; expect to administer one quarter of usual oxycodone dose. Herbal: None known. Food: None known.

DIAGNOSTIC TEST EFFECTS
May increase serum amylase and lipase levels.

SIDE-EFFECTS
Frequent: Somnolence, dizziness, hypotension (including orthostatic hypotension),

anorexia. **Occasional:** Confusion, diaphoresis, facial flushing, urine retention, constipation, dry mouth, nausea, vomiting, headache. **Rare:** Allergic reaction, depression, paradoxic CNS hyperactivity or nervousness in children, paradoxic excitement and restlessness in elderly or debilitated patients

CRITICAL CARE CONSIDERATIONS

ADMINISTRATION/HANDLING

PO ALERT

- **Side effects:** Oxycodone's side effects are dependent on the dosage.
- Ambulatory patients and those not in severe pain are more likely to experience dizziness, hypotension, nausea, and vomiting than supine patients or those in severe pain.
- Give oxycodone without regard to food.
- Crush immediate-release tablets as needed.
- Swallow controlled-release tablets (OxyContin) whole because crushing, breaking, or chewing them may lead to the rapid release and absorption of a potentially fatal dose.

PRECAUTIONS

HEALTH-RELATED

- Use oxycodone with extreme caution in patients with acute alcoholism, anoxia, CNS depression, hypercapnia, respiratory depression or dysfunction, seizures, shock, or untreated myxedema.
- Use oxycodone cautiously in patients with acute abdominal conditions, Addison's disease, chronic obstructive pulmonary disease (COPD), hypothyroidism, hepatic impairment, increased intracranial pressure, prostatic hypertrophy, or urethral stricture.
- **Cytochrome P450 enzyme metabolism:** Drug is metabolized in part by CYP2D6. Elimination of oxycodone may be blocked by other medications using this pathway.

AGE-RELATED

- **Children:** Children are more prone to experience paradoxic excitement; those under 2 yr are more susceptible to respiratory depression.
- **Elderly:** Age-related renal impairment may increase the risk of urinary retention; elderly are more susceptible to respiratory depression.

PREGNANCY/LACTATION-RELATED

- Pregnancy category B (category D if used for prolonged periods or in high doses at term); excreted into breast milk.

MONITORING

- **Baseline assessment:** Assess the duration, location, onset, and type of pain. Obtain vital signs before administering oxycodone. If patient is being treated for cough, assess the frequency, severity, and type of cough.
- **Baseline lab work:** Biochemical profile including liver (AST [SGOT], ALT [SGPT], alkaline phosphatase, bilirubin, GGT) and renal (BUN, creatinine) function tests.
- **Persistent pain:** Oxycodone's effect is reduced if the full pain response recurs before the next dose. Instruct to report when pain begins to return. It is inappropriate to tell patients in pain it is not yet time for medication. Medication should be provided at the proper frequency/dosage to keep patients comfortable.
- **Autonomic nervous system depression:** Monitor vital signs for bradycardia, hypotension, and bradypnea. If respiratory rate is consistently below 10 breaths/min or very shallow, pulse rate is consistently below 50 beats/min, and BP is consistently below 85 mmHg systolic, with difficulty awakening patients or keeping patients awake, consider reducing medication dose or frequency of administration unless patients are receiving end-of-life comfort care.
- **Ventilation/oxygenation:** Monitor pulse oximetry (SpO_2) continuously on patients receiving high doses or continuous IV or epidural medication infusions. Use reading to augment assessment of ventilation and oxygenation rather than in place of the assessment. Low readings may be corrected using supplemental oxygen and/or noninvasive positive pressure ventilation (bilevel positive airway pressure [BiPAP] or continuous positive airway pressure [CPAP]) on nonintubated/mechanically ventilated patients if drug dosage reduction results in patients experiencing severe pain.
- **Pulmonary hygiene:** Initiate deep-breathing and coughing exercises, particularly in patients with impaired respiratory function.
- **Constipation:** Assess pattern of daily bowel activity and stool consistency, especially with long-term use.

O

- **Therapeutic response:** Assess for clinical improvement and record the onset of pain relief.
- **Tolerance and drug dependence:** Monitor usage pattern for development of tolerance and assess for physical dependence.
- **Patient education:** Instruct to alert a health care provider when pain starts to return; oxycodone is less effective if a full pain response recurs before the next dose. Strongly warn that oxycodone has a potential for abuse and that accidental overdose may result in death. Urge avoidance of alcohol during oxycodone therapy. Inform that oxycodone may cause drowsiness, dizziness, and dry mouth. Warn to avoid tasks that require mental alertness and motor skills until response to the drug is known. Instruct to change positions slowly to avoid orthostatic hypotension. Instruct not to break, chew, or crush controlled-release tablets (OxyContin).

SERIOUS ADVERSE REACTIONS

- **Drug tolerance:** Drug tolerance is common when managing chronic pain patients and requires increasing doses of medication or combinations of medications to provide pain relief.
- **Drug dependence:** Addiction to narcotics occurs infrequently compared with drug tolerance, but chronic pain patients are often viewed as addicted when tolerance has occurred. Patients with cancer pain or other severe pain may require extraordinary doses to attain pain relief due to drug tolerance or low pain tolerance, rather than addiction. Do not withhold medication from patients based on dosage norms when dealing with patients in severe, persistent pain.
- **Cumulative effect:** Oxycodone may have a prolonged duration of action and cumulative effect in patients with hepatic or renal impairment.

OVERDOSE/TOXICITY

- **Hepatotoxicity:** May occur with overdose of the acetaminophen component of fixed-combination products.
- **Overdose:** Respiratory depression, skeletal muscle flaccidity, cold or clammy skin, cyanosis, and extreme somnolence progressing to seizures, stupor, and coma.
- **Management:** Initiate Advanced Cardiac Life Support (ACLS) guidelines for respiratory depression and management of bradycardia and hypotension, if present.
- **GI decontamination:** No specific recommendations.

ANTIDOTE/DIALYSIS

- **Antidote:** Naloxone 0.4-2 mg IV, subcutaneously, or IM; may repeat if ineffective. Well absorbed IM and subcutaneously in noncirculatory-impaired patients. Use with caution in patients with cardiovascular disease to avoid compromise if opiates rapidly displace from receptors. Hypertension, tachypnea, and return of extreme pain may immediately return causing extreme increases in myocardial oxygen consumption.
- **Dialysis:** No data are available on removal of oxycodone by hemodialysis, high-permeability hemodialysis, or peritoneal dialysis.

oxymorphone

See Opioid Analgesics (p. 980)

paclitaxel

pak-li-tax'-el

Classes

Chemical: antimitotic, taxus baccarata derivative

Therapeutic: antineoplastic

Pregnancy Category: D

Trade Names

Prescription: Abraxane, Onxol, Taxol

Do not confuse paclitaxel with Paxil.

CLINICAL PHARMACOLOGY

Mechanism of Action

An antimitotic agent in the taxoid family that disrupts the microtubular cell network, which is essential for cellular function. Blocks cells in the late G_2 phase and M phase of the cell cycle. **Therapeutic Effect:** Inhibits cellular mitosis and replication.

PHARMACOKINETICS

Does not readily cross the blood-brain barrier. Protein binding: 89%-98%. Metabolized in the liver to active metabolites; eliminated by bile. Not removed by hemodialysis. **Half-life:** 1.3-8.6 hr.

AVAILABILITY

Injection (Abraxane): 100-mg vial.
Injection (Onxol, Taxol): 6 mg/mL.

INDICATIONS AND DOSAGE

Ovarian cancer

IV

Adults: 135-175 mg/m^2/dose over 3 hr every 3 wk or 135 mg/m^2 over 24 hr every 3 wk; 50-80 mg/m^2 over 1-3 hr weekly; or 1.4-4 mg/m^2 continuous infusion for 14 days given every 4 wk.

Breast carcinoma

IV (Onxol, Taxol)

Adults, Elderly: 175-250 mg/m^2 over 3 hr every 3 wk, or 50-80 mg/m^2 weekly or 1.4-4 mg/m^2/day continuous infusion for 14 days given every 4 wk.

IV (Abraxane)

Adults, Elderly: 260 mg/m^2 over 30 min every 3 wk.

Non–small-cell lung carcinoma

IV

Adults, Elderly: 135 mg/m^2 over 24 hr, followed by cisplatin 75 mg/m^2 every 3 wk.

Kaposi's sarcoma

IV

Adults, Elderly: 135 mg/m^2/dose over 3 hr every 3 wk or 100 mg/m^2/dose over 3 hr every 2 wk.

Dosage in hepatic impairment

Note: These recommendations are based on the first course of therapy, where the usual dose would be 135 mg/m^2 dose over 24 hr or the 175 mg/m^2 dose over 3 hr in patients with normal hepatic function. Dosage in subsequent courses should be based on individual tolerance. Adjustments for other regimens are not available.

24-hr infusion:

If transaminase levels less than 2 times upper limit of normal (ULN) and bilirubin level less than or equal to 1.5 mg/dL, 135 mg/m^2.

If transaminase levels 2 less than 10 times ULN and bilirubin level less than or equal to 1.5 mg/dL, 100 mg/m^2.

If transaminase levels less than 10 times ULN and bilirubin level 1.6-7.5 mg/dL, 50 mg/m^2.

If transaminase levels greater than 10 times ULN and bilirubin level greater than or equal to 7.5 mg/dL, avoid use.

3-hr infusion:

If transaminase levels less than 10 times ULN and bilirubin level less than or equal to 1.25 times ULN, 175 mg/m^2.

If transaminase levels less than 10 times ULN and bilirubin level 1.26-2 times ULN, 135 mg/m^2.

If transaminase levels less than 10 times ULN and bilirubin level 2.01-5 times ULN, 90 mg/m^2.

If transaminase levels greater than or equal to 10 times ULN and bilirubin level greater than 5 times ULN; avoid use.

OFF-LABEL USES

Treatment of upper GI tract adenocarcinoma, head and neck cancer, hormone-refractory prostate cancer, metastatic breast cancer, non-Hodgkin's lymphoma, small-cell-lung cancer, transitional cell cancer of urothelium

CONTRAINDICATIONS

Baseline neutropenia (neutrophil count 1500 cells/mm^3), hypersensitivity to paclitaxel or drugs developed with Cremophor EL (polyoxyethylated castor oil), neutropenia (less than 1000 cells/m^2) for Kaposi's sarcoma

INTERACTIONS

Drug: Bone marrow depressants: May increase myelosuppression. **Live-virus vaccines:** May potentiate virus replication, increase vaccine side effects, and decrease antibody response to the vaccine. **Herbal:** None known. **Food:** None known.

P

DIAGNOSTIC TEST EFFECTS

May elevate serum alkaline phosphatase, bilirubin, AST (SGOT), and ALT (SGPT) levels. Decreases blood Hgb and Hct levels and platelet, RBC, and WBC counts.

IV INCOMPATIBILITIES

Amphotericin B complex (Abelcet, AmBisome, Amphotec), *chlorproMAZINE (Thorazine), *DOXOrubicin liposomal (Doxil), *hydrOXYzine (Vistaril), *methylPREDNISolone (Solu-Medrol), mitoxantrone (Novantrone)

IV COMPATIBILITIES

Carboplatin (Paraplatin), cisplatin (Platinol AQ), cyclophosphamide (Cytoxan), cytarabine (Cytosar), dacarbazine (DTIC-Dome), dexamethasone (Decadron), *diphenhydrAMINE (Benadryl), *DOXOrubicin (Adriamycin), etoposide (VePesid), gemcitabine (Gemzar), granisetron (Kytril), hydromorphone (Dilaudid), magnesium sulfate, mannitol, methotrexate, morphine, ondansetron (Zofran), potassium chloride, *vinBLAStine (Velban), *vinCRIStine (Oncovin)

SIDE-EFFECTS

Expected (90%-70%): Diarrhea, alopecia, nausea, vomiting. **Frequent (48%-46%):** Myalgia or arthralgia, peripheral neuropathy. **Occasional (20%-13%):** Mucositis, hypotension during infusion, pain or redness at injection site. **Rare (3%):** Bradycardia

P

CRITICAL CARE CONSIDERATIONS

ADMINISTRATION/HANDLING

IV ALERT

- **Pretreatment:** Pretreat with corticosteroids (dexamethasone 20 mg PO/IV at 14 hr, then 7 hr before paclitaxel), *diphenhydrAMINE (50 mg IV 30-60 min before dose), and H_2 antagonists (famotidine 20 mg IV 30-60 min before dose).
- Paclitaxel may be carcinogenic, mutagenic, or teratogenic; gloves should be worn when handling the drug. If contact with skin occurs, wash the skin thoroughly with soap and water; if drug contacts mucous membranes, flush area with water.
- **Neutrophil counts:** Paclitaxel should not be given to patients with solid tumors who have baseline neutrophil counts of less than 1500 cells/mm^3 and may be given to patients with AIDS-related Kaposi's sarcoma if baseline neutrophil count is less than 1000 cells/mm^3.
- **Storage:** Refrigerate unopened vials. Store diluted solutions in bottles or plastic bags; administer through polyethylene-lined administration sets. Avoid storing diluted solutions in plasticized polyvinyl chloride equipment or devices.
- **Stability:** Reconstituted solution is stable at room temperature for up to 24 hr. Dilute with 0.9% NaCl or D_5W to a final concentration of 0.3-1.2 mg/mL.
- **Administration:** Administer through in-line filter not greater than 0.22 microns.

PRECAUTIONS

HEALTH-RELATED

- Use paclitaxel cautiously in patients with hepatic impairment, peripheral neuropathy, or severe neutropenia.

AGE-RELATED

- **Children:** Safety and efficacy of paclitaxel have not been established in children.
- **Elderly:** No age-related precautions have been noted.

PREGNANCY/LACTATION-RELATED

- Pregnancy category D; breast-feeding should be discontinued while using paclitaxel

MONITORING

- **Baseline assessment:** Assess for history of cancer and onset of symptoms; assess prior chemotherapy; assess vital signs before administration.
- **Baseline/ongoing lab work:** CBC with WBC differential, including neutrophil and platelet counts, before each course of paclitaxel and as clinically indicated. Biochemical panel including hepatic function (AST [SGOT], ALT [SGPT], alkaline phosphatase, GGT, bilirubin) tests.
- **Baseline diagnostic tests:** Baseline 12-lead ECG to assess baseline rhythm.
- **Aseptic technique:** Use strict aseptic technique during care.
- **Infection:** Assess for and protect patients from infection.
- **Dysrhythmias:** Continuous cardiac monitoring for critically ill patients to assess for dysrhythmias, including sinus tachycardia, premature ventricular contractions, ST-T wave changes; bradycardia is indicative of hypersensitivity if it occurs with hypotension; other bradycardia is relatively uncommon.
- **Hematologic toxicity:** Monitor for toxicity including excessive fatigue and weakness, ecchymosis, fever, signs of local infection, sore throat, and unusual bleeding.

- **Hypotension:** Monitor vital signs during the infusion, especially during the first hr; tachycardia and hypotension are possible.
- **Diarrhea:** Assess pattern of bowel movements and consistency.
- **Bleeding precautions:** Initiate bleeding precautions including avoiding IM injections, starting additional IV lines, taking rectal temperatures, and performing traumatic procedures that may induce bleeding.
- **Neutropenic precautions:** Initiate neutropenic precautions as nadir approaches.
- **Post-administration:** Apply pressure to the IV site for a full 5 min after administration.
- **Patient education:** Patients should be instructed to report immediately signs of infection including fever and flulike symptoms, and to report promptly if nausea and vomiting continue at home to a health care provider. Teach recognition of symptoms of peripheral neuropathy. Urge not to receive vaccinations and to avoid contact with crowds and people with known infections. Warn to avoid pregnancy during paclitaxel therapy. Teach various contraception methods; nonhormonal methods are recommended. Inform that alopecia is reversible but that new hair may have a different color or texture. Offer support to patients and families.

SERIOUS ADVERSE REACTIONS

- **Neutropenia:** Neutropenic nadir occurs at approximately day 11 of paclitaxel therapy.
- **Hematologic:** Anemia and leukopenia are common; thrombocytopenia occurs occasionally.
- **Hypersensitivity:** Severe reaction, including dyspnea, severe hypotension, angioedema, and generalized urticaria, occurs rarely. Fatal reactions have occurred despite premedication.

OVERDOSE/TOXICITY

- **Hematologic:** Severe neutropenia with infection, anemia, thrombocytopenia with bleeding.
- **Management:** Platelets and/or packed RBCs may be needed to manage anemia and bleeding. Medications such as filgrastim (Neupogen, G-CSF) or pegfilgrastim (Neulasta) may be used to help reverse neutropenia; oprelvekin (Neumega) may be used to help reverse thrombocytopenia; severe anemia may be managed with darbepoetin (Aranesp) or epoetin alfa (Epogen).
- **GI decontamination:** No specific recommendations.

ANTIDOTE/DIALYSIS

- **Antidote:** No specific recommendations.
- **Dialysis:** Paclitaxel is not removed by hemodialysis and is unlikely to be removed by peritoneal dialysis. No data are available on removal by high-permeability hemodialysis.

palonosetron hydrochloride

pal-oh-noe'-se-tron hye-droe-klor'-ide

Classes
Chemical: isoquinoline derivative
Therapeutic: antiemetic

Pregnancy Category: B

Trade Names
Prescription: Aloxi

CLINICAL PHARMACOLOGY

Mechanism of Action

A 5-HT_3 receptor antagonist that acts centrally in the chemoreceptor trigger zone and peripherally at the vagal nerve terminals. **Therapeutic Effect:** Prevents nausea and vomiting associated with chemotherapy.

PHARMACOKINETICS

Protein binding: 62%. Metabolized in liver. Eliminated in urine. **Half-life:** 40 hr.

AVAILABILITY

Injection: 0.25 mg/5 mL.

INDICATIONS AND DOSAGE

Chemotherapy-induced nausea and vomiting

IV

Adults, Elderly: 0.25 mg as a single dose 30 min before starting chemotherapy. Should not be given more than once per wk.

OFF-LABEL USES

Prevention of postoperative bleeding

CONTRAINDICATIONS

Hypersensitivity to palonosetron

INTERACTIONS

Drug: Apomorphine: May cause profound hypotension, altered consciousness. **Herbal:** None known. **Food:** None known.

P

DIAGNOSTIC TEST EFFECTS
May transiently increase serum bilirubin, AST (SGOT), and ALT (SGPT) levels.

IV INCOMPATIBILITIES
Do not mix palonosetron with any other drugs.

SIDE-EFFECTS
Occasional (22%-5%): Headache, constipation, pruritis (8%-22%). **Rare (less than 1%):** Diarrhea, dizziness, fatigue, abdominal pain, insomnia

CRITICAL CARE CONSIDERATIONS

ADMINISTRATION/HANDLING

IV ALERT
- **Storage:** Store vials at room temperature. The solution normally appears clear and colorless. Discard if it appears cloudy or contains precipitate.
- **IV push:** Give palonosetron undiluted as an IV push over 30 sec. Flush the IV line with 0.9% NaCl before and after administration.

PRECAUTIONS

HEALTH-RELATED
- Use palonosetron cautiously in patients with a history of cardiovascular disease.

AGE-RELATED
- **Children:** Safety and efficacy of palonosetron have not been established in children.
- **Elderly:** No age-related precautions have been noted.

PREGNANCY/LACTATION-RELATED
- Pregnancy category B; excretion into breast milk unknown; use caution in nursing mothers.

MONITORING
- **Baseline assessment:** Assess patients experiencing severe vomiting for dehydration (dry mucous membranes, furrows in the tongue, poor skin turgor).
- **Baseline lab work:** Biochemical profile to assess fluid and electrolyte balance.
- **Diarrhea:** Assess daily bowel activity and stool consistency.
- **Patient education:** Inform that nausea and vomiting should be relieved shortly after drug administration. Instruct to report promptly if vomiting persists to a health care provider. Urge avoidance of alcohol and barbiturates during palonosetron therapy. Teach other methods of reducing nausea and vomiting, including lying quietly and avoiding strong odors. Provide support and encouragement.

SERIOUS ADVERSE REACTIONS
- **CNS effects:** Tremors or weakness.
- **Cardiovascular:** Tachycardia or bradycardia, chest discomfort, heart failure.

OVERDOSE/TOXICITY
- **Overdose:** May produce a combination of CNS stimulant and depressant effects.
- **GI decontamination:** No specific recommendations.

ANTIDOTE/DIALYSIS
- **Antidote:** No specific recommendations.
- **Dialysis:** No data are available on removal of palonosetron using hemodialysis, high-permeability hemodialysis, or peritoneal dialysis.

pamidronate disodium

pa-mi-droe'-nate dye-soe'-dee-um

Classes
Chemical: pyrophosphate analog
Therapeutic: bisphosphonate, bone resorption inhibitor

Pregnancy Category: D

Trade Names
Prescription: Aredia, Pamidronate Disodium Novaplus

Do not confuse Aredia with Adriamcyin.

CLINICAL PHARMACOLOGY

Mechanism of Action
A bisphosphate that binds to bone and inhibits osteoclast-mediated calcium resorption. **Therapeutic Effect:** Lowers serum calcium concentrations.

PHARMACOKINETICS

Route	Onset	Peak	Duration
IV	24-48 hr	5-7 days	N/A

After IV administration, rapidly absorbed by bone. Slowly excreted unchanged in urine. Unknown if removed by hemodialysis. **Half-life:** bone, 300 days; unmetabolized, 21-35 hr.

AVAILABILITY
Powder for injection (Aredia, Pamidronate Disodium Novaplus): 30 mg, 90 mg. **Injection solution:** 3 mg/mL, 6 mg/mL, 9 mg/mL.

INDICATIONS AND DOSAGE

Hypercalcemia

IV Infusion

Adults, Elderly: Moderate hypercalcemia (corrected serum calcium level 12-13.5 mg/dL), 60-90 mg. Severe hypercalcemia (corrected serum calcium level greater than 13.5 mg/dL), 90 mg.

Paget's disease

IV Infusion

Adults, Elderly: 30 mg/day for 3 days.

Osteolytic bone lesion

IV Infusion

Adults, Elderly: 90 mg over 2-4 hr once per mo.

CONTRAINDICATIONS

Hypersensitivity to pamidronate or other bisphosphonates, such as etidronate, tiludronate, risedronate, and alendronate

INTERACTIONS

Drug: **Calcium-containing medications, vitamin D:** May antagonize effects of pamidronate in treatment of hypercalcemia. **Herbal:** None known. **Food:** **High calcium-containing foods (such as dairy):** May antagonize effects of pamidronate in treatment of hypercalcemia.

DIAGNOSTIC TEST EFFECTS

May decrease serum phosphate, magnesium, calcium, and potassium levels.

IV INCOMPATIBILITIES

Calcium-containing IV fluids

SIDE-EFFECTS

Frequent (greater than 10%): Temperature elevation (at least 1°C) 24-48 hr after administration (27%); redness, swelling, induration, pain at catheter site in patients receiving 90 mg (18%); anorexia, nausea, fatigue. **Occasional (10%-1%):** Constipation, rhinitis

CRITICAL CARE CONSIDERATIONS

ADMINISTRATION/HANDLING

IV ALERT

- **Storage:** Store parenteral form at room temperature.
- **Stability:** Reconstituted vial is stable for 24 hr when refrigerated; IV solution is stable for 24 hr after dilution.
- **Reconstitution/dilution:** Reconstitute each 30-mg vial with 10 mL sterile water for injection to provide concentration of 3 mg/mL. Allow drug to dissolve before withdrawing. Further dilute with 1000 mL sterile 0.45% or 0.9% NaCl or D_5W.
- **IV infusion:** Administer as IV infusion over 2-24 hr for treatment of hypercalcemia and over 2-4 hr for other indications.
- **Retreatment:** Allow at least 7 days between initial treatment and retreatment for hypercalcemia.

PRECAUTIONS

HEALTH-RELATED

- **Heart or renal failure:** Use pamidronate cautiously in patients with cardiac failure or renal impairment. Adequate hydration is essential during administration. Avoid overhydration in patients with the potential for heart failure.
- **Second-generation bisphosphonate:** Has potential advantages over etidronate; inhibits bone resorption at doses that do not impair bone mineralization; less likely than etidronate to produce osteomalacia.

AGE-RELATED

- **Children:** Safety and efficacy of pamidronate have not been established in children.
- **Elderly:** May become overhydrated and require careful monitoring of fluid and electrolytes. Dilute drug in a smaller volume for elderly patients.

PREGNANCY/LACTATION-RELATED

- Pregnancy category D; use caution with administration to a nursing mother.

MONITORING

- **Baseline assessment:** Assess vital signs before treatment and for history of heart and kidney disease. Assess hydration status. Cancer patients with hypercalcemia are often dehydrated and must be rehydrated (orally or IV) before receiving pamidronate.
- **Lab work:** CBC with WBC differential and platelet count, biochemical panel, including BUN, creatinine, potassium, magnesium, phosphate, and calcium. Low phosphate levels usually require treatment. Monitor Hct, Hgb, magnesium, phosphate, and creatinine levels. Monitor alkaline phosphatase if patients have Paget's disease.
- **Hydration:** Provide adequate hydration; avoid overhydrating. Monitor fluid intake and output carefully. Hydration with saline is preferred to facilitate excretion of calcium.

- **Fluid retention or overload:** Auscultate lungs for crackles and examine for dependent edema, indicative of possible heart failure.
- **Dysrhythmias:** Monitor continuous ECG when administering in an intensive care unit environment for dysrhythmias related to hypokalemia and hypomagnesemia.
- **IV insertion site:** Assess site for pain, redness, and swelling.
- **Constipation:** Assess pattern of daily bowel activity and stool consistency.
- **Patient education:** Explain need for follow-up testing and to avoid drugs containing calcium and vitamin D (antacids), which may antagonize effects of pamidronate. Diet may need restriction in calcium- and vitamin D-containing foods. Advise on use of appropriate contraceptives to prevent pregnancy. Instruct to report promptly abdominal cramps, confusion, chills, fever, sore throat, or muscle spasms to a health care provider.

SERIOUS ADVERSE REACTIONS

- **Electrolyte imbalance:** Hypophosphatemia, hypokalemia, hypomagnesemia, and hypocalcemia occur more frequently with higher dosages.
- **90-mg dose-related:** Anemia, hypertension, tachycardia, atrial fibrillation, and somnolence occur more frequently with 90-mg doses.
- **Hypersensitivity:** Allergic reactions including dyspnea, angioedema, anaphylaxis, and hypotension occur rarely.
- **Heart failure:** Dyspnea, shortness of breath, peripheral edema, activity intolerance secondary to overhydration.
- **Management:** Severely depleted potassium, phosphorous, and magnesium may need replacement. Mild depletion may normalize within 10 days without replacement. Calcium gluconate may be needed if symptomatic hypocalcemia is present. Monitor serum calcium and rehydrate with or without diuretics for 2-3 days.

OVERDOSE/TOXICITY

- **Hematologic:** Anemia, thrombocytopenia, leukopenia, lymphopenia with high fever, chills, and sore throat.
- **Nephrotoxicity:** Elevated BUN and creatinine, edema, nausea, vomiting, weight gain, fluid retention, oliguria, or anuria. Renal tubular necrosis may occur.
- **Management:** Discontinue pamidronate immediately. High fever may respond to steroids. RBC transfusion may be needed to manage anemia.
- **GI decontamination:** No specific recommendations.

ANTIDOTE/DIALYSIS

- **Antidote:** No specific antidote. Calcium gluconate may be used to manage hypocalcemia. Serum albumin must be monitored along with calcium.
- **Dialysis:** No data are available on removal of pamidronate using hemodialysis, high-permeability hemodialysis, or peritoneal dialysis.

pancreatin/pancrelipase

pan-kree-ah'-tin/pan-kre-lye'-pase

Classes

Chemical: pancreatic enzymes
Therapeutic: digestant

Pregnancy Category: C

Trade Names

Prescription: (pancreatin) Ku-Zyme, Pancreatin; (pancrelipase) Cotazym-S, Creon 5, Creon 10, Creon 20, Ilozyme, Kutrase, Ku-Zyme, Ku-Zyme HP, Lipram, Lipram-CR, Lipram-CR 5, Lipram-CR 20, Lipram-PN, Lipram-UL 12, Lipram-UL 18, Lipram-UL 20, Panase, Pancrease, Pancrease MT 4, Pancrease MT 20, Pancreatic EC, Pancreatil-UL 12, Pancrecarb MS-4, Pancrecarb MS-8, Pangestyme CN 10, Pangestyme CN 20, Pangestyme EC, Pangestyme MT 16, Pangestyme NL 18, Panokase, Plaretase, Protilase, Ultrase, Ultrase MT 12, Ultrase MT 18, Ultrase MT 20, Viokase, Viokase 8, Viokase 16, Zymase

CLINICAL PHARMACOLOGY

Mechanism of Action

Digestive enzymes that replace endogenous pancreatic enzymes. **Therapeutic Effect:** Assist in digestion of protein, starch, and fats.

PHARMACOKINETICS

Not absorbed systemically. Released at the duodenojejunal junction.

AVAILABILITY

Capsules: 15,000 units-12,000 units-15,000 units (Ku-Zyme), 30,000 units-24,000 units-30,000 units (Kutrase), 30,000 units-8000 units-30,000 units (Panokase, Cotazym, Ku-Zyme HP).

Capsules (extended release): 33,200 units-10,000 units-37,500 units (Creon 10, Lipram-CR), 30,000 units-10,000 units-30,000 units (Pangestyme CN 10, Lipram, Pancrease MT 10), 39,000 units-12,000 units-39,000 units (Lipram-UL 12, Pancreatil-UL 12, Ultrase MT 12), 12,000 units-4000 units-12,000 units (Pancrease MT 4), 48,000 units-16,000 units-48,000 units (Lipram-PN, Pancrease MT 16, Pangestyme MT 16), 16,600 units-5000 units-18,750 units (Creon 5, Lipram-CR5), 59,000 units-18,000 units-59,000 units (Pangestyme NL 18, Lipram-UL 18, Ultrase MT 18), 20,000 units-5000 units-20,000 units (Cotazym-S), 66,400 units-20,000 units-75,000 units (Creon 20, Lipram-CR 20), 20,000 units-4500 units-25,000 units (Lipram, Pancrease, Pangestyme EC, Ultrase), 56,000 units-20,000 units-44,000 units (Lipram-PN, Pancrease MT 20), 65,000 units-20,000 units-65,000 units (Lipram-UL 20, Pangestyme NL 18, Pangestyme CN 20, Ultrase MT 20), 20,000 units-4000 units-25,000 units (Panase, Pancreatic EC, Protilase), 25,000 units-4000 units-25,000 units (Pancrecarb MS-4), 40,000 units-8000 units-45,000 units (Pancrecarb MS-8).
Powder for reconstitution, oral (Viokase): 70,000 units-16,800 units-70,000 units/ 0.7 gm.
Tablets: 30,000 units-11,000 units-30,000 units (Ilozyme), 60,000 units-16,000 units-60,000 units (Viokase 16), 30,000 units-8000 units-30,000 units (Panokase, Plaretase, Viokase 8).

INDICATIONS AND DOSAGE

Pancreatic enzyme replacement or supplement when enzymes are absent or deficient, such as with chronic pancreatitis, cystic fibrosis, or ductal obstruction from cancer of the pancreas or common bile duct; to reduce malabsorption; treatment of steatorrhea associated with bowel resection or postgastrectomy syndrome

PO

Adults, Elderly: 1-3 capsules or tablets before or with meals or snacks. May increase to 8 tablets/dose. **Children:** 1-2 tablets with meals or snacks.

OFF-LABEL USES

Treatment of occluded feeding tubes

CONTRAINDICATIONS

Acute pancreatitis; exacerbation of chronic pancreatitis; hypersensitivity to pancreatin, pancrelipase, or pork protein

INTERACTIONS

Drug: Antacids: May decrease the effects of pancreatin and pancrelipase. **Iron supplements:** May decrease the absorption of iron supplements. **Herbal:** None known. **Food:** None known.

DIAGNOSTIC TEST EFFECTS

May increase serum uric acid level.

SIDE-EFFECTS

Rare: Allergic reaction, mouth irritation, shortness of breath, wheezing

CRITICAL CARE CONSIDERATIONS

ADMINISTRATION/HANDLING

PO ALERT

- Give pancreatin or pancrelipase before or with meals or snacks.
- Do not crush enteric-coated form.
- Crush tablets as needed.
- Spilling Viokase powder on the hands may irritate skin. Inhaling powder may irritate mucous membranes and produce bronchospasm.

PRECAUTIONS

HEALTH-RELATED

- Use pancreatin and pancrelipase cautiously because inhalation of the powder form may precipitate an asthma attack.

AGE-RELATED

- **Children:** No information is available on pancreatin or pancrelipase use in children.
- **Elderly:** No age-related precautions have been noted.

PREGNANCY/LACTATION-RELATED

- Pregnancy category C; unknown if distributed in breast milk.

MONITORING

- **Baseline assessment:** Assess nutritional status before beginning and regularly throughout therapy. Determine allergy to pork because hypersensitivity to pancreatin and pancrelipase may exist.
- **Baseline lab work:** Biochemical profile to assess nutritional status and fluid and electrolyte balance.
- **Therapeutic response:** Evaluate for relief of GI symptoms/indigestion.
- **Patient education:** Instruct not to chew capsules or tablets to minimize irritation to the mouth, lips, and tongue. If patients cannot swallow capsules, instruct to open

P

capsules and spread contents over applesauce, mashed fruit, or rice cereal. Advise not to change brands of the drug without first consulting the physician. Warn not to spill Viokase powder on the hands because it may irritate the skin. Instruct to avoid inhaling powder because it may irritate mucous membranes and produce bronchospasm.

SERIOUS ADVERSE REACTIONS

- **Hypersensitivity:** Urticaria, rash, itching, respiratory distress.

OVERDOSE/TOXICITY

- **Overdose:** Excessive dosage may produce nausea, cramping, and diarrhea. Hyperuricosuria and hyperuricemia have occurred with extremely high dosages.
- **GI decontamination:** No specific recommendations.

ANTIDOTE/DIALYSIS

- **Antidote:** No specific recommendations.
- **Dialysis:** No data are available on removal of pancrelipase by hemodialysis, peritoneal dialysis, or high-permeability hemodialysis.

pancuronium bromide

pan-cure-own'-ee-um broe'-mide

Classes

Chemical: non-depolarizing neuromuscular blocking agent

Therapeutic: skeletal muscle relaxant, paralytic agent

Pregnancy Category: C

Trade Names

Prescription: Pavulon

CLINICAL PHARMACOLOGY

Mechanism of Action

A nondepolarizing skeletal muscle relaxant that blocks neural transmission at the myoneural junction by binding with cholinergic receptor sites. **Therapeutic Effect:** Produces skeletal muscle relaxation.

PHARMACOKINETICS

Onset of action is dose dependent and occurs within 2-3 min. Duration of action is 60-100 min. Metabolized in liver. Excreted in urine. **Half-life:** 110 min (half-life is double in patients with renal failure).

AVAILABILITY

Injection: 1 mg/mL, 2 mg/mL (Pavulon).

INDICATIONS AND DOSAGE

Adjunct to general anesthesia; to facilitate endotracheal intubation and to provide skeletal muscle relaxation during surgery or mechanical ventilation

IV

Adults, Elderly, Children: Initially, a bolus dose of 0.06-0.1 mg/kg is recommended. Later, incremental doses starting at 0.01 mg/kg may be used every 25-60 min. Dosage must be individualized. Neuromuscular blockade/intensive care unit: 0.06-0.1 mg/kg bolus, then 0.8-1.7 mcg/kg/min continuous infusion. **Infants:** Neonates are especially sensitive to pancuronium during the first month of life. It is recommended that a test dose of 0.02 mg/kg be given first in this group to measure responsiveness. Later, incremental doses of 0.01 mg/kg IV every 20-40 min. Maximum: 0.1 mg. **Infants, Neonates:** 0.1 mg/kg every 30-60 min as needed or as continuous infusion of 0.02-0.04 mg/kg/hr or 0.4-0.6 mcg/kg/min. **Children:** 0.15 mg/kg every 30-60 min as needed or as continuous infusion of 0.03-0.1 mg/kg/hr or 0.5-1.7 mcg/kg/min.

CONTRAINDICATIONS

Hypersensitivity to pancuronium, bromide, or any component of the formulation

INTERACTIONS

Drug: Isoflurane, halothane, aminoglycosides, polymyxins, lithium, magnesium salts, procainamide, and quinidine: May enhance neuromuscular blockade, which may lead to respiratory depression and paralysis. **Muscle relaxants:** May block the effects of pancuronium. **Succinylcholine:** May accelerate the onset and/or increase the depth of neuromuscular blockade induced by pancuronium. **Herbal: St. John's wort:** May increase the risk of cardiovascular collapse and/or delay emergence from anesthesia. **Food:** None known.

DIAGNOSTIC TEST EFFECTS

None known.

IV INCOMPATIBILITIES

Incompatible when mixed with diazepam at a Y-site injection.

SIDE-EFFECTS

Frequency not defined: Excessive salivation, flushing, bradycardia, allergic reactions, rash, urticaria, reaction at injection site, inadequate or prolonged block, hypotension, tachycardia

CRITICAL CARE CONSIDERATIONS

ADMINISTRATION/HANDLING

IV ALERT

- Do not give pancuronium as IM injection because of the potential for tissue irritation.
- Pancuronium should be administered by adequately trained individuals familiar with its actions, characteristics, and hazards.
- **IV push direct injection:** May be administered undiluted by rapid IV injection.
- **Dilution:** Infusion solutions may be prepared by admixing pancuronium with an appropriate diluent (D_5W, 0.9% NaCl, D_5NS, or lactated Ringer's solution).
- **Stability:** Pancuronium will remain stable in solution for 48 hr. Unused solutions should be discarded.
- **Storage:** Vials of pancuronium should be refrigerated. Pancuronium is stable for up to 6 mo at room temperature.

PRECAUTIONS

HEALTH-RELATED

- Use cautiously in patients with electrolyte disturbances, hypothermia, myasthenia gravis, Eaton-Lambert syndrome, amyotrophic lateral sclerosis, respiratory acidosis, severe obesity, dystrophia myotonica, or impaired renal or liver function.

AGE-RELATED

- **Children:** Children under 1 mo are extremely sensitive to pancuronium. Test dose is 0.02 mg/kg with assessment of responsiveness. Has caused rare severe skeletal muscle weakness in mechanically ventilated neonates.
- **Elderly:** No age-related precautions have been noted.

PREGNANCY/LACTATION-RELATED

- Pregnancy category C; use with extreme caution in breast-feeding women; breast-feeding by mothers undergoing neuromuscular blockade is unusual.

MONITORING

- **Baseline assessment:** Assess vital signs, ventilation status, and pain and anxiety management.
- **Baseline and ongoing lab work:** Biochemical profile with renal (BUN, creatinine) and liver (AST [SGOT], ALT [SGPT], alkaline phosphatase, bilirubin) function studies.
- **Sedation and analgesia:** Patients undergoing neuromuscular blockade with pancuronium should be sedated and have appropriate pain management provided because patients are unable to express anxiety and discomfort during neuromuscular blockade. Pancuronium produces apnea and paralysis.
- **Ongoing assessment:** Monitor heart rate, BP, and respiratory rate. Try to assess level of pain. Assess renal and liver function if in the intensive care unit.
- **Sedation and neuromuscular blockade:** Monitor the degree of neuromuscular blockade using the train of four technique with a peripheral nerve stimulator and sedation with a bispectral brain wave analysis device (bispectral index monitoring). Adjust pancuronium and other medications to keep patients still, well ventilated, and as comfortable as possible. Because patients are totally dependent on health care providers to anticipate all needs and provide all care, most patients would rather not have awareness of the neuromuscular blockade experience.
- **Mechanical ventilation:** Assess ventilation status using lung assessment, vital signs, pulse oximetry, and end tidal CO_2 monitoring.
- **Weaning neuromuscular blockade:** Sedation with propofol (Diprivan), benzodiazepine infusion (lorazepam/Ativan), or morphine may provide enough relaxation to be able to wean pancuronium without compromising critically ill patients' ventilatory status. Confirm recovery with 5-second head lift and grip strength once pancuronium is weaned.
- **Patient education:** Explain that they will be unable to speak, open eyes, and move when full neuromuscular blockade is in place. When weaning pancuronium, explain it will be difficult to talk because of head and neck muscle blockade.

SERIOUS ADVERSE REACTIONS

- Dysrhythmias, edema, and hypotension may occur.
- Anaphylaxis and hypersensitivity reactions occur rarely.

OVERDOSE/TOXICITY

- **Symptoms:** Prolonged apnea, respiratory depression, inability to maintain patent airway to move extremities, speak, or open eyes. May occur more often when agents that potentiate pancuronium are given concomitantly. Seizures have been

P

reported in critically ill patients, but cause may be multifactorial. Cardiovascular collapse occurs rarely.

- **Management:** Continue to keep patients endotracheally intubated and mechanically ventilated until patients are fully able to maintain breathing and respiration effectively. Antidote may be administered if needed. Resuscitate per Advanced Cardiac Life Support (ACLS) guidelines for cardiac arrest.
- **GI decontamination:** No specific recommendations.

ANTIDOTE/DIALYSIS

- **Antidote:** Edrophonium (Enlon) or neostigmine (Prostigmin) given with atropine reverses muscle relaxation in most patients, but may aggravate severe overdosage. Ensure that patients are endotracheally intubated and mechanical or manual ventilation is in place.
- **Dialysis:** No data is available on removal of pancuronium by hemodialysis, high-permeability hemodialysis, or peritoneal dialysis.

pantoprazole sodium

See Acid Secretion Inhibitors (p. 884)

P

paricalcitol

par-i-kal'-si-trole

Classes

Chemical: vitamin D analog
Therapeutic: vitamin

Pregnancy Category: C

Trade Names

Prescription: Zemplar

CLINICAL PHARMACOLOGY

Mechanism of Action

A fat-soluble vitamin that is essential for absorption, utilization of calcium phosphate, and normal calcification of bone. **Therapeutic Effect:** Stimulates calcium and phosphate absorption from small intestine, promotes secretion of calcium from bone to blood, promotes renal tubule phosphate resorption, acts on bone cells to stimulate skeletal growth and on parathyroid gland to suppress hormone synthesis and secretion.

PHARMACOKINETICS

Protein binding: more than 99%. Metabolized in liver. Primarily eliminated in feces; minimal excretion in urine. Not removed by hemodialysis. **Half-life:** 14-15 hr.

AVAILABILITY

Injection: 2 mcg/mL, 5 mcg/mL
Capsule: 1 mg, 2 mg, 4 mg

INDICATIONS AND DOSAGE

Hypoparathyroidism

IV

Adults, Elderly, Children: 0.04-0.1 mcg/kg (2.8-7 mcg) given as a bolus dose no more frequently than every other day at any time during dialysis; dose as high as 0.24 mcg/kg (16.8 mcg) have been administered safely. Usually start with 0.04 mcg/kg 3 times/wk as a bolus, increased by 0.04 mcg/kg every 2 wk. Dose adjustment based on serum parathyroid hormone (PTH) levels: **Same or increasing serum PTH level;** increase dose. **Serum PTH level decreased by less than 30%;** increase dose. **Serum PTH level decreased by greater than 30% and less than 60%;** maintain dose. **Serum PTH level decreased by greater than 60%;** decrease dose. **Serum PTH level 1.5-3 times upper limit of normal;** maintain dose

PO

Adults, Elderly: Initial dose based on baseline serum PTH: **PTH level less than or equal to 500 pg/mL;** 1 mcg/day or 2 mcg 3 times/wk. **PTH level greater than 500 pg/mL;** 2 mcg/day or 4 mcg 3 times/wk. Dosage adjustment based on PTH level relative to baseline, adjust dose at 2-4 wk intervals: **Same or increasing serum PTH level;** increase dose by 1 mcg/day or 2 mcg 3 times/wk. **Serum PTH level decreased by less than 30%;** increase dose by 1 mcg/day or 2 mcg 3 times/wk. **Serum PTH level decreased by greater than or equal to 30% or less than or equal to 60%;** maintain dose. **Serum PTH level decreased by greater than 60%;** decrease dose by 1 mcg/day* or 2 mcg 3 times/wk. **Serum PTH level less than 60 pg/mL;** decrease dose by 1 mcg/day* or 2 mcg 3 times/wk *If patients are taking the lowest dose on a once-daily regimen, but further dose reduction is needed, decrease dose to 1 mcg 3 times/wk. If further dose reduction is required, withhold drug as needed and restart at a lower dose. If applicable, calcium phosphate binder dosing may also be adjusted or withheld, or switch to noncalcium-based binder.

CONTRAINDICATIONS

Hypercalcemia, malabsorption syndrome, vitamin D toxicity, hypersensitivity to paricalcitol or other vitamin D products or analogs

INTERACTIONS

Drug: Aluminum-containing antacid (long-term use): May increase aluminum concentration and aluminum bone toxicity. **Calcium-containing preparations, thiazide diuretics:** May increase the risk of hypercalcemia. **Digoxin:** May increase the risk of digitalis toxicity. **Magnesium-containing antacids:** May increase magnesium concentration. **Herbal:** None known. **Food:** None known.

DIAGNOSTIC TEST EFFECTS

May decrease serum alkaline phosphatase.

SIDE-EFFECTS

Occasional (5%-13%): Edema (7%), nausea (6%-13%), vomiting (6%-8%), headache (5%), dizziness (5%). **Rare:** Palpitations

CRITICAL CARE CONSIDERATIONS

ADMINISTRATION/HANDLING

IV ALERT

- **Storage:** Store unopened vials at controlled room temperature.
- **Dilution:** May give paricalcitol undiluted.
- **IV direct injection:** Administer as a bolus. Discard any unused portion.

PO ALERT

- May give paricalcitol without regard to food.

PRECAUTIONS

HEALTH-RELATED

- Use paricalcitol cautiously in patients with contrary artery disease, kidney stones, and renal impairment.
- **Digoxin:** Hypercalcemia produced by paricalcitol may potentiate digoxin toxicity.

AGE-RELATED

- **Children:** May be more sensitive to the effects of paricalcitol.
- **Elderly:** No age-related precautions have been noted.

PREGNANCY/LACTATION-RELATED

- Pregnancy category C; use caution in nursing mothers.

MONITORING

- **Baseline assessment:** Assess for history of parathyroid disease. Paricalcitol therapy should begin at the lowest possible dosage.
- **Baseline lab work:** Biochemical profile including BUN, creatinine, alkaline phosphatase, magnesium, phosphate, calcium, and phosphorus levels; obtain baseline parathyroid hormone (PTH) and urinary calcium level.
- **Ongoing lab work:** Serum calcium and phosphorus twice weekly during initial phase of therapy, then at least monthly once dosage has been established; if an elevated calcium level or a Ca × P product greater than 75 is noted, immediately reduce or interrupt dosage until parameters are normalized, then reinitiate at lower dose; intact PTH assay every 3 mo (target range in CRF patients is the non-uremic upper limit of normal).
- **Therapeutic serum calcium level:** 9 to 10 mg/dL.
- **Dysrhythmias:** Patients taking digitalis must be closely monitored for dysrhythmias; hypercalcemia prompts shortening of the ST segment and QT intervals; PR interval may be prolonged; ventricular dysrhythmias may occur.
- **Dietary calcium:** Estimate the daily dietary calcium intake. Adhere to a dietary regimen of calcium supplementation and phosphorus restriction; avoid excessive use of aluminum-containing compounds.
- **Hydration:** Maintain adequate oral and IV fluid intake.
- **Hyperphosphatemia:** Phosphate-binding compounds may be needed to control serum phosphorus levels.
- **Patient education:** Encourage consumption of foods rich in vitamin D, including eggs, leafy vegetables, margarine, meats, milk, vegetable oils, and vegetable shortening. Warn not to take mineral oil during paricalcitol therapy. Advise dialysis patients not to take magnesium-containing antacids during therapy. Encourage drinking plenty of liquids.

SERIOUS ADVERSE REACTIONS

- **Hypercalcemia:** Occurs rarely and requires an immediate reduction of the dose or temporarily stopping therapy. Low-calcium diet, increased exercise, stopping calcium and vitamin D supplements, and monitoring for magnesium, phosphate, and potassium imbalance is helpful.

P

- **Digitalis toxicity:** May occur if patients become hypercalcemic.

OVERDOSE/TOXICITY

- **Early signs:** Weakness, headache, somnolence, nausea, vomiting, dry mouth, constipation, muscle and bone pain, and metallic taste sensation.
- **Later signs:** Polyuria, polydipsia, anorexia, weight loss, nocturia, photophobia, rhinorrhea, pruritus, disorientation, hallucinations, hyperthermia, hypertension, and ventricular dysrhythmias.
- **Management:** IV isotonic saline administered rapidly helps increase calcium excretion; steroids compete with vitamin D, which helps reduce intestinal calcium absorption.
- **GI decontamination:** No specific recommendations.

ANTIDOTE/DIALYSIS

- **Antidote:** No specific recommendations.
- **Dialysis:** Paricalcitol is not removed by hemodialysis. No data are available on removal by peritoneal dialysis or high-permeability hemodialysis.

paroxetine

See Antidepressants (p. 906)

peginterferon alfa 2a

See Immunologics (p. 968)

peginterferon alfa 2b

See Immunologics (p. 968)

pegfilgrastim

peg-fil-gra'-stim

Classes

Chemical: amino acid glycoprotein
Therapeutic: hematopoietic agent

Pregnancy Category: C

Trade Names

Prescription: Neulasta

Do not confuse Neulasta with Neumega.

CLINICAL PHARMACOLOGY

Mechanism of Action

A colony-stimulating factor that regulates production of neutrophils within bone marrow. Also a glycoprotein that primarily affects neutrophil progenitor proliferation, differentiation, and selected end-cell functional activation. **Therapeutic Effect:** Increases phagocytic ability and antibody-dependent destruction; decreases incidence of infection.

PHARMACOKINETICS

Readily absorbed after subcutaneous administration. **Half-life:** 15-80 hr.

AVAILABILITY

Solution for injection: 6 mg/0.6 mL syringe.

INDICATIONS AND DOSAGE

Myelosuppression

Subcutaneous

Adults, Elderly: Give as a single 6-mg injection once per chemotherapy cycle.

CONTRAINDICATIONS

Hypersensitivity to pegfilgrastim or *Escherichia coli*–derived proteins; do not administer within 14 days before and 24 hr after cytotoxic chemotherapy

INTERACTIONS

Drug: Lithium: May potentiate the release of neutrophils. **Herbal:** None known. **Food:** None known.

DIAGNOSTIC TEST EFFECTS

May increase LDH concentrations, leukocyte alkaline phosphatase scores, and serum alkaline phosphatase and uric acid levels.

SIDE-EFFECTS

Frequent (72%-12%): Bone pain (31%-57%), vomiting (13%), constipation (12%), arthralgia (16%), generalized weakness (13%), peripheral edema (12%)

CRITICAL CARE CONSIDERATIONS

ADMINISTRATION/HANDLING

SUBCUTANEOUS ALERT

- **Storage:** Store in refrigerator but may warm to room temperature up to 48 hr before use. Discard if left at room temperature for longer than 48 hr. Protect from light. Avoid freezing, but if accidentally frozen, may thaw in refrigerator before administration. Discard if freezing takes place a second time. Discard if discoloration or precipitate is present.

- **Chemotherapy:** Do not administer from 14 days before to 24 hr after cytotoxic chemotherapy.

PRECAUTIONS

HEALTH-RELATED

- Use pegfilgrastim cautiously in patients who concurrently use medications with mycelioid properties and in those with sickle cell disease.

AGE-RELATED

- **Children:** Safety and efficacy of pegfilgrastim have not been established in children; use should be avoided in infants, children, and adolescents weighing less than 45 kg.
- **Elderly:** No age-related precautions have been noted.

PREGNANCY/LACTATION-RELATED

- Pregnancy category C; breast milk excretion unknown; use caution in nursing mothers.

MONITORING

- **Baseline assessment:** Assess history of cancer and plans for chemotherapy. Pegfilgrastim should not be given less than 14 days before chemotherapy.
- **Lab work:** CBC with WBC differential and platelet count before initiation of pegfilgrastim therapy and routinely thereafter.
- **Baseline diagnostic testing:** Chest x-ray.
- **Hypersensitivity:** Monitor for allergic reactions.
- **Fluid retention:** Examine for peripheral edema, particularly behind the medial malleolus.
- **Mucositis:** Assess mucous membranes for evidence of mucositis (red mucous membranes, white patches, and extreme mouth soreness) and stomatitis.
- **Muscle weakness:** Evaluate muscle strength.
- **Diarrhea:** Assess pattern of daily bowel activity and stool consistency.
- **Immunosuppression:** Evaluate for increased work of breathing in patients with sepsis, which may indicate the onset of acute respiratory distress syndrome (ARDS).
- **Patient education:** Explain possible side effects of pegfilgrastim, as well as the symptoms of allergic reactions. Stress the importance of compliance with pegfilgrastim regimen, including regular monitoring of blood counts.

SERIOUS ADVERSE REACTIONS

- **Hypersensitivity:** Allergic reactions including anaphylaxis, rash, and urticaria (rare).
- **ARDS:** May occur with sepsis.

OVERDOSE/TOXICITY

- **Cytopenia:** Poor bone marrow response resulting from an antibody response to growth factors occurs rarely.
- **Splenomegaly:** Left upper abdominal or shoulder pain (rare).
- **GI decontamination:** No specific recommendations.

ANTIDOTE/DIALYSIS

- **Antidote:** No specific recommendations.
- **Dialysis:** Pegfilgrastim is unlikely to be removed by hemodialysis, high-permeability hemodialysis, or peritoneal dialysis.

pegvisomant

peg-vi'-soe-mant

Classes

Chemical: recombinant human peptide
Therapeutic: growth hormone receptor antagonist

Pregnancy Category: B

Trade Names

Prescription: Somavert

Do not confuse Somavert with somatrem or somatropin.

CLINICAL PHARMACOLOGY

Mechanism of Action

A protein that selectively binds to growth hormone (GH) receptors on cell surfaces, blocking the binding of endogenous growth hormones and interfering with GH signal transduction. **Therapeutic Effect:** Decreases serum concentrations of insulinlike growth factor 1 (IGF-1) and other GH-responsive serum proteins.

PHARMACOKINETICS

Not distributed extensively into tissues after subcutaneous administration. Less than 1% excreted in urine. **Half-life:** 6 days.

AVAILABILITY

Powder for injection: 10-mg, 15-mg, 20-mg vials.

P

INDICATIONS AND DOSAGE

Acromegaly

Subcutaneous

Adults, Elderly: Initially, 40 mg, as a loading dose, then 10 mg daily. After 4-6 wk, adjust dosage in 5-mg increments if serum IGF-1 level is still elevated or in 5-mg decrements if IGF-1 level has decreased below the normal range. Maximum: 30 mg daily.

CONTRAINDICATIONS

Latex allergy (stopper on vial contains latex), hypersensitivity to pegvisomant

INTERACTIONS

Drug: Insulin, oral antidiabetics: May enhance effects of these drugs, possibly resulting in hypoglycemia. Dosage should be decreased when initiating pegvisomant therapy. **Opioids:** Decrease serum pegvisomant level. **Herbal:** None known. **Food:** None known.

DIAGNOSTIC TEST EFFECTS

Interferes with measurement of serum growth hormone concentration. May increase AST (SGOT), ALT (SGPT), and transaminase levels. Decreases effect of insulin on carbohydrate metabolism.

SIDE-EFFECTS

Frequent (23%): Infection (cold symptoms, upper respiratory tract infection, blister, ear infection). **Occasional (8%-5%):** Back pain, dizziness, injection site reaction, peripheral edema, sinusitis, nausea. **Rare (less than 5%):** Diarrhea, paresthesia

CRITICAL CARE CONSIDERATIONS

ADMINISTRATION/HANDLING

SUBCUTANEOUS ALERT

- **Storage:** Store unreconstituted vials in the refrigerator.
- **Preparation:** Withdraw 1 mL sterile water for injection and inject it into the vial of pegvisomant, aiming the stream against the glass wall. Hold the vial between the palms of both hands and roll it gently to dissolve the powder; do not shake.
- **Stability:** Administer the drug within 6 hr of reconstitution. The solution normally appears clear after reconstitution. Discard the solution if it appears cloudy or contains particles.
- Administer only one dose from each vial.

PRECAUTIONS

HEALTH-RELATED

- **Tumor growth:** May cause expansion of growth hormone secreting pituitary tumors, which may impose on the optic chiasm.
- **Glucose metabolism:** Growth hormone increases insulin sensitivity, resulting in hypoglycemia. Dose of hypoglycemic agents (diabetes medications) and insulin may have to be reduced in diabetic patients.
- **Liver impairment:** If initial liver enzymes are found to be elevated 3 times normal, a complete liver workup should be done before initiating pegvisomant.
- **Growth hormone deficiency:** A functional growth hormone deficiency may result from use of pegvisomant, despite normal growth hormone blood levels. IGF-1 levels should be used to assess drug efficacy.

AGE-RELATED

- **Children:** Safety and efficacy of pegvisomant have not been established in children.
- **Elderly:** Treatment should begin at the low end of the dosage range due to age-related organ impairment.

PREGNANCY/LACTATION-RELATED

- Pregnancy category B; unknown if distributed in breast milk.

MONITORING

- **Baseline assessment:** Assess history of growth pattern, including acromegalic changes.
- **Baseline lab work:** Biochemical profile including liver function tests (alkaline phosphatase, bilirubin, AST [SGOT], and ALT [SGPT] levels).
- **Baseline diagnostic tests:** CT scan or MRI of tumor area.
- **Ongoing lab work:** Obtain serum IGF-1 concentrations 4-6 wk after therapy begins and periodically thereafter. Adjust the drug dosage based on these results, not on growth hormone assays. Pegvisomant interferes with measurement of growth hormone concentrations done using commercially available GH assays.
- **Ongoing diagnostic tests:** For patients with tumors that secrete growth hormone, monitor for progressive tumor growth with periodic imaging scans of the sella turcica.

- **Hypoglycemia:** Monitor diabetic patients for hypoglycemia.
- **Growth deficit:** Monitor for signs of functional growth deficit, despite presence of normal blood levels of growth hormone.
- **Patient education:** Inform that routine monitoring of liver function is essential during pegvisomant treatment. Instruct to report promptly yellowing of the skin or sclera of eyes or any other adverse effects to a health care provider. Review symptoms and treatment of hypoglycemia with diabetic patients.

SERIOUS ADVERSE REACTIONS

- **Elevated liver enzymes:** Pegvisomant use may markedly elevate liver function test results, including serum transaminase levels. If transaminase levels become 3 times normal, pegvisomant should be discontinued and liver enzymes monitored. If enzymes normalize, evaluate for reinitiation of drug.
- **Weight gain:** Substantial weight gain occurs rarely.

OVERDOSE/TOXICITY

- **Hepatotoxicity:** Jaundice, fatigue, nausea, vomiting, right upper quadrant pain, ascites, unexplained edema, easy bruising.
- **Management:** Discontinue pegvisomant upon confirmed liver injury. Manage symptoms according to current standard of care for liver injury.
- **GI decontamination:** No specific recommendations.

ANTIDOTE/DIALYSIS

- **Antidote:** No specific recommendations.
- **Dialysis:** Pegvisomant is unlikely to be removed by hemodialysis, high-permeability hemodialysis, or peritoneal dialysis.

pemoline

pem'-oh-leen

DEA Schedule: IV

Classes

Chemical: oxazolidinone derivative

Therapeutic: anorexiant, central nervous system stimulant

Pregnancy Category: B

Trade Names

Prescription: Cylert, PemADD, PemADD CT

CLINICAL PHARMACOLOGY

Mechanism of Action

A CNS stimulant that blocks the reuptake mechanism present in dopaminergic neurons in the cerebral cortex and subcortical structures. **Therapeutic Effect:** Reduces motor restlessness and fatigue, increases alertness, elevates mood.

PHARMACOKINETICS

Rapidly absorbed from GI tract. Protein binding: 50%. Metabolized in liver. Primarily excreted in urine. **Half-life:** 12 hr.

AVAILABILITY

Tablets (Cylert, PemADD): 18.75 mg, 37.5 mg, 75 mg.

Tablets (chewable [Cylert, PemADD CT]): 37.5 mg.

INDICATIONS AND DOSAGE

Attention-deficit/hyperactivity disorder (ADHD)

PO

Children 6 yr and older: Initially, 37.5 mg/day as a single dose in morning. May increase by 18.75 mg at weekly intervals until therapeutic response is achieved. Range: 56.25-75 mg/day. Maximum: 112.5 mg/day.

CONTRAINDICATIONS

Family history of Tourette's syndrome, hepatic impairment, motor tics, hypersensitivity to pemoline

INTERACTIONS

Drug: **Other CNS stimulants:** May increase CNS stimulation. **Herbal:** None known. **Food:** None known.

DIAGNOSTIC TEST EFFECTS

May increase serum LDH, AST (SGOT), and ALT (SGPT) levels.

SIDE-EFFECTS

Frequent: Anorexia, insomnia. **Occasional:** Nausea, abdominal discomfort, diarrhea, headache, dizziness, somnolence

CRITICAL CARE CONSIDERATIONS

ADMINISTRATION/HANDLING

PO ALERT

- Store at controlled room temperature.
- **Reassessment for need:** Patients should be taken off pemoline periodically to see if behavioral symptoms return.

PRECAUTIONS

HEALTH-RELATED

- Use pemoline cautiously in patients with hypertension, psychosis, renal impairment, seizures, or a history of drug abuse.
- Pemoline should not be used for patients with increased liver enzymes. All patients should sign a consent indicating understanding of the possibility of significant liver disease, including liver failure.

AGE-RELATED

- **Children:** Safety and efficacy of pemoline have not been established in children under 6 yr.
- **Elderly:** Age-related organ impairment may prompt a dosage adjustment.

PREGNANCY/LACTATION-RELATED

- Pregnancy category B; unknown if excreted in breast milk.

MONITORING

- **Baseline assessment:** Obtain baseline height and weight; weigh regularly to detect delayed growth in children.
- **Baseline lab work:** Biochemical profile including hepatic function tests (AST [SGOT], ALT [SGPT], alkaline phosphatase, GGT, bilirubin) before and periodically during pemoline therapy.
- **Therapeutic effect:** Observe over time for increase in attention span, reduced hyperactivity, stabilization of emotions, and improved impulse control.
- **Patient education:** Warn to avoid tasks that require mental alertness or motor skills until response to the drug is known. Explain that pemoline may be habit forming. Caution against abruptly discontinuing the drug. Instruct to report promptly dark urine, GI complaints, loss of appetite, or yellow skin to a health care provider. Urge avoidance of alcohol and caffeine during pemoline therapy.

SERIOUS ADVERSE REACTIONS

- **Neurologic effects:** Visual disturbances, rash, and dyskinetic movements of the tongue, lips, face, and extremities have occurred.
- **CNS stimulation:** Large doses of pemoline may produce extreme nervousness and tachycardia.
- **Growth delay:** Prolonged administration to children with ADHD may temporarily delay growth in children.

OVERDOSE/TOXICITY

- **Hepatotoxicity:** Hepatitis and jaundice appear to be reversible when the drug is discontinued. Pemoline should be discontinued if serum ALT (SGPT) is increased greater than 2 times the upper limit of normal or if clinical signs and symptoms suggest liver failure.
- **Management:** Discontinue medication and observe for improvement. Provide supportive care tailored to liver dysfunction. If patients fail to improve, consider evaluation for liver transplantation.
- **GI decontamination:** No specific recommendations.

ANTIDOTE/DIALYSIS

- **Antidote:** No specific recommendations.
- **Dialysis:** Pemoline is removed by hemodialysis and is likely to be removed by high-permeability hemodialysis. It is not removed by peritoneal dialysis.

penbutolol

See Beta-Adrenergic Blockers (p. 943)

penicillin G benzathine

pen-i-sill'-in gee ben'-za-theen

Classes

Chemical: penicillin
Therapeutic: antibiotic, antibacterial

Pregnancy Category: B

Trade Names

Prescription: Bicillin C-R, Bicillin LA, Isoject Permapen, Wycillin

Do not confuse penicillin G benzathine with penicillin G potassium or penicillin G procaine.

CLINICAL PHARMACOLOGY

Mechanism of Action

A penicillin that inhibits bacterial cell wall synthesis by binding to one or more of the penicillin-binding proteins of bacteria. **Therapeutic Effect:** Bactericidal.

PHARMACOKINETICS

Slow absorption following IM administration. Protein binding: 60%. Metabolized in the liver. Primarily excreted in urine. **Half-life:** Unknown.

AVAILABILITY

Injection (prefilled syringe [Bicillin LA, Isoject Permapen]): 300,000 units/mL, 600,000 units/mL.

Injection (Bicillin C-R): 150,000 units G benzathine-150,000 units procaine/mL, 900,000 units G benzathine-300,000 units procaine/2 mL.
Injection, G procaine (Wycillin): 600,000 units/mL.

INDICATIONS AND DOSAGE

Group A streptococcal infections

IM

Adults, Elderly: 1.2 million units as a single dose. **Children:** 25,000-50,000 units/kg as a single dose. Maximum: 1.2 million units.

Prevention of rheumatic fever

IM

Adults, Elderly: 1.2 million units every 3-4 wk or 600,000 units twice monthly. **Children:** 25,000-50,000 units/kg every 3-4 wk. Maximum: 1.2 million units.

Early syphilis

IM

Adults, Elderly: 2.4 million units divided and administered in two separate injection sites.

Congenital syphilis

IM

Children: 50,000 units/kg as a single dose.

Syphilis of more than 1 year's duration

IM

Adults, Elderly: 2.4 million units divided and administered in two separate injection sites weekly for 3 wk.

CONTRAINDICATIONS

Hypersensitivity to penicillin G or any penicillin

INTERACTIONS

Drug: Erythromycin: May antagonize effects of penicillin. **Probenecid:** Increases serum concentration of penicillin. **Herbal:** None known. **Food:** None known.

DIAGNOSTIC TEST EFFECTS

May cause a positive Coombs' test.

SIDE-EFFECTS

Occasional: Lethargy, fever, dizziness, rash, pain at injection site. **Rare:** Seizures, interstitial nephritis

CRITICAL CARE CONSIDERATIONS

ADMINISTRATION/HANDLING

IM ALERT

- Store prefilled syringes in the refrigerator. Do not freeze.
- **Administration:** Administer the drug undiluted by deep IM injection.
- **IM only:** Do not administer penicillin G benzathine IV, intraarterially, or subcutaneously because doing so may cause heart attack, severe neurovascular damage, thrombosis, and death.

PRECAUTIONS

HEALTH-RELATED

- Use penicillin G benzathine cautiously in patients with a hypersensitivity to cephalosporins, impaired cardiac or renal function, or seizure disorders.

AGE-RELATED

- **Children:** No age-related precautions have been noted. Drug is indicated for managing rheumatic fever and chorea in children.
- **Elderly:** Age-related organ impairment may prompt a dosage adjustment.

PREGNANCY/LACTATION-RELATED

- Pregnancy category B; use with caution in breast-feeding mothers; may cause diarrhea, candidiasis, or allergic reaction in nursing infants.

MONITORING

- **Baseline assessment:** Determine history of allergies, particularly to cephalosporins or penicillins before beginning drug therapy.
- **Baseline lab work:** CBC with WBC differential, biochemical profile with renal function tests (BUN, creatinine), and urinalysis.
- **IM injection:** Check the IM injection site for pain and swelling. Inform that IM injections may cause discomfort. Care must be taken to give IM injection appropriately to avoid serious cardiac complications including cardiac arrest.
- **Therapeutic effect:** Assess for improvement in underlying disease process (venereal disease, rheumatic fever, or chorea).
- **Patient education:** Inform that they may experience temporary pain at the injection site. Instruct to immediately report chills, fever, rash, or any other unusual symptoms to a health care provider.

SERIOUS ADVERSE REACTIONS

- **Hypersensitivity reactions:** Ranging from chills, fever, and rash, to anaphylaxis.
- **Management:** Maintain patent airway and support ventilation. Endotracheal intubation should be done promptly for signs of respiratory distress following administration. Hypotension should be managed with IV fluids and then, vasopressors. Epinephine and *diphenhydrAMINE are used to help control allergic reaction. Corticosteroids are used if other measures do not provide complete relief of symptoms.

OVERDOSE/TOXICITY
- **Hematologic:** Hemolytic anemia.
- **Neurotoxicity:** Neuropathy.
- **Nephrotoxicity:** Elevated BUN, creatinine, oliguria, nausea, edema.
- **GI decontamination:** No specific recommendations.

ANTIDOTE/DIALYSIS
- **Antidote:** No specific recommendations.
- **Dialysis:** Penicillin is removed by hemodialysis and is likely to be removed by high-permeability hemodialysis. It is not removed by peritoneal dialysis.

penicillin G potassium
See Antibiotics (p. 892)

penicillin G procaine
See Antibiotics (p. 892)

penicillin V potassium
pen-i-sill'-in vee poe-tass'-ee-um

Classes
Chemical: penicillin
Therapeutic: antibiotic, antibacterial

Pregnancy Category: B

Trade Names
Prescription: Apo-Pen-VK ♣, Beepen-VK, Nadopen-V ♣, Novopen-VK ♣, PC Pen VK, Pen-V, Truxcillin VK, Veetids

CLINICAL PHARMACOLOGY
Mechanism of Action
A penicillin that inhibits cell wall synthesis by binding to bacterial cell membranes. **Therapeutic Effect:** Bactericidal.

PHARMACOKINETICS
Moderately absorbed from the GI tract. Protein binding: 80%. Widely distributed. Metabolized in the liver. Primarily excreted in urine. **Half-life:** 1 hr (increased in impaired renal function).

AVAILABILITY
Tablets: 250 mg (PC Pen VK, Pen-V, Veetids), 500 mg (Pen-V, Veetids, Truxcillin VK). **Powder for oral solution:** 125 mg/5 mL (Veetids), 250 mg/5 mL (Beepen-VK, Veetids).

INDICATIONS AND DOSAGE
Mild to moderate respiratory tract or skin or skin structure infections, otitis media, necrotizing ulcerative gingivitis
PO
Adults, Elderly, Children 12 yr and older: 125-500 mg every 6-8 hr. **Children younger than 12 yr:** 25-50 mg/kg/day in divided doses every 6-8 hr. Maximum: 3 g/day.
Primary prevention of rheumatic fever
PO
Adults, Elderly: 500 mg 2-3 times per day for 10 days. **Children:** 250 mg 2-3 times per day for 10 days.
Recurrent rheumatic fever, prophylaxis or prevention
PO
Adults, Elderly, Children: 250 mg twice per day.
Dosage in renal impairment
Dosage interval is modified based on creatinine clearance.

Creatinine Clearance	Dosage Interval
10-50 mL/min	Every 8-12 hr
Less than 10 mL/min	Every 12-16 hr

CONTRAINDICATIONS
Hypersensitivity to penicillin V or any penicillin

INTERACTIONS
Drug: Probenecid: May increase penicillin blood concentration and risk of toxicity. **Herbal:** None known. **Food:** None known.

DIAGNOSTIC TEST EFFECTS
May cause a positive Coombs' test.

SIDE-EFFECTS
Frequent: Mild hypersensitivity reaction (chills, fever, rash), nausea, vomiting, diarrhea. **Rare:** Bleeding, allergic reaction

CRITICAL CARE CONSIDERATIONS

ADMINISTRATION/HANDLING
PO ALERT
- Give penicillin V potassium on an empty stomach 1 hr before or 2 hr after meals.
- Store tablets at room temperature.
- After reconstitution, oral solution is stable for 14 days if refrigerated.
- Space drug doses evenly around the clock.

PRECAUTIONS

HEALTH-RELATED

- Use penicillin V potassium cautiously in patients with renal impairment, a history of seizures, or a history of allergies, particularly to cephalosporins.

AGE-RELATED

- **Children:** Use of penicillin V potassium may lead to allergic sensitization, candidiasis, diarrhea, and rash in infants. Use caution when giving penicillin V to neonates and young infants; immature renal function may delay drug excretion.
- **Elderly:** Age-related renal impairment may require a dosage adjustment.

PREGNANCY/LACTATION-RELATED

- Pregnancy category B; use with caution in breast-feeding women; may cause diarrhea, candidiasis, or allergic reaction in the nursing infant.

MONITORING

- **Baseline assessment:** Determine history of allergies, particularly to aspirin, cephalosporins, or penicillins before beginning drug therapy.
- **Baseline lab work:** CBC with WBC differential, biochemical profile with renal function tests (BUN, creatinine), and urinalysis.
- **Rash or diarrhea:** Withhold penicillin V potassium if rash or diarrhea occurs. Although rash is a common side effect of penicillin, it may also indicate hypersensitivity. Severe diarrhea with abdominal pain, blood or mucus in stools, and fever may indicate antibiotic-associated colitis.
- **Nephrotoxicity:** Monitor intake and output, renal function test results, and urinalysis results for signs of nephrotoxicity.
- **Anemia/bleeding:** Review blood Hgb levels. Check for signs of bleeding, including ecchymosis, overt bleeding, and swelling of tissue.
- **Superinfection:** Assess for signs and symptoms of superinfection such as anal or genital pruritus, black hairy tongue, oral ulceration or pain, diarrhea, increased fever, sore throat, and vomiting.
- **Evenly spaced doses:** Space doses evenly around the clock.
- **Patient education:** Instruct to report immediately chills, fever, rash, or any other unusual symptoms to a health care provider. Advise to space doses evenly and to continue taking the drug for the full course of treatment. Instruct to promptly report bleeding, bruising, diarrhea, rash, or any other new symptoms to a health care provider.

SERIOUS ADVERSE REACTIONS

- **Hypersensitivity reactions:** Ranging from chills, fever, and rash to anaphylaxis.
- **Management:** Maintain patent airway and support ventilation. Endotracheal intubation should be done promptly for signs of respiratory distress following administration. Hypotension should be managed with IV fluids and then, vasopressors. Epinephrine and *diphenhydrAMINE are used to help control allergic reaction. Corticosteroids are used if other measures do not provide complete relief of symptoms.
- **Antibiotic-associated colitis:** Antibiotic-associated colitis and other superinfections may result from high dosages or prolonged therapy.

OVERDOSE/TOXICITY

- **Hematologic:** Hemolytic anemia, thrombocytopenia, leukopenia.
- **Neurotoxicity:** Neuropathy, hyperreflexia, seizures, coma.
- **Nephrotoxicity:** Elevated BUN, creatinine, oliguria, nausea, edema.
- **GI decontamination:** No specific recommendations.

ANTIDOTE/DIALYSIS

- **Antidote:** No specific recommendations.
- **Dialysis:** Penicillin is removed by hemodialysis and is likely to be removed by high-permeability hemodialysis. It is not removed by peritoneal dialysis.

pentamidine isethionate

pen-tam'-i-deen eyes-eth'-ee-oh-nate

Classes

Chemical: aromatic diamidine derivative
Therapeutic: antiprotozoal

Pregnancy Category: C

Trade Names

Prescription: NebuPent, Pentam 300

CLINICAL PHARMACOLOGY

Mechanism of Action

An antiinfective that interferes with nuclear metabolism and incorporation of nucleotides, inhibiting DNA, RNA, phospholipid, and protein synthesis. **Therapeutic Effect:** Produces antibacterial and antiprotozoal effects.

PHARMACOKINETICS

Well absorbed after IM administration; minimally absorbed after inhalation. Widely distributed. Primarily excreted in urine. Not removed by hemodialysis. **Half-life:** 6.5 hr (increased in impaired renal function).

AVAILABILITY

Injection (Pentam-300): 300 mg.
Powder for nebulization (NebuPent): 300 mg.

INDICATIONS AND DOSAGE

***Pneumocystis carinii* pneumonia (PCP)**

IV, IM

Adults, Elderly: 4 mg/kg/day once per day for 14 days. **Children:** 4 mg/kg/day once per day for 10-14 days.

Prevention of PCP

Inhalation

Adults, Elderly: 300 mg once every 4 wk. **Children 5 yr and older:** 300 mg every 3-4 wk. **Children younger than 5 yr:** 8 mg/kg/dose once every 3-4 wk.

OFF-LABEL USES

Treatment of African trypanosomiasis, cutaneous or visceral leishmaniasis

CONTRAINDICATIONS

Hypersensitivity to pentamidine

INTERACTIONS

Drug: Blood dyscrasia-producing medications, bone marrow depressants: May increase the abnormal hematologic effects of pentamidine. **Didanosine:** May increase the risk of pancreatitis. **Foscarnet:** May increase the risk of hypocalcemia, hypomagnesemia, and nephrotoxicity of pentamidine. **Nephrotoxic medications:** May increase the risk of nephrotoxicity. **Herbal:** None known. **Food:** None known.

DIAGNOSTIC TEST EFFECTS

May increase BUN and serum alkaline phosphatase, bilirubin, creatinine, AST (SGOT), and ALT (SGPT) levels. May decrease serum calcium and magnesium levels. May alter blood glucose levels.

IV INCOMPATIBILITIES

Cefazolin (Ancef), cefotaxime (Claforan), ceftazidime (Fortaz), ceftriaxone (Rocephin), fluconazole (Diflucan), foscarnet (Foscavir), interleukin (Proleukin), cefoxitin (Mefoxin), linezolid (Zyvox)

IV COMPATIBILITIES

Diltiazem (Cardizem), gatifloxacin (Tequin) total parenteral nutrition (TPN), zidovudine (Retrovir)

SIDE-EFFECTS

Frequent: Injection (greater than 10%): Abscess, pain at injection site, hypotension, rash, nausea, vomiting, diarrhea, hypoglycemia, hyperglycemia. **Inhalation (greater than 5%):** Fatigue, metallic taste, shortness of breath, decreased appetite, dizziness, rash, cough, chest pain, rash. **Occasional: Injection (10%-1%):** Nausea, decreased appetite, hypotension, fever, rash, altered taste, confusion. **Inhalation (5%-1%):** Diarrhea, headache, anemia, muscle pain. **Rare: Injection (less than 1%):** Neuralgia, thrombocytopenia, phlebitis, dizziness

CRITICAL CARE CONSIDERATIONS

ADMINISTRATION/HANDLING

IV ALERT

- **Storage:** Store vials at room temperature.
- **Reconstitution/dilution:** Reconstitute each vial with 3-5 mL D_5W or sterile water for injection. Withdraw the desired dose and further dilute with 50-250 mL D_5W. IV solution is stable at room temperature for 48 hr.
- **IV intermittent infusion (piggyback):** Infuse over 60 min. Discard any unused portion. Do not give the drug by IV injection or rapid IV infusion because this increases the risk of severe hypotension.
- **Risk of life-threatening hypotension:** Place patients in a supine position during administration; check BP frequently throughout administration; have resuscitative equipment readily available.

IM ALERT

- **Reconstitution:** Reconstitute each 300-mg vial with 3 mL sterile water for injection to provide a concentration of 100 mg/mL.
- **Risk of life-threatening hypotension:** Place in a supine position during administration. Check BP frequently throughout administration. Have resuscitative equipment readily available.

AEROSOL (NEBULIZER) ALERT

- **Storage:** Store the aerosol at room temperature for 48 hr.
- **Reconstitution:** Reconstitute each 300-mg vial with 6 mL sterile water for injection. Avoid using 0.9% NaCl because it may cause a precipitate to form.

- **Nebulize separately:** Do not mix pentamidine with other medications in the nebulizer reservoir.
- **Respirgard nebulizer:** Do not use the respirgard nebulizer to administer bronchodilating medications.

PRECAUTIONS

HEALTH-RELATED

- **PCP:** Pentamidine should only be used if patients are not successfully treated by sulfamethoxazole-trimethoprim, the drug of choice for PCP. Patients should have a confirmed diagnosis of PCP before initiating pentamidine.
- Use pentamidine cautiously in patients with diabetes mellitus, hypoglycemia, hyperglycemia, hypertension, hypotension, thrombocytopenia, leukopenia, anemia, renal or hepatic impairment, history of ventricular tachycardia, pancreatitis, or Stevens–Johnson syndrome.

AGE-RELATED

- **Children:** No age-related precautions have been noted in children.
- **Elderly:** Little information is available; age-related organ impairment may prompt a dosage adjustment.

PREGNANCY/LACTATION-RELATED

- Pregnancy category C. Because aerosolized pentamidine results in very low systemic concentrations, fetal exposure to the drug is probably negligible. Breast milk levels following aerosolized administration are likely nil.

MONITORING

- **Baseline assessment:** Assess for history of HIV or other immunosuppressive process/medications. Determine whether patients are receiving nephrotoxic drugs and avoid concurrent use. Measure vital signs and point of care blood glucose reading.
- **Baseline lab work:** CBC with WBC differential and platelet count, biochemical profile including glucose and calcium values, renal (BUN, creatinine) and liver (AST [SGOT], ALT [SGPT], alkaline phosphatase, GGT, bilirubin) function tests. Obtain specimens for diagnostic tests before giving the first dose of pentamidine.
- **Ongoing lab work:** Monitor CBC with WBC differential; biochemical profile with renal and liver function tests may be done daily.
- **Diagnostic tests:** 12-lead ECG to assess for myocardial ischemia and underlying dysrhythmias.
- **Dysrhythmias:** Monitor ECG continuously to assess for tachycardia, ventricular dysrhythmias, and life-threatening ventricular dysrhythmias.
- **Hypotension:** Monitor BP closely and keep supine until stable during both IM and IV pentamidine administration. Hypotension can be fatal.
- **Blood glucose changes:** Check blood glucose levels and assess for hypoglycemia (diaphoresis, double vision, headache, incoordination, lightheadedness, nervousness, numbness of lips, palpitations, tachycardia, and tremor) and hyperglycemia (abdominal pain, headache, malaise, nausea, polydipsia, polyphagia, polyuria, visual changes, and vomiting); can be fatal.
- **Bronchospasm:** Inhaled pentamidine may cause respiratory distress secondary to bronchospasms in patients with history of asthma or smoking.
- **Injection sites:** Evaluate IM sites for induration, pain, and redness.
- **IV sites:** Evaluate IV sites for evidence of phlebitis, such as heat, pain, and red streaking over the vein.
- **Rash:** Examine skin for rash.
- **Patient education:** Teach to remain flat in bed during pentamidine administration and to get up slowly with assistance when stable. Instruct to report immediately lightheadedness, palpitations, shakiness, or sweating, or shortness of breath to a health care provider. Instruct to report cough, fever, unusual bruising or bleeding to a health care provider. Inform that drowsiness, decreased appetite, and increased thirst and urination may develop in the months following therapy. Instruct to drink plenty of water to maintain adequate hydration. Urge avoidance of alcohol during therapy.

SERIOUS ADVERSE REACTIONS

- **Risk of death:** Pentamidine administration has resulted in fatalities from hypotension, hypoglycemia, and cardiac dysrhythmias during the first dose.
- **Hypersensitivity:** Rash, urticaria, anaphylactic shock, Stevens–Johnson syndrome, and toxic epidural necrolysis.
- **Cardiovascular decompensation:** Life-threatening or fatal hypotension, dysrhythmias including ventricular tachycardia.

- **Hyperglycemia/hypoglycemia:** Blood glucose changes are common during therapy and may become life threatening if unmanaged; hyperglycemia and insulin-dependent diabetes mellitus (often permanent) may occur even months after therapy has stopped.
- **Bronchospasm:** If respiratory distress consistently occurs, patients may benefit from using an inhaled bronchodilator prior to pentamidine administration.
- **Incidence of side effects:** Over 50% of patients experience side effects, which may be life threatening.

OVERDOSE/TOXICITY

- **Nephrotoxicity:** Elevated BUN and creatinine, oliguria, nausea, edema, nephritis.
- **Hepatotoxicity:** Elevated liver enzymes, nausea, right upper quadrant pain, dark urine, edema, hepatitis (rare).
- **Pancreatitis:** Abdominal pain, nausea, vomiting; hyperglycemia and diabetes mellitus; pancreatic necrosis with high plasma insulin levels and hypoglycemia.
- **Hematologic:** Anemia, leukopenia, thrombocytopenia leading to abnormal bleeding and further immunosuppression.
- **Management:** Discontinue pentamidine if life-threatening side effects occur. Provide supportive care and resuscitation according to accepted guidelines.
- **GI decontamination:** No specific recommendations.

ANTIDOTE/DIALYSIS

- **Antidote:** No specific recommendations.
- **Dialysis:** Pentamidine is not removed by hemodialysis or peritoneal dialysis. No data are available on removal by high-permeability hemodialysis.

pentazocaine

See Opioid Analgesics (p. 980)

pergolide mesylate

per'-go-lide mes'-sil-ate

Classes

Chemical: ergoline derivative
Therapeutic: anti-Parkinson's agent, dopaminergic

Pregnancy Category: B

Trade Names

Prescription: Permax

Do not confuse Permax with Pentrax or Pernox.

CLINICAL PHARMACOLOGY

Mechanism of Action

A centrally active dopamine agonist that directly stimulates dopamine receptors. **Therapeutic Effect:** Decreases signs and symptoms of Parkinson's disease.

PHARMACOKINETICS

Well absorbed from the GI tract. Protein binding: 90%. Undergoes extensive first-pass metabolism in the liver. Primarily excreted in urine. **Half-life:** 27 hr.

AVAILABILITY

Tablets: 0.05 mg, 0.25 mg, 1 mg.

INDICATIONS AND DOSAGE

Parkinsonism

PO

Adults, Elderly: Initially, 0.05 mg/day for 2 days. May increase by 0.1-0.15 mg/day every 3 days over the next 12 days; afterward may increase by 0.25 mg/day every 3 days. Range: 2-3 mg/day in 3 divided doses. Maximum: 5 mg/day.

OFF-LABEL USES

Chronic motor or vocal tic disorder, Tourette's disorder

CONTRAINDICATIONS

Hypersensitivity to pergolide or other ergot derivatives

INTERACTIONS

Drug: Haloperidol, loxapine, methyldopa, metoclopramide, phenothiazines: May decrease the effectiveness of pergolide. **Hypotension-producing medications:** May increase the hypotensive effect. **Herbal:** None known. **Food:** None known.

DIAGNOSTIC TEST EFFECTS

May increase the serum growth hormone level.

SIDE-EFFECTS

Frequent (24%-10%): Nausea, dizziness, hallucinations, constipation, rhinitis, dystonia, confusion, somnolence. **Occasional (9%-3%):** Orthostatic hypotension, insomnia, dry mouth, peripheral edema, anxiety, diarrhea, dyspepsia, abdominal pain, headache, abnormal vision, anorexia, tremor, depression, rash. **Rare (less than 2%):** Urinary frequency, vivid dreams, neck pain, hypotension, vomiting

CRITICAL CARE CONSIDERATIONS

ADMINISTRATION/HANDLING

PO ALERT

- Pergolide is usually given in 3 divided doses daily.
- Crush scored tablets as needed.
- Give pergolide without regard to food.

PRECAUTIONS

HEALTH-RELATED

- Use pergolide cautiously in patients with preexisting cardiac dysrhythmias, confusion, or hallucinations.

AGE-RELATED

- **Children:** Safety and efficacy of pergolide have not been established in children.
- **Elderly:** Age-related renal impairment may prompt a dosage adjustment.

PREGNANCY/LACTATION-RELATED

- Pregnancy category B; may interfere with lactation.

MONITORING

- **Baseline assessment:** Monitor BP and heart rate for hypotension and irregularities indicative of dysrhythmias. Assess other medications used to manage Parkinson's disease. Assess neurological and mental status.
- **Baseline lab work:** Biochemical profile including renal (BUN, creatinine) function tests.
- **Baseline diagnostic tests:** 12-lead ECG for patients with a history of cardiac disease.
- **Neurologic effects:** Monitor for agitation, headache, lethargy, confusion, tremors, and dyskinesia.
- **Cardiovascular effects:** Monitor continuous ECG in critically ill patients and monitor for hypotension. Monitor for myocardial and cerebral ischemia.
- **Therapeutic effect:** Assess for relief of parkinsonian symptoms including improvement of masklike facial expression, muscular rigidity, shuffling gait, and resting tremors of the hands and head.
- **Patient education:** Inform that dizziness, drowsiness, and dry mouth are expected side effects of pergolide. Warn to avoid tasks that require mental alertness or motor skills until response to the drug is known. Urge to avoid alcoholic beverages during therapy.

SERIOUS ADVERSE REACTIONS

- **Hypotension:** Approximately 10% of patients taking pergolide in clinical trials experienced symptomatic hypotension.
- **Parkinson's disease:** Visual or auditory hallucinations.
- **Long-term therapy:** May produce rhinorrhea, syncope, GI hemorrhage, peptic ulcer, severe abdominal pain, confusion, and psychosis.
- **Acute vasospastic crisis:** May result in cerebral, myocardial, or mesenteric ischemia.
- **Inflammation and fibrosis:** Rare case reports include pleuritis, pleural effusion, pulmonary fibrosis, pericarditis, pericardial effusion, cardiac valvulopathy, and retroperitoneal fibrosis.

OVERDOSE/TOXICITY

- **Overdose:** Symptoms may vary from CNS depression (sedation, apnea, "sleep attacks," cardiovascular collapse, and death) to severe paradoxic reactions (hallucinations, tremor, and seizures).
- **Management:** Maintain patent airway and support ventilation. Support BP with IV fluids and then vasopressors if necessary. Monitor and manage dysrhythmias, acid/base and fluid/electrolyte imbalance.
- **GI decontamination:** Activated charcoal may be more effective than ipecac for emesis or gastric lavage for overdose.

ANTIDOTE/DIALYSIS

- **Antidote:** Cyprohepadine, alprotadil, and epoprostenol have been used to manage ergot-induced vasospasms.
- **Dialysis:** Pergolide is unlikely to be removed by hemodialysis or peritoneal dialysis. No data are available on removal using high-permeability hemodialysis.

perindopril erbumine

See ACE Inhibitors (p. 883)

perphenazine

See Anticonvulsants (p. 903)

phenelzine sulfate

fen'-el-zeen sul'-fate

Classes
Chemical: hydrazine derivative
Therapeutic: antidepressant, MAOI

Pregnancy Category: C

Trade Names
Prescription: Nardil

CLINICAL PHARMACOLOGY

Mechanism of Action

An MAOI that inhibits the activity of the enzyme monoamine oxidase at CNS storage sites, leading to increased levels of the neurotransmitters epinephrine, norepinephrine, serotonin, and dopamine at neuronal receptor sites. **Therapeutic Effect:** Relieves depression.

PHARMACOKINETICS

Well absorbed from GI tract. Metabolized in the liver. Primarily excreted in urine. **Half-life:** 11 hr.

AVAILABILITY

Tablets: 15 mg.

INDICATIONS AND DOSAGE

Depression refractory to other antidepressants or electroconvulsive therapy

PO

Adults: 15 mg 3 times per day. May increase to 60-90 mg/day. **Elderly:** Initially, 7.5 mg/day. May increase by 7.5-15 mg/day every 3-4 days up to 60 mg/day in 3-4 divided doses.

OFF-LABEL USES

Treatment of panic disorder, selective mutism, vascular or tension headaches

CONTRAINDICATIONS

Cardiovascular or cerebrovascular disease, hepatic or renal impairment, pheochromocytoma, hypersensitivity to phenelzine, uncontrolled hypertension, heart failure, ethanol, meperidine, buproprion, guanethidine, general anesthesia, spinal anesthesia, foods high in tyramine, tryptophan, *DOPamine, chocolate, caffeine

INTERACTIONS

Drug: Alcohol, other CNS depressants: May increase CNS depression. ***BusPIRone:** May increase BP. **Caffeine-containing medications:** May increase the risk of cardiac dysrhythmias and hypertension. **Carbamazepine, cyclobenzaprine, maprotiline, other MAOIs:** May precipitate hypertensive crisis. ***DOPamine, tryptophan:** May cause sudden, severe hypertension. **Fluoxetine, trazodone, tricyclic antidepressants:** May cause serotonin syndrome. **Insulin, oral antidiabetics:** May increase the effects of these drugs. **Meperidine, other opioid analgesics:** May produce diaphoresis, immediate excitation, rigidity, and severe hypertension or hypotension, sometimes leading to severe respiratory distress, vascular collapse, seizures, coma, and death. **Methylphenidate:** May increase the CNS stimulant effects of methylphenidate. **Sympathomimetics:** May increase the cardiac stimulant and vasopressor effects of phenelzine. **Herbal:** None known. **Food: Caffeine, chocolate, tyramine-containing foods (such as aged cheese):** May cause hypertensive crisis. These foods are contraindicated when using Nardil (phenelzine).

DIAGNOSTIC TEST EFFECTS

None known.

SIDE-EFFECTS

Frequent: Orthostatic hypotension, restlessness, GI upset, insomnia, dizziness, headache, lethargy, asthenia, dry mouth, peripheral edema. **Occasional:** Flushing, diaphoresis, rash, urinary frequency, increased appetite, transient impotence. **Rare:** Visual disturbances

CRITICAL CARE CONSIDERATIONS

ADMINISTRATION/HANDLING

PO ALERT

- Store phenelzine tablets at room temperature. Do not freeze.
- Administer phenelzine with food or milk to alleviate GI symptoms.
- Avoid pickled herring, liver, dry sausage (e.g., salami, pepperoni, Lebanon bologna), fava or other broad-bean pods, cheese (may have cottage and cream cheeses), yogurt, beer, wine, excessive chocolate and caffeine, products containing brewer's yeast.
- Tablets may be crushed if patients have difficulty swallowing; give with food or fluids.

PRECAUTIONS

HEALTH-RELATED

- Use phenelzine cautiously in patients with cardiac dysrhythmias, frequent or severe headaches, hypertension, and suicidal tendencies.
- Use phenelzine cautiously within several hr of ingestion of a contraindicated substance, such as tyramine-containing foods (avocados, bananas, broad beans, figs, papayas, raisins, sour cream, soy sauce, beer, wine, yeast extracts, meat tenderizers, and smoked or pickled meats).

AGE-RELATED

- **Children:** Safety and efficacy of phenelzine have not been established in children under 16 yr.
- **Elderly:** Age-related organ impairment may warrant a dosage adjustment.

PREGNANCY/LACTATION-RELATED

- Pregnancy category C; unknown if excreted in breast milk.

MONITORING

- **Baseline assessment:** Assess BP and heart rate. Determine history of hypertension, heart disease, and liver disease. Ensure patients understand it is necessary to avoid a number of foods and OTC medications while taking phenelzine.
- **Baseline and ongoing lab work:** Biochemical profile including renal (BUN, creatinine) and liver (AST [SGOT], ALT [SGPT], alkaline phosphatase, GGT, bilirubin) function tests. Perform periodically throughout therapy.
- **Baseline diagnostic tests:** 12-lead ECG to assess for myocardial ischemia; chest x-ray to evaluate for heart failure.
- **Ongoing monitoring:** Monitor BP, heart rate, diet, and weight.
- **Therapeutic effect:** Monitor continuous ECG in critically ill patients and monitor for hypotension. Monitor for myocardial and cerebral ischemia.
- **Therapeutic effect:** Assess for improved appearance, behavior, level of interest, mood, and sleep pattern.
- **Suicidal patients:** Closely supervise suicidal patients during early therapy. As depression lessens, energy level improves, increasing the suicide potential.
- **Hypertensive crisis:** Monitor for occipital headache radiating frontally and neck stiffness or soreness, which may be the first symptoms of an impending hypertensive crisis. If hypertensive crisis occurs, administer phentolamine 5-10 mg IV.
- **Patient education:** Explain that depression may start to lift during the first wk of therapy; phenelzine's full therapeutic effect may require 2-6 wk of therapy. Instruct to report promptly headache or neck soreness or stiffness to a health care provider. Urge avoidance of foods that require bacteria or molds for their preparation or preservation (such as yogurt and aged cheese); foods containing tyramine (including avocados, bananas, broad beans, figs, papayas, raisins, sour cream, soy sauce, beer, wine, yeast extracts, meat tenderizers, and smoked or pickled meats); and excessive amounts of caffeine-containing foods or beverages (such as chocolate, coffee, and tea). Warn to avoid using OTC preparations for colds, hay fever, and weight reduction (cold and cough medications, nasal decongestants including nose drops and spray, sinus medications, asthma inhalants, appetite suppressants, "high energy" formulas used for fatigue and weight loss, L-tryptophan containing formulas).

SERIOUS ADVERSE REACTIONS

- **Hypertensive crisis:** Severe hypertension, occipital headache radiating frontally, neck stiffness or soreness, nausea, vomiting, diaphoresis, fever or chilliness, clammy skin, dilated pupils, palpitations, tachycardia or bradycardia, and constricting chest pain.
- **Tyramine reaction:** Reaction is variable, but hallmark sign is occipital or temporal headache associated with hypertension, palpitations, neck stiffness, diaphoresis, excitation, and chest discomfort. Rare fatalities have been reported from intracranial hemorrhage or myocardial infarction.
- **Management:** For hypertension associated with crisis and tyramine reaction, administer phentolamine 5-10 mg IV. Avoid betablockers which may worsen hypertension.

OVERDOSE/TOXICITY

- **Two distinct MAOI overdose characteristics:** The difference between a therapeutic dose and lethal dose is less with MAOIs than with other antidepressants; less than twice the therapeutic dose may be toxic. Second, the symptoms of toxicity are delayed far beyond the normal observation period for patients taking other antidepressants.

- **Overdose symptoms:** May be nonspecific. There is no typical presentation or progression of symptoms. There may be a latent period followed by rapid deterioration with life-threatening symptoms.
- **Initial/mild symptoms of toxicity:** Initial symptoms include headache, agitation, irritability, tremor, nausea, and palpitations. Patients may experience tachycardia, hyperreflexia, drowsiness, hyperactivity, mydriasis, fasciculations, hyperventilation, flushing, and nystagmus with mild toxicity.
- **Moderate toxicity:** Muscle rigidity, opisthonos, marked hyperthermia, diaphoresis, hypertension, chest pain, diarrhea, hallucinations, confusion, combativeness and "ping-pong gaze" with bilateral horizontal eye movements.
- **Severe toxicity:** Bradycardia, hypotension, respiratory failure, cardiac arrest, seizures. Hyperkalemia, metabolic acidosis, and rhabdomyolysis are possible. Hypotension is resistant to management.
- **Management:** No well-controlled studies on management of overdose. Provide supportive care. Onset is gradual and may be delayed to 24 hr following ingestion. Provide patent airway and support ventilation.
- **GI decontamination:** Syrup of ipecac is contraindicated. Activated charcoal should be administered in a single dose. Gastric lavage may be attempted if patients present within 1 hr of ingestion.

ANTIDOTE/DIALYSIS

- **Antidote:** No specific recommendations.
- **Dialysis:** No data are available on removal of phenylzine by hemodialysis, high-permeability hemodialysis, or peritoneal dialysis. One source stated hemodialysis, hemoperfusion, and peritoneal dialysis have no established role in management of MAOI overdose.

phenindomine

See Antihistamines (p. 925)

phenobarbital

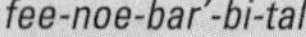

fee-noe-bar'-bi-tal

DEA Schedule: IV

Classes

Chemical: barbituric acid derivative

Therapeutic: anticonvulsant, sedative/hypnotic

Pregnancy Category: D

Trade Names

Prescription: Luminal

Combinations

Prescription: with atropine, hyoscyamine, scopolamine (Donnatal); with belladonna, ergotamine (Bellergal Spacetabs)

Do not confuse phenobarbital with pentobarbital, or Luminal with Tuinal.

CLINICAL PHARMACOLOGY

Mechanism of Action

A barbiturate that enhances the activity of gamma-aminobutyric acid (GABA) by binding to the GABA receptor complex. **Therapeutic Effect:** Depresses CNS activity.

PHARMACOKINETICS

Route	Onset	Peak	Duration
PO	20-60 min	N/A	6-10 hr
IV	5 min	30 min	4-10 hr

Well absorbed after PO or parenteral administration. Protein binding: 35%-50%. Rapidly and widely distributed. Metabolized in the liver. Primarily excreted in urine. Removed by hemodialysis. **Half-life:** 53-140 hr.

AVAILABILITY

Elixir: 15 mg/5 mL, 20 mg/5 mL.

Tablets: 15 mg, 30 mg, 32.4 mg, 60 mg, 64.8 mg, 97.2 mg, 100 mg.

Injection: 30 mg/mL, 60 mg/mL, 65 mg/mL, 130 mg/mL.

INDICATIONS AND DOSAGE

Status epilepticus

IV

Adults, Elderly: Initially, 300-800 mg, then 120-240 mg/dose at 20 min intervals until seizures are controlled or total dose of 1-2 g administered. **Children, Infants:** 10-20 mg/kg. May administer additional 5 mg/kg/dose every 15-30 min until seizures controlled or total dose of 40 mg/kg administered.

Seizure control

PO, IV

Adults, Elderly, Children older than 12 yr: 1-3 mg/kg/day or 50-100 mg 2-3 times per day. **Children 6-12 yr:** 4-6 mg/kg/day in 1-2 divided doses. **Children 1-5 yr:** 6-8 mg/kg/day in 1-2 divided doses.

Children younger than 1 yr: 5-8 mg/kg/day in 1-2 divided doses. **Neonates:** 3-4 mg/kg/day as a single dose.

Sedation

PO, IM

Adults, Elderly: 30-120 mg/day in 2-3 divided doses.

PO

Children: 2 mg/kg 3 times per day.

Hypnotic

PO, IV, IM, Subcutaneous

Adults, Elderly: 100-320 mg at bedtime. **Children:** 3-5 mg/kg at bedtime.

OFF-LABEL USES

Prevention and treatment of febrile seizures in children and hyperbilirubinemia, management of sedative or hypnotic withdrawal

CONTRAINDICATIONS

Hypersensitivity to phenobarbital or other barbiturates, porphyria, preexisting CNS depression, severe pain, severe respiratory disease

INTERACTIONS

Drug: Alcohol, other CNS depressants: May increase the effects of phenobarbital. **Carbamazepine:** May increase the metabolism of carbamazepine. **Digoxin, glucocorticoids, metronidazole, oral anticoagulants, quinidine, tricyclic antidepressants:** May decrease the effects of these drugs. **Valproic acid:** Increases the blood concentration and risk of toxicity of phenobarbital. **Herbal:** None known. **Food:** None known.

DIAGNOSTIC TEST EFFECTS

May decrease serum bilirubin level. Therapeutic serum level is 10-40 mcg/mL; toxic serum level is greater than 40 mcg/mL.

IV INCOMPATIBILITIES

Amphotericin B complex (Abelcet, AmBisome, Amphotec), hydrocortisone (Solu-Cortef), hydromorphone (Dilaudid), insulin

IV COMPATIBILITIES

Calcium gluconate, enalapril (Vasotec), fentanyl (Sublimaze), fosphenytoin (Cerebyx), morphine, propofol (Diprivan)

SIDE-EFFECTS

Occasional (3%-1%): Somnolence, lethargy. **Rare (less than 1%):** Confusion; paradoxic CNS reactions, such as hyperactivity or nervousness in children and excitement or restlessness in the elderly (generally noted during first 2 wk of therapy, particularly in the presence of uncontrolled pain)

CRITICAL CARE CONSIDERATIONS

ADMINISTRATION/HANDLING

PO ALERT

- Give phenobarbital without regard to food.
- May crush tablets as needed.
- Elixir may be mixed with fruit juice, milk, or water.

IV ALERT

- **Storage:** Store vials at room temperature.
- **Hydration:** Adequately hydrate patients before and immediately after infusion to decrease the risk of adverse renal effects.
- **Preparation:** Phenobarbital may be given undiluted or may be diluted with NaCl, D_5W, or lactated Ringer's solution.
- **IV infusion:** Do not exceed an injection rate of 30 mg/min for children and 60 mg/min for adults (weighing more than 60 kg). Injecting too rapidly may produce marked respiratory depression and severe hypotension.
- **Maintenance dose:** Administer maintenance dose 12 hr after the loading dose.
- **Accidental intraarterial injection:** Inadvertent intraarterial injection may result in arterial spasm with severe pain and tissue necrosis; extravasation in subcutaneous tissue may produce redness, tenderness, and tissue necrosis. For either, inject 0.5% procaine solution into the affected area and apply moist heat.

IM ALERT

- Do not inject more than 5 mL in any one injection site; may cause tissue irritation. Inject the drug deep intramuscularly.

PRECAUTIONS

HEALTH-RELATED

- Use phenobarbital cautiously in patients with hepatic or renal impairment.

AGE-RELATED

- **Children:** Phenobarbital use may cause paradoxic excitement in children.
- **Elderly:** Age-related organ impairment may prompt a reduced dose. May exhibit confusion, excitement, and mental depression; more likely to cause barbiturate induced hypothermia.

PREGNANCY/LACTATION-RELATED

- Pregnancy category D. Risks to fetus include minor congenital defects, hemorrhage at

P

birth, addiction. Risk to mother may be greater if seizure control is lost due to stopping drug; use at lowest possible level to control seizures. Excreted into breast milk; has caused major adverse effects in some nursing infants; use caution in nursing women.

MONITORING

- **Baseline assessment:** Assess BP, pulse rate, and respiratory rate immediately before giving phenobarbital. Review the seizure patient history of the seizure disorder (duration, frequency, and intensity of seizures).
- **Baseline and ongoing lab work:** Biochemical profile with renal (BUN, creatinine) and liver (AST [SGOT], ALT [SGPT], alkaline phosphatase, GGT, bilirubin) function studies.
- **Seizure precautions:** Initiate seizure precautions and observe frequently for a recurrence of seizure activity. Status epilepticus can occur from too rapid withdrawal of phenobarbital.
- **Drug as hypnotic:** Provide conditions conducive to sleep, such as a quiet environment with low lighting. Raise the bed rails as a safety precaution.
- **Response to drug:** Monitor for hypotension, respiratory depression, level of consciousness, and seizure activity. Phenobarbital levels should be monitored.
- **Drug levels:** Therapeutic phenobarbital level is 10-40 mcg/mL; toxic phenobarbital level is greater than 40 mcg/mL.
- **Patient education:** Caution against discontinuing phenobarbital abruptly to avoid withdrawal. Urge avoidance of alcohol consumption and limiting caffeine intake while taking phenobarbital. Inform that phenobarbital may be habit forming. Warn to avoid tasks that require mental alertness or motor skills until response to the drug is known. Advise always carrying an identification card or wearing an identification bracelet to display the seizure disorder and anticonvulsant therapy.

SERIOUS ADVERSE REACTIONS

- **Abrupt withdrawal after prolonged use:** May produce increased dreaming, nightmares, insomnia, tremor, diaphoresis, nausea and vomiting, hallucinations, delirium, seizures, and status epilepticus.
- **Hypersensitivity reaction:** Rash, urticaria, angioedema, anaphylaxis.
- **Hypocalcemia:** Occurs rarely.

OVERDOSE/TOXICITY

- **Overdose:** Respiratory depression, Cheyne-Stokes respirations, apnea, pulmonary edema, cyanosis, tachycardia, delirium, coma, hypotension, hypothermia, severe CNS depression, flat EEG (reversible unless hypoxic damage has occurred), sluggish or absent reflexes.
- **Nephrotoxicity:** Elevated BUN, creatinine, oliguria, nausea, edema, nephritis.
- **Hepatotoxicity:** Elevated liver enzymes, right upper quadrant pain, edema, nausea, vomiting, jaundice.
- **Hematologic:** Thrombocytopenia, thrombocytopenic purpura.
- **Management:** Maintain patent airway and support ventilation. Endotracheal intubation and mechanical ventilation may be needed. Support BP with IV fluids, then vasopressors if needed. Keep warm. Diuretics may promote elimination of the drug.
- **GI decontamination:** No specific recommendations.

ANTIDOTE/DIALYSIS

- **Antidote:** No specific recommendations.
- **Dialysis:** Phenobarbital is removed by hemodialysis, high-permeability hemodialysis, and peritoneal dialysis.

phensuximide

See Anticonvulsants (p. 903)

phentolamine mesylate

fen-tole'-a-meen meh'-sil-ate

Classes

Chemical: imidazoline derivative
Therapeutic: pheochromocytoma agent, sympatholytic

Pregnancy Category: C

Trade Names

Prescription: Regitine

CLINICAL PHARMACOLOGY

Mechanism of Action

An alpha-adrenergic blocking agent that produces peripheral vasodilation and cardiac stimulation. **Therapeutic Effect:** Decreases BP.

PHARMACOKINETICS

Poorly absorbed from the GI tract. Protein binding: 72%. Metabolized in liver. Eliminated in urine and feces. **Half-life:** 19 min.

AVAILABILITY

Injection: 5 mg/mL (Regitine).

INDICATIONS AND DOSAGE

Extravasation—norepinephrine

Subcutaneous

Adults, Elderly: Infiltrate area with a small amount (1 mL) of solution (made by diluting 5-10 mg in 10 mL of normal saline [NS]) within 12 hr of extravasation. Do not exceed 0.1-0.2 mg/kg or 5 mg total. If dose is effective, normal skin color should return to the blanched area within 1 hr. **Children:** Infiltrate area with a small amount (1 mL) of solution (made by diluting 5-10 mg in 10 mL of NS) within 12 hr of extravasation. Do not exceed 0.1-0.2 mg/kg or 5 mg total.

Diagnosis of pheochromocytoma

IM/IV

Adults, Elderly: 5 mg as a single dose. **Children:** 0.05-0.1 mg/kg/dose. Maximum single dose: 5 mg.

Surgery for pheochromocytoma: Hypertension

IM/IV

Adults, Elderly: 5 mg given 1-2 hr before procedure and repeated as needed every 2-4 hr. **Children:** 0.05-0.1 mg/kg/dose given 1-2 hr before procedure. Repeat as needed every 2-4 hr until hypertension is controlled. Maximum single dose: 5 mg.

Hypertensive crisis

IV

Adults, Elderly: 5-20 mg as a single dose.

OFF-LABEL USES

Treatment of pralidoxime-induced hypertension, dysrhythmias, asthma, bladder instability, cardiac diseases, diabetes mellitus, erectile dysfunction, extravasation (*DOPamine and epinephrine), hyperhidrosis, myocardial infarction, Raynaud's phenomenon, surgery, sympathetic pain

CONTRAINDICATIONS

Renal impairment, coronary or cerebral arteriosclerosis, concurrent use with phosphodiesterase-5 (PDE-5) inhibitors including sildenafil (greater than 25 mg), tadalafil, or vardenafil, hypersensitivity to phentolamine or related compounds.

INTERACTIONS

Drug: Alcohol: May increase the risk of disulfiram-type reactions. **Beta-blockers:** May exaggerate hypotensive effects. **Epinephrine, ephedrine:** May decrease the effects of phentolamine. **Sildenafil, tadalafil, vardenafil:** May increase BP-lowering effects. **Herbal:** None known. **Food:** None known.

DIAGNOSTIC TEST EFFECTS

May increase liver function tests.

IV INCOMPATIBILITIES

Iron

IV COMPATIBILITIES

Amiodarone (Cordarone), *DOBUTamine (Dobutrex), norepinephrine (Levophed), papaverine (Papacon), verapamil

SIDE-EFFECTS

Occasional: Hypotension, tachycardia, dysrhythmia, flushing, orthostatic hypotension, weakness, dizziness, nausea, vomiting, diarrhea, nasal congestion, pulmonary hypertension

CRITICAL CARE CONSIDERATIONS

ADMINISTRATION/HANDLING

IV ALERT

- **Allocation or distribution:** Phentolamine is available only in limited supply via the manufacturer (Novartis). Hospitals are required to fax requests for additional medication to Novartis with a copy of the physician's order for the drug. This drug should not be routinely used for BP control; alternatives are available.
- **Epinephrine and ephedrine:** Phentolamine antagonizes effects of both drugs.
- **Necrosis prevention:** May add 5 mg to every 500 mL vasopressor infusion bag (e.g., norepinephrine) to help prevent necrosis if IV infiltrates/extravasation.
- **Off-label uses:** Treatment of heart failure, rebound hypertension occurring after an antihypertensive medication is discontinued or hypertensive crisis secondary to MAOI use in patients who received catecholamine infusions.

SUBCUTANEOUS ALERT

- **IV infiltration/vasopressor extravasation:** Infiltrate the entire area of alpha adrenergic catecholamine (i.e., *DOPamine, epinephrine, neosynephrine, norepinephrine) extravasation with multiple small injections using only 27- or 30-gauge needles. Change the needle between each skin entry. One source stated if IV catheter is still in place, phentolamine may be injected through the catheter if the care

P

provider is certain the IV has moved out of the vein into the subcutaneous tissues.

- **Dilution:** Reconstitute each 5 mg with 1 mL sterile water or saline. May be further diluted with 5-10 mL of sterile water or saline. Prepare immediately before use.

PRECAUTIONS

HEALTH-RELATED

- Use cautiously in patients with gastritis or peptic ulcer, tachycardia, or history of dysrhythmias. Normal sinus rhythm is the preferred rhythm when drug is used.
- **Pheochromocytoma diagnosis:** Consider urinary tests for VMA (vanillylmandelic acid) as a safer, effective alternative. Phentolamine should be used only if alternative testing is not possible.

AGE-RELATED

- **Children:** No age-related precautions in children have been noted.
- **Elderly:** May be more sensitive to the hypotensive effects of phentolamine.

PREGNANCY/LACTATION-RELATED

- Pregnancy category C; safety for use in breast-feeding mothers has not been established.

MONITORING

- **Baseline assessment:** Assess vital signs. Examine IV site thoroughly if patients had a vasopressor extravasation. If using drug for BP reduction, assess hydration, and cardiac and renal status before starting medication.
- **Baseline lab work:** Biochemical profile including BUN and creatinine.
- **Baseline diagnostic tests:** 12-lead ECG to check for myocardial ischemia and dysrhythmias.
- **Hypotension:** Monitor for excessive hypotension. Monitor vital signs every 2 min throughout IV administration. Phentolamine is a potent vasodilator. Patients should be monitored closely for at least 20 min following use. Assist with ambulation if dizziness or lightheadedness occurs.
- **Dysrhythmias:** Continuously monitor ECG for all types of tachycardia and ventricular dysrhythmias. Significant changes in rhythm may occur within 2-5 min. Monitor for ST segment depression and elevation.
- **Stroke:** Monitor for headache and deterioration in neurologic status.
- **Acute MI:** Monitor ECG for ST segment elevation and for chest discomfort, shortness of breath, nausea, and diaphoresis.
- **Patient education:** Instruct to report promptly dizziness or palpitations to a health care provider. Warn to avoid tasks requiring mental alertness or motor skills for 12-24 hr after receiving the dose.

SERIOUS ADVERSE REACTIONS

- Mixed alpha- and beta-adrenergic agents, such as epinephrine, may cause more hypotension.

OVERDOSE/TOXICITY

- **Overdose:** Tachycardia, severe hypotension, shock, vomiting (possibly during anesthesia), dizziness; acute myocardial infarction, and acute stroke.
- **Management:** For hypotension, IV fluids and plasma expanders (hetastarch, albumin). Elevate legs. Avoid catecholamines if possible, but epinephrine and ephedrine should definitely NOT be used. If catecholamines are needed, norepinephrine (Levophed) or phenylephrine (Neosynephrine) may be attempted. Avoid use of digitalis drugs (e.g., Lanoxin, digoxin) to manage dysrhythmias.
- **GI decontamination:** No specific recommendations.

ANTIDOTE/DIALYSIS

- **Antidote:** No specific recommendations.
- **Dialysis:** No data are available on removal of phentolamine by hemodialysis, peritoneal dialysis, or high-permeability hemodialysis.

P

phenylephrine hydrochloride

fen-ill-eh'-frin hye-droe-klor'-ide

Classes

Chemical: synthetic catecholamine alpha adrenergic agonist
Therapeutic: decongestant vasopressor

Pregnancy Category: C

Trade Names

Prescription: AK-Dilate, AD-Nephrin, Despec-SF, Mydfrin, Neo-Synephrine, Neo-Synephrine Ophthalmic, Ocu-Phrin, Phenoptic, Prefrin, Rectasol, Sudafed PE Nasal Decongestant

CLINICAL PHARMACOLOGY

Mechanism of Action

A sympathomimetic alpha receptor stimulant that acts on the alpha-adrenergic receptors of vascular smooth muscle. Causes vasoconstriction of arterioles of nasal mucosa or conjunctiva, activates dilator muscle of the pupil to cause contraction, produces systemic arterial vasoconstriction. **Therapeutic Effect:** Decreases mucosal blood flow and relieves congestion and increases systolic BP.

PHARMACOKINETICS

Route	Onset	Peak	Duration
IV	Immediate	N/A	15-30 min
IM	10-15 min	N/A	0.5-2 hr
Subcutaneous	10-15 min	N/A	1 hr

Minimal absorption after intranasal and ophthalmic administration. Metabolized in the liver and GI tract. Primarily excreted in urine. **Half-life:** 2.5 hr.

AVAILABILITY

Injection: 1% (10 mg/mL).
Nasal solution drops (Neo-Synephrine): 0.5%, 1%.
Nasal spray (Neo-Synephrine): 0.25%, 0.5%, 1%.
Ophthalmic solution: 0.12% (AK-Nephrin), 2.5% (AK-Dilate, Mydfrin, Neofrin, Neo-Synephrine Ophthalmic, Ocu-Phrin, Phenoptic), 10% (AK-Dilate, Ocu-Phrin, Neo-Synephrine).
Oral liquid (Despec-SF): 5 mg/5 mL.
Tablets (Sudafed PE nasal decongestant): 10 mg.

INDICATIONS AND DOSAGE

Nasal decongestant

Nasal Spray, Nasal Solution, Nasal Tablet

Adults, Elderly, Children 12 yr and older: 1-2 drops or 1-2 sprays of 0.25%-0.5% solution into each nostril every 4 hr as needed, or 10-20 mg every 4 hr as needed (not more than 6 doses/24 hr). **Children 6-11 yr:** 1-2 drops or 1-2 sprays of 0.25% solution into each nostril every 4 hr as needed for up to 3 days maximum. **Children younger than 6 yr:** 1 drop of 0.125% solution (dilute 0.5% solution with 0.9% NaCl to achieve 0.125%) in each nostril. Repeat every 2-4 hr as needed. Do not use for more than 3 days.

Conjunctival congestion, itching, and minor irritation; whitening of sclera

Ophthalmic

Adults, Elderly, Children 12 yr and older: 1-2 drops of 0.12% solution every 3-4 hr.

Hypotension, shock

IM, Subcutaneous

Adults, Elderly: 2-5 mg/dose every 1-2 hr. Maximum: 10 mg. **Children:** 0.1 mg/kg/dose every 1-2 hr. Maximum: 5 mg.

IV Bolus

Adults, Elderly: 0.1-0.5 mg/dose every 10-15 min as needed. **Children:** 5-20 mcg/kg/dose every 10-15 min.

IV Infusion

Adults, Elderly: 100-180 mcg/min. When BP is stabilized, maintenance rate: 40-60 mcg/min. **Children:** 0.1-0.5 mcg/kg/min. Titrate to desired effect.

CONTRAINDICATIONS

Heart disease, hepatitis, narrow-angle glaucoma, pheochromocytoma, severe hypertension, thrombosis, ventricular tachycardia, hypersensitivity to phenylephrine, use within 14 days of MAOIs.

INTERACTIONS

Drug: Beta-blockers: May have mutually inhibitory effects. **Digoxin:** May increase risk of dysrhythmias. **Ergonovine, oxytocin:** May increase vasoconstriction. **MAOIs:** May increase vasopressor effects. **Maprotiline, tricyclic antidepressants:** May increase cardiovascular effects. **Methyldopa:** May decrease effects of methyldopa. **Herbal:** None known. **Food:** None known.

DIAGNOSTIC TEST EFFECTS

None known.

IV INCOMPATIBILITIES

Thiopentothal (Pentothal)

IV COMPATIBILITIES

Amiodarone (Cordarone), *DOBUTamine (Dobutrex), lidocaine, potassium chloride, propofol (Diprivan)

SIDE-EFFECTS

Frequent: Nasal: Rebound nasal congestion due to overuse, especially when used longer than 3 days. **Occasional:** Mild CNS stimulation (restlessness, nervousness, tremors, headache, insomnia, particularly in those hypersensitive to sympathomimetics, such as elderly patients). **Nasal:** Stinging, burning, drying of nasal mucosa. **Ophthalmic:** Transient burning or stinging, brow ache, blurred vision

CRITICAL CARE CONSIDERATIONS

ADMINISTRATION/HANDLING

NASAL ALERT

- **Administration:** Clear nasal passages (blow nose) before giving the medication. Administer nasal spray into each nostril

P

with the head erect. Tilt the head back and instill the drops in 1 nostril. Sniff briskly while squeezing container; stay in the same position; wait 5 min before applying drops in other nostril. Wait 3-5 min before blowing nose gently. Rinse tip of spray bottle.

OPHTHALMIC ALERT

- **Instillation:** Tilt the head backward and look up. With a gloved finger, gently pull the lower eyelid down to form a pouch. Instill medication into the pouch. Do not touch tip of applicator to eyelids or any surface. When lower eyelid is released, keep the eye open without blinking for at least 30 sec. Apply gentle finger pressure to lacrimal sac, located at the bridge of the nose at inside corner of the eye, for 1-2 min. Remove excess solution around eye with tissue. Wash hands immediately to remove medication on hands.

IV ALERT

- **Storage:** Store vials at room temperature. Protect from light.
- **IV push:** Dilute 1 mL of 10-mg/mL solution with 9 mL sterile water for injection to provide a concentration of 1 mg/mL. Give over 20-30 sec to treat supraventricular tachycardia.
- **IV infusion:** Dilute 10-mg vial with 500 mL D_5W or 0.9% NaCl to provide a concentration of 2 mcg/mL. Maximum concentration: 500 mg/250 mL to help maintain BP during shock states.

P

PRECAUTIONS

HEALTH-RELATED

- Use phenylephrine cautiously in patients with bradycardia, heart block, hyperthyroidism, or severe heart or vascular disease.
- **Sulfite allergy:** Phenylephrine contains bisulfites.
- If phenylephrine 10% ophthalmic is instilled into denuded or damaged corneal epithelium, corneal clouding may result.

AGE-RELATED

- **Children:** May exhibit increased absorption and toxicity with nasal preparation. No age-related precautions have been noted with systemic use in children.
- **Elderly:** More likely to experience adverse effects. Use with extreme caution.

PREGNANCY/LACTATION-RELATED

- Pregnancy category C; safety for use during breast-feeding has not been established.

MONITORING

- **Baseline assessment:** Obtain vital signs, noting heart rate and BP. Assess for irritation of nasal mucosa before administering nasal preparation. Assess for cause of shock state when using IV infusion; dehydration or volume depletion should be corrected before starting, or during infusion.
- **Baseline lab work:** Biochemical profile including renal (BUN, creatinine) function studies.
- **Baseline diagnostic tests:** Consider placement of a pulmonary artery catheter (Swan Ganz catheter) to help with differential diagnosis and management of shock.
- **Nasal congestion:** Monitor for relief of nasal congestion when using nasal preparations.
- **Redness of eyes:** Monitor for decreased redness and itching of eyes when using ophthalmic preparation.
- **Drug effects:** Phenylephrine, unlike many other catecholamines, slows heart rate and increases stroke volume.
- **Dysrhythmias:** Monitor continuous ECG for tachycardia, bradycardia, and ventricular dysrhythmias.
- **Hypotension:** Assess for continued hypotension; if present, assess if patients may tolerate additional IV fluids for volume expansion; either administer IV fluid bolus or increase hourly IV fluid infusion rate.
- **IV infiltration:** If phenylephrine has been given in a peripheral vein and IV infiltrates, area must be treated with phentolamine immediately to prevent tissue necrosis. Phentolamine is injected with a fine sterile needle throughout the area of infiltration (demarcated by pallor and/or gray appearance).
- **Peripheral vasoconstriction:** Large IV doses can cause extreme vasoconstriction in feet and hands. Correcting dehydration helps abate loss of perfusion to small, distal peripheral blood vessels.
- **Patient education:** Instruct not to use the drug for nasal decongestion longer than 5 days because of the risk of rebound nasal congestion. Instruct to report promptly to a health care provider if dizziness, feeling of irregular heartbeat, insomnia, tremor, or weakness occurs; drug should be discontinued. Explain the different preparations of the drug and the common side effects associated with each. Warn to discontinue ophthalmic medication and report redness, swelling of eyelids, or itching to a health care provider.

SERIOUS ADVERSE REACTIONS

- **Cardiovascular:** Large doses may produce tachycardia and palpitations (particularly in those with cardiac disease), lightheadedness, nausea, and vomiting.
- **Nasal preparations:** Prolonged nasal use may produce chronic swelling of nasal mucosa and rhinitis.
- **Tissue necrosis:** Will occur if IV infiltrates and infiltrated area is not managed with phentolamine (Regitine).

OVERDOSE/TOXICITY

- **Overdose:** Tachycardia, ventricular tachycardia, peripheral vasoconstriction, headache, dizziness, hypertension; in those over 60 yr, may cause hallucinations, CNS depression, and seizures.
- **Management:** Reduce phenylephrine infusion rate or turn off medication. Provide supportive care according to accepted guidelines.
- **GI decontamination:** No specific recommendations.

ANTIDOTE/DIALYSIS

- **Antidote:** Phentolamine (Regitine) for IV infiltration given directly into affected tissues with a fine hypodermic needle. Phentolamine may also be used to manage hypertension associated with use of phenylephrine.
- **Dialysis:** No data are available on removal of phenylephrine by hemodialysis, high-permeability hemodialysis, or peritoneal dialysis.

phenytoin

fen'-i-toyn

Classes

Chemical: hydantoin
Therapeutic: anticonvulsant

Pregnancy Category: D

Trade Names

Prescription: Dilantin, Epamin, Phenytek

Do not confuse phenytoin with mephenytoin, or Dilantin with Dilaudid.

CLINICAL PHARMACOLOGY

Mechanism of Action

A hydantoin anticonvulsant that stabilizes neuronal membranes in the motor cortex by decreasing sodium and calcium ion influx into the neurons. Also acts as an antidysrhythmic agent by decreasing abnormal ventricular automaticity and shortening the refractory period, QT interval, and action potential duration. **Therapeutic Effect:** Limits the spread of seizure activity. Restores normal cardiac rhythm.

PHARMACOKINETICS

Slowly and variably absorbed after PO administration; slowly but completely absorbed after IM administration. Protein binding: 90%-95%. Widely distributed. Metabolized in the liver. Primarily excreted in urine. **Half-life:** 22 hr.

AVAILABILITY

Capsules (prompt release): 100 mg.
Capsules (extended release [Dilantin]): 30 mg.
Capsules (extended release [Phenytek]): 200 mg, 300 mg.
Oral suspension (Dilantin): 125 mg/5 mL.
Tablets (chewable [Dilantin]): 50 mg.
Injection: 50 mg/mL.

INDICATIONS AND DOSAGE

Status epilepticus

IV

Adults, Elderly, Children: 15-20 mg/kg. Maintenance dose: 300 mg/day in 2-3 divided doses for adults and elderly; 6-7 mg/kg/day (for children 10-16 yr); 7-8 mg/kg/day (for children 7-9 yr); 7.5-9 mg/kg/day (for children 4-6 yr); 8-10 mg/kg/day (for children 6 mo-3 yr). **Neonates:** Loading dose: 15-20 mg/kg. Maintenance dose: 5-8 mg/kg/day.

Seizure control

PO

Adults, Elderly, Children: Loading dose: 15-20 mg/kg in 3 divided doses 2-4 hr apart. Maintenance dose: Same as for status epilepticus.

Dysrhythmias

PO

Adults, Elderly: Loading dose: 250 mg 4 times per day for 1 day, then 250 mg twice per day for 2 days. Maintenance dose: 300-400 mg/day 1-4 times per day. **Children:** Maintenance dose: 5-10 mg/kg/day in 2-3 divided doses.

IV

Adults, Elderly, Children: Loading dose: 1.25 mg/kg every 5 min. May repeat up to total dose of 15 mg/kg. **Children:** Maintenance dose: 5-10 mg/kg/day in 2-3 divided doses.

OFF-LABEL USES

Adjunctive treatment of tricyclic antidepressant toxicity; treatment of muscle hyperirritability, digoxin-induced dysrhythmias, and trigeminal neuralgia

CONTRAINDICATIONS

Hypersensitivity to phenytoin and other hydantoins, seizures due to hypoglycemia
IV: Adam-Stokes syndrome, second- and third-degree AV block, sinoatrial block, sinus bradycardia

INTERACTIONS

Drug: **Alcohol, other CNS depressants:** May increase CNS depression. **Amiodarone, anticoagulants, cimetidine, disulfiram, fluoxetine, isoniazid, sulfonamides:** May increase phenytoin blood concentration, effects, and risk of toxicity. **Antacids:** May decrease phenytoin absorption. **Fluconazole, ketoconazole, miconazole:** May increase phenytoin blood concentration. **Glucocorticoids:** May decrease the effects of glucocorticoids. **Lidocaine, propranolol:** May increase cardiac depressant effects. **Valproic acid:** May decrease the metabolism and increase the blood concentration of phenytoin. **Xanthines:** May increase the metabolism of these drugs. **Herbal:** None known. **Food:** None known.

DIAGNOSTIC TEST EFFECTS

May increase blood glucose level and serum GGT and alkaline phosphatase levels. Therapeutic serum level is 10-20 mcg/mL; toxic serum level is greater than 20 mcg/mL.

IV INCOMPATIBILITIES

Diltiazem (Cardizem), *DOBUTamine (Dobutrex), enalapril (Vasotec), heparin, hydromorphone (Dilaudid), insulin, lidocaine, morphine, nitroglycerin, norepinephrine (Levophed), potassium chloride, propofol (Diprivan)

SIDE-EFFECTS

Frequent: Drowsiness, lethargy, confusion, slurred speech, irritability, gingival hyperplasia, hypersensitivity reaction (including fever, rash, and lymphadenopathy), constipation, dizziness, nausea. **Occasional:** Headache, hirsutism, coarsening of facial features, insomnia, muscle twitching

CRITICAL CARE CONSIDERATIONS

ADMINISTRATION/HANDLING

PO ALERT

- Give phenytoin with food if GI distress occurs.
- Do not chew, open, or break capsules. Tablets may be chewed.
- Shake the oral suspension well before using.

IV ALERT

- **Storage/stability:** If refrigerated, the solution may form a precipitate that dissolves at room temperature. Do not use the cloudy solution. A slight yellow discoloration of the solution does not affect potency.
- **Dilution:** Phenytoin may be given undiluted or may be diluted with 0.9% NaCl.
- **Direct IV injection:** Give phenytoin by IV push. For adults, do not exceed an injection rate of 50 mg/min for adults to avoid cardiovascular collapse and severe hypotension. For elderly patients, administer 50 mg over 2-3 min. For neonates, do not exceed 1-3 mg/kg/min.
- **Maintenance dose:** Usually given 12 hr after the loading dose.
- **Following administration:** To minimize injection site pain from chemical irritation of the vein, flush catheter with IV saline after each dose of phenytoin.

PRECAUTIONS

HEALTH-RELATED

- Use IV phenytoin extremely cautiously in patients with heart failure, myocardial damage/infarction or respiratory depression.
- Use phenytoin cautiously in patients with hyperglycemia, hypotension, hepatic or renal impairment, or severe myocardial insufficiency.

AGE-RELATED

- **Children:** More susceptible to coarsening of facial hair, hirsutism, and gingival hyperplasia.
- **Elderly:** Lower dosages are recommended; no age-related precautions are noted.

PREGNANCY/LACTATION-RELATED

- Pregnancy category D; discontinue breastfeeding during phenytoin therapy.

MONITORING

- **Baseline assessment:** Assess for history of dysrhythmias. Take vital signs before drug administration. Assess seizure patients' LOC, and review the history of the seizure disorder, including the duration, frequency, and intensity of seizures. Initiate seizure precautions.
- **Baseline/ongoing lab work:** CBC with WBC differential; biochemical profile

including renal (BUN, creatinine) and liver (AST [SGOT], ALT [SGPT], alkaline phosphatase, GGT, bilirubin) function studies. Repeat CBC 2 wk after beginning phenytoin therapy and 2 wk after maintenance dose is established.

- **Baseline diagnostic tests:** 12-lead ECG to diagnose dysrhythmias and to check for myocardial ischemia.
- **Dysrhythmias:** Monitor continuous ECG for bradycardia, heart block, ventricular fibrillation, and asystole.
- **Hypotension:** Monitor for hypotension when using IV phenytoin.
- **Seizures:** Observe frequently for recurrence of seizure activity.
- **Serum drug levels:** Therapeutic drug level is 10-20 mcg/mL. Toxic serum drug level is greater than 20 mcg/mL. Assess for phenytoin toxicity which may lead to cardiovascular collapse and CNS depression.
- **Therapeutic effect:** Assess for improvement, such as decreased frequency or intensity of seizures.
- **CNS effects:** Assist with ambulation for drowsiness, dizziness, or lethargy.
- **Patient education:** Caution against abruptly discontinuing phenytoin after long-term use to avoid recurrence of seizures or dysrhythmias; strict maintenance of drug therapy is essential for control. Inform that IV injection may cause pain. Encourage maintenance of good oral hygiene (gum massage and regular dental visits), to prevent gingival hyperplasia (bleeding, swollen, tender gums). Instruct to undergo a CBC every month for 1 yr after the maintenance dose is established and every 3 mo thereafter. Warn to avoid tasks requiring mental alertness or motor skills until response to the drug is known. Inform that drowsiness usually diminishes with continued therapy. Instruct to report fever, swollen glands, sore throat, a skin reaction, or signs of hematologic toxicity (such as a bleeding tendency, bruising, fatigue, or fever). Urge avoidance of alcohol while taking phenytoin. Advise carrying an identification card or wearing a medical alert ID bracelet that displays the seizure disorder and anticonvulsant therapy.

SERIOUS ADVERSE REACTIONS

- **Abrupt withdrawal:** May precipitate status epilepticus.
- **Hematologic/immunologic:** Blood dyscrasias, lymphadenopathy, and osteomalacia (caused by impaired vitamin D metabolism).

OVERDOSE/TOXICITY

- **CNS effects:** Toxic phenytoin blood concentration (25 mcg/mL or more) may produce ataxia, nystagmus, or diplopia. At higher levels, extreme lethargy may lead to coma. Tonic seizures have been reported.
- **Cardiopulmonary:** Complete heart block, bradycardia, respiratory distress, respiratory arrest, ventricular fibrillation, asystole, shock.
- **Hematologic toxicity:** Bleeding tendency, bruising, fatigue, or fever.
- **Management:** Maintain patent airway and support ventilation. Heart block and bradycardia generally respond to IV atropine or epinephrine infusion. Resuscitate according to Advanced Cardiac Life Support (ACLS) guidelines.
- **GI decontamination:** No specific recommendations.

ANTIDOTE/DIALYSIS

- **Antidote:** No specific recommendations.
- **Dialysis:** Phenytoin is removed by high-permeability hemodialysis but not by regular hemodialysis or peritoneal dialysis.

phosphates

fos'-fates

Classes

Chemical: phosphorous derivatives, nonvalent anion
Therapeutic: electrolyte replenisher, antihypophosphatemic, laxative

Pregnancy Category: C

Trade Names

Prescription: Fleet Enema, Fleet Phospho-Soda, K-Phos MF, K-Phos Neutral, Neutra-Phos, Neutra-Phos-K, Uro-KP-Neutral

CLINICAL PHARMACOLOGY

Mechanism of Action

Electrolytes that participate in bone deposition, calcium metabolism, and utilization of B complex vitamins and act as a buffer in maintaining acid-base balance. Also exert an osmotic effect in small intestine, producing distention and promoting peristalsis. **Therapeutic Effect:** Correct hypophosphatemia, acidify urine in urinary tract infections, help prevent calcium deposits in urinary tract, and promote evacuation of the bowel.

P

PHARMACOKINETICS

Poorly absorbed after PO administration. PO form excreted in feces; IV form excreted in urine.

AVAILABILITY

Oral solution (Fleet Phospho-Soda): 4 mmol phosphate per mL.
Powder (Neutra-Phos, Neutra-Phos-K): 250 mg (8 mmol) phosphate.
Tablets: 125 mg (4 mmol) phosphate, 250 mg (8 mmol) phosphate (K-Phos MF, K-Phos Neutral, Uro-KP-Neutral).
Enema (Fleet Enema): 2.25 oz, 4.5 oz.
Injection (potassium phosphate): 3 mmol phosphate and 4.4 mEq potassium per mL.
Injection (sodium phosphate): 3 mmol phosphate and 4 mEq sodium per mL.

INDICATIONS AND DOSAGE

Hypophosphatemia

PO (Neutra-Phos, Neutra-Phos-K, K-Phos MF, K-Phos Neutral, Uro-KP-Neutral)

Adults, Elderly: 50-150 mmol/day. **Children:** 2-3 mmol/kg/day.

IV

Adults, Elderly: 50-70 mmol/day. **Children:** 0.5-1.5 mmol/kg/day.

Laxative

PO (Neutra-Phos, Neutra-Phos-K, Uro-KP-Neutral)

Adults, Elderly, Children 4 yr and older: 1-2 capsules/packets 4 times per day. **Children younger than 4 yr:** 1 capsule/packet 4 times per day.

Rectal

Adults, Elderly, Children 12 yr and older: 4.5-oz enema as single dose. May repeat. **Children younger than 12 yr:** 2.25-oz enema as single dose. May repeat.

Urine acidification

PO

Adults, Elderly: 8 mmol 4 times per day.

OFF-LABEL USES

Prevention of calcium renal calculi

CONTRAINDICATIONS

Abdominal pain or fecal impaction (from rectal dosage form), ascitic conditions, heart failure, hyperkalemia, hypernatremia, hyperphosphatemia, hypocalcemia, hypomagnesemia, paralytic ileus, phosphate renal calculi, severe renal impairment, hypersensitivity to phosphate or any component of the product

INTERACTIONS

Drug: ACE inhibitors, NSAIDs, potassium-containing medications, potassium-sparing diuretics, salt substitutes containing potassium phosphate: May increase potassium blood concentration. **Antacids:** May decrease the absorption of phosphates. **Calcium-containing medications:** May increase the risk of calcium deposition in soft tissues and decrease phosphate absorption. **Digoxin:** May increase the risk of heart block caused by hyperkalemia when given with potassium phosphates. **Glucocorticoids:** May cause edema when given with sodium phosphate. **Phosphate-containing medications:** May increase the risk of hyperphosphatemia. **Sodium-containing medications:** May increase the risk of edema when given with sodium phosphate. **Herbal:** None known. **Food:** None known.

DIAGNOSTIC TEST EFFECTS

None known.

IV INCOMPATIBILITIES

*DOBUTamine (Dobutrex)

IV COMPATIBILITIES

Diltiazem (Cardizem), enalapril (Vasotec), famotidine (Pepcid), magnesium sulfate, metoclopramide (Reglan)

SIDE-EFFECTS

Frequent: Mild laxative effect (in first few days of therapy). **Occasional:** Diarrhea, nausea, abdominal pain, vomiting. **Rare:** Headache; dizziness; confusion; heaviness of lower extremities; fatigue; muscle cramps; paresthesia; peripheral edema; dysrhythmias, weight gain; thirst

CRITICAL CARE CONSIDERATIONS

ADMINISTRATION/HANDLING

PO ALERT

- Dissolve tablets in water.
- Give phosphates after meals or with food to decrease GI upset. Maintain high fluid intake to prevent renal calculi.

IV ALERT

- **Storage:** Store vials at room temperature.
- **Dilution:** Dilute the drug in a larger volume of IV solution before using; soluble in commonly used IV solutions except for Ringer's products (e.g., lactated Ringer's, D_5RL, Ringer's).
- **Infusion:** Infuse at a maximum rate of 0.06 mmol phosphate/kg/hr.

P

PRECAUTIONS

HEALTH-RELATED

- Use phosphates cautiously in patients with adrenal insufficiency, cirrhosis, or renal impairment and in those receiving potassium-sparing drugs concurrently.

AGE-RELATED

- **Children:** No age-related precautions have been noted in children.
- **Elderly:** No age-related precautions have been noted.

PREGNANCY/LACTATION-RELATED

- Pregnancy category C; use with caution in breast-feeding women.

MONITORING

- **Baseline assessment for laxatives:** Assess for abdominal pain including pattern, duration, quality, intensity, location, radiation, and factors that relieve or worsen it. If using phosphates as a laxative, assess pattern of daily bowel activity, amount, color, and consistency of stools; auscultate bowel sounds for peristalsis. Determine history of recent abdominal surgery, nausea, vomiting, and weight loss.
- **Baseline assessment for acute hypophosphatemia:** Assess for confusion, seizures, coma, chest discomfort (poor oxygenation of the myocardium), muscle pain, weakness, poor coordination, difficulty weaning from mechanical ventilation. Chronic low phosphorous causes memory loss, weakness, bone pain. Respiratory alkalosis may result in hypophosphatemia. Assess for history of alcoholism, diabetes/DKA, sepsis; postoperative patients, postrenal transplant patients, those with severe burns and mechanically-ventilated patients may be hypophosphatemic.
- **Baseline and ongoing lab work:** Biochemical profile including phosphate, sodium, chloride, calcium, magnesium, and potassium levels; AST (SGOT), ALT (SGPT), phosphatase, bilirubin; urinalysis including urinary pH. Hypophosphatemic patients need an ABG to assess for metabolic/lactic acidosis due to cellular level lack of ability to produce ATP and 2,3 DPG without phosphates.
- **Hypocalcemia:** Monitor for hypocalcemia (numbness/tingling of fingers, hyperactive reflexes, muscle cramps, tetany, seizures); calcium may be reduced in response to phosphate infusion.
- **Dysrhythmias:** Monitor ECG continuously for prolonged QT interval.
- **Hemodynamic changes:** Severely hypophosphatemic patients may have depressed myocardial contractility reflected as elevated pulmonary capillary wedge pressures, decreased cardiac output, hypotension with poor response to medications. Cardiac performance should improve from phosphate infusion.
- **Patient education:** Instruct to report diarrhea, nausea, or vomiting. If acutely hypophosphatemic, instruct patients to report chest discomfort, shortness of breath, muscle pain throughout phosphate infusion. If patients have been constipated, encourage increased fluid and fiber intake, along with a walking or exercise program. Instruct hypophosphatemic patients to consume foods high in phosphates, including dairy products, nuts, dried beans/peas, fish, meats (especially organ meats), poultry, eggs, seeds (pumpkin, sunflower, sesame), and whole grains (oatmeal, barley, bran).

SERIOUS ADVERSE REACTIONS

- Hyperphosphatemia may produce calcification in the joints, arteries, and soft tissues leading to oliguria, irregular heart rate, corneal haziness, and papular lesions.

OVERDOSE/TOXICITY

- **Hyperphosphatemia (with resultant hypocalcemia):** Anorexia, nausea, vomiting, muscle weakness, hyperreflexia, tetany, and tachycardia. Potassium may shift out of cells as phosphorous shifts into cells, resulting in hyperkalemia with flaccid paralysis, weakness, confusion, paresthesias, and low energy level.
- **Management:** Discontinue phosphates. Give calcium gluconate or calcium chloride to restore calcium level, which decreases in response to higher phosphorous level. Help shift potassium back into cells with glucose and insulin. Correct acidosis with sodium bicarbonate. If hypernatremia is present or results from treatment, diuretics may be used to reduce sodium level.
- **GI decontamination:** No specific recommendations.

ANTIDOTE/DIALYSIS

- **Antidote:** Calcium gluconate or calcium chloride.
- **Dialysis:** Phosphates are removed by hemodialysis, high-permeability hemodialysis, and peritoneal dialysis.

pimozide

See Antipsychotics (p. 934)

pioglitazone hydrochloride 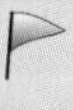

pye-oh-gli'-ta-zone hye-droe-klor'-ide

Classes

Chemical: thiazolidinedione
Therapeutic: antidiabetic, hypoglycemic, insulin resistance reducer

Pregnancy Category: C

Trade Names

Prescription: Actos

CLINICAL PHARMACOLOGY

Mechanism of Action

An antidiabetic that improves target-cell response to insulin without increasing pancreatic insulin secretion. Decreases hepatic glucose output and increases insulin-dependent glucose utilization in skeletal muscle. **Therapeutic Effect:** Lowers blood glucose concentration.

PHARMACOKINETICS

Rapidly absorbed. Highly protein bound (99%), primarily to albumin. Metabolized in the liver. Excreted in urine. Unlikely to be removed by hemodialysis. **Half-life:** 16-24 hr.

AVAILABILITY

Tablets: 15 mg, 30 mg, 45 mg.

INDICATIONS AND DOSAGE

Diabetes mellitus, combination therapy

PO

Adults, Elderly: *With insulin*—Initially 15-30 mg once per day, continuing current insulin dosage, then decrease insulin dosage by 10%-25% if hypoglycemia occurs or plasma glucose level decreases to less than 100 mg/dL. Maximum: 45 mg/day. *With sulfonylureas*—Initially 15-30 mg/day. Decrease sulfonylurea dosage if hypoglycemia occurs. *With metformin*—Initially, 15-30 mg/day.

Diabetes mellitus, monotherapy

PO

Adults, Elderly: Monotherapy is not to be used if patient is well controlled with diet and exercise alone. Initially 15-30 mg/day. May increase dosage in increments until 45 mg/day is reached.

CONTRAINDICATIONS

Active hepatic disease; diabetic ketoacidosis; increased serum transaminase levels, including ALT (SGPT) greater than 2.5 times normal serum level; type 1 diabetes mellitus, hypersensitivity to pioglitazone

INTERACTIONS

Drug: Gemfibrizol: May increase the effect and toxicity of pioglitazone. **Ketoconazole:** May significantly inhibit metabolism of pioglitazone. **Oral contraceptives:** May alter the effects of oral contraceptives. **Food:** None known. **Herbal:** None known.

DIAGNOSTIC TEST EFFECTS

May increase creatine kinase (CK) level. May decrease Hgb levels by 2% to 4% and serum alkaline phosphatase, bilirubin, and ALT (SGPT) levels. Less than 1% of patients experience ALT (SGPT) values 3 times the normal level.

SIDE-EFFECTS

Frequent (13%-9%): Headache, upper respiratory tract infection, weight gain. **Occasional (6%-5%):** Sinusitis, myalgia, pharyngitis, aggravated diabetes mellitus

CRITICAL CARE CONSIDERATIONS

ADMINISTRATION/HANDLING

PO ALERT

- Give pioglitazone without regard to meals.

PRECAUTIONS

HEALTH-RELATED

- Use pioglitazone cautiously in patients with heart failure, edema, and hepatic impairment; drug causes fluid retention and hepatotoxicity; pioglitazone should not be used on patients with preexisting AST(SGOT)/ALT(SGPT) level 2.5 times upper limit of normal.
- **Cytochrome P450 enzyme metabolism:** Drug is metabolized by a series of CYP 450 enzyme substrates, which produces numerous drug interactions.

AGE-RELATED

- **Children:** Safety and efficacy of pioglitazone have not been established in children.
- **Elderly:** No age-related precautions have been noted.

PREGNANCY/LACTATION-RELATED

- Pregnancy category C. Abnormally high glucose levels during pregnancy associated with higher incidence of congenital anomalies, morbidity, and mortality. Insulin monotherapy or sulfonylurea are preferred agents. Breast milk excretion unknown.

P

MONITORING

- **Baseline assessment:** Assess pattern of blood glucose control and dietary and exercise habits. Proper diet and exercise are essential for control of blood glucose. Insulin is the drug of choice for hyperglycemia in the critically ill.
- **Baseline lab work:** CBC, HbA_{1c}, biochemical profile including blood glucose and liver function tests (AST [SGOT], ALT [SGPT], alkaline phosphatase, GGT, bilirubin). Hb/Hct, and ALT (SGPT) levels should be monitored every 2 mo for the first yr of therapy. HbA_{1c} levels should be monitored periodically to assess for glycemic control.
- **Hypoglycemia:** Assess for anxiety, cool wet skin, diplopia, dizziness, headache, hunger, numbness in mouth, tachycardia, tremors. Continuous ECG monitoring may reveal ST segment changes along with heart rate changes.
- **Hyperglycemia:** Assess for deep rapid breathing, visual disturbance, fatigue, nausea, polydipsia, polyphagia, polyuria, vomiting. Be alert to conditions that alter blood glucose requirements, such as fever, increased activity, stress, or a surgical procedure. Stressors increase blood glucose, while increased activity or exercise decreases blood glucose. Consider use of an insulin infusion to control hyperglycemia.
- **Patient education:** Ensure additional education if patients or families do not thoroughly understand diabetes management or blood glucose testing technique. Encourage patients to self-monitor or have monitored a HbA_{1c} level to assess overall glycemic control. Stress that prescribed diet and exercise are a principal part of treatment. Warn not to skip or delay meals. Make sure patients are aware of symptoms of hypoglycemia and hyperglycemia. Instruct about need to carry candy, sugar packets, or other sugar supplements for immediate response to hypoglycemia. Urge avoidance of alcohol. Instruct to report promptly abdominal or chest pain, dark urine or light stool, hypoglycemic reactions, fever, nausea, palpitations, rash, vomiting, or yellowing of the eyes or skin to a health care provider.

SERIOUS ADVERSE REACTIONS

- **Heart failure:** Fluid retention may prompt heart failure in susceptible patients. Weight gain and edema are relatively common.
- **Ovulation:** Pioglitazone may prompt ovulation in previously anovulatory women, which increases chance of pregnancy.
- **Anemia:** Decreased hemoglobin and hematocrit may manifest during the first 4-12 wk of therapy and remain at the same lower levels thereafter.

OVERDOSE/TOXICITY

- **Hepatotoxicity:** Elevated liver enzymes with rare occurrence of hepatitis, hepatic necrosis, liver failure, need for liver transplantation; can be fatal.
- **Management:** If liver enzymes (particularly ALT [SGPT]) becomes elevated 2.5 times the upper limit of normal, liver enzyme monitoring should be done more frequently. If ALT (SGPT) levels remain 3 times normal or patient becomes jaundiced, drug should be discontinued.
- **GI decontamination:** No specific recommendations.

ANTIDOTE/DIALYSIS

- **Antidote:** No specific recommendations.
- **Dialysis:** Pioglitazone is unlikely to be removed by hemodialysis or peritoneal dialysis. No data are available on removal by high-permeability hemodialysis.

pindolol

See Beta-Adrenergic Blockers (p. 943)

pipracillin

See Antibiotics (p. 892)

piroxicam

peer-ox'-i-kam

Classes

Chemical: oxicam derivative

Therapeutic: NSAID, antipyretic, nonnarcotic analgesic

Pregnancy Category: C, D (3rd trimester)

Trade Names

Prescription: Apo-Piroxicam ♣, Feldene, Novopirocam ♣, Nu-Pirox ♣

Do not confuse Feldene with Seldane.

CLINICAL PHARMACOLOGY

Mechanism of Action

An NSAID that produces analgesic and antiinflammatory effects by inhibiting prostaglandin synthesis. **Therapeutic Effect:**

Reduces inflammatory response and intensity of pain.

PHARMACOKINETICS

Well absorbed following oral administration. Protein binding: 99%. Extensively metabolized in liver. Primarily excreted in urine; small amount eliminated in feces. **Half-life:** 50 hr.

AVAILABILITY

Capsules: 10 mg, 20 mg.

INDICATIONS AND DOSAGE

Acute or chronic rheumatoid arthritis and osteoarthritis

PO

Adults, Elderly: Initially, 10-20 mg/day as a single dose or in divided doses. Some patients may require up to 30-40 mg/day. **Children:** 0.2-0.3 mg/kg/day. Maximum: 15 mg/day.

OFF-LABEL USES

Treatment of acute gouty arthritis, ankylosing spondylitis, dysmenorrhea

CONTRAINDICATIONS

Active peptic ulcer disease, chronic inflammation of the GI tract, GI bleeding or ulceration, history of hypersensitivity to aspirin or NSAIDs

INTERACTIONS

Drug: **Antihypertensives, diuretics:** May decrease the effects of these drugs. **Aspirin, other salicylates:** May increase the risk of GI side effects such as bleeding. **Bone marrow depressants:** May increase the risk of hematologic reactions. **Heparin, oral anticoagulants, thrombolytics:** May increase the effects of these drugs. **Lithium:** May increase the blood concentration and risk of toxicity of lithium. **Methotrexate:** May increase the risk of methotrexate toxicity. **Probenecid:** May increase the piroxicam blood concentration. **Herbal:** **Feverfew:** May decrease the effects of feverfew. **Ginkgo biloba:** May increase the risk of bleeding. **St. John's wort:** May increase the risk of phototoxicity. **Food:** None known.

DIAGNOSTIC TEST EFFECTS

May increase AST (SGOT) and ALT (SGPT) levels. May decrease serum uric acid levels.

SIDE-EFFECTS

Frequent (9%-4%): Dyspepsia, nausea, dizziness, rash, abdominal cramps. **Occasional (3%-1%):** Diarrhea, constipation, abdominal cramps or pain, flatulence, stomatitis. **Rare (less than 1%):** Hypertension, urticaria, dysuria, ecchymosis, blurred vision, insomnia, phototoxicity

CRITICAL CARE CONSIDERATIONS

ADMINISTRATION/HANDLING

PO ALERT

- Do not crush or break capsules.
- Give piroxicam with food, milk, or antacids if GI distress occurs.

PRECAUTIONS

HEALTH-RELATED

- Use piroxicam cautiously in patients with GI disease, hypertension, or impaired cardiac or hepatic function, and in patients using anticoagulants concurrently.

AGE-RELATED

- **Children:** Safety and efficacy of piroxicam have not been established in children.
- **Elderly:** Age-related renal changes may prompt a dosage adjustment.

PREGNANCY/LACTATION-RELATED

- Pregnancy category C (D if used in third trimester or near delivery). Excreted into breast milk at approximately 1% of mother's serum levels; should not present a risk to nursing infant.

MONITORING

- **Baseline assessment:** Assess the duration, location, onset, and type of inflammation or pain. Inspect arthritic joints for deformity, immobility, and skin condition.
- **Baseline lab work:** CBC with WBC differential; biochemical profile including renal (BUN, creatinine) and liver (AST [SGOT], ALT [SGPT] levels, alkaline phosphatase, bilirubin) function studies.
- **GI side effects:** Monitor for GI distress and nausea. Assess pattern of daily bowel activity and stool consistency.
- **Edema:** Examine for edema, including behind the medial malleolus.
- **Therapeutic response:** Evaluate for evidence of improved grip strength, increased joint mobility, and decreased pain, tenderness, stiffness, and swelling.
- **Patient education:** Instruct to take piroxicam with food, milk, or antacids if GI upset occurs. Warn to avoid tasks requiring mental alertness or motor skills until response to the drug is known. Caution

P

to avoid alcohol and aspirin to lower risk of GI bleeding. Advise female patients to inform the physician of pregnancy or plans to become pregnant.

SERIOUS ADVERSE REACTIONS

- **GI effects:** Rare reactions with long-term use include peptic ulcer disease, GI bleeding, gastritis.
- **Severe hypersensitivity reaction:** Fever, chills, bronchospasm, anaphylaxis.

OVERDOSE/TOXICITY

- **Hepatotoxicity:** Cholestasis, jaundice, elevated liver enzymes, hepatitis.
- **Nephrotoxicity:** Dysuria, hematuria, edema, proteinuria, nephrotic syndrome.
- **Hematologic sensitivity:** Anemia, leukopenia, eosinophilia, thrombocytopenia.
- **Overdose:** Hypotonia, muscle fasciculations, twitching, bone marrow suppression, metabolic acidosis, nausea, vomiting, diarrhea, GI bleeding, abdominal pain, volume depletion with secondary hypotension, tachycardia, pulmonary edema and acute respiratory distress syndrome, acute psychosis, seizures, CNS depression following agitation.
- **Management:** Discontinue piroxicam and provide supportive care. Maintain patent airway, support ventilation, manage acidosis, provide IV volume infusion to support BP and vasopressors if needed, manage seizures with benzodiazepines.
- **GI decontamination:** No specific recommendations.

ANTIDOTE/DIALYSIS

- **Antidote:** No specific recommendations.
- **Dialysis:** Piroxicam is unlikely to be removed by hemodialysis or peritoneal dialysis. No data are available on removal by high-permeability hemodialysis.

piruterol

See Bronchodilators (p. 947)

polycarbophil

pol-ee-car'-boe-fil

Classes

Chemical: polyacrylic acid with divinyl glycol

Therapeutic: bulk-forming laxative, antidiarrheal, intestinal absorbent

Pregnancy Category: C

Trade Names

Prescription: Equalactin, Fibercon, Fiber-Lax, Konsyl Fiber, Phillips Fibercaps

CLINICAL PHARMACOLOGY

Mechanism of Action

A bulk-forming laxative and antidiarrheal. As a laxative, retains water in the intestine and opposes dehydrating forces of the bowel. **Therapeutic Effect:** Promotes well-formed stools. As an antidiarrheal, absorbs fecal-free water, restores normal moisture level, and provides bulk.

PHARMACOKINETICS

Route	Onset	Peak	Duration
PO	12-72 hr	N/A	N/A

Polycarbophil is not absorbed following oral administration. Acts in small and large intestines.

AVAILABILITY

Tablets: 500 mg, 625 mg.
Tablets (chewable): 500 mg.

INDICATIONS AND DOSAGE

Constipation, diarrhea

PO

Adults, Elderly, Children 12 yr and older: 1-1.25 g 1-4 times per day, or as needed. Maximum: 4 g/24 hr. **Children 6-11 yr:** 500-625 mg 1-4 times per day, or as needed. Maximum: 2 g/24 hr. **Children younger than 6 yr:** Consult product labeling.

CONTRAINDICATIONS

Abdominal pain, dysphagia, fecal impaction, nausea, partial bowel obstruction, symptoms of appendicitis, vomiting, hypersensitivity to polycarbophil or any component of the product

INTERACTIONS

Drug: Digoxin, oral anticoagulants, salicylates, tetracyclines: May decrease the effects of digoxin, salicylates, and tetracyclines. **Potassium-sparing diuretics, potassium supplements:** May interfere with the effects of potassium-sparing diuretics and potassium supplements. **Herbal:** None known. **Food:** None known.

P

DIAGNOSTIC TEST EFFECTS

May increase blood glucose level. May decrease serum potassium levels.

SIDE-EFFECTS

Occasional: Epigastric fullness, flatulence. **Rare:** Some degree of abdominal discomfort, nausea, mild cramps, griping, syncope/near syncope

CRITICAL CARE CONSIDERATIONS

ADMINISTRATION/HANDLING

PO ALERT

- For severe diarrhea, give every half hr up to maximum daily dosage; for constipation, give with 8 oz liquid.

PRECAUTIONS

HEALTH-RELATED

- Use cautiously in dehydrated patients, those with history of a bowel obstruction, and those at risk for a bowel obstruction.

AGE-RELATED

- **Children:** Polycarbophil use is not recommended in children under 6 yr.
- **Elderly:** No age-related precautions have been noted.

PREGNANCY/LACTATION-RELATED

- Pregnancy category C; compatible with breast-feeding.

MONITORING

- **Baseline assessment:** Before polycarbophil administration, assess abdomen for signs of tenderness, rigidity, and presence of bowel sounds. Determine last bowel movement, the amount, and consistency. Determine diet, exercise, and fluid intake habits.
- **Baseline lab work:** CBC with WBC differential, biochemical profile. Monitor serum electrolyte levels periodically in patients with excessive and/or prolonged use of polycarbophil.
- **Baseline diagnostic tests:** Abdominal x-ray if last bowel movement occurred more than a week ago.
- **Hydration:** Provide or encourage adequate fluid intake.
- **Bowel obstruction:** Assess bowel sounds for peristalsis in all four quadrants. Assess pattern of daily bowel activity and stool consistency.
- **Patient education:** Instruct about measures to promote defecation such as increasing fluid intake, exercising, and eating a high-fiber diet. Advise to drink 6-8 glasses of water per day when using polycarbophil as a laxative to aid in stool softening.

SERIOUS ADVERSE REACTIONS

- **Esophageal or bowel obstruction:** May occur if administered with less than 250 mL or 1 full glass of liquid.

OVERDOSE/TOXICITY

- No systemic toxicities; drug is not absorbed into the bloodstream.
- **GI decontamination:** No specific recommendations.

ANTIDOTE/DIALYSIS

- **Antidote:** No specific recommendations.
- **Dialysis:** Polycarbophil is not systemically absorbed, so removal by dialysis is not possible.

polyethylene glycol-electrolyte solution (PEG-ES)

pol-ee-eth'-i-leen glye'-col

Classes

Chemical: polyethylene glycol derivative
Therapeutic: laxative

Pregnancy Category: C

Trade Names

Prescription: CoLyte, CoLyte 4 Flavor, CoLyte Flavored, GlycoLax, GoLYTELY, MiraLax, NuLytely, NuLytely Cherry, NuLytely Lemon Lime, NuLytely Orange, TriLyte

CLINICAL PHARMACOLOGY

Mechanism of Action

A laxative that has an osmotic effect. **Therapeutic Effect:** Induces diarrhea and cleanses bowel without depleting electrolytes.

PHARMACOKINETICS

Route	Onset	Peak	Duration
PO (bowel cleansing)	1-2 hr	N/A	N/A
PO (constipation)	2-4 days	N/A	N/A

AVAILABILITY

Powder for reconstitution: (CoLyte, CoLyte Flavored, Colyte 4 Flavor, GlycoLax, GoLYTELY, MiraLax, NuLytely, NuLytely Cherry, NuLytely Lemon Lime, NuLytely Orange, TriLyte).

INDICATIONS AND DOSAGE

Bowel cleansing

PO

Adults, Elderly: Before GI examination: 240 mL (8 oz) every 10 min until 4 L consumed or rectal effluent clear. Nasogastric (NG) tube: 20-30 mL/min until 4 L given. **Children:** 25-40 mL/kg/hr until rectal effluent clear.

Constipation

PO (MiraLax)

Adults: 17 g or 1 heaping tbsp per day.

CONTRAINDICATIONS

Bowel perforation, gastric retention, GI obstruction, megacolon, toxic colitis, toxic ileus, hypersensitivity to polyethylene glycol

INTERACTIONS

Drug: Oral medications: May decrease the absorption of oral medications if given within 1 hr because they may be flushed from GI tract. **Herbal:** None known. **Food:** None known.

DIAGNOSTIC TEST EFFECTS

None known.

SIDE-EFFECTS

Frequent (50%): Some degree of abdominal fullness, nausea, bloating. **Occasional (10%-1%):** Abdominal cramping, vomiting, anal irritation. **Rare (less than 1%):** Urticaria, rhinorrhea, dermatitis

CRITICAL CARE CONSIDERATIONS

ADMINISTRATION/HANDLING

PO ALERT

- **Storage:** Refrigerate reconstituted solutions; use within 48 hr.
- **Preparation:** May use tap water to prepare solution. Shake vigorously for several minutes to ensure complete dissolution of powder. Give nothing by mouth 3 hr or more before ingestion of solution.
- Give only clear liquids after administration. Rapid drinking preferred. Chilled solution is more palatable.
- May give via NG tube; do not chill NG solutions.

PRECAUTIONS

HEALTH-RELATED

- Use polyethylene cautiously in patients with ulcerative colitis.

AGE-RELATED

- **Children:** No age-related precautions have been noted in children.
- **Elderly:** No age-related precautions have been noted.

PREGNANCY/LACTATION-RELATED

- Pregnancy category C; unknown if distributed in breast milk.

MONITORING

- **Baseline assessment:** Do not give oral medication within 1 hr of the initiation of polyethylene therapy because the oral medication may not be adequately absorbed before GI cleansing. Assess for history of hyperglycemia or diabetes.
- **Baseline lab work:** Biochemical profile and CBC with WBC differential; monitor urine osmolality. If elevated, patients may be dehydrated.
- **Bowel obstruction:** Assess bowel sounds for peristalsis. Assess the pattern of daily bowel activity and stool consistency. Monitor for abdominal pain, tenderness, and distention.
- **Dehydration:** Monitor for excessive fluid loss via diarrhea and electrolyte imbalance secondary to fluid imbalance. Solution does not usually result in electrolyte imbalance.
- **Patient education:** Chill the solution to make it more palatable; encourage fast ingestion unless solution is given by enteral (NG) tube. Patients should understand they will be unable to eat or drink for 3 hr before taking the drug and will ingest only clear liquids afterward. Instruct to report promptly severe abdominal pain or bloating to a health care provider.

SERIOUS ADVERSE REACTIONS

- **Hypersensitivity reaction:** Urticaria, dermatitis, rash.

OVERDOSE/TOXICITY

- No data are available.
- **GI decontamination:** No specific recommendations.

ANTIDOTE/DIALYSIS

- **Antidote:** No specific recommendations.
- **Dialysis:** Polyethylene glycol electrolyte solution is unlikely to be removed by hemodialysis, peritoneal dialysis, or high-permeability hemodialysis.

P

polysaccharide iron complex

See Hematinic Iron Preparations (p. 960)

polythiazide

See Diuretics (p. 956)

poractant alfa

poor-ak'-tant al'-fah

Classes

Chemical: phospholipid
Therapeutic: lung surfactant, porcine

Trade Names

Prescription: Curosurf

CLINICAL PHARMACOLOGY

Mechanism of Action

A pulmonary surfactant that reduces alveolar surface tension during ventilation and stabilizes the alveoli against collapse that may occur at resting transpulmonary pressures. **Therapeutic Effect:** Improves lung compliance and respiratory gas exchange.

PHARMACOKINETICS

The pharmacokinetics of poractant alfa are not fully understood.

P

AVAILABILITY

Intratracheal suspension: 1.5 mL (120 mg), 3 mL (240 mg).

INDICATIONS AND DOSAGE

Respiratory distress syndrome (RDS)

Intratracheal

Infants: Initially, 2.5 mL/kg of birth weight. May give up to 2 subsequent doses of 1.25 mL/kg of birth weight at 12-hr intervals. Maximum: 5 mL/kg (total dose).

OFF-LABEL USES

Adult RDS due to viral pneumonia or near-drowning, *Pneumocystis carinii* pneumonia in HIV-infected patients, prevention of RDS

CONTRAINDICATIONS

Hypersensitivity to poractant alfa or any component of the product

INTERACTIONS

Drug: None known. **Herbal:** None known. **Food:** None known.

DIAGNOSTIC TEST EFFECTS

None known.

SIDE-EFFECTS

Frequent: Transient bradycardia, oxygen (O_2) desaturation, increased carbon dioxide (CO_2) retention. **Occasional:** Endotracheal tube reflux. **Rare:** Hypotension or hypertension, pallor, vasoconstriction

CRITICAL CARE CONSIDERATIONS

ADMINISTRATION/HANDLING

INTRATRACHEAL ALERT

- **Storage:** Refrigerate vials. Unopened, unused vials may be returned to the refrigerator only once after having been warmed to room temperature.
- **Preparation of solution:** Warm vial by letting it stand at room temperature for 20 min or by warming it in the hand for 8 min. Turn vial upside down and gently swirl it to obtain a uniform suspension. Do not shake the vial.
- **Instillation:** Withdraw the entire contents of the vial into a 3- or 5-mL plastic syringe through a large-gauge needle (20 gauge or larger). Attach the syringe to a catheter inserted into the infant's endotracheal tube, and instill the solution through the catheter. Be prepared to stop the procedure if bradycardia and decreased oxygen saturation (SaO_2) occurs during administration. Ensure infants stabilize before reinstituting therapy.

PRECAUTIONS

HEALTH-RELATED

- Use poractant cautiously in patients at risk for circulatory overload.

AGE-RELATED

- **Neonates:** Poractant alfa is for use only in neonates. No age-related precautions have been noted.

PREGNANCY/LACTATION-RELATED

- This drug is not indicated for use in pregnant women; drug is for use only in neonates.

MONITORING

- **Baseline assessment:** Assess for and manage acidosis, anemia, hypoglycemia, hypotension, and hypothermia before beginning poractant alfa administration.
- **Baseline lab work:** CBC, biochemical profile.

- **Ventilator adjustments:** Change ventilator settings to 40-60 breaths/min, inspiratory time 0.5 sec, and supplemental O_2 sufficient to maintain arterial SaO_2 greater than 92% immediately before administering drug.
- **Critical care:** Clinicians caring for the neonate must be experienced with intubation and ventilator management. Administer poractant in a supervised setting. Monitor oxygenation and ventilation using arterial or transcutaneous measurement of systemic O_2 and CO_2.
- **Assessment:** Monitor heart rate and auscultate breath sounds for crackles and rhonchi.
- **Limit visitation:** Limit visitors during treatment; monitor for hand washing and other infection control measures to minimize the risk of nosocomial infections.
- **Support:** Offer emotional support to the parents.
- **Patient education:** Tell parents the purpose of the treatment and the expected outcome.

SERIOUS ADVERSE REACTIONS

- Apnea, endotracheal tube blockage, severe bradycardia.

OVERDOSE/TOXICITY

- No data are available.
- **GI decontamination:** No specific recommendations.

ANTIDOTE/DIALYSIS

- **Antidote:** No specific recommendations.
- **Dialysis:** No data are available on removal of poractant alfa by hemodialysis, high-permeability hemodialysis, or peritoneal dialysis.

porfimer sodium

pour'-fim-er soe'-dee-um

Classes

Chemical: dihematoporphyrin ether
Therapeutic: photosensitizing agent, cytotoxic

Pregnancy Category: C

Trade Names

Prescription: Photofrin

CLINICAL PHARMACOLOGY

Mechanism of Action

A photosensitizing agent (not cytotoxic until activated by light). Selective accumulation mainly in abnormally active tissues (e.g., cancer, organs of reticuloendothelial system). Tissues containing porfimer when activated by light cause a photochemical reaction. **Therapeutic Effect:** Produces cell damage and death by oxidation.

PHARMACOKINETICS

Protein binding: 90%. Metabolic fate is unknown. Eliminated primarily in feces; minimal excretion in urine. **Half-life:** 21 days.

AVAILABILITY

Powder for injection: 75 mg.

INDICATIONS AND DOSAGE

Esophageal cancer, lung cancer

IV injection

Adults, Elderly: 2 mg/kg. Illuminate with laser light (630-nm wavelength) 40-50 hr following injection with porfimer. A second laser light application may be given 96-120 hr after initial light application. May be preceded by gentle debridement of tumor via endoscopy. A second course of photodynamic therapy with porfimer may be given no earlier than 30 days after initial therapy, up to 3 courses. Each course should be separated by 30-day rest periods.

CONTRAINDICATIONS

Existing tracheoesophageal or bronchoesophageal fistula, tumors eroding into a major blood vessel, emergency treatment of patients with severe acute respiratory distress caused by an obstructing endobronchial lesion, esophageal or gastric varices, or patients with esophageal ulcers greater than 1 cm in diameter, porphyria or known allergies to porphyrins, hypersensitivity to porfimer sodium

P

INTERACTIONS

Drug: **Photosensitizing agents (e.g., tetracyclines, sulfonamides, phenothiazines, sulfonylurea hypoglycemic agents, thiazide diuretics, griseofulvin, and fluoroquinolones):** May increase the photosensitivity reaction. **Herbal:** None known. **Food:** None known.

DIAGNOSTIC TEST EFFECTS

None known.

SIDE-EFFECTS

Expected (100%): Photosensitivity (extreme reaction to light exposure). **Frequent (greater than 10%):** Photosensitivity reaction to sunlight, bright indoor light (mild erythema on face and hands), fever, nausea, constipation, chest pain, dyspnea, abdominal pain, vomiting, insomnia, back pain. **Occasional (10%-5%):** Dysphagia, respiratory insufficiency, decrease in weight, anorexia, confusion, moniliasis, esophageal disturbances, urinary tract infection. **Rare (5% or less):** Diarrhea, esophagitis, ocular discomfort

CRITICAL CARE CONSIDERATIONS

ADMINISTRATION/HANDLING

IV ALERT

- **Photodynamic therapy:** Should be supervised by a physician who has been trained to administer porfimer, operate the laser system, and respond to any emergency that may arise related to the procedure.
- **Storage:** Porfimer freeze-dried cake or powder should be stored at room temperature.
- **Reconstitution:** Reconstitute vial with 31.8 mL of D_5W or NS to yield final concentration of 2.5 mg/mL. Reconstituted porfimer is an opaque solution; detection of particulate matter by visual inspection is extremely difficult. Reconstituted product should be protected from bright light and used immediately.
- **IV direct injection:** Administer as a single slow IV injection over 3-5 min. Use rubber gloves and eye protection. Avoid any skin or eye contact with porfimer. Dispose of contaminated objects/cloths in a polyethylene bag to protect others from accidental exposure.
- **Extravasation:** Avoid extravasation; if it occurs, protect area from light.

PRECAUTIONS

HEALTH-RELATED

- All patients who receive porfimer sodium will be photosensitive and must observe precautions to avoid exposure of skin and eyes to direct sunlight or bright indoor light (from examination lamps, including dental lamps, operating room lamps, unshaded light bulbs at close proximity, etc.) for at least 30 days.
- Use porfimer cautiously in patients with chest pain, esophageal strictures, or respiratory distress.
- Photodynamic therapy with porfimer is indicated for palliation of patients with completely obstructing esophageal cancer, or with partially obstructing esophageal cancer who cannot be satisfactorily treated with thermal or yttrium aluminum garnet (YAG) laser therapy; for reduction of obstruction and palliation of symptoms in patients with completely or partially obstructing endobronchial non–small cell lung cancer (NSCLC); for treatment of microinvasive endobronchial NSCLC in patients for whom surgery and radiotherapy are not indicated; and for ablation of high-grade dysplasia in Barrett's esophagus patients who do not undergo esophagectomy.

AGE-RELATED

- **Children:** Safety and efficacy of porfimer have not been established in children.
- **Elderly:** No age-related precautions have been noted.

PREGNANCY/LACTATION-RELATED

- Pregnancy category C; breast-feeding should be discontinued.

MONITORING

- **Baseline assessment:** Assess vital signs; determine prior treatments for cancer and patient response. Determine whether patients understand the need to keep skin fully covered for 30 days following administration.
- **Baseline lab work:** CBC with WBC differential. Assess for anemia (excessive fatigue, weakness).
- **Anemia:** Assess for excessive fatigue, weakness, tachycardia, and hypotension.
- **Dysrhythmias:** Monitor ECG continuously for tachycardias, atrial fibrillation, and ST depression indicative of myocardial ischemia.
- **Bleeding:** Vigorous tumor debriding may cause bleeding. Evaluate for blood in sputum or GI secretions. Monitor for anemia. Hemoptysis may indicate tumor has eroded into the pulmonary artery.
- **Respiratory distress:** Monitor for tachypnea, increased work of breathing and stridor in patients with endobronchial cancer, which may indicate airway obstruction. Immediate bronchoscopy may be needed to relieve airway obstruction created by necrotic debris, mucositis, or inflammation.
- **Photosensitivity:** Keep the skin completely covered and avoid exposure to direct sunlight in room. Indoor light is beneficial (inactivates remaining drug). Patients should not be kept continuously in a darkened room. Evaluate for photosensitivity (redness, blistering, swelling).
- **Chest pain:** Assess for chest discomfort following therapy; pain may warrant the

short-term prescription of opiate analgesics. Perform 12-lead ECG if chest discomfort is reported; may be myocardial ischemia.

- **Patient education:** Explain that therapy is a two-step process involving an IV injection of porfimer followed in 40-50 hr by endoscopic/bronchscopic administration of laser light with debridement of tumor. A second light application may be done 4-5 days following injection. Up to 3 courses may be done, but should be at least 30 days apart. Instruct to avoid exposure of skin and eyes to direct sunlight or bright indoor light (from examination lamps, including dental lamps, operating room lamps, unshaded light bulbs at close proximity, etc.) for at least 30 days (can last up to 90 days). Explain that ocular discomfort, such as sensitivity to sun, bright lights, or car headlights, may occur. Explain that sunscreen is ineffective, because photosensitivity is to all visible light rather than UV rays only. Several wk after therapy, test for residual photosensitivity by exposing a small area (not the face) to bright indoor light for 10 min. Note if redness, swelling, or blistering occurs. Wait 2 wk between tests if reaction occurs. Advise women of child-bearing age to practice an effective method of contraception to avoid pregnancy.

SERIOUS ADVERSE REACTIONS

- Anemia has been reported secondary to bleeding from the tumor following treatment.
- Atrial fibrillation and heart failure occur rarely.
- Airway obstruction from necrotic tumor debris, inflammation, or mucositis. Immediate bronchoscopy may be needed. Stent placement may be needed if endobronchial stricture is present.

OVERDOSE/TOXICITY

- **Overdose management:** Do not provide laser light therapy, which will prompt increased damage to normal tissues and more profound side effects.
- **GI decontamination:** No specific recommendations.

ANTIDOTE/DIALYSIS

- **Antidote:** No specific recommendations.
- **Dialysis:** Porfimer is not removed by hemodialysis. No data are available on removal by high-permeability hemodialysis or peritoneal dialysis.

potassium salts 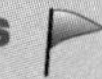

poe-tass'-i-um

Classes

Chemical: monovalent cation
Therapeutic: electrolyte supplement

Pregnancy Category: C, A

Trade Names

Prescription: (potassium bicarbonate-citrate) Effer K, Klor-Con EF, K-Lyte, K-Lyte DS; (potassium chloride) Cena K, Ed K+10, K+Care, K-8, K-10, Kaochlor, Kaon-Cl, Kaon-CL 10, Kaon-CL 20%, Kato, Kay Ciel, KCl-20, KCl-40, K-Dur, K-Dur 10, K-Dur 20, K-Lor, K-Lor-Con M 15, Klor-Con, Klor-Con 8, Klor-Con 10, Klor-Con/25, Klor-Con M10, Klor-Con M15, Klor-Con M20, Klotrix, K-Norm, K-Sol, K-Tab, Kaon-Cl, Micro-K, Micro-K 10, Rum-K; (potassium gluconate) Kaon

Do not confuse K-dur with Cardura.

CLINICAL PHARMACOLOGY

Mechanism of Action

An electrolyte that is necessary for multiple cellular metabolic processes. Primary action is intracellular. **Therapeutic Effect:** Needed for nerve impulse conduction and contraction of cardiac, skeletal, and smooth muscle; maintains normal renal function and acid-base balance.

PHARMACOKINETICS

Well absorbed from the GI tract. Enters cells by active transport from extracellular fluid. Primarily excreted in urine.

AVAILABILITY

Potassium Acetate

Injection: 2 mEq/mL.

Potassium Bicarbonate and Potassium Citrate

Tablets for solution: 25 mEq (Klor-Con EF, Effer-K, K-Lyte), 50 mEq (K-Lyte DS).

Potassium Chloride

Capsules (controlled release [Micro-K]): 8 mEq, 10 mEq.
Liquid: 20 mEq/15 mL (Kaochlor), 40 mEq/15 mL (Kaon-Cl).
Powder for oral solution (K-Lor): 20 mEq.
Powder for Reconstitution (K+Care): 20 mEq
Injection: 2 mEq/mL.
Tablets (extended release): 8 mEq (K-8, Klor-Con, Klor-Con 8, Klor-Con M10, Micro-K, Micro-K10), 10 mEq (K-8, Kaon-CL,

Kaon-CL 10, K-Dur, Klor-Con, Klor-Con 8, Klor-Con M10, Klotrix, K-Tab, Micro-K, Micro-K 10), 20 mEq (K-Dur).

Potassium Gluconate

Elixir (Kaon): 20 mEq/15 mL.

INDICATIONS AND DOSAGE

Prevention of hypokalemia (in patients on diuretic therapy)

PO

Adults, Elderly: 20-40 mEq/day in 1-2 divided doses. **Children:** 1-2 mEq/kg/day divided in 1-2 divided doses.

Treatment of hypokalemia

PO

Adults, Elderly: 40-80 mEq/day; further doses based on laboratory values. **Children:** 2-5 mEq/day; further doses based on laboratory values.

IV

Adults, Elderly: 5-10 mEq/hr. Maximum: 400 mEq/day. **Children:** 1 mEq/kg over 1-2 hr.

CONTRAINDICATIONS

Concurrent use of potassium-sparing diuretics, digitalis toxicity, heat cramps, hyperkalemia, postoperative oliguria, severe burns, severe renal impairment, shock with dehydration or hemolytic reaction, untreated Addison's disease, hypersensitivity to components of potassium products

INTERACTIONS

Drug: **ACE inhibitors, beta-adrenergic blockers, heparin, NSAIDs, potassium-containing medications, potassium-sparing diuretics, salt substitutes:** May increase potassium blood concentration. **Anticholinergics:** May increase the risk of GI lesions. **Herbal:** None known. **Food:** None known.

DIAGNOSTIC TEST EFFECTS

None known.

IV INCOMPATIBILITIES

Amphotericin B complex (Abelcet, AmBisome, Amphotec), *methylPREDNISolone (Solu-Medrol), phenytoin (Dilantin)

IV COMPATIBILITIES

Aminophylline, amiodarone (Cordarone), atropine, aztreonam (Azactam), calcium gluconate, cefepime (Maxipime), ciprofloxacin (Cipro), clindamycin (Cleocin), dexamethasone (Decadron), digoxin (Lanoxin), diltiazem (Cardizem), *diphenhydrAMINE (Benadryl), *DOBUTamine (Dobutrex), *DOPamine (Intropin), enalapril (Vasotec), famotidine (Pepcid), fluconazole (Diflucan), furosemide (Lasix), granisetron (Kytril), heparin, hydrocortisone (Solu-Cortef), insulin, lidocaine, lorazepam (Ativan), magnesium sulfate, *methylPREDNISolone (Solu-Medrol), metoclopramide (Reglan), midazolam (Versed), milrinone (Primacor), morphine, norepinephrine (Levophed), ondansetron (Zofran), oxytocin (Pitocin), piperacillin and tazobactam (Zosyn), procainamide (Pronestyl), propofol (Diprivan), propranolol (Inderal)

SIDE-EFFECTS

Occasional: Nausea, vomiting, diarrhea, flatulence, abdominal discomfort with distention, phlebitis with IV administration (particularly when potassium concentration of greater than 40 mEq/L is infused). **Rare:** Rash

CRITICAL CARE CONSIDERATIONS

ADMINISTRATION/HANDLING

PO ALERT

- Give potassium during or after meals with full glass of water to decrease GI upset.
- Mix effervescent tablets, liquids, and powders with juice or water and let them dissolve before administering.
- Instruct to swallow the tablets whole, not to chew or crush. Potassium dosage must be individualized.

IV ALERT

- **Storage:** Store vials at room temperature.
- **Dilution:** Common dilution is 40 mEq/L; 80 mEq/L is the usual maximum concentration and must be administered with caution; mix well before IV infusion. Avoid adding potassium to a hanging IV line unless solution can be well mixed and concentration is safe in the volume of the infusion.
- *Never* give by direct IV injection. Direct IV injection of concentrated potassium solution may cause immediate cardiac arrest and death.
- **Infusion rate:** Infuse the drug slowly at a rate not exceeding 20 mEq/hr. Potassium dosage must be individualized. Up to 100 mEq/100 mL has been infused through a central IV line for replacement therapy using an infusion pump to ensure patient the proper dose is received.
- **IV site care:** Check the IV site closely during the infusion for phlebitis (hardness of vein; heat, pain, red streaking of skin

over vein) and extravasation (cool skin, little or no blood return, pain, and swelling). Higher concentrations of potassium should be administered through a central IV line to avoid phlebitis.

PRECAUTIONS

HEALTH-RELATED

- Use potassium cautiously in patients with cardiac or renal disease and in those with adrenal insufficiency and tartrazine sensitivity (common in those with aspirin hypersensitivity).
- Alkalyzing potassiums (e.g., citrate, acetate) may be more effective in hypokalemic patients with renal tubular acidosis. Use with caution in patients with alkalosis (respiratory or metabolic). Some potassium acetate formulations contain aluminum, which may reach toxic levels in renal impaired patients, especially neonates.

AGE-RELATED

- **Children:** No age-related precautions have been noted in children.
- **Elderly:** May be at increased risk for hyperkalemia because of an impaired ability to excrete potassium.

PREGNANCY/LACTATION-RELATED

- Pregnancy category C (A for potassium chloride); use with caution in breastfeeding women.

MONITORING

- **Baseline assessment:** Assess for causes of hypokalemia including overuse of diuretics without potassium replacement, increased loss via diarrhea or diaphoresis, dialysis, or hyperaldosteronism. Note muscle weakness, cramps, soft and flabby muscles, nausea, vomiting, and paresthesias.
- **Baseline lab work:** Biochemical profile including potassium, sodium, BUN, creatinine, magnesium, and calcium levels.
- **Renal impairment:** Monitor the potassium level throughout replacement therapy, particularly in those with renal impairment. Be alert for decreased urine output, which may be an indication of renal insufficiency.
- **Dysrhythmias:** Continuous ECG monitoring for patients receiving IV potassium replacement for hypokalemia; note ST segment depression, flattened T wave, presence of U wave, ventricular dysrhythmias, increased P wave amplitude, prolonged PR and QT intervals with widened QRS complexes indicative of hypokalemia.
- **Nausea/vomiting:** If GI upset is experienced, dilute the IV preparation further or give oral forms with meals.
- **Constipation:** Assess for decreased bowel sounds. Ileus may be present with severe hypokalemia.
- **Hyperkalemia:** As infusion progresses, assess for cold skin, feeling of heaviness in lower extremities, paresthesia, and skin pallor. ECG rhythm may reflect loss of P wave or progressive widening of QRS with elevated T waves. Progressive hyperkalemia may lead to cardiac arrest. Those with renal impairment and adrenal insufficiency can develop hyperkalemia quickly.
- **Patient education:** Give a list of foods rich in potassium, including apricots, avocados, bananas, beans, beef, broccoli, brussel sprouts, cantaloupe, chicken, dates, fish, ham, lentils, milk, molasses, potatoes, prunes, raisins, spinach, turkey, watermelon, veal, and yams. Instruct to report a feeling of heaviness in the lower extremities and paresthesia.

SERIOUS ADVERSE REACTIONS

- **Hyperkalemia:** More common in elderly and those with impaired renal function; may be manifested as paresthesia, feeling of heaviness in the lower extremities, cold skin, grayish pallor, hypotension, confusion, irritability, flaccid paralysis, and cardiac dysrhythmias.
- **Management:** Cation exchange resins (e.g., sodium polystyrene sulfonate [Kayexelate]) given by mouth or by retention enema exchanges potassium for sodium in the GI tract. Oral Kayexelate is combined with sorbitol to induce diarrhea, which helps eliminate additional potassium. Use with caution in digitalized patients; rapid potassium loss may induce digitalis toxicity.

OVERDOSE/TOXICITY

- **Cardiac arrest:** Direct IV injection of concentrated potassium can result in immediate death from severe hyperkalemia.
- **Management:** IV calcium gluconate helps counteract the cardiac and neuromuscular effects of hyperkalemia. Serum potassium levels will remain elevated. IV dextrose 50% one amp followed by IV dextrose (10%-20%) and insulin (one unit for every 3 g dextrose) helps shift

P

potassium into the cells to temporarily reduce potassium. Sodium bicarbonate helps shift potassium temporarily into the cells. Beta-2 adrenergic agonists (e.g., albuterol) shifts potassium into the cells temporarily. Resuscitate according to Advanced Cardiac Life Support (ACLS) guidelines.

- **GI decontamination:** No specific recommendations.

ANTIDOTE/DIALYSIS

- **Antidote:** IV calcium gluconate; IV dextrose and insulin; IV sodium bicarbonate; beta-2 adrenergic agonists (e.g., albuterol). Use with caution in digitalized patients; rapid potassium loss may induce digitalis toxicity.
- **Dialysis:** Potassium salts are removed by hemodialysis, high-permeability hemodialysis, and peritoneal dialysis.

pramipexole dihydrochloride

pra-mi-pex'-ole dye-hye-droe-klor'-ide

Classes

Chemical: benzothiazolamine derivative
Therapeutic: antiparkinson's agent, dopaminergic

Pregnancy Category: C

Trade Names

Prescription: Mirapex

Do not confuse Mirapex with Mifeprex or MiraLax.

CLINICAL PHARMACOLOGY

Mechanism of Action

An antiparkinson agent that stimulates dopamine receptors in the striatum. Therapeutic Effect: Relieves signs and symptoms of Parkinson's disease.

PHARMACOKINETICS

Rapidly and extensively absorbed after PO administration. Protein binding: 15%. Widely distributed. Steady-state concentrations achieved within 2 days. Primarily eliminated in urine. Not removed by hemodialysis. Half-life: 8 hr (12 hr in patients older than 65 yr).

AVAILABILITY

Tablets: 0.125 mg, 0.25 mg, 0.5 mg, 1 mg, 1.5 mg.

INDICATIONS AND DOSAGE

Parkinson's disease

PO

Adults, Elderly: Initially, 0.375 mg/day in 3 divided doses. Do not increase dosage more frequently than every 5-7 days. Maintenance: 1.5-4.5 mg/day in 3 equally divided doses.

Dosage in renal impairment

Dosage and frequency are modified based on creatinine clearance.

Creatinine Clearance	Initial Dose	Maximum Dose
Greater than 60 mL/min	0.125 mg 3 times per day	1.5 mg 3 times per day
35-60 mL/min	0.125 mg twice per day	1.5 mg twice per day
15-34 mL/min	0.125 mg once per day	1.5 mg once per day

OFF-LABEL USES

Depression (due to bipolar disorder), fibromyalgia, restless leg syndrome

CONTRAINDICATIONS

History of hypersensitivity to pramipexole

INTERACTIONS

Drug: **Carbidopa and levodopa, levodopa:** May increase plasma level of levodopa. **Cimetidine:** Increases pramipexole plasma concentration and half-life. May decrease pramipexole clearance. **Diltiazem, quinidine, quinine, ranitidine, triamterene, verapamil:** May decrease pramipexole clearance. Herbal: None known. Food: **All food:** Delays peak drug plasma levels by 1 hr but does not affect drug absorption.

DIAGNOSTIC TEST EFFECTS

None known.

SIDE-EFFECTS

Frequent: **Early Parkinson's disease (28%-10%):** Nausea, asthenia, dizziness, somnolence, insomnia, constipation. **Advanced Parkinson's disease (53%-17%):** Orthostatic hypotension, extrapyramidal reactions, insomnia, dizziness, hallucinations. Occasional: **Early Parkinson's disease (5%-2%):** Edema, malaise, confusion, amnesia, akathisia, anorexia, dysphagia, peripheral edema, vision changes, impotence. **Advanced Parkinson's disease (10%-7%):** Asthenia, somnolence, confusion, constipation, abnormal gait, dry mouth. Rare: **Advanced Parkinson's disease (6%-2%):** General edema, malaise, chest pain, amnesia, tremor, urinary frequency or incontinence, dyspnea, rhinitis, vision changes

CRITICAL CARE CONSIDERATIONS

ADMINISTRATION/HANDLING

PO ALERT

- Give pramipexole without regard to food.

PRECAUTIONS

HEALTH-RELATED

- Use pramipexole cautiously in patients with hallucinations, syncope, renal impairment, history of orthostatic hypotension; in those using CNS depressants concurrently.

AGE-RELATED

- **Children:** Safety and efficacy of pramipexole have not been established in children.
- **Elderly:** Are at increased risk for hallucinations.

PREGNANCY/LACTATION-RELATED

- Pregnancy category C; inhibits prolactin secretion. Excretion into breast milk unknown.

MONITORING

- **Baseline assessment:** Obtain vital signs.
- **Baseline lab work:** Biochemical profile including renal function (BUN, creatinine) studies. Renal function guides dosage.
- **Hypotension:** Instruct to change positions slowly to prevent orthostatic hypotension. Assist with ambulation if experiencing dizziness.
- **Constipation:** Assess pattern of bowel elimination and stool consistency.
- **Therapeutic effect:** Assess for improvement of masklike facial expression, muscular rigidity, shuffling gait, and resting tremors of the hands and head.
- **Patient education:** Instruct to take pramipexole with food if nausea is a problem. Caution against abruptly discontinuing pramipexole. Inform (especially if elderly) that the drug may cause hallucinations. Explain that orthostatic hypotension occurs more commonly during initial therapy. Warn to avoid tasks requiring mental alertness or motor skills until response to the drug is known.

SERIOUS ADVERSE REACTIONS

- **Rhabdomyolysis:** Dark urine, severe generalized muscle pain, acute renal failure (very rare).
- **Dyskinesia:** Pramipexole may potentiate the dopaminergic effects of levodopa and may worsen preexisting dykinesia.
- **Falling asleep during activities of daily living:** Patients have fallen asleep while driving a motor vehicle resulting in a motor vehicle crash.

OVERDOSE/TOXICITY

- **Overdose:** Delirium, hallucinations, nausea, vomiting, hypotension, possible paranoia, lethargy.
- **Management:** Supportive care, including maintaining patent airway and supporting ventilation; providing calm support and prevent patients from injuring themselves.
- **GI decontamination:** No specific recommendations.

ANTIDOTE/DIALYSIS

- **Antidote:** No specific recommendations.
- **Dialysis:** Pramipexole is not removed by hemodialysis and is unlikely to be removed by peritoneal dialysis. No data are available on removal by high-permeability hemodialysis.

pramlintide

See Antidiabetics (p. 911)

pravastatin

pra′-va-stat-in

Classes

Chemical: substituted hexahydronaphthalene
Therapeutic: HMG-CoA reductase inhibitor, antilipemic

Pregnancy Category: X

Trade Names

Prescription: Pravachol

Do not confuse pravastatin with Prevacid, or Pravachol with propranolol.

CLINICAL PHARMACOLOGY

Mechanism of Action

An HMG-CoA reductase inhibitor that interferes with cholesterol biosynthesis by preventing the conversion of hydroxy methyglutaryl-CoA reductase to mevalonate, a precursor to cholesterol. **Therapeutic Effect:** Lowers serum LDL and very low-density lipoprotein cholesterol and plasma triglyceride levels; increases serum HDL concentration.

P

PHARMACOKINETICS
Poorly absorbed from the GI tract. Protein binding: 50%. Metabolized in the liver (minimal active metabolites). Primarily excreted in feces via the biliary system. Not removed by hemodialysis. **Half-life:** 2.7 hr.

AVAILABILITY
Tablets: 10 mg, 20 mg, 40 mg, 80 mg.

INDICATIONS AND DOSAGE
Hyperlipidemia, primary and secondary prevention of cardiovascular events in patients with elevated cholesterol levels
PO

Adults, Elderly: Initially, 40 mg/day. Titrate to desired response. Range: 10-80 mg/day. **Children 14-18 yr:** 40 mg/day. **Children 8-13 yr:** 20 mg/day.

Dosage in hepatic and renal impairment
For adults, give 10 mg/day initially. Titrate to desired response.

CONTRAINDICATIONS
Active hepatic disease or unexplained, persistent elevations of liver function test results, hypersensitivity to pravastatin

INTERACTIONS
Drug: *CycloSPORINE, erythromycin, gemfibrozil, immunosuppressants, niacin: Increases the risk of acute renal failure and rhabdomyolysis. **Herbal:** None known. **Food:** None known.

P

DIAGNOSTIC TEST EFFECTS
May increase serum creatine kinase (CK) and transaminase concentrations.

SIDE-EFFECTS
Pravastatin is generally well tolerated. Side effects are usually mild and transient. **Occasional (7%-4%):** Nausea, vomiting, diarrhea, constipation, abdominal pain, headache, rhinitis, rash, pruritus. **Rare (3%-2%):** Heartburn, myalgia, dizziness, cough, fatigue, flulike symptoms

CRITICAL CARE CONSIDERATIONS

ADMINISTRATION/HANDLING
PO ALERT
- Give pravastatin without regard to meals and administer in the evening.
- Patients should be placed on a standard cholesterol-lowering diet for a minimum of 3-6 mo before beginning pravastatin therapy. Diet should continue throughout pravastatin therapy.

PRECAUTIONS
HEALTH-RELATED
- Use pravastatin cautiously in patients with a history of hepatic disease or severe electrolyte, endocrine, or metabolic disorders and in those who consume a substantial amount of alcohol.
- Withholding or discontinuing pravastatin may be necessary when patients are at risk for renal failure secondary to rhabdomyolysis.

AGE-RELATED
- **Children:** Safety and efficacy of pravastatin have not been established in children.
- **Elderly:** No age-related precautions have been noted.

PREGNANCY/LACTATION-RELATED
- Pregnancy category X; small amounts excreted in breast milk; should probably not be used by women who are nursing.

MONITORING
- **Baseline assessment:** Assess dietary and exercise habits, history of liver disease and assess for pregnancy before beginning pravastatin therapy.
- **Baseline and ongoing lab work:** Biochemical profile including liver function tests (alkaline phosphatase, bilirubin, AST [SGOT], and ALT [SGPT] levels). Assess baseline laboratory serum cholesterol and triglyceride levels. Monitor cholesterol and triglycerides for therapeutic response and liver enzymes every 12 wk after initial therapy and each time dosage is adjusted. Semiannual monitoring may be appropriate for patients on fixed doses with good response.
- **Therapeutic response:** Monitor for reduced cholesterol and triglyceride levels.
- **Common side effects:** Constipation, abdominal pain, dyspepsia, flatulence. May require symptom specific management to control.
- **Myalgias:** CPK level may be measured for patients with unexplained myalgias. Urine will appear brown if myoglobin is present.
- **Renal failure:** Monitor BUN, creatinine, and potassium levels if patients manifest myalgia or brown urine indicative of myoglobinuria. Urinalysis is used to diagnose myoglobinuria.

- **Hypersensitivity:** Assess for pruritus and rash.
- **Impending rhabdomyolysis:** Assess for malaise and muscle cramping, or weakness. If these conditions occur and are accompanied by fever, pravastatin should be discontinued.
- **Patient education:** Advise to follow the prescribed diet; explain that the diet is an important part of treatment. Stress that periodic laboratory tests are an essential part of therapy. Instruct patients to promptly report muscle pain or weakness, especially if accompanied by fever or malaise, to a health care provider. Advise avoidance of tasks requiring mental alertness or motor skills until response to the drug is known. Urge females during child-bearing years to use nonhormonal contraceptives while taking pravastatin. Explain that pravastatin is pregnancy risk category X.

SERIOUS ADVERSE REACTIONS

- **Hypersensitivity:** Urticaria, rash, angioedema occurs rarely.
- **Musculoskeletal pain:** Myopathy, arthralgia, myalgia, which may indicate impending rhabdomyolysis.
- Malignancy and cataracts may occur.

OVERDOSE/TOXICITY

- **Nephrotoxicity:** Acute renal failure ensues when rhabdomyolysis is present.
- **Hepatotoxicity:** Liver enzyme elevation indicative of impending liver failure.
- **Rhabdomyolysis:** Rare cases; can lead to acute renal failure. Markedly elevated serum CK and possible myoglobinuria indicate the condition may be present. Should be managed according to accepted guidelines, which include aggressive volume replacement, hemodialysis, or continuous veno-venous hemofiltration to support patients during acute renal failure. Use of bicarbonate to induce alkaline diuresis or mannitol for osmotic diuresis has not been well studied. Hyperkalemia and hyperphosphatemia are commonly seen with rhabdomyolysis and may require aggressive management.
- **GI decontamination:** No specific recommendations.

ANTIDOTE/DIALYSIS

- **Antidote:** No specific recommendations.
- **Dialysis:** Pravastatin is not removed by hemodialysis. No data are available on removal by high-permeability hemodialysis or peritoneal dialysis.

prazosin hydrochloride 

pra'-zoe-sin hye-droe-klor'-ide

Classes

Chemical: quinazoline derivative
Therapeutic: antihypertensive, α1-adrenergic blocker

Pregnancy Category: C

Trade Names

Prescription: Minipress

Combinations

Prescription: with polythiazide (Minizide)

CLINICAL PHARMACOLOGY

Mechanism of Action

An antidote, antihypertensive, and vasodilator that selectively blocks $alpha_1$-adrenergic receptors, decreasing peripheral vascular resistance. **Therapeutic Effect:** Produces vasodilation of veins and arterioles, decreases total peripheral resistance, and relaxes smooth muscle in bladder neck and prostate.

PHARMACOKINETICS

Well absorbed following oral administration. Protein binding: 92%-97%. Metabolized in liver. Primarily excreted in feces. **Half-life:** 2-4 hr.

AVAILABILITY

Capsules: 1 mg, 2 mg, 5 mg.

INDICATIONS AND DOSAGE

Mild to moderate hypertension

PO

Adults, Elderly: Initially, 1 mg 2-3 times per day. Maintenance: 3-15 mg/day in divided doses. Maximum: 20 mg/day. **Children:** 5 mcg/kg/dose every 6 hr. Gradually increase up to 25 mcg/kg/dose.

OFF-LABEL USES

Treatment of benign prostatic hyperplasia, heart failure, ergot alkaloid toxicity, pheochromocytoma, Raynaud's phenomenon

CONTRAINDICATIONS

Hypersensitivity to prazosin or other quinazolines

INTERACTIONS

Drug: **Estrogen, NSAIDs, other sympathomimetics:** May decrease the effects of prazosin. **Hypotension-producing medications, such as antihypertensives and diuretics:** May increase the effects of prazosin. **Herbal:** **Licorice:** Causes sodium and water retention, potassium loss. **Food:** None known.

DIAGNOSTIC TEST EFFECTS
None known.

SIDE-EFFECTS
Frequent (10%-7%): Dizziness, somnolence, headache, asthenia (loss of strength, energy). **Occasional (5%-4%):** Palpitations, nausea, dry mouth, nervousness. **Rare (less than 1%):** Angina, urinary urgency

CRITICAL CARE CONSIDERATIONS

ADMINISTRATION/HANDLING

PO ALERT
- Give prazosin without regard to food.
- Administer the first dose at bedtime to minimize the risk of fainting from first-dose syncope.

PRECAUTIONS

HEALTH-RELATED
- Use prazosin cautiously in patients with chronic renal failure or impaired hepatic function.
- May cause syncope with sudden loss of consciousness.

AGE-RELATED
- **Children:** Safety and efficacy of prazosin have not been established in children.
- **Elderly:** Age-related organ impairment may warrant a dosage reduction.

PREGNANCY/LACTATION-RELATED
- Pregnancy category C; unknown if distributed in breast milk.

MONITORING
- **Baseline assessment:** Assess vital signs immediately before each dose and every 15-30 min thereafter until BP is stabilized.
- **Baseline lab work:** Biochemical profile with renal (BUN, creatinine) and liver (AST [SGOT], ALT [SGPT], alkaline phosphatase, bilirubin, GGT) tests.
- **First dose syncope:** Give the first prazosin dose at bedtime. If the initial dose is given during the day, keep patients recumbent for 3-4 hr. Monitor BP and pulse frequently because first-dose syncope may be preceded by tachycardia.
- **Dysrhythmias:** Monitor ECG continuously for tachycardia and supraventricular tachycardia in critically ill patients who receive prazosin.
- **Diarrhea or constipation:** Assess pattern of daily bowel activity and stool consistency.
- **Dizziness:** Assist with ambulation if dizziness occurs.
- **Patient education:** Warn to avoid tasks requiring mental alertness or motor skills until response to the drug is known, and to use caution when rising from a sitting or lying position. Instruct to report promptly to a health care provider if dizziness or palpitations become bothersome.

SERIOUS ADVERSE REACTIONS
- **First dose syncope:** Hypotension with sudden loss of consciousness may occur 30-90 min following initial dose of more than 2 mg, following a too-rapid increase in dosage, or adding another antihypertensive agent to therapy. First-dose syncope may be preceded by tachycardia.
- **Cardiovascular:** Edema, dyspnea, orthostatic hypotension, tachycardia.
- **Management:** Manage blood pressure initially with IV fluid infusion. Larger doses of alpha adrenergic vasopressors may be required to override the alpha-adrenergic blocking effects of prazosin.

OVERDOSE/TOXICITY
- **Hepatotoxicity:** Elevated liver enzymes, right upper quadrant pain, jaundice.
- **GI decontamination:** No specific recommendations.

ANTIDOTE/DIALYSIS
- **Antidote:** No specific recommendations.
- **Dialysis:** Prazosin is not removed by hemodialysis or peritoneal dialysis. No data are available on removal by high-permeability hemodialysis.

*prednisoLONE
See Corticosteroids (p. 953)

*predniSONE
pred'-ni-sone

Classes
Chemical: glucocorticoid, synthetic
Therapeutic: corticosteroid, systemic

Pregnancy Category: C, D (if used in 1st trimester)

Trade Names
Prescription: Apo-Prednisone ♣, Deltasone, Liquid Pred, Meticorten, Prednicen-M,

P

Prednicot, Prednisone Intensol, Sterapred, Sterapred DS

Do not confuse *predniSONE with *prednisoLONE or primidone.

CLINICAL PHARMACOLOGY

Mechanism of Action

An adrenocortical steroid that inhibits accumulation of inflammatory cells at inflammation sites, phagocytosis, lysosomal enzyme release and synthesis, and release of mediators of inflammation. **Therapeutic Effect:** Prevents or suppresses cell-mediated immune reactions. Decreases or prevents tissue response to inflammatory process.

PHARMACOKINETICS

Well absorbed from the GI tract. Protein binding: 70%-90%. Widely distributed. Metabolized in the liver and converted to *prednisoLONE. Primarily excreted in urine. Not removed by hemodialysis. **Half-life:** 2.5-3.5 hr.

AVAILABILITY

Oral concentrate (Prednisone Intensol): 5 mg/mL.
Oral solution (Liquid Pred): 5 mg/5 mL.
Tablets: 1 mg (Sterapred), 2.5 mg (Deltasone), 5 mg (Deltasone, Prednicen-M, Sterapred), 10 mg (Deltasone, Sterapred), 20 mg (Deltasone), 50 mg (Deltasone).

INDICATIONS AND DOSAGE

Substitution therapy in deficiency states: acute or chronic adrenal insufficiency, congenital adrenal hyperplasia, and adrenal insufficiency secondary to pituitary insufficiency; nonendocrine disorders: arthritis; rheumatic carditis; allergic, collagen, intestinal tract, liver, ocular, renal, skin diseases; bronchial asthma; cerebral edema; malignancies

PO

Adults, Elderly: 5-60 mg/day in divided doses. **Children:** 0.05-2 mg/kg/day in 1-4 divided doses.

CONTRAINDICATIONS

Acute superficial herpes simplex keratitis, systemic fungal infections, varicella, hypersensitivity to *predniSONE

INTERACTIONS

Drug: **Amphotericin:** May increase hypokalemia. **Digoxin:** May increase the risk of digoxin toxicity caused by hypokalemia **Diuretics, insulin, oral hypoglycemics, potassium supplements:** May decrease the effects of these drugs. **Hepatic enzyme inducers:** May decrease the effects of *predniSONE. **Live-virus vaccines:** May decrease antibody response to vaccine, increase vaccine side effects, and potentiate virus replication. **Herbal:** None known. **Food:** None known.

DIAGNOSTIC TEST EFFECTS

May increase blood glucose and serum lipid, amylase, and sodium levels. May decrease serum calcium, potassium, and thyroxine levels.

SIDE-EFFECTS

Frequent: Insomnia, heartburn, nervousness, abdominal distention, increased sweating, acne, mood swings, increased appetite, facial flushing, delayed wound healing, increased susceptibility to infection, diarrhea or constipation. **Occasional:** Headache, edema, change in skin color, frequent urination. **Rare:** Tachycardia, allergic reaction (including rash and hives), psychologic changes, hallucinations, depression

CRITICAL CARE CONSIDERATIONS

ADMINISTRATION/HANDLING

PO ALERT

- Give *predniSONE without regard to meals; give with food if GI upset occurs.
- Give single doses before 9 AM; give multiple doses at evenly spaced intervals.

PRECAUTIONS

HEALTH-RELATED

- Use *predniSONE cautiously in patients with heart failure, cirrhosis, hypertension, hyperthyroidism, myasthenia gravis, ocular herpes simplex, osteoporosis, peptic ulcer disease, thromboembolic disorders, or ulcerative colitis.

AGE-RELATED

- **Children:** Prolonged treatment or high dosages may decrease the cortisol secretion and short-term growth rate in children.
- **Elderly:** May be more susceptible to developing hypertension or osteoporosis.

P

PREGNANCY/LACTATION-RELATED

- Pregnancy category C (D if used in first trimester). Distributed in breast milk; breast-feeding is not recommended.

MONITORING

- **Baseline assessment:** Monitor vital signs including BP, height and body weight. Determine hypersensitivity to corticosteroids.
- **Baseline lab work:** Biochemical profile including blood glucose and serum electrolyte levels. Determine whether diabetes mellitus is present; increase antidiabetic drug regimen because of raised blood glucose level. If digoxin is being taken, draw serum digoxin levels.
- **Diagnostic tests:** Evaluate results of tuberculosis skin test, x-rays, and ECG.
- **Live virus vaccines:** Patients taking *predniSONE should never be given live virus vaccines (e.g., smallpox vaccine).
- **Weight gain/BP elevation:** Monitor for salt and retention-induced weight gain, edema, and increase in BP.
- **Hypokalemia:** Monitor ECG for dysrhythmias induced by increased potassium excretion such as premature ventricular beats, and ventricular and supraventricular tachycardias.
- **Electrolyte imbalance:** Monitor for hypocalcemia (muscle twitching, cramps, and positive Chvostek's or Trousseau's signs), or hypokalemia (ECG changes, nausea and vomiting, irritability, weakness and muscle cramps, numbness and tingling, especially in lower extremities).
- **Hyperglycemia:** Consider insulin infusion if blood glucose remains elevated.
- **Adrenal insufficiency:** Wean *predniSONE slowly when discontinuing either short- or long-term therapy to avoid adrenal insufficiency.
- **Sleep disturbance and emotional lability:** Assess sleep pattern and emotional status, since drug may cause sleeplessness, euphoria, high energy, or labile emotional state. Inform that *predniSONE often causes mood swings.
- **Immunosuppression:** Assess the mouth daily for candidal infection (white patches, painful mucous membranes and tongue).
- **Patient education:** Instruct to report fever, muscle aches, sore throat, and sudden weight gain, or swelling promptly to a health care provider. Urge avoidance of alcohol and limiting caffeine intake during *predniSONE therapy. Caution against abruptly discontinuing the drug without physician approval. Instruct to avoid exposure to chicken pox or measles. Explain that steroids often cause mood swings ranging from euphoria to depression.

SERIOUS ADVERSE REACTIONS

- **Long-term therapy:** May cause hypocalcemia, hypokalemia, hyperglycemia, muscle wasting (especially in the arms and legs), osteoporosis, spontaneous fractures, impaired wound healing, development of Cushingoid state, amenorrhea, cataracts, glaucoma, peptic ulcer disease, and heart failure. "Steroid-induced" diabetes mellitus may occur.
- **Pediatric patients:** Growth suppression.
- **Abrupt withdrawal after long-term use:** May cause anorexia, nausea, fever, headache, severe or sudden joint pain, rebound inflammation, fatigue, weakness, lethargy, dizziness, and orthostatic hypotension.
- **Sudden discontinuation:** May be fatal.

OVERDOSE/TOXICITY

- **Severe behavioral changes:** Extreme euphoria, personality changes, severe depression, frank psychosis (more likely in patients with mental health history).
- **Edema/weight gain:** Significant weight gain (over 15 lb), sodium retention, pitting edema, heart failure, difficulty breathing.
- **GI bleeding:** Hematemesis, bloody stools, expectoration of blood.
- **Severe infection:** Patients who have underlying infection or acquire a significant infection may develop fatal septic shock.
- **Negative nitrogen balance:** Due to protein catabolism.
- **GI decontamination:** No specific recommendations.

ANTIDOTE/DIALYSIS

- **Antidote:** No specific recommendations.
- **Dialysis:** *PredniSONE is not removed by hemodialysis or peritoneal dialysis. No data are available on removal by high-permeability hemodialysis.

pregabalin

See Anticonvulsants (p. 903)

primidone

See Anticonvulsants (p. 903)

procainamide hydrochloride

proe-kane'-a-mide hye-droe-klor'-ide

Classes

Chemical: para-aminobenzoic acid derivative

Therapeutic: antidysrhythmic, class IA

Pregnancy Category: C

Trade Names

Prescription: Procanbid, Procan-SR, Pronestyl, Pronestyl-SR

Do not confuse with Procanbid with probenecid, or Pronestyl with Ponstel.

CLINICAL PHARMACOLOGY

Mechanism of Action

An antidysrhythmic that increases the electrical stimulation threshold of the ventricles and His-Purkinje system. Decreases myocardial excitability and conduction velocity and depresses myocardial contractility. Exerts direct cardiac effects. **Therapeutic Effect:** Suppresses dysrhythmias.

PHARMACOKINETICS

Rapidly, completely absorbed from the GI tract. Protein binding: 15%-20%. Widely distributed. Metabolized in the liver to active metabolite. Primarily excreted in urine. Removed by hemodialysis. **Half-life:** 2.5-4.5 hr; metabolite, 6 hr.

AVAILABILITY

Capsules (Pronestyl): 250 mg, 500 mg.
Tablets (extended release [Pronestyl-SR]): 500 mg.
Tablets (extended release [Procanbid]): 500 mg, 750 mg, 1000 mg.
Injection (Pronestyl): 100 mg/mL, 500 mg/mL.

INDICATIONS AND DOSAGE

Maintenance of normal sinus rhythm after conversion of atrial fibrillation or flutter; treatment of premature ventricular contractions, paroxysmal atrial tachycardia, atrial fibrillation, and ventricular tachycardia

PO

Adults, Elderly: 250-500 mg of immediate-release tablets every 3-6 hr. 0.5-1 g of extended-release tablets every 6 hr. 1-2 g of Procanbid every 12 hr. **Children:** 15-50 mg/kg/day of immediate-release tablets in divided doses every 3-6 hr. Maximum: 4 g/day.

IV

Adults, Elderly: Loading dose: 50-100 mg. May repeat every 5-10 min or 15-18 mg/kg (maximum: 1-1.5 g). Then maintenance infusion of 3-4 mg/min. Range: 1-6 mg/min. **Children:** Loading dose: 3-6 mg/kg over 5 min (maximum: 100 mg). May repeat every 5-10 min to maximum total dose of 15 mg/kg. Then maintenance dose of 20-80 mcg/kg/min. Maximum: 2 g/day.

Dosage in renal impairment

Dosage interval is modified based on creatinine clearance.

Creatinine Clearance	Dosage Interval
10-50 mL/min	Every 6-12 hr
Less than 10 mL/min	Every 8-24 hr

OFF-LABEL USES

Conversion and management of atrial fibrillation

CONTRAINDICATIONS

Complete heart block, myasthenia gravis, preexisting QT prolongation, second-degree heart block, systemic lupus erythematosus, torsades de pointes, hypersensitivity to procainamide

INTERACTIONS

Drug: Antihypertensives (IV procainamide), neuromuscular blockers: May increase the effects of these drugs. May decrease antimyasthenic effect on skeletal muscle. **Other antidysrhythmics, pimozide:** May increase cardiac effects. **Herbal:** None known. **Food:** None known.

DIAGNOSTIC TEST EFFECTS

May cause ECG changes and positive antinuclear antibody (ANA) titers and Coombs' test. May increase AST (SGOT), ALT (SGPT), serum alkaline phosphatase, serum bilirubin, and serum LDH levels. Therapeutic serum level is 4-8 mcg/mL; toxic serum level is greater than 10 mcg/mL.

IV INCOMPATIBILITIES

Milrinone (Primacor)

IV COMPATIBILITIES

Amiodarone (Cordarone), *DOBUTamine (Dobutrex), heparin, lidocaine, potassium chloride

SIDE-EFFECTS

Frequent: PO: Abdominal pain or cramping, nausea, diarrhea, vomiting. **Occasional:** Dizziness, giddiness, weakness, hypersensitivity reaction (rash, urticaria, pruritus,

P

flushing). **IV:** Transient but at times marked hypotension. Rare: Confusion, mental depression, psychosis

CRITICAL CARE CONSIDERATIONS

ADMINISTRATION/HANDLING

PO ALERT

- Do not crush or break sustained-release tablets used for maintenance therapy.

IM ALERT

- **Injectate:** Solution normally appears clear and colorless to light yellow. Discard if solution darkens or appears discolored or if precipitate forms.

IV ALERT

- **Dilution:** When diluted with D_5W, solution is stable for 24 hr at room temperature or for 7 days if refrigerated; should appear clear, colorless, or light yellow.
- **IV push dilution:** Dilute with 5-10 mL D_5W.
- **IV push:** With patients in the supine position, administer at a rate not exceeding 25-50 mg/min.
- **Initial IV push infusion loading dose:** Add 1 g to 50 mL D_5W to provide a concentration of 20 mg/mL. Infuse 1 mL/min for up to 25-30 min.
- **IV maintenance infusion:** Add 1 g to 250-500 mL D_5W to provide concentration of 2 to 4 mg/mL. The maximum concentration is 4 g/250 mL. Infuse at 1-6 mg/min.

PROCAINAMIDE DOSAGE/RATE INFUSION TABLE

Dose	1000 mg/250 mL D_5W		1000 mg/500 mL D_5W	
(mg/min)	Rate mL/hr	mg/hr	Rate mL/hr	mg/hr
1	15	60	30	60
2	30	120	60	120
3	45	180	90	180
4	60	240	120	240
5	75	300	150	300
6	90	360	180	360

PRECAUTIONS

HEALTH-RELATED

- Use procainamide cautiously in patients with bundle-branch block, heart failure, hepatic or renal impairment, marked AV-conduction disturbances, severe digoxin toxicity, or supraventricular tachydysrhythmias.
- Procainamide dosage and the interval of administration are individualized based on age, clinical response, renal and liver function, and underlying heart disease.
- Prolonged administration may prompt patients to develop a positive antinuclear antibody test (ANA), which may or may not be associated with symptoms of systemic lupus erythematosus.
- Patients with myasthenia gravis may experience worsened symptoms due to the procainelike effect on decreasing acetylcholine release at skeletal motor neuron terminals; anticholinesterase medications may need dosage adjustment.

AGE-RELATED

- **Children:** No age-related precautions have been noted.
- **Elderly:** Are more susceptible to hypotensive effects; age-related renal impairment may require dosage adjustment.

PREGNANCY/LACTATION-RELATED

- Pregnancy category C; compatible with breast-feeding; long-term effects in nursing infant unknown.

MONITORING

- **Baseline assessment:** Check baseline vital signs including BP and heart rate. Patients should be on a continuous ECG monitor when IV procainamide is used. Heart rate/rhythm should be checked thoroughly for 1 min when patients are on oral maintenance therapy off the cardiac monitor.
- **Lab work:** CBC with WBC differential and biochemical profile including renal (BUN, creatinine) and liver (AST [SGOT], ALT [SGPT], alkaline phosphatase, GGT, bilirubin) function studies.
- **Hypotension:** Check BP every 5-10 min during IV infusion. If BP drops rapidly, slow infusion rate. If BP does not recover with slowed infusion, infusion should be discontinued.
- **Dysrhythmias:** Monitor ECG continuously for changes including widened QRS, prolonged PR and QT intervals. Infusion rate may need to be reduced if QRS widens by 50% or PR interval exceeds 0.20 sec. Heart block may progress to complete heart block. Continuously monitor BP to assess if dysrhythmias prompt hypotension. Ventricular dysrhythmias may progress to ventricular fibrillation and/or asystole.
- **Atrial fibrillation/flutter:** Patients should be digitalized or cardioverted before

P

procainamide administration to avoid possible tachycardia.

- **Pretoxicity side effects:** Monitor for bruising, bleeding, chills, confusion, dizziness, hallucinations, fever, loss of appetite, tremors, joint pain, vomiting and weakness, which may indicate serum drug level is high.
- **Hypersensitivity:** Assess skin for urticaria, flushing, itching, rash, especially in patients receiving high-dose therapy.
- **Serum drug levels:** Monitor for a therapeutic serum level of 4-8 mcg/mL. Discontinue procainamide for a level of greater than 10 mcg/mL.
- **N-acetyl procainamide (NAPA) level:** Monitor for NAPA, an active metabolite, in renal impaired patients and those receiving more than 3 mg/min for more than 24 hr.
- **Patient education:** Advise to space oral doses evenly around the clock. Instruct to report promptly fever, joint pain or stiffness, or upper respiratory tract infection to a health care provider. Caution against abruptly discontinuing procainamide; compliance with therapy is essential to control dysrhythmias. Explain that nasal decongestants or OTC cold preparations, especially those containing stimulants, should not be taken without prior health care provider approval. Warn to avoid performing tasks that require mental alertness or motor skills until response to the drug is known.

SERIOUS ADVERSE REACTIONS

- **Dysrhythmias:** Paradoxic, extremely rapid ventricular rate may occur during treatment of atrial fibrillation or flutter. Prolonged PR and QT intervals and flattened T waves occur less frequently.
- **Myasthenic crisis:** May occur in patients with myasthenia gravis.
- **Hypersensitivity:** Procainamide injection contains sulfites and may prompt an allergic reaction in sensitive patients.

OVERDOSE/TOXICITY

- **Hematologic toxicity:** Agranulocytosis, bone marrow suppression, neutropenia, thrombocytopenia, and hypoplastic anemia.
- **Cardiotoxicity:** Occurs most commonly with IV administration; includes conduction changes 50% widening of QRS complex, frequent ventricular premature contractions, ventricular tachycardia, ventricular fibrillation, torsades de pointes, complete AV block and asystole.
- **Systemic lupus erythematosus-like syndrome:** Fever, myalgia, and pleuritic chest pain may occur with prolonged therapy.
- **Management:** Procainamide should be discontinued and an alternative agent identified to manage the dysrhythmia. Another class 1 antidysrhythmic (lidocaine) or possibly a class 3 agent (amiodarone, sotalol) may be effective without causing toxicity or serious side effects. Other class IA antidysrhythmics (quinidine) may prompt further deterioration of ventricular dysrhythmias. Supportive care should be provided to maintain patent airway and support ventilation. Hypotension may be managed with IV fluids and then vasopressors if BP does not respond to fluid challenges. Transcutaneous or transvenous pacing may help manage heart block or asystole. Manage ventricular fibrillation using defibrillation according to Advanced Cardiac Life Support (ACLS) guidelines. Torsades de pointes may respond to magnesium sulfate or epinephrine infusion (isoproterenol is an older drug used for torsades) along with defibrillation.
- **GI decontamination:** No specific recommendations.

ANTIDOTE/DIALYSIS

- **Antidote:** Infusion of 1/6 M sodium lactate may help manage cardiotoxic effects. Urinary acidifiers may increase clearance.
- **Dialysis:** Procainamide and NAPA are removed by hemodialysis and are likely removed by high-permeability hemodialysis. No data are available on removal by peritoneal dialysis.

prochlorperazine

See Antipsychotics (p. 934)

promethazine hydrochloride

proe-meth'-a-zeen hye-droe-klor'-ide

DEA Schedule: V

Classes

Chemical: ethylamine phenothiazine derivative

Therapeutic: antiemetic, antihistamine, antitussive, antivertigo agent, sedative

P

Pregnancy Category: C

Trade Names

Prescription: Adgan, Anergan 50, Antinaus 50, Pentazine, Phenadoz, Phenergan, Phenoject-50, Promacot, Promethegan

Combinations

Prescription: with codeine (Phenergan with Codeine Syrup); with dextromethorphan (Phenergan with Dextromethorphan Syrup)

Do not confuse promethazine with promazine.

CLINICAL PHARMACOLOGY

Mechanism of Action

A phenothiazine that acts as an antihistamine, antiemetic, and sedative-hypnotic. As an antihistamine, inhibits histamine at histamine receptor sites. As an antiemetic, diminishes vestibular stimulation, depresses labyrinthine function, and act on the chemoreceptor trigger zone. As a sedative-hypnotic, produces CNS depression by decreasing stimulation to the brain stem reticular formation. **Therapeutic Effect:** Prevents allergic responses mediated by histamine, such as rhinitis, urticaria, and pruritus. Prevents and relieves nausea and vomiting.

PHARMACOKINETICS

Route	Onset	Peak	Duration
PO	20 min	N/A	2-8 hr
IV	3-5 min	N/A	2-8 hr
IM	20 min	N/A	2-8 hr
Rectal	20 min	N/A	2-8 hr

Well absorbed from the GI tract after IM administration. Widely distributed. Metabolized in the liver. Primarily excreted in urine. Not removed by hemodialysis. **Half-life:** 16-19 hr.

AVAILABILITY

Syrup (Pentazine, Phenergan): 6.25 mg/mL.

Tablets (Phenergan, Promacot): 12.5 mg, 25 mg, 50 mg.

Injection: 25 mg/mL (Phenergan), 50 mg/mL (Adgan, Anergan 50, Antinaus 50, Phenergan, Phenoject-50, Promacot).

Suppositories: 12.5 mg (Phenergan, Promethegan), 25 mg (Phenadoz, Phenergan, Promethegan), 50 mg (Phenergan, Promethegan).

INDICATIONS AND DOSAGE

Alert: Contraindicated in children 2 yr and younger.

Allergic symptoms

PO

Adults, Elderly: 6.25-12.5 mg 3 times per day plus 25 mg at bedtime. **Children:** 0.1 mg/kg/dose (maximum: 12.5 mg) 3 times per day plus 0.5 mg/kg/dose (maximum: 25 mg) at bedtime.

IV, IM

Adults, Elderly: 25 mg. May repeat in 2 hr.

Motion sickness

PO

Adults, Elderly: 25 mg 30-60 min before departure; may repeat in 8-12 hr, then every morning on rising and before evening meal. **Children:** 0.5 mg/kg 30-60 min before departure; may repeat in 8-12 hr, then every morning on rising and before evening meal.

Prevention of nausea, and vomiting

PO, IV, IM, Rectal

Adults, Elderly: 12.5-25 mg every 4-6 hr as needed. **Children:** 0.25-1 mg/kg every 4-6 hr as needed. Maximum: 25 mg per dose.

Preoperative and postoperative sedation; adjunct to analgesics

IV, IM

Adults, Elderly: 25-50 mg. **Children:** 12.5-25 mg.

Sedative

PO, IV, IM, Rectal

Adults, Elderly: 25-50 mg/dose. May repeat every 4-6 hr as needed. **Children:** 0.5-1 mg/kg/dose every 6 hr as needed. Maximum: 50 mg/dose.

CONTRAINDICATIONS

Angle-closure glaucoma, children 2 yr and younger, GI or GU obstruction, hypersensitivity to phenothiazines, severe CNS depression or coma, hypersensitivity to promethazine

INTERACTIONS

Drug: Alcohol, other CNS depressants: May increase CNS depressant effects. **Anticholinergics:** May increase anticholinergic effects. **MAOIs:** May intensify and prolong the anticholinergic and CNS depressant effects of promethazine. **Herbal:** None known. **Food:** None known.

DIAGNOSTIC TEST EFFECTS

May suppress wheal and flare reactions to antigen skin testing unless the drug is discontinued 4 days before testing.

IV INCOMPATIBILITIES

Allopurinol (Aloprim), amphotericin B complex (Abelcet, AmBisome, Amphotec), heparin, ketorolac (Toradol), nalbuphine (Nubain), piperacillin and tazobactam (Zosyn)

IV COMPATIBILITIES

Atropine, *diphenhydrAMINE (Benadryl), glycopyrrolate (Robinul), hydromorphone (Dilaudid), *hydrOXYzine (Vistaril), meperidine (Demerol), midazolam (Versed), morphine, prochlorperazine (Compazine)

SIDE-EFFECTS

Expected: Somnolence, disorientation; in elderly, hypotension, confusion, syncope. **Frequent:** Dry mouth, nose, or throat; urine retention; thickening of bronchial secretions. **Occasional:** Epigastric distress, flushing, visual disturbances, hearing disturbances, wheezing, paresthesia, diaphoresis, chills. **Rare:** Dizziness, urticaria, photosensitivity, nightmares

CRITICAL CARE CONSIDERATIONS

ADMINISTRATION/HANDLING

PO ALERT

- Give promethazine without regard to food.
- Crush scored tablets as needed.

IV ALERT

- **Storage:** Store vials at room temperature.
- **Dilution:** Promethazine may be given undiluted or diluted with 0.9% NaCl; final dilution should not exceed 25 mg/mL.
- **IV push/direct injection:** Inject promethazine at a rate of 25 mg/min through the tubing of an infusing IV solution; injecting drug too rapidly may cause a transient drop in BP, orthostatic hypotension, and reflex tachycardia.

IM ALERT

- Significant tissue necrosis may occur if promethazine is given subcutaneously. Inject the drug carefully because inadvertent intraarterial injection may produce severe arteriospasm, possibly resulting in gangrene.
- **Administration:** Inject deep into a large muscle mass.

RECTAL ALERT

- **Storage:** Refrigerate suppositories.
- **Preparation:** Moisten the suppository with cold water before inserting it well into the rectum.

PRECAUTIONS

HEALTH-RELATED

- Use promethazine cautiously in patients with asthma, history of seizures, cardiovascular disease, hepatic or renal impairment, peptic ulcer disease, sleep apnea, or possible Reye's syndrome.

AGE-RELATED

- **Children:** More likely to experience paradoxic reactions, such as increased excitement, nervousness, and tremor. Promethazine is not recommended for children under 2 yr.
- **Elderly:** More sensitive to the anticholinergic effects (dry mouth, confusion, dizziness, hypotension, syncope, and sedation).

PREGNANCY/LACTATION-RELATED

- Pregnancy category C; passage of drug into breast milk should be expected.

MONITORING

- **Baseline assessment:** Assess severely vomiting patients for dehydration (dry mucous membranes, longitudinal furrows in the tongue, and poor skin turgor). Assess appearance, behavior, emotional status, response to the environment, speech pattern, and thought content of psychotic patients. Discontinue drug 4 days before antigen skin testing.
- **Lab work:** CBC with WBC differential, biochemical profile including renal (BUN, creatinine) and liver (AST [SGOT], ALT [SGPT], alkaline phosphatase, GGT, bilirubin) function tests. Monitor CBC for blood dyscrasias.
- **Hypotension:** Monitor for low BP.
- **Extrapyramidal symptoms:** Assess for involuntary movements including tremors and jerking movements of extremities or facial muscles.
- **Tardive dyskinesia:** Observe for rapid tongue movement, which may be an early sign of tardive dyskinesia.
- **Suicidal patients:** Closely supervise suicidal psychotic patients during early therapy. As depression lessens, energy level generally improves, which increases the suicide potential.
- **Therapeutic response:** Assess psychotic patients for improvement in self-care, increased ability to concentrate, more interest in surroundings, and a more relaxed facial expression.
- **Patient education:** Urge avoidance of alcohol and limiting caffeine intake while taking promethazine. Warn to avoid tasks

requiring mental alertness or motor skills until response to the drug is known. Inform that drowsiness and dry mouth are expected side effects of promethazine. Drinking coffee or tea may help reduce drowsiness and sipping tepid water and chewing sugarless gum may relieve dry mouth. Instruct to report visual disturbances promptly to a health care provider.

SERIOUS ADVERSE REACTIONS

- Children may experience paradoxic reactions, such as excitation, nervousness, tremor, hyperactive reflexes, and seizures.
- Infants and young children have experienced CNS depression manifested as respiratory depression, sleep apnea, and sudden infant death syndrome.

OVERDOSE/TOXICITY

- **Neuroleptic malignant syndrome:** Hyperpyrexia, muscle rigidity, altered mental status, autonomic instability (irregular pulse, labile BP, cardiac dysrhythmias, tachycardia, diaphoresis).
- **Extrapyramidal symptoms:** Dose-related and divided into three categories: akathisia (including inability to sit still, tapping of feet); parkinsonian symptoms (such as masklike face, tremors, shuffling gait, hypersalivation); and acute dystonias (including torticollis, opisthotonos, and oculogyric crisis). A dystonic reaction may also produce diaphoresis and pallor.
- **Cardiac dysrhythmias:** Tachycardia, heart block, ST depression, T wave and U wave abnormalities, prolonged QT interval (quinidine like), supraventricular and ventricular dysrhythmias, hypotension.
- **Blood dyscrasias:** Most often agranulocytosis and mild leukopenia. Hemolytic anemia, aplastic anemia, thrombocytopenic purpura, and pancytopenia have been reported.
- **Respiratory depression:** Slow, shallow, irregular, ineffective breathing.
- **Seizures:** Promethazine may lower the seizure threshold prompting from petit mal to grand mal seizures.
- **Hepatotoxicity:** Jaundice and elevated serum transaminases occur most often between the second and fourth wk of therapy.
- **Management:** Supportive treatment including endotracheal intubation, mechanical ventilation, support of BP with fluids and vasopressors, possible trial of naloxone. Avoid Class 1A antidysrhythmic agents (procainamide, quinidine), IC agents (propafenone) and Class III agents (amiodarone), which may worsen conduction problems. Torsade de pointes is treated per Advanced Cardiac Life Support (ACLS) guidelines.
- **GI decontamination:** Activated charcoal if ingestion is within 3 hr. Because gut motility is slowed, charcoal is often effective longer following ingestion. Gastric lavage is not recommended. Multiple-dose activated charcoal is NOT recommended.

ANTIDOTE/DIALYSIS

- **Antidote:** No antidote for all drug effects. Physostigmine to control agitation and delirium. Benzodiazepines (diazepam, lorazepam) for seizures.
- **Dialysis:** Promethazine is not removed by hemodialysis. No data are available on removal by high-permeability hemodialysis or peritoneal dialysis.

propafenone hydrochloride

proe-pa-feh'-none hye-droe-klor'-ide

Classes

Chemical: 3-phenylpropiophenone derivative

Therapeutic: antidysrhythmic, class IC

Pregnancy Category: C

Trade Names

Prescription: Rythmol, Rythmol SR

CLINICAL PHARMACOLOGY

Mechanism of Action

An antidysrhythmic that decreases the fast sodium current in Purkinje or myocardial cells. Decreases excitability and automaticity; prolongs conduction velocity and the refractory period. **Therapeutic Effect:** Suppresses dysrhythmias.

PHARMACOKINETICS

Nearly completely absorbed following oral administration. Protein binding: 85%-97%. Metabolized in liver; undergoes first-pass metabolism. Primarily excreted in feces. **Half-life:** 2-10 hr.

AVAILABILITY

Tablets (Rythmol): 150 mg, 225 mg, 300 mg.

Capsules (extended release [Rythmol SR]): 225 mg, 325 mg, 425 mg.

INDICATIONS AND DOSAGE

Documented, life-threatening ventricular dysrhythmias, such as sustained ventricular tachycardia

PO

Adults, Elderly: Initially, 150 mg every 8 hr; may increase at 3- to 4-day intervals to 225 mg every 8 hr, then to 300 mg every 8 hr. Maximum: 900 mg/day.

PO (Extended Release)

Adults, Elderly: Initially, 225 mg every 12 hr. May increase at 5-day intervals. Maximum: 425 mg every 12 hr.

OFF-LABEL USES

Treatment of supraventricular dysrhythmias

CONTRAINDICATIONS

Bradycardia; bronchospastic disorders; cardiogenic shock; electrolyte imbalance; sinoatrial, AV, and intraventricular impulse generation or conduction disorders, such as sick sinus syndrome or AV block, without the presence of a pacemaker; uncontrolled heart failure, hypersensitivity to propafenone

INTERACTIONS

Drug: *CycloSPORINE: May increase risk of *cycloSPORINE toxicity. **Desipramine:** May increase risk of cardiotoxicity. **Digoxin, propranolol:** May increase concentrations of these drugs. **Local anesthetics:** May increase risk of CNS side effects. **Rifampin:** May decrease propafenone effectiveness. **Warfarin:** May increase warfarin effects. **Herbal:** None known. **Food:** None known.

DIAGNOSTIC TEST EFFECTS

May cause ECG changes, such as QRS widening and PR interval prolongation, and positive antinuclear antibodies (ANA) titers.

SIDE-EFFECTS

Frequent (13%-7%): Dizziness, nausea, vomiting, altered taste, constipation. **Occasional (6%-3%):** Headache, dyspnea, blurred vision, dyspepsia (heartburn, indigestion, epigastric pain). **Rare (less than 2%):** Rash, weakness, dry mouth, diarrhea, edema, hot flashes

CRITICAL CARE CONSIDERATIONS

ADMINISTRATION/HANDLING

PO ALERT

- Give propafenone without regard to meals.

PRECAUTIONS

HEALTH-RELATED

- Use propafenone cautiously in patients with bundle-branch block, heart failure, hepatic or renal impairment, marked AV-conduction disturbances, severe digoxin toxicity, recent MI, or supraventricular tachydysrhythmias.
- Propafenone dosage and the interval of administration are individualized based on age, clinical response, renal and liver function, and underlying heart disease.
- Prolonged administration may prompt patients to develop a positive antinuclear antibody (ANA) test, which may or may not be associated with symptoms of systemic lupus erythematosus.
- Patients with myasthenia gravis may experience worsened symptoms; anticholinesterase medications may need dosage adjustment.

AGE-RELATED

- **Children:** Safety and efficacy of propafenone have not been established in children.
- **Elderly:** Age-related organ impairment may prompt a dosage reduction.

PREGNANCY/LACTATION-RELATED

- Pregnancy category C; unknown if distributed in breast milk.

MONITORING

- **Baseline assessment:** Assess history of cardiac disease and symptoms of the dysrhythmia.
- **Baseline and ongoing lab work:** Biochemical profile including renal (BUN, creatinine) and liver (AST [SGOT], ALT [SGPT], alkaline phosphatase, GGT, bilirubin) function tests; correct electrolyte imbalances before beginning propafenone therapy. Monitor serum electrolyte levels.
- **Dysrhythmias:** Monitor continuous ECG for widening of the QRS complex and prolongation of the PR interval. Assess pulse quality and irregularity. Monitor for symptoms associated with changing ECG, including hypotension and chest discomfort.
- **Atrial fibrillation/flutter:** Patients should be digitalized or cardioverted before propafenone administration to avoid possible tachycardia.
- **Common side effects:** Assess for GI upset, constipation, headache, dizziness, unsteadiness, or visual disturbances.
- **Therapeutic drug serum level:** Monitor for therapeutic serum level; 0.06-1 mcg/mL.
- **Patient education:** Stress that compliance with the therapy regimen is essential to

P

control dysrhythmias. Advise that altered taste sensation may be present while taking propafenone. Instruct to report promptly blurred vision or headache to a health care provider. Recommend avoiding tasks that require mental alertness or motor skills until response to the drug is known.

SERIOUS ADVERSE REACTIONS

- **Proarrhythmia:** Propafenone may produce or worsen existing dysrhythmias.
- **Myasthenic crisis:** May occur in patients with myasthenia gravis.
- **Impaired spermatogenesis:** Reversible disorders have been reported.

OVERDOSE/TOXICITY

- **Hematologic toxicity:** Agranulocytosis, bone marrow suppression, neutropenia, thrombocytopenia, and hypoplastic anemia.
- **Cardiotoxicity:** Occurs most commonly with IV administration; includes conduction changes 50% widening of QRS complex, frequent ventricular premature contractions, ventricular tachycardia, ventricular fibrillation, torsades de pointes, complete AV block and asystole.
- **Systemic lupus erythematosus-like syndrome:** Fever, myalgia, pleuritic chest pain may occur with prolonged therapy.
- **Management:** Propafenone should be discontinued and an alternative agent identified to manage the dysrhythmia. A Class 1 antidysrhythmic (lidocaine) or possibly another Class 3 agent (amiodarone, sotalol) may be effective without causing toxicity or serious side effects. Supportive care should be provided to maintain patent airway and support ventilation. Hypotension may be managed with IV fluids and then, vasopressors if BP does not respond to fluid challenges. Transcutaneous or transvenous pacing may help manage heart block or asystole. Manage ventricular fibrillation using defibrillation according to Advanced Cardiac Life Support (ACLS) guidelines. Torsades de pointes may respond to magnesium sulfate, epinephrine infusion (isoproterenol is an older drug used for torsades) along with defibrillation.
- **GI decontamination:** No specific recommendations.

ANTIDOTE/DIALYSIS

- **Antidote:** No specific recommendations.
- **Dialysis:** Propafenone is not removed by hemodialysis or peritoneal dialysis. No data are available on removal by high-permeability hemodialysis.

P

propofol

proe'-po-fole

Classes

Chemical: disopropylphenol
Therapeutic: general anesthetic, anesthesia adjunct, sedative-hypnotic

Pregnancy Category: B

Trade Names

Prescription: Diprivan

CLINICAL PHARMACOLOGY

Mechanism of Action

A rapidly acting general anesthetic that inhibits sympathetic vasoconstrictor nerve activity and decreases vascular resistance. **Therapeutic Effect:** Produces hypnosis rapidly.

PHARMACOKINETICS

Route	Onset	Peak	Duration
IV	30 sec	N/A	3-10 min

Rapidly and extensively distributed. Protein binding: 97%-99%. Metabolized in the liver. Primarily excreted in urine. Unlikely to be removed by hemodialysis. **Half-life:** 3-12 hr.

AVAILABILITY

Injection: 10 mg/mL.

INDICATIONS AND DOSAGE

Anesthesia

IV

Adults, Elderly: Induction, 20-40 mg every 10 sec until induction onset, then infusion of 50-200 mcg/kg/min with 20-50 mg bolus as needed. **Children 3-16 yr:** Induction, 2.5-3.5 mg/kg over 20-30 sec, then infusion of 125-300 mcg/kg/min.

Intensive care unit (ICU) sedation

IV

Adults, Elderly: Initially, 5 mcg/kg/min for 5 min, then titrate to 5-50 mcg/kg/min in 5-10 mcg/kg/min increments allowing a minimum of 5 min between dose adjustments.

CONTRAINDICATIONS

Impaired cerebral circulation, increased intracranial pressure (ICP), hypersensitivity to propofol

INTERACTIONS

Drug: **Alcohol, other CNS depressants:** May increase hypotensive and CNS and respiratory depressant effects of propofol. **Herbal:** None known. **Food:** None known.

DIAGNOSTIC TEST EFFECTS

None known.

IV INCOMPATIBILITIES

Amikacin (Amikin), amphotericin B complex (Abelcet, AmBisome, Amphotec), bretylium (Bretylol), calcium chloride, ciprofloxacin (Cipro), diazepam (Valium), digoxin (Lanoxin), *DOXOrubicin (Adriamycin), gentamicin (Garamycin), *methylPREDNISolone (Solu-Medrol), minocycline (Minocin), phenytoin (Dilantin), tobramycin (Nebcin), verapamil (Isoptin)

IV COMPATIBILITIES

Acyclovir (Zovirax), bumetanide (Bumex), calcium gluconate, ceftazidime (Fortaz), *DOBUTamine (Dobutrex), *DOPamine (Intropin), enalapril (Vasotec), fentanyl, heparin, insulin, labetalol (Normodyne, Trandate), lidocaine, lorazepam (Ativan), magnesium, milrinone (Primacor), nitroglycerin, norepinephrine (Levophed), potassium chloride, vancomycin (Vancocin)

SIDE-EFFECTS

Frequent: Involuntary muscle movements, apnea (common during induction; lasts longer than 60 sec), hypotension, nausea, vomiting, IV site burning or stinging. **Occasional:** Twitching, bucking, jerking, thrashing, headache, dizziness, bradycardia, hypertension, fever, abdominal cramps, paresthesia, coldness, cough, hiccups, facial flushing, greenish-colored urine. **Rare:** Rash, dry mouth, agitation, confusion, myalgia, thrombophlebitis

CRITICAL CARE CONSIDERATIONS

ADMINISTRATION/HANDLING

IV ALERT

- Do not give propofol through the same IV line as blood or plasma.
- **Anesthesia:** Apnea lasting up to a full minute may occur during induction. Severe bradycardia may occur from increased vagal tone during surgery or use of succinylcholine.
- **Monitored anesthesia care sedation:** Infusion rate when initiated should be individualized; dose is approximately 25% of anesthesia.
- **Mechanically ventilated ICU patients:** Administer initially at 5 mcg/kg/min over 5 min. Increase dosage slowly over 5-10 min (5 mcg/kg/min increments no more frequently than every 5 min) to avoid hypotension, up to 50 mcg/kg/min (maximum for sedation).
- **ICU sedation:** Average maintenance dose is 38 mcg/kg/min for patients under 55 yr old; 20 mcg/kg/min for those over 55 yr old; post-open-heart surgical patients require an average of 11 mcg/kg/min because of high doses of intraoperative analgesics.
- **Storage:** Store propofol at room temperature. Do not use propofol if the emulsion separates. Discard any unused portions of drug.
- **Preparation:** Shake well before using.
- **Dilution:** Propofol may be given undiluted, or it may be diluted only with D_5W to a concentration of no less than 2 mg/mL (2 mg/mL is 4 mL D_5W to 1 mL propofol).
- **Administration rate:** Too-rapid IV administration of propofol may produce irregular muscle movements, respiratory depression, and severe hypotension.
- **Intraarterial injection:** Observe for signs of inadvertent intraarterial injection, such as delayed onset of drug action, pain or discolored skin near the injection site, or blue or white discoloration of the hand if hand or arm IV site is used.

PRECAUTIONS

HEALTH-RELATED

- Use propofol cautiously in debilitated patients; patients with circulatory, hepatic, lipid metabolism (pancreatitis), renal, or respiratory disorders; those with history of epilepsy.
- **Impaired cerebral circulation:** Use with caution in patients with ICP, stroke or cerebrovascular insufficiency; decreased mean arterial pressure may prompt reduced cerebral perfusion.

AGE-RELATED

- **Children:** Safety and efficacy of propofol have not been established in children. However, the Food and Drug Administration has approved the drug for use in children 2 mo and older. Anesthesia induction is approved only for children at least 3 yr. In children 2 mo to 3 yr, anesthesia induction is done using another agent to supplement propofol (possibly 60%-70% nitrous oxide).
- **Elderly:** Lower propofol dosages are recommended; for ICU sedation in mechanically ventilated patients, average dose is 20 mcg/kg/min. For monitored anesthesia care (MAC) sedation, average maintenance dose is 20-60 mcg/kg/min.

P

PREGNANCY/LACTATION-RELATED

- Pregnancy category B; not recommended for use during breast-feeding.

MONITORING

- **Baseline assessment:** Obtain vital signs before giving propofol. Have resuscitative equipment, suction equipment, and oxygen available. If patients will have short-term sedation for a procedure, pain medication should also be used. Thoroughly assess cause of agitation or need for continuous sedation if used as a continuous infusion not related to a procedure; evaluate for hypoxemia. If patients cannot communicate or if propofol used as an adjunct to neuromuscular blockade, patients may need regular doses of pain medication. Evaluate for dehydration and correct fluid volume deficit before administration, if possible.
- **Baseline lab work:** CBC with WBC differential; biochemical panel including renal (BUN, creatinine), liver (AST [SGOT], ALT [SGPT], alkaline phosphatase, GGT, bilirubin), lipid and triglyceride levels if propofol is given for longer than 24 hr; possible arterial blood gases to evaluate respiratory status.
- **Ongoing evaluation:** Monitor SpO_2 (pulse oximetry) continuously, continuous ECG, BP, heart and respiratory rates, depth of sedation, and need for pain medication.
- **Pain management:** If patients are unable to communicate and have reason to have pain, medicate with an appropriate dose of medication for the condition (surgery, trauma, pancreatitis, bowel obstruction, rhabdomyolysis, back pain, peripheral vascular occlusion, vasculitis, pressure ulcer, rib fractures, etc.).
- **"Wake-up" assessment:** Perform a wake-up assessment (or "sedation vacation") daily to assess level of consciousness with low-level sedation. Propofol should not be turned off to do wake-up assessment, but dose should be reduced to the point where the patient can awaken. Wake-up assessments are not done on patients undergoing neuromuscular blockade.
- **Ventilator weaning:** Reduce dose of propofol as ventilator is being weaned. Propofol should be reduced before patients are challenged to breathe more "on their own" with less support from the ventilator.
- **Neuromuscular blockade:** Evaluate for pain and use train of four technique to evaluate patient comfort in addition to sedation. Consider use of bispectral analysis or other objective means to evaluate comfort.
- **Hypotension:** If patients become hypotensive, reduce the infusion rate; if constantly hypotensive, consider use of another sedative (lorazepam or midazolam infusion). If alternatives are ineffective, use vasopressors and fluid infusion to help control hypotension.
- **Long-term sedation:** All patients on long-term sedation with propofol should be evaluated for change to another sedative (lorazepam, midazolam) or an analgesic with sedative effects (morphine, fentanyl).
- **Total parenteral nutrition with additional lipid infusion:** Nutritional lipid infusions should be discontinued during long-term propofol administration to avoid severe hyperlipidemia.
- **Patient education:** Inform patients and families that propofol may turn urine green. Advise to avoid drinking alcohol or taking other CNS depressants (benzodiazepines, antihistamines) for 24 hr following anesthesia.

SERIOUS ADVERSE REACTIONS

- **Continuous or repeated intermittent infusions:** May result in extreme somnolence, respiratory depression, and circulatory depression.
- **Too-rapid IV administration:** May produce severe hypotension, respiratory depression, and involuntary muscle movements.
- **Acute allergic reaction:** Abdominal pain, anxiety, restlessness, dyspnea, erythema, hypotension, pruritus, rhinitis, and urticaria.
- **Hyperlipidemia:** Elevated triglyceride level which may complicate cardiovascular disease; more likely in patients with lipid metabolism disorders (pancreatitis, diabetic hyperlipidemia, primary hyperlipoproteinemia).

OVERDOSE/TOXICITY

- **Overdose:** Apnea, hypotension, hypoxemia with notable desaturation, airway obstruction.
- **Management:** Dose should be immediately reduced or propofol stopped. All patients receiving propofol should have an endotracheal tube in place, tracheostomy, or other secured, controlled airway in place. Provide manual or mechanical ventilation. Support BP with IV fluids

P

and then vasopressors if needed. If bradycardia ensues, manage with atropine or glycopyrrolate. Resuscitate as needed per Advanced Cardiac Life Support (ACLS) guidelines.
- **GI decontamination:** No specific recommendations.

ANTIDOTE/DIALYSIS
- **Antidote:** No specific recommendations.
- **Dialysis:** Propofol is unlikely to be removed by hemodialysis or peritoneal dialysis. No data are available on removal using high-permeability hemodialysis.

propoxyphene hydrochloride/ propoxyphene napsylate

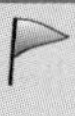

See Opioid Analgesics (p. 980)

propranolol hydrochloride

proe-pran'-oh-lole hye-droe-klor'-ide

Classes
Chemical: β-adrenergic blocker, nonselective
Therapeutic: antianginal; antidysrhythmic, class II; antiglaucoma agent; antihypertensive; antimigraine agent

Pregnancy Category: C (1st trimester), D (2nd and 3rd trimesters)

Trade Names
Prescription: Apo-Propranolol ♣, Inderal, Inderal LA, InnoPran XL, Propranolol Intensol

Combinations
Prescription: with HCTZ (Inderide)

Do not confuse Inderal with Adderall or Isordil, or propranolol with Pravachol.

CLINICAL PHARMACOLOGY
Mechanism of Action
An antihypertensive, antianginal, antidysrhythmic, and antimigraine agent that blocks $beta_1$- and $beta_2$-adrenergic receptors. Decreases oxygen requirements. Slows AV conduction and increases refractory period in AV node. Large doses increase airway resistance. Therapeutic Effect: Slows sinus heart rate; decreases cardiac output, BP, and myocardial ischemia severity. Exhibits antidysrhythmic activity.

PHARMACOKINETICS

Route	Onset	Peak	Duration
PO	1-2 hr	N/A	6 hr

Well absorbed from the GI tract. Protein binding: 93%. Widely distributed. Metabolized in the liver. Primarily excreted in urine. Not removed by hemodialysis. Half-life: 3-5 hr.

AVAILABILITY
Tablets (Inderal): 10 mg, 20 mg, 40 mg, 60 mg, 80 mg.
Capsules (extended release): 60 mg (Inderal LA), 80 mg (Inderal LA, InnoPran XL), 120 mg (Inderal LA, InnoPran XL), 160 mg (Inderal LA).
Oral solution (Inderal): 20 mg/5 mL, 40 mg/5 mL.
Oral concentrate (Propranolol Intensol): 80 mg/mL.
Injection (Inderal): 1 mg/mL.

INDICATIONS AND DOSAGE
Hypertension
PO
Adults, Elderly: Initially, 40 mg twice per day. May increase dose every 3-7 days. Range: Up to 320 mg/day in divided doses. Maximum: 640 mg/day. **Children:** Initially 0.5-1 mg/kg/day in divided doses every 6-12 hr. May increase at 5- to 7-day intervals. Usual dose: 1-5 mg/kg/day. Maximum: 16 mg/kg/day.

Angina
PO
Adults, Elderly: 80-320 mg/day in divided doses. Long acting: Initially, 80 mg/day. Maximum: 320 mg/day.

Dysrhythmias
IV
Adults, Elderly: 1 mg/dose. May repeat every 5 min. Maximum: 5 mg total dose. **Children:** 0.01-0.1 mg/kg. Maximum: infants, 1 mg; children, 3 mg.
PO
Adults, Elderly: Initially 10-20 mg every 6-8 hr. May gradually increase dose. Range: 40-320 mg/day. **Children:** Initially, 0.5-1 mg/kg/day in divided doses every 6-8 hr. May increase every 3-7 days. Usual dosage: 2-4 mg/kg/day. Maximum: 16 mg/kg/day or 60 mg/day.

Life-threatening dysrhythmias
IV
Adults, Elderly: 0.5-3 mg. Repeat once in 2 min. Give additional doses at intervals of at least 4 hr. **Children:** 0.01-0.1 mg/kg.

P

Hypertrophic subaortic stenosis

PO

Adults, Elderly: 20-40 mg in 3-4 divided doses. Or 80-160 mg/day as extended-release capsule.

Adjunct to alpha-blocking agents to treat pheochromocytoma

PO

Adults, Elderly: 60 mg/day in divided doses with alpha-blocker for 3 days before surgery. Maintenance (inoperable tumor): 30 mg/day with alpha-blocker.

Migraine headache

PO

Adults, Elderly: 80 mg/day in divided doses. Or 80 mg once daily as extended-release capsule. Increase up to 160-240 mg/day in divided doses. **Children:** 0.6-1.5 mg/kg/day in divided doses every 8 hr. Maximum: 4 mg/kg/day.

Reduction of cardiovascular mortality and reinfarction in patients with previous MI

PO

Adults, Elderly: 180-240 mg/day in divided doses.

Essential tremor

PO

Adults, Elderly: Initially, 40 mg twice per day increased up to 120-320 mg/day in 3 divided doses.

OFF-LABEL USES

Treatment adjunct for anxiety, mitral valve prolapse syndrome, thyrotoxicosis

P

CONTRAINDICATIONS

Asthma, bradycardia, cardiogenic shock, chronic obstructive pulmonary disease (COPD), heart block, Raynaud's syndrome, uncompensated heart failure; hypersensitivity to propranolol

INTERACTIONS

Drug: **Diuretics, other antihypertensives:** May increase hypotensive effect. **Insulin, oral hypoglycemics:** May mask symptoms of hypoglycemia and prolong the hypoglycemic effect of insulin and oral hypoglycemics. **IV phenytoin:** May increase cardiac depressant effect. **NSAIDs:** May decrease antihypertensive effect. **Sympathomimetics, xanthines:** May mutually inhibit effects. **Herbal:** None known. **Food:** None known.

DIAGNOSTIC TEST EFFECTS

May increase serum antinuclear antibody titer and BUN, serum LDH, serum lipoprotein, serum alkaline phosphatase, serum bilirubin, serum creatinine, serum potassium, serum uric acid, AST (SGOT), ALT (SGPT), and serum triglyceride levels.

IV INCOMPATIBILITIES

Amphotericin B complex (Abelcet, AmBisome, Amphotec)

IV COMPATIBILITIES

Alteplase (Activase), heparin, milrinone (Primacor), potassium chloride, propofol (Diprivan)

SIDE-EFFECTS

Frequent: Diminished sexual ability, drowsiness, difficulty sleeping, unusual fatigue or weakness. **Occasional:** Bradycardia, depression, sensation of coldness in extremities, diarrhea, constipation, anxiety, nasal congestion, nausea, vomiting. **Rare:** Altered taste, dry eyes, pruritus, paresthesia

CRITICAL CARE CONSIDERATIONS

ADMINISTRATION/HANDLING

PO ALERT

- Crush scored tablets if necessary.
- Give propranolol at same time each day.

IV ALERT

- **Storage:** Store at room temperature.
- **IV push/direct injection:** Give undiluted for IV push; do not exceed 1 mg/min injection rate.
- **IV infusion:** May dilute each 1 mg in 10 mL D_5W; give 1 mg over 10-15 min.

PRECAUTIONS

HEALTH-RELATED

- **Heart block:** Use propranolol cautiously in patients who are also receiving calcium channel blockers, especially when giving IV, because heart block is possible.
- Use cautiously in patients with diabetes (may mask signs of hypoglycemia and may promote hyperglycemia over time) or hepatic or renal impairment.
- **COPD patients:** Propranolol is contraindicated because it is a nonselective beta-blocker (blocks both beta-1 and -2 receptors); when beta-2 receptors are blocked, respiratory medications (bronchodilators) may lose effectiveness prompting respiratory distress in the COPD (bronchial asthma, bronchitis, emphysema) patient. Other selective (beta-1-only blocked) beta-blocking agents are less likely to cause respiratory distress.

AGE-RELATED

- **Children:** Safety and efficacy of propranolol have not been established in children.
- **Elderly:** Age-related peripheral vascular disease and organ impairment may increase susceptibility to decreased peripheral circulation and reduced clearance; decreased doses may be needed.

PREGNANCY/LACTATION-RELATED

- Pregnancy category C (D if used in second or third trimester). Similar drug, atenolol, frequently used in the third trimester for treatment of hypertension (many studies of efficacy and safety of atenolol in pregnancy-induced hypertension). Long-term use has been associated with intrauterine growth retardation. Milk levels approximately half of peak plasma levels and considered insignificant; compatible with breast-feeding.

MONITORING

- **Baseline assessment:** Assess heart rate and BP immediately before giving propranolol. If heart rate is less than 60 or systolic BP is less than 90 mmHg, may withhold the medication if this is a significant change in vital signs. If used for chest pain, document the onset, type (sharp, dull, or squeezing), radiation, location, intensity, and duration, discomfort and precipitating factors.
- **Baseline lab work:** Biochemical profile including renal (BUN, creatinine) and liver (AST [SGOT], ALT [SGPT], alkaline phosphatase, GGT, bilirubin) function tests; CBC with WBC differential to evaluate for anemia and infection.
- **Dysrhythmias:** Monitor continuous ECG for bradycardia and heart block. Dose may need to be reduced or drug discontinued if dysrhythmias occur.
- **Heart failure:** Monitor intake, output, and weight. An increase in weight or a decrease in urine output may indicate heart failure. Evaluate for distended neck veins, dyspnea (on exertion or lying down), night cough, and peripheral edema.
- **Hypertension:** Measure BP near the end of the dosing interval to determine if BP is controlled throughout the day.
- **Ventricular tachycardia:** Monitor for resolution of ventricular tachycardia if propranolol is used to manage VT induced by catecholamine infusions; drug is ineffective to manage VT induced by other mechanisms.
- **Raynaud's syndrome:** Examine the fingers for lack of color and numbness, which may indicate Raynaud's syndrome.
- **Hypoglycemia:** Sympathetic nervous system responses (tachycardia, sweating) to low blood glucose are blocked by propranolol. Altered mental status may be the most overt sign in hypoglycemia in patients taking beta blocking drugs.
- **Common side effects:** Assess for behavioral changes, fatigue, and rash.
- **Therapeutic effect:** Once propranolol is begun, therapeutic effect occurs a few days to several wk.
- **Patient education:** Caution against discontinuing propranolol. Stress that compliance with the therapy regimen is essential to control anginal pain, dyshythmias, and hypertension; if a dose is missed, only the next scheduled dose should be taken (should not double the dose). Teach to rise slowly from a lying to sitting position and to pause before standing to avoid orthostatic hypotension. Advise not to take nasal decongestants and OTC cold preparations, especially those containing stimulants, without prior health care provider approval. Urge limiting alcohol and salt intake. Advise avoidance of tasks requiring mental alertness or motor skills until response to the drug is known. Warn to report dizziness, excessively slow pulse rate (less than 60 beats/min), or peripheral numbness.

P

SERIOUS ADVERSE REACTIONS

- Propranolol administration may precipitate heart failure and MI in patients with cardiac disease; thyroid storm in those with hyperthyroidism (drug may prompt thyroid storm by masking ineffective drug management and is used off label to manage thyroid storm once it occurs); and peripheral ischemia in those with existing peripheral vascular disease.
- **Hypoglycemia:** Propranolol may mask symptoms of hypoglycemia and potentiate insulin-induced hypoglycemia in diabetic patients. Hypoglycemia may occur in patients with previously controlled diabetes.
- **Respiratory distress/bronchospasms:** Bronchodilator-dependent COPD patients do not tolerate propranolol without increasing doses of bronchodilators; because

bronchodilators often cause tachycardia and increased BP, this may defeat the purpose of using propranolol to reduce heart rate or BP.

- **Abrupt withdrawal:** May cause angina, acute MI, sweating, palpitations, headache, tremulousness, and lethal ventricular dysrhythmias if not withdrawn gradually unless patient is toxic.

OVERDOSE/TOXICITY

- **Overdose:** Profound hypotension, heart failure, bradycardia, heart block, dizziness, syncope, drowsiness, breathing difficulty, nausea, vomiting, pallor, central cyanosis, bluish fingernails or palms of hands, somnolence, speech disorders, weakness, hypo- or hyperglycemia, and seizures.
- **Management:** Maintain patent airway and support ventilation. Treat bradycardia and heart block initially with atropine 0.5 mg-1 mg IV push. If patient is unresponsive to atropine, catecholamine infusions (epinephrine, *DOPamine, or with caution, isoproterenol) may be used. If BP does not increase when heart rate increases, vasopressors (norepinephrine) may be used along with fluid infusion, if fluids are not contraindicated because of heart failure. Unresponsive bradycardia and hypotension may be managed with glucagon 5-10 mg IV over 30 sec followed by a continuous infusion at 5 mg/hr. Manage blood glucose according to accepted standard. Manage bronchospasms with bronchodilator aerosols or infusion (isoproterenol or aminophylline), if aerosol is ineffective. Nitroglycerin and diuretics may be effective in supporting heart failure.
- **GI decontamination:** No specific recommendations.

ANTIDOTE/DIALYSIS

- **Antidote:** No specific antidote, but catecholamine infusions and glucagons may help resolve bradycardia and hypotension.
- **Dialysis:** Propranolol is not removed by hemodialysis or peritoneal dialysis. No data are available on removal by high-permeability hemodialysis.

P

propylthiouracil

proe-pill-thye-oh-yoor'-a-sill

Classes

Chemical: thioamide derivative
Therapeutic: antithyroid agent

Pregnancy Category: D

Trade Names

Prescription: Propylthiouracil, Propyl-Thyracil ♣

CLINICAL PHARMACOLOGY

Mechanism of Action

A thiourea derivative that blocks oxidation of iodine in the thyroid gland and blocks synthesis of thyroxine and triiodothyronine. **Therapeutic Effect:** Inhibits synthesis of thyroid hormone.

PHARMACOKINETICS

Readily absorbed from GI tract. Protein binding: 80%. Metabolized in liver. Excreted in urine. **Half-life:** 1-4 hr.

AVAILABILITY

Tablets: 50 mg.

INDICATIONS AND DOSAGE

Hyperthyroidism

PO

Adults, Elderly: Initially 300-450 mg/day in divided doses every 8 hr. Maintenance: 100-150 mg/day in divided doses every 8-12 hr. **Children:** Initially 5-7 mg/kg/day in divided doses every 8 hr. Maintenance: 33%-66% of initial dose in divided doses every 8-12 hr. **Neonates:** 5-10 mg/kg/day in divided doses every 8 hr.

CONTRAINDICATIONS

Breast-feeding mothers, hypersensitivity to propylthiouracil

INTERACTIONS

Drug: **Amiodarone, iodinated glycerol, iodine, potassium iodide:** May decrease response of propylthiouracil. **Digoxin:** May increase digoxin blood concentration as patient becomes euthyroid. **I^{131}:** May decrease thyroid uptake of I^{131}. **Oral anticoagulants:** May decrease the effects of oral anticoagulants. **Herbal:** None known. **Food:** None known.

DIAGNOSTIC TEST EFFECTS

May increase LDH, serum alkaline phosphatase, bilirubin, AST (SGOT), and ALT (SGPT) levels and prothrombin time.

SIDE-EFFECTS

Frequent: Urticaria, rash, pruritus, nausea, skin pigmentation, hair loss, headache, paresthesia. **Occasional:** Somnolence, lymphadenopathy, vertigo. **Rare:** Drug fever, lupuslike syndrome

CRITICAL CARE CONSIDERATIONS

ADMINISTRATION/HANDLING

PO ALERT

- Store at controlled room temperature.

PRECAUTIONS

HEALTH-RELATED

- Use propylthiouracil cautiously in patients over 40 yr and in patients taking propylthiouracil with other agranulocytosis-inducing drugs.

AGE-RELATED

- **Children:** Use cautiously in children because of the risk of hepatic dysfunction.
- **Elderly:** Age-related organ impairment may require dosage adjustment to avoid agranulocytosis and other adverse reactions.

PREGNANCY/LACTATION-RELATED

- Pregnancy category D; considered drug of choice for medical treatment of hyperthyroidism during pregnancy. Excreted into breast milk in low amounts; breastfeeding should be discontinued.

MONITORING

- **Baseline assessment:** Obtain vital signs, height, and weight. Assess history of hyperthyroidism including presence of goiter, thyroid nodules, or patients with a recent stressful experience including pregnancy, labor, and delivery. If acute thyrotoxicosis is present, assess for confusion, disorientation, fever, hyperglycemia, tremors, and exopthalmos.
- **Baseline lab work:** Review thyroid studies (serum TSH, free T3 [thyroxine triiodothyronine] and T4). CBC with WBC differential; biochemical profile including liver function tests (LDH, serum alkaline phosphatase, bilirubin, AST [SGOT], and ALT [SGPT] levels); coagulation studies including prothrombin time and international normalized ratio (INR).
- **Therapeutic effect:** Monitor for decreased heart rate and weight loss daily.
- **Side effects:** Assess skin for eruptions, itching, and swollen lymph glands.
- **Bleeding and immunosuppression:** Monitor CBC for bone marrow suppression, and assess for easy bruising, fever and cough.
- **Hepatitis:** Assess for somnolence, jaundice, nausea, and vomiting.
- **Patient education:** Instruct to space doses evenly around the clock. Teach how to take a resting pulse daily to monitor results. Instruct to report a pulse rate of less than 60 beats/min. Urge restricted consumption of iodine products and seafood. Instruct to report immediately cold intolerance, depression, and weight gain to a health care provider.

SERIOUS ADVERSE REACTIONS

- **Hematologic:** Agranulocytosis as long as 4 mo after therapy, pancytopenia, granulocytopenia, and thrombocytopenia.
- **Lupuslike syndrome:** Splenomegaly, hepatitis, periarteritis, hypoprothrombinemia, and bleeding.
- **Interstitial pneumonitis and erythema nodosum:** Have been reported.

OVERDOSE/TOXICITY

- **Hepatotoxicity:** Elevated liver enzymes, right upper quadrant pain, nausea, jaundice, hepatitis, hepatic necrosis, and death.
- **Nephrotoxicity:** Nephritis, increased BUN and creatinine.
- **Overdose:** Hypothyroidism with possible myxedema coma including low energy level, depression, bradycardia, somnolence, hypothermia, low BP, hypoglycemia, hyponatremia, possible heart failure with respiratory distress.
- **Management:** Discontinue propylthiouracil. Provide patent airway and support ventilation. Diuretics may be needed to manage heart failure or fluid retention leading to respiratory distress. Thyroid hormones given rapidly IV along with steroids to reduce the possibility of creating hyperadrenalism. Hypoglycemia is managed with IV D50 (50% dextrose). Restrict fluids and consider 3% saline to manage hyponatremia. IV solutions used should be isotonic (0.9% saline or lactated Ringer's solution). External rewarming should be avoided, as it may prompt vasodilation leading to vascular collapse.
- **GI decontamination:** No specific recommendations.

ANTIDOTE/DIALYSIS

- **Antidote:** Thyroid hormones (IV thyroxine).
- **Dialysis:** Propylthiouracil is not removed by hemodialysis. No data are available on removal by high-permeability hemodialysis or peritoneal dialysis.

P

protriptyline

See Antidepressants (p. 906)

psyllium

sil'-i-yum

Classes

Chemical: psyllium colloid
Therapeutic: laxative

Pregnancy Category: B

Trade Names

Over the Counter: Fiberall, Hydrocil, Konsyl, Metamucil, Perdiem

Combinations

Over the Counter: with senna (Perdiem)

CLINICAL PHARMACOLOGY

Mechanism of Action

A bulk-forming laxative that dissolves and swells in water providing increased bulk and moisture content in stool. **Therapeutic Effect:** Promotes peristalsis and bowel motility.

PHARMACOKINETICS

Route	Onset	Peak	Duration
PO	12-24 hr	2-3 days	N/A

Acts in small and large intestines.

P

AVAILABILITY

Powder (Fiberall, Hydrocil, Konsyl, Metamucil): 3.4 g/dose.
Wafer (Metamucil): 3.4 g/dose.
Capsules (Metamucil): 0.52 g.
Granules (Perdiem): 4 g/5 mL.

INDICATIONS AND DOSAGE

Constipation, irritable bowel syndrome

PO

Alert: 3.4 g powder equals 1 rounded tsp, 1 packet, or 1 wafer. **Adults, Elderly:** 2-5 capsules/dose 1-3 times per day. 1-2 tsp granules 1-2 times per day. 1 rounded tsp or 1 tbsp of powder 1-3 times per day. 2 wafers 1-3 times per day. **Children 6-11 yr:** 0.5-1 tsp powder in water 1-3 times per day.

CONTRAINDICATIONS

Fecal impaction, GI obstruction, undiagnosed abdominal pain, hypersensitivity to psyllium

INTERACTIONS

Drug: Digoxin, oral anticoagulants, salicylates: May decrease the effects of digoxin, oral anticoagulants, and salicylates by decreasing absorption. **Potassium-sparing diuretics, potassium supplements:** May interfere with the effects of potassium-sparing diuretics and potassium supplements. **Herbal:** None known. **Food:** None known.

DIAGNOSTIC TEST EFFECTS

May increase blood glucose level. May decrease serum potassium level.

SIDE-EFFECTS

Rare: Some degree of abdominal discomfort, nausea, mild abdominal cramps, griping, faintness

CRITICAL CARE CONSIDERATIONS

ADMINISTRATION/HANDLING

PO ALERT

- Psyllium may decrease effects of other medications; administer at least 2 hr before or after other medication administration.
- Drink 6-8 glasses of water per day to aid in stool softening. Drugs should not be swallowed in dry form but should be mixed with at least 1 full glass (8 oz) of liquid and then followed by 8 ounces of liquid.

PRECAUTIONS

HEALTH-RELATED

- Use psyllium cautiously in patients with esophageal strictures, intestinal adhesions, stenosis, or ulcers.

AGE-RELATED

- **Children:** Safety and efficacy of psyllium have not been established in children under 6 yr.
- **Elderly:** No age-related precautions have been noted.

PREGNANCY/LACTATION-RELATED

- Pregnancy category B; not systemically absorbed. Exposure of fetus or nursing infant unlikely; compatible with breastfeeding.

MONITORING

- **Baseline assessment:** Before psyllium administration, assess abdomen for tenderness, rigidity, and the presence of bowel sounds. Try to determine when last bowel movement occurred; find out the amount and consistency. Psyllium is not used for patients with a bowel obstruction.
- **Baseline lab work:** CBC with differential and biochemical profile to rule out anemia

(may indicate GI bleeding) or significant digestive system disease.
- **Fluids:** Provide adequate PO and/or IV fluid intake.
- **Bowel obstruction:** Assess bowel sounds in all 4 abdominal quadrants for peristalsis. Assess pattern of daily bowel activity and stool consistency. Monitor for abdominal pain and tenderness.
- **Electrolyte imbalance:** Monitor serum electrolyte levels in patients with excessive, frequent, or prolonged use of psyllium.
- **Patient education:** When using psyllium outside the hospital, instruct to institute measures to promote defecation such as increasing fluid intake, exercising, and eating a high-fiber diet. Instruct on taking each dose with a full glass (at least 250 mL) of water. Warn that taking psyllium with an inadequate amount of fluid may cause GI obstruction.

SERIOUS ADVERSE REACTIONS
- Esophageal or bowel obstruction may occur if administered less than 250 mL of liquid.

OVERDOSE/TOXICITY
- Psyllium is not systemically absorbed.
- **GI decontamination:** No specific recommendations.

ANTIDOTE/DIALYSIS
- **Antidote:** No specific antidote. Water by mouth or enteral tube is often helpful in correcting acute constipation if patients have not taken enough water with psyllium.
- **Dialysis:** Psyllium is not systemically absorbed; all modes of dialysis are ineffective in removing psyllium because it is not in the bloodstream.

pyrazinamide

peer-a-zin'-a-mide

Classes
Chemical: niacinamide derivative
Therapeutic: antituberculosis agent

Pregnancy Category: C

Trade Names
Prescription: Pyrazinamide, Tebrazid ♣

CLINICAL PHARMACOLOGY
Mechanism of Action
An antitubercular whose exact mechanism of action is unknown. **Therapeutic Effect:** Either bacteriostatic or bactericidal, depending on the drug's concentration at the infection site and the susceptibility of infecting bacteria.

PHARMACOKINETICS
Nearly completely absorbed from GI tract. Protein binding: 5%-10%. Excreted in urine. **Half-life:** 10 hr.

AVAILABILITY
Tablets: 500 mg.

INDICATIONS AND DOSAGE
Tuberculosis (in combination with other antituberculars)
PO
Adults: 15-30 mg/kg/day based on lean body weight in 1-4 doses. Maximum: 2 g/day. Other dosage regimes (2-3 times/wk) are available. **Children:** 20-40 mg/kg/day in 1 or 2 doses. Maximum: 2 g/day.

CONTRAINDICATIONS
Severe hepatic dysfunction, hypersensitivity to pyrazinamide

INTERACTIONS
Drug: Allopurinol, colchicine, probenecid, sulfinpyrazone: May decrease the effects of these drugs. **Herbal:** None known. **Food:** None known.

DIAGNOSTIC TEST EFFECTS
May increase AST (SGOT), ALT (SGPT), and serum uric acid concentrations.

SIDE-EFFECTS
Frequent: Arthralgia, myalgia (usually mild and self-limiting). **Rare:** Hypersensitivity reaction (rash, pruritus, urticaria), photosensitivity, gouty arthritis

CRITICAL CARE CONSIDERATIONS

ADMINISTRATION/HANDLING
PO ALERT
- Pyrazinamide should be used with at least one other effective antituberculosis agent.

PRECAUTIONS
HEALTH-RELATED
- Use pyrazinamide cautiously in patients with diabetes mellitus, renal impairment, or a history of gout.
- Use pyrazinamide cautiously in patients with a hypersensitivity to ethionamide, isoniazid, or niacin.

P

AGE-RELATED

- **Children:** Safety and efficacy of pyrazinamide have not been established in children.
- **Elderly:** Age-related organ impairment may prompt a dosage reduction.

PREGNANCY/LACTATION-RELATED

- Pregnancy category C; excreted into human breast milk.

MONITORING

- **Baseline assessment:** Determine hypersensitivity to pyrazinamide, ethionamide, isoniazid, or niacin before beginning pyrazinamide therapy.
- **Lab work:** Ensure that specimens for culture and sensitivity tests have been obtained before beginning drug therapy. CBC with WBC differential; biochemical profile including blood glucose, liver (AST [SGOT], ALT [SGPT], alkaline phosphatase, GGT, bilirubin) function tests, and serum uric acid levels.
- **Hepatotoxicity:** Monitor liver function test results and for anorexia, fever, jaundice, liver tenderness, malaise, nausea, and vomiting. If such reactions occur, stop the drug.
- **Hyperuricemia:** Check serum uric acid levels and assess for gout (hot, painful, swollen joints, especially the ankle, big toe, or knee).
- **Hyperglycemia:** Evaluate blood glucose levels, especially in patients with diabetes mellitus, because pyrazinamide administration may make diabetes management difficult.
- **Bone marrow suppression:** Monitor CBC for anemia and thrombocytopenia.
- **Skin:** Assess for a rash or skin eruptions.
- **Patient education:** Instruct to take pyrazinamide with food to reduce GI upset. Advise not to skip drug doses and to complete the full course of therapy, which may take months or years. Explain that follow-up physician office visits and laboratory tests are essential parts of treatment. Encourage reduced exposure to the sun or ultraviolet light to prevent photosensitivity reactions. Instruct to report any new symptoms, especially fever; hot, painful, or swollen joints; unusual fatigue; or jaundice.

SERIOUS ADVERSE REACTIONS

- **Hyperglycemia:** Elevated blood glucose leading to dehydration, hyperosmolality, and possibly acidosis if not managed. Patients are more likely to acquire infections and have higher morbidity and mortality rates when glucose is elevated.
- **Hyperuricemia:** May result in development of gouty arthritis.

OVERDOSE/TOXICITY

- **Hepatotoxicity:** Elevated liver enzymes, right upper quadrant pain, nausea, confusion, jaundice, hepatitis, hepatic necrosis; possible death.
- **Bone marrow suppression:** Anemia, thrombocytopenia.
- **GI decontamination:** No specific recommendations.

ANTIDOTE/DIALYSIS

- **Antidote:** No specific recommendations.
- **Dialysis:** No data are available on removal of pyrazinamide by hemodialysis, high-permeability hemodialysis, or peritoneal dialysis.

pyridostigmine bromide

peer-id-oh-stig'-meen broe'-mide

Classes

Chemical: cholinesterase inhibitor, quaternary ammonium derivative
Therapeutic: cholinergic

Pregnancy Category: B

Trade Names

Prescription: Mestinon, Mestinon-SR ♣, Mestinon Timespan

Do not confuse pyridostigmine with physostigmine, or Mesitonin with Mesantoin or Metatensin.

CLINICAL PHARMACOLOGY

Mechanism of Action

A cholinergic that prevents destruction of acetylcholine by inhibiting the enzyme acetylcholinesterase, thus enhancing impulse transmission across the myoneural junction. **Therapeutic Effect:** Produces miosis; increases tone of intestinal and skeletal muscle tone; stimulates salivary and sweat gland secretions.

PHARMACOKINETICS

Not protein bound. Excreted unchanged in urine. **Half-life:** Unknown.

AVAILABILITY

Syrup (Mestinon): 60 mg/5 mL.
Tablets (Mestinon): 60 mg.

P

Tablets (extended release [Mestinon Timespan]): 180 mg.
Injection (Mestinon): 5 mg/mL.

INDICATIONS AND DOSAGE

Myasthenia gravis

PO

Adults, Elderly: Initially, 60 mg 3 times per day. Dosage increased at 48-hr intervals. Maintenance: 60 mg-1.5 g per day.

PO (Extended Release)

Adults, Elderly: 180-540 mg once or twice per day with at least a 6-hr interval between doses.

IV, IM

Adults, Elderly: 2 mg every 2-3 hr. **Children, Neonates:** 0.05-0.15 mg/kg/dose. Maximum single dose: 10 mg.

Reversal of nondepolarizing neuromuscular blockade

IV

Adults, Elderly: 10-20 mg with or shortly after 0.6-1.2 mg atropine sulfate or 0.3-0.6 mg glycopyrrolate. **Children:** 0.1-0.25 mg/kg/dose preceded by atropine or glycopyrrolate.

CONTRAINDICATIONS

Mechanical GI or urinary tract obstruction, hypersensitivity to pyridostigmine or other anticholinesterase agents

INTERACTIONS

Drug: Anticholinergics: Prevent or reverse the effects of pyridostigmine. **Cholinesterase inhibitors:** May increase the risk of toxicity. **Neuromuscular blockers:** Antagonizes the effects of these drugs. **Procainamide, quinidine:** May antagonize the action of pyridostigmine. **Herbal:** None known. **Food:** None known.

DIAGNOSTIC TEST EFFECTS

None known.

IV INCOMPATIBILITIES

Do not mix pyridostigmine with any other medications.

SIDE-EFFECTS

Frequent: Miosis, increased GI and skeletal muscle tone, bradycardia, constriction of bronchi and ureters, diaphoresis, increased salivation. **Occasional:** Headache, rash, temporary decrease in diastolic BP with mild reflex tachycardia, short periods of atrial fibrillation (in hyperthyroid patients), marked drop in BP (in hypertensive patients)

CRITICAL CARE CONSIDERATIONS

ADMINISTRATION/HANDLING

PO ALERT

- **3 dosage forms available:** Syrup, conventional tablets, and timespan (extended-release) tablets.
- May crush conventional tablets as needed; timespan tablets may not be crushed or chewed but may be broken in half.
- **Vary dosage:** Give larger doses at times of increased fatigue, for example 30-45 min before meals for patients with difficulty chewing. Drug dosage and frequency of administration depend on the daily clinical response, including exacerbations, physical and emotional stress, and remissions.

IM, IV ALERT

- Give large parenteral doses concurrently with 0.6-1.2 mg atropine sulfate IV to minimize side effects.

PRECAUTIONS

HEALTH-RELATED

- Use pyridostigmine cautiously in patients with bradycardia, bronchial asthma, cardiac dysrhythmias, epilepsy, hyperthyroidism, peptic ulcer disease, recent MI, or vagotonia.

AGE-RELATED

- **Children:** Very important to differentiate between myasthenic and cholinergic crises in neonates; both conditions manifest as muscle weakness but are treated very differently.
- **Elderly:** Age-related renal impairment may require a dosage adjustment. Pyridostigmine is eliminated unchanged by the kidney and may accumulate with decreased renal function.

PREGNANCY/LACTATION-RELATED

- Pregnancy category B. Would not be expected to cross the placenta because it is ionized at physiologic pH. Although apparently safe for the fetus, may cause transient muscle weakness in the newborn. Use with caution in breast-feeding women.

MONITORING

- **Baseline assessment:** Assess muscle strength before and after drug administration. Before beginning therapy, determine whether patient has reduced GI motility or megacolon, because these patients should not receive large doses.

- **Baseline lab work:** CBC with WBC differential; biochemical panel including renal (BUN, creatinine) and liver (AST [SGOT], ALT [SGPT], alkaline phosphatase, bilirubin, LDH) function tests.
- **Baseline diagnostic tests:** If differentiation between myasthenic and cholinergic crisis is needed, edrophonium may be used ("Tensilon test") to help distinguish between the conditions; 12-lead ECG to evaluate for cardiac disease.
- **Respiratory distress:** Monitor respirations closely when dosage is increased.
- **Cholinergic reaction:** Monitor for progressively increased muscle weakness when dose is given.
- **Dysrhythmias:** Monitor for bradycardia in patients with myasthenic crisis; use atropine cautiously in patients with history of dysrhythmias.
- **GI side effects:** Atropine may also be used to reduce gastrointestinal side effects.
- **Therapeutic response:** Monitor for decreased fatigue, improved chewing, easier swallowing, and increased muscle strength.
- **Patient education:** Inform that regular tablets may be crushed if needed and extended-release tablets may be broken in half but not chewed or crushed. Instruct to report diarrhea, difficulty breathing, profuse salivation or sweating, irregular heartbeat, muscle weakness, severe abdominal pain, or nausea and vomiting. Tell to keep a log of their energy level and muscle strength to help guide drug dosing.

SERIOUS ADVERSE REACTIONS

- **Muscarinic effects:** Nausea, vomiting, diarrhea, abdominal cramps, increased peristalsis, increased salivation and secretions, miosis, and diaphoresis.
- **Nicotinic effects:** Muscle cramps, fasciculations, and weakness.

OVERDOSE/TOXICITY

- **Overdose:** May produce a cholinergic crisis, manifested as increasingly severe muscle weakness that appears first in muscles involving chewing and swallowing, followed by muscle weakness of the shoulder girdle, and upper extremities and respiratory muscle pelvis girdle and leg muscle paralysis.
- **Management:** Stop all cholinergic drugs and immediately administer 1-4 mg atropine sulfate IV for adults or 0.01 mg/kg for infants and children under 12 yr.
- **GI decontamination:** No specific recommendations.

ANTIDOTE/DIALYSIS

- **Antidote:** Atropine counteracts muscarinic effects but may mask the signs of overdosage.
- **Dialysis:** No data are available on removal of pyridostigmine by hemodialysis, peritoneal dialysis, or high-permeability hemodialysis.

pyridoxine hydrochloride (vitamin B_6)

peer-i-dox'-een hye-droe-klor'-ide

Classes

Chemical: vitamin B complex
Therapeutic: antidote, hydralazine/isoniazid; vitamin

Pregnancy Category: A

Trade Names

Prescription: Aminoxin, Beesix, Doxine, Nestrex, Pryi, Rodex, Vitabee 6, Vitamin B6

Do not confuse pyridoxine with paroxetine, pralidoxime, or Pyridium.

CLINICAL PHARMACOLOGY

Mechanism of Action

Acts as a coenzyme for various metabolic functions, including metabolism of proteins, carbohydrates, and fats. Aids in the breakdown of glycogen and in the synthesis of gamma-aminobutyric acid in the CNS. **Therapeutic Effect:** Prevents pyridoxine deficiency. Increases the excretion of certain drugs, such as isoniazid, that are pyridoxine antagonists.

PHARMACOKINETICS

Readily absorbed primarily in jejunum. Stored in the liver, muscle, and brain. Metabolized in the liver. Primarily excreted in urine. **Half-life:** 15-20 days.

AVAILABILITY

Capsules: 250 mg.

P

Tablets: 25 mg, 50 mg, 100 mg, 250 mg, 500 mg.
Tablets (enteric-coated [Aminoxin]): 20 mg.
Injection (Vitamin B6): 100 mg/mL.

INDICATIONS AND DOSAGE

Pyridoxine deficiency

PO

Adults, Elderly: Initially 2.5-10 mg/day, then 2.5 mg/day when clinical signs are corrected. **Children:** Initially 5-25 mg/day for 3 wk, then 1.5-2.5 mg/day.

Pyridoxine-dependent seizures

PO, IV, IM, Subcutaneous

Infants: Initially 10-100 mg/day. Maintenance: PO: 2-100 mg/day.

Drug-induced neuritis

PO (treatment)

Adults, Elderly: 100-300 mg/day in divided doses. **Children:** 10-50 mg/day.

PO (prophylaxis)

Adults, Elderly: 25-100 mg/day. **Children:** 1-2 mg/kg/day.

CONTRAINDICATIONS

Hypersensitivity to components of pyridoxine products

INTERACTIONS

Drug: Immunosuppressants, isoniazid, penicillamine: May antagonize pyridoxine, causing anemia or peripheral neuritis. **Levodopa:** Reverses the effects of levodopa. **Herbal:** None known. **Food:** None known.

DIAGNOSTIC TEST EFFECTS

None known.

IV INCOMPATIBILITIES

Do not mix pyridoxine with any other medications.

SIDE-EFFECTS

Occasional: Stinging at IM injection site. **Rare:** Headache, nausea, somnolence; sensory neuropathy (paresthesia, unstable gait, clumsiness of hands) with high doses

CRITICAL CARE CONSIDERATIONS

ADMINISTRATION/HANDLING

PO ALERT

- Give pyridoxine orally unless malabsorption, nausea, or vomiting occurs.
- Do not crush/break extended-release capsules and tablets. Avoid chewing capsules or tablets.
- Avoid doses exceeding the recommended daily allowance (RDA) unless directed by a clinician.

IV ALERT

- **Dilution:** Pyridoxine may be given undiluted or may be added to IV solutions and given as an infusion.
- Avoid IV use in cardiac patients.

PRECAUTIONS

HEALTH-RELATED

- Vitamin B_6 deficiency can cause an abnormal EEG.
- Need for pyridoxine increases with the amount of protein in the diet.

AGE-RELATED

- **Children:** Safety of pyridoxine in children has not been established.
- **Elderly:** No age-related precautions have been noted.

PREGNANCY/LACTATION-RELATED

- Pregnancy category A. Deficiency during pregnancy is common in unsupplemented women. Excreted in human breast milk; RDA for lactating women is 2.3-2.5 mg.

MONITORING

- **Baseline assessment:** Before and during therapy, assess for pyridoxine deficiency including CNS abnormalities (anxiety, depression, insomnia, motor difficulty, peripheral numbness, tremors) and skin lesions (glossitis, seborrhea-like lesions around eyes, mouth, nose).
- **Baseline lab work:** Biochemical profile to help rule out other conditions associated with symptoms of vitamin B_6 deficiency.
- **Therapeutic effects:** Observe for improvement of deficiency symptoms, including CNS abnormalities and skin lesions.
- **Diet:** Evaluate for adequate B_6 intake in diet.
- **Vital signs:** Monitor respiratory rate, heart rate, BP during large IV doses.
- **Patient education:** Inform that IM injection may cause discomfort. Encourage consuming foods rich in pyridoxine, including avocados, bananas, bran, carrots, eggs, organ meats, tuna, shrimp, hazelnuts, legumes, soybeans, sunflower seeds, and wheat germ.

SERIOUS ADVERSE REACTIONS

- Seizures have occurred after IV megadoses.
- Withdrawal seizures occur in infants born of mothers taking high pyridoxine doses.

OVERDOSE/TOXICITY

- **Neurotoxicity:** Long-term megadoses (2-6 g over more than 2 mo) may produce sensory neuropathy (reduced deep tendon reflexes, profound impairment of sense of position in distal limbs, gradual sensory ataxia).
- **Management:** Toxic symptoms subside when drug is discontinued.
- **GI decontamination:** No specific recommendations.

ANTIDOTE/DIALYSIS

- **Antidote:** No specific recommendations.
- **Dialysis:** Pyridoxine is removed by high-permeability hemodialysis. No data are available on removal by hemodialysis or peritoneal dialysis.

P

quetiapine fumarate

kwe-tye'-a-peen fyoo'-muh-rate

Classes
Chemical: dibenzothiazepine derivative
Therapeutic: antipsychotic

Pregnancy Category: C

Trade Names
Prescription: Seroquel

CLINICAL PHARMACOLOGY

Mechanism of Action
A dibenzothiazepine derivative that antagonizes dopamine, serotonin, histamine, and $alpha_1$-adrenergic receptors. **Therapeutic Effect:** Diminishes manifestations of psychotic disorders. Produces moderate sedation, few extrapyramidal effects, and no anticholinergic effects.

PHARMACOKINETICS

Well absorbed after PO administration. Protein binding: 83%. Widely distributed in tissues; CNS concentration exceeds plasma concentration. Undergoes extensive first-pass metabolism in the liver. Primarily excreted in urine. **Half-life:** 6 hr.

AVAILABILITY

Tablets: 25 mg, 50 mg, 100 mg, 200 mg, 300 mg, 400 mg.

INDICATIONS AND DOSAGE

To manage manifestations of psychotic disorders
PO
Adults, Elderly: Initially, 25 mg twice per day, then 25-50 mg 2-3 times per day on the second and third days, up to 300-400 mg/day in divided doses 2-3 times per day by the fourth day. Further adjustments of 25-50 mg twice per day may be made at intervals of 2 days or longer. Maintenance: 300-800 mg/day (adults); 50-200 mg/day (elderly).
Mania in bipolar disorder
PO
Adults, Elderly: Initially, 50 mg twice per day for 1 day. May increase in increments of 100 mg/day to 200 mg twice per day on day 4. May increase in increments of 200 mg/day to 800 mg/day on day 6. Range: 400-800 mg/day.
Dosage in hepatic impairment, elderly or debilitated patients, and those predisposed to hypotensive reactions
These patients should receive a lower initial dose and lower dosage increases.

OFF-LABEL USES

Autism, psychosis (children)

CONTRAINDICATIONS

Hypersensitivity to quetiapine

INTERACTIONS

Drug: Alcohol, other CNS depressants: May increase CNS depression. **Antihypertensives:** May increase the hypotensive effects of these drugs. **Hepatic enzyme inducers (such as phenytoin):** May increase quetiapine clearance. **Herbal:** None known. **Food:** None known.

DIAGNOSTIC TEST EFFECTS

May decrease serum total and free thyroxine (T_4) serum levels. May increase serum cholesterol, triglyceride, AST (SGOT), and ALT (SGPT) levels. May produce a false-positive pregnancy test result.

SIDE-EFFECTS

Frequent (19%-10%): Headache, somnolence, dizziness. **Occasional (9%-3%):** Constipation, orthostatic hypotension, tachycardia, dry mouth, dyspepsia, rash, asthenia, abdominal pain, rhinitis. **Rare (2%):** Back pain, fever, weight gain

CRITICAL CARE CONSIDERATIONS

ADMINISTRATION/HANDLING

PO ALERT
- Give quetiapine without regard to food.
- Dosage adjustments should occur at 2-day intervals.
- When restarting therapy for patients off quetiapine for more than 1 wk, follow the initial titration schedule. When restarting therapy for patients who have been off quetiapine for less than 1 wk, titration is not required; maintenance dose can be reinstituted.

PRECAUTIONS

HEALTH-RELATED
- Use quetiapine cautiously in patients with Alzheimer's disease, cardiovascular disease (heart failure or prior MI), cerebrovascular disease, seizures, hepatic impairment, dehydration, hypothyroidism, hypovolemia, a history of breast cancer, or history of drug abuse or dependence.

AGE-RELATED
- **Children:** Safety and efficacy of quetiapine have not been established in children.

- **Elderly:** No age-related precautions have been noted; however, lower initial and target dosages may be necessary.

PREGNANCY/LACTATION-RELATED

- Pregnancy category C; excretion into breast milk unknown; breast-feeding is not recommended.

MONITORING

- **Baseline assessment:** Assess appearance, behavior, emotional status, response to environment, speech pattern, and thought content.
- **Baseline lab work:** CBC with WBC differential; biochemical profile including liver (AST [SGOT], ALT [SGPT], alkaline phosphatase, GGT, bilirubin) function tests.
- **Fall prevention:** Assist with ambulation if dizziness is experienced.
- **Suicidal patients:** Closely supervise suicidal patients during early therapy. As depression lessens, energy level improves, causing increased suicide potential.
- **Hypotension:** Monitor for hypotension and tachycardia, especially if the drug dosage has been increased rapidly.
- **Constipation:** Assess pattern of daily bowel activity and stool consistency.
- **Therapeutic response:** Assess for evidence of a therapeutic response, such as improvement in self-care, increased interest in surroundings and ability to concentrate, and relaxed facial expression.
- **Patient education:** Instruct to take quetiapine as prescribed. Caution against abruptly discontinuing the drug or increasing the dosage. Inform that drowsiness generally subsides during continued therapy. Warn to avoid tasks that require mental alertness or motor skills until response to the drug is known. Recommend changing positions slowly to reduce the hypotensive effect of quetiapine. Urge avoidance of alcohol and exposure to extreme heat. Advise to drink lots of fluids, especially during physical activity.

SERIOUS ADVERSE REACTIONS

- Weight gain of more than 7% of baseline weight.
- Tachycardia and postural hypotension.

OVERDOSE/TOXICITY

- **Overdose:** May produce heart block, hypotension, hypokalemia, and tachycardia.
- **GI decontamination:** No specific recommendations.

ANTIDOTE/DIALYSIS

- **Antidote:** No specific recommendations.
- **Dialysis:** No data are available on removal of quetiapine by hemodialysis, high-permeability hemodialysis, or peritoneal dialysis.

quinapril hydrochloride

See ACE Inhibitors (p. 883)

quinethazone

See Diuretics (p. 956)

quinidine gluconate

kwin'-i-deen glue'-kun-ate

Classes

Chemical: quinine isomer, dextrorotatory
Therapeutic: antidysrhythmic, class IA; antimalarial

Pregnancy Category: C

Trade Names

Prescription: Apo-Quin-G, BioQuin Durules, Quinaglute Dura-Tabs, Quinidex Extentabs

Do not confuse quinidine with clonidine or quinine.

CLINICAL PHARMACOLOGY

Mechanism of Action

An antidysrhythmic that decreases sodium influx during depolarization, potassium efflux during repolarization, and reduces calcium transport across the myocardial cell membrane. Decreases myocardial excitability, conduction velocity, and contractility. **Therapeutic Effect:** Suppresses dysrhythmias.

PHARMACOKINETICS

Almost completely absorbed after PO administration. Protein binding: 80%-90%. Metabolized in liver. Excreted in urine. Not removed by hemodialysis. **Half-life:** 6-8 hr.

AVAILABILITY

Injection: 80 mg/mL.
Tablets: 200 mg, 300 mg.
Tablets (extended release): 300 mg (Quinidex Extentabs) 324 mg (Quinaglute Dura-Tabs).

INDICATIONS AND DOSAGE

Maintenance of normal sinus rhythm after conversion of atrial fibrillation or flutter; prevention of premature atrial, AV, and ventricular contractions; paroxysmal atrial tachycardia; paroxysmal AV junctional rhythm; atrial fibrillation; atrial flutter; paroxysmal ventricular tachycardia not associated with complete heart block

PO

Adults, Elderly: 100-600 mg every 4-6 hr. Long-acting: 324-972 mg every 8-12 hr. **Children:** 30 mg/kg/day in divided doses every 4-6 hr.

IV

Adults, Elderly: 200-400 mg every 4 hr. **Children:** 2-10 mg/kg every 3-6 hr.

OFF-LABEL USES

Treatment of malaria (IV only)

CONTRAINDICATIONS

Complete AV block, development of thrombocytopenic purpura during prior therapy with quinidine or quinine, intraventricular conduction defects (widening of QRS complex), hypersensitivity to quinidine

INTERACTIONS

Drug: Antimyasthenics: May decrease effects of these drugs on skeletal muscle. **Digoxin:** May increase digoxin serum concentration. **Other antidysrhythmics, pimozide:** May increase cardiac effects. **Neuromuscular blockers, oral anticoagulants:** May increase effects of these drugs. **Urinary alkalizers such as antacids:** May decrease quinidine renal excretion. **Herbal:** None known. **Food:** None known.

DIAGNOSTIC TEST EFFECTS

None known. Therapeutic serum level is 2-5 mcg/mL; toxic serum level is greater than 5 mcg/mL.

IV INCOMPATIBILITIES

Furosemide (Lasix), heparin

IV COMPATIBILITIES

Milrinone (Primacor)

SIDE-EFFECTS

Frequent: Abdominal pain and cramps, nausea, diarrhea, vomiting (can be immediate, intense). **Occasional:** Mild cinchonism (ringing in ears, blurred vision, hearing loss) or severe cinchonism (headache, vertigo, diaphoresis, lightheadedness, photophobia, confusion, delirium). **Rare:** Hypotension (particularly with IV administration), hypersensitivity reaction (fever, anaphylaxis, photosensitivity reaction)

CRITICAL CARE CONSIDERATIONS

ADMINISTRATION/HANDLING

PO ALERT

- Do not crush or chew sustained-release tablets.
- Give quinidine with food to reduce GI upset.

IV ALERT

- **Stability:** Solution is stable for 24 hr at room temperature when diluted with D_5W. Use only clear, colorless solution.
- **IV infusion:** Dilute 800 mg with 40 mL D_5W to provide concentration of 16 mg/mL. Give at rate of 1 mL (16 mg)/min because a rapid rate may markedly decrease arterial pressure. Administer with patients in supine position.

PRECAUTIONS

HEALTH-RELATED

- Use quinidine cautiously in patients with digoxin toxicity, incomplete AV block, hepatic or renal impairment, myasthenia gravis, myocardial depression, and sick sinus syndrome.

AGE-RELATED

- **Children:** Safety and efficacy of quinidine have not been established in children.
- **Elderly:** Age-related organ impairment may prompt a dosage adjustment.

PREGNANCY/LACTATION-RELATED

- Pregnancy category C. Use during pregnancy has been classified in reviews of cardiovascular drugs as relatively safe for the fetus. High doses can produce oxytocic properties and potential for abortion. Excreted in breast milk; use cautiously in breast-feeding women.

MONITORING

- **Baseline assessment:** Check vital signs. Place patients on a cardiac monitor.
- **Baseline and ongoing lab work:** CBC with WBC differential and biochemical profile including renal (BUN, creatinine) and liver (serum alkaline phosphatase, bilirubin, creatinine, AST [SGOT], ALT [SGPT]) function tests in patients receiving long-term therapy.

- **Baseline diagnostic tests:** 12-lead ECG to assess baseline heart rhythm and to assess for myocardial ischemia.
- **Drug levels:** Quinidine's therapeutic serum level is 2-5 mcg/mL. Toxic level is greater than 5 mcg/mL.
- **Dysrhythmias:** Continuously monitor BP and ECG during IV administration; adjust the rate of infusion as appropriate to minimize dysrhythmias and hypotension. Monitor ECG for prolongation of PR or QT interval and widening of the QRS complex, which may signal heart block is ensuing.
- **Diarrhea:** Assess pattern of daily bowel activity and stool consistency.
- **Hypotension:** Monitor BP for hypotension, especially in patients receiving high-dose therapy. Discontinue quinidine if quinidine-induced syncope develops.
- **Patient education:** Instruct to report fever, ringing in the ears, or visual disturbances. Advise that quinidine may cause a photosensitivity reaction. Urge avoidance of direct sunlight or artificial light.

SERIOUS ADVERSE REACTIONS

- **Drug-induced syncope:** May occur with the usual quinidine dosage.
- **Severe hypotension:** May result from high dosages.
- Patients with atrial flutter and fibrillation may experience a paradoxic, extremely rapid ventricular rate that may be prevented by prior digitalization.

OVERDOSE/TOXICITY

- **Cardiotoxic effects:** Occur most commonly with IV administration using high concentrations; observed as conduction changes (50% widening of QRS complex, prolonged QT interval, flattened T waves, and disappearance of P wave), ventricular tachycardia or flutter, frequent premature ventricular contractions (PVCs), or complete AV block.
- **Hepatotoxicity:** Elevated liver enzymes with jaundice due to drug hypersensitivity may occur.
- **Hematologic toxicity:** Agranulocytosis, bone marrow suppression, neutropenia, thrombocytopenia, and hypoplastic anemia.
- **Management:** Quinidine should be discontinued and an alternative agent identified to manage the dysrhythmia. Another Class 1 antidysrhythmic (lidocaine) or possibly a Class 3 agent (amiodarone, sotalol) may be effective without causing toxicity or serious side effects. Supportive care should be provided to maintain patent airway and support ventilation. Hypotension may be managed with IV fluids and then, vasopressors if BP does not respond to fluid challenges. Transcutaneous or transvenous pacing may help manage heart block or asystole. Manage ventricular fibrillation using defibrillation according to Advanced Cardiac Life Support (ACLS) guidelines. Torsades de pointes may respond to magnesium sulfate, epinephrine infusion (isoproterenol is an older drug used for torsades), along with defibrillation.
- **GI decontamination:** No specific recommendations.

ANTIDOTE/DIALYSIS

- **Antidote:** No specific recommendations.
- **Dialysis:** Quinidine is not removed by hemodialysis or peritoneal dialysis. No data are available on removal by high-permeability hemodialysis.

quinine sulfate

kwye'-nine sul'-fate

Classes

Chemical: cinchona alkaloid
Therapeutic: antimalarial

Pregnancy Category: X

Trade Names

Prescription: Quinine

Do not confuse quinine with quinidine.

CLINICAL PHARMACOLOGY

Mechanism of Action

A cinchone alkaloid that relaxes skeletal muscle by increasing the refractory period, decreasing excitability of motor end plates (curarelike), and affecting distribution of calcium with muscle fiber. Antimalaria: Depresses oxygen uptake, carbohydrate metabolism, elevates pH in intracellular organelles of parasites. **Therapeutic Effect:** Relaxes skeletal muscle; produces parasite death.

PHARMACOKINETICS

Rapidly absorbed mainly from upper small intestine. Protein binding: 70%-95%. Metabolized in liver. Excreted in feces, saliva, and urine. **Half-life:** 8-14 hr (adults), 6-12 hr (children).

AVAILABILITY

Capsules: 200 mg, 325 mg (Quinine).
Tablets: 260 mg (Quinine).

INDICATIONS AND DOSAGE

Nocturnal leg cramps

PO

Adults, Elderly: 260-300 mg at bedtime as needed.

Treatment of malaria

PO

Adults, Elderly: 260-650 mg 3 times per day for 6-12 days. **Children:** 10 mg/kg every 8 hr for 5-7 days.

Dosage in renal impairment

Creatinine Clearance	Dosage Interval
10-50 mL/min	75% of normal dose or every 12 hr
Less than 10 mL/min	30%-50% of normal dose or every 24 hr

CONTRAINDICATIONS

Hypersensitivity to quinine (possible cross-sensitivity to quinidine), G-6-PD deficiency, tinnitus, optic neuritis, history of thrombocytopenia during previous quinine therapy, blackwater fever

INTERACTIONS

Drug: Amiodarone, alkalinizing agents, cimetidine, verapamil: May increase quinine serum concentrations. **Beta-blockers:** May increase bradycardia. **Digoxin:** May increase blood concentration of digoxin. **Mefloquine:** May increase risk of seizures and ECG abnormalities. **Phenobarbital, phenytoin, rifampin:** May decrease quinine serum concentrations. **Warfarin:** May increase anticoagulant effect. **Herbal: St. John's wort:** May decrease quinine levels. **Food:** None known.

DIAGNOSTIC TEST EFFECTS

May interfere with 17-OH steroid determinations. May result in positive Coombs' test.

SIDE-EFFECTS

Frequent: Nausea, headache, tinnitus, slight visual disturbances (mild cinchonism). **Occasional:** Extreme flushing of skin with intense generalized pruritus is most typical hypersensitivity reaction; also rash, wheezing, dyspnea, angioedema. **Prolonged therapy:** Cardiac conduction disturbances, decreased hearing

CRITICAL CARE CONSIDERATIONS

ADMINISTRATION/HANDLING

PO ALERT

- Do not crush tablets or capsules to avoid bitter taste.
- Give quinine with food.

PRECAUTIONS

HEALTH-RELATED

- Use quinine cautiously in patients with cardiovascular disease, myasthenia gravis, and asthma.

AGE-RELATED

- **Children:** No age-related precautions have been noted in children.
- **Elderly:** Age-related renal impairment may require a dosage adjustment.

PREGNANCY/LACTATION-RELATED

- Pregnancy category X; excreted into breast milk; use cautiously in breast-feeding women; use caution in infants at risk for G-6-PD deficiency

MONITORING

- **Baseline assessment:** Determine possibility of pregnancy before initiating therapy. Question for hypersensitivity to quinine and/or quinidine.
- **Baseline lab work:** CBC with WBC differential to monitor for blood dyscrasias; biochemical profile including blood glucose.
- **Baseline diagnostic tests:** 12-lead ECG.
- **Hypersensitivity:** Monitor for flushing, rash/urticaria, itching, dyspnea, wheezing.
- **Cinchonism:** Assess level of hearing, visual acuity, presence of headache/tinnitus, and nausea.
- **Infection:** Assess for fever, sore throat, bleeding and bruising, or unusual tiredness and weakness.
- **Dysrhythmias:** Assess continuous ECG for dysrhythmias including prolongation of the QT interval.
- **Hypoglycemia:** Check point of care capillary glucose (e.g., Accuchek); assess for hypoglycemia such as cold sweating, tremors, tachycardia, hunger, anxiety.
- **Patient education:** Instruct to use appropriate nonhormonal contraceptive measures. Instruct to report promptly visual or hearing difficulties, shortness of breath,

Q

rash, itching, or nausea to a health care provider. Inform that periodic lab tests are essential for safe, successful therapy. Advise to take with food. May cause blurred vision; use caution driving. Discontinue quinine if flushing, itching, rash, fever, stomach pain, difficult breathing, ringing in ears, or visual disturbances occur.

SERIOUS ADVERSE REACTIONS

- **Blood dyscrasias:** Hypoprothrombinemia, thrombocytopenic purpura, hemoglobinuria, agranulocytosis are rare.
- **Hypersensitivity:** Flushing, rash/urticaria, itching, dyspnea, wheezing.
- Asthma, hypoglycemia, deafness, and optic atrophy occur rarely.

OVERDOSE/TOXICITY

- **Cinchonism:** Severe cinchonism may result in cardiovascular effects, severe headache, intestinal cramps with vomiting and diarrhea, apprehension, confusion, seizures, blindness, and respiratory depression.
- **GI decontamination:** No specific recommendations.

ANTIDOTE/DIALYSIS

- **Antidote:** No specific recommendations.
- **Dialysis:** Quinine is not removed by hemodialysis or peritoneal dialysis. No data are available on removal by high-permeability hemodialysis.

quinupristin; dalfopristin

kwin-yoo'-pris-tin; dal-foh'-pris-tin

Classes
Chemical: streptogramin combination
Therapeutic: antibiotic

Pregnancy Category: B

Trade Names
Prescription: Synercid

CLINICAL PHARMACOLOGY

Mechanism of Action
Two chemically distinct compounds that, when given together, bind to different sites on bacterial ribosomes, inhibiting protein synthesis. **Therapeutic Effect:** Bactericidal.

PHARMACOKINETICS

After IV administration, both are extensively metabolized in the liver, with dalfopristin to active metabolite. Protein binding: quinupristin, 23%-32%; dalfopristin, 50%-56%. Primarily eliminated in feces. **Half-life:** quinupristin, 0.85 hr; dalfopristin, 0.7 hr.

AVAILABILITY

Injection: 500-mg vial (150 mg quinupristin/350 mg dalfopristin); 600-mg vial (180 mg quinupristin/420 mg dalfopristin).

INDICATIONS AND DOSAGE

Infections caused by vancomycin-resistant *Enterococcus faecium*
IV
Adults, Elderly: 7.5 mg/kg/dose every 8 hr.
Skin and skin structure infections
IV
Adults, Elderly: 7.5 mg/kg/dose every 12 hr.

CONTRAINDICATIONS

Hypersensitivity to pristinamycin, virginiamycin, quinupristin, or dalfopristin

INTERACTIONS

Drug: Pimozide: May increase risk of cardiotoxicity. **Herbal:** None known. **Food:** None known.

DIAGNOSTIC TEST EFFECTS

May increase serum bilirubin, creatinine, LDH, AST (SGOT), and ALT (SGPT) levels.

IV INCOMPATIBILITIES

Heparin, sodium chloride

IV COMPATIBILITIES

Aztreonam (Azactam), ciprofloxacin (Cipro), fluconazole (Diflucan), haloperidol (Haldol), metoclopramide (Reglan), morphine, potassium chloride

SIDE-EFFECTS

Frequent: Mild erythema, pruritus, pain, or burning at infusion site (with doses greater than 7 mg/kg). **Occasional:** Headache, diarrhea. **Rare:** Vomiting, arthralgia, myalgia

CRITICAL CARE CONSIDERATIONS

ADMINISTRATION/HANDLING

IV ALERT

- **Storage:** Refrigerate unopened vials.
- **Reconstitution:** Slowly add 5 mL D_5W or sterile water for injection to each vial to yield a concentration of 100 mg/mL. Gently swirl vial contents to minimize foaming.
- **Futher dilution:** Dilute with D_5W to a final concentration of 2 mg/mL (5 mg/mL if using a central line).

- **Stability:** Reconstituted vials are stable for 1 hr at room temperature. Diluted infusion bags are stable for 6 hr at room temperature or 54 hr if refrigerated.
- **IV intermittent infusion (piggyback):** Infuse the solution over 60 min.
- **Following infusion:** Flush the line with D_5W to minimize vein irritation. Do not flush with 0.9% NaCl; it is incompatible with quinupristin and dalfopristin.

PRECAUTIONS

HEALTH-RELATED

- Use quinupristin-dalfopristin cautiously in patients with renal or hepatic dysfunction.

AGE-RELATED

- **Children:** Safety and efficacy of quinupristin-dalfopristin have not been established in children.
- **Elderly:** No age-related precautions have been noted. Age-related organ impairment may prompt a dosage adjustment.

PREGNANCY/LACTATION-RELATED

- Pregnancy category B; breast milk excretion unknown.

MONITORING

- **Baseline assessment:** Assess BP, body temperature, pulse, and respiratory rate.
- **Baseline and ongoing lab work:** CBC with WBC differential, biochemical profile including renal (BUN, creatinine) and liver function test results (AST [SGOT], ALT [SGPT], alkaline phosphatase, GGT, bilirubin) and urinalysis results.
- **Diarrhea:** Withhold quinupristin-dalfopristin if diarrhea occurs. Diarrhea with abdominal pain, fever, and mucus or blood in stools may indicate antibiotic-associated colitis.
- **IV site:** Evaluate the IV site for redness, vein irritation, burning, pruritus, mild erythema, and pain.
- **Superinfections:** Assess the mouth for white patches on the mucous membranes or tongue and for severe mouth or tongue soreness; assess for severe anal or genital pruritus or discharge.
- **Possible *Clostridium difficile* colitis:** Assess pattern of daily bowel activity and stool consistency. Although mild GI effects may be tolerable, severe symptoms including abdominal pain or cramping, moderate to severe diarrhea may indicate the onset of antibiotic-associated colitis.
- **Hand washing:** If *C. difficile* (antibiotic-associated) colitis develops, wash hands with antibacterial soap. Alcohol-based foam is ineffective against *C. difficile* spores.
- **Nephrotoxicity and hepatotoxicity:** Monitor for fluid retention (edema, positive fluid balance); run liver and renal function test results to assess for toxicity.
- **Patient education:** Advise to report immediately pain, redness, or swelling at the infusion site to a health care provider. Warn to report immediately severe diarrhea and to avoid taking antidiarrheals until instructed to use them.

SERIOUS ADVERSE REACTIONS

- **Hypersensitivity:** Patients with a history of allergies are at increased risk for developing a severe hypersensitivity reaction marked by severe pruritus, angioedema, bronchospasm, and anaphylaxis.
- **Management of hypersensitivity:** May require treatment with epinephrine and other emergency measures including oxygen, endotracheal intubation, mechanical ventilation, IV fluids, IV antihistamines, corticosteroids, and vasopressors.

OVERDOSE/TOXICITY

- **Nephrotoxicity:** Increased BUN and creatinine, decreased urine output, anuria, possible hyperkalemia, fluid overload indicative of acute renal failure.
- **Superinfection:** Antibiotic-associated colitis (pseudomembranous colitis) and other superinfections may result from altered bacterial balance.
- **Manage pseudomembraneous colitis:** Fluids, electrolytes, protein supplements, oral vancomycin (Vancocin) or IV metronidazole (Flagyl).
- **Hepatotoxicity, leukopenia, thrombocytopenia:** Occur rarely.
- **GI decontamination:** No specific recommendations.

ANTIDOTE/DIALYSIS

- **Antidote:** No specific recommendations.
- **Dialysis:** Quinupristin-dalfopristin is not removed by peritoneal dialysis. No data are available on removal using hemodialysis or high-permeability hemodialysis.

Q

rabeprazole sodium

See Acid Secretion Inhibitors (p. 884)

raloxifene

ral-ox'-i-feen

Classes

Chemical: benzothiophene derivative
Therapeutic: antiosteoporotic, selective estrogen receptor modulator (SERM)

Pregnancy Category: X

Trade Names

Prescription: Evista

Do not confuse raloxifene with propoxyphene.

CLINICAL PHARMACOLOGY

Mechanism of Action

A selective estrogen receptor modulator that affects some receptors similarly to estrogen. **Therapeutic Effect:** Like estrogen, prevents bone loss and improves lipid profiles.

PHARMACOKINETICS

Rapidly absorbed after PO administration. Highly bound to plasma proteins (greater than 95%) and albumin. Undergoes extensive first-pass metabolism in liver. Excreted mainly in feces and, to a lesser extent, in urine. **Half-life:** 30 hr.

AVAILABILITY

Tablets: 60 mg.

INDICATIONS AND DOSAGE

Prevention or treatment of osteoporosis

PO

Adults, Elderly: 60 mg per day.

OFF-LABEL USES

Prevention of fractures, treatment of breast cancer in postmenopausal women

CONTRAINDICATIONS

Active or history of venous thromboembolic events, such as deep vein thrombosis (DVT), pulmonary embolism, and retinal vein thrombosis; women who are or may become pregnant; hypersensitivity to raloxifene

INTERACTIONS

Drug: Cholestyramine: Reduce raloxifene absorption. **Hormone replacement therapy, systemic estrogen:** Do not use raloxifene concurrently with these drugs. **Warfarin:** May decrease prothrombin time and the effects of warfarin. **Herbal:** None known. **Food:** None known.

DIAGNOSTIC TEST EFFECTS

Lowers serum total cholesterol and LDL levels but does not affect HDL or triglyceride levels. Slightly decreases platelet count and serum inorganic phosphate, albumin, calcium, and protein levels.

SIDE-EFFECTS

Frequent (29%-10%): Hot flashes, flulike symptoms, arthralgia, sinusitis. **Occasional (9%-5%):** Weight gain, nausea, myalgia, pharyngitis, cough, dyspepsia, leg cramps, rash, depression. **Rare (4%-3%):** Vaginitis, urinary tract infection, peripheral edema, flatulence, vomiting, fever, migraine, diaphoresis

CRITICAL CARE CONSIDERATIONS

ADMINISTRATION/HANDLING

PO ALERT

- Give raloxifene without regard to food at any time of day.
- Discontinue raloxifene 72 hr before and during prolonged immobilization (postoperative recovery and prolonged bed rest). Resume therapy only after patients are fully ambulatory.

PRECAUTIONS

HEALTH-RELATED

- Use raloxifene cautiously in patients with cardiovascular disease, hepatic or renal impairment, or a history of cervical or uterine cancer.
- Raloxifene may increase risk of venous thromboembolism in all women; not recommended for use in premenopausal females.

AGE-RELATED

- **Children:** Raloxifene is not used in children.
- **Elderly:** No age-related precautions have been noted.

PREGNANCY/LACTATION-RELATED

- Pregnancy category X; abortion and fetal anomalies noted in animal studies. Unknown if excreted in milk.

MONITORING

- **Baseline assessment:** Determine pregnancy before starting raloxifene therapy.

- **Baseline lab work:** CBC with platelet count, biochemical profile including total and LDL cholesterol serum levels before beginning raloxifene therapy and routinely thereafter. Monitor platelet count and serum levels of inorganic phosphate, calcium, total and LDL cholesterol, and protein.
- **Baseline diagnostic tests:** Bone density scan to evaluate for osteopenia and osteoporosis.
- **Patient education:** Warn to avoid prolonged immobility during travel because limited movement increases the risk of venous thromboembolic events. Instruct how to take supplemental calcium and vitamin D if daily dietary intake is inadequate. Encourage avoidance of alcohol and cigarette smoking during raloxifene therapy to reduce probability of thrombus formation. Instruct to exercise regularly.

SERIOUS ADVERSE REACTIONS

- Pneumonia, gastroenteritis, chest pain, vaginal bleeding, hot flashes, and breast pain occur rarely.

OVERDOSE/TOXICITY

- **Thrombosis:** If patients experience leg cramps, raloxifene should be discontinued.
- **GI decontamination:** No specific recommendations.

ANTIDOTE/DIALYSIS

- **Antidote:** No specific recommendations.
- **Dialysis:** Raloxifene is unlikely to be removed by hemodialysis or peritoneal dialysis. No data are available on removal by high-permeability hemodialysis.

ramipril

See ACE Inhibitors (p. 883)

ranitidine hydrochloride/ ranitidine bismuth citrate

ra-ni'-ti-deen

Classes

Chemical: aminoalkyl furan derivative
Therapeutic: antiulcer agent

Pregnancy Category: B

Trade Names

Prescription: Apo-Ranitidine ♣, Zantac, Zantac-150, Zantac-300, Zantac EFFERdose, Zantac-25 EFFERdose, Zantac-150 EFFERdose
Over the Counter: Zantac 75

Do not confuse Zantac with Xanax, Ziac, or Zyrtec.

CLINICAL PHARMACOLOGY

Mechanism of Action

An antiulcer agent that inhibits histamine action at histamine-2 receptors of gastric parietal cells. **Therapeutic Effect:** Inhibits gastric acid secretion when fasting, at night, or when stimulated by food, caffeine, or insulin. Reduces volume and hydrogen ion concentration of gastric juice.

PHARMACOKINETICS

Rapidly absorbed from the GI tract. Protein binding: 15%. Widely distributed. Metabolized in the liver. Primarily excreted in urine. **Half-life:** PO, 2.5-3 hr; IV, 2-2.5 hr (increased up to 5 hr with impaired renal function).

AVAILABILITY

Tablets (effervescent): 25 mg (Zantac-25 EFFERdose), 150 mg (Zantac-150 EFFERdose).
Capsules (Zantac): 150 mg, 300 mg.
Granules (Zantac EFFERdose): 150 mg.
Syrup (Zantac): 15 mg/mL.
Tablets: 75 mg (Zantac-75), 150 mg (Zantac-150, Zantac-150 Maximum Strength), 300 mg (Zantac-300).
Injection (Zantac): 25 mg/mL.

INDICATIONS AND DOSAGE

Duodenal ulcers, gastric ulcers, gastroesophageal reflux disease

PO

Adults, Elderly: 150 mg twice per day or 300 mg at bedtime. Maintenance: 150 mg at bedtime. **Children 1 mo to 16 yr:** 2-4 mg/kg/day in divided doses twice per day. Maximum: 300 mg/day.

Duodenal ulcers associated with *Helicobacter pylori* infection

PO

Adults, Elderly: 150 mg twice per day for 4 wk in combination with clarithromycin 500 mg 2-3 times per day for the first 2 wk.

Erosive esophagitis

PO

Adults, Elderly: 150 mg 4 times per day. Maintenance: 150 mg twice per day or 300 mg at bedtime. **Children:** 4-10 mg/kg/day in 2 divided doses. Maximum: 600 mg/day.

R

Hypersecretory conditions
PO
Adults, Elderly: 150 mg twice per day. May increase up to 6 g/day.
OTC use
PO
Adults, Elderly: 75 mg 30-60 min before eating food or drinking beverages that cause heartburn. Maximum: 150 mg per 24 hr period and/or longer than 14 days.
Usual parenteral dosage
IV, IM
Adults, Elderly: 50 mg/dose every 6-8 hr.
Children: 2-4 mg/kg/day in divided doses every 6-8 hr. Maximum: 200 mg/day.
Usual neonatal dosage
PO
Neonates less than 1 mo: 2 mg/kg/day in divided doses every 12 hr.
IV
Neonates: Initially 1.5 mg/kg/dose; then 1.5-2 mg/kg/day in divided doses every 12 hr.
Dosage in renal impairment
For patients with creatinine clearance less than 50 mL/min, give 150 mg PO every 24 hr or 50 mg IV or IM every 18-24 hr.

OFF-LABEL USES

Prevention of aspiration pneumonia, treatment of recurrent postoperative ulcer, upper GI bleeding, prevention of acid aspiration pneumonitis during surgery, prevention of stress-induced ulcers.

CONTRAINDICATIONS

History of acute porphyria, hypersensitivity to ranitidine

INTERACTIONS

Drug: Antacids: May decrease the absorption of ranitidine. **Triazolam:** May increase triazolam concentration by 10%-30%. **Herbal:** None known. **Food:** None known.

DIAGNOSTIC TEST EFFECTS

Interferes with skin tests using allergen extracts. May increase hepatic function enzyme, gamma-glutamyl transpeptidase, and serum creatinine levels.

IV INCOMPATIBILITIES

Amphotericin B complex (Abelcet, AmBisome, Amphotec), regular insulin

IV COMPATIBILITIES

Diltiazem (Cardizem), *DOBUTamine (Dobutrex), *DOPamine (Intropin), heparin, hydromorphone (Dilaudid), insulin, lidocaine, lorazepam (Ativan), morphine, norepinephrine (Levophed), potassium chloride, propofol (Diprivan)

SIDE-EFFECTS

Occasional (2%): Diarrhea. **Rare (1%):** Constipation, headache (may be severe)

CRITICAL CARE CONSIDERATIONS

ADMINISTRATION/HANDLING

PO ALERT

- Give ranitidine without regard to meals; best given after meals or at bedtime.
- Do not administer ranitidine within 1 hr of magnesium- or aluminum-containing antacids because they decrease ranitidine absorption by 33%.

IV ALERT

- **Stability:** IV infusion (piggyback) is stable for 48 hr at room temperature. Discard if discolored or precipitate forms. IV solutions normally appear clear and are colorless to yellow; slight darkening does not affect potency.
- **IV push:** Dilute each 50 mg with 20 mL 0.9% NaCl or D_5W. Administer IV push over a minimum of 5 min to prevent dysrhythmias and hypotension.
- **Intermittent IV infusion (piggyback):** Dilute each 50 mg with 50 mL 0.9% NaCl or D_5W. Infuse IV piggyback over 15-20 min.
- **IV infusion:** Dilute with 250-1000 mL 0.9% NaCl or D_5W. Infuse IV infusion over 24 hr.

IM ALERT

- **Dilution:** May be given undiluted.
- **Administration:** Give deep IM into large muscle mass, such as the gluteus maximus.

PRECAUTIONS

HEALTH-RELATED

- Use ranitidine cautiously in elderly patients, diabetics on sulfonylureas (glyburide, glipizide), and those with impaired hepatic and renal function.

AGE-RELATED

- **Children:** Safety of ranitidine for use in neonates under 1 mo has not been established; limited data suggest drug may be effective in infants at risk of GI bleeding.
- **Elderly:** More likely to experience confusion, especially those with hepatic or renal impairment; half life is prolonged.

PREGNANCY/LACTATION-RELATED

- Pregnancy category B; unknown if distributed in breast milk.

MONITORING

- **Baseline assessment:** Assess history of GI distress, including whether pain is related to meals.
- **Baseline lab work:** Biochemical profile including renal (BUN, creatinine) and liver (serum alkaline phosphatase, bilirubin, AST [SGOT], and ALT [SGPT]) function tests.
- **Baseline diagnostic tests:** Endoscopy if GI symptoms have persisted for a long time despite use of antacid therapy.
- **GI bleeding:** Assess for GI bleeding in stool and hematemesis. Instruct to notify a health care provider if blood is noted in emesis or stool or if stool is dark and tarry.
- **Confusion:** Check the mental status in elderly and severely ill patients and in those with impaired renal function.
- **Injection site:** Monitor for transient discomfort and redness at the injection site.
- **Antacids:** Do not administer antacids within 1 hr of oral ranitidine administration.
- **Patient education:** Inform that smoking decreases the effectiveness of ranitidine. Advise not to take ranitidine within 1 hr of magnesium- or aluminum-containing antacids. Warn that transient burning or itching may occur with IV administration. Instruct to report headache promptly to a health care provider. Urge avoidance of alcohol and aspirin, both of which may cause GI distress during ranitidine therapy.

SERIOUS ADVERSE REACTIONS

- **Rapid IV administration:** May produce bradycardia, tachycardia, premature ventricular contractions, and hypotension.

OVERDOSE/TOXICITY

- **Hematologic:** Granulocytopenia, anemia, leukopenia, thrombocytopenia.
- **Hepatotoxicity:** Reversible hepatitis.
- **Central anticholinergic syndrome:** Agitation, altered mental status, anxiety, ataxia, coma, delirium, dysarthria, extrapyramidal reactions, auditory and visual hallucinations, paranoia, psychosis, seizures, cardiopulmonary arrest.
- **GI decontamination:** No specific recommendations.

ANTIDOTE/DIALYSIS

- **Antidote:** No specific antidote. Physostigmine may be used to reverse anticholinergic effects.
- **Dialysis:** Ranitidine is removed by high-permeability hemodialysis. Ranitidine is not removed by hemodialysis or peritoneal dialysis.

remifentanil

See Opioid Analgesics (p. 980)

repaglinide

re-pag'-lin-ide

Classes

Chemical: meglitinide
Therapeutic: antidiabetic, hypoglycemic

Pregnancy Category: C

Trade Names

Prescription: GlucoNorm ♣, Prandin

CLINICAL PHARMACOLOGY

Mechanism of Action

A hypoglycemic that stimulates release of insulin from beta cells of the pancreas by depolarizing beta cells, leading to an opening of calcium channels. Resulting calcium influx induces insulin secretion. **Therapeutic Effect:** Lowers blood glucose concentration.

PHARMACOKINETICS

Rapidly, completely absorbed from the GI tract. Protein binding: 98%. Metabolized in the liver to inactive metabolites. Excreted primarily in feces with a lesser amount in urine. Unlikely to be removed by hemodialysis. **Half-life:** 1 hr.

AVAILABILITY

Tablets: 0.5 mg, 1 mg, 2 mg.

INDICATIONS AND DOSAGE

Diabetes mellitus

PO

Adults, Elderly: 0.5-4 mg 2-4 times per day. Patients not previously treated or HbA_{1c} less than 8%: 0.5 mg before each meal. Patients previously treated or HbA_{1c} more than 8%: 1-2 mg before each meal. Maximum: 16 mg/day.

CONTRAINDICATIONS

Diabetic ketoacidosis, type 1 diabetes mellitus, hypersensitivity to repaglinide

R

INTERACTIONS

Drug: Beta-blockers, chloramphenicol, gemfibrozil, MAOIs, NSAIDs, probenecid, salicylates, sulfonamides, warfarin: May increase the effects of repaglinide. **Herbal:** None known. **Food:** Decreases repaglinide plasma concentration.

DIAGNOSTIC TEST EFFECTS

None known.

SIDE-EFFECTS

Frequent (10%-6%): Upper respiratory tract infection, headache, rhinitis, bronchitis, back pain. **Occasional (5%-3%):** Diarrhea, dyspepsia, sinusitis, nausea, arthralgia, urinary tract infection. **Rare (2%):** Constipation, vomiting, paresthesia, allergy

CRITICAL CARE CONSIDERATIONS

ADMINISTRATION/HANDLING

PO ALERT

- Give repaglinide ideally within 15 min of a meal; may be given as long as 30 min before a meal or directly before eating.

PRECAUTIONS

HEALTH-RELATED

- Use repaglinide cautiously in patients with hepatic or renal impairment.

AGE-RELATED

- **Children:** Safety and efficacy of repaglinide have not been established in children.
- **Elderly:** No age-related precautions have been noted; hypoglycemia may be more difficult to recognize in this patient population.

R

PREGNANCY/LACTATION-RELATED

- Pregnancy category C; excretion into breast milk unknown. Because of the potential for hypoglycemia in the infant, use with caution in nursing mothers.

MONITORING

- **Baseline assessment:** Assess history of diabetes, cardiovascular risk factors, diet and exercise patterns, and knowledge of hypoglycemia.
- **Baseline lab work:** Biochemical profile including blood glucose. Check fasting blood glucose level and hemoglobin A_{1c} periodically to determine the minimum effective dosage of repaglinide.
- **Hyperglycemia in the intensive care unit:** Treat hyperglycemia in critically ill patients with insulin infusion until improvement is seen. Blood glucose goal of 80-140 mg/dL or 80-110 is recommended. Oral agents should be discontinued when insulin is used.
- **Dosage adjustments:** Allow at least 1 wk to elapse to assess the response to the drug before a new dosage adjustment is made.
- **Diet:** Monitor carbohydrate intake. When patients are eating, meals should include only four servings of carbohydrates.
- **Hypoglycemia:** Assess for anxiety, tachycardia, cool and wet skin, diplopia, dizziness, headache, hunger, numbness in mouth, tremors. Patients receiving beta blocking drugs do not exhibit classic symptoms of hypoglycemia. Elderly diabetics are also less likely to have acute symptoms. Altered level of consciousness and lack of energy may signal low blood glucose.
- **Hyperglycemia:** Assess for deep rapid breathing, blurred vision, fatigue, nausea, polydipsia, polyphagia, polyuria, vomiting.
- **Insulin resistance:** Be alert to conditions that may increase blood glucose, including stress or a surgical procedure.
- **Fever:** Ensure that patients are well hydrated if fever is present.
- **Patient education:** Stress that the prescribed diet is a principal part of treatment. Warn not to skip or delay meals. Teach typical signs and symptoms of hypoglycemia and hyperglycemia. Urge wearing of medical alert identification identifying diabetes. Instruct to report to a health care provider when blood glucose may be altered, such as with fever, heavy physical activity, infection, stress, or trauma. Explain that diabetes mellitus requires lifelong control. Urge adherence to dietary instructions, a regular exercise program, and regular testing of blood glucose. Tell patients taking repaglinide with insulin or a sulfonylurea to always have a source of glucose available to treat symptoms of low blood sugar.

SERIOUS ADVERSE REACTIONS

- Hypoglycemia occurs in 16%-31% of patients.
- Elevated liver enzymes.
- **Cardiovascular disease:** If blood glucose is not controlled, studies reveal a higher incidence of stroke, heart attack, and limb ischemia. Chest pain occurs rarely.

OVERDOSE/TOXICITY

- **Hematologic:** Thrombocytopenia and leukopenia (rare).
- **Hypoglycemia:** Tachycardia, hypotension, seizures. Blood glucose may require aggressive treatment to recover if large doses of repaglinide were ingested.
- **Management:** Administer D50 (50% dextrose) IV. Maintain patent airway and support ventilation. Seizures, tachycardia and hypotension are generally transient and will resolve when blood glucose is normalized.
- **GI decontamination:** No specific recommendations.

ANTIDOTE/DIALYSIS

- **Antidote:** D50 (50% dextrose) solution 25 mL given IV if blood glucose is less than 50 mg/dL. May repeat as needed every 15 min until glucose is at leat 80 mg/dL. Do not raise blood glucose above 140 mg/dL when managing hypoglycemia, if possible.
- **Dialysis:** Repaglinide is unlikely to be removed by hemodialysis or peritoneal dialysis, and is not removed by high-permeability hemodialysis.

reteplase, recombinant

re'-te-plays

Classes

Chemical: tissue plasminogen activator (tPA)
Therapeutic: thrombolytic

Pregnancy Category: C

Trade Names

Prescription: Retavase

Do not confuse reteplase or Retavase with Restasis.

CLINICAL PHARMACOLOGY

Mechanism of Action

A tissue plasminogen activator that activates the fibrinolytic system by directly cleaving plasminogen to generate plasmin, an enzyme that degrades the fibrin of the thrombus. **Therapeutic Effect:** Exerts thrombolytic action.

PHARMACOKINETICS

Rapidly cleared from plasma. Eliminated primarily by the liver and kidney. **Half-life:** 13-16 min.

AVAILABILITY

Powder for injection: 10.4 units (18.1 mg).

INDICATIONS AND DOSAGE

Acute MI, heart failure

IV Bolus

Adults, Elderly: 10 units over 2 min; repeat in 30 min.

OFF-LABEL USES

Occluded catheters

CONTRAINDICATIONS

Active internal bleeding, AV malformation or aneurysm, bleeding diathesis, history of cerebrovascular accident (CVA), intracranial neoplasm, recent intracranial or intraspinal surgery or trauma, severe uncontrolled hypertension, hypersensitivity to reteplase

INTERACTIONS

Drug: Heparin, platelet aggregation antagonists (such as abciximab, aspirin, dipyridamole), warfarin: Increase the risk of bleeding. **Herbal: Ginkgo biloba:** May increase the risk of bleeding. **Food:** None known.

DIAGNOSTIC TEST EFFECTS

May decrease fibrinogen and serum plasminogen levels.

IV INCOMPATIBILITIES

Do not mix with other medications.

SIDE-EFFECTS

Frequent: Bleeding at superficial sites (4.6%-48.6%), such as venous injection sites, catheter insertion sites, venous cutdowns, arterial punctures, and sites of recent surgical procedures, gingival bleeding

R

CRITICAL CARE CONSIDERATIONS

ADMINISTRATION/HANDLING

IV ALERT

- **Storage:** Kit should remain sealed, protected from light, and stored at controlled room temperature.
- **Stability:** Use within 4 hr of reconstitution. Discard any unused portion.
- **Reconstitution:** Reconstitute only with sterile water for injection immediately before use; reconstituted solution contains 1 unit/mL; do not shake the vial; slight foaming may occur; let stand for a few minutes to allow bubbles to dissipate.

- **Administration:** Give through a dedicated IV line.
- **IV direct injection/first bolus:** Give as a 10-unit plus 10-unit double bolus, with each IV bolus administered over 2 min. Do not add other medications to the bolus injection solution. Do not give second IV bolus if serious bleeding or anaphylaxis or bleeding is experienced after first bolus.
- **Second IV bolus:** Give the second bolus 30 min after the first bolus injection.

PRECAUTIONS

HEALTH-RELATED

- Use reteplase cautiously in patients with acute pericarditis; bacterial endocarditis; cerebrovascular disease; diabetic retinopathy; hepatic or renal impairment; hypertension; major surgery, including coronary artery bypass graft, obstetric delivery, and organ biopsy; mitral stenosis with atrial fibrillation; occluded AV cannula at an infected site; ophthalmic hemorrhage; recent GI or GU bleeding; or septic thrombophlebitis.
- Use cautiously in patients of advanced age and in patients receiving oral anticoagulants.

AGE-RELATED

- **Children:** Safety and efficacy of reteplase have not been established in children.
- **Elderly:** Are more susceptible to bleeding; use with caution.

PREGNANCY/LACTATION-RELATED

- Pregnancy category C; unknown if distributed in breast milk.

R

MONITORING

- **Baseline assessment:** Obtain vital signs. Assess for risk of bleeding before administering reteplase. If risk factors for bleeding are present, do not administer.
- **Baseline lab work:** CBC; biochemical profile including cardiac enzymes (CPK) and isoenzymes (troponins and CKMB). Assess aPTT, Hct, plasminogen, and fibrinogen levels, platelet count, prothrombin time, and thrombin time before therapy starts. Type, screen, and hold blood sample for possible RBC transfusion.
- **Baseline diagnostic tests:** 12-lead ECG to assess for myocardial infarction and chest x-ray to rule out other causes of chest discomfort. Serial 12-lead ECGs should be performed on patients with acute coronary syndrome/acute MI. Absence of ST segment elevation on 12-lead ECG does not negate the need for thrombolysis if cardiac enzymes are strongly positive.
- **Bleeding precautions:** Minimize invasive procedures during and following initiation of reteplase. Carefully monitor all needle puncture sites and catheter insertion sites for bleeding. Avoid procedures such as injections and shaving.
- **Dysrhythmias:** Perform continuous cardiac monitoring for dysrhythmias, ST segment elevation, and/or depression and reperfusion dysrhythmias. If patients are not unstable with dysrhythmias, use of antidysrhythmic drugs should be avoided.
- **Hemodynamic stability:** Monitor for hypotension, tachycardia, tachypnea, increased work of breathing, and desaturation using pulse oximetry.
- **Heart failure:** Evaluate for rales/bubbly breath sounds and diminished pulse quality.
- **Chest pain:** Monitor for relief of chest pain. Note intensity, location, and quality of pain. Recurrance of chest pain may indicate reocclusion of the affected coronary artery and extension of myocardial infarction.
- **Patient education:** Advise to use an electric razor and soft toothbrush to prevent bleeding during drug therapy. Instruct to report black or red stool, coffee-ground vomitus, dark or red urine, red-speckled mucus from cough, or other signs of bleeding if not under constant direct observation. Instruct to report immediately chest pain, headache, palpitations, or shortness of breath.

SERIOUS ADVERSE REACTIONS

- **Reperfusion dysrhythmias:** Lysis or coronary thrombi may produce atrial or ventricular dysrhythmias.
- **Allergic reactions:** Nausea, vomiting, hypotension, fever.
- **Cholesterol embolization:** May be fatal.

OVERDOSE/TOXICITY

- **Hemorrhage:** Bleeding at internal sites may occur, including intracranial (stroke), retroperitoneal, GI, GU, and respiratory sites.
- **Management:** If bleeding occurs, withhold the second dose if not given. Discontinue heparin therapy, if used. Apply direct pressure to external bleeding sites. Administer blood products (whole blood, packed RBCs, fresh frozen plasma, cryoprecipitate) for severe bleeding.

Administer desmopressin, aminocaproic acid (Amicar), and tranexamic acid as needed. Protamine may be used to reverse effects of heparin. If neurologic deterioration occurs, use CT scan to help diagnose possible stroke and monitor for signs of increased intracranial pressure.

- **GI decontamination:** No specific recommendations.

ANTIDOTE/DIALYSIS

- **Antidote:** No specific recommendations.
- **Dialysis:** No data are available on removal of reteplase by hemodialysis, high-permeability hemodialysis, or peritoneal dialysis.

ribavirin

See Antivirals (p. 937)

rifabutin

rif-a-byoo'-tin

Classes

Chemical: rifamycin S derivative
Therapeutic: antibiotic

Pregnancy Category: B

Trade Names

Prescription: Mycobutin

Do not confuse rifabutin with rifampin.

CLINICAL PHARMACOLOGY

Mechanism of Action

An antitubercular that inhibits DNA-dependent RNA polymerase, an enzyme in susceptible strains of *Escherichia coli* and *Bacillus subtilis*. Rifabutin has a broad spectrum of antimicrobial activity, including against mycobacteria such as *Mycobacterium avium* complex (MAC). **Therapeutic Effect:** Prevents MAC disease.

PHARMACOKINETICS

Readily absorbed from the GI tract (high-fat meals delay absorption). Protein binding: 85%. Widely distributed. Crosses the blood-brain barrier. Extensive intracellular tissue uptake. Metabolized in the liver to active metabolite. Excreted in urine; eliminated in feces. **Half-life:** 16-69 hr.

AVAILABILITY

Capsules: 150 mg.

INDICATIONS AND DOSAGE

Prevention of MAC disease (first episode)

PO

Adults, Elderly: 300 mg as a single dose or in 2 divided doses if GI upset occurs.

Prevention of recurrent MAC disease

PO

Adults, Elderly: 300 mg/day (in combination)

Dosage in renal impairment

Dosage is modified based on creatinine clearance. If creatinine clearance is less than 30 mL/min, reduce dosage by 50%.

OFF-LABEL USES

Part of multidrug regimen for treatment of MAC

CONTRAINDICATIONS

Active tuberculosis; hypersensitivity to other rifamycins, including rifampin, coadministration of voriconazole

INTERACTIONS

Drug: Clarithromycin, delavirdine, fosamprenavir, fluconazole, indinivir, lopinavir, nelfinavir, neotrapine, ritonavir, tipranavir: May increase rifabutin toxicity. **Oral contraceptives:** May decrease contraceptive effectiveness. **Zidovudine:** May decrease blood concentration of zidovudine, but does not affect the drug's inhibition of HIV. **Dapsone, delavirdine, clarithromycin, itraconazole, saquinavir, sirolimus, trimatrexate, warfarin:** Rifabutin may decrease effectiveness of these drugs. **Clarithromycin, imatinib:** Rifabutin may lower plasma levels of these drugs. **Efavirenz:** May decrease rifabutin concentration and efficacy. **Sulfamethoxazole:** Rifabutin may increase sulfamethoxazole concentration. **Herbal:** None known. **Food:** None known.

DIAGNOSTIC TEST EFFECTS

May increase serum alkaline phosphatase, AST (SGOT), and ALT (SGPT) levels.

SIDE-EFFECTS

Frequent (30%): Red-orange or red-brown discoloration of urine, feces, saliva, skin, sputum, sweat, or tears. **Occasional (11%-3%):** Rash, nausea, abdominal pain, diarrhea, dyspepsia, belching, headache, altered taste, uveitis, corneal deposits. **Rare (less than 2%):** Anorexia, flatulence, fever, myalgia, vomiting, insomnia

R

CRITICAL CARE CONSIDERATIONS

ADMINISTRATION/HANDLING

PO ALERT

- Give rifabutin with food only if GI irritation occurs. Administration on an empty stomach is preferred. Mix the drug with applesauce if patients cannot swallow capsules whole.

PRECAUTIONS

HEALTH-RELATED

- Use rifabutin cautiously in patients with hepatic or renal impairment.

AGE-RELATED

- **Children:** Safety and efficacy of rifabutin have not been established in children.
- **Elderly:** No age-related precautions have been noted.

PREGNANCY/LACTATION-RELATED

- Pregnancy category B; unknown if excreted in breast milk.

MONITORING

- **Baseline assessment:** Assess for symptoms of infection.
- **Baseline and ongoing lab work:** CBC with WBC differential, biochemical profile including liver (AST [SGOT], ALT [SGPT], bilirubin, alkaline phosphatase) function tests; blood or sputum cultures.
- **Baseline diagnostic tests:** Patients should undergo a biopsy of suspicious nodes if present, and a chest x-ray to rule out active tuberculosis. Tuberculosis is common in HIV-positive patients and may present with atypical or extrapulmonary findings.
- **Bleeding precautions:** Avoid giving IM injections, taking rectal temperature, and any other traumatic procedures that may induce bleeding.
- **Side effects:** Check body temperature and notify the physician of flulike symptoms, GI intolerance, or rash.
- **Patient education:** Inform that urine, feces, perspiration, saliva, skin, sputum, and tears may become reddish brown or reddish orange during drug therapy and that soft contact lenses may become permanently discolored. Caution female patients who use oral contraceptives that rifabutin may decrease their effectiveness. Teach alternative methods of contraception. Advise to avoid crowds and those with known infection. Instruct to report promptly dark urine, flulike symptoms, nausea or vomiting, unusual bleeding or bruising, or any visual disturbances to a health care provider.

SERIOUS ADVERSE REACTIONS

- Hepatitis occurs rarely.

OVERDOSE/TOXICITY

- **Hematologic:** Anemia, thrombocytopenia, and neutropenia may occur.
- **GI decontamination:** No specific recommendations.

ANTIDOTE/DIALYSIS

- **Antidote:** No specific recommendations.
- **Dialysis:** Rifabutin is unlikely to be removed by hemodialysis or peritoneal dialysis. No data are available on removal by high-permeability hemodialysis.

R

rifampin

rif-am'-pin

Classes

Chemical: rifamycin B derivative
Therapeutic: antituberculosis agent

Pregnancy Category: C

Trade Names

Prescription: Rifadin, Rifadin IV, Rimactane

Do not confuse rifampin with rifabutin, Rifamate, rifapentine, or Ritalin.

CLINICAL PHARMACOLOGY

Mechanism of Action

An antitubercular that interferes with bacterial RNA synthesis by binding to DNA-dependent RNA polymerase, thus preventing its attachment to DNA and blocking RNA transcription. **Therapeutic Effect:** Bactericidal in susceptible microorganisms.

PHARMACOKINETICS

Well absorbed from the GI tract (food delays absorption). Protein binding: 80%. Widely distributed. Metabolized in the liver to active metabolite. Primarily eliminated by the biliary system. Not removed by hemodialysis. **Half-life:** 3-5 hr (increased in hepatic impairment), 1.8-11 hr (end-stage renal disease).

AVAILABILITY

Capsules: 150 mg (Rifadin), 300 mg (Rifadin, Rimactane).

Injection, powder for reconstitution (Rifadin IV): 600 mg.

INDICATIONS AND DOSAGE

Tuberculosis

PO, IV

Adults, Elderly: 10 mg/kg/day. Maximum: 600 mg/day. **Children:** 10-20 mg/kg/day in divided doses every 12-24 hr.

Prevention of meningococcal infections

PO, IV

Adults, Elderly: 600 mg every 12 hr for 2 days. **Children 1 mo and older:** 20 mg/kg/day in divided doses every 12-24 hr. Maximum: 600 mg/dose. **Infants younger than 1 mo:** 10 mg/kg/day in divided doses every 12 hr for 2 days.

Staphylococcal infections

PO, IV

Adults, Elderly: 600 mg once per day. **Children:** 15 mg/kg/day in divided doses every 12 hr for 5-10 days.

Staphylococcus aureus infections (in combination with other antiinfectives)

PO

Adults, Elderly: 300-600 mg twice per day. **Neonates:** 5-20 mg/kg/day in divided doses every 12 hr.

Prevention of *Haemophilus influenzae* infection

PO

Adults, Elderly: 600 mg/day for 4 days. **Children 1 mo and older:** 20 mg/kg/day (one dose) for 4 days. **Children younger than 1 mo:** 10 mg/kg/day (one dose) for 4 days.

OFF-LABEL USES

Prophylaxis of *H. influenzae* type B infection; treatment of atypical mycobacterial infection and serious infections caused by *Staphylococcus* species

CONTRAINDICATIONS

Concomitant therapy with amprenavir, hypersensitivity to rifampin or other rifamycins

INTERACTIONS

Drug: Alcohol, hepatotoxic medications, ritonavir, saquinavir: May increase the risk of hepatotoxicity. **Aminophylline, theophylline:** May increase clearance of these drugs. **Chloramphenicol, digoxin, disopyramide, fluconazole, methadone, mexiletine, oral anticoagulants, oral antidiabetics, phenytoin, quinidine, tocainide, verapamil:** May decrease the effects of these drugs. **Oral contraceptives:** May decrease oral contraceptive effectiveness. **Herbal:** None known. **Food:** None known.

DIAGNOSTIC TEST EFFECTS

May increase serum alkaline phosphatase, bilirubin, uric acid, AST (SGOT), and ALT (SGPT) levels.

IV INCOMPATIBILITIES

Diltiazem (Cardizem)

SIDE-EFFECTS

Expected: Red-orange or red-brown discoloration of urine, feces, saliva, skin, sputum, sweat, or tears. **Occasional (5%-2%):** Hypersensitivity reaction (such as flushing, pruritus, or rash). **Rare (less than 2%):** Diarrhea, dyspepsia, nausea, candida as evidenced by sore mouth or tongue

CRITICAL CARE CONSIDERATIONS

ADMINISTRATION/HANDLING

PO ALERT

- **Combination therapy:** A three-drug regimen to control tuberculosis including rifampin, isoniazid (INH), and pyrazinamide is recommended for initial management; either streptomycin or ethambutol is also recommended unless probability of INH resistance is low.
- If possible, give rifampin with 8 oz of water 1 hr before or 2 hr after a meal. Rifampin may be given with food to decrease GI upset, but this will delay its absorption. Mix the capsule contents with applesauce or jelly if patients cannot swallow capsules whole.
- Give rifampin at least 1 hr before administering antacids, especially antacids containing aluminum.

IV ALERT

- Administer rifampin by IV infusion only. Avoid IM and subcutaneous administration.
- **Stability:** Reconstituted vial is stable for 24 hr. Once the reconstituted vial is further diluted, it is stable for 4 hr in D_5W or 24 hr in 0.9% NaCl.
- **Reconstitution/further dilution:** Reconstitute each 600-mg vial with 10 mL of sterile water for injection to provide a concentration of 60 mg/mL. Withdraw the desired dose and further dilute with 500 mL of D_5W.
- **Infusion:** Infuse the solution over 3 hr (or over 30 min if diluted with 100 mL of D_5W).

R

PRECAUTIONS

HEALTH-RELATED

- Use rifampin cautiously in patients with active alcoholism, a history of alcohol abuse, or hepatic dysfunction.
- **Cytochrome P450 enzyme induction:** Rifampin induces certain cytochrome enzymes that will increase metabolism of other medications metabolized by these enzymes, which creates numerous drug interactions.
- **Coumadin:** Rifampin also increases the requirement of coumadin anticoagulants.

AGE-RELATED

- **Children:** No age-related precautions have been noted in children.
- **Elderly:** Risk of hepatitis is increased in patients over 50 yr. Symptomatic hepatitis or fulminant liver failure are seen almost exclusively in elderly.

PREGNANCY/LACTATION-RELATED

- Pregnancy category C; compatible with breast-feeding; distributed in breast milk.

MONITORING

- **Baseline assessment:** Determine hypersensitivity to rifampin or other rifamycins before beginning drug therapy.
- **Baseline and ongoing lab work:** CBC with WBC differential and platelet count; biochemical profile including liver (AST [SGOT], ALT [SGPT], bilirubin, GGT, alkaline phosphatase) function tests; collect specimens for culture and sensitivity tests before beginning drug therapy; initial and daily prothrombin time and international normalized ratio on patients taking coumadin. There are no commercially available tests to detect rifampin-dependent antibodies.
- **Extravasation:** Assess IV site at least hourly during the infusion for local inflammation and irritation. At the first sign of extravasation, restart the IV line at another site.
- **Hepatitis:** Monitor liver function test results and assess for hepatitis symptoms including anorexia, fatigue, nausea and vomiting, jaundice and weakness; if present, withhold rifampin.
- **Hypersensitivity reactions:** Assess for flulike symptoms and skin eruptions.
- **Colitis:** Severe diarrhea with abdominal pain, blood or mucus in stools, and fever may indicate antibiotic-associated colitis.
- **Bleeding:** Monitor for bleeding, ecchymosis, infection (manifested as a fever or sore throat), and unusual fatigue and weakness.
- **Patient education:** Instruct to take rifampin with 8 oz of water 1 hr before or 2 hr after a meal. If GI upset occurs, instruct to take rifampin with food. Encourage to avoid alcohol while taking this drug. Instruct not to take any other medications, including antacids, while taking rifampin without first consulting with a health care provider. Advise taking rifampin at least 1 hr before taking an antacid. Inform that urine, feces, sputum, sweat, and tears may become reddish orange or reddish brown during therapy and that soft contact lenses may become permanently stained. Skin may be washed clean of the discoloration. Instruct to report fatigue, fever, flulike symptoms, nausea, vomiting, unusual bleeding or bruising, weakness, yellow eyes and skin, or any other new symptoms. Caution female patients taking oral contraceptives to check with the physician because rifampin may decrease the effectiveness of oral contraceptives; teach such patients alternative methods of contraception.

SERIOUS ADVERSE REACTIONS

- **Stevens–Johnson syndrome:** Severe anaphylactoid reaction is rare.
- **Colitis:** Antibiotic-associated colitis, pseudomembranous colitis, or *Clostridium difficile* colitis, and other superinfections may result from altered bacterial balance.
- **Cerebral hemorrhage:** Has occurred when drug treatment is continued or resumed in thrombocytopenic patients with purpura.
- **Hyperglycemia:** Diabetes may become more difficult to control.

OVERDOSE/TOXICITY

- **Hepatotoxicity:** Hepatitis, hepatic encephalopathy, jaundice, and death have occurred when rifampin has been given with other hepatotoxic agents including isoniazid, alcohol, or halothane. One of the hepatotoxic agents should be discontinued if liver dysfunction ensues. Brownish red discoloration of urine, sweat, feces, tears, and saliva are directly related to the amount of the overdose.
- **Nephrotoxicity:** Acute renal failure, which may rapidly progress to glomerulonephritis, acute interstitial nephritis, and light chain proteinuria.
- **Lupuslike syndrome:** Seen when rifampin is used with clarithromycin or ciprofloxacin; may be autoantibody mediated.

- **Blood dyscrasias:** Hemolytic anemia, thrombocytopenia, ecchymosis, purpura; may be antibody mediated.
- **Fatal overdose:** Dysrhythmias, hypotension, seizures, and cardiac arrest.
- **GI decontamination:** No specific recommendations.

ANTIDOTE/DIALYSIS

- **Antidote:** No specific antidote. Forced diuresis facilitates excretion.
- **Dialysis:** Rifampin is not removed by hemodialysis, high-permeability hemodialysis, or peritoneal dialysis.

rifapentine

rif-a-pen'-teen

Classes

Chemical: rifamycin B derivative
Therapeutic: antituberculosis agent

Pregnancy Category: C

Trade Names

Prescription: Priftin

Do not confuse rifapentine with rifampin.

CLINICAL PHARMACOLOGY

Mechanism of Action

An antitubercular that inhibits bacterial RNA synthesis by binding to DNA-dependent RNA polymerase in *Mycobacterium tuberculosis*. This action prevents the enzyme from attaching to DNA, thereby blocking RNA transcription. **Therapeutic Effect:** Bactericidal.

PHARMACOKINETICS

Rapidly and well absorbed from the GI tract. Protein binding: 97.7%. Metabolized in liver. Primarily eliminated in feces; partial excretion in urine. Unlikely to be removed by hemodialysis. **Half-life:** 14-17 hr.

AVAILABILITY

Tablets: 150 mg.

INDICATIONS AND DOSAGE

Tuberculosis

PO

Adults, Elderly: Intensive phase: 600 mg twice weekly for 2 mo (interval between doses no less than 3 days). Continuation phase: 600 mg weekly for 4 mo.

CONTRAINDICATIONS

History of hypersensitivity to rifapentine or any rifamycins (e.g., rifampin and rifabutin)

INTERACTIONS

Drug: Alcohol: May increase the risk of hepatotoxicity. **Indinavir:** May decrease its effect. **Oral contraceptives, warfarin:** May decrease the effects of these drugs.
Herbal: None known. **Food:** None known.

DIAGNOSTIC TEST EFFECTS

May increase serum AST (SGOT), ALT (SPGT), and bilirubin levels.

SIDE-EFFECTS

Rare (less than 4%): Red-orange or red-brown discoloration of urine, feces, saliva, skin, sputum, sweat, or tears; arthralgia, pain, nausea, vomiting, headache, dyspepsia, hypertension, dizziness, diarrhea

CRITICAL CARE CONSIDERATIONS

ADMINISTRATION/HANDLING

PO ALERT

- **Combination therapy:** Rifapentine is used only in combination with another antitubercular.
- **Storage:** Store at controlled room temperature. Avoid extreme heat and humidity.

PRECAUTIONS

HEALTH-RELATED

- Use rifapentine cautiously in alcoholic patients and patients with hepatic impairment. Drug should not be used in patients with porphyria.
- Rifapentine produces a red-orange discoloration of all secretions, excretions, sweat, tears, teeth, and skin.
- **Cytochrome P450 metabolism:** Rifapentine is a stronger inducer of CYP3A4 and CYP2C8/9, which creates the potential for multiple drug interactions. Rifapentine administration increases the metabolism of other drugs metabolized by these enzyme pathways within 4 days of first dose; effect stops within 14 days following the last dose.

AGE-RELATED

- **Children:** Safety and efficacy of rifapentine in children under 12 yr have not been established.
- **Elderly:** Age-related organ impairment may prompt a dosage reduction.

PREGNANCY/LACTATION-RELATED

- Pregnancy category C (teratogenic in rats); excreted in breast milk but compatible with breast-feeding.

MONITORING

- **Baseline assessment:** Assess exposure pattern to pulmonary tuberculosis and whether other treatment has been provided; assess for liver disease; evaluate for patient compliance with initial intensive phase of therapy with rifapentine, especially if liver disease is present. If compliance is not possible, other medication may be more effective.
- **Baseline and ongoing lab work:** CBC with WBC differential; biochemical profile including liver (AST [SGOT], ALT [SGPT], bilirubin, alkaline phosphatase) function tests. Monitor hepatic enzyme levels every 2-4 wk throughout therapy.
- **GI effects:** Evaluate for diarrhea, GI upset, nausea, or vomiting.
- **Patient education:** Emphasize that all doses of rifapentine and other antituberculosis medications must be taken to avoid relapse. Inform that urine, feces, sputum, skin, teeth, sweat, and tears may become red-orange or red-brown during therapy and that soft contact lenses may become permanently stained. Instruct to report promptly dark urine, decreased appetite, fever, nausea or vomiting, or pain or swelling of the joints to a health care provider. Caution if taking oral contraceptives, to check with the prescriber because rifapentine may decrease the effectiveness of oral contraceptives; inform about alternative methods of contraception.

SERIOUS ADVERSE REACTIONS

- **Lab:** Hyperuricemia, hyperbilirubinemia, hyperkalemia, LDH, and alkaline phosphatase increase.
- **Skin:** Urticaria, rash, skin, and dental discoloration.
- **Renal:** Proteinuria, hematuria.
- **Gastrointestinal:** Constipation, esophagitis, gastritis, pancreatitis.

OVERDOSE/TOXICITY

- **Hepatotoxicity:** Elevated liver enzymes, decreased appetite, fever, right upper quadrant pain, nausea, vomiting, edema, abdominal distention, jaundice, hepatitis, hepatic encephalopathy.
- **Hematologic:** Neutropenia, thrombocytopenia, leukocytosis, purpura.
- **Management:** Rifapentine should be stopped and supportive care provided.
- **GI decontamination:** No specific recommendations.

ANTIDOTE/DIALYSIS

- **Antidote:** No specific recommendations.
- **Dialysis:** Rifapentine is unlikely to be removed by hemodialysis or peritoneal dialysis. No data are available on removal by high-permeability hemodialysis.

riluzole

ril'-yoo-zole

Classes

Chemical: benzothiazolamine derivative
Therapeutic: amyotrophic lateral sclerosis agent

Pregnancy Category: C

Trade Names

Prescription: Rilutek

CLINICAL PHARMACOLOGY

Mechanism of Action

An amyotrophic lateral sclerosis (ALS) agent that inhibits presynaptic glutamate release in the CNS and interferes postsynaptically with the effects of excitatory amino acids. **Therapeutic Effect:** Extends survival of ALS patients.

PHARMACOKINETICS

Well absorbed following PO administration. High-fat meals decrease absorption. Protein binding: 96%. Extensively metabolized in liver. Excreted in urine. **Half-life:** 12 hr.

AVAILABILITY

Tablets: 50 mg.

INDICATIONS AND DOSAGE

ALS

PO

Adults, Elderly: 50 mg every 12 hr.

CONTRAINDICATIONS

Hypersensitivity to riluzole

INTERACTIONS

Drug: Alcohol: May increase CNS depression. **Amiodarone, amitriptyline, quinolones, theophylline:** May increase the effects and risk of toxicity of riluzole. **Carbamazepine, fluvoxamine, omeprazole, rifampin:** May decrease the effects of riluzole. **Herbal:** None known. **Food: Caffeine:** May increase the effects and risk of toxicity of riluzole. **High-fat meals:** May decrease the absorption and effects of riluzole.

DIAGNOSTIC TEST EFFECTS

May increase liver function test results.

R

SIDE-EFFECTS

Frequent (greater than 10%): Nausea (12%-21%), reduced respiratory function (10%-16%), weakness (15%-20%). **Occasional (less than 10%):** Edema, tachycardia, headache, dizziness, somnolence, depression, vertigo, tremor, pruritus, alopecia, abdominal pain, diarrhea, anorexia, dyspepsia, vomiting, stomatitis, increased cough

CRITICAL CARE CONSIDERATIONS

ADMINISTRATION/HANDLING

PO ALERT

- Administer riluzole at least 1 hr before or 2 hr after a meal.
- Riluzole is a substrate of CYP4501A2.

PRECAUTIONS

HEALTH-RELATED

- Use riluzole cautiously in patients with renal or hepatic impairment.

AGE-RELATED

- **Children:** Safety and efficacy of riluzole have not been established in children.
- **Elderly:** Age-related organ impairment may prompt a dosage reduction.

PREGNANCY/LACTATION-RELATED

- Pregnancy category C; excretion into breast milk unknown; use caution in nursing mothers.

MONITORING

- **Baseline assessment:** Evaluate history of amyotrophic lateral sclerosis (ALS or Lou Gehrig's disease), including prior treatments. Evaluate for liver disease. Take vital signs, including temperature.
- **Baseline and ongoing lab work:** Biochemical profile including liver (AST [SGOT], ALT [SGPT], GGT, bilirubin, alkaline phosphatase) function tests; CBC including WBC differential. Discontinue riluzole if the ALT level exceeds 10 times the upper normal limit. All patients receiving the drug will have liver enzyme elevation.
- **Therapeutic effect:** Helps abate progression of weakness and need for tracheostomy.
- **Patient education:** Instruct to take riluzole at least 1 hr before or 2 hr after a meal and at the same times each day. Inform that riluzole may cause drowsiness, dizziness, or vertigo. Warn to avoid tasks requiring mental alertness or motor skills until response to the drug is known. Urge avoidance of alcohol during therapy. Instruct to report fever promptly to a health care provider, because it may prompt a repeat CBC to evaluate for neutropenia.

SERIOUS ADVERSE REACTIONS

- **Hepatitis:** All patients have liver enzyme elevation, but condition must be monitored to ensure that patients are not experiencing extensive liver damage.

OVERDOSE/TOXICITY

- **Hepatotoxicity:** Elevated liver enzymes, decreased appetite, fever, right upper quadrant pain, nausea, vomiting, edema, abdominal distention, jaundice, hepatitis, hepatic encephalopathy.
- **Hematologic:** Neutropenia associated with fever.
- **Management:** Riluzole should be stopped and supportive care provided.
- **GI decontamination:** No specific recommendations.

ANTIDOTE/DIALYSIS

- **Antidote:** No specific recommendations.
- **Dialysis:** Riluzole is unlikely to be removed by hemodialysis, high-permeability hemodialysis, or peritoneal dialysis.

rimantadine hydrochloride

See Antivirals (p. 937)

R

risperidone

ris-per'-i-done

Classes

Chemical: benzisoxazole derivative

Therapeutic: antipsychotic

Pregnancy Category: C

Trade Names

Prescription: Risperdal, Risperdal Consta, Risperdol M-Tabs

Do not confuse risperidone with reserpine.

CLINICAL PHARMACOLOGY

Mechanism of Action

A benzisoxazole derivative that may antagonize dopamine and serotonin receptors.

Therapeutic Effect: Suppresses psychotic behavior.

PHARMACOKINETICS

Well absorbed from the GI tract; unaffected by food. Protein binding: 90%. Extensively metabolized in the liver to active metabolite. Primarily excreted in urine. **Half-life:** 3-20 hr; metabolite: 21-30 hr (increased in elderly).

AVAILABILITY

Oral solution (Risperdal): 1 mg/mL.
Tablets (Risperdal): 0.25 mg, 0.5 mg, 1 mg, 2 mg, 3 mg, 4 mg.
Tablets (orally disintegrating [Risperdal M-Tabs]): 0.5 mg, 1 mg, 2 mg.
Injection (Risperdal Consta): 25 mg, 37.5 mg, 50 mg.

INDICATIONS AND DOSAGE

Schizophrenia

PO

Adults: 0.5-1 mg twice per day. May increase dosage by 2 mg/day to target dose of 6 mg/day. Range: 4-8 mg/day. **Elderly:** Initially, 0.5 mg twice per day. May increase dosage in increments of no more than 0.5 mg twice daily. Range: 2-6 mg/day.

IM

Adults, Elderly: 25 mg every 2 wk. Adjust dose every 4 wk. Maximum: 50 mg every 2 wk.

Mania

PO

Adults, Elderly: Initially, 2-3 mg as a single daily dose. May increase at 24-hr intervals of 1 mg/day. Range: 1-6 mg/day.

Dosage in renal impairment

Initial dosage for adults and elderly patients is 0.5 mg twice per day. Dosage is titrated slowly to desired effect.

OFF-LABEL USES

Autism in children, behavioral symptoms associated with dementia, Tourette's disorder

CONTRAINDICATIONS

Hypersensitivity to risperidone

INTERACTIONS

Drug: Alcohol, other CNS depressants: May increase CNS depression. **Carbamazepine:** May decrease the risperidone blood concentration. **Clozapine:** May increase the risperidone blood concentration. **Dopamine agonists, levodopa:** May decrease the effects of these drugs. **Paroxetine:** May increase the risperidone blood concentration and the risk of extrapyramidal symptoms.
Herbal: None known. **Food:** None known.

DIAGNOSTIC TEST EFFECTS

May increase serum prolactin, creatinine, alkaline phosphatase, uric acid, AST (SGOT), ALT (SGPT), and triglyceride levels. May increase blood glucose, decrease serum potassium, protein, and sodium levels. May cause ECG changes.

SIDE-EFFECTS

Frequent (26%-13%): Agitation, anxiety, insomnia, headache, constipation. **Occasional (10%-4%):** Dyspepsia, rhinitis, somnolence, dizziness, nausea, vomiting, rash, abdominal pain, dry skin, tachycardia. **Rare (3%-2%):** Visual disturbances, fever, back pain, pharyngitis, cough, arthralgia, angina, aggressive behavior, orthostatic hypotension, breast swelling

CRITICAL CARE CONSIDERATIONS

ADMINISTRATION/HANDLING

PO ALERT

- Give risperidone without regard to food. Mix the oral solution with water, orange juice, coffee, or low-fat milk, but not with cola (Coke, Pepsi) or tea.

IM ALERT

- **Reconstitution of suspension:** Use only the diluent and needle supplied in the dose pack; all the components in the dose pack for administration are needed. Do not substitute any components. Prepare suspension according to manufacturer's directions. If 2 min pass before the injection, reconstitute the solution by shaking the upright vial vigorously back and forth for as long as it takes to resuspend the microspheres.
- **Stability:** Risperidone may be given up to 6 hr after reconstitution, but immediate administration is recommended.
- **Storage:** Store the drug below 77°F (25°C) once reconstituted.
- **Administration:** Inject the drug IM into the upper outer quadrant of the gluteus maximus. Do not administer the drug by the IV route.

PRECAUTIONS

HEALTH-RELATED

- Use risperidone cautiously in suicidal patients; patients with cardiac disease,

R

breast cancer, hepatic or renal impairment, seizure disorders, or recent MI and in those at risk for aspiration pneumonia.
- Use risperidone cautiously in patients with dementia because the drug may increase the risk of stroke in these patients.
- Risperidone use may increase the risk of hyperglycemia.

AGE-RELATED

- **Children:** Safety and efficacy of risperidone have not been established in children.
- **Elderly:** Are more susceptible to orthostatic hypotension. Elderly may require a dosage adjustment because of age-related renal or hepatic impairment.

PREGNANCY/LACTATION-RELATED

- Pregnancy category C; excreted in breast milk.

MONITORING

- **Baseline assessment:** Assess appearance, behavior, emotional status, response to environment, speech pattern, and thought content. Note vital signs, results of 12-lead ECG, and weight.
- **Baseline lab work:** Biochemical profile including renal (BUN, creatinine) and liver (AST [SGOT], ALT [SGPT], GGT, alkaline phosphatase, bilirubin) function tests.
- **Baseline diagnostic tests:** 12-lead ECG to evaluate for dysrhythmias and myocardial ischemia.
- **Tardive dyskinesia:** Observe for fine tongue movement, which may be the first sign of irreversible tardive dyskinesia.
- **ECG monitoring:** Observe for sinus tachycardia; prolongation of the PR, QRS, and QT intervals; ST depression; T wave and U wave notching or inversion; heart block; may lead to torsades de pointes secondary to prolonged QT syndrome.
- **BP changes:** Monitor for hypertension or hypotension, which may indicate the onset of an adverse drug reaction.
- **Neurologic changes:** Observe for involuntary movements, tremors, drowsiness, restlessness, agitation, confusion, fatigue, visual disturbances, sweating, excessive salivation.
- **Suicidal patients:** Closely supervise during early therapy. As depression lessens, energy level improves, which increases the suicide potential.
- **Therapeutic response:** Assess for increased interest in surroundings and ability to concentrate, improvement in self-care, and relaxed facial expression.
- **Abrupt withdrawal:** Do not discontinue risperidone abruptly to avoid recurrence of psychotic symptoms.
- **Anticholinergic effects:** Monitor for urinary retention, constipation, and dry mouth.
- **Neuroleptic malignant syndrome:** Monitor for altered mental status, fever, irregular BP or pulse, and muscle rigidity.
- **Patient education:** Inform that risperidone may cause dizziness or drowsiness. Warn to avoid tasks that require mental alertness or motor skills until response to the drug is known. Instruct to promptly report altered gait, difficulty breathing, palpitations, pain or swelling in breasts, severe dizziness or fainting, trembling fingers, unusual movements, rash, or visual changes to a health care provider. Teach how to change positions slowly to minimize the hypotensive effects. Urge avoidance of alcohol during risperidone therapy.

SERIOUS ADVERSE REACTIONS

- **Seizures:** Occur infrequently.
- **Neurologic:** Extrapyramidal symptoms, akathisia, tardive dyskinesia, and neuroleptic malignant syndrome occur rarely.
- **Tardive dyskinesia:** Tongue protrusion, puffing of the cheeks, and chewing or puckering of the mouth.
- **Ventricular dysrhythmias:** Prolonged QT syndrome resulting in torsades de pointes. Manage according to Advanced Cardiac Life Support (ACLS) guidelines, include magnesium infusion and drugs to increase conduction velocity (epinephrine, possibly isoproterenol if QT interval is severely prolonged). Defibrillate as needed.

OVERDOSE/TOXICITY

- **Symptoms:** CNS depression (sedation, coma, and delirium), hypersalivation, seizures, agranulocytosis, respiratory depression, respiratory arrest, fatal myocarditis, dysrhythmias, orthostatic hypotension, cardiac arrest.
- **Neuroleptic malignant syndrome (NMS):** Hyperpyrexia, muscle rigidity, change in mental status, irregular pulse or BP, tachycardia, diaphoresis, cardiac dysrhythmias, rhabdomyolysis, and acute renal failure.
- **NMS management:** Discontinue risperidone immediately, aggressive management of BP, heart rate, and dysrhythmias according to accepted ACLS guidelines; manage other associated medical problems per accepted guidelines. When reintroducing

risperidone, monitor carefully to avoid recurrent NMS.

- **GI decontamination:** No specific recommendations.

ANTIDOTE/DIALYSIS

- **Antidote:** No specific antidote. Physostigmine has been used for overdose for other neuroleptic agents.
- **Dialysis:** No data are available on removal of risperidone by hemodialysis, high-permeability hemodialysis, or peritoneal dialysis.

ritonavir

See HIV Medications (p. 961)

rivastigmine tartrate

riv-a-stig'-meen tar'-trate

Classes

Chemical: carbamate derivative, cholinesterase inhibitor
Therapeutic: acetylcholinesterase inhibitor

Pregnancy Category: B

Trade Names

Prescription: Exelon

CLINICAL PHARMACOLOGY

Mechanism of Action

A cholinesterase inhibitor that inhibits the enzyme acetylcholinesterase, thus increasing the concentration of acetylcholine at cholinergic synapses and enhancing cholinergic function in the CNS. **Therapeutic Effect:** Slows the progression of symptoms of Alzheimer's disease.

PHARMACOKINETICS

Rapidly and completely absorbed. Protein binding: 40%. Widely distributed throughout the body. Rapidly and extensively metabolized. Primarily excreted in urine. **Half-life:** 1.5 hr.

AVAILABILITY

Capsules: 1.5 mg, 3 mg, 4.5 mg, 6 mg.
Oral solution: 2 mg/mL.

INDICATIONS AND DOSAGE

Alzheimer's disease

PO

Adults, Elderly: Initially 1.5 mg twice per day. May increase at intervals of least 2 wk to 3 mg twice per day, then 4.5 mg twice per day, and finally 6 mg twice per day. Maximum: 6 mg twice per day.

CONTRAINDICATIONS

Hypersensitivity to rivastigmine or other carbamate derivatives

INTERACTIONS

Drug: Anticholinergics: May decrease the effects of rivastigmine or anticholinergics. **Beta-adrenergic blockers:** May increase incidence of bradycardia. **Bethanecol:** May increase the effects of rivastigmine or bethanecol. **Calcium channel blockers:** May increase incidence of bradycardia. **Digoxin:** May increase incidence of bradycardia. **Herbal:** None known. **Food:** None known.

DIAGNOSTIC TEST EFFECTS

None known.

SIDE-EFFECTS

Frequent (47%-17%): Nausea, vomiting, dizziness, diarrhea, headache, anorexia. **Occasional (13%-6%):** Abdominal pain, insomnia, dyspepsia (heartburn, indigestion, epigastric pain), confusion, urinary tract infection, depression. **Rare (5%-3%):** Anxiety, somnolence, constipation, malaise, hallucinations, tremor, flatulence, rhinitis, hypertension, flulike symptoms, weight loss, syncope

CRITICAL CARE CONSIDERATIONS

ADMINISTRATION/HANDLING

PO ALERT

- Give rivastigmine with morning and evening meals.
- When administering the oral solution, withdraw the prescribed amount of rivastigmine from the container, using the oral syringe provided by the manufacturer. Drug may be slowly placed in the mouth directly from the syringe or mixed in a small glass of water, cold fruit juice, or soda. Use the solution within 4 hr of mixing.

PRECAUTIONS

HEALTH-RELATED

- Use rivastigmine cautiously in patients with asthma, bradycardia, chronic obstructive pulmonary disease (COPD), peptic ulcer disease, history of seizures, sick sinus syndrome, or urinary obstruction.

R

- Use rivastigmine cautiously in patients taking NSAIDs concurrently.

AGE-RELATED

- **Children:** Safety and efficacy of rivastigmine have not been established in children.
- **Elderly:** Age-related renal impairment may prompt a dosage adjustment.

PREGNANCY/LACTATION-RELATED

- Pregnancy category B; excretion into human breast milk unknown.

MONITORING

- **Baseline assessment:** Obtain baseline vital signs. Determine history of asthma, COPD, peptic ulcer disease, or renal insufficiency, urinary obstruction. Assess behavioral, cognitive, and functional deficits.
- **Baseline lab work:** Biochemical profile including renal (BUN, creatinine) function studies.
- **Cholinergic reaction:** Monitor for diaphoresis, dizziness, excessive salivation, facial warmth, abdominal cramps or discomfort, lacrimation, pallor, and urinary urgency.
- **GI effects:** Monitor for diarrhea, nausea, vomiting, heartburn; note coffee-ground materials in secretions, or frank bleeding.
- **Neurologic effects:** Monitor for headache, seizures, and insomnia.
- **Cardiac:** Continuous ECG monitoring in critically ill patients may reveal bradycardia, as drug increases vagal tone.
- **Patient education:** Instruct to take rivastigmine with morning and evening meals. Teach to swallow capsules whole, not to break, chew, or crush. For oral solution, explain the prescribed amount of drug should be withdrawn into the syringe and sipped directly from the syringe or mixed with a small glass of water, cold fruit juice, or soda. Instruct to promptly report diarrhea, excessive sweating or salivation, dizziness, nausea and vomiting, or severe abdominal pain to a health care provider. Inform patients and families that rivastigmine is not a cure for Alzheimer's disease but may slow the progression of its symptoms. Refer families to the local chapter of the Alzheimer's Disease Association for a guide to available services.

SERIOUS ADVERSE REACTIONS

- **Gastrointestinal:** Nausea, vomiting, anorexia and weight loss; increased gastric acid secretions leading to GI bleeding.

OVERDOSE/TOXICITY

- **Cholinergic crisis:** Severe nausea and vomiting, increased salivation, diaphoresis, bradycardia, hypotension, respiratory depression, and seizures.
- **Management:** Maintain patent airway and support ventilation. Manage hypotension with IV fluids and then, vasopressors if needed. Bradycardia is managed with atropine 0.6 mg IV. Seizures are managed with benzodiazepines.
- **GI decontamination:** No specific recommendations.

ANTIDOTE/DIALYSIS

- **Antidote:** No specific recommendations.
- **Dialysis:** No data are available on removal of rivastigmine by hemodialysis, high-permeability hemodialysis, or peritoneal dialysis.

rizatriptan benzoate

See Triptans (p. 984)

ropinirole hydrochloride

ro-pin'-i-role hye-droe-klor'-ide

Classes

Chemical: dipropylaminoethyl indolone derivative

Therapeutic: antiparkinson's agent, dopaminergic

Pregnancy Category: C

Trade Names

Prescription: Requip

CLINICAL PHARMACOLOGY

Mechanism of Action

An antiparkinson's agent that stimulates dopamine receptors in the striatum. **Therapeutic Effect:** Relieves signs and symptoms of Parkinson's disease.

PHARMACOKINETICS

Rapidly absorbed after PO administration. Protein binding: 40%. Extensively distributed throughout the body. Extensively metabolized. Steady-state concentrations achieved within 2 days. Eliminated in urine. Unlikely to be removed by hemodialysis. **Half-life:** 6 hr.

AVAILABILITY

Tablets: 0.25 mg, 0.5 mg, 1 mg, 2 mg, 3 mg, 4 mg, 5 mg.

INDICATIONS AND DOSAGE

Parkinson's disease

PO

Adults, Elderly: Initially, 0.25 mg 3 times per day. May increase dosage by 0.25 mg per dose every 7 days.

Restless leg syndrome

PO

Adults, Elderly: 0.25 mg for days 1 and 2; 0.5 mg for days 3-7; 1 mg for wk 2; 1.5 mg for wk 3; 2 mg for wk 4; 2.5 mg for wk 5; 3 mg for wk 6; 4 mg for wk 7. All doses to be given 1-3 hr before bedtime.

CONTRAINDICATIONS

Hypersensitivity to ropinirole

INTERACTIONS

Drug: Ciprofloxacin: Increases ropinirole blood concentration by 60%. **CNS depressants:** May increase CNS depressant effects. **Estrogens:** Reduce the clearance of ropinirole by 36%. **Levodopa:** Increases the blood concentration of levodopa. **Herbal: Kava kava:** May decrease the effectiveness of ropinirole. **Food: All food:** Delays peak plasma levels by 1 hr but does not affect drug absorption.

DIAGNOSTIC TEST EFFECTS

May increase serum alkaline phosphatase level.

SIDE-EFFECTS

Frequent (60%-40%): Nausea, dizziness, somnolence. **Occasional (12%-5%):** Syncope, vomiting, fatigue, viral infection, dyspepsia, diaphoresis, asthenia, orthostatic hypotension, abdominal discomfort, pharyngitis, abnormal vision, dry mouth, hypertension, hallucinations, confusion. **Rare (less than 4%):** Anorexia, peripheral edema, memory loss, rhinitis, sinusitis, palpitations, impotence

R

CRITICAL CARE CONSIDERATIONS

ADMINISTRATION/HANDLING

PO ALERT

- **Gradually increase dosage schedule:** Wk 1, 0.25 mg 3 times per day to total daily dose of 0.75 mg; wk 2, 0.5 mg 3 times per day to total daily dose of 1.5 mg; wk 3, 0.75 mg 3 times per day to total daily dose of 2.25 mg; wk 4, 1 mg 3 times per day to total daily dose of 3 mg, as prescribed. After wk 4, dosage may be increased every wk if needed by 1.5-3 mg/day to a total dose of 24 mg/day.
- **Discontinue ropinirole gradually by 7-day intervals:** For the first 4 days, decrease the frequency to twice per day (from 3 times per day); for the remaining 3 days, decrease the frequency to once per day before complete withdrawal.

PRECAUTIONS

HEALTH-RELATED

- Use ropinirole cautiously in patients with hallucinations (especially the elderly), syncope, or a history of orthostatic hypotension, and in patients who take CNS depressants concurrently.

AGE-RELATED

- **Children:** Safety and efficacy of ropinirole have not been established in children.
- **Elderly:** No age-related precautions have been noted, but elderly are more likely than other age groups to experience hallucinations.

PREGNANCY/LACTATION-RELATED

- Pregnancy category C; inhibits lactation.

MONITORING

- **Baseline assessment:** Assess for parkinsonian extrapyramidal symptoms.
- **Baseline lab work:** Biochemical profile including renal (BUN, creatinine) and liver (AST [SGOT], ALT [SGPT], GGT, alkaline phosphatase, bilirubin) function tests.
- **Baseline diagnostic tests:** 12-lead ECG to evaluate for dysrhythmias and myocardial ischemia.
- **ECG:** Observe for sinus tachycardia, prolongation of the PR, QRS and QT intervals, ST depression, T wave and U wave notching or inversion, heart block; may lead to torsades de pointes secondary to prolonged QT syndrome.
- **BP changes:** Monitor for hypertension or hypotension, which may indicate the onset of an adverse drug reaction. Assist patients with ambulation if dizziness occurs.
- **Neurologic changes:** Observe for involuntary movements, tremors, drowsiness,

restlessness, agitation, confusion, fatigue, visual disturbances, sweating, excessive salivation.

- **GI side effects:** Monitor for nausea, vomiting, dyspepsia, and abdominal pain.
- **Abrupt withdrawal:** Do not abruptly discontinue ropinirole to avoid exacerbation of parkinsonian symptoms.
- **Therapeutic effect:** Monitor for improvement of masklike facial expression, muscular rigidity, shuffling gait, and resting tremors of the hands and head.
- **Patient education:** Instruct to take ropinirole with food if nausea is a problem. Inform that dizziness, drowsiness, and orthostatic hypotension are common initial responses to the drug. Advise changing positions slowly to help prevent orthostatic hypotension. Warn avoidance of tasks that require mental alertness or motor skills until response to the drug is known. Inform patients (especially elderly) that ropinirole may cause hallucinations and extreme somnolence.

SERIOUS ADVERSE REACTIONS

- **Severe drowsiness:** Falling asleep during activities of daily living increases risk of falls and motor vehicle crashes.
- **Syncope:** May be associated with bradycardia.
- **Symptomatic hypotension:** Postural or orthostatic hypotension.
- **Hallucinations:** May be severe enough to warrant discontinuation of therapy.

OVERDOSE/TOXICITY

- **Symptoms reflecting dopamine receptor overstimulation:** Nausea, vomiting, dizziness, lethargy, sweating, hypotension, agitation, hallucinations, and dyskinesias. Seizures are possible.
- **Management:** If patients experience visual disturbances, headache, and hypertension, discontinue ropinirole to avoid seizures.
- **GI decontamination:** No specific recommendations.

ANTIDOTE/DIALYSIS

- **Antidote:** No specific recommendations.
- **Dialysis:** Ropinirole is unlikely to be removed by hemodialysis or peritoneal dialysis. No data are available on removal by high-permeability hemodialysis.

rosiglitazone maleate 

roz-ih-gli'-ta-zone mal'-ee-ate

Classes

Chemical: thiazolidinedione
Therapeutic: antidiabetic, hypoglycemic, insulin resistance reducer

Pregnancy Category: C

Trade Names

Prescription: Avandia

Combinations

Prescription: with metformin (Avandamet); with glimepiride (Avandaryl)

Do not confuse Avandia with Avalide, Avinza, or Prandin.

CLINICAL PHARMACOLOGY

Mechanism of Action

An antidiabetic that improves target-cell response to insulin without increasing pancreatic insulin secretion. Increases insulin-dependent glucose utilization in skeletal muscle. **Therapeutic Effect:** Lowers blood glucose concentration.

PHARMACOKINETICS

Rapidly absorbed. Protein binding: 99%. Metabolized in the liver. Excreted primarily in urine, with a lesser amount in feces. Not removed by hemodialysis. **Half-life:** 3-4 hr.

AVAILABILITY

Tablets: 2 mg, 4 mg, 8 mg.

INDICATIONS AND DOSAGE

Diabetes mellitus, combination therapy

PO (with sulfonylureas, metformin)

Adults, Elderly: Initially, 4 mg as a single daily dose or in divided doses twice per day. May increase to 8 mg/day after 12 wk of therapy if fasting glucose level is not adequately controlled.

PO (with insulin)

Adults, Elderly: Initially, 4 mg/day in 1 or 2 doses and reduce insulin dose by 10-25%. If hypoglycemia occurs or plasma glucose falls to less than 100 mg/dL, doses of rosiglitazone greater than 4 mg are not recommended.

Diabetes mellitus, monotherapy

Adults, Elderly: Initially, 4 mg as single daily dose or in divided doses twice per day. May increase to 8 mg/day after 12 wk of therapy.

CONTRAINDICATIONS

Active hepatic disease, diabetic ketoacidosis, increased serum transaminase levels, including ALT (SGPT) greater than 2.5 times the normal serum level, type 1 diabetes mellitus, hypersensitivity to rosiglitazone

INTERACTIONS

Drug: **Gemfibrozil:** May increase plasma concentrations of rosiglitazone. **Rifampin:** May decrease effectiveness of rosiglitazone. Herbal: **Bitter melon, eucalyptus, fenugreek, ginseng, guar gum, St. John's wort:** May increase the risk of hypoglycemia. **Glucosamine, licorice:** May reduce the effectiveness of rosiglitazone. Food: None known.

DIAGNOSTIC TEST EFFECTS

May decrease Hct and Hgb and serum alkaline phosphatase, bilirubin, and AST (SGOT) levels. Less than 1% of patients experience ALT (SGPT) values that are 3 times the normal level.

SIDE-EFFECTS

Frequent (9%): Upper respiratory tract infection. Occasional (4%-2%): Headache, edema, back pain, fatigue, sinusitis, diarrhea

CRITICAL CARE CONSIDERATIONS

ADMINISTRATION/HANDLING

PO ALERT

- Give rosiglitazone without regard to meals.

PRECAUTIONS

HEALTH-RELATED

- Use rosiglitazone cautiously in patients with anemia, heart failure, edema, or hepatic impairment.

AGE-RELATED

- **Children:** Safety and efficacy of rosiglitazone have not been established in children.
- **Elderly:** No age-related precautions have been noted.

PREGNANCY/LACTATION-RELATED

- Pregnancy category C. No adequate and well-controlled studies in pregnant women available. Abnormally high glucose levels during pregnancy are associated with higher incidence of congenital anomalies, morbidity, and mortality. Insulin is the monotherapy preferred agent. Drug detected in lactating rats; no information in humans.

MONITORING

- **Baseline assessment:** Assess history of type II diabetes, metabolic syndrome, diet, exercise, and treatments.
- **Baseline and ongoing lab work:** CBC, biochemical profile including blood glucose and liver (AST [SGOT], ALT [SGPT], GGT, alkaline phosphatase, bilirubin) function tests; hemoglobin A_{1c} to assess blood glucose control over the past 2 mo. Liver enzymes should be monitored every 2 mo for 1 yr. Patients with ALT (SGPT) level greater than 2.5 times normal should not receive rosiglitazone.
- **Hypoglycemia:** Assess for anxiety, cool wet skin, diplopia, dizziness, headache, hunger, numbness in mouth, tachycardia, tremors.
- **Hyperglycemia:** Assess for deep and rapid breathing, blurred vision, fatigue, nausea, polydipsia, polyphagia, polyuria, and vomiting. Insulin infusion is recommended for management of hyperglycemia in the critically ill. Blood glucose should be maintained 80-140 mg/dL or 80-110 mg/dL. Rosiglitazone should be discontinued if IV insulin infusion is begun.
- **Increased insulin resistance:** Be alert to conditions that may increase blood glucose, including stress or a surgical procedure.
- **Increased glucose uptake:** Note conditions that may lower blood glucose, such as fever or increased activity.
- **Patient education:** Stress that prescribed diet is a principal part of treatment; meals should not be skipped and carbohydrates should be controlled. Teach the signs and symptoms of hypoglycemia and hyperglycemia. Instruct to carry candy, sugar packets, or other sugar supplements for immediate response to hypoglycemia, especially if taking rosiglitazone with insulin or a sulfonylurea. Urge wearing medical alert identification identifying diabetes. Recommend avoidance of alcohol. Instruct to report promptly abdominal or chest pain, dark urine or light stool, hypoglycemic reactions, fever, nausea, palpitations, rash, vomiting, and yellowing of the eyes or skin to a health care provider. Ensure follow-up instruction if patients or families do not thoroughly understand diabetes management or blood

glucose-testing technique. Instruct those taking rosiglitazone with insulin or a sulfonylurea to always have a source of glucose available to treat symptoms of low blood sugar.

SERIOUS ADVERSE REACTIONS

- **Heart failure:** Fluid retention may lead to weight gain, followed by activity intolerance, shortness of breath, and dependent edema. Increased plasma volume may decrease measurable hemoglobin, white blood cells, and electrolytes due to hemodilution. Acute MI is possible.

OVERDOSE/TOXICITY

- **Hypoglycemia:** Tremors, tachycardia, diaphoresis, anxiety, hypotension, altered mental status, dysrhythmias, seizures; manage with D50 given IV.
- **Hepatotoxicity:** Elevated liver enzymes, loss of appetite, fever, abdominal pain, nausea, vomiting, edema, fatigue, dark urine, jaundice, hepatitis; liver failure, need for liver transplant, and death have been reported.
- **Management:** If ALT (SGPT) levels remain more than 3 times normal after recheck, rosiglitazone should be discontinued. Supportive care for liver dysfunction should be provided.
- **GI decontamination:** No specific recommendations.

ANTIDOTE/DIALYSIS

- **Antidote:** D50 (50% dextrose) 25 mL IV may be given for blood glucose below 50 mg/dL and repeated until blood glucose is at least 80 mg/dL, but not over 140 mg/dL.
- **Dialysis:** Rosiglitazone is not removed by hemodialysis and is unlikely to be removed by peritoneal dialysis. No data is available on removal by high permeability hemodialysis.

rosuvastatin calcium

roe-soo'-va-sta-tin kal'-see-um

Classes

Chemical: substituted heptenoic acid derivative

Therapeutic: HMG-CoA reductase inhibitor, antilipemic

Pregnancy Category: X

Trade Names

Prescription: Crestor

CLINICAL PHARMACOLOGY

Mechanism of Action

An antihyperlipidemic that interferes with cholesterol biosynthesis by inhibiting the conversion of the enzyme hydroxymethylglutaryl-CoA (HMG-CoA) to mevalonate, a precursor to cholesterol. **Therapeutic Effect:** Decreases LDL cholesterol, very low density lipoprotein, and plasma triglyceride levels, increases HDL concentration.

PHARMACOKINETICS

Protein binding: 88%. Minimal hepatic metabolism. Primarily eliminated in the feces. **Half-life:** 19 hr (increased in patients with severe renal dysfunction).

AVAILABILITY

Tablets: 5 mg, 10 mg, 20 mg, 40 mg.

INDICATIONS AND DOSAGE

Hyperlipidemia, dyslipidemia

PO

Adults, Elderly: 5-40 mg/day. Usual starting dosage is 10 mg/day, with adjustments based on lipid levels; monitor every 2-4 wk until desired level is achieved. A lower starting dose of 5 mg is recommended in patients of Asian descent. Consider initial dose of 20 mg if LDL cholesterol is more than 190 mg/dL. Maximum: 40 mg/day.

Renal impairment (creatinine clearance less than 30 mL/min)

PO

Adults, Elderly: 5 mg/day; do not exceed 10 mg/day.

Concurrent cyclosporine use

PO

Adults, Elderly: 5 mg/day.

Concurrent gemfibrozil use

PO

Adults, Elderly: 10 mg/day.

CONTRAINDICATIONS

Active hepatic disease, breast-feeding, pregnancy, unexplained persistent elevations of serum transaminase levels, hypersensitivity to rosuvastatin

INTERACTIONS

Drug: ***CycloSPORINE, gemfibrozil, niacin:** Increases the risk of myopathy with *cycloSPORINE, gemfibrozil, and niacin. **Erythromycin:** Reduces the plasma concentration of erythromycin. **Ethinylestradiol, norgestrel:** Increases the plasma concentrations of ethinylestradiol and norgestrel. **Warfarin:** Enhances anticoagulant effect. **Herbal:** **St. John's wort:** May reduce the effectiveness of rosuvastatin. **Food:** None known.

DIAGNOSTIC TEST EFFECTS

May increase serum creatine kinase (CK) and transaminase concentrations. May produce hematuria and proteinuria.

SIDE-EFFECTS

Rosuvastatin is generally well tolerated. Side effects are usually mild and transient. **Occasional (9%-3%):** Pharyngitis, headache, diarrhea, dyspepsia, including heartburn and epigastric distress, nausea. **Rare (less than 3%):** Myalgia, asthenia or unusual fatigue and weakness, back pain, jaundice

CRITICAL CARE CONSIDERATIONS

ADMINISTRATION/HANDLING

PO ALERT

- Give rosuvastatin without regard to meals and administer in the evening.

PRECAUTIONS

HEALTH-RELATED

- Use rosuvastatin cautiously in patients with a history of hepatic disease; hypotension; severe acute infection; severe electrolyte, endocrine, or metabolic imbalances or disorders; trauma; or uncontrolled seizures.
- Use cautiously in patients on anticoagulant therapy, in those who consume a substantial amount of alcohol, and in patients who have had recent major surgery.

AGE-RELATED

- **Children:** Safety and efficacy of rosuvastatin have not been established in children.
- **Elderly:** No age-related precautions have been noted.

PREGNANCY/LACTATION-RELATED

- Pregnancy category X; not recommended for nursing mothers.

MONITORING

- **Baseline assessment:** Determine pregnancy before beginning rosuvastatin therapy. Patients should be on a standard cholesterol-lowering diet for a minimum of 3-6 mo prior to beginning rosuvastatin therapy; diet should be continued throughout rosuvastatin therapy.
- **Baseline and ongoing lab work:** Biochemical profile including liver (AST [SGOT], ALT [SGPT], GGT, alkaline phosphatase, bilirubin) function tests, serum cholesterol and triglyceride levels. Monitor cholesterol, and triglycerides for therapeutic response and liver enzymes every 12 wk after initial therapy and each time dosage is adjusted. Semiannual monitoring may be appropriate for patients on fixed doses with good response. Periodic laboratory tests are an essential part of ongoing therapy.
- **Therapeutic effect:** Monitor for decreased cholesterol and triglyceride levels.
- **Common side effects:** Constipation, abdominal pain, dyspepsia, flatulence. May require symptom specific management to control.
- **Myalgias:** CPK level may be measured for patients with unexplained myalgias. Urine will appear brown if myoglobin is present.
- **Renal failure:** Monitor BUN, creatinine, and potassium levels if patients manifest myalgia or brown urine indicative of myoglobinuria. Urinalysis is used to diagnose myoglobinuria.
- **Diet instruction:** Patients must follow the prescribed diet because diet is an important part of lowering cholesterol and triglycerides.
- **Other medications:** When therapy is continued outside the hospital, warn patients not to take other medications without prescriber approval.
- **Patient education:** Instruct to continue a cholesterol-lowering diet, which is an important part of treatment. Tell patients of child-bearing age to use appropriate contraceptive measures during rosuvastatin therapy. Explain that rosuvastatin is pregnancy risk category X. Stress that periodic laboratory tests are an essential part of therapy.

SERIOUS ADVERSE REACTIONS

- Lens opacities may occur.
- **Hypersensitivity:** Urticaria, rash, angioedema.
- **Musculoskeletal pain:** Myopathy, arthralgia, myalgia, which may indicate impending rhabdomyolysis. Rosuvastatin should be discontinued if patients develop myopathy and/or rhabdomyolysis.
- **Hypocalcemia:** Must be managed cautiously with rhabdomyolysis because calcium infusion may increase the deposition of calcium in the injured muscles.

R

OVERDOSE/TOXICITY

- **Rhabdomyolysis:** Rare cases; can lead to acute renal failure. Markedly elevated serum creatine kinase and possible myoglobinuria indicate the condition may be present. Should be managed according to accepted guidelines, which include aggressive volume replacement, hemodialysis, or continuous hemofiltration (CVVH) to support patients during acute renal failure. Use of bicarbonate to induce alkaline diuresis or mannitol for osmotic diuresis has not been well studied. Hyperkalemia and hyperphosphatemia are commonly seen with rhabdomyolysis and may require aggressive management.
- **Renal failure:** Acute renal failure ensues when rhabdomyolysis is present.
- **Liver failure:** Liver enzyme elevation indicative of impending liver failure.
- **GI decontamination:** No specific recommendations.

ANTIDOTE/DIALYSIS

- **Antidote:** No specific recommendations.
- **Dialysis:** Rosuvastatin is not removed by hemodialysis. No data are available on removal by peritoneal dialysis or high-permeability hemodialysis.

salmeterol xinafoate 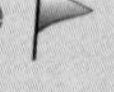

See Bronchodilators (p. 947)

salsalate

See Salicylates (p. 982)

saquinavir

See HIV Medications (p. 961)

sargramostim (granulocyte macrophage colony-stimulating factor, GM-CSF)

sar-gram'-oh-stim

Classes
Chemical: hematinic
Therapeutic: colony stimulating factor

Pregnancy Category: C

Trade Names
Prescription: Leukine

Do not confuse Leukine with Leukeran.

CLINICAL PHARMACOLOGY

Mechanism of Action
A colony-stimulating factor that stimulates proliferation and differentiation of hematopoietic cells to activate mature granulocytes and macrophages. **Therapeutic Effect:** Assists bone marrow in making new WBCs and increases their chemotactic, antifungal, and antiparasitic activity. Increases cytoneoplastic cells and activates neutrophils to inhibit tumor cell growth.

PHARMACOKINETICS

Effect	Onset	Peak	Duration
Increase WBCs	7-14 days	N/A	1 wk

Detected in serum within 5 min after subcutaneous administration. **Half-life:** IV, 1 hr; subcutaneous, 3 hr.

AVAILABILITY

Injection solution: 500 mcg/mL.
Injection powder for reconstitution: 250 mcg.

INDICATIONS AND DOSAGE

Myeloid recovery following bone marrow transplant (BMT)
IV Infusion
Adults, Elderly: Usual parenteral dosage: 250 mcg/m^2/day for 21 days (as 2-hr infusion). Begin 2-4 hr after autologous bone marrow infusion and not less than 24 hr after last dose of chemotherapy or not less than 12 hr after last radiation treatment. Discontinue if blast cells appear or underlying disease progresses.

BMT failure, engraftment delay
IV Infusion
Adults, Elderly: 250 mcg/m^2/day for 14 days. Infuse over 2 hr. May repeat after 7 days off therapy if engraftment has not occurred with 500 mcg/m^2/day for 14 days.

Stem cell transplant
IV, Subcutaneous
Adults: 250 mcg/m^2/day.

OFF-LABEL USES

Treatment of AIDS-related neutropenia; chronic, severe neutropenia; drug-induced neutropenia; myelodysplastic syndrome

CONTRAINDICATIONS

Twelve hours before or after radiation therapy; 24 hr before or after chemotherapy; excessive leukemic myeloid blasts in bone marrow or peripheral blood (greater than 10%); known hypersensitivity to sargramostim or yeast-derived products

INTERACTIONS

Drug: Lithium, steroids: May increase the effects of sargramostim. **Herbal:** None known. **Food:** None known.

DIAGNOSTIC TEST EFFECTS

May increase serum bilirubin, creatinine, and hepatic enzyme levels. May decrease serum albumin level.

IV INCOMPATIBILITIES

Acyclovir, amphotericin B complex (Abelcet, AmBisome, Amphotec), ampicillin, ampicillin/sulbactam, cefoperazone, *chlorproMAZINE, ganciclovir, haloperidol, hydrocortisone sodium phosphate, hydrocortisone sodium succinate, hydromorphone (Dilaudid), *hydrOXYzine, imipenem/cilastatin, lorazepam (Ativan), *methylPREDNISolone sodium succinate, mitomycin, morphine, nalbuphine, ondansetron, piperacillin, sodium bicarbonate, tobramycin

IV COMPATIBILITIES

Amikacin, aminophylline, aztreonam, bleomycin, butorphanol, calcium gluconate, carboplatin, carmustine, cefazolin, cefepime, cefotaxime, cefotetan, ceftizoxime, ceftriaxone, cefuroxime, cimetidine, dexamethasone sodium phosphate, *diphenhydrAMINE, *DOPamine (Intropin), *DOXOrubicin, doxycycline, droperidol, etoposide, famotidine, fentanyl, floxuridine, fluconazole, fluorouracil, furosemide, gentamicin, granisetron, heparin, idarubicin, ifosfamide, immune globulin, magnesium sulfate, mannitol, mechlorethamine, meperidine, mesna, methotrexate, metoclopramide, metronidazole, minocycline, mitoxantrone, netilmicin, pentostatin, piperacillin/tazobactam, potassium chloride, prochlorperazine edisylate, promethazine, ranitidine, teniposide, ticarcillin, ticarcillin/clavulanate, *vinBLAStine, *vinCRIStine, zidovudine

SIDE-EFFECTS

Frequent (10%-89%): GI disturbances, including nausea, diarrhea, vomiting, stomatitis, anorexia, and abdominal pain; arthralgia or myalgia; headache; malaise; rash; pruritus. **Occasional (less than 10%):** Peripheral edema, weight gain, dyspnea, asthenia, fever, leukocytosis, capillary leak syndrome (such as fluid retention, irritation at local injection site, and peripheral edema). **Rare:** Rapid or irregular heartbeat, thrombophlebitis

CRITICAL CARE CONSIDERATIONS

ADMINISTRATION/HANDLING

IV ALERT

- **Storage:** Refrigerate all forms of sargramostim (powder, reconstituted solution, and diluted solution for injection). Do not shake. Do not use past expiration date.
- **Reconstitution:** Add 1 mL preservative-free sterile water for injection to 250-mcg or 500-mcg vial. Direct sterile water for injection to side of vial and gently swirl contents to avoid foaming. Do not shake or vigorously agitate. Use one dose/vial; do not reenter vial. Reconstituted solution is normally clear and colorless; use within 6 hr; discard unused portion.
- **Further dilution:** After reconstitution, further dilute with 0.9% NaCl. To prevent drug adsorption into the IV tubing system, if final concentration will be less than 10 mcg/mL, before adding sargramostim, add 1 mL of 5% albumin for every 50 mL saline to provide a final albumin concentration of 0.1%.
- **Administration:** Give each single dose over 2, 4, or 24 hr.

PRECAUTIONS

HEALTH-RELATED

- Use sargramostim cautiously in patients with heart failure, hypoxia, impaired hepatic or renal function, heart disease, fluid retention, or pulmonary infiltrates.
- Sargramostim can promote growth of any myeloid malignancies.
- Sargramostim may be less effective for patients who have had intensive chemotherapy or radiation therapy; patients may develop antibodies in response to drug, which may inhibit therapeutic effects.

AGE-RELATED

- **Children:** Safety and efficacy of sargramostim have not been established in children, but drug has been successfully used in more than 100 children (4 mo to 18 yr). Liquefied product contains benzyl alcohol and should not be used in premature infants.
- **Elderly:** No age-related precautions have been noted.

PREGNANCY/LACTATION-RELATED

- Pregnancy category C; unknown if distributed in breast milk.

MONITORING

- **Baseline assessment:** Assess for history of heart, lung, kidney, and liver disease. Obtain vital signs and weight.
- **Baseline and ongoing lab work:** CBC with WBC differential; biochemical profile with renal (BUN, creatinine) and liver (AST [SGOT], ALT [SGPT], alkaline phosphatase, GGT, bilirubin) function tests. CBC should be obtained twice weekly to monitor for leukocytosis or absolute neutrophil counts greater than 20,000 cells/mm^3. If blast cells are noted or disease is progressing, drug should be discontinued.
- **Baseline diagnostic tests:** 12-lead ECG to evaluate for myocardial ischemia, chest x-ray to evaluate for lung disease.
- **Dysrhythmias:** Monitor ECG continuously for supraventricular dysrhythmias

during administration, especially if the patient has a history of heart disease.

- **Respiratory distress:** Assess closely for dyspnea during and immediately after infusion, particularly if the history of lung disease is present. Slow the infusion rate by half if dyspnea occurs during infusion. Stop the infusion immediately if dyspnea continues.
- **Fluid retention:** Assess for peripheral edema; assess chest x-ray for pleural and/or pericardial effusions.
- **First dose:** Monitor for flushing, syncope, and hypotension; may occur with subsequent doses; reduce infusion rate or stop infusion.
- **Patient education:** Explain that frequent follow-up blood tests are needed to evaluate the effectiveness of drug therapy. Instruct to report promptly chest pain, chills, fever (or other signs of infection), palpitations, or dyspnea to a health care provider. Advise to avoid situations that offer risk of contracting an infectious disease (e.g., influenza).

SERIOUS ADVERSE REACTIONS

- **Effusions:** Pleural or pericardial effusion occurs rarely after infusion.
- **Hypersensitivity:** Rash, urticaria, injection site reactions, allergic reactions, and anaphylaxis.

OVERDOSE/TOXICITY

- **Leukocytosis/thrombocytosis:** WBC count greater than 50,000 cells/mm^3, absolute neutrophil count exceeds 20,000 cells/mm^3 or platelet count exceeds 500,000/mm^3; stop the infusion or reduce the rate by half, based on clinical condition. Blood counts will return to normal or to baseline 3-7 days after discontinuation of therapy.
- **Hepatotoxicity:** Elevated liver enzymes, fever, abdominal pain, nausea, vomiting, dark urine, jaundice; symptoms should resolve when drug is discontinued.
- **Nephrotoxicity:** Elevated liver enzymes, fever, abdominal pain, nausea, vomiting, dark urine, jaundice; symptoms should resolve when drug is discontinued.
- **GI decontamination:** No specific recommendations.

ANTIDOTE/DIALYSIS

- **Antidote:** No specific recommendations.
- **Dialysis:** No data is available on removal of sargramostim by hemodialysis, high-permeability hemodialysis, or peritoneal dialysis.

S

scopolamine

skoe-pol'-a-meen

Classes

Chemical: belladonna alkaloid
Therapeutic: anticholinergic, antiemetic, antivertigo agent, cycloplegic, mydriatic

Pregnancy Category: C

Trade Names

Prescription: Transdermal: Transderm-Scop; Ophth: Isopto Hyoscine; Oral: Scopace

CLINICAL PHARMACOLOGY

Mechanism of Action

An anticholinergic that reduces excitability of labyrinthine receptors, depressing conduction in the vestibular cerebellar pathway. **Therapeutic Effect:** Prevents motion-induced nausea and vomiting.

PHARMACOKINETICS

Well absorbed percutaneously. Crosses blood-brain barrier. Metabolized in liver. Excreted in urine. **Half-life:** 9.5 hr (transdermal). Onset: 0.5-1 hr (PO, IM); 10 min (IV). Peak: 24 hr (transdermal); other routes unknown. Duration: 4-6 hr (PO, IM); 2 hr (IV).

AVAILABILITY

Transdermal system (Transderm-Scop): 1.5 mg.

INDICATIONS AND DOSAGE

Prevention of motion sickness

Transdermal

Adults: 1 system every 72 hr. Apply behind the ear at least 4 hr before exposure. Best if applied 12 hr before exposure.

Postoperative nausea or vomiting

Transdermal

Adults, Elderly: One system no sooner than 1 hr before surgery and removed 24 hr after surgery.

CONTRAINDICATIONS

Angle-closure glaucoma, GI or GU obstruction, myasthenia gravis, paralytic ileus, tachycardia, thyrotoxicosis, hypersensitivity to scopolamine

INTERACTIONS

Drug: **Antihistamines, tricyclic antidepressants:** May increase the anticholinergic effects of scopolamine. **CNS depressants:** May increase CNS depression. **Herbal:** None known. **Food:** None known.

DIAGNOSTIC TEST EFFECTS

May interfere with gastric secretion test.

SIDE-EFFECTS

Frequent (greater than 15%): Dry mouth, somnolence, blurred vision. **Rare (5%-1%):** Dizziness, restlessness, hallucinations, confusion, difficulty urinating, rash

CRITICAL CARE CONSIDERATIONS

ADMINISTRATION/HANDLING

IM/IV/SUBCUTANEOUS ALERT

- **Antiparkinsonian effects:** Suddenly stopping scopolamine in patients with parkinsonism may cause withdrawal-like symptoms including sweating, vomiting, and malaise; addiction does not occur, however.

PO ALERT

- **Altered mental status:** Many people are sensitive to scopolamine and easily develop symptoms of toxicity including complete disorientation and active delirium.

OPHTHALMIC ALERT

- **Administration:** Do not touch dropper to any surface to avoid introducing bacteria into the solution. The lacrimal sac should be compressed by digital pressure for 2-3 min following instillation to prevent excessive absorption.
- **Glaucoma:** Therapy in patients with open-angle (wide-angle) glaucoma may experience increased intraocular pressure.

TRANSDERMAL ALERT

- **Application:** Apply patch to the hairless area behind one ear. Replace the patch after 72 hr or if it becomes dislodged.
- **Glaucoma:** Therapy in patients with open-angle (wide-angle) glaucoma may experience increased intraocular pressure.

PRECAUTIONS

HEALTH-RELATED

- Use scopolamine cautiously in patients with cardiac disease, renal or hepatic impairment, psychoses, or seizures.

AGE-RELATED

- **Children:** Safety and efficacy of scopolamine are established for children over 6 mo for all forms except oral and transdermal; children are more susceptible to behavioral alterations and poisoning.
- **Elderly:** Are more susceptible to behavioral alterations and poisoning; may require a dosage reduction; use cautiously.

PREGNANCY/LACTATION-RELATED

- Pregnancy category C; no reports of adverse effects reported; compatible with breast-feeding.

MONITORING

- **Baseline assessment:** Determine whether other CNS depressants or drugs with anticholinergic action are being used. Determine history of angle-closure glaucoma. Instruct patients to urinate before giving drug to reduce risk of urinary retention.
- **Baseline lab work:** Biochemical profile including renal (BUN, creatinine) and liver (AST [SGOT], ALT [SGPT], alkaline phosphatase, bilirubin) function tests.
- **Tachycardia:** Monitor patients with heart disease for tachycardia.
- **Dehydration:** Assess skin turgor and mucous membranes to evaluate status. Assess for dry mouth and thirst. Encourage drinking fluids unless patients are NPO (cannot eat or drink) before a procedure.
- **Constipation:** Assess for diminished bowel sounds; drug is sometimes effective in managing diarrhea.
- **Urinary retention:** Monitor intake and output; palpate the bladder to assess for urinary retention.
- **Patient education:** Teach how to administer scopolamine properly (apply the patch, instill eye drops). For transdermal, instruct how to use only one patch at a time and not to cut it. Advise to wash hands after applying the patch. Warn to avoid tasks requiring mental alertness or motor skills until response to the drug is known.

SERIOUS ADVERSE REACTIONS

- **Cardiac:** Tachycardia, palpitations.
- **Integumentary:** Hot, dry, or flushed skin with dry mouth.
- **Gastrointestinal:** Absence of bowel sounds, nausea, vomiting.
- **Neurologic:** Confusion, restlessness, somnolence, slurred speech, dizziness, agitation, visual hallucinations, paranoid behavior, and delusions.
- **Respiratory:** Tachypnea.
- **Visual:** Blurred vision with dilated pupils.

OVERDOSE/TOXICITY

- **Anticholinergic syndrome symptoms:** Tachycardia; palpitations; hot, dry, or flushed skin; fever without sweating; absence of bowel sounds; dilated pupils;

blurred vision; possible seizures; increased respiratory rate; nausea; vomiting; confusion; somnolence; slurred speech; dizziness; and CNS stimulation.

- **Anticholinergic syndrome behaviors:** Psychosis as evidenced by excitement, agitation, restlessness, rambling speech, visual hallucinations, paranoid behavior, and delusions, followed by depression.
- **Management:** Diazepam, phenobarbital, or chloral hydrate may be used to manage excitement. *ChlorproMAZINE should be avoided because it has anticholinergic properties. Severe hyperthermia (temperature above 40°C) should be managed by rapid cooling with a hypothermia blanket, cool water immersion, cold water irrigation of the stomach, rectum, or peritoneal cavity. Rhabdomyolysis may occur secondary to marked agitation, increased muscle tone, or severe hyperthermia and may lead to acute renal failure. Intubation and mechanical ventilation may be needed to manage respiratory distress.
- **GI decontamination:** No specific recommendations.

ANTIDOTE/DIALYSIS

- **Antidote:** Physostigmine reverses most cardiovascular and CNS effects, but may cause bradycardia, seizures, or asystole. Neostigmine is the alternate antidote choice. Administer pilocarpine until the mouth is moist.
- **Dialysis:** No data are available on removal of scopolamine by hemodialysis, peritoneal dialysis, or high-permeability hemodialysis.

selegiline hydrochloride

se-le'-ji-leen high-droe-klor'-ide

Classes

Chemical: phenethylamine derivative
Therapeutic: antiparkinson's agent

Pregnancy Category: C

Trade Names

Prescription: Eldepryl, Emsam

Do not confuse selegiline with Stelazine, or Eldepryl with enalapril.

CLINICAL PHARMACOLOGY

Mechanism of Action

An antiparkinson agent that irreversibly inhibits the activity of monoamine oxidase type B, the enzyme that breaks down dopamine, thereby increasing dopaminergic action. **Therapeutic Effect:** Relieves signs and symptoms of Parkinson's disease.

PHARMACOKINETICS

Rapidly absorbed from the GI tract. Crosses the blood-brain barrier. Metabolized in the liver to the active metabolites. Primarily excreted in urine. **Half-life:** 10 hr (PO), 18-25 hr (transdermal).

AVAILABILITY

Capsules: 5 mg.
Tablets: 5 mg.
Tablets, orally disintegrating: 1.25 mg.
Transdermal: 6 mg/24 hr, 9 mg/24 hr, 12 mg/24 hr.

INDICATIONS AND DOSAGE

Major depressive disorder

Transdermal

Adults, Elderly: Initially, 6 mg/24 hr. May increase in 3 mg in 24-hr increments at a minimum of 2 wk. Maximum: 12 mg/24 hr.

Adjunctive treatment for parkinsonism

PO

Adults: 10 mg/day in divided doses, such as 5 mg at breakfast and lunch, given concomitantly with each dose of carbidopa and levodopa. **Elderly:** Initially 5 mg in the morning. May increase up to 10 mg/day.

OFF-LABEL USES

Treatment of Alzheimer's disease, attention-deficit/hyperactivity disorder, depression, early Parkinson's disease, extrapyramidal symptoms, negative symptoms of schizophrenia

CONTRAINDICATIONS

Concurrent use with meperidine, hypersensitivity to selegiline. **Orally disintegrating form:** Concurrent use of dextromethorphan, methadone, propoxyphene, tramadol, oral selegiline, other MAOIs. **Transdermal form:** Pheochromocytoma; concurrent use of bupropion, selective or dual serotonin reuptake inhibitors (including selective serotonin reuptake inhibitors [SSRIs] and serotonin and norepinephrine reuptake inhibitors), tricyclic antidepressants, *busPIRone, tramadol, propoxyphene, methadone, dextromethorphan, St. John's wort, mirtazapine, cyclobenzaprine, oral selegiline, and other MAOIs; sympathomimetic amines (e.g., pseudoephedrine), carbamazepine, and oxcarbazepine; elective surgery requiring general anesthesia, local anesthesia containing sympathomimetic vasoconstrictors.

INTERACTIONS

Drug: **Amphetamines, CNS stimulants, cyclic antidepressants, dextromethorphan, fluoxetine, methadone, propoxyphene, sibutramine, SSRIs, tramadol, venlafaxine, trazadone:** May cause serotonin syndrome. ***BusPIRone:** May increase BP; avoid use if possible. **Meperidine:** May cause a diaphoresis, excitation, hypertension or hypotension, coma, and even death. **Alpha-adrenergic catecholmaines (*DOPamine, phenylephrine, pseudoephedrine):** May increase BP; avoid use if possible. **Herbal:** **Kava, kava, St. John's wort, valerian:** May increase sedation. **Food:** **Caffeine, tyramine-rich foods:** Large amounts of these substances may produce a severe hypertensive reaction.

DIAGNOSTIC TEST EFFECTS

None known.

SIDE-EFFECTS

Frequent (10%-4%): Nausea, dizziness, lightheadedness, syncope, abdominal discomfort, headache, insomnia, application site reaction (transdermal). **Occasional (3%-2%):** Confusion, hallucinations, dry mouth, vivid dreams, dyskinesia. **Rare (1%):** Headache, myalgia, anxiety, diarrhea, insomnia

CRITICAL CARE CONSIDERATIONS

ADMINISTRATION/HANDLING

PO ALERT

- Administer selegiline with carbidopa and levodopa; begin selegiline with the lowest dosage, then increase gradually over 3-4 wk.

PRECAUTIONS

HEALTH-RELATED

- Use selegiline cautiously in patients with cardiac dysrhythmias, dementia, peptic ulcer disease, profound tremor, psychosis, or tardive dyskinesia.

AGE-RELATED

- **Children:** Safety and efficacy of selegiline have not been established in children.
- **Elderly:** No age-related precautions have been noted.

PREGNANCY/LACTATION-RELATED

- Pregnancy category C; excretion in breast milk unknown.

MONITORING

- **Baseline assessment:** Obtain vital signs; selegiline may cause hypotension.
- **Baseline lab work:** Biochemical profile.
- **Baseline diagnostic tests:** 12-lead ECG to evaluate for myocardial ischemia and dysrhythmias.
- **Neurologic effects:** Monitor for agitation, headache, lethargy, dyskinesia, and confusion. Meperidine, tramadol, and dextromethorphan may prompt adverse neurologic effects.
- **Therapeutic effect:** Assess for improvement of masklike facial expression, muscular rigidity, shuffling gait, and resting tremor of the hands and head.
- **Patient education:** Inform that dizziness, drowsiness, lightheadedness, and dry mouth are common side effects of selegiline but will diminish or disappear with continued treatment. Instruct to change positions slowly and to pause momentarily before standing to reduce the drug's hypotensive effect. Warn to avoid tasks that require mental alertness or motor skills until response to the drug is known. Urge avoidance of alcoholic beverages. Instruct to avoid tyramine-rich foods, such as wine and aged cheese, to prevent a hypertensive reaction.

SERIOUS ADVERSE REACTIONS

- **Neurologic/behavioral:** Involuntary movements, impaired motor coordination, loss of balance, blepharospasm, facial grimaces, feeling of heaviness in the lower extremities, depression, nightmares, delusions, overstimulation, sleep disturbance, and anger.

OVERDOSE/TOXICITY

- **Serotonin syndrome (SS):** Diaphoresis, confusion, myoclonus, hyperreflexia, muscle rigidity, extreme tremor, restlessness, ataxia, hyperthermia, hypertension, tachycardia, tachypnea, coma, seizures, hypotension (poor prognostic sign); flushed skin, diarrhea, abdominal pain, and salivation occur relatively infrequently. Dilated pupils and "ping-pong" (side-to-side) gaze have been noted.
- **Management:** Prognosis is favorable. Provide supportive care, discontinue all serotoninergic drugs, consider giving antiserotoninergic drugs, manage airway and ventilation (with endotracheal intubation and mechanical ventilation if needed). Manage hyperthermia with a hypothermia blanket, cool-water immersion, packing

S

axillae and groin with ice, cold water via nasogastric tube or rectal tube, or peritoneal irrigation. Benzodiazepines are first-line therapy for muscle rigidity. Phenytoin is not expected to be effective.

- **GI decontamination:** May attempt gastric lavage and activated charcoal if patients present early following an acute overdose, but airway must be protected. Multiple doses of activated charcoal have not proven effective.

ANTIDOTE/DIALYSIS

- **Antidote:** No specific antidote, but animal studies reveal *chlorproMAZINE, cyproheptadine, methysergide, and propranolol are helpful in preventing SS, and case reports support use to treat SS. Cyproheptadine seems to be the most consistent antiseritonergic drug in humans.
- **Dialysis:** No data are available on removal of selegiline by hemodialysis, high-permeability hemodialysis, or peritoneal dialysis.

senna

sen'-na

Classes

Chemical: anthraquinone derivative
Therapeutic: laxative, stimulant

Pregnancy Category: C

Trade Names

Prescription: Ex-Lax, Perdiem, Senexon, Senna-Gen, Sennatural, Senokot, X-Prep

CLINICAL PHARMACOLOGY

Mechanism of Action

A GI stimulant that has a direct effect on intestinal smooth musculature by stimulating the intramural nerve plexi. **Therapeutic Effect:** Increases peristalsis and promotes laxative effect.

PHARMACOKINETICS

Route	Onset	Peak	Duration
PO	6-12 hr	N/A	N/A
Rectal	0.5-2 hr	N/A	N/A

Minimal absorption after oral administration. Hydrolyzed to active form by enzymes of colonic flora. Absorbed drug metabolized in the liver. Eliminated in feces via biliary system.

AVAILABILITY

Granules (Senokot): 15 mg/tsp.
Liquid (X-Prep): 8.8 mg/5 mL.
Syrup (Senokot): 8.8 mg/5 mL.
Tablets (Perdiem): 15 mg.
Tablets (Sennatural, Senokot, Senexon, Senna-Gen): 8.6 mg, 15 mg.
Tablets (Ex-Lax): 15 mg, 25 mg

INDICATIONS AND DOSAGE

Constipation

PO (Tablets)

Adults, Elderly, Children 12 yr and older: 2 tablets at bedtime. Maximum: 4 tablets twice per day. **Children 6-11 yr:** 1 tablet at bedtime. Maximum: 2 tablets twice per day. **Children 2-5 yr:** Half tablet at bedtime. Maximum: 1 tablet twice per day.

PO (Syrup)

Adults, Elderly, Children 12 yr and older: 10-15 mL at bedtime. Maximum: 15 mL twice per day. **Children 6-11 yr:** 5-7.5 mL at bedtime. Maximum: 7.5 mL twice per day. **Children 2-5 yr:** 2.5-3.75 mL at bedtime. Maximum: 3.75 mL twice per day. **Children 1 mo-2 yr:** 1.25-2.5 mL at bedtime. Maximum: 5 mL/day.

PO (Granules)

Adults, Elderly, Children 12 yr and older: 1 tsp at bedtime. Maximum: 2 tsp twice per day. **Children 6-11 yr:** One half ½ tsp at bedtime up to 1 tsp 2 times/day. **Children 2-5 yr:** One quarter ¼ tsp at bedtime up to one half ½ teaspoon 2 times/day.

Bowel evacuation

PO

Adults, Elderly, Children older than 12 yr: 75 mL between 2 PM and 4 PM on day before procedure (x-ray prep).

CONTRAINDICATIONS

Abdominal pain, appendicitis, intestinal obstruction, nausea, vomiting, hypersensitivity to senna

INTERACTIONS

Drug: **Oral medications:** May decrease transit time of concurrently administered oral medications, decreasing absorption of senna. **Herbal:** None known. **Food:** None known.

DIAGNOSTIC TEST EFFECTS

May increase blood glucose level. May decrease serum potassium level.

SIDE-EFFECTS

Frequent: Pink-red, red-violet, red-brown, or yellow-brown discoloration of urine. **Occasional:** Some degree of abdominal discomfort, nausea, mild cramps, griping, faintness

S

CRITICAL CARE CONSIDERATIONS

ADMINISTRATION/HANDLING

PO ALERT

- Give senna on an empty stomach for faster results. Offer at least 6-8 glasses of water per day to aid in stool softening.
- Avoid giving within 1 hr of other oral medications because drug absorption is decreased.

PRECAUTIONS

HEALTH-RELATED

- Use senna cautiously for extended periods (greater than 1 wk).

AGE-RELATED

- **Children:** Safety and efficacy of senna have not been established in children under 6 yr.
- **Elderly:** No age-related precautions have been noted; elderly should be monitored for dehydration and electrolyte loss.

PREGNANCY/LACTATION-RELATED

- Pregnancy category C; unknown if distributed in breast milk.

MONITORING

- **Baseline assessment:** Before senna administration, assess for abdominal tenderness, rigidity, and the presence of bowel sounds. Determine when last bowel movement occurred; determine amount and consistency.
- **Baseline lab work:** Biochemical profile to check for fluid and electrolyte imbalance from laxative abuse. Monitor serum electrolyte levels in patients with excessive, frequent, or prolonged use of senna.
- **Hydration:** Encourage adequate fluid intake.
- **Constipation:** Assess bowel sounds for peristalsis. Assess pattern of daily bowel activity and stool consistency and record time of evacuation.
- **Patient education:** Explain that senna may turn urine pink-red, red-violet, red-brown, or yellow-brown. Instruct to institute measures to promote defecation, such as increasing fluid intake, exercising, and eating a high-fiber diet. Instruct not to take other oral medications within 1 hr of taking senna because these substances may decrease the effectiveness of senna. Advise that oral senna generally produces a laxative effect in 6-12 hr but that it may take 24 hr.

SERIOUS ADVERSE REACTIONS

- **Long-term use:** May result in laxative dependence, chronic constipation, and loss of normal bowel function.
- **Hypersensitivity:** Rash, urticaria.

OVERDOSE/TOXICITY

- **Prolonged use or overdose:** May result in electrolyte and metabolic disturbances (such as hypokalemia, hypocalcemia, and metabolic acidosis or alkalosis), vomiting, muscle weakness, persistent diarrhea, malabsorption, and weight loss.
- **GI decontamination:** No specific recommendations.

ANTIDOTE/DIALYSIS

- **Antidote:** No specific recommendations.
- **Dialysis:** No data are available on removal of senna by hemodialysis, high-permeability hemodialysis, or peritoneal dialysis.

sertraline hydrochloride

ser'-tra-leen hy-droe-klor'-ide

Classes

Chemical: naphthalenamine derivative
Therapeutic: antidepressant, selective serotonin reuptake inhibitor (SSRI)

Pregnancy Category: C

Trade Names

Prescription: Zoloft

Do not confuse sertraline with Serentil.

CLINICAL PHARMACOLOGY

Mechanism of Action

An antidepressant, anxiolytic, and obsessive-compulsive disorder (OCD) adjunct that blocks the reuptake of the neurotransmitter serotonin at CNS neuronal presynaptic membranes, increasing its availability at postsynaptic receptor sites. **Therapeutic Effect:** Relieves depression, reduces obsessive-compulsive behavior, decreases anxiety.

PHARMACOKINETICS

Incompletely and slowly absorbed from the GI tract; food increases absorption. Protein binding: 98%. Widely distributed. Undergoes extensive first-pass metabolism in the liver to active compound. Excreted in urine and feces. Not removed by hemodialysis. **Half-life:** 26 hr.

S

AVAILABILITY

Oral concentrate: 20 mg/mL.
Tablets: 25 mg, 50 mg, 100 mg.

INDICATIONS AND DOSAGE

Depression

PO

Adults: Initially 50 mg/day. May increase by 50 mg/day at 7-day intervals up to 200 mg/day. **Elderly:** Initially 25 mg/day. May increase by 25-50 mg/day at 7-day intervals up to 200 mg/day.

OCD

PO

Adults, Children 13-17 yr: Initially 50 mg/day with morning or evening meal. May increase by 50 mg/day at 7-day intervals. **Elderly, Children 6-12 yr:** Initially 25 mg/day. May increase by 25-50 mg/day at 7-day intervals. Maximum: 200 mg/day.

Panic disorder, posttraumatic stress disorder, social anxiety disorder

PO

Adults, Elderly: Initially, 25 mg/day. May increase by 50 mg/day at 7-day intervals. Range: 50-200 mg/day. Maximum: 200 mg/day.

Premenstrual dysphoric disorder

PO

Adults: Initially, 50 mg/day. May increase up to 150 mg/day in 50-mg increments.

OFF-LABEL USES

Eating disorders, generalized anxiety disorder (GAD), impulse control disorders

CONTRAINDICATIONS

Use within 14 days of MAOIs, hypersensitivity to sertraline, pimozide, disulfiram syrup (contains 12% alcohol)

INTERACTIONS

Drug: Highly protein-bound medications (such as digoxin and warfarin): May increase the blood concentration and risk of toxicity of these drugs. **Linezolid:** May increase risk of serotonin syndrome. **MAOIs:** May cause neuroleptic malignant syndrome, hypertensive crisis, hyperpyrexia, seizures, and serotonin syndrome (marked by diaphoresis, diarrhea, fever, mental changes, restlessness, and shivering). **Herbal: St. John's wort:** May increase the risk of adverse effects. **Food:** None known.

DIAGNOSTIC TEST EFFECTS

May increase serum total cholesterol, triglyceride, AST (SGOT), and ALT (SGPT) levels. May decrease serum uric acid level.

SIDE-EFFECTS

Frequent (26%-12%): Headache, nausea, diarrhea, insomnia, somnolence, dizziness, fatigue, rash, dry mouth. **Occasional (6%-4%):** Anxiety, nervousness, agitation, tremor, dyspepsia, diaphoresis, vomiting, constipation, abnormal ejaculation, visual disturbances, altered taste. **Rare (less than 3%):** Flatulence, urinary frequency, paresthesia, hot flashes, chills

CRITICAL CARE CONSIDERATIONS

ADMINISTRATION/HANDLING

PO ALERT

- Make sure at least 14 days elapse between the use of MAOIs and sertraline.
- Give sertraline with food or milk if GI distress occurs.

PRECAUTIONS

HEALTH-RELATED

- Use sertraline cautiously in patients with cardiac disease, hepatic impairment, or seizure disorders; in patients who have had a recent MI; and in suicidal patients.

AGE-RELATED

- **Children:** No age-related precautions have been noted in children over 6 yr; children may require lower doses because of their more efficient drug metabolism.
- **Elderly:** Lower initial sertraline dosages are recommended although no age-related precautions have been noted in this age group.

PREGNANCY/LACTATION-RELATED

- Pregnancy category C; excretion into breast milk unknown; use caution in nursing mothers.

MONITORING

- **Baseline assessment:** Assess appearance, behavior, level of interest, mood, and sleep pattern.
- **Baseline lab work:** CBC and biochemical profile including renal (BUN, creatinine) and liver (AST [SGOT], ALT [SGPT], alkaline phosphatase, GGT, bilirubin) function tests. Liver and renal function tests are performed periodically during long-term therapy.
- **Baseline diagnostic tests:** 12-lead ECG to evaluate for myocardial ischemia.
- **Suicidal patients:** Closely supervise suicidal patients during early therapy. As

depression lessens, energy level improves, increasing suicide potential.

- **Therapeutic effect:** Assess for improvement in appearance, behavior, level of interest, mood, and sleep pattern before and during therapy.
- **Diarrhea:** Monitor pattern of daily bowel activity and stool consistency.
- **Dizziness:** Assist with ambulation if dizziness is experienced.
- **Patient education:** Advise to take sertraline with food if nauseated. Instruct female patients to notify the prescriber if newly pregnant. Instruct to report fatigue, headache, sexual dysfunction, or tremor. Recommend avoidance of tasks that require mental alertness or motor skills until response to the drug is known. Urge avoidance of alcohol while taking sertraline. Caution not to take OTC medications without consulting the prescriber.

SERIOUS ADVERSE REACTIONS

- **MAOIs:** Use of sertraline with MAOIs has resulted in fatalities. Symptoms of this drug interaction include hyperthermia, rigidity, myoclonus, confusion, irritability, extreme agitation progressing to delirium and coma.
- **Hyponatremia:** Possibly related to syndrome of inappropriate antidiuretic hormone.
- **Platelet dysfunction:** Rare abnormal bleeding and purpura reported, but role of sertraline remains unclear in these reactions.

OVERDOSE/TOXICITY

- **Serotonin syndrome (SS):** Diaphoresis, confusion, myoclonus, hyperreflexia, muscle rigidity, extreme tremor, restlessness, ataxia, hyperthermia, hypertension, tachycardia, tachypnea, coma, seizures, hypotension (poor prognostic sign); flushed skin, diarrhea, abdominal pain, and salivation occur relatively infrequently. Dilated pupils and "ping-pong" (side-to-side) gaze have been noted.
- **Management:** Prognosis is favorable. Provide supportive care, discontinue all serotoninergic drugs, consider giving antiserotoninergic drugs, manage airway and ventilation (with endotracheal intubation and mechanical ventilation if needed). Manage hyperthermia with a hypothermia blanket, cool-water immersion, packing axillae and groin with ice, cold water via nasogastric tube or rectal tube, or peritoneal irrigation. Benzodiazepines are first-line therapy for muscle rigidity. Phenytoin is not expected to be effective.
- **GI decontamination:** May attempt gastric lavage and activated charcoal if patients present early following an acute overdose, but airway must be protected. Multiple doses of activated charcoal have not proven effective.

ANTIDOTE/DIALYSIS

- **Antidote:** No specific recommendations.
- **Dialysis:** Sertraline is not removed by hemodialysis and is unlikely to be removed by peritoneal dialysis. No data are available on removal by high-permeability hemodialysis.

sevelamer hydrochloride

seh-vel'-ah-mer hye-droe-klor'-ide

Classes

Chemical: allylamine
Therapeutic: phosphate adsorbent

Pregnancy Category: C

Trade Names

Prescription: Renagel

Do not confuse Renagel with Reglan or Regonol.

CLINICAL PHARMACOLOGY

Mechanism of Action

An antihyperphosphatemia agent that binds with dietary phosphorus in the GI tract, thus allowing phosphorus to be eliminated through the normal digestive process and decreasing the serum phosphorus level. **Therapeutic Effect:** Decreases incidence of hypercalcemic episodes in patients receiving calcium acetate treatment.

PHARMACOKINETICS

Not absorbed systemically.

AVAILABILITY

Capsules: 403 mg.
Tablets: 400 mg, 800 mg.

INDICATIONS AND DOSAGE

Hyperphosphatemia

PO

Adults, Elderly: 800-1600 mg with each meal, depending on severity of hyperphosphatemia. Phosphate level 5.5-7.4: 800 mg 3 times per day. Phosphate level 7.5-8.9: 1200-1600 mg 3 times per day.

S

Phosphate level greater than 9 mg/dL: 1600 mg 3 times per day.

CONTRAINDICATIONS

Bowel obstruction, hypophosphatemia, hypersensitivity to sevelamer

INTERACTIONS

Drug: Ciprofloxacin: May decrease ciprofloxacin bioavailability to 50%. **Herbal:** None known. **Food:** None known.

DIAGNOSTIC TEST EFFECTS

None known.

SIDE-EFFECTS

Frequent (20%-11%): Infection, pain, hypotension, diarrhea, dyspepsia, nausea, vomiting, rash (13%), limb pain (13%). **Occasional (10%-1%):** Headache, constipation, hypertension, thrombosis, increased cough

CRITICAL CARE CONSIDERATIONS

ADMINISTRATION/HANDLING

PO ALERT

- Give sevelamer with food.
- Do not break capsules apart; the contents expand in water.
- Give other medications at least 1 hr before or 3 hr after sevelamer.
- **Dosage titration:** Dose should be adjusted gradually, using serum phosphorous levels as a guide; goal should be to lower phosphorous to 5.5 mg/dL or less. Dose may be increased or decreased by 1 tablet or capsule per meal at 2-wk intervals.

PRECAUTIONS

HEALTH-RELATED

- Use sevelamer cautiously in patients with dysphagia, severe GI tract motility disorders, or swallowing disorders and in those who have undergone major GI tract surgery.
- Has not been studied in end-stage renal disease patients not on hemodialysis; all chronic renal failure patients studied had hemodialysis.
- Compared with calcium acetate, may reduce the risk of developing hypercalcemia.

AGE-RELATED

- **Children:** Safety and efficacy of sevelamer have not been established in children.
- **Elderly:** No age-related precautions have been noted.

PREGNANCY/LACTATION-RELATED

- Pregnancy category C; use caution in nursing mothers because of potential for reductions in serum levels of various vitamins.

MONITORING

- **Baseline assessment:** Assess for signs of bowel obstruction, including absent bowel sounds, abdominal distention, and pain. Drug is contraindicated in patients with history of bowel obstruction.
- **Lab work:** Biochemical profile including renal (BUN, creatinine) function tests and baseline serum phosphorus, bicarbonate, chloride, and calcium levels. Monitor the serum bicarbonate, chloride, calcium, and phosphorus levels during therapy.
- **Diet:** Ensure that patients are on a renal diet, low in phosphorous and potassium.
- **Hypotension:** Monitor for low BP, dizziness, and persistent headache.
- **Phosphate imbalance:** Assess for hypophosphatemia (confusion, seizures, coma, chest pain, muscle weakness, numbness/tingling in fingers and on face/lips), and hyperphosphatemia (hyperactive reflexes, muscle cramps, tetany, seizures, altered mental status, prolonged QT interval on ECG tracing). Hyperphosphatemia is associated with hypocalcemia and hypermagnesemia, and hypophosphatemia is associated with hypercalcemia and hypomagnesemia.
- **Vitamin deficiencies:** A daily multivitamin supplement may prevent reduction in serum levels of fat soluble vitamins D, E, K, and folic acid
- **Patient education:** Instruct to take sevelamer with food and to swallow capsules or tablets whole and to take other medications at least 1 hr before or 3 hr after sevelamer. Instruct to report diarrhea, signs of hypotension (such as lightheadedness), nausea or vomiting, or a persistent headache. Remind that a daily vitamin supplement may help reduce vitamin deficiencies.

SERIOUS ADVERSE REACTIONS

- Thrombosis occurs rarely.

OVERDOSE/TOXICITY

- **Hypophosphatemia:** Confusion, difficulty speaking, seizures, coma, muscle weakness; paralysis of respiratory muscles may lead to respiratory failure. Hypomagnesemia and hypercalcemia may prompt nausea, vomiting, decreased deep tendon reflexes, shortened ST segment and QT interval, possible heart block on ECG. Bruising and bleeding may occur secondary to platelet dysfunction. Rhabdomyolysis, hemolysis, and myocardial depression may be present. Patients' lactate levels will be elevated, and ABG will reflect metabolic acidosis and respiratory alkalosis (hyperventilation may occur to help normalize pH).

- **Management:** Moderate hypophosphatemia may be treated with oral phosphate supplements (Neutra-Phos or Phospho-Soda). Administration of IV sodium phosphate or potassium phosphate is needed to manage severe hypophosphatemia or when the GI tract is dysfunctional.
- **GI decontamination:** No specific recommendations.

ANTIDOTE/DIALYSIS

- **Antidote:** Oral or IV phosphorous supplements.
- **Dialysis:** Sevelamer is unlikely to be removed by hemodialysis, high-permeability hemodialysis, or peritoneal dialysis.

sibutramine hydrochloride

sih-byoo'-tra-meen high-droe-klor'-ide

DEA Schedule: IV

Classes

Chemical: cyclobutanemethamine derivative

Therapeutic: anorexiant

Pregnancy Category: C

Trade Names

Prescription: Meridia

CLINICAL PHARMACOLOGY

Mechanism of Action

A CNS stimulant that inhibits reuptake of serotonin (enhancing satiety) and norepinephrine (raises metabolic rate) centrally. **Therapeutic Effect:** Induces and maintains weight loss.

PHARMACOKINETICS

Rapidly absorbed from the GI tract. Protein binding: 95%-97%. Metabolized in liver, undergoes first-pass metabolism. Primarily excreted in urine, minimal elimination in feces. **Half-life:** 1.1 hr.

AVAILABILITY

Capsules: 5 mg, 10 mg, 15 mg (Meridia).

INDICATIONS AND DOSAGE

Weight loss

PO

Adults 16 yr and older: Initially, 10 mg/day. May increase up to 15 mg/day. Maximum: 20 mg/day.

CONTRAINDICATIONS

Anorexia nervosa, concomitant MAOI use, concomitant use of centrally acting appetite suppressants, hypersensitivity to sibutramine or any component of the formulation

INTERACTIONS

Drug: **CNS-acting appetite suppressants:** May increase risk of hypertension and tachycardia. **Dextromethorphan, dihydroergotamine, ergotamine, fentanyl, lithium, meperidine, MAOIs, pentazocine, selective serotonin reuptake inhibitors, serotonin agonists, tryptophan:** May increase risk of serotonin syndrome. **Herbal:** **St. John's wort:** May decrease sibutramine levels. **Yohimbine:** May increase risk of adverse cardiovascular effects. **Food:** None known.

DIAGNOSTIC TEST EFFECTS

None known.

SIDE-EFFECTS

Frequent (10%-30%): Headache (30%), dry mouth (17%), anorexia (13%), constipation (11%), insomnia (10%), rhinitis, pharyngitis. **Occasional (less than 10%):** Back pain, flu syndrome, dizziness, nausea, asthenia (loss of strength, energy), arthralgia, nervousness, dyspepsia, sinusitis, abdominal pain, anxiety, dysmenorrheal. **Rare:** Depression, rash, cough, sweating, tachycardia, migraine, increased BP, paresthesia, altered taste

S

CRITICAL CARE CONSIDERATIONS

ADMINISTRATION/HANDLING

PO ALERT

- Give sibutramine with or without food, usually in the morning. Administer sibutramine with a low-calorie diet.

PRECAUTIONS

HEALTH-RELATED

- **Patient selection:** Sibutramine is intended for obese patients with an initial body mass index greater than or equal to 30 kg/m^2 or greater than or equal to 27 kg/m^2 in the presence of other risk factors such as hypertension, diabetes, or dyslipidemia.

- **Hypertension:** Sibutramine may significantly increase BP in some patients. Regular monitoring of BP is necessary.
- **Primary pulmonary hypertension and cardiac valve disorders:** Have been associated with other centrally acting weight loss agents that cause release of serotonin from nerve terminals; although sibutramine has not been associated with these effects in premarketing clinical studies, patients should be informed of the potential for these side effects and monitored closely for their occurrence.
- Use cautiously in patients with cardiac dysrhythmias, heart failure, coronary artery disease, gallstones, hypertension (uncontrolled or poorly controlled), narrow-angle glaucoma, seizures, severe liver or renal impairment, and stroke.
- Maintenance of weight loss beyond 18 mo has not been studied.
- **Cytochrome P450 inhibitors:** Patients taking other medications metabolized by cytochrome P4503A4 may have drug interactions. Medications include phenytoin, carbamazepine, haloperidol, clozapine, alprazolam, lithium, and tryptophan.

AGE-RELATED

- **Children:** Safety and efficacy of sibutramine have not been established in children under 16 yr.
- **Elderly:** Sibutramine is not recommended for use in the elderly.

PREGNANCY/LACTATION-RELATED

- Pregnancy category C; excretion into breast milk unknown; not recommended in nursing mothers.

MONITORING

- **Baseline assessment:** Obtain patient history and allergies, baseline weight, BP, and heart rate. Hypertensive patients require close monitoring of BP.
- **Lab work:** Biochemical profile including renal (BUN, creatinine) and liver (AST [SGOT], ALT [SGPT], alkaline phosphatase, bilirubin) function tests and lipid profile.
- **Diagnostic testing:** 12-lead ECG to evaluate for myocardial ischemia.
- **Hemodynamic monitoring:** Assess for pulmonary hypertension (elevated pulmonary artery pressures) and for abnormal V waves on pressure tracings to evaluate for mitral valve changes if critical care is required.
- **Vital signs:** Monitor for tachycardia and hypertension. If there are increases in BP or heart rate, discontinue sibutramine use.
- **Therapeutic effect:** Monitor for weight loss.
- **Patient education:** Urge to avoid alcohol while on sibutramine therapy. Explain that sibutramine may be habit-forming. Caution against abruptly discontinuing the medication. Warn not to take any OTC medications before consulting with the prescriber. Patients should have BP and heart rate monitored frequently and should be reminded of the importance of keeping follow-up appointments.

SERIOUS ADVERSE REACTIONS

- **Hypersensitivity:** Rash, hives, urticaria, pruritis.
- **Interstitial nephritis:** Very rarely occurs.
- **Serotonin syndrome:** May occur with concomitant use of drugs that increase serotonin.
- Seizures, thrombocytopenia, and deaths have been reported.
- Abnormal ECG, hypertension, palpitations.

OVERDOSE/TOXICITY

- **Serotonin syndrome (SS):** Altered cognition, abnormal behavior, and possibly neuromuscular dysfunction (myoclonus, hyperreflexia, muscle rigidity, extreme tremor), which can lead to seizures, hyperthermia, coma, disseminated intravascular coagulation (DIC), hypotension, ventricular tachycardia, and metabolic acidosis. May occur when given with another serotoninergic (fluoxetine [Prozac], sertraline [Zoloft, Paxil], fluvoxamine [Fluvox], citalopram [Celexa], and escitalopram [Celexa]). May occur when sibutramine is given within 14 days of an MAOI (phenelzine [Nardil], tranylcypromine [Parnate]).
- **GI decontamination:** No specific recommendations.

ANTIDOTE/DIALYSIS

- **Antidote:** No specific antidote. Cyproheptadine is the most consistently effective antiserotoninergic agent in humans. *ChlorproMAZINE may be effective. Benzodiazepines may be used as adjunctive agents to control muscle rigidity.
- **Dialysis:** Sibutramine is unlikely to be removed by hemodialysis or peritoneal dialysis. No data are available on removal by high-permeability hemodialysis.

sildenafil citrate

sill-den'-a-fill sye'-trate

Classes

Chemical: cGMP-specific phosphodiesterase inhibitor
Therapeutic: antiimpotence agent

Pregnancy Category: B

Trade Names

Prescription: Revatio, Viagra

Do not confuse Viagra with Vaniqa.

CLINICAL PHARMACOLOGY

Mechanism of Action

An erectile dysfunction agent that inhibits phosphodiesterase type 5, the enzyme responsible for degrading cyclic guanosine monophosphate in the corpus cavernosum of the penis, pulmonary vascular smooth muscle, resulting in smooth muscle relaxation and increased blood flow. Therapeutic Effects: Facilitates an erection, produces pulmonary vasodilation.

PHARMACOKINETICS

Rapidly absorbed from the GI tract. Protein binding: greater than 96%. Metabolized in the liver. Excreted primarily in the feces, urine, and semen. Half-life: 4 hr.

AVAILABILITY

Tablets: 20 mg (Revatio), 25 mg (Viagra), 50 mg (Viagra), 100 mg (Viagra).

INDICATIONS AND DOSAGE

Erectile dysfunction

PO

Adults: 50 mg (30 min-4 hr before sexual activity). Range: 25-100 mg. Maximum dosing frequency is once daily. Dose may be reduced to 25 mg if patients are using a potent CYP4503A4 inhibitor (e.g., erythromycin, itraconazole, ketoconazole) or alpha-adrenergic blockers (e.g., terazosin, doxazosin). **Elderly older than 65 yr:** Consider starting dose of 25 mg.

Pulmonary arterial hypertension

PO

Adults, Elderly: 20 mg 3 times per day.

OFF-LABEL USES

Treatment of diabetic gastroparesis, sexual dysfunction associated with the use of selective serotonin reuptake inhibitors

CONTRAINDICATIONS

Concurrent use of sodium nitroprusside, nitroglycerin, or nitrates in any form; hypersensitivity to sildenafil

INTERACTIONS

Drug: **Cimetidine, erythromycin, itraconazole, ketoconazole:** May increase sildenafil plasma concentration up to 200%. **Nitrates:** Potentiates the hypotensive effects of nitrates. **Ritonavir, saquinavir:** May cause hypotension and visual changes; increased plasma concentration of sildenafil. Herbal: None known. Food: **High-fat meals:** Delay drug's maximum effectiveness by 1 hr.

DIAGNOSTIC TEST EFFECTS

None known.

SIDE-EFFECTS

Frequent: Headache (16%), flushing (10%). Occasional (7%-3%): Dyspepsia, nasal congestion, urinary tract infection, abnormal vision, diarrhea. Rare (2%): Dizziness, rash

CRITICAL CARE CONSIDERATIONS

ADMINISTRATION/HANDLING

PO ALERT

- Sildenafil (Viagra) is usually taken 1 hr before sexual activity but may be taken anywhere from 4 hr to 30 min beforehand.
- Revatio (for pulmonary hypertension) may be given with or without food.

PRECAUTIONS

HEALTH-RELATED

- Use sildenafil cautiously in patients with an anatomic deformity of the penis; cardiac, hepatic, or renal impairment; or conditions that increase the risk of priapism, including leukemia, multiple myeloma, and sickle cell anemia.

AGE-RELATED

- **Children:** Safety and efficacy of sildenafil have not been established in children.
- **Elderly:** No age-related precautions have been noted in the elderly but have been noted to have higher drug levels than patients under 65 yr. Elderly with activity restrictions related to heart disease are advised not to use sildenafil.

S

PREGNANCY/LACTATION-RELATED

- Pregnancy category B; use not recommended in women.

MONITORING

VIAGRA

- **Baseline assessment:** Determine presence of other medical conditions, including angina, cardiac disease, and benign prostatic hypertrophy.
- **Lab work:** Biochemical profile including renal (BUN, creatinine) and liver (AST [SGOT], ALT [SGPT], bilirubin, alkaline phosphatase) function tests.
- **Patient education:** Explain that sildenafil is not effective without sexual stimulation. Warn to seek treatment immediately if an erection lasts longer than 4 hr. Instruct to avoid using nitrate drugs concurrently with sildenafil. Inform that high-fat meals may affect the drug's absorption rate and effectiveness.

REVATIO

- **Baseline assessment:** Obtain history of dyspnea, activity intolerance, and/or chest discomfort.
- **Lab work:** Obtain baseline ABGs; biochemical profile including renal (BUN, creatinine) and liver (AST [SGOT], ALT [SGPT], bilirubin, alkaline phosphatase) function tests.
- **Diagnostic tests:** Pulmonary function tests, 12-lead ECG to evaluate for myocardial ischemia, echocardiogram to evaluate right and left cardiac output and pulmonary artery pressures.
- **Hemodynamic monitoring:** Monitor pulmonary artery pressures for decrease in pressures and decreased right ventricular stroke work index.
- **Vital signs:** Assess for systemic hypotension and tachycardia. Patients may experience vasodilation.
- **Therapeutic response:** Assess for improvement in pulmonary function, decreased dyspnea on exertion, fatigue, syncope, chest pain, pulmonary vascular resistance, and pulmonary arterial pressure.
- **Patient education:** Instruct to report promptly dizziness, chest discomfort, increased shortness of breath and racing heart, or palpitations to a health care provider.

SERIOUS ADVERSE REACTIONS

- **Prolonged erections:** Erections lasting more than 4 hr and priapism (painful erections lasting over 6 hr) occur rarely.
- **Neurologic/behavioral:** Seizures and anxiety.
- **Ophthalmic:** Ocular swelling with pressure, diplopia, temporary loss of vision, vitreous detachment, paramacular edema, ocular burning, and reddened or bloodshot eyes.

OVERDOSE/TOXICITY

- **Vascular events:** Acute MI, sudden cardiac death, ventricular dysrhythmias, ischemic and hemorrhagic stroke, transient ischemic attack, epistaxis, hematuria and pulmonary hemorrhage have been reported primarily in patients with preexisting risk factors for adverse vascular events. Most events occurred during sexual activity; some occurred after sexual activity (up to days after), and some were unrelated to sexual activity.
- **GI decontamination:** No specific recommendations.

ANTIDOTE/DIALYSIS

- **Antidote:** No specific recommendations.
- **Dialysis:** Sildenafil is unlikely to be removed by hemodialysis or peritoneal dialysis. No data are available on removal by high-permeability hemodialysis.

simethicone

sye-meth'-i-kone

Classes

Chemical: siloxane polymer
Therapeutic: antiflatulent

Pregnancy Category: C

Trade Names

Over the Counter: Alka-Seltzer Gas Relief, Gas-X, Genasyme, Infant Mylicon, Mylanta Gas, Phazyme

Combinations

Over the Counter: with calcium carbonate (Titralac Plus); with aluminum hydroxide, magnesium hydroxide (Mylanta Gelisil, Maalox Extra Strength); with calcium carbonate, magnesium hydroxide (Tempo, Rolaids); with magaldrate, (Riopan Plus); with charcoal (Charcoal Plus, Flatulex)

CLINICAL PHARMACOLOGY

Mechanism of Action

An antiflatulent that changes surface tension of gas bubbles, allowing easier elimination of gas. **Therapeutic Effect:** Drug dispersal, prevents formation of gas pockets in the GI tract.

PHARMACOKINETICS

Does not appear to be absorbed from GI tract. Excreted unchanged in feces.

AVAILABILITY

Oral drops (Infant Mylicon): 40 mg/0.6 mL. **Softgel:** 125 mg (Alka-Seltzer Gas Relief, Gas-Z, Mylanta Gas), 180 mg (Phazyme). **Tablets (chewable):** 80 mg (Gas-X, Genasyme, Mylanta Gas), 125 mg (Gas-X, Mylanta Gas).

INDICATIONS AND DOSAGE

Antiflatulent

PO

Adults, Elderly, Children 12 yr and older: 40-360 mg after meals and at bedtime. Maximum: 500 mg/day. **Children 2-11 yr:** 40 mg 4 times per day after meals and at bedtime. Maximum: 240 mg/day. **Children younger than 2 yr:** 20 mg 4 times per day after meals and at bedtime. Maximum: 240 mg/day.

OFF-LABEL USES

Adjunct to bowel radiography and gastroscopy

CONTRAINDICATIONS

Hypersensitivity to simethicone, known or suspected intestinal perforation and obstruction

INTERACTIONS

Drug: None known. **Herbal:** None known. **Food:** None known.

DIAGNOSTIC TEST EFFECTS

None known.

SIDE-EFFECTS

Occasional: GI effects including diarrhea (5.5%), nausea (3.4%), and vomiting (2.1%)

CRITICAL CARE CONSIDERATIONS

ADMINISTRATION/HANDLING

PO ALERT

- Give simethicone after meals and at bedtime as needed. Chew tablets thoroughly before swallowing.
- Shake suspension well before using.

PRECAUTIONS

HEALTH-RELATED

- Use cautiously in patients with history of bowel obstruction.

AGE-RELATED

- **Children:** Simethicone may be used safely in children.
- **Elderly:** No age-related precautions have been noted.

PREGNANCY/LACTATION-RELATED

- Pregnancy category C; unknown if distributed in breast milk.

MONITORING

- **Baseline assessment:** Before simethicone administration, assess abdomen for tenderness, rigidity, and the presence of bowel sounds. Determine when last bowel movement occurred; determine amount and consistency.
- **Therapeutic effect:** Evaluate for relief of abdominal bloating and flatulence.
- **Patient education:** Urge avoidance of carbonated beverages during simethicone therapy. Instruct to chew tablets thoroughly before swallowing.

SERIOUS ADVERSE REACTIONS

- None known.

OVERDOSE/TOXICITY

- Unlikely to be life-threatening.
- **GI decontamination:** No specific recommendations.

ANTIDOTE/DIALYSIS

- **Antidote:** No specific recommendations.
- **Dialysis:** Simethicone is unlikely to be removed by hemodialysis, high-permeability hemodialysis, or peritoneal dialysis.

S

simvastatin

sim'-va-sta-tin

Classes

Chemical: substituted hexahydronaphthalene

Therapeutic: hydromethylglutyral (HMG)-CoA reductase inhibitor, antilipemic

Pregnancy Category: X

Trade Names

Prescription: Zocor

Combinations

Prescription: with ezetimibe (Vytorin)

Do not confuse Zocor with Cozaar.

CLINICAL PHARMACOLOGY

Mechanism of Action

A HMG-CoA reductase inhibitor that interferes with cholesterol biosynthesis by inhibiting the conversion of the enzyme HMG-CoA to mevalonate. **Therapeutic Effect:** Decreases serum LDL, cholesterol, VLDL, and plasma triglyceride levels; slightly increases serum HDL concentration.

PHARMACOKINETICS

Route	Onset	Peak	Duration
PO to reduce cholesterol	2 wk	4-6 wk	N/A

Well absorbed from the GI tract. Protein binding: 95%. Undergoes extensive first-pass metabolism. Hydrolyzed to active metabolite. Primarily eliminated in feces.

AVAILABILITY

Tablets: 5 mg, 10 mg, 20 mg, 40 mg, 80 mg.

INDICATIONS AND DOSAGE

Prevention of cardiovascular events, hyperlipidemias

PO

Adults, Elderly: 20-40 mg once daily. Range: 5-80 mg/day.

Homozygous familial hypercholesterol

PO

Adults, Elderly: 40 mg once every evening or 80 mg/day in divided doses (20 mg morning, 20 mg afternoon, 40 mg evening).

Heterozygous familial hypercholesterol

PO

Children 10-17 yr: 10 mg once daily in evening. Range: 5-40 mg/day. Give 5 mg/day with *cycloSPORINE, danazol, or immunosuppressive drugs (maximum 10 mg/day). Maximum: 10 mg/day with gemfibrozil and 20 mg/day with amiodarone or verapamil.

S

CONTRAINDICATIONS

Active hepatic disease or unexplained, persistent elevations of liver function test results, age younger than 18 yr, pregnancy, hypersensitivity to simvastatin

INTERACTIONS

Drug: Amiodarone: May increase risk of rhabdomyolysis. ***CycloSPORINE, erythromycin, gemfibrozil, immunosuppressants, niacin:** Increases the risk of acute renal failure and rhabdomyolysis. **Erythromycin, itraconazole, ketoconazole:** May increase simvastatin blood concentration and cause muscle inflammation, myalgia, or weakness. **Herbal:** None known. **Food: Grapefruit, grapefruit juice:** Large amounts of grapefruit juice may increase the risk of side effects, such as myalgia and weakness.

DIAGNOSTIC TEST EFFECTS

May increase serum creatine kinase (CK) and serum transaminase concentrations.

SIDE-EFFECTS

Simvastatin is generally well tolerated. Side effects are usually mild and transient. **Occasional (3%-2%):** Headache, abdominal pain or cramps, constipation, upper respiratory tract infection. **Rare (less than 2%):** Diarrhea, flatulence, asthenia (loss of strength and energy), nausea or vomiting

CRITICAL CARE CONSIDERATIONS

ADMINISTRATION/HANDLING

PO ALERT

- Patients should be placed on a standard cholesterol-lowering diet for a minimum of 3-6 mo before starting simvastatin therapy and should continue the diet throughout therapy.
- Give simvastatin without regard to meals and administer in the evening.
- Simvastatin should not be given with grapefruit juice.

PRECAUTIONS

HEALTH-RELATED

- Use simvastatin cautiously in patients with hepatic disease, hypotension, major surgery, severe acute infection, substantial alcohol consumption, uncontrolled seizures, severe endocrine, electrolyte, or metabolic disorders or trauma.
- **Cytochrome P450 enzyme metabolism:** Simvastatin is a substrate for CYP3A4, which creates the potential for numerous drug interactions.
- **Serious illness:** Simvastatin should be temporarily withheld or discontinued in acutely ill patients to avoid increased probability of development of a myopathy.
- **Increased probability of myopathy:** Increased when used concomitantly with *cycloSPORINE, erthyromycin, fibric acid derivatives, immunosuppressive drugs, niacin, and azole antifungal agents.

Withholding or discontinuing simvastatin may be necessary when patients are at risk for acute renal failure secondary to rhabdomyolysis.

AGE-RELATED

- **Children:** Safety and efficacy of simvastatin have not been established in children.
- **Elderly:** No age-related precautions have been noted.

PREGNANCY/LACTATION-RELATED

- Pregnancy category X. Breast milk excretion unknown; other drugs in this class are excreted in small amounts. Manufacturer recommends breast-feeding should be discontinued.

MONITORING

- **Baseline assessment:** Determine pregnancy or hypersensitivity to simvastatin before beginning drug therapy. If overweight, evaluate for metabolic syndrome.
- **Baseline and ongoing lab work:** Biochemical profile including serum cholesterol, hepatic enzymes (AST [SGOT], ALT [SGPT], alkaline phosphatase, GGT, bilirubin), and triglyceride levels. Monitor cholesterol and triglycerides for therapeutic response and liver enzymes every 12 wk after initial therapy and each time dosage is adjusted. Semiannual monitoring may be appropriate for patients on fixed doses with good response. Periodic laboratory tests are an essential part of ongoing therapy.
- **Baseline diagnostic tests:** 12-lead ECG to evaluate for myocardial ischemia.
- **Common side effects:** Constipation, abdominal pain, dyspepsia, and flatulence. May require symptom specific management to control.
- **Myalgias:** CPK level may be measured for patients with unexplained myalgias. Urine will appear brown if myoglobin is present.
- **Renal failure:** Monitor BUN, creatinine, and potassium levels if myalgia or brown urine indicative of myoglobinuria are manifested. Urinalysis is used to diagnose myoglobinuria.
- **Diet instruction:** Patients must follow the prescribed diet because diet is an important part of lowering cholesterol and triglycerides.
- **Patient education:** Advise to use appropriate contraceptive measures while taking simvastatin. Explain that the drug is pregnancy risk category X. Stress that periodic laboratory tests are an essential part of therapy. When therapy is continued outside the hospital, warn to consult a health care provider before taking new medications.

SERIOUS ADVERSE REACTIONS

- Lens opacities may occur.
- Hypersensitivity reaction and hepatitis occur rarely.
- **Musculoskeletal pain:** Myopathy, arthralgia, myalgia, which may indicate impending rhabdomyolysis.

OVERDOSE/TOXICITY

- **Hepatotoxicity:** Liver enzyme elevation indicative of impending liver failure.
- **Nephrotoxicity:** Acute renal failure ensues when rhabdomyolysis is present.
- **Rhabdomyolysis:** Rare cases; can lead to acute renal failure. Markedly elevated serum creatine kinase and possible myoglobinuria indicate the condition may be present. Should be managed according to accepted guidelines, which include aggressive volume replacement, hemodialysis or continuous hemofiltration (CVVH) to support patients during acute renal failure. Use of bicarbonate to induce alkaline diuresis or mannitol for osmotic diuresis has not been well studied. Hyperkalemia and hyperphosphatemia are commonly seen with rhabdomyolysis and may require aggressive management.
- **Hypocalcemia:** Must be managed cautiously with rhabdomyolysis because calcium infusion may increase the deposition of calcium in the injured muscles.
- **Medication discontinuation:** Simvastatin should be discontinued if patients develop myopathy and/or rhabdomyolysis.
- **GI decontamination:** No specific recommendations.

ANTIDOTE/DIALYSIS

- **Antidote:** No specific recommendations.
- **Dialysis:** Simvastatin is unlikely to be removed by hemodialysis or peritoneal dialysis. No data are available on removal by high-permeability hemodialysis.

simvastatin/ezetimibe

See Antihyperlipidemics (p. 928)

sirolimus

sir-oh'-li-mus

Classes
Chemical: macrolide derivative
Therapeutic: immunosuppressant

Pregnancy Category: C

Trade Names
Prescription: Rapamune

CLINICAL PHARMACOLOGY

Mechanism of Action

An immunosuppressant that inhibits T-lymphocyte proliferation induced by stimulation of cell surface receptors, mitogens, alloantigens, and lymphokines. Prevents activation of the enzyme target of rapamycin, a key regulatory kinase in cell cycle progression. Therapeutic Effect: Inhibits proliferation of T and B cells, essential components of the immune response; prevents organ transplant rejection.

PHARMACOKINETICS

Rapidly absorbed from the GI tract. Protein binding: 92%. Extensively metabolized in the liver. Primarily eliminated in feces; minimal excretion in urine. Half-life: 57-63 hr.

AVAILABILITY

Oral solution: 1 mg/mL.
Tablets: 1 mg, 2 mg, 5 mg.

INDICATIONS AND DOSAGE

Prevention of organ transplant rejection

PO

Adults: Loading dose: 6 mg. Maintenance: 2 mg/day. **Children 13 yr and older weighing less than 40 kg:** Loading dose: 3 mg/m^2. Maintenance: 1 mg/m^2/day.

S

OFF-LABEL USES

Immunosuppression of other organ transplants

CONTRAINDICATIONS

Hypersensitivity to sirolimus (Rapamune)

INTERACTIONS

Drug: ***CycloSPORINE, diltiazem, ketoconazole, fluconazole, itraconazole, voriconazole:** May increase the blood concentration and risk of toxicity of sirolimus. **Rifampin:** May decrease the blood concentration and effects of sirolimus. Herbal: None known. Food: **Grapefruit, grapefruit juice:** May decrease the metabolism of sirolimus.

DIAGNOSTIC TEST EFFECTS

May decrease blood Hgb level, Hct, and platelet count. May increase serum cholesterol, creatinine, and triglyceride levels.

SIDE-EFFECTS

Occasional: Hypercholesterolemia, hyperlipidemia, hypertension, rash; with high doses (5 mg/day): anemia, arthralgia, diarrhea, hypokalemia, and thrombocytopenia. Rare: Peripheral edema, hypertension

CRITICAL CARE CONSIDERATIONS

ADMINISTRATION/HANDLING

PO ALERT

- **Dosage equivalency:** Tablets and solution are not bioequivalent. Tablet has 27% greater bioavailability; however, 2-mg tablets are clinically equivalent to 2-mg oral solution; not known if higher doses of oral solution are clinically equivalent to higher doses of tabs; IV formulation is under development.
- **Storage:** Oral solution bottles and pouches should be protected from light and refrigerated. Open containers should be used within 1 mo. Pouches may be stored for 24 hr at controlled room temperature; bottles can be stored up to 15 days at controlled room temperature. Oral solution may develop a slight haze, which may resolve as drug is exposed to room temperature or slightly shaken. Haze does not impair the quality of the drug.
- Use of sirolimus should allow for lower dosage of *cycloSPORINE to be effective in controlling transplant rejection.
- Experience is limited for use as rescue therapy.
- African American patients had higher rejection rates (56% vs. 13%) than non–African Americans given same regimen; no significant differences in trough sirolimus concentrations at equal doses between African Americans and non–African Americans.
- **Experienced prescribers only:** Patients should be managed by facilities with a properly equipped laboratory, with staff and physicians trained in immunosuppressive therapy and management of transplant patients.
- **Cytochrome P450 enzyme metabolism:** Sirolimus is a substrate for CYP3A4 and P-glycoprotein, prompting drug interactions

with *cycloSPORINE, diltiazem, ketoconazole, and rifampin.

PRECAUTIONS

HEALTH-RELATED

- Use sirolimus cautiously in patients with chicken pox, herpes zoster, hepatic impairment, or an infection.
- Increased susceptibility to infection and development of lymphoma and other malignancies may be prompted by immunosuppression.

AGE-RELATED

- **Children:** Safety and efficacy of sirolimus have not been established in children under 13 yr.
- **Elderly:** No age-related precautions have been noted.

PREGNANCY/LACTATION-RELATED

- Pregnancy category C; excretion into breast milk unknown; use caution in nursing mothers.

MONITORING

- **Baseline assessment:** Determine presence of chicken pox, herpes zoster, an infection, or a malignancy; or if other medications, especially *cycloSPORINE, diltiazem, ketoconazole, and rifampin are being taken. Determine whether female patients are pregnant or breast-feeding.
- **Lab work:** Baseline and ongoing CBC with WBC differential and platelet count; biochemical profile including liver (AST [SGOT], ALT [SGPT], alkaline phosphatase, bilirubin) and renal (BUN, creatinine) function tests and serum lipid profile. Whole-blood sirolimus levels (drawn 1 hr before next dose), are done 5-7 days after initiation or dose change. Maintain levels at 10-15 ng/mL for first mo, then consider increasing to 15-20 ng/mL, especially in patients receiving lower doses of *cycloSPORINE.
- **Infection versus rejection:** Dosing of immunosuppressive medications is a delicate balance between development of a serious infection (overly immunosuppressed) and rejection of the transplanted organ (not receiving enough immunosuppression). Fluid volume excess is common during rejection.
- **Organ rejection:** Assess for organ rejection. Signs of organ rejection are organ-specific, but all patients may have low-grade, persistent fevers. With acute rejection, fevers may be higher (100-104°F). Symptoms of organ rejection will reflect failure of the affected organ. Appropriate testing should include the same evaluation done to assess for failure of the transplanted organ.
- **Patient education:** Instruct to take sirolimus at the same time each day with regard to timing of meals and other medications and to report missed doses to the prescriber. Tell to avoid drinking grapefruit or grapefruit juice during therapy and to avoid coming in contact with people with colds or other infections. Remind that strict monitoring is an essential part of identifying and preventing symptoms of organ rejection in sirolimus therapy. Advise to limit UV/sunlight exposure, wear protective clothing, and use sunsreen because of increased risk of skin cancer.

SERIOUS ADVERSE REACTIONS

- **Renal transplant patients:** Use of sirolimus may prompt increased serum cholesterol and triglycerides requiring treatment.
- **Liver transplant patients:** Use of sirolimus in combination with tacrolimus was associated with excess mortality and graft loss to de novo liver transplant patients; use with *cycloSPORINE and tacrolimus resulted in hepatic artery thrombosis.
- **Lung transplant patients:** Cases of fatal bronchial anastamotic dehiscence have been linked to use of sirolimus in de novo lung transplant patients.

OVERDOSE/TOXICITY

- **Infection:** Herpes zoster, mycobacterial infections, Epstein-Barr virus infection.
- **Hematologic:** Anemia, leukopenia, thrombocytopenia, pancytopenia.
- **Hepatotoxicity:** Occurs rarely.
- **Pancreatitis:** Occurs rarely.
- **GI decontamination:** No specific recommendations.

ANTIDOTE/DIALYSIS

- **Antidote:** No specific recommendations.
- **Dialysis:** Sirolimus is unlikely to be removed by hemodialysis. No data are available on removal by high-permeability hemodialysis or peritoneal dialysis.

sodium bicarbonate 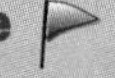

soe'-dee-um bye-car'-bon-ate

Classes

Chemical: monosodium salt of carbonic acid
Therapeutic: alkalinizing agent, systemic/urinary; antacid; electrolyte supplement

Pregnancy Category: C

Trade Names

Prescription: Neut

Combinations

Over the Counter: with alginic acid, (AlOH, Mg Trisilicate Gastrocote); with sodium citrate (Citrocarbonate)

CLINICAL PHARMACOLOGY

Mechanism of Action

An alkalinizing agent that dissociates to provide bicarbonate ion. Therapeutic Effect: Neutralizes hydrogen ion concentration, raises blood and urinary pH.

PHARMACOKINETICS

Route	Onset	Peak	Duration
PO	15 min	N/A	1-3 hr
IV	Immediate	N/A	8-10 min

After administration, sodium bicarbonate dissociates to sodium and bicarbonate ions. With increased hydrogen ion concentrations bicarbonate ions combine with hydrogen ions to form carbonic acid, which then dissociates to CO_2, which is excreted by the lungs.

AVAILABILITY

Tablets: 325 mg, 650 mg.
Injection: 4%, 0.5 mEq/mL (4.2%), 0.6 mEq/mL (5%), 0.9 mEq/mL (7.5%), 1 mEq/mL (8.4%).

INDICATIONS AND DOSAGE

Cardiac arrest

IV

Adults, Elderly: Initially 1 mEq/kg (as 7.5%-8.4% solution). May repeat with 0.5 mEq/kg every 10 min during continued cardiopulmonary arrest. Use in the postresuscitation phase is based on arterial blood pH, partial pressure of carbon dioxide in arterial blood ($PaCO_2$), and base deficit calculation. **Children, Infants:** Initially, 1 mEq/kg.

Metabolic acidosis (not severe)

IV

Adults, Elderly, Children: 2-5 mEq/kg over 4-8 hr. May repeat based on laboratory values.

Metabolic acidosis (associated with chronic renal failure)

PO

Adults, Elderly: Initially 20-36 mEq/day in divided doses.

Renal tubular acidosis (distal)

PO

Adults, Elderly: 0.5-2 mEq/kg/day in 4-6 divided doses. **Children:** 2-3 mEq/kg/day in divided doses.

Renal tubular acidosis (proximal)

PO

Adults, Elderly, Children: 5-10 mEq/kg/day in divided doses.

Urine alkalinization

PO

Adults, Elderly: Initially, 4 g, then 1-2 g every 4 hr. Maximum: 16 g/day. **Children:** 84-840 mg/kg/day in divided doses.

Antacid

PO

Adults, Elderly: 300 mg to 2 g 1-4 times per day.

Hyperkalemia

IV

Adults, Elderly: 1 mEq/kg over 5 min.

CONTRAINDICATIONS

Excessive chloride loss because of diarrhea, diuretics, GI suctioning, or vomiting; hypocalcemia; metabolic or respiratory alkalosis; hypersensitivity to components of sodium bicarbonate products

INTERACTIONS

Drug: **Calcium-containing products:** May result in milk-alkali syndrome. **Corticosteroids:** May cause edema and hypertension. **Lithium, salicylates:** May increase the excretion of these drugs. **Methenamine:** May decrease the effects of methenamine. Herbal: None known. Food: **Milk, other dairy products:** May result in milk-alkali syndrome.

DIAGNOSTIC TEST EFFECTS

May increase serum and urinary pH.

IV INCOMPATIBILITIES

Ascorbic acid, calcium chloride, diltiazem (Cardizem), *DOBUtamine (Dobutrex), *DOPamine (Intropin), hydromorphone (Dilaudid), magnesium sulfate, midazolam (Versed), morphine, norepinephrine (Levophed), total parenteral nutrition (TPN)

IV COMPATIBILITIES

Aminophylline, furosemide (Lasix), heparin, insulin, lidocaine, mannitol, milrinone (Primacor), morphine, phenylephrine (Neo-Synephrine), phenytoin (Dilantin), potassium chloride, propofol (Diprivan), vancomycin (Vancocin)

SIDE-EFFECTS

Frequent: Abdominal distention, flatulence, belching

CRITICAL CARE CONSIDERATIONS

ADMINISTRATION/HANDLING

PO ALERT

- Give sodium bicarbonate 1-3 hr after meals.
- Do not give other oral drugs within 2 hr of sodium bicarbonate administration.

IV ALERT

- **Storage:** Store vials at room temperature.
- **Dilution:** Sodium bicarbonate may be given undiluted. Use a 0.5 mEq/mL concentration for direct IV administration to neonates and infants.
- **IV push:** Give up to 1 mEq/kg over 1-3 min for cardiac arrest.
- **IV infusion:** Do not exceed an infusion rate of 50 mEq/hr. For children under 2 yr, premature infants, and neonates, do not infuse more than 8 mEq/min.
- **Dosage:** Dosage is individualized based on age, weight, clinical conditions, electrolyte levels, and severity of acidosis; administer sodium bicarbonate when plasma bicarbonate level is less than 15 mEq/L. Metabolic alkalosis may result if the bicarbonate deficit is fully corrected during the first 24 hr.

PRECAUTIONS

HEALTH-RELATED

- Use sodium bicarbonate cautiously in patients with heart failure, renal insufficiency, edema, and in those receiving concurrent corticosteroid therapy.

AGE-RELATED

- **Children:** No age-related precautions have been noted; however, sodium bicarbonate should not be used as an antacid in children under 6 yr.
- **Elderly:** Age-related renal or cardiovascular impairment may require cautious use; contains sodium which increases fluid retention.

PREGNANCY/LACTATION-RELATED

- Pregnancy category C; may be distributed in breast milk and produce hypernatremia and increased deep tendon reflexes in the neonate or fetus if the mother was given chronically high doses.

MONITORING

- **Baseline assessment:** Assess for signs of metabolic acidosis, including disorientation, hyperventilation, and weakness. For those using oral bicarbonate, assess for GI symptoms, including flatulence and abdominal distention.
- **Baseline and ongoing lab work:** Biochemical panel including electrolytes, BUN, creatinine, magnesium, calcium, phosphates and uric acid; ABG for pH, $PaCO_2$ and CO_2, plasma bicarbonate; urine sample for urinary pH.
- **Fluid retention:** Observe for fluid overload and metabolic alkalosis.
- **Metabolic acidosis:** Assess for clinical improvement of metabolic acidosis, including relief from disorientation, hyperventilation, and weakness.
- **Dyspepsia:** Assess for relief of gastric distress.
- **Hypochloremia:** Assess pattern of daily bowel activity, stool consistency, and vomiting. Bicarbonate is not recommended for correction of acidosis because of excessive chloride losses due to excessive diarrhea, GI suction, or vomiting.
- **Patient education:** Advise patients considering breast-feeding to consult a health care provider before taking sodium bicarbonate. Encourage to consult with the prescriber before taking any OTC drugs because they may contain sodium.

SERIOUS ADVERSE REACTIONS

- **Fluid overload:** Headache, weakness, blurred vision, behavioral changes, incoordination, muscle twitching, elevated BP, bradycardia, tachypnea, wheezing, coughing, and distended neck veins.
- **Extravasation:** May occur at the IV site, resulting in tissue necrosis and ulceration.

S

OVERDOSE/TOXICITY

- **Excessive or chronic use:** May produce metabolic alkalosis characterized by irritability, twitching, paresthesias, cyanosis, slow or shallow respirations, headache, thirst, nausea, and tetany.
- **Management:** Discontinue sodium bicarbonate. Administration of a balanced electrolyte solution (Normosol-M, Plasmalyte-56) with added sodium and potassium chloride may be used to help correct pH, but additional sodium may be undesirable. Ammonium chloride may help lower pH. Treat tetany with calcium gluconate.
- **GI decontamination:** No specific recommendations.

ANTIDOTE/DIALYSIS

- **Antidote:** No specific recommendations.
- **Dialysis:** Hemodialysis, high-permeability hemodialysis, and peritoneal dialysis are not able to isolate sodium bicarbonate for removal, but may be used as adjunctive strategies to manage pH and electrolyte imbalance.

sodium chloride

soe'-dee-um klor'-ide

Classes

Chemical: monovalent cation
Therapeutic: electrolyte supplement, irrigant, moisturizing agent

Pregnancy Category: C

Trade Names

Over the Counter: Muro 128, Nasal Mist, Nasal Moist, Ocean, SalineX, SeaMist, Slo-Salt

CLINICAL PHARMACOLOGY

Mechanism of Action

Sodium is a major cation of extracellular fluid that controls water distribution, fluid and electrolyte balance, and osmotic pressure of body fluids; it also maintains acid-base balance.

PHARMACOKINETICS

Well absorbed from the GI tract. Widely distributed. Primarily excreted in urine.

AVAILABILITY

Tablets (OTC): 1 g.
Injection (concentrate): 23.4% (4 mEq/mL).
Injection: 0.45%, 0.9%, 3%.
Irrigation: 0.45%, 0.9%.
Nasal Gel (Nasal Moist): 0.65%.
Nasal solution (OTC): 0.4% (SalineX), 0.65% (Nasal Moist, SeaMist).
Ophthalmic solution (OTC [Muro 128]): 5%.
Ophthalmic ointment (OTC [Muro 128]): 5%.

INDICATIONS AND DOSAGE

Prevention and treatment of sodium and chloride deficiencies; source of hydration
IV
Adults, Elderly: 1-2 L/day 0.9% or 0.45% or 100 mL 3% or 5% over 1 hr; assess serum electrolyte levels before giving additional fluid.

Prevention of heat prostration and muscle cramps from excessive perspiration
PO
Adults, Elderly: 1-2 g 3 times per day.

Relief of dry and inflamed nasal membranes
Intranasal
Adults, Elderly: Use as needed.

Diagnostic aid in ophthalmoscopic exam, treatment of corneal edema
Ophthalmic solution
Adults, Elderly: Apply 1-2 drops every 3-4 hr.
Ophthalmic ointment
Adults, Elderly: Apply once per day or as directed.

CONTRAINDICATIONS

Fluid retention, hypernatremia, hypersensitivity to sodium chloride products

INTERACTIONS

Drug: **Hypertonic saline solution, oxytocics:** May cause uterine hypertonus, ruptures, or lacerations. **Herbal:** None known. **Food:** None known.

DIAGNOSTIC TEST EFFECTS

None known.

SIDE-EFFECTS

Frequent: Facial flushing. **Occasional:** Fever; irritation, phlebitis, or extravasation at injection site
Ophthalmic: Temporary burning or irritation

CRITICAL CARE CONSIDERATIONS

ADMINISTRATION/HANDLING

PO ALERT

- Do not crush or break enteric-coated or slow-release tablets.
- Administer tablets with a full glass of water.

NASAL ALERT

- Instruct to begin inhaling slowly just before releasing the drug into nose. Teach how to inhale slowly and exhale gently through the mouth. Have patients continue this technique for 20-30 sec after administration.

IV ALERT

- **Hypertonic solutions (3% or 5%):** Administer through a large vein at a rate not exceeding 100 mL/hr. Avoid infiltration.

- **Dilution:** Dilute vials containing 2.5 to 4 mEq/mL (concentrated NaCl) with D_5W or $D_{10}W$ before administration.
- **Dosage:** Based on acid-base status, age, weight, clinical condition, and fluid and electrolyte status.
- **Hypotonic solutions (0.45%):** May be used for hydration in patients who need water replacement, but without the full amount of sodium.
- **Normotonic solutions (0.9%):** May be used for hydration in conjunction with blood transfusions or as a flush to keep IV lines patent, as a diluent for drugs, to help manage metabolic alkalosis, and as an antidote for drug-induced hypercalcemia.

OPHTHALMIC ALERT

- **Administration:** Place a gloved finger on the lower eyelid; pull it out until a pocket is formed between the eye and lower lid. Hold the dropper above the pocket and instill the prescribed number of drops (or apply a thin strip of ointment) in the pocket. Close eyes gently so the drug is not squeezed out of the sac. Apply gentle finger pressure to the lacrimal sac for 1 to 2 min to reduce systemic absorption. Release the lower lid; keep the affected eye open without blinking for at least 30 sec and roll the eyeball to distribute the drug.

PRECAUTIONS

HEALTH-RELATED

- Use sodium chloride cautiously in patients with cirrhosis, heart failure, hypertension, or renal impairment.

AGE-RELATED

- **Children:** Safety and efficacy of sodium chloride for use in children have not been established. Do not administer sodium and chloride preserved with benzyl alcohol to neonates.
- **Elderly:** Age-related renal or cardiovascular disease may prompt a dosage reduction.

PREGNANCY/LACTATION-RELATED

- Pregnancy category C; distributed in breast milk.

MONITORING

- **Baseline assessment:** Assess weight and fluid balance; examine for edema; auscultate breath sounds to determine if heart failure may be present.
- **Baseline lab work:** Biochemical profile to assess electrolytes; if used for metabolic alkalosis, ABG to determine pH, pCO_2, HCO_3; calcium level if used to manage hypercalcemia.
- **Extravasation:** Assess the IV site for extravasation. If present, aspirate available solution (up to 5 mL) though the needle still in place, remove needle, and apply warm compresses.
- **Fluid/electrolyte/acid-base balance:** Monitor for fluid retention, developing acidosis, change in BP, hypernatremia (edema, hypertension, weight gain); hyponatremia (dry mucous membranes, muscle cramps, nausea, vomiting), and hyperchloremia (may lead to acidosis).
- **Patient education:** For ophthalmic preparations, inform that temporary burning or irritation may be noted after instillation of the ophthalmic drug. Instruct to discontinue the ophthalmic medication and promptly report acute redness of eyes, floating spots, severe eye pain or pain on exposure to light, a rapid change in vision (side and straight ahead), or headache to a health care provider.

SERIOUS ADVERSE REACTIONS

- **Fluid retention:** Too-rapid administration may produce peripheral edema, heart failure, and pulmonary edema.

OVERDOSE/TOXICITY

- **Excessive dosage:** Hypokalemia, hypervolemia, hypernatremia, and hyperchloremia.
- **GI decontamination:** No specific recommendations.

ANTIDOTE/DIALYSIS

- **Antidote:** No specific recommendations.
- **Dialysis:** Sodium chloride may be removed by hemodialysis, high-permeability hemodialysis, or peritoneal dialysis.

S

sodium ferric gluconate

soe'-dee-um fer'-ric glue'-kun-ate

Pregnancy Category: B

Trade Names

Prescription: Ferrlecit

CLINICAL PHARMACOLOGY

Mechanism of Action

A trace element that repletes total iron content in the body. Replaces iron found in

Hgb, myoglobin, and specific enzymes; allows oxygen transport via Hgb. **Therapeutic Effect:** Prevents and corrects iron deficiency.

PHARMACOKINETICS

Half-life: 1 hr.

AVAILABILITY

Ampules: 12.5 mg/mL elemental iron.

INDICATIONS AND DOSAGE

Iron deficiency anemia

IV Infusion

Adults, Elderly: 125 mg in 100 mL 0.9% NaCl infused over 1 hr. Minimum cumulative dose 1 g elemental iron given over 8 sessions at sequential dialysis treatments. May be given during dialysis session. **Children 6 yr and older:** 1.5 mg/kg diluted in 25 mL 0.9% NaCl administered over 60 min at sequential dialysis sessions. Maximum: 125 mg/dose.

CONTRAINDICATIONS

All anemias not associated with iron deficiency, hypersensitivity to iron products

INTERACTIONS

Drug: Aluminum-, calcium-, magnesium-containing drugs: May decrease iron effectiveness. **Ibandronate, levodopa, quinolone antibiotics:** May decrease the effectiveness of these drugs. **Herbal:** None known. **Food: High calcium foods (e.g., dairy products):** May decrease iron effectiveness.

DIAGNOSTIC TEST EFFECTS

None known.

IV INCOMPATIBILITIES

Do not mix with other medications.

S

SIDE-EFFECTS

Frequent (greater than 3%): Flushing, hypotension, hypersensitivity reaction. **Occasional (3%-1%):** Injection site reaction, headache, abdominal pain, chills, flulike syndrome, dizziness, leg cramps, dyspnea, nausea, vomiting, diarrhea, myalgia, pruritus, edema

CRITICAL CARE CONSIDERATIONS

ADMINISTRATION/HANDLING

IV ALERT

- **Test dose:** Administer a 25-mg test dose; dilute in 50 mL 0.9% NaCl; infuse over 1 hr.
- **Slow IV injection:** May give undiluted as slow IV injection without test dose.
- **Storage:** Store at room temperature.
- **Dilution:** Standard recommended dose is 125 mg (10 mL) diluted with 100 mL 0.9% NaCl. Use immediately after dilution. Infuse over 1 hr.
- Do not give concurrently with oral iron. Excessive iron intake may produce excessive iron storage (hemosiderosis).

PRECAUTIONS

HEALTH-RELATED

- Use sodium ferric gluconate complex cautiously in patients with asthma, iron overload, hepatic impairment, rheumatoid arthritis, or significant allergies.
- Renal impaired patients may not respond to iron without receiving erythropoetin, in addition to iron therapy for anemia.

AGE-RELATED

- **Children:** Safety and efficacy of sodium ferric gluconate complex have not been established in children.
- **Elderly:** No age-related precautions have been noted; however, lower initial dosages of sodium ferric gluconate complex are recommended.

PREGNANCY/LACTATION-RELATED

- Pregnancy category B; unknown if distributed in breast milk.

MONITORING

- **Baseline assessment:** Assess nutritional status, dietary iron intake, and vital signs.
- **Baseline lab work:** CBC and serum iron concentrations. Test results may not be meaningful for 3 wk after beginning sodium ferric gluconate complex therapy.
- **Hypotension:** Have patients remain lying down throughout and after infusion; hypotension may be related to hemodialysis treatment or too rapid infusion rate.
- **Hypersensitivity reaction:** Monitor for urticaria, respiratory distress, and flushing throughout infusion. Patients should receive a test dose before infusion.
- **Acute joint pain:** Assess patients with rheumatoid arthritis or iron deficiency anemia for acute exacerbation of joint pain and swelling.
- **Patient education:** Advise that stools may become black during iron therapy; this effect is harmless. Instruct to report abdominal cramping, pain with red streaking and

sticky consistency of stool. Inform that the drug may be administered during dialysis treatments.

SERIOUS ADVERSE REACTIONS

- **Hypersensitivity reaction:** Dyspnea, angioedema, urticaria, bronchospasm, cardiovascular collapse, and cardiac arrest; rare.
- **Rapid administration:** May cause hypotension associated with flushing, lightheadedness, fatigue, weakness, or severe pain in the chest, back, or groin.

OVERDOSE/TOXICITY

- **Overdose:** Nausea, vomiting, diarrhea, abdominal pain, possible GI bleeding followed by altered mental status, pallor or cyanosis, drowsiness, metabolic acidosis, hyperventilation (secondary to acidosis), iatrogenic hemosiderosis, hypotension, cardiac arrest. Patients may develop acute respiratory distress syndrome.
- **Management:** Discontinue infusion or reduce infusion rate; manage hypotension with plasma expanders (hetastarch, albumin, dextran). Provide supportive care; resuscitate according to Advanced Cardiac Life Support (ACLS) guidelines.
- **GI decontamination:** No specific recommendations.

ANTIDOTE/DIALYSIS

- **Antidote:** Deferoxamine is the specific chelator for iron poisoning and should be initiated as early as possible. After combining with free iron (iron outside of hemoglobin, myoglobin, transferrin, or ferritin), it forms ferrioxamine, which is excreted in urine. Deferoxamine also promotes effective clearance of intracellular iron.
- **Dialysis:** Sodium ferric gluconate complex is not removed by hemodialysis, high-permeability hemodialysis, or peritoneal dialysis.

sodium nitrate

See Antidotes (p. 918)

sodium polystyrene sulfonate

soe'-dee-um po-lee-stye'-reen sul'-foe-nate

Classes

Chemical: cation exchange resin
Therapeutic: antihyperkalemic

Pregnancy Category: C

Trade Names

Prescription: Kayexalate, Kionex, SPS

CLINICAL PHARMACOLOGY

Mechanism of Action

An ion-exchange resin that releases sodium ions in exchange primarily for potassium ions. **Therapeutic Effect:** Moves potassium from the blood into the intestine so it can be expelled from the body.

PHARMACOKINETICS

Not absorbed from GI tract. Not metabolized. Completely excreted in feces.

AVAILABILITY

Suspension (SPS): 15 g/60 mL.
Powder for suspension (Kayexalate, Kionex): 454 g.
Rectal enema: 15 g/60 mL, 50 g/200 mL.

INDICATIONS AND DOSAGE

Hyperkalemia

PO

Adults, Elderly: 60 mL (15 g) 1-4 times per day. **Children:** 1 g/kg/dose every 6 hr.

Rectal

Adults, Elderly: 30-50 g as needed every 6 hr. **Children:** 1 g/kg/dose every 2-6 hr.

CONTRAINDICATIONS

Hypokalemia, hypernatremia, intestinal obstruction or perforation, hypersensitivity to sodium polystyrene sulfonate

INTERACTIONS

Drug: Cation-donating antacids, laxatives (such as magnesium hydroxide): May decrease effect of sodium polystyrene sulfonate, and cause systemic alkalosis in patients with renal impairment. **Herbal:** None known. **Food:** None known.

DIAGNOSTIC TEST EFFECTS

May decrease serum calcium and magnesium levels.

SIDE-EFFECTS

Frequent: High dosage: Anorexia, nausea, vomiting, constipation

High dosage in elderly: Fecal impaction characterized by severe stomach pain with nausea or vomiting. **Occasional:** Diarrhea, sodium retention marked by decreased urination, peripheral edema, and increased weight

CRITICAL CARE CONSIDERATIONS

ADMINISTRATION/HANDLING

PO ALERT

- Give with 20-100 mL sorbitol to aid in potassium removal, facilitate passage of resin through intestinal tract, and prevent constipation.
- Do not mix sodium polystyrene sulfonate with foods or liquids containing potassium.

RECTAL ALERT

- **Preparation:** After initial cleansing enema, insert large rubber tube well into sigmoid colon and tape in place.
- **Retention enema:** Introduce suspension with 100 mL sorbitol by gravity. Flush with 50-100 mL fluid and clamp. Enema should be retained for 30 min to several hr, if possible. Irrigate colon with a non-sodium-containing solution to remove resin.

PRECAUTIONS

HEALTH-RELATED

- Use sodium polystyrene sulfonate cautiously in patients with edema, hypertension, or severe heart failure.

AGE-RELATED

- **Children:** No age-related precautions have been noted in children.
- **Elderly:** May be at increased risk for fecal impaction.

PREGNANCY/LACTATION-RELATED

- Pregnancy category C; excretion in breast milk not expected.

MONITORING

- **Baseline assessment:** Assess severity of hyperkalemia. Sodium polystyrene sulfonate does not rapidly correct severe hyperkalemia (it may take hours to days). Consider other measures such as dialysis, IV glucose and insulin, IV calcium, and IV sodium bicarbonate to correct severe hyperkalemia in a medical emergency.
- **Lab work:** Biochemical profile including potassium, calcium, and magnesium levels. Monitor serum potassium level frequently. Monitor serum calcium and magnesium levels with at least every other potassium level.
- **Dysrhythmias:** Hyperkalemia can cause loss of P wave, widening of the QRS complex and prolongation of the QT interval. Assess clinical condition and ECG, which is valuable in determining when treatment should be discontinued.
- **Constipation:** Assess pattern of daily bowel activity and stool consistency. Fecal impaction may occur in patients receiving high dosages of sodium polystyrene sulfonate, particularly the elderly.
- **Ongoing hyperkalemia management:** Consult a dietician to provide dietary instructions about potassium.
- **Patient education:** Instruct to drink the entire amount of the resin for best results. Urge patients receiving sodium polystyrene sulfonate rectally to try to retain the solution for several hours, if possible. Instruct about which foods are rich in potassium.

SERIOUS ADVERSE REACTIONS

- **Hypocalcemia:** Abdominal or muscle cramps occur occasionally.
- **Fluid overload:** May occur due to absorption of sodium from the drug, which can result in fluid retention.
- **Dysrhythmias:** Hyperkalemia and hypokalemia cause ECG and heart rhythm changes. Hyperkalemic patients can become hypokalemic with aggressive treatment. Potassium imbalance also affects magnesium and calcium levels, which may prompt additional dysrhythmias.

OVERDOSE/TOXICITY

- **Hypokalemia:** Potassium deficiency may occur. Early signs of hypokalemia include confusion, delayed thought processes, extreme weakness, irritability, and ECG changes (including prolonged QT interval; QRS widening, flattening, or inversion of T wave; and prominent U waves).
- **Management:** Careful administration of IV potassium supplements if patients are symptomatic.

S

- **GI decontamination:** No specific recommendations.

ANTIDOTE/DIALYSIS

- **Antidote:** Potassium replacement with a well-diluted IV potassium chloride infusion.
- **Dialysis:** Sodium polystyrene sulfonate is unlikely to be removed by hemodialysis, high-permeability hemodialysis, or peritoneal dialysis.

sodium thiosulfate

soe'-dee-um thye-oh-sul'-fate

Classes
Chemical: sodium hyposulfite
Therapeutic: antidote, antineoplastic adjunct

Pregnancy Category: C

Trade Names
Prescription: Cyanide Antidote Package

CLINICAL PHARMACOLOGY

Mechanism of Action
An antidote for cyanide poisoning that converts cyanide to the nontoxic thiocyanate ion and involves the enzyme rhodanese (thiosulfate: cyanide sulfurtransferase). **Therapeutic Effect:** Cyanide detoxification.

PHARMACOKINETICS

Excreted unchanged in urine. **Half-life:** 80 min.

AVAILABILITY

Intravenous solution: 10%, 25%.

INDICATIONS AND DOSAGE

Cyanide poisoning
IV
Adults: 12.5 g over 10 min after giving sodium nitrite 300 mg. Repeat as needed with 6.25 g over 10 min after sodium nitrite 150 g. **Children:** 7 g per square meter of body surface area administered at 0.625-1.25 g/min IV. Maximum: 12.5 g.

CONTRAINDICATIONS

Hypersensitivity to sodium thiosulfate

INTERACTIONS

Drug: None known. **Herbal:** None known. **Food:** None known.

DIAGNOSTIC TEST EFFECTS

None known.

SIDE-EFFECTS

Occasional: Diarrhea

CRITICAL CARE CONSIDERATIONS

ADMINISTRATION/HANDLING

IV ALERT

- **Risk of death:** Delays in administering sodium thiosulfate should be avoided; death from cyanide poisoning occurs rapidly.
- **Storage:** Store at room temperature. Inspect visually for particulate matter and discoloration before administering.
- **IV push/direct injection:** Administer slowly over 10 min.
- **Recurrent symptoms:** If symptoms return, sodium thiosulfate dosage should be repeated at one-half the original dose.

PRECAUTIONS

HEALTH-RELATED

- **Cyanide poisoning:** Death occurs rapidly. Sodium thiosulfate should be given promptly following diagnosis of cyanide toxicity. Renal impaired patients are more likely to develop cyanide toxicity. Cyanide toxicity should be considered when CNS dysfunction, metabolic acidosis, and cardiovascular dysfunction are present. Patients exposed to nitriles (used as solvents, intermediates in chemical synthesis, in nylon production and other industrial uses) may be asymptomatic when cyanide toxicity is present.
- **Sodium nitroprusside toxicity:** Patients receiving nitroprusside at greater than 4 mcg/kg/min are at risk of developing both cyanide toxicity and thiocyanate toxicity. Nitroprusside infusions should be limited to 1-2 days in patients with renal insufficiency and 6-7 days in those with normal kidneys. Doses should not exceed 0.5-1.5 mg/kg to avoid cyanide toxicity. Circulating cyanide levels start increasing in 2-3 hr at doses of about 2 mcg/kg/min.

AGE-RELATED

- **Children:** No age-related precautions have been noted. Children and neonates have been successfully managed following sodium nitroprusside (Nipride)-induced cyanide toxicity.
- **Elderly:** No age-related precautions have been noted. Cyanide toxicity is more common in older patients receiving nitroprusside (Nipride) because of age-related renal dysfunction.

S

PREGNANCY/LACTATION-RELATED

- Pregnancy category C; unknown if distributed in breast milk.

MONITORING

- **Baseline assessment for nitroprusside toxicity:** Assess patients receiving sodium nitroprusside (Nipride, SNP) for toxicity (agitation, confusion, coma, seizures, cerebral death, tachycardia, bradycardia, hypotension, or early hypertension). Metabolic acidosis is present in cyanide-poisoned patients but not present in those with thiocyanate toxicity more commonly seen with nitroprusside toxicity. Avoid delays in administering the antidote.
- **Baseline assessment for industry, work-related, and smoke-related cyanide poisoning:** Assess for exposure to the 3 main sources of cyanide: hydrogen cyanide, inorganic cyanide salts, and cyanogens (compounds that release cyanide or undergo metabolism to cyanide after absorption; nitriles are the most common industry-related cyanogens). Smoke, including cigarette smoke, contains hydrogen cyanide. Cyanide poisoning may cause death from smoke inhalation, especially if plastics were involved in the fire.
- **Lab work:** Thiocyanate (SCN-) level to determine thiocyanate toxicity. Serum or plasma thiocyanate concentrations are nontoxic in most patients with cyanide toxicity and are not diagnostic for cyanide poisoning. Whole blood cyanide concentrations are not analyzed quickly enough to be helpful in managing cyanide poisoning. Biochemical profile including renal (BUN, creatinine) function tests helps identify patients at higher risk for cyanide toxicity. Diagnosis is most often based on clinical findings. Moderate/severe thiocyanate toxicity is asymptomatic until thiocyanate levels are greater than 150-200 mg/L (15-20 mg/dL).
- **SNP (Nipride) cyanide prevention:** Keep drug well protected from sunlight to avoid cyanide release. When nitroprusside (Nipride) is exposed to direct sunlight, drug decomposes rapidly to release cyanide. The drug does not decompose in response to artificial indoor lighting.
- **Hemodynamic monitoring:** Cyanide or thiocyanate toxic patients may have low systemic vascular resistance and decreased oxygen consumption. Low systemic vascular resistance, decreased oxygen consumption, anion gap metabolic acidosis, and elevated lactate levels are also seen with sepsis, liver failure, systemic inflammatory response syndrome, and toxic shock syndrome.
- **Concommitant infusions:** Patients receiving both nitroprusside and sodium thiosulfate (may help reduce possibility of SNP-induced cyanide poisoning) form thiocyanate more quickly. If nitroprusside infusion is limited to 1-2 days with renal-impaired patients and 6-7 days with normal patients, thiocyanate toxicity should be avoided.
- **Recurrent toxicity:** Monitor patients closely for 24 to 48 hr for symptoms of cyanide poisoning to reappear.
- **Patient education:** Instruct to report agitation, blurred vision, hallucinations (seeing, hearing, or feeling things that are not there), mental changes, muscle cramps, nausea and vomiting, pain in the joints, or ringing in the ears.

SERIOUS ADVERSE REACTIONS

- Reactions are difficult to assess because cyanide and/or thiocyanate toxicity are present when patients are being managed with sodium thiosulfate.

OVERDOSE/TOXICITY

- **Cyanide poisoning antidote kit:** Includes sodium thiosulfate, sodium nitrite, and amyl nitrite available for use in management of cyanide poisoning and in nitroprusside-induced cyanide toxicity.
- **GI decontamination:** No specific recommendations.

ANTIDOTE/DIALYSIS

- **Antidote:** There is no antidote for sodium thiosulfate, which is the antidote for cyanide toxicity.
- **Dialysis:** Thiocyanate resulting from nitroprusside toxicity is effectively removed by hemodialysis. No data are available on removal by high-permeability hemodialysis or peritoneal dialysis. No data are available specifically on removal of sodium thiosulfate by dialysis.

somatrem

soe'-ma-trem

Pregnancy Category: C

Trade Names

Prescription: Protropin

Do not confuse somatrem with somatropin, or Protropin with Proloprim, Protamine, or Protopam.

CLINICAL PHARMACOLOGY

Mechanism of Action

A polypeptide hormone that increases the number and size of muscle cells and increases red blood cell (RBC) mass. Affects carbohydrate metabolism by antagonizing action of insulin, increasing the mobilization of fats, and increasing cellular protein synthesis. **Therapeutic Effect:** Stimulates linear growth.

PHARMACOKINETICS

Well absorbed after subcutaneous or IM administration. Localized primarily in the kidneys and liver. **Half-life:** IV: 20-30 min; subcutaneous, IM: 3-5 hr.

AVAILABILITY

Powder for injection: 5 mg, 10 mg.

INDICATIONS AND DOSAGE

Long-term treatment of children who have growth failure due to endogenous growth hormone deficiency

IM/Subcutaneous

Children: Weekly dose of 0.3 mg/kg divided into daily IM or subcutaneous doses.

CONTRAINDICATIONS

Hypersensitivity to somatrem, active neoplasia, acute critical illness due to complications following open-heart or abdominal surgery, acute respiratory failure, patients with closed epiphyses who have multiple accidental trauma

INTERACTIONS

Drug: Corticosteroids: May inhibit growth response. **Herbal:** None known. **Food:** None known.

DIAGNOSTIC TEST EFFECTS

May increase serum parathyroid hormone levels, serum alkaline phosphatase, and inorganic phosphorus levels.

SIDE-EFFECTS

Frequent (30%): Persistent antibodies to growth hormone but generally does not cause failure to respond to somatrem. **Occasional:** Headache, muscle pain, weakness, mild hyperglycemia, allergic reaction, including rash and itching, pain and swelling at injection site, pain in hip or knee

CRITICAL CARE CONSIDERATIONS

ADMINISTRATION/HANDLING

IM/SUBCUTANEOUS ALERT

- **Storage:** Store in refrigerator. Do not freeze.
- **Stability:** Use reconstituted vial within 14 days. Do not use if solution is cloudy.
- **Reconstitution:** Reconstitute each 5-mg vial of somatrem with 1-5 mL bacteriostatic water for injection or each 10-mg vial with 1-10 mL bacteriostatic water for injection (contains benzyl alcohol). Aim stream of diluent toward side of vial; swirl gently to dissolve completely. Do not shake; solution should be clear immediately after reconstitution; if solution is cloudy, do not use.
- **Reconstitution for neonates:** Use only sterile water for injection; the preservative benzyl alcohol is associated with fatal toxicities (gasping syndrome) in premature infants. Use only 1 dose per vial; discard unused portion.

PRECAUTIONS

HEALTH-RELATED

- Use cautiously in patients with diabetes mellitus, malignancy, and untreated hypothyroidism.

AGE-RELATED

- **Children:** No age-related precautions have been noted. Neonates have had fatal toxicity from benzyl alcohol, the preservative used in bacteriostatic water used for reconstitution.
- **Elderly:** No age-related precautions have been noted.

PREGNANCY/LACTATION-RELATED

- Pregnancy category C; unknown if distributed in breast milk.

MONITORING

- **Baseline assessment:** Assess height, weight, and growth pattern.
- **Baseline and ongoing lab work:** Biochemical profile including blood glucose levels, renal (BUN, creatinine) function studies, calcium, and phosphorous; thyroid and parathyroid function studies.
- **Therapeutic effect:** Monitor for increased bone density and growth rate.
- **AIDS/HIV-positive patients:** Assess for decreased muscle wasting.
- **Injection site:** Monitor for skin changes indicative of lipodystrophy at injection sites.
- **Patient education:** Instruct patients or caregivers in the correct reconstitution procedure for IM/subcutaneous administration. Teach safe handling and disposal of needles. Stress the importance of regular follow-up appointments with the precriber.

S

SERIOUS ADVERSE REACTIONS

- **Promotes growth of tumors:** Tumors may be undiagnosed at the time of treatment.
- **Hypersensitivity:** Neonates and other patients may be allergic to benzyl alcohol.
- **Intracranial hypertension:** May be present if patients have history of intracranial lesion.
- **Pancreatitis:** Abdominal pain, nausea, vomiting, abdominal distention.

OVERDOSE/TOXICITY

ACUTE OVERDOSE

- **Hypoglycemia:** Anxiety; altered mental status; blurred vision; diaphoresis; confusion; cool, pale skin; difficulty concentrating; drowsiness; polyphagia; tachycardia; headache; nausea; nervousness; nightmares; restless sleep; shakiness; slurred speech; unusual tiredness or weakness.
- **Hyperglycemia:** Blurred vision; drowsiness; dry mouth; flushed, dry skin; fruity breath odor; polyuria, polydipsia; ketonuria; anorexia; nausea or vomiting; tiredness; increased work of breathing (Kussmaul respirations); unconsciousness.

CHRONIC OVERDOSE

- **Acromegaly:** Back pain; blurred vision; excessive sweating; weakness; headache; increased hat, glove, or shoe size; joint pain; pain in extremities; polydipsia; polyuria.

ANTIDOTE/DIALYSIS

- **Antidote:** No specific recommendations.
- **Dialysis:** Somatrem is unlikely to be removed by hemodialysis or peritoneal dialysis. No data are available on removal by high-permeability hemodialysis.

S

somatropin, biosynthetic

soe-ma-troe'-pin

Classes

Chemical: glycoprotein hormone
Therapeutic: human growth hormone replacement

Pregnancy Category: C

Trade Names

Prescription: Genotropin, Humatrope, Norditropin, Nutropin, Nutropin AQ, Nutropin Depot, Omnitrope

Do not confuse somatropin with somatrem or sumatriptan.

CLINICAL PHARMACOLOGY

Mechanism of Action

A polypeptide hormone that increases the number and size of muscle cells and increases red blood cell (RBC) mass. Affects carbohydrate metabolism by antagonizing action of insulin, increasing the mobilization of fats, and increasing cellular protein synthesis. **Therapeutic Effect:** Stimulates linear growth.

PHARMACOKINETICS

Well absorbed after subcutaneous or IM administration. Localized primarily in the kidneys and liver. **Half-life:** IV: 20-30 min; subcutaneous, IM: 3-5 hr.

AVAILABILITY

Injection: 0.2 mg, 0.4 mg, 0.6 mg, 0.8 mg, 1 mg, 1.2 mg, 1.4 mg, 1.5 mg, 1.6 mg, 1.8 mg, 2 mg, 4 mg, 5 mg, 5.8 mg, 8 mg, 10 mg, 12 mg, 13.5 mg, 13.8 mg, 18 mg, 22.5 mg, 24 mg.
Injection (depot): 13.5 mg, 18 mg, 22.5 mg.

INDICATIONS AND DOSAGE

Growth hormone deficiency

IM/Subcutaneous

Children: Humatrope—0.18 mg/kg/wk divided into equal doses and given on 3 alternate days, 6 times per wk, or daily. Maximum: 0.3 mg/kg/wk.

Subcutaneous

Adults: Genotropin—Initially not more than 0.04 mg/kg/wk; increase at 4- to 8-wk intervals to a maximum of 0.08 mg/kg/wk. **Adults:** Humatrope—Initially not more than 0.006 mg/kg/day; may increase to a maximum of 0.0125 mg/kg/day. **Adults:** Norditropin—0.024-0.034 mg/kg/wk divided into equal doses and given 6-7 times per wk. **Adults:** Norditropin—Initially not more than 0.004 mg/kg/day; may increase to a maximum of 0.016 mg/kg/day after approximately 6 wk. **Adults:** Nutropin, Nutropin AQ—Initially not more than 0.006 mg/kg given as daily injections; may increase to a maximum of 0.025 mg/kg daily in patients under 35 yr or to a maximum of 0.0125 mg/kg daily in patients over 35 yr. **Adults:** Nutropin depot—1.5 mg/kg/mo (same day each mo) or 0.75 mg/kg twice each mo (same days each mo); some patients will require more than 1 injection/dose. **Adults:** Omnitrope—Initially not more than 0.04 mg/kg/wk given as a daily divided dose, preferably in the evening. Increase at 4- to 8-wk intervals to a maximum of 0.08 mg/kg/wk. **Children:** Genotropin—0.16-0.24 mg/kg/wk divided into 6-7 doses per wk.

Children: Nutropin, Nutropin AQ—0.3 mg/kg/wk divided into equal doses and given daily; a dose of 0.7 mg/kg/wk subcutaneously may be used for pubertal patients. **Children:** Nutropin depot—1.5 mg/kg/mo (same day each mo) or 0.75 mg/kg twice each mo (same days each mo); some patients will require more than 1 injection/dose. **Children:** Omnitrope—0.16-0.24 mg/kg/wk given as a daily divided dose, preferably in the evening.

Renal function impairment with growth failure

Subcutaneous

Adults: Nutropin, Nutropin AQ—Up to 0.35 mg/kg/wk divided into equal daily doses; may continue up to time of renal transplantation.

Turner's syndrome

Subcutaneous

Children: Humatrope, Nutropin, Nutropin AQ—Up to 0.375 mg/kg/wk divided over 3-7 days/wk. **Children:** Genotropin—0.33 mg/kg/wk divided over 6-7 days/wk.

Dwarfism, idiopathic

Subcutaneous

Children: Humatrope—Weekly dosage range of up to 0.37 mg/kg divided and given 6-7 times/wk.

Dwarfism, short-stature homeobox-containing gene (SHOX) deficiency

Subcutaneous

Children: Humatrope—Weekly dosage of 0.35 mg/kg of body weight divided into equal daily doses.

Small for gestational age fetus

Subcutaneous

Children: Genotropin—0.48 mg/kg/wk divided into equal doses given on 6 or 7 days/wk.

Prader-Willi syndrome

Subcutaneous

Children: Genotropin—0.24 mg/kg/wk divided into equal doses given on 6 or 7 days/wk.

CONTRAINDICATIONS

Hypersensitivity to somatotropin products; active malignancy; acute critical illness resulting from open heart surgery, GI surgery, or multiple trauma; acute respiratory failure; diabetic retinopathy; Prader-Willi syndrome; pediatric patients with closed epiphyses

INTERACTIONS

Drug: Corticosteroids: May inhibit growth response. **Herbal:** None known. **Food:** None known.

DIAGNOSTIC TEST EFFECTS

May increase serum parathyroid hormone levels, serum alkaline phosphatase and inorganic phosphorus levels.

SIDE-EFFECTS

Frequent: Development of persistent antibodies to growth hormone, generally does not cause failure to respond to somatropin; hypercalciuria during first 2-3 mo of therapy. **Occasional:** Headache, muscle pain, weakness, mild hyperglycemia, allergic reaction, including rash and itching, pain or swelling at injection site, pain in hip or knee

CRITICAL CARE CONSIDERATIONS

ADMINISTRATION/HANDLING

IM/SUBCUTANEOUS ALERT

- **Storage:** Store in refrigerator. Do not freeze.
- **Stability:** Use reconstituted vial within 14 days if bacteriostatic water was used for reconstitution; use drug within 24 hr if reconstituted with sterile water for injection. Do not use if solution is cloudy.
- **Humatrope reconstitution:** Reconstitute vials with 1.5-5 mL of diluent provided. Aim stream of diluent toward side of vial; swirl gently to dissolve completely. Do not shake; solution should be clear immediately after reconstitution; if solution is cloudy, do not use. For Humatrope cartridges, use only the diluent syringe and diluent connector; do not use diluent provided with Humatrope vials.
- **Nutropin reconstitution:** Reconstitute each 5-mL vial with 1-5 mL bacteriostatic water for injection (contains benzyl alcohol). Aim stream of diluent toward side of vial; swirl gently to dissolve completely. Do not shake; solution should be clear immediately after reconstitution; if solution is cloudy, do not use.
- **Reconstitution for neonates:** Use only sterile water for injection; the preservative benzyl alcohol is associated with fatal toxicities (gasping syndrome) in premature infants. Use only 1 dose per vial; discard unused portion.

PRECAUTIONS

HEALTH-RELATED

- Use cautiously in patients with diabetes mellitus, malignancy, and untreated hypothyroidism.

AGE-RELATED

- **Children:** No age-related precautions have been noted. Neonates have had fatal toxicity from benzyl alcohol, the preservative

S

used in bacteriostatic water used for reconstitution.
- **Elderly:** No age-related precautions have been noted.

PREGNANCY/LACTATION-RELATED
- Pregnancy category C; unknown if distributed in breast milk.

MONITORING
- **Baseline assessment:** Assess height, weight, and growth pattern.
- **Baseline and ongoing lab work:** Biochemical profile including blood glucose levels, renal (BUN, creatinine) function studies, calcium, and phosphorous; thyroid and parathyroid function studies.
- **Therapeutic effect:** Monitor for increased bone density and growth rate.
- **AIDS/HIV-positive patients:** Assess for decreased muscle wasting.
- **Injection site:** Monitor for skin changes indicative of lipodystrophy at injection sites.
- **Patient education:** Instruct patients or caregivers in the correct reconstitution procedure for IM/subcutaneous administration. Teach safe handling and disposal of needles. Stress the importance of regular follow-up appointments with the prescriber.

SERIOUS ADVERSE REACTIONS
- **Promotes growth of tumors:** Tumors may be undiagnosed at the time of treatment.
- **Hypersensitivity:** Neonates and other patients may be allergic to benzyl alcohol.
- **Intracranial hypertension:** May be present if patients have history of intracranial lesion.
- **Pancreatitis:** Abdominal pain, nausea, vomiting, abdominal distention.

OVERDOSE/TOXICITY

S

ACUTE OVERDOSE
- **Hypoglycemia:** Anxiety; altered mental status; blurred vision; diaphoresis; confusion; cool, pale skin; difficulty concentrating; drowsiness; polyphagia; tachycardia; headache; nausea; nervousness; nightmares; restless sleep; shakiness; slurred speech; unusual tiredness or weakness.
- **Hyperglycemia:** Blurred vision; drowsiness; dry mouth; flushed, dry skin; fruity breath odor; polyuria, polydipsia; ketonuria; anorexia; nausea or vomiting; tiredness; increased work of breathing (Kussmaul respirations); unconsciousness.

CHRONIC OVERDOSE
- **Acromegaly:** Back pain; blurred vision; excessive sweating; weakness; headache; increased hat, glove, or shoe size; joint pain; pain in extremities; polydipsia; polyuria.

ANTIDOTE/DIALYSIS
- **Antidote:** No specific recommendations.
- **Dialysis:** Somatropin is unlikely to be removed by hemodialysis or peritoneal dialysis. No data are available on removal by high-permeability hemodialysis.

sotalol hydrochloride 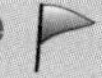

soe'-ta-lole hye-droe-klor'-ide

Classes
Chemical: β-adrenergic blocker, nonselective
Therapeutic: antidysrhythmic, class III

Pregnancy Category: B

Trade Names
Prescription: Betapace, Betapace AF, Sorine, Sotacor ♣

Do not confuse sotalol with Stadol.

CLINICAL PHARMACOLOGY
Mechanism of Action
A beta-adrenergic blocking agent that prolongs action potential, effective refractory period, and QT interval. Decreases heart rate and AV node conduction; increases AV node refractoriness. **Therapeutic Effect:** Produces antidysrhythmic activity.

PHARMACOKINETICS
Well absorbed from the GI tract. Protein binding: None. Widely distributed. Primarily excreted unchanged in urine. Removed by hemodialysis. **Half-life:** 12 hr (increased in the elderly and patients with impaired renal function).

AVAILABILITY
Tablets: 80 mg (Betapace, Betapace AF, Sorine), 120 mg (Betapace, Betapace AF, Sorine), 160 mg (Betapace, Betapace AF, Sorine), 240 mg (Betapace, Sorine).

INDICATIONS AND DOSAGE
Documented, life-threatening dysrhythmias
PO (Betapace, Sorine)
Adults, Elderly: Initially, 80 mg twice per day. May increase gradually at 2- to 3-day intervals. Range: 240-320 mg/day.

Atrial fibrillation, atrial flutter
PO (Betapace AF)
Adults, Elderly: 80 mg twice per day.

Dosage in renal impairment

Betapace, Sorine

Dosage interval is modified based on creatinine clearance.

Creatinine Clearance	Dosage Interval
31-60 mL/min	24 hr
10-30 mL/min	36-48 hr
Less than 10 mL/min	Individualized

Betapace AF

Creatinine Clearance	Dosage Interval
Greater than 60 mL/min	12 hr
40-60 mL/min	24 hr
Less than 40 mL/min	Contraindicated

OFF-LABEL USES

Maintenance of normal heart rhythm in chronic or recurring atrial fibrillation or flutter; treatment of anxiety, chronic angina pectoris, hypertension, hypertrophic cardiomyopathy, MI, mitral valve prolapse syndrome, pheochromocytoma, thyrotoxicosis, tremors

CONTRAINDICATIONS

Bronchial asthma, cardiogenic shock, prolonged QT syndrome (more than 450 milliseconds unless functioning pacemaker is present), second- and third-degree heart block, sinus bradycardia, uncontrolled cardiac failure, hypersensitivity to sotalol, creatinine clearance less than 40 mL/min, concurrent use of QTc-prolonging drugs (for Betapace AF only)

INTERACTIONS

Drug: Antidysrhythmics, phenothiazine, tricyclic antidepressants: May prolong QT interval. **Calcium channel blockers:** May increase effect on AV conduction and BP. **Clonidine:** May potentiate rebound hypertension after clonidine is discontinued. **Digoxin:** May increase risk of proarrhythmias. **Insulin, oral hypoglycemics:** May mask signs of hypoglycemia and prolong the effects of insulin and oral hypoglycemics. **Sympathomimetics:** May inhibit the effects of sympathomimetics. **Herbal:** None known. **Food:** None known.

DIAGNOSTIC TEST EFFECTS

May increase blood glucose, serum alkaline phosphatase, serum LDH, serum lipoprotein, AST (SGOT), ALT (SGPT), and serum triglyceride levels.

SIDE-EFFECTS

Frequent (more than 10%): Diminished sexual function, drowsiness, insomnia, unusual fatigue or weakness, bradycardia (16%), chest pain (16%), palpitations (14%), dizziness (20%), dyspnea (20%). **Occasional (1%-10%):** Depression, cold hands or feet, diarrhea, constipation, anxiety, nasal congestion, nausea, vomiting. **Rare:** Altered taste, dry eyes, itching, numbness of fingers, toes, or scalp

CRITICAL CARE CONSIDERATIONS

ADMINISTRATION/HANDLING

PO ALERT

- Give sotalol without regard to food.
- Some patients may require 480-640 mg/day. Sotalol has a long half-life, and administering the drug more than 2 times per day is usually not necessary. Avoid abrupt withdrawal.

PRECAUTIONS

HEALTH-RELATED

- Use sotalol cautiously in patients with cardiomegaly, heart failure, diabetes mellitus, QT-interval prolongation, history of ventricular tachycardia, hypokalemia, hypomagnesemia, severe and prolonged diarrhea, sick sinus syndrome, or ventricular fibrillation.
- **Hyperthyroidism:** Use cautiously in patients who may develop thyrotoxicosis.
- **Transitioning to sotalol:** Other antidysrhythmic therapy should be gradually withdrawn (wait 2-3 plasma half-lives of other drug if tolerated) before starting sotalol (Betapace); if on amiodarone, sotalol should not be initiated until QT interval normalizes.
- **Atrial fibrillation/flutter:** Patients on Betapace should be transitioned to Betapace AF for enhanced patient safety.

AGE-RELATED

- **Children:** Safety and efficacy of soatalol have not been established in children.
- **Elderly:** Age-related peripheral vascular disease may increase susceptibility to decreased peripheral circulation.

PREGNANCY/LACTATION-RELATED

- Pregnancy category B. A similar drug, atenolol, is frequently used in the third trimester for treatment of hypertension (many studies of efficacy and safety of

S

atenolol in pregnancy-induced hypertension). Long-term use has been associated with intrauterine growth retardation. Concentrated in breast milk (levels 3-5 times those of plasma); symptoms of beta-blockade possible in infant but considered compatible with breast-feeding.

MONITORING

- **Baseline assessment:** Assess for history of dysrhythmias, including medications used and prior electrophysiologic testing; obtain vital signs
- **Baseline lab work:** Biochemical profile including potassium and magnesium levels.
- **Baseline diagnostic tests:** 12-lead ECG to establish baseline heart rhythm. Institute continuous cardiac monitoring when beginning sotalol therapy.
- **Bradycardia:** If heart rate is 60 beats/min or less, monitor closely for instability; if unstable, discontinue the drug. Monitor diligently for dysrhythmias. If QT prolongation ensues, patients are at risk for developing torsades de pointes.
- **Prolonged QT syndrome:** Patients transitioning to Betapace AF must have a QT interval less than 450 milliseconds. If continuous ECG monitoring reveals QT interval exceeds 500 milliseconds, drug should be discontinued or dosage reduced.
- **Heart failure:** Evaluate for decreased urine output, distended neck veins, dyspnea, jugular vein distention, peripheral edema, rales, and weight gain.
- **Hemodynamic monitoring:** Cardiac index may be reduced by nearly 25% with a simultaneous increase in pulmonary capillary wedge pressure.
- **Patient education:** Caution against abruptly discontinuing the drug without prescriber's approval. Warn to avoid tasks that require mental alertness or motor skills until response to the drug is known. Explain that periodic laboratory tests and ECGs are a necessary part of therapy.

SERIOUS ADVERSE REACTIONS

- Bronchospasms, hypoglycemia.
- **Thyrotoxicosis:** Use of beta-blocking drugs may mask tachycardia associated with hyperthyroidism; if hyperthyroidism is present, sotalol and other beta-blockers must be withdrawn gradually to avoid thyroid crisis.

OVERDOSE/TOXICITY

- **Cardiotoxicity:** Bradycardia, heart failure, hypotension, prolonged QT interval, premature ventricular complexes, ventricular tachycardia, and torsades de pointes may occur.
- **Management:** Manage dysrhythmias according to Advanced Cardiac Life Support (ACLS) guidelines.
- **GI decontamination:** No specific recommendations.

ANTIDOTE/DIALYSIS

- **Antidote:** No specific recommendations.
- **Dialysis:** Sotalol is removed by hemodialysis and is likely removed by high-permeability hemodialysis. No data are available on removal by peritoneal dialysis.

sparfloxacin

See Antibiotics (p. 892)

spironolactone

speer-on-oh-lak'-tone

Classes

Chemical: aldosterone antagonist
Therapeutic: antihypertensive; diuretic, potassium-sparing

Pregnancy Category: C

Trade Names

Prescription: Aldactone

Combinations

Prescription: with hydrochlorothiazide (Aldactazide)

Do not confuse Aldactone with Aldactazide.

CLINICAL PHARMACOLOGY

Mechanism of Action

A potassium-sparing diuretic that interferes with sodium reabsorption by competitively inhibiting the action of aldosterone in the distal tubule, thus promoting sodium and water excretion and increasing potassium retention. **Therapeutic Effect:** Produces diuresis; lowers BP; diagnostic aid for primary aldosteronism.

PHARMACOKINETICS

Route	Onset	Peak	Duration
PO	24-48 hr	48-72 hr	48-72 hr

S

Well absorbed from the GI tract (absorption increased with food). Protein binding: 91%-98%. Metabolized in the liver to active metabolite. Primarily excreted in urine. **Half-life:** 1-1.5 hr.

AVAILABILITY

Tablets: 25 mg, 50 mg, 100 mg.

INDICATIONS AND DOSAGE

Edema

PO

Adults, Elderly: 25-200 mg/day as a single dose or in 2 divided doses. **Children:** 1.5-3.3 mg/kg/day in divided doses every 6-24 hr. **Neonates:** 1-3 mg/kg/day in 1-2 divided doses.

Hypertension

PO

Adults, Elderly: 25-50 mg/day in 1-2 doses/day. **Children:** 1.5-3.3 mg/kg/day in divided doses every 6-24 hr.

Hypokalemia

PO

Adults, Elderly: 25-100 mg/day as a single dose or in 2 divided doses.

Male hirsutism

PO

Adults, Elderly: 50-200 mg/day as a single dose or in 2 divided doses.

Primary aldosteronism

PO

Adults, Elderly: 100-400 mg/day as a single dose or in 2 divided doses. **Children:** 100-400 mg/m^2/day as a single dose or in 2 divided doses.

Heart failure

PO

Adults, Elderly: Initially 100 mg/day in single or divided dose. Adjusted based on patient response and evidence of hyperkalemia after 5 days, if needed. Range: 25-200 mg/day.

Dosage in renal impairment

Dosage interval is modified based on creatinine clearance.

Creatinine Clearance	Interval
10-50 mL/min	Usual dose every 12-24 hr
Less than 10 mL/min	Avoid use

OFF-LABEL USES

Treatment of edema and hypertension in children; female acne, hirsutism, polycystic ovary disease

CONTRAINDICATIONS

Acute renal insufficiency, anuria, BUN and serum creatinine levels more than twice normal values, hyperkalemia, hypersensitivity to spironolactone

INTERACTIONS

Drug: ACE inhibitors (such as captopril), potassium-containing medications, potassium supplements: May increase the risk of hyperkalemia. **Anticoagulants, heparin:** May decrease the effects of these drugs. **Digoxin:** May increase the half-life of digoxin. **Lithium:** May decrease the clearance and increase the risk of toxicity of lithium. **NSAIDs:** May decrease the antihypertensive effect of spironolactone. **Herbal:** None known. **Food:** None known.

DIAGNOSTIC TEST EFFECTS

May increase urinary calcium excretion; BUN and blood glucose levels; serum creatinine, magnesium, potassium, and uric acid levels. May decrease serum sodium level.

SIDE-EFFECTS

Frequent: Hyperkalemia (in patients with renal insufficiency and those taking potassium supplements), dehydration, hyponatremia, lethargy. **Occasional:** Nausea, vomiting, anorexia, abdominal cramps, diarrhea, headache, ataxia, somnolence, confusion, fever. **Male:** Gynecomastia, impotence, decreased libido. **Female:** Menstrual irregularities (including amenorrhea and postmenopausal bleeding), breast tenderness. **Rare:** Rash, urticaria, hirsutism

CRITICAL CARE CONSIDERATIONS

ADMINISTRATION/HANDLING

PO ALERT

- Give spironolactone with food to enhance its absorption.
- Crush scored tablets as needed.
- Suspension containing crushed tablets in cherry syrup is stable for up to 30 days if refrigerated.

PRECAUTIONS

HEALTH-RELATED

- Use spironolactone cautiously in patients with hyponatremia or hepatic or renal impairment, dehydrated patients, and those who take potassium supplements.

AGE-RELATED

- **Children:** No age-related precautions have been noted in children.

S

- **Elderly:** May be more susceptible to hyperkalemia; age-related renal impairment may require a dosage reduction.

PREGNANCY/LACTATION-RELATED

- Pregnancy category C. Feminization occurs in male rat fetuses. Active metabolite excreted in breast milk; compatible with breast-feeding but alternate options preferred. Therapy for existing hypertension can be continued throughout pregnancy with minimal risk. Initiating for simple edema not recommended; few unequivocal indications for diuretic therapy in pregnancy except for pulmonary edema or congestive heart failure.

MONITORING

- **Baseline assessment:** Monitor vital signs, including pulse quality; note extent and location of edema; evaluate for dehydration. Obtain baseline weight.
- **Baseline and ongoing lab work:** Biochemical profile including electrolytes, renal (BUN, creatinine) and liver (AST [SGOT], ALT [SGPT], GGT, alkaline phosphatase, bilirubin) function tests; urinalysis.
- **Baseline diagnostic tests:** 12-lead ECG to assess for myocardial ischemia and dysrhythmias.
- **Hyperkalemia:** Monitor ECG continuously for dysrhythmias, colic, diarrhea, and muscle twitching, followed by paralysis and weakness. Monitor fluid intake and output. Obtain a 12-lead ECG if hyperkalemia is severe.
- **Hyponatremia:** Assess for cold and clammy skin, confusion, drowsiness, dry mouth, and thirst.
- **Dehydration:** Perform daily weights, monitor intake/output for edema as well as developing poor skin turgor.
- **Patient education:** Advise to expect an increase in the frequency and volume of urination. Inform that therapeutic effect takes several days to begin and can last for several days once the drug is discontinued (unless also taking a potassium-losing drug concomitantly). Caution to avoid consuming potassium supplements and foods high in potassium, including apricots, bananas, raisins, orange juice, potatoes, legumes, meat, and whole grains (such as cereals). Instruct to report promptly irregular heartbeat, diarrhea, muscle twitching, cold and clammy skin, confusion, drowsiness, dry mouth, or excessive thirst to a health care provider. Recommend avoiding tasks that require mental alertness or motor skills until response to the drug is known.

SERIOUS ADVERSE REACTIONS

- Cirrhosis patients are at risk for hepatic decompensation if dehydration or hyponatremia occurs.
- Primary aldosteronism patients may experience rapid weight loss and severe fatigue during high-dose therapy.

OVERDOSE/TOXICITY

- **Severe hyperkalemia:** Dysrhythmias, bradycardia, and ECG changes (tented T waves, widening QRS complex and ST segment depression), which may proceed to cardiac standstill or ventricular fibrillation.
- **Management:** Initiate cation exchange resins (Kayexelate) orally or given by retention enema; if life-threatening, give IV calcium gluconate to counteract neuromuscular and cardiac effects; IV glucose and insulin shifts K+ into the cells. IV sodium bicarbonate shifts potassium into cells. Beta$_2$-agonists (albuterol) shift K+ into the cells.
- **GI decontamination:** No specific recommendations.

ANTIDOTE/DIALYSIS

- **Antidote:** Calcium gluconate and/or sodium bicarbonate given IV.
- **Dialysis:** Spironolactone is unlikely to be removed by hemodialysis or peritoneal dialysis. No data are available on removal by high-permeability hemodialysis.

stavudine

See HIV Medications (p. 961)

streptokinase

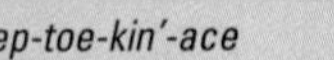

strep-toe-kin'-ace

Classes

Chemical: betahemolytic streptococcus filtrate, purified
Therapeutic: thrombolytic

Pregnancy Category: C

Trade Names

Prescription: Kabikinase, Streptase

CLINICAL PHARMACOLOGY

Mechanism of Action

An enzyme that activates the fibrinolytic system by converting plasminogen to plasmin, an enzyme that degrades fibrin clots. Acts indirectly by forming a complex with plasminogen, which converts plasminogen to plasmin. Action occurs within the thrombus, on its surface, and in circulating blood. **Therapeutic Effect:** Destroys thrombi.

PHARMACOKINETICS

Rapidly cleared from plasma by antibodies and the reticuloendothelial system. Route of elimination unknown. Duration of action continues for several hours after drug has been discontinued. **Half-life:** 23 min. Anticoagulant effect: 12-24 hr.

AVAILABILITY

Powder for injection (Kabikinase, Streptase): 250,000 units, 750,000 units, 1.5 million units.

INDICATIONS AND DOSAGE

Acute evolving transmural MI for coronary artery thrombi (given as soon as possible after symptoms occur)

IV Infusion

Adults, Elderly: (1.5 million units diluted to 45 mL)—1.5 million units infused over 60 min.

Intracoronary Infusion

Adults, Elderly: (250,000 units diluted to 125 mL)—Initially 20,000 units (10-mL) bolus; then 2000 units/min for 60 min. Total dose: 140,000 units.

Pulmonary embolism, deep vein thrombosis (DVT), arterial thrombosis and embolism (given within 7 days of onset)

IV Infusion

Adults, Elderly: (1.5 million units diluted to 90 mL)—Initially 250,000 units infused over 30 min; then 100,000 units/hr for 24 hr for arterial thrombosis or embolism, and pulmonary embolism, 72 hr for DVT.

Intraarterial Infusion

Adults, Elderly: (1.5 million units diluted to 45 mL)—Initially a single dose of 250,000 units infused over 30 min; then 100,000 units/hr for maintenance for 24-72 hr.

CONTRAINDICATIONS

Carcinoma of the brain, cerebrovascular accident, internal bleeding, intracranial surgery within 2 mo, recent streptococcal infection, severe hypertension, hypersensitivity to streptokinase, AV malformation, known bleeding diathesis

INTERACTIONS

Drug: **Anticoagulants, heparin:** May increase the risk of hemorrhage. **Platelet aggregation inhibitors such as aspirin:** May increase the risk of bleeding. **Herbal:** None known. **Food:** None known.

DIAGNOSTIC TEST EFFECTS

Decreases serum plasminogen and fibrinogen level during infusion, decreasing clotting time and confirming presence of lysis

IV INCOMPATIBILITIES

Do not mix with medications other than *DOBUTamine (Dobutrex), *DOPamine (Intropin), heparin, lidocaine, and nitroglycerin.

SIDE-EFFECTS

Frequent: Fever, superficial bleeding at puncture sites, decreased BP. **Occasional:** Allergic reaction, including rash and wheezing; ecchymosis

CRITICAL CARE CONSIDERATIONS

ADMINISTRATION/HANDLING

IV ALERT

- **Filter:** An inline 0.45-micron filter should be used.
- **Timing of dosage:** Streptokinase must be administered within 12-14 hr of clot formation. It has little effect on older, organized clots.
- **Repeat administration:** Do not use within 5 days to 6 mo of previous streptokinase treatment if administered for streptococcal infection, such as acute glomerulonephritis secondary to streptococcal infection, pharyngitis, and rheumatic fever.
- **Storage:** Store unopened vials at room temperature. Refrigerate reconstituted solution and use within 24 hr.
- **Reconstitution:** Reconstitute vial with 5 mL D_5W or 0.9% NaCl (preferred). Add diluent slowly to side of vial; roll and tilt to avoid foaming. Do not shake vial. May dilute further with 50-500 mL of D_5W or 0.9% NaCl in 45-mL increments.
- **Direct intracoronary administration of coronary artery thrombi:** Give 20,000 unit bolus dose over 25-30 sec using coronary catheter. Follow with 2000 units/min for 60 min.

PRECAUTIONS

HEALTH-RELATED

- Use streptokinase cautiously in patients with GI bleeding or recent trauma and in those who have had major surgery within past 10 days.

AGE-RELATED

- **Children:** Safety and efficacy of streptokinase have not been established in children.
- **Elderly:** May have an increased risk of intracranial hemorrhage. Streptokinase should be used cautiously in the elderly.

PREGNANCY/LACTATION-RELATED

- Pregnancy category C; no data available for breast-feeding.

MONITORING

- **Baseline assessment:** Assess for risk of bleeding. Discontinue heparin (if heparin is a component of treatment) before giving streptokinase. Prothrombin time or aPTT should be less than twice normal value before therapy starts. Determine usual discharge amount during menses in female patients.
- **Lab work:** CBC and coagulation profile including aPTT, Hct, fibrinogen level, platelet count, and prothrombin time before therapy starts. Monitor Hgb and Hct, platelet count, aPTT, fibrinogen level, prothrombin time, and thrombin every 4 hr after therapy begins.
- **Diagnostic tests:** 12-lead ECG or appropriate perfusion studies for target area.
- **Hypotension:** Monitor BP continuously or frequently during infusion. Severe hypotension occurs in 1%-10% of patients. Infusion rate may need to be reduced for low BP (reduced by more than 25 mmHg).
- **Fever:** Temperature increases of up to 2° F are relatively common.
- **Therapeutic effect:** Assess peripheral pulses to evaluate for reperfusion of affected target area. If using for coronary artery disease, continuous ECG monitoring is essential for recognition and management of dysrhythmias. Assess the area of peripheral thromboembolus for color and temperature.
- **Bleeding:** Handle patients carefully and as infrequently as possible to prevent bleeding and ecchymosis. Do not obtain BP in lower extremities if a deep vein thrombus may be present. Examine stool for occult blood. Assess for abdominal or back pain, decreased BP, an increased heart rate, and severe headache, which may indicate hemorrhage. Monitor females for increased menstrual flow. Assess skin for bruises and petechiae and urine for hematuria. Examine for excessive bleeding from minor cuts and scratches and other signs of bleeding.
- **Patient education:** Advise to use an electric razor and soft toothbrush to prevent bleeding during drug therapy. Instruct to report chest pain, headache, palpitations, or shortness of breath immediately, and promptly to report black or red stool, coffee-ground vomitus, dark or red urine, red-speckled mucus from cough, or other signs of bleeding to a health care provider.

SERIOUS ADVERSE REACTIONS

- **Reperfusion dysrhythmias:** Lysis of coronary thrombi may produce life-threatening dysrhythmias. Manage according to Advanced Cardiac Life Support (ACLS) recommendations for management of symptomatic dysrhythmias.
- **Hypersensitivity:** Allergic reactions including anaphylaxis occur somewhat often. Ensure a patent airway, provide oxygen and ventilatory support as needed. Corticosteroids and epinephrine may be needed to manage shock, along with fluid infusions and vasopressors. Streptokinase should be discontinued if anaphylaxis occurs.

OVERDOSE/TOXICITY

- **Hemorrhage:** Severe internal hemorrhage may occur.
- **Management:** Discontinue the infusion immediately if uncontrolled hemorrhage occurs. Be aware that slowing the rate of infusion instead of discontinuing it may produce worsening hemorrhage. Do not use dextran to control hemorrhage. Packed RBCs, platelets, cryoprecipitate, fresh frozen plasma, desmopressin, tranexamic acid, and aminocaproic acid may help control bleeding. Protamine may be used to reverse bleeding secondary to heparin.
- **GI decontamination:** No specific recommendations.

ANTIDOTE/DIALYSIS

- **Antidote:** No specific recommendations.
- **Dialysis:** Streptokinase is unlikely to be removed by hemodialysis, high-permeability hemodialysis, or peritoneal dialysis.

streptomycin sulfate

See Antibiotics (p. 892)

succinylcholine chloride

suk-se-nil-koe'-leen klor'-ide

Classes

Chemical: depolarizing neuromuscular blocking agent

Therapeutic: skeletal muscle relaxant, paralytic agent

Pregnancy Category: C

Trade Names

Prescription: Anectine, Quelicin

CLINICAL PHARMACOLOGY

Mechanism of Action

A depolarizing skeletal muscle relaxant that combines with the cholinergic receptors of the motor end plate to produce depolarization. **Therapeutic Effect:** Produces skeletal muscle relaxation.

PHARMACOKINETICS

Following administration, neuromuscular blockade develops in 30-60 sec; maximum blockade may persist for about 4-6 min. The onset of effect of succinylcholine given IM is usually observed in about 2-3 min. Rapidly hydrolyzed by plasma cholinesterase to succinylmonocholine and then more slowly to succinic acid and choline. IM duration: 10-30 min. Excreted in urine. **Half-life:** Unknown.

AVAILABILITY

Intravenous solution: 20 mg/mL or 50 mg/mL (Quelicin, Anectine), 100 mg/mL (Quelicin).

INDICATIONS AND DOSAGE

General anesthesia, adjunct (short surgical procedures)

IV

Adults: 0.6 mg/kg. The optimum dose will vary among individuals and may be 0.3-1.1 mg/kg. **Children:** For emergency tracheal intubation or in instances where immediate securing of the airway is necessary, the IV dose of succinylcholine is 2 mg/kg for infants and small children; for older children and adolescents, the dose is 1 mg/kg.

IM

Adults, Children: A dose of up to 3-4 mg/kg may be given, but not more than 150 mg total dose should be administered by this route.

General anesthesia, adjunct (long surgical procedures)

IV

Adults: The average rate ranges between 2.5 and 4.3 mg/min. Solutions containing from 1-2 mg/mL succinylcholine have commonly been used for continuous infusion. The more dilute solution (1 mg/mL) is probably preferable from the standpoint of ease of control of the rate of administration of the drug and, hence, of relaxation. This IV solution containing 1 mg/mL may be administered at a rate of 0.5 mg (0.5 mL) to 10 mg (10 mL) per min to obtain the required amount of relaxation. Intermittent IV injections of succinylcholine may also be used to provide muscle relaxation for long procedures. An IV injection of 0.3-1.1 mg/kg may be given initially, followed, at appropriate intervals, by further injections of 0.04-0.07 mg/kg to maintain the degree of relaxation required.

CONTRAINDICATIONS

Personal or familial history of malignant hyperthermia, skeletal muscle myopathies, after the acute phase of injury following major burns, multiple trauma, extensive denervation of skeletal muscle, or upper motor neuron injury, hypersensitivity to succinylcholine

INTERACTIONS

Drug: **Aprotinin, beta-blockers, certain MAOIs, certain nonpenicillin antibiotics, chloroquine, desflurane, diethylether, glucocorticoids, isoflurane, lidocaine, lithium carbonate, magnesium salts, metoclopramide, oral contraceptives, oxytocin, procainamide, promazine, quinidine, quinine, terbutaline, trimethaphan:** May enhance the neuromuscular blocking action of succinylcholine. **Other neuromuscular blocking agents:** May cause synergistic or antagonistic effect. **Herbal:** None known. **Food:** None known.

DIAGNOSTIC TEST EFFECTS

None known.

SIDE-EFFECTS

Frequency not defined: Cardiac arrest, malignant hyperthermia, dysrhythmias, bradycardia, tachycardia, hypertension, hypotension, hyperkalemia, prolonged respiratory depression or apnea, increased intraocular pressure, muscle fasciculation, jaw rigidity, postoperative muscle pain, rhabdomyolysis with possible myoglobinuric acute renal failure, excessive salivation, rash

S

CRITICAL CARE CONSIDERATIONS

ADMINISTRATION/HANDLING

IV ALERT

- **Storage:** Store in refrigerator.
- **Stability:** Succinylcholine is acidic and should not be mixed with alkaline solutions having a pH greater than 8.5 (e.g., barbiturate solutions). Anectine injection is stable for 24 hr after dilution to a final concentration of 1-2 mg/mL in 5% dextrose injection or 0.9% sodium chloride injection.
- **Admixtures of succinylcholine:** Should be prepared for single-patient use only. The unused portion of diluted succinylcholine should be discarded.
- **Dosage:** Should be individualized. The dose of succinylcholine administered by infusion depends on the duration of the surgical procedure and the need for muscle relaxation.
- **Test dose:** A 5- to 10-mg test dose injected over 30 sec may be used to determine the sensitivity of the patient and the individual recovery time.
- **Intermittent IV injections:** May also be used to provide muscle relaxation for long procedures.
- **Skilled providers only:** Succinylcholine should be administered by adequately trained individuals familiar with its actions, characteristics, and hazards.
- **Unconsciousness:** Do not administer before unconsciousness has been induced.

IM ALERT

- Succinylcholine may be given intramuscularly to infants, older children, or adults when a suitable vein is inaccessible.

S

PRECAUTIONS

HEALTH-RELATED

- May cause serious or lethal dysrhythmias in patients who are digitalized, those receiving quinidine, those with electrolyte imbalance including hyperkalemia, or in cases of severe trauma.
- Use cautiously in patients with fractures or muscle spasm.
- May increase intragastric pressure, which could result in regurgitation and possible aspiration of stomach contents.
- Neuromuscular blockade may be prolonged in patients with hypokalemia or hypocalcemia.

AGE-RELATED

- **Children:** Children are more likely to experience bradycardia with repeat dosing; there are rare reports of ventricular dysrhythmias and cardiac arrest secondary to acute rhabdomyolysis with hyperkalemia in apparently healthy children who receive succinylcholine.
- **Elderly:** No age-related precautions have been noted.

PREGNANCY/LACTATION-RELATED

- Pregnancy category C; unknown if distributed in breast milk; use extreme caution with breast-feeding women.

MONITORING

- **Baseline assessment:** Assess baseline vital signs. Assess for electrolyte imbalance. Assess past exposure to sedation, analgesia, and neuromuscular blockade. Assess for prior problems with anesthesia, including problems with endotracheal intubation.
- **Lab work:** Baseline biochemical profile including calcium and potassium levels.
- **Sedation and analgesia:** Patients undergoing neuromuscular blockade with succinylcholine should be sedated and have appropriate pain management provided because they are unable to express anxiety and discomfort during neuromuscular blockade. Succinylcholine produces apnea and paralysis.
- **Ongoing assessment:** Monitor heart rate, BP, and respiratory rate. Try to assess level of pain. Assess for muscle paralysis.
- **Sedation and neuromuscular blockade monitoring:** If repeated dosing of succinylcholine is necessary, monitor the degree of neuromuscular blockade and consider switching to an IV infusion of a nondepolarizing neuromuscular blocking agent (atracurium cistatracurium, vecuronium). Use "train of four" technique with a peripheral nerve stimulator and sedation with a bispectral brain wave analysis device. Provide dose of succinylcholine and other medications to keep patients still, well-ventilated, and as comfortable as possible. Because patients are totally dependent on health care providers to anticipate all needs and provide all care, most patients would rather not have awareness of the neuromuscular blockade experience. During surgical procedures, anesthesia awareness is considered unacceptable.
- **Mechanical ventilation:** Assess ventilation status using lung assessment, vital

signs, pulse oximetry, and end tidal CO_2 monitoring.

- **Ongoing monitoring:** Monitor BP, heart rate, oxygen saturation, and respiratory rate.
- **Continuous cardiac monitoring:** Monitor ECG for dysrhythmias, especially if calcium, potassium, or other electrolytes are imbalanced. Observe for peaked T wave (indicative of hyperkalemia), which may signal onset of skeletal muscle myopathy.
- **Increased intragastric pressure:** Monitor pressure with tonometry if available to predict patients who are at risk of vomiting/aspirating.
- **Weaning neuromuscular blockade:** Sedation or anesthesia with propofol (Diprivan) and pain management with fentanyl may provide enough sedation/analgesia to be able to wean succinylcholine without compromising critically ill patients' ventilatory status. If repeated doses of succinylcholine are required for long-term and/or effective sedation, an infusion of a nondepolarizing neuromuscular blocking agent may be used.
- **Patient education:** Explain that patients will be unable to speak, open eyes, or move when full neuromuscular blockade is in place. When weaning succinylcholine, inform that it will be difficult to talk because of head and neck muscle blockade. Instruct to report if muscle pain after surgery or trouble breathing occurs.

SERIOUS ADVERSE REACTIONS

- **Acute rhabdomyolysis with hyperkalemia:** Reported rarely but followed by ventricular dysrhythmias, cardiac arrest, and death after administration of succinylcholine to apparently healthy children who were subsequently found to have undiagnosed skeletal muscle myopathy, most frequently Duchenne's muscular dystrophy.
- **Hypersensitivity reactions:** Anaphylaxis, may occur in rare instances.
- **Malignant hyperthermia:** Jaw muscle spasm, muscle rigidity rather than relaxation, tachycardia unresponsive to medications.

OVERDOSE/TOXICITY

- **Overdosage:** May be manifested by skeletal muscle weakness, bradycardia, decreased respiratory reserve, hyperthermia, hyperkalemia, low tidal volume, or prolonged apnea with phase II block.
- **Management:** Discontinue succinylcholine immediately. An anesthesiologist should manage the treatment, which should include endotracheal intubation or tracheostomy to protect the airway/provide ventilation. Atropine should be used to manage bradycardia. Hyperthermia or malignant hyperthermia should be managed with cooling, hydration with IV fluids, restoration of electrolyte balance, and maintenance of urinary output, especially if myoglobinuria is present. Sodium bicarbonate and/or dantrolene may be indicated. IV calcium, bicarbonate, glucose with insulin and possibly beta-adrenergic drugs (albuterol) may be used to manage hyperkalemia.
- **GI decontamination:** No specific recommendations.

ANTIDOTE/DIALYSIS

- **Antidote:** Pyridostigmine (Mestinon) or neostigmine (Prostigmin) given with atropine reverses muscle relaxation in most patients but may aggravate severe overdosage. Muscle twitch should have returned for at least 20 min before using antidotes. Peripheral nerve stimulator should be used to assess patients for presence of level II block. Ensure patients are endotracheally intubated and mechanical or manual ventilation is in place.
- **Dialysis:** Succinylcholine is not effectively removed by hemodialysis, peritoneal dialysis, or high-permeability hemodialysis because very little of the drug is naturally excreted by the kidney.

sucralfate

soo-kral'-fate

Classes

Chemical: aluminum complex of sulfated sucrose

Therapeutic: antiulcer agent

Pregnancy Category: B

Trade Names

Prescription: Carafate, Sulcrate ♣

Do not confuse Carafate with Cafergot.

CLINICAL PHARMACOLOGY

Mechanism of Action

An antiulcer agent that forms an ulcer-adherent complex with proteinaceous exudate, such as albumin, at ulcer site. Also forms a viscous adhesive barrier on the surface of intact mucosa of the stomach or duodenum.

Therapeutic Effect: Protects damaged mucosa from further destruction by absorbing gastric acid, pepsin, and bile salts.

PHARMACOKINETICS

Minimally absorbed from the GI tract. Eliminated in feces, with small amount excreted in urine. Not removed by hemodialysis.

AVAILABILITY

Oral suspension: 1 g/10 mL.
Tablets: 1 g.

INDICATIONS AND DOSAGE

Active duodenal ulcers

PO

Adults, Elderly: 1 g 4 times per day (before meals and at bedtime) for up to 8 wk.

Maintenance therapy after healing of acute duodenal ulcers

PO

Adults, Elderly: 1 g twice per day.

OFF-LABEL USES

Prevention and treatment of stress-related mucosal damage, especially in acutely or critically ill patients; treatment of gastric ulcer and rheumatoid arthritis; relief of GI symptoms associated with NSAIDs; treatment of gastroesophageal reflux disease

CONTRAINDICATIONS

Hypersensitivity to sucralfate

INTERACTIONS

Drug: Antacids: May interfere with binding of sucralfate. **Digoxin, phenytoin, quinolones, such as ciprofloxacin, theophylline:** May decrease the absorption of these drugs. **Herbal:** None known. **Food:** None known.

DIAGNOSTIC TEST EFFECTS

None known.

SIDE-EFFECTS

Frequent (2%): Constipation. **Occasional (less than 2%):** Dry mouth, backache, diarrhea, dizziness, somnolence, nausea, indigestion, rash, hives, itching, abdominal discomfort

CRITICAL CARE CONSIDERATIONS

ADMINISTRATION/HANDLING

PO ALERT

- Administer 1 hr before meals and at bedtime.
- Tablets may be crushed or dissolved in water.
- Do not give antacids within 30 min of sucralfate.
- **Drug binding:** Do not give digoxin, phenytoin, quinolones, or theophylline within 2 to 3 hr of sucralfate.
- **Dosage:** 1 g equals 10 mL suspension.

PRECAUTIONS

HEALTH-RELATED

- Aluminum toxicity may result if patients are receiving other medications containing aluminum; renal impaired patients are at higher risk of aluminum toxicity; duodenal ulcers may reoccur following successful healing using sucralfate.

AGE-RELATED

- **Children:** Safety and efficacy of sucralfate have not been established in children.
- **Elderly:** No age-related precautions have been noted.

PREGNANCY/LACTATION-RELATED

- Pregnancy category B; little systemic absorption, so minimal, if any, excretion into milk expected.

MONITORING

- **Baseline assessment:** Before sucralfate administration, assess abdomen for tenderness, rigidity, and the presence of bowel sounds. Determine when the last bowel movement occurred; note the amount and consistency.
- **Lab work:** Biochemical profile including renal function (BUN, creatinine) studies.
- **Constipation:** Assess pattern of daily bowel activity and stool consistency.
- **Patient education:** Instruct to take sucralfate on an empty stomach. Teach that antacids should not be taken for 30 min before or after sucralfate because the formation of sucralfate gel is activated by stomach acid. Suggest to take sips of tepid water or suck on sour hard candy to relieve dry mouth.

SERIOUS ADVERSE REACTIONS

- None known when recommended doses are taken.

OVERDOSE/TOXICITY

- **Aluminum toxicity:** Osteodystrophy, osteomalacia, and encephalopathy are possible in renal impaired patients receiving other medications containing aluminum, such as some antacids.
- **GI decontamination:** No specific recommendations.

ANTIDOTE/DIALYSIS

- **Antidote:** No specific recommendations.
- **Dialysis:** Sucralfate is not removed by hemodialysis or peritoneal dialysis. No data are available on removal by high-permeability hemodialysis.

sufentanil citrate

soo-fen'-tah-nil sih'-trayt

DEA Schedule: II

Classes

Chemical: proprionolide citrate

Therapeutic: anesthesia adjunct, analgesic, narcotic

Pregnancy Category: C

Trade Names

Prescription: Sufenta

CLINICAL PHARMACOLOGY

Mechanism of Action

A synthetic opioid analgesic that binds at opiate receptor sites within the CNS, reducing stimuli from sensory nerve endings. **Therapeutic Effect:** Increases pain threshold, alters pain reception, inhibits ascending pain pathways.

PHARMACOKINETICS

Protein binding: 93%. The liver and small intestine are the major sites of metabolism. Excreted in urine. **Half-life:** 164 min.

AVAILABILITY

Intravenous solution: 50 mcg/mL.

INDICATIONS AND DOSAGE

General anesthesia, primary agent

IV

Adults: 8-30 mcg/kg with 100% oxygen and a muscle relaxant, then 0.5-10 mcg/kg as needed in response to signs of lightening of anesthesia. Maximum: 30 mcg/kg/procedure. **Children up to 12 yr:** Procedure on cardiovascular system: 10-25 mcg/kg with 100% oxygen, additional doses up to 25-50 mcg for maintenance of anesthesia.

General anesthesia, adjunct for anesthesia

IV

Adults: 1-8 mcg/kg. Give 75% before intubation, then incrementally as 10-50 mcg in response to signs of lightening of analgesia.

Analgesia for labor and delivery

Epidural

Adults: 10-15 mcg administered with 10 mL bupivacaine 0.125% with or without epinephrine. Sufentanil citrate and bupivacaine should be mixed together before administration. Doses can be repeated twice (for a total of 3 doses) at not less than 1-hr intervals until delivery.

CONTRAINDICATIONS

Hypersensitivity to sufentanil, intolerance of opioid agonists

INTERACTIONS

Drug: **Benzodiazepines:** May decrease arterial pressure and systemic vascular resistance. **Beta-blockers, calcium channel blockers:** May increase the risk of bradycardia and hypotension. **CNS depressants:** May increase CNS and cardiovascular effects. **Neuromuscular blocking agents:** May increase the risk of bradycardia and hypotension. **Herbal:** None known. **Food:** None known.

DIAGNOSTIC TEST EFFECTS

May increase serum amylase and lipase concentrations.

SIDE-EFFECTS

Frequent (greater than 9%): Pruritus, hypotension, bradycardia, somnolence, nausea, vomiting. **Occasional (3%-9%):** Confusion, blurred vision, orthostatic hypotension, chest wall rigidity, somnolence, nausea, vomiting. **Rare (less than 3%):** Skeletal muscle rigidity of neck and extremities, dysrhythmia, tachycardia, chills, erythema, apnea, bronchospasm, postoperative respiratory depression, intraoperative muscle movement

CRITICAL CARE CONSIDERATIONS

ADMINISTRATION/HANDLING

IV ALERT

- **Skilled providers only:** Sufentanil citrate should be given only by those specially trained in the use of IV anesthetics, including management of respiratory depression. Opioid antagonist, resuscitative and endotracheal intubation equipment, and oxygen should be readily available.
- **Anesthesiologist/anesthetist:** Before IV catheter insertion, those administering sufentanil should be familiar with patient conditions (such as bleeding disorders, current use of anticoagulants and infection) so that appropriate risk-benefit assessment can be performed before drug is given.
- **Dosage reduction:** If benzodiazepines, barbiturates, inhalation agents, other

S

opioids or other CNS depressants are used concomitantly, the dose of sufentanil and/or these agents should be reduced.

- **Dosage:** Sufentanil citrate dosage should be individualized according to body weight, physical status, underlying pathologic condition, use of other drugs, type of surgical procedure, and anesthesia.

EPIDURAL ALERT

- **Use during labor and delivery:** Proper placement of the needle or catheter in the epidural space should be verified before sufentanil citrate is injected to avoid unintentional IV injection, which can result in overdose.

PRECAUTIONS

HEALTH-RELATED

- Use cautiously in patients with bradycardia, head injuries, impaired consciousness, and liver, renal, or respiratory disease.
- **Sedation and analgesia:** If sedation is needed for management of anxiety, agitation, or mechanical ventilation, give fentanyl before sedation to ensure pain relief rather than having sedation mask response to pain.

AGE-RELATED

- **Children:** No age-related precautions have been noted in children.
- **Elderly:** Are more susceptible to the respiratory depressant effects of sufentanil. The initial dose should be appropriately reduced in these patients.

PREGNANCY/LACTATION-RELATED

- Pregnancy category C; use with extreme caution in breast-feeding women.

S

MONITORING

- **Baseline assessment:** Assess vital signs. Assess the duration, intensity, location, and type of pain experienced. For epidural use, ensure proper placement of epidural catheter or needle before injection of sufentanil (by the person specially trained in use of anesthetic medications).
- **Respiratory depression:** Monitor for hypotension, tachycardia/tachypnea, bradycardia/bradypnea, and hypoxemia. Early signs of hypoxemia reflect sympathetic nervous system stimulation while late signs reflect central nervous system depression secondary to hypoxemia.
- **Cardiac:** Monitor ECG continuously for dysrhythmias.
- **Bedridden patients:** Assist to cough, turn, and breathe deeply every 2 hr. If able to sit or get out of bed, assist with ambulation.
- **Therapeutic effect:** Assess for relief of pain. If patients cannot communicate, note tachycardia, hypertension, increased level of agitation, and grimacing, which may indicate pain is not relieved.
- **Patient education:** Urge to avoid alcohol and not to take any other medications during therapy. Tasks requiring mental alertness or motor skills should be avoided.

SERIOUS ADVERSE REACTIONS

- **Respiratory depression:** Slow respiratory rate (less than 8 breaths/min), shallow respirations, decreasing pulse oximetry reading, decreasing heart rate, bradycardia, ventricular dysrhythmias. Patients should be intubated before IV use. If epidural patients experience respiratory depression, position of the catheter/needle should be validated as well as dose. All patients with respiratory distress should be endotracheally intubated and should be resuscitated as needed according to Advanced Cardiac Life Support (ACLS) guidelines.

OVERDOSE/TOXICITY

- **Overdose:** Overdosage may result in severe respiratory depression, skeletal and thoracic muscle rigidity resulting in apnea, laryngospasm, bronchospasm, cold and clammy skin, cyanosis, coma, and cardiac arrest.
- **Management:** Resuscitate according to ACLS guidelines. Maintain patent airway using endotracheal tube, manual or mechanical ventilation, support of heart rate and BP with inotropes, chronotropes, and vasopressors. Administer naloxone to reverse narcotic effects, keeping in mind patients will require alternate form of pain management when conscious.
- **GI decontamination:** No specific recommendations.

ANTIDOTE/DIALYSIS

- **Antidote:** Naloxone given IV is effective in reversing the effects of sufentanil and other opioid narcotics. May require repeated administration.
- **Dialysis:** Sufentanil is unlikely to be removed with hemodialysis or peritoneal dialysis. No data are available regarding removal using high-permeability hemodialysis.

sulfamethoxazole and trimethoprim (co-trimoxazole)

sul-fa-meth-ox'-a-zole; trye-meth'-oh-prim

Classes

Chemical: dihydrofolate reductase inhibitor (trimethoprim), sulfonamide derivative (sulfamethoxazole)
Therapeutic: antibiotic

Pregnancy Category: C

Trade Names

Prescription: Apo-Sulfatrim ♣, Bactrim, Bactrim DS, Bactrim Pediatric, Bethaprim, Bethaprim Pediatric, Cotrim, Comoxol, Novotrimel ♣, Septra, Septra DS, Sulfatrim Pediatric, Sulfatrim Suspension, Uroplus, Uroplus DS

Do not confuse Bactrim with bacitracin, co-trimoxazole with clotrimazole, or Septra with Sectral or Septa.

CLINICAL PHARMACOLOGY

Mechanism of Action

A sulfonamide and folate antagonist that blocks bacterial synthesis of essential nucleic acids. **Therapeutic Effect:** Bactericidal in susceptible microorganisms.

PHARMACOKINETICS

Rapidly and well absorbed from the GI tract. Protein binding: 45%-60%. Widely distributed. Metabolized in the liver. Excreted in urine. **Half-life:** sulfamethoxazole 6-12 hr, trimethoprim 8-10 hr (increased in impaired renal function).

AVAILABILITY

Alert: All dosage forms have same 5:1 ratio of sulfamethoxazole (SMX) to trimethoprim (TMP).
Oral Suspension (Bactrim Pediatric, Bethaprim Pediatric, Septra, Sulfatrim, Sulfatrim Pediatric): SMX 200 mg and TMP 40 mg per 5 mL.
Tablets (Bactrim, Septra, Uroplus): SMX 400 mg and TMP 80 mg.
Tablets (double strength [Bactrim DS, Septra DS, Uroplus DS]): SMX 800 mg and TMP 160 mg.
Injection: SMX 80 mg and TMP 16 mg per mL.

INDICATIONS AND DOSAGE

Chronic bronchitis

PO

Adults, Elderly: 1 double-strength or 2 single-strength tablets or 20 mL suspension every 12 hr for 14 days.

Pneumocystis Carinii pneumonia (PCP) prophylaxis

PO

Adults, Elderly: 1 double-strength tablet daily or 3 times per wk or 1 single-strength tablet daily. **Children 1 mo and older:** 150 mg/m^2 as trimethoprim each day in 2 divided doses 3 times per wk on consecutive days.

PCP Treatment

PO, IV

Adults, Elderly, Children 2 mo and older: 15-20 mg/kg as trimethoprim per day in 4 divided doses for 14-21 days.

Shigellosis

PO

Adults, Elderly: 1 double-strength tablet or 2 single-strength tablets or 20 mL suspension every 12 hr for 5 days.

IV

Children: 8-10 mg/kg as trimethoprim per day in 2-4 divided doses for up to 5 days.

Otitis media

PO

Children 2 mo and older: 8 mg/kg trimethoprim per day every 12 hr for 10 days.

Urinary tract infections

PO

Adults, Elderly: 1 double-strength or 2 single-strength tablets or 20-mL suspension every 12 hr for 10-14 days. **Children 2 mo and older:** 8 mg/kg as trimethoprim per day in 2 divided doses for 10 days.

Travelers' diarrhea

PO

Adults, Elderly: 1 double-strength or 2 single-strength tablets or 20-mL suspension every 12 hr for 5 days.

Dosage in renal impairment

Dosage and frequency are modified based on creatinine clearance, the severity of the infection, and the serum concentration of the drug. For those with creatinine clearance of 15-30 mL/min, a 50% dosage reduction is recommended.

OFF-LABEL USES

Treatment of bacterial endocarditis; gonorrhea; meningitis; septicemia; sinusitis; and biliary tract, bone, joint, chancroid, chlamydial, intraabdominal, skin and soft-tissue infections

S

CONTRAINDICATIONS

Hypersensitivity to trimethoprim or any sulfonamides, infants younger than 2 mo old, megaloblastic anemia due to folate deficiency, nursing mothers, pregnant women

INTERACTIONS

Drug: Hemolytics: May increase the risk of toxicity. **Hepatotoxic medications:** May increase the risk of hepatotoxicity. **Hydantoin anticonvulsants, oral antidiabetics, warfarin:** May increase or prolong the effects of these drugs and increase their risk of toxicity. **Methenamine:** May form a precipitate. **Methotrexate:** May increase the effects of methotrexate. **Herbal:** None known. **Food:** None known.

DIAGNOSTIC TEST EFFECTS

May increase BUN and serum alkaline phosphatase, creatinine, potassium, AST (SGOT), and ALT (SGPT) levels.

IV INCOMPATIBILITIES

Fluconazole (Diflucan), foscarnet (Foscavir), midazolam (Versed), vinorelbine (Navelbine), total parenteral nutrition (TPN)

IV COMPATIBILITIES

Diltiazem (Cardizem), heparin, hydromorphone (Dilaudid), lorazepam (Ativan), magnesium sulfate, morphine

SIDE-EFFECTS

Frequent: Anorexia, nausea, vomiting, rash (generally 7-14 days after therapy begins), urticaria. **Occasional:** Diarrhea, abdominal pain, pain or irritation at the IV infusion site. **Rare:** Headache, vertigo, insomnia, seizures, hallucinations, depression

CRITICAL CARE CONSIDERATIONS

ADMINISTRATION/HANDLING

PO ALERT

- Store tablets and oral suspension at room temperature.
- Give the oral form with 8 oz water on an empty stomach. Have patients drink several additional glasses of water each day.
- Drug potency is expressed in terms of trimethoprim content.

IV ALERT

- **Stability:** Discard the solution if it is cloudy or contains a precipitate. IV infusion solution (piggyback) is stable for 2-6 hr. Use the solution immediately.
- **IV intermittent (piggyback) infusion:** Dilute each 5-mL vial with 75-125 mL D_5W. Do not mix co-trimoxazole with other drugs or solutions. Infuse the solution over 60-90 min. Avoid bolus or rapid infusion and IM injection.

PRECAUTIONS

HEALTH-RELATED

- Use co-trimoxazole cautiously in patients with impaired renal or hepatic function or glucose-6-phosphate dehydrogenase deficiency.

AGE-RELATED

- **Children:** Co-trimoxazole use is contraindicated in children under 2 mo; if given to newborns, it may produce kernicterus.
- **Elderly:** Have an increased risk of developing myelosuppression, decreased platelet count, and severe skin reactions.

PREGNANCY/LACTATION-RELATED

- Pregnancy category C; contraindicated in pregnant women and nursing mothers. *Do not use at term.* May cause kernicterus in the neonate. Not recommended in the neonatal nursing period because sulfonamides excreted in breast milk may cause kernicterus.

MONITORING

- **Baseline assessment:** Determine history of bronchial asthma, hypersensitivity to trimethoprim or any sulfonamide, or sulfite sensitivity before beginning drug therapy. Assess for dehydration, which should be corrected early.
- **Lab work:** Baseline CBC with WBC differential, biochemical panel including renal (BUN, creatinine) and liver (AST [SGOT], ALT [SGPT], bilirubin, alkaline phosphatase) function tests. Monitor CBC with differential and renal and liver function tests.
- **Hydration:** Monitor intake and output. Ensure adequate hydration.
- **Diarrhea:** Assess pattern of daily bowel activity and stool consistency. Uncontrolled diarrhea may lead to dehydration, which may prompt renal and liver insufficiency.
- **Phlebitis:** Check the IV site for redness and flow rate.
- **CNS symptoms:** Evaluate patients for such symptoms as hallucinations, headache, insomnia, and vertigo.
- **Adverse reactions:** Discontinue co-trimoxazole at the first sign of skin rash, pallor, purpura, cough, shortness of breath, ecchymosis, overt bleeding, or edema.

- **Patient education:** Instruct to take oral co-trimoxazole doses with 8 oz of water and to drink several extra glasses of water each day. Advise spacing drug doses evenly around the clock and to continue taking co-trimoxazole for the full course of treatment. Instruct to report new symptoms promptly, especially bleeding, bruising, fever, sore throat, and a rash or other skin changes to a health care provider.

SERIOUS ADVERSE REACTIONS

- Rash, fever, sore throat, pallor, purpura, cough, and shortness of breath may be early signs of serious adverse reactions.
- **Hypersensitivity:** Stevens–Johnson syndrome, toxic epidermal necrolysis, severe dermatologic reactions (especially in the elderly).
- **Management:** Co-trimoxazole should be discontinued at the first sign of skin rash or any adverse reaction. Supportive care should be provided according to current standards.

OVERDOSE/TOXICITY

- **Hematologic:** Thrombocytopenia, agranulocytosis, aplastic anemia, generalized myelosuppression, and other blood dyscrasias; some are fatal.
- **Hepatotoxicity:** Elevated liver enzymes, fever, right upper quadrant pain, fulminant hepatic necrosis; has been fatal.
- **Nephrotoxicity:** Increased BUN, creatinine, nausea, vomiting, flank pain, possible hematuria and hyperkalemia.
- **GI decontamination:** No specific recommendations.

ANTIDOTE/DIALYSIS

- **Antidote:** No specific recommendations.
- **Dialysis:** Sulfamethoxazole and trimethoprim are removed by hemodialysis and are likely removed by high-permeability hemodialysis. They are not removed by peritoneal dialysis.

sulfasalazine

sul-fa-sal'-a-zeen

Classes

Chemical: salicylate derivative, sulfonamide derivative

Therapeutic: disease-modifying antirheumatic drug (DMARD), gastrointestinal antiinflammatory

Pregnancy Category: B, D (near or at term)

Trade Names

Prescription: Azulfidine, Azulfidine EN-Tabs, Salazopyrin ♣, Salazopyrin-EN ♣

Do not confuse Azulfidine with azathioprine, or sulfasalazine with sulfadiazine or sulfisoxazole.

CLINICAL PHARMACOLOGY

Mechanism of Action

A sulfonamide that inhibits prostaglandin synthesis, acting locally in the colon. **Therapeutic Effect:** Decreases inflammatory response, interferes with GI secretion.

PHARMACOKINETICS

Poorly absorbed from the GI tract. Cleaved in colon by intestinal bacteria, forming sulfapyridine and mesalamine (5-ASA). Absorbed in colon. Widely distributed. Metabolized in the liver. Primarily excreted in urine. **Half-life:** sulfapyridine, 6-14 hr; 5-ASA, 0.6-1.4 hr.

AVAILABILITY

Tablets (Azulfidine): 500 mg.

Tablets (delayed release [Azulfidine EN-Tabs]): 500 mg.

INDICATIONS AND DOSAGE

Ulcerative colitis

PO

Adults, Elderly: 1 g 3-4 times per day in divided doses every 4-6 hr. Maintenance: 2 g/day in divided doses every 6-12 hr. Maximum: 6 g/day. **Children more than 2 yr:** 40-75 mg/kg/day in divided doses every 4-6 hr. Mild exacerbation: 40-50 mg/kg/day. Moderate to severe exacerbation: 50-75 mg/kg/day. Maintenance: 30-50 mg/kg/day in divided doses every 4-8 hr. Maximum: 6 g/day.

Rheumatoid arthritis

PO

Adults, Elderly: Initially, 0.5-1 g/day for 1 wk. Increase by 0.5 g/wk, up to 3 g/day.

Juvenile rheumatoid arthritis

PO

Children: Initially, 10 mg/kg/day. May increase by 10 mg/kg/day at weekly intervals. Range: 30-50 mg/kg/day. Maximum: 2 g/day.

OFF-LABEL USES

Treatment of ankylosing spondylitis, collagenous colitis, Crohn's disease, juvenile chronic arthritis, psoriasis, psoriatic arthritis

CONTRAINDICATIONS

Children younger than 2 yr; hypersensitivity to sulfasalazine, carbonic anhydrase inhibitors, local anesthetics, salicylates, sulfonamides, sulfonylureas, sunscreens containing PABA, or thiazide or loop diuretics; intestinal or urinary tract obstruction; porphyria; pregnancy at term; severe hepatic or renal dysfunction

INTERACTIONS

Drug: Anticonvulsants, methotrexate, oral anticoagulants, oral antidiabetics: May increase the effects of these drugs. **Hemolytics:** May increase the toxicity of sulfasalazine. **Hepatotoxic medications:** May increase the risk of hepatotoxicity. **Herbal:** None known. **Food:** None known.

DIAGNOSTIC TEST EFFECTS

None known.

SIDE-EFFECTS

Frequent (33%): Anorexia, nausea, vomiting, headache, oligospermia (generally reversed by withdrawal of drug). **Occasional (3%):** Hypersensitivity reaction (rash, urticaria, pruritus, fever, anemia). **Rare (less than 1%):** Tinnitus, hypoglycemia, diuresis, photosensitivity

CRITICAL CARE CONSIDERATIONS

ADMINISTRATION/HANDLING

PO ALERT

- Space drug doses evenly at intervals less than 8 hr.
- Administer sulfasalazine after meals to prolong intestinal passage.
- Swallow delayed-release tablets whole without chewing or crushing.
- Give sulfasalazine with 8 oz of water.

PRECAUTIONS

HEALTH-RELATED

- Use sulfasalazine cautiously in patients with bronchial asthma, G6PD deficiency, impaired hepatic or renal function, or severe allergies.
- Sulfasalazine may produce infertility and oligospermia in men.

AGE-RELATED

- **Children:** No age-related precautions for children over 2 yr.
- **Elderly:** No age-related precautions have been noted.

PREGNANCY/LACTATION-RELATED

- Pregnancy category B, D (at or near term); excreted into breast milk; should be given to nursing mothers with caution because significant adverse effects (bloody diarrhea) may occur in some nursing infants.

MONITORING

- **Baseline assessment:** Determine hypersensitivity to medications, including carbonic anhydrase inhibitors, local anesthetics, salicylates, sulfonamides, sulfonylureas, thiazide or loop diuretics, and sunscreens containing PABA, before beginning drug therapy.
- **Lab work:** CBC; biochemical profile including liver and renal function studies; urinalysis test results.
- **Oliguria:** Monitor intake and output, renal function and urinalysis test results. Ensure that patients drink plenty of water to maintain adequate hydration (minimum output 1500 mL/24 hr) and prevent nephrotoxicity.
- **Hypersensitivity:** Examine skin for rash. Withhold sulfasalazine at the first sign of rash.
- **Diarrhea:** Assess pattern of daily bowel activity and stool consistency. The drug dosage may need to be increased if diarrhea continues or recurs.
- **Bone marrow suppression:** Closely monitor CBC with differential; check for bleeding, ecchymosis, fever, jaundice, pallor, purpura, pharyngitis, and weakness.
- **Patient education:** Instruct to take sulfasalazine after food with 8 oz of water and to drink several glasses of water between meals. Advise to space drug doses around the clock and to continue sulfasalazine therapy for the full course of treatment. Explain that the drug therapy may need to continue even after symptoms are relieved. Stress the importance of complying with follow-up and laboratory tests. Instruct to inform the dentist or surgeon of sulfasalazine therapy if planning dental or other surgical procedures. Urge to avoid exposure to sun and ultraviolet light until photosensitivity is determined; photosensitivity may last for months after the last dose of sulfasalazine.

SERIOUS ADVERSE REACTIONS

- **Hypersensitivity:** Anaphylaxis, Stevens–Johnson syndrome, exfoliative dermatitis, epidermal necrolysis, lupuslike syndrome, pericarditis, pneumonitis.

S

- **Gastrointestinal:** Hepatitis, pancreatitis, bloody diarrhea, diarrhea.
- **Central nervous system:** Seizures, transverse myelitis, meningitis, peripheral neuropathy, hallucinations, tinnitus.
- **Urinary tract infection:** Dysuria, pyuria, hematuria.

OVERDOSE/TOXICITY

- **Hematologic toxicity:** Leukopenia, agranulocytosis.
- **Hepatotoxicity:** Nausea, vomiting, abdominal and/or right upper quadrant pain, fever, elevated liver enzymes, jaundice. Patients have required liver transplant.
- **Nephrotoxicity:** Oliguria, elevated BUN and creatinine, nausea, proteinuria, hematuria, nephrotic syndrome, hemolytic-uremic syndrome.
- **GI decontamination:** No specific recommendations.

ANTIDOTE/DIALYSIS

- **Antidote:** No specific recommendations.
- **Dialysis:** Sulfasalazine is unlikely to be removed by hemodialysis, high-permeability hemodialysis, or peritoneal dialysis.

sulindac

See NSAIDs and Cox-2 Inhibitors (p. 976)

sumatriptan succinate

soo-ma-trip'-tan suk'-si-nate

Classes

Chemical: serotonin derivative
Therapeutic: antimigraine agent

Pregnancy Category: C

Trade Names

Prescription: Imitrex, Imitrex Nasal, Imitrex Statdose, Imitrex Statdose Refill

Do not confuse sumatriptan with somatropin.

CLINICAL PHARMACOLOGY

Mechanism of Action

A serotonin receptor agonist that binds selectively to vascular receptors, producing a vasoconstrictive effect on cranial blood vessels. **Therapeutic Effect:** Relieves migraine headache.

PHARMACOKINETICS

Route	Onset	Peak	Duration
Nasal	15 min	2 hr	Unknown
PO	1-2 hr	2 hr	4 hr
Subcutaneous	10 min	1 hr	Unknown

Rapidly absorbed after subcutaneous administration. Absorption after PO administration is incomplete, with significant amounts undergoing hepatic metabolism, resulting in low bioavailability (about 14%). Protein binding: 10%-21%. Widely distributed. Undergoes first-pass metabolism in the liver. Excreted in urine. **Half-life:** 2 hr.

AVAILABILITY

Tablets (Imitrex): 25 mg, 50 mg, 100 mg.
Injection (Imitrex, Imitrex Statdose): 4-mg prefilled cartridge, 6 mg/0.5 mL.
Nasal spray (Imitrex Nasal): 5 mg, 20 mg.

INDICATIONS AND DOSAGE

Acute migraine attack

PO

Adults, Elderly: 25-100 mg. Dose may be repeated after at least 2 hr. Maximum: 100 mg/single dose; 200 mg/24 hr.

Subcutaneous

Adults, Elderly: 6 mg. Maximum: Two 6-mg injections/24 hr (separated by at least 1 hr).

Intranasal

Adults, Elderly: 5-20 mg; may repeat in 2 hr. Maximum: 40 mg/24 hr.

CONTRAINDICATIONS

Cerebrovascular accident (CVA), ischemic heart disease (including angina pectoris, history of MI, silent ischemia, and Prinzmetal's angina), severe hepatic impairment, transient ischemic attack, uncontrolled hypertension, use within 14 days of MAOIs, use within 24 hr of ergotamine preparations, hypersensitivity to sumatriptan

INTERACTIONS

Drug: Ergotamine-containing medications: May produce vasospastic reaction. **MAOIs:** May increase sumatriptan blood concentration and half-life. **Herbal:** None known. **Food:** None known.

DIAGNOSTIC TEST EFFECTS

None known.

SIDE-EFFECTS

Frequent: Oral (10%-5%): Tingling, nasal discomfort. **Subcutaneous (greater than**

S

10%): Injection site reactions, tingling, warm or hot sensation, dizziness, vertigo. **Nasal (greater than 10%):** Bad or unusual taste, nausea, vomiting. **Occasional: Oral (5%-1%):** Flushing, asthenia, visual disturbances. **Subcutaneous (10%-2%):** Burning sensation, numbness, chest discomfort, drowsiness, asthenia. **Nasal (5%-1%):** Nasopharyngeal discomfort, dizziness. **Rare: Oral (less than 1%):** Agitation, eye irritation, dysuria. **Subcutaneous (less than 2%):** Anxiety, fatigue, diaphoresis, muscle cramps, myalgia. **Nasal (less than 1%):** Burning sensation

CRITICAL CARE CONSIDERATIONS

ADMINISTRATION/HANDLING

PO ALERT

- Swallow tablets whole with a full glass of water; do not crush.

SUBCUTANEOUS ALERT

- **Autoinjection:** Follow manufacturer's instructions to use autoinjection device.
- **Not for IV use:** Sumatriptan succinate injection should not be given IV because of risk of coronary vasospasm.

NASAL ALERT

- Do not test before use; each unit contains only 1 spray.
- **Preparation:** Blow the nose gently to clear nasal passages. With the head upright, close one of the nostrils with an index finger and breathe gently through the mouth.
- **Administration:** Insert the nozzle about a half inch into the open nostril. Close the mouth, breathe through the nose, and depress the blue plunger to release the spray. Remove nozzle from the nose and shallowly breathe in through the nose and out through the mouth for 10-20 sec.

PRECAUTIONS

HEALTH-RELATED

- Sumatriptan should only be used when a clear diagnosis of migraines is established.
- Sumatriptan should not be used in patients with hemiplegic or basilar migraines.
- Use sumatriptan cautiously in patients with cardiovascular risk factors, mild to moderate hepatic impairment, epilepsy, or a hypersensitivity to sulfonamides.
- The prescriber should be aware that patients with cluster headaches often have at least one predictive risk factor for coronary artery disease (CAD). All patients who use sumatriptan long term should undergo evaluation of cardiovascular status periodically, particularly males over 40 yr with cluster headaches.
- If decision is made to use sumatriptan in a patient with CAD risk factors, manufacturer recommends the first dose be given in an environment with appropriate medical staffing and ability to respond to emergencies.

AGE-RELATED

- **Children:** Safety and efficacy of sumatriptan have not been established in children.
- **Elderly:** No age-related precautions have been noted.

PREGNANCY/LACTATION-RELATED

- Pregnancy category C; excreted in breast milk in animals, no data for humans.

MONITORING

- **Baseline assessment:** Determine history of hepatic disease, renal impairment, peripheral vascular disease, pregnancy or planned pregnancy. Assess the onset, location, and duration of migraines and possible precipitating factors. Obtain a baseline BP for evidence of uncontrolled hypertension, a contraindication.
- **Lab work:** Baseline biochemical profile including renal (BUN, creatinine) and liver (AST [SGOT], ALT [SGPT], alkaline phosphatase, bilirubin, GGT) function tests. If chest discomfort is experienced during treatment, perform a cardiac profile (CPK, creatine kinase-MB and troponins).
- **Diagnostic tests:** Baseline 12-lead ECG to evaluate for myocardial ischemia.
- **Therapeutic effect:** Assess for relief of migraines and associated symptoms, including nausea and vomiting, photophobia, and phonophobia. Patients may go to sleep as headache resolves.
- **Environment:** Have patients lie in a dark, quiet room until headache subsides.
- **Vomiting:** Migraine headaches may induce sudden onset, projectile vomiting. Have personal protective equipment readily available.
- **Dysrhythmias:** Monitor ECG rhythm continuously for ST depression or elevation and ventricular dysrhythmias if used while patients are in a critical care unit.

S

- **Cardiovascular crisis:** Monitor for changes in neurologic status, chest discomfort, severe abdominal pain, low urine output and limb ischemia. Vasospasms may be severe and create end-organ ischemia and peripheral ischemia leading to tissue damage.
- **Patient education:** Teach how to load the autoinjector properly, inject the medication, and discard the syringe. Instruct on how to inject the drug into an area with adequate subcutaneous tissue because the needle will penetrate the skin and adipose tissue as deeply as 6 mm; patients are not to administer more than two subcutaneous injections during any 24-hr period and should allow at least 1 hr between injections. Instruct to report immediately palpitations, a rash, wheezing, pain or tightness in the chest or throat, or facial edema to a health care provider. Advise to lie down in dark, quiet room for additional benefit after taking sumatriptan. Recommend avoidance of tasks that require mental alertness or motor skills until response to the drug is known. Urge female patients of childbearing age to use contraceptives during therapy and to inform the physician if pregnancy is suspected.

SERIOUS ADVERSE REACTIONS

- **Cardiovascular instability:** Hypertension, chest discomfort, angina, dyspnea, ventricular dysrhythmias; seen more often in patients with hypertension, diabetes, or a strong family history of coronary artery disease; obese patients; and smokers.
- **Neurovascular instability:** Confusion, disorientation, weakness, slurred speech, inability to speak or to communicate clearly; pain in or paresis or paralysis of one or more extremities; loss of peripheral pulses.
- **Excessive dosage:** May produce tremor, red extremities, reduced respirations, cyanosis, seizures, and paralysis.

OVERDOSE/TOXICITY

- **Cardiovascular crisis:** Coronary artery vasospasm, acute MI, cerebral vasospasm, CVA/stroke. Vasospasm-related reactions and intracranial hemorrhage occur rarely but are more common in patients with cardiovascular risk factors (hypertension, diabetes, strong family history of coronary artery disease, obesity, smokers, males aged over 40 yr, and postmenopausal women).
- **Ophthalmologic disturbances:** May bind to the melanin in the eye, causing visual impairment or corneal opacities.
- **Death:** Significant cardiovascular events have resulted in death.
- **GI decontamination:** No specific recommendations.

ANTIDOTE/DIALYSIS

- **Antidote:** No specific antidote. Animal studies have had positive results using *chlorproMAZINE, cyproheptadine, and propranolol as serotonin antagonists for serotonin syndrome, but these drugs may not have direct effects on vasospasms.
- **Dialysis:** No data are available regarding removal of sumatriptan using hemodialysis, high-permeability hemodialysis, or peritoneal dialysis.

S

tacrine hydrochloride

tak'-reen hye-droe-klor'-ide

Classes
Chemical: cholinesterase inhibitor, monoamine acridine derivative
Therapeutic: antidementia agent

Pregnancy Category: C

Trade Names
Prescription: Cognex

CLINICAL PHARMACOLOGY

Mechanism of Action
A cholinesterase inhibitor that inhibits the enzyme acetylcholinesterase, thus increasing the concentration of acetylcholine at cholinergic synapses and enhancing cholinergic function in the CNS. **Therapeutic Effect:** Slows the progression of Alzheimer's disease.

PHARMACOKINETICS

Rapidly absorbed following PO administration. Protein binding: 55%. Extensively metabolized in liver. Negligible amounts excreted in urine. **Half-life:** 2-4 hr.

AVAILABILITY

Capsules: 10 mg, 20 mg, 30 mg, 40 mg.

INDICATIONS AND DOSAGE

Alzheimer's disease
PO
Adults, Elderly: Initially, 10 mg 4 times per day for 6 wk, followed by 20 mg 4 times per day for 6 wk, 30 mg 4 times per day for 12 wk, then 40 mg 4 times per day if needed.

Dosage in hepatic impairment
For patients with ALT (SGPT) greater than 3-5 times normal, decrease the dose by 40 mg/day and resume the normal dose when ALT (SGPT) returns to normal. For patients with ALT (SGPT) greater than 5 times normal, stop treatment and resume it when ALT (SGPT) returns to normal.

CONTRAINDICATIONS

Known hypersensitivity to tacrine, patients previously treated with tacrine who developed jaundice

INTERACTIONS

Drug: Anticholinergics: May decrease the effects of tacrine or anticholinergics. **Cimetidine:** May increase the tacrine blood concentration. **NSAIDs:** May increase the adverse effects of NSAIDs. **Theophylline:** May increase the theophylline blood concentration. **Herbal:** None known. **Food:** None known.

DIAGNOSTIC TEST EFFECTS

Increases AST (SGOT) and ALT (SGPT) levels. Alters blood Hgb, Hct, and serum electrolyte levels.

SIDE-EFFECTS

Frequent (28%-11%): Headache, nausea, vomiting, diarrhea, dizziness. **Occasional (9%-4%):** Fatigue, chest pain, dyspepsia, anorexia, abdominal pain, flatulence, constipation, confusion, agitation, rash, depression, ataxia, insomnia, rhinitis, myalgia. **Rare (less than 3%):** Weight loss, anxiety, cough, facial flushing, urinary frequency, back pain, tremor

CRITICAL CARE CONSIDERATIONS

ADMINISTRATION/HANDLING

PO ALERT

- Give tacrine without regard to food.
- **Rechallenge:** If tacrine therapy is stopped because of liver enzyme elevation less than 10 times upper limit of normal (ULN), check liver enzymes and reinstitute therapy if transaminases (AST [SGOT], ALT [SGPT]) have normalized. Patients with jaundice, elevated bilirubin (more than 3 mg/dL), and/or 10 times ULN elevations should not be rechallenged.

PRECAUTIONS

HEALTH-RELATED

- Use tacrine cautiously in patients with alcohol abuse, asthma, bradycardia, cardiac dysrhythmias, chronic obstructive pulmonary disease, peptic ulcer disease, hyperthyroidism, hepatic dysfunction, or a history of seizures.
- **Cytochrome P450 enzyme metabolism:** Tacrine is metabolized by this enzyme pathway, which may prompt drug interactions with other medications that are metabolized by these enzymes. Noted interactions include theophylline, cimetidine, anticholinergic medications, and drugs that increase or decrease cholinergic activity.

AGE-RELATED

- **Children:** Safety and efficacy of tacrine have not been established in children.
- **Elderly:** No age-related precautions have been noted.

PREGNANCY/LACTATION-RELATED

- Pregnancy category C; excretion into breast milk unknown.

MONITORING

- **Baseline assessment:** Assess behavioral, cognitive, and functional deficits related to Alzheimer's disease and other diagnoses.
- **Baseline and ongoing lab work:** Biochemical profile including liver function (AST [SGOT], ALT [SGPT], alkaline phosphatase, GGT, bilirubin) tests.
- **Diagnostic tests:** Obtain baseline 12-lead ECG to evaluate for myocardial ischemia.
- **Therapeutic effect:** Monitor for improvement in behavioral, cognitive, and functional status.
- **BP:** Monitor for significant elevations/decreases in BP.
- **Dysrhythmias:** Continuous ECG monitoring in the intensive care unit, periodically evaluate a 12-lead ECG and rhythm strips of patients with underlying dysrhythmias.
- **Respiratory distress:** Assess for increased work of breathing or respiratory distress in patients with obstructive lung disease, including asthma.
- **Heartburn/abdominal pain:** Assess for GI irritation (coffee-ground flecks in nasogastric tube secretions, dark and tarry stools, blood in stool or emesis).
- **Patient education:** Instruct to take tacrine at regular intervals between meals; drug may be taken with meals if GI upset occurs. Caution against abruptly discontinuing tacrine or adjusting the drug dosage. Urge smoking cessation during tacrine therapy; smoking reduces the drug's blood level. Inform patients and families that tacrine is not a cure for Alzheimer's disease but may slow the progression of its symptoms. Refer families to the local chapter of the Alzheimer's Disease Association for a guide to available services.

SERIOUS ADVERSE REACTIONS

- **Anesthesia:** Tacrine is likely to increase succinylcholine-related muscle relaxation.
- **Dysrhythmias:** May cause bradycardia and prompt exacerbation of sick sinus syndrome due to vagal stimulation properties; increases when underlying cardiac disease is present.
- **Gastric hyperacidity:** Drug increases gastric acid secretion due to increased cholinergic activity; risk of ulcer development increases.
- **Liver dysfunction:** Liver enzyme elevation is common in patients without prior liver disease and may lead to severe liver dysfunction in those with prior history of liver disease.
- **Abrupt withdrawal:** Drug dosage should be gradually reduced in order to prevent a sudden worsening of cognition or marked change in behavior.

OVERDOSE/TOXICITY

- **Cholinergic crisis:** Abdominal discomfort or cramps, nausea, vomiting, diarrhea, possible shock, flushing, facial warmth, excessive salivation, diaphoresis, urinary incontinence or urgency, lacrimation, pallor, bradycardia or tachycardia, hypotension, bronchospasm, blurred vision, miosis, and fasciculation (involuntary muscular contractions visible under the skin).
- **Management:** Endotracheal intubation, support of ventilation, possible mechanical ventilation, management of hypotension with IV fluids and vasopressors if IV fluids are ineffective, management of heart rate using Advanced Cardiac Life Support (ACLS) guidelines. Atropine, often given before neostigmine, may mask the symptoms of overdose.
- **GI decontamination:** No specific recommendations.

ANTIDOTE/DIALYSIS

- **Antidote:** Atropine sulfate 0.6 mg given IV should reverse side effects; may repeat every 3-10 min. Pralidoxime chloride (PAM) 2 g IV may be required to reactivate cholinesterase and reverse paralysis.
- **Dialysis:** No data are available on removal of tacrine by hemodialysis, peritoneal dialysis, or high-permeability hemodialysis.

T

tacrolimus

ta-kroe-li'-mus

Classes

Chemical: macrolide derivative
Therapeutic: immunosuppressant

Pregnancy Category: C

Trade Names

Prescription: Prograf, Protopic

Do not confuse Protopic with Protonix, Protopam, or Protopin.

CLINICAL PHARMACOLOGY

Mechanism of Action

An immunologic agent that inhibits T-lymphocyte activation by binding to intracellular proteins, forming a complex, and inhibiting phosphatase activity. Therapeutic Effect: Suppresses the immunologically mediated inflammatory response; prevents organ transplant rejection.

PHARMACOKINETICS

Variably absorbed after PO administration (food reduces absorption). Protein binding: 75%-97%. Extensively metabolized in the liver. Excreted in urine. Not removed by hemodialysis. Half-life: 11 hr.

AVAILABILITY

Capsules (Prograf): 0.5 mg, 1 mg, 5 mg.
Injection (Prograf): 5 mg/mL.
Ointment (Protopic): 0.03%, 0.1%.

INDICATIONS AND DOSAGE

Prevention of liver transplant rejection

PO

Adults, Elderly: 0.1-0.15 mg/kg/day in 2 divided doses 12 hr apart. **Children:** 0.15-0.2 mg/kg/day in 2 divided doses 12 hr apart.

IV

Adults, Elderly, Children: 0.03-0.05 mg/kg/day as a continuous infusion.

Prevention of kidney transplant rejection

PO

Adults, Elderly: 0.2 mg/kg/day in 2 divided doses 12 hr apart.

IV

Adults, Elderly: 0.03-0.05 mg/kg/day as continuous infusion.

Atopic dermatitis

Topical

Adults, Elderly, Children 2 yr and older: Apply 0.03% ointment to affected area twice per day. 0.1% ointment may be used in adults and the elderly. Continue until 1 wk after symptoms have cleared.

OFF-LABEL USES

Prevention of organ rejection in patients receiving allogeneic bone marrow, heart, pancreas, pancreatic island cell, or small-bowel transplant, treatment of autoimmune disease, severe recalcitrant psoriasis

CONTRAINDICATIONS

Concurrent use with *cycloSPORINE (increases the risk of nephrotoxicity), hypersensitivity to tacrolimus or HCO-60 polyoxyl 60 hydrogenated castor oil (used in solution for injection)

INTERACTIONS

Drug: **Aminoglycosides, amphotericin B, cisplatin:** May increase the risk of renal dysfunction. **Antacids:** May decrease the absorption of tacrolimus. **Antifungals, bromocriptine, calcium channel blockers, cimetidine, clarithromycin, *cycloSPORINE, danazol, diltiazem, erythromycin, *methylPREDNISolone, metoclopramide:** Increase tacrolimus blood concentration. **Carbamazepine, phenobarbital, phenytoin, rifamycin:** Decrease tacrolimus blood concentration. ***CycloSPORINE:** Increases the risk of nephrotoxicity. **Live-virus vaccines:** May potentiate virus replication, increase vaccine side effects, and decrease the patient's antibody response to the vaccine. **Other immunosuppressants:** May increase the risk of infection or lymphomas. Concurrent use with sirolimus has resulted in higher mortality and graft loss in liver transplant patients. Herbal: **Echinacea:** May decrease the effects of tacrolimus. Food: **Grapefruit, grapefruit juice:** May alter the effects of the drug.

DIAGNOSTIC TEST EFFECTS

May increase blood glucose, BUN, and serum creatinine levels, as well as WBC count. May decrease serum magnesium level and RBC and thrombocyte counts. May alter serum potassium level.

IV INCOMPATIBILITIES

Manufacturer recommends drug should not be mixed with solutions that are highly base, with a pH of 9 or above (i.e., acyclovir [Zovirax] or ganciclovir [Cytovene]).

IV COMPATIBILITIES

Calcium gluconate, dexamethasone (Decadron), *diphenhydrAMINE (Benadryl), *DOBUtamine (Dobutrex), *DOPamine (Intropin), furosemide (Lasix), heparin, hydromorphone (Dilaudid), insulin, leucovorin, lorazepam (Ativan), morphine, nitroglycerin, potassium chloride

SIDE-EFFECTS

Frequent (greater than 30%): Headache, tremor, insomnia, paresthesia, diarrhea, nausea, constipation, vomiting, abdominal pain, hypertension. Occasional (29%-10%): Rash, pruritus, anorexia, asthenia, peripheral edema, photosensitivity

CRITICAL CARE CONSIDERATIONS

ADMINISTRATION/HANDLING

PO ALERT

- Administer tacrolimus on an empty stomach.
- Do not give tacrolimus while eating grapefruit or drinking grapefruit juice.
- Do not give tacrolimus within 2 hr of antacids.

IV ALERT

- For patients unable to take capsules, initiate therapy with IV infusion. Give oral dose 8 to 12 hr after discontinuing IV infusion. Titrate dosage based on clinical assessments of rejection and patient tolerance. For patients with hepatic or renal impairment, give the lowest IV and oral doses as prescribed. Plan to delay administration for 48 hr or longer in patients with postoperative oliguria.
- **Storage:** Store diluted solution in a glass or polyethylene container and discard it after 24 hr. Do not store in a polyvinyl chloride container because the container may absorb the drug or affect its stability.
- **Emergency preparation:** Keep oxygen and an aqueous solution of epinephrine 1:1000 available at the bedside before beginning the IV infusion.
- **Dilution:** Dilute the drug with 250 to 1000 mL 0.9% NaCl or D_5W, depending on the desired dose, to provide a concentration of 0.004-0.02 mg/mL.
- **Continuous IV infusion:** Administer tacrolimus as a continuous IV infusion. Monitor continuously for the first 30 min of the infusion and at frequent intervals thereafter. Stop the infusion immediately at the first sign of a hypersensitivity reaction.

TOPICAL ALERT

- Tacrolimus ointment is for external use only.
- Rub the ointment gently and completely into clean, dry skin.
- Do not cover the treated area with an occlusive dressing.

PRECAUTIONS

HEALTH-RELATED

- Use tacrolimus cautiously in patients with immunosuppression or hepatic or renal impairment.
- There is a potential cancer risk from use of topical Protopic ointment.
- African American patients may need higher doses in kidney transplant.

AGE-RELATED

- **Neonates:** Hyperkalemia and renal dysfunction have been noted in neonates.
- **Children:** May require a higher dosage because of decreased bioavailability and increased clearance of the drug. Posttransplant lymphoproliferative disorder is more common in children, especially children under 3 yr.
- **Elderly:** Age-related renal impairment may require a dosage reduction.

PREGNANCY/LACTATION-RELATED

- Pregnancy category C; excreted in breast milk; avoid nursing.

MONITORING

- **Baseline assessment:** Assess drug history, especially for other immunosuppressants, and medical history, especially renal function.
- **Baseline lab work:** CBC; biochemical profile including renal (BUN, creatinine) and liver (AST [SGOT], ALT [SGPT], bilirubin, alkaline phosphatase) function studies.
- **Ongoing lab work:** Closely monitor patients with impaired renal function. Obtain a CBC weekly during the first mo of therapy, twice monthly during the second and third mo of treatment, then monthly for the rest of the first yr. Also monitor liver function test results and serum creatinine and potassium levels. Whole blood tacrolimus concentrations as measured by enzyme-linked immunoabsorbent assay may be helpful in assessing rejection and toxicity, median trough concentrations measured after the second wk of therapy ranged from 9.8-19.4 mg/mL.
- **Fluid balance:** Measure accurate intake and output to assess for fluid volume excess, an early sign of rejection.
- **Infection versus rejection:** Dosing of immunosuppressive medications is a delicate balance between development of a serious infection (overly immunosuppressed) and rejection of the transplanted organ (not receiving enough immunosuppression). Fluid volume excess is common during rejection.
- **Organ rejection:** Assess for organ rejection. Signs of organ rejection are organ-specific, but all patients may have low-grade, persistent fevers. With acute rejection, fevers may be higher (100-104°F). Symptoms of

T

organ rejection will reflect failure of the affected organ. Appropriate testing should include the same evaluation done to assess for failure of the transplanted organ.

- **Patient education:** Instruct to take tacrolimus at the same time each day with regard to timing of meals and other medications and to report missed doses to the prescriber. Caution to avoid eating grapefruit or drinking grapefruit juice during therapy and to avoid coming in contact with people with colds or other infections. Remind that strict monitoring is an essential part of identifying and preventing symptoms of organ rejection in tacrolimus therapy. Limit UV/sunlight exposure, wear protective clothing, and use sunscreen because of increased risk of photosensitivity reaction and skin cancer. Instruct to report promptly chest pain, dizziness, headache, decreased urination, rash, respiratory infection, or unusual bleeding or bruising to a health care provider. Drug is also known as FK 506.

SERIOUS ADVERSE REACTIONS

- **Hypersensitivity:** Rash, urticaria, respiratory distress.
- **Pleural effusion:** Commonly seen adverse reaction.
- Thrombocytopenia, leukocytosis, anemia, atelectasis, sepsis, and infection occur occasionally.

OVERDOSE/TOXICITY

- **Nephrotoxicity:** Increased serum creatinine level and decreased urine output.
- **Neurotoxicity:** Tremor, headache, and mental status changes.
- **GI decontamination:** No specific recommendations.

ANTIDOTE/DIALYSIS

- **Antidote:** No specific recommendations.
- **Dialysis:** Tacrolimus is not removed by hemodialysis and is unlikely to be removed by peritoneal dialysis. No data are available on removal by high-permeability hemodialysis.

T

tamoxifen citrate 

ta-mox'-i-fen sit'-trate

Classes

Chemical: estrogen agonist-antagonist, triphenylethylene derivative
Therapeutic: antineoplastic

Pregnancy Category: D

Trade Names

Prescription: Istubol ♣, Nolvadex, Soltamox

CLINICAL PHARMACOLOGY

Mechanism of Action

A nonsteroidal antiestrogen that competes with estradiol for estrogen-receptor binding sites in the breasts, uterus, and vagina. **Therapeutic Effect:** Inhibits DNA synthesis and estrogen response.

PHARMACOKINETICS

Well absorbed from the GI tract. Metabolized in the liver. Primarily eliminated in feces by biliary system. **Half-life:** 7 days.

AVAILABILITY

Tablets (Nolvadex): 10 mg, 20 mg.
Oral liquid (Soltamox): 10 mg/5 mL

INDICATIONS AND DOSAGE

Adjunctive treatment of breast cancer

PO

Adults, Elderly: 20-40 mg/day. Give doses greater than 20 mg/day in divided doses.

Prevention of breast cancer in high-risk women

PO

Adults, Elderly: 20 mg/day.

OFF-LABEL USES

Treatment of mastalgia, gynecomastia, pancreatic carcinoma, ovulation induction, treatment of precocious puberty in females

CONTRAINDICATIONS

Concomitant coumarin-type therapy when used in the treatment of breast cancer in high-risk women, history of deep vein thrombosis or pulmonary embolism in high-risk women, pregnancy, hypersensitivity to tamoxifen

INTERACTIONS

Drug: Anticoagulants: May increase the risk of bleeding. **Estrogens:** May decrease the effects of tamoxifen. **Herbal: Red clover, St. John's wort:** May decrease tamoxifen's effectiveness. **Food:** None known.

DIAGNOSTIC TEST EFFECTS

May increase serum cholesterol, calcium, and triglyceride levels.

SIDE-EFFECTS

Frequent: Women (greater than 10%): Hot flashes, nausea, vomiting. **Occasional:**

Women (9%-1%): Changes in menstruation, genital itching, vaginal discharge, endometrial hyperplasia or polyps. **Men:** Impotence, decreased libido. **Men and women:** Headache, nausea, vomiting, rash, bone pain, confusion, weakness, somnolence

CRITICAL CARE CONSIDERATIONS

ADMINISTRATION/HANDLING

PO ALERT

- Give tamoxifen without regard to food.

PRECAUTIONS

HEALTH-RELATED

- Use tamoxifen cautiously in patients with leukopenia or thrombocytopenia.
- Treatment duration greater than 5 yr may provide no further benefit and increase risk of endometrial cancer for some women; reevaluate the need for continued therapy.
- The Gail Model Risk Assessment Tool is available to health care professionals by calling (800) 456-3669 (ext. 3838).

AGE-RELATED

- **Children:** Tamoxifen use is safe and effective in girls aged 2-10 yr with McCune Albright syndrome and precocious puberty.
- **Elderly:** No age-related precautions have been noted.

PREGNANCY/LACTATION-RELATED

- Pregnancy category D; excretion into breast milk unknown.

MONITORING

- **Baseline assessment:** Assess for history of pulmonary embolism, stroke, deep vein thrombosis, and use of coumadin (or other coumarin derivatives). These conditions/drugs are contraindications. Assess for prior treatment of cancer or management of other estrogen-related problems. Discuss risks and benefits of tamoxifen use for prevention of breast cancer, as drug has caused fatalities in high risk for breast cancer patients trying to reduce risk of cancer.
- **Lab work:** Check estrogen receptor assay test before beginning tamoxifen therapy. Monitor CBC with WBC differential and biochemical profile including serum calcium levels before and periodically during tamoxifen therapy.
- **Thromboembolism:** Assess for deep vein thrombosis, sudden increase in work of breathing, other cardiovascular and oncologic risk factors for thromboembolism. Assess neurologic status and monitor for altered level of consciousness, weakness, difficulty swallowing, which may indicate a stroke occurred.
- **Bone pain:** Assess for increased bone pain and provide pain relief.
- **Diuresis:** Monitor intake and output and weight.
- **Edema:** Assess for dependent edema.
- **Hypercalcemia:** Assess for constipation, deep bone or flank pain, excessive thirst, hypotonicity of muscles, increased urine output, nausea and vomiting, and renal calculi.
- **Patient education:** Instruct to immediately report leg cramps, weakness, weight gain, or vaginal bleeding, itching, or discharge to a health care provider. Explain that there may be increased bone and tumor pain, which appears to indicate a good tumor response to tamoxifen. Instruct to call the prescriber if nausea and vomiting continue at home. Urge to use nonhormonal contraception during tamoxifen treatment. Monitor for weight loss and weight gain. Instruct to report unexpected vaginal bleeding; endometrial biopsy is indicated for abnormal vaginal bleeding.

SERIOUS ADVERSE REACTIONS

- Endometrial changes including malignancies, thromboembolic events including stroke and pulmonary embolism, and uterine malignancies while using tamoxifen.
- **Hypersensitivity:** Rare Stevens–Johnson syndrome, erythema multiforme, and angioedema.
- **Hyperlipidemia:** Rare cases of elevated serum triglyceride levels with or without pancreatitis have been reported.

OVERDOSE/TOXICITY

- **Ophthalmic:** Retinopathy, corneal opacity, and decreased visual acuity have been noted in patients receiving extremely high dosages (240-320 mg/day) for longer than 17 mo.
- **Hepatocellular carcinoma:** Rare cases of liver cancer were reported in clinical trials.

- **GI decontamination:** No specific recommendations.

ANTIDOTE/DIALYSIS

- **Antidote:** No specific recommendations.
- **Dialysis:** No data are available on removal of tamoxifen by hemodialysis, high-permeability hemodialysis, or peritoneal dialysis.

tamsulosin hydrochloride

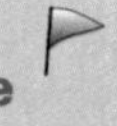

tam-soo-loe'-sin hye-droe-klor'-ide

Classes

Chemical: quinazoline
Therapeutic: α1-adrenergic blocker

Pregnancy Category: B

Trade Names

Prescription: Flomax

Do not confuse Flomax with Fosamax or Volmax.

CLINICAL PHARMACOLOGY

Mechanism of Action

An $alpha_1$ antagonist that targets receptors around bladder neck and prostate capsule. **Therapeutic Effect:** Relaxes smooth muscle and improves urinary flow and symptoms of prostatic hyperplasia.

PHARMACOKINETICS

Well absorbed and widely distributed. Protein binding: 94%-99%. Metabolized in the liver. Primarily excreted in urine. **Half-life:** 9-13 hr.

AVAILABILITY

Capsules: 0.4 mg.

T

INDICATIONS AND DOSAGE

Benign prostatic hyperplasia

PO

Adults: 0.4 mg once per day, approximately 30 min after same meal each day. May increase dosage to 0.8 mg if inadequate response in 2-4 wk.

CONTRAINDICATIONS

Concurrent use of sildenafil, tadalafil, or vardenafil; hypersensitivity to tamsulosin

INTERACTIONS

Drug: Other alpha-adrenergic blocking agents (such as cimetidine, doxazosin, prazosin, terazosin): May increase the alpha-blockade effects of both drugs. **Warfarin:** May alter the effects of warfarin. **Herbal:** None known. **Food:** None known.

DIAGNOSTIC TEST EFFECTS

None known.

SIDE-EFFECTS

Frequent (21%-8%): Headache (19%-21%), orthostatic hypotension (16%-19%), dizziness (15%-17%), rhinitis (13%-18%), abnormal ejaculation (8%-18%). **Occasional (6%-3%):** Somnolence (3%-4%), anxiety, diarrhea (4%-6%), nausea (3%-4%). **Rare (less than 2%):** Nasal congestion, pharyngitis, insomnia, nausea, vertigo, impotence

CRITICAL CARE CONSIDERATIONS

ADMINISTRATION/HANDLING

PO ALERT

- Give tamsulosin at the same time each day, 30 min after the same meal.
- Do not crush or open capsule unless absolutely necessary. Prescribers should be aware if patients require alteration of capsule before ingestion.

PRECAUTIONS

HEALTH-RELATED

- Use tamsulosin cautiously in patients with renal impairment.

AGE-RELATED

- **Children:** Tamsulosin is not indicated for use in women or children.
- **Elderly:** No age-related precautions have been noted.

PREGNANCY/LACTATION-RELATED

- Pregnancy category B; not indicated for use in women.

MONITORING

- **Baseline assessment:** Determine hypersensitivity to tamsulosin and whether other alpha-adrenergic blocking agents or warfarin (Coumadin) are being used.
- **Baseline lab work:** Biochemical profile including renal (BUN, creatinine) function studies. Monitor for renal insufficiency.
- **Postural hypotension:** Assist with ambulation if dizziness occurs.
- **Patient education:** Instruct to take tamsulosin at the same time each day, 30 min after the same meal. Teach not to chew,

crush, or open the capsules. Advise to use caution when getting up from a sitting or lying position. Warn to avoid tasks that require mental alertness or motor skills until response to the drug is known. Inform patients that ejaculation may be abnormal.

SERIOUS ADVERSE REACTIONS

- **First-dose syncope:** Hypotension with sudden loss of consciousness may occur within 30-90 min after administration of initial dose; may be preceded by tachycardia (120-160 beats/min).
- **Hypersensitivity:** Pruritis, angioedema of the tongue, lips, and face; urticaria with a positive rechallenge in some cases.

OVERDOSE/TOXICITY

- **Hypotension:** Markedly decreased BP, headache, tachycardia, shocklike symptoms, which may lead to symptoms of renal insufficiency (low urine output, nausea, vomiting, elevated BUN, and creatinine).
- **Management:** Administer IV fluid bolus; if ineffective, consider use of vasopressors. Tachycardia will resolve with fluid administration if due to relative hypovolemia.
- **GI decontamination:** No specific recommendations.

ANTIDOTE/DIALYSIS

- **Antidote:** No specific recommendations.
- **Dialysis:** Tamsulosin is unlikely to be removed by hemodialysis or peritoneal dialysis. No data are available on removal by high-permeability hemodialysis.

telithromycin

See Antibiotics (p. 892)

telmisartan

tel-mi-sar'-tan

Classes

Chemical: angiotensin II receptor antagonist
Therapeutic: antihypertensive

Pregnancy Category: C (1st trimester), D (2nd and 3rd trimester)

Trade Names

Prescription: Micardis

CLINICAL PHARMACOLOGY

Mechanism of Action

An angiotensin II receptor, type AT_1, antagonist that blocks vasoconstrictor and aldosterone-secreting effects of angiotensin II, inhibiting the binding of angiotensin II to the AT_1 receptors. **Therapeutic Effect:** Causes vasodilation, decreases peripheral resistance, and decreases BP.

PHARMACOKINETICS

Rapidly and completely absorbed after PO administration. Protein binding: greater than 99%. Undergoes metabolism in the liver to inactive metabolite. Excreted in feces. **Half-life:** 24 hr.

AVAILABILITY

Tablets: 20 mg, 40 mg, 80 mg.

INDICATIONS AND DOSAGE

Hypertension

PO

Adults, Elderly: 40 mg once per day. Range: 20-80 mg/day.

OFF-LABEL USES

Treatment of heart failure

CONTRAINDICATIONS

Hypersensitivity to telmisartan

INTERACTIONS

Drug: Digoxin: Increases digoxin plasma concentration. **Warfarin:** Slightly decreases warfarin plasma concentration. **Herbal:** None known. **Food:** None known.

DIAGNOSTIC TEST EFFECTS

May increase serum creatinine level. May decrease blood Hgb and Hct levels.

SIDE-EFFECTS

Occasional (7%-3%): Upper respiratory tract infection, sinusitis, back or leg pain, diarrhea. **Rare (1%):** Dizziness, headache, fatigue, nausea, heartburn, myalgia, cough, peripheral edema

CRITICAL CARE CONSIDERATIONS

ADMINISTRATION/HANDLING

PO ALERT

- Give telmisartan without regard to meals.
- Telmisartan may be given concurrently with other antihypertensives. If BP is not controlled by telmisartan alone, a diuretic may be added.

PRECAUTIONS

HEALTH-RELATED

- Use telmisartan cautiously in patients with hepatic and renal impairment, renal artery stenosis (bilateral or unilateral), and volume depletion.

AGE-RELATED

- **Children:** Safety and efficacy of telmisartan have not been established in children.
- **Elderly:** No age-related precautions have been noted.

PREGNANCY/LACTATION-RELATED

- Pregnancy category C, first trimester; category D, second and third trimesters. Drugs acting directly on the renin-angiotensin-aldosterone system are documented to cause fetal harm (hypotension, oligohydramnios, neonatal anemia, hyperkalemia, neonatal skull hypoplasia, anuria, and renal failure); neonatal limb contractures, craniofacial deformities, and hypoplastic lung development.

MONITORING

- **Baseline assessment:** Assess vital signs, heart rate, and BP immediately before each telmisartan dose and regularly throughout therapy. Assess medication history, especially for diuretics. Determine history of hepatic or renal impairment or renal artery stenosis. Assess hydration.
- **Lab work:** Baseline and periodic CBC with WBC differential; biochemical profile including renal (BUN, creatinine) and liver (AST [SGOT], ALT [SGPT], alkaline phosphatase, GGT, bilirubin) function tests.
- **Labile BP:** Monitor BP regularly for fluctuations in heart rate and BP. If hypotension occurs, place in the supine position with legs elevated and consider if an IV fluid volume infusion may be needed.
- **Patient education:** Encourage to drink fluids frequently to maintain proper hydration. Advise female patients of the consequences of second- and third-trimester exposure to telmisartan. Emphasize the importance of immediately reporting pregnancy to the prescriber. Urge avoidance of tasks that require mental alertness or motor skills until response to the drug is known. Instruct to report promptly symptoms of infection, including fever and sore throat. Explain that telmisartan must be taken throughout life to control hypertension. Caution against excessive exertion during hot weather to avoid dehydration and hypotension.

SERIOUS ADVERSE REACTIONS

- **Hypotension:** In volume-depleted and/or salt-depleted patients.
- **Hypersensitivity:** Dermatitis, rash, eczema, pruritis; rare angioedema.
- **Hepatic:** Elevated liver enzymes (rare).

OVERDOSE/TOXICITY

- **Cardiovascular:** Hypotension and tachycardia. Bradycardia occurs less often.
- **Acute renal failure:** Progressive renal dysfunction may be seen in patients whose renal function may depend on the renin-angiotensin-aldosterone system, such as heart failure patients.
- **Management:** Fluid resuscitation, discontinue medication. If patients do not respond to fluids, vasopressors may be needed to maintain BP.
- **GI decontamination:** No specific recommendations.

ANTIDOTE/DIALYSIS

- **Antidote:** No specific recommendations.
- **Dialysis:** Telmisartan is not removed by hemodialysis and is unlikely to be removed by peritoneal dialysis. No data are available on removal by high-permeability hemodialysis.

temazepam

te-maz'-e-pam

DEA Schedule: IV

Classes

Chemical: benzodiazepine
Therapeutic: hypnotic

Pregnancy Category: X

Trade Names

Prescription: Restoril

Do not confuse Restoril with Vistaril or Zestril.

CLINICAL PHARMACOLOGY

Mechanism of Action

A benzodiazepine that enhances the action of the inhibitory neurotransmitter gamma-aminobutyric acid, resulting in CNS depression. **Therapeutic Effect:** Induces sleep.

PHARMACOKINETICS

Well absorbed from the GI tract. Protein binding: 96%. Widely distributed. Crosses the blood-brain barrier. Metabolized in the liver.

Primarily excreted in urine. Not removed by hemodialysis. Half-life: 9 hr.

AVAILABILITY

Capsules: 7.5 mg, 15 mg, 22.5 mg, 30 mg.

INDICATIONS AND DOSAGE

Insomnia

PO

Adults, Children 18 yr and older: 15-30 mg at bedtime. **Elderly, debilitated:** 7.5-15 mg at bedtime.

OFF-LABEL USES

Treatment of anxiety, depression, panic attacks

CONTRAINDICATIONS

Pregnancy or breast-feeding, hypersensitivity to temazepam or other benzodiazepines

INTERACTIONS

Drug: **Alcohol, other CNS depressants:** May increase CNS depression. Herbal: **Kava kava, valerian:** May increase CNS depression. Food: None known.

DIAGNOSTIC TEST EFFECTS

None known.

SIDE-EFFECTS

Frequent: Somnolence, sedation, rebound insomnia (may occur for 1-2 nights after drug is discontinued), dizziness, confusion, euphoria. Occasional: Asthenia, anorexia, diarrhea. Rare: Paradoxic CNS excitement or restlessness (particularly in elderly or debilitated patients)

CRITICAL CARE CONSIDERATIONS

ADMINISTRATION/HANDLING

PO ALERT

- May open temazepam capsules and mix the contents with food.

PRECAUTIONS

HEALTH-RELATED

- Use temazepam cautiously in patients with CNS depression, mental impairment, or the potential for drug dependence.

AGE-RELATED

- **Children:** Temazepam use is not recommended for children under 18 yr.
- **Elderly:** Administer small doses initially and increase dosage gradually to avoid ataxia or excessive sedation.

PREGNANCY/LACTATION RELATED

- Pregnancy category X; may cause sedation and poor feeding in nursing infant.

MONITORING

- **Baseline assessment:** Determine pregnancy before beginning temazepam therapy. Assess BP, pulse, and respirations immediately before beginning temazepam administration. Assess baseline sleep pattern, including time needed to fall asleep and number of nocturnal awakenings.
- **Baseline lab work:** CBC with WBC differential, platelet count. Biochemical profile with BUN, creatinine, and liver function studies. For long-term therapy, perform tests periodically.
- **Environment:** Provide patients with an environment conducive to sleep. For example, offer a back rub, low lighting, and a quiet environment.
- **Paradoxic reactions:** Assess elderly or debilitated patients for paradoxic CNS reactions (increased agitation), particularly early in therapy.
- **Pain management:** Assess for pain in patients who are unable to communicate well. Patients in pain are sometimes given large doses of sedatives/hypnotics to control restlessness/sleeplessness that is due to pain.
- **Respiratory status:** Assess for patent airway, secretions control and effective breathing, especially following seizures and when dosage is increased.
- **Hypotension:** Assess for hypotension and tachycardia if patients are in an environment where they do not have to be awakened to perform assessment.
- **Therapeutic response:** Evaluate for a decrease in number of nocturnal awakenings and a longer duration of sleep.
- **Patient education:** Caution not to stop taking temazepam abruptly after long-term therapy. Instruct to take temazepam about 30 min before bedtime. Inform that temazepam may cause daytime drowsiness. Warn to avoid tasks that require mental alertness or motor skills until response to the drug is known. Urge avoidance of smoking, drinking alcoholic beverages, and taking other CNS depressants. Explain that smoking reduces the effectiveness of temazepam, while alcohol and CNS depressants increase sedation. Urge female patients on long-term therapy to use effective contraception during therapy and to report pregnancy or suspected pregnancy immediately to a health care provider.

SERIOUS ADVERSE REACTIONS

- **Abrupt or too-rapid withdrawal:** May result in pronounced restlessness, irritability, insomnia, hand tremor, abdominal or muscle cramps, vomiting, diaphoresis, and seizures.
- **Paradoxic reactions:** Some patients are intolerant of benzodiazepines and respond to the drug with increased agitation rather than sedation or sleeping.

OVERDOSE/TOXICITY

- **Severe sedation:** Overdose results in somnolence, confusion, diminished reflexes, ataxia, coma, respiratory depression.
- **Management:** Supportive care including providing a patent airway and ventilation, nasogastric tube to help protect against aspiration, IV fluids for hydration. Advanced Cardiac Life Support (ACLS) guidelines should be followed for other resuscitative efforts.
- **GI decontamination:** No specific recommendations.

ANTIDOTE/DIALYSIS

- **Antidote:** Cautiously use flumazenil (Romazicon) 0.2 mg (2 mL) over 30 sec; may repeat after 30 sec with 0.3 mg (3 mL) over 30 sec. Further doses may be given up to 0.5 mg (5 mL) up to a total of 3 mg (30 mL). Flumazenil reverses CNS depressive effects. Naloxone (Narcan) should be considered in addition to flumazenil if patients have significant respiratory depression.
- **Dialysis:** Temazepam is not removed by hemodialysis and is unlikely to be removed by peritoneal dialysis. No data are available on removal by high-permeability hemodialysis.

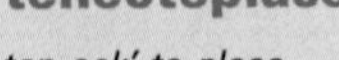

tenecteplase

ten-eck'-te-plase

Classes

Chemical: recombinant tissue plasminogen activator
Therapeutic: thrombolytic agent

Pregnancy Category: C

Trade Names

Prescription: TNKase

CLINICAL PHARMACOLOGY

Mechanism of Action

A tissue plasminogen activator produced by recombinant DNA that binds to fibrin and converts plasminogen to plasmin. Initiates fibrinolysis by degrading fibrin clots, fibrinogen, other plasma proteins. **Therapeutic Effect:** Exerts thrombolytic action.

PHARMACOKINETICS

Extensively distributed to tissues. Completely eliminated by hepatic metabolism. **Half-life:** 20-24 min.

AVAILABILITY

Powder for injection: 50 mg.

INDICATIONS AND DOSAGE

Acute MI

IV

Adults: Dosage is based on weight. Treatment should be initiated as soon as possible after onset of symptoms.

Weight (kg)	(mg)	(mL)
90 or more	50	10
80 to 89	45	9
70 to 79	40	8
60 to 69	35	7
Less than 60	30	6

CONTRAINDICATIONS

Active internal bleeding, aneurysm, AV malformation, bleeding diathesis, history of cerebrovascular accident (CVA), intracranial or intraspinal surgery or trauma within past 2 mo, intracranial neoplasm, severe uncontrolled hypertension, hypersensitivity to tenecteplase

INTERACTIONS

Drug: **Anticoagulants (such as heparin, warfarin), aspirin, dipyridamole, glycoprotein IIb/IIIa inhibitors:** Increase the risk of bleeding. **Herbal:** **Ginkgo biloba:** May increase the risk of bleeding. **Food:** None known.

DIAGNOSTIC TEST EFFECTS

Decreases plasminogen and fibrinogen levels during infusion, decreasing clotting time, and confirming presence of lysis. Decreases Hct and Hgb.

IV INCOMPATIBILITIES

Do not mix with other medications.

SIDE-EFFECTS

Frequent: Bleeding (major, 4.7%; minor, 21.8%)

CRITICAL CARE CONSIDERATIONS

ADMINISTRATION/HANDLING

IV ALERT

- **Storage:** Store at room temperature. Tenecteplase is normally a colorless to pale-yellow solution. Do not use if solution is discolored or contains particulates.
- **Reconstitution:** Add 10 mL sterile water for injection without preservative to vial to provide concentration of 5 mg/mL. Gently swirl until dissolved. Do not shake. If foaming occurs, allow vial to sit undisturbed for several min. Ideally use immediately after reconstitution, but may refrigerate for up to 8 hr. Discard after 8 hr.
- **IV direct injection (bolus):** Flush line with saline before and after administration. Give as a single IV bolus over 5 seconds. Precipitate may occur when given in an IV line containing dextrose.

PRECAUTIONS

HEALTH-RELATED

- Use tenecteplase cautiously in patients who have previously received tenecteplase and in patients with severe hepatic impairment.

AGE-RELATED

- **Children:** Safety and efficacy of tenecteplase have not been established in children.
- **Elderly:** May have an increased risk of intracranial hemorrhage, major bleeding, and stroke. Tenecteplase should be used cautiously in elderly patients.

PREGNANCY/LACTATION-RELATED

- Pregnancy category C; unknown if distributed in breast milk.

MONITORING

- **Baseline assessment:** Assess for risk of bleeding, vital signs, and record actual weight after weighing, if possible (rather than estimated weight or weight reported from patients). Evaluate history of chest discomfort and whether aspirin, nitroglycerin, or morphine have been taken. Evaluate 12-lead ECG, cardiac enzyme concentrations, and electrolyte levels.
- **Lab work:** CBC with WBC differential and platelet count, biochemical profile including cardiac enzymes and isoenzymes (Creatinine Kinease-MB and troponins). Assess coagulation studies (prothrombin time/international normalized ratios, aPTT, fibrinogen level, and thrombin time) before therapy starts. Type and hold blood sample. Monitor aPTT per protocol.
- **Diagnostic tests:** Evaluate 12-lead ECG for ST segment elevation and possibly, 15- or 18-lead ECG if symptoms reflect possible MI that is not apparent on 12-lead ECG. Echocardiogram may also be used to evaluate cardiac output, pressures within the heart, and ventricular wall motion.
- **Door to needle time:** Patients should have the full assessment including lab work and diagnostic tests finished in no longer than 30 min, so tenecteplase can be given within 30 min of arrival in the emergency dept or onset of symptoms within the hospital. Thrombolysis is given only to patients with documented myocardial infarction, rather than patients with myocardial ischemia.
- **Door to balloon time:** If patients are not a candidate for thrombolytic therapy or coronary angioplasty is chosen as the reperfusion strategy, patients should arrive in the cardiac cath lab in a timely fashion so the angioplasty balloon is able to be inflated within the obstructed artery within 90 min of arrival in the emergency dept or onset of symptoms within the hospital.
- **Dysrhythmias:** Perform continuous cardiac monitoring for ST segment changes and various dysrhythmias. Reperfusion dysrhythmias are common and should not be managed unless patients become unstable (hypotensive with chest discomfort or altered mental status).
- **Vital signs:** BP, pulse, and respiration rates every 15 min until patients are stable, then hourly.
- **Cardiovascular assessment:** Evaluate heart sounds for murmurs, S3 or S4, breath sounds for crackles, congestion or wheezing and for palpable peripheral pulses. Monitor for relief of chest pain. Additional evaluation may be needed if pain recurs, as MI may be extending. Note the intensity, location, and quality of pain.
- **Bleeding:** Assess all invasive sites and for blood in secretions, stool, and urine. Perform a thorough neurologic assessment to evaluate for stroke. If intracranial hemorrhage is suspected, if heparin is infusing, discontinue heparin immediately.

Avoid procedures that might increase the risk of bleeding, such as injections and shaving. Have patients stay in bed throughout reperfusion therapy. Control minor bleeding using pressure directly to the bleeding site.

- **Patient education:** Instruct to report immediately chest pain, headache, palpitations, or shortness of breath. Instruct to report black or red stool, coffee-ground vomitus, dark or red urine, red-speckled mucus from cough, or other signs of bleeding if not immediately noted by health care providers.

SERIOUS ADVERSE REACTIONS

- **Reperfusion dysrhythmias:** Lysis of coronary thrombi may produce reperfusion related atrial or ventricular dysrhythmias. Symptomatic dysrhythmias should be managed according to Advanced Cardiac Life Support (ACLS) guidelines.
- **Hypersensitivity:** Anaphylaxis, angioedema, laryngeal edema, rash, and urticaria have been reported (rarely).
- **Cardiogenic shock:** If treatment is not successful and MI is large, patients may experience shock because of inability of the heart to eject blood effectively (low cardiac output). Intraaortic balloon pump therapy may be needed if heart failure is not manageable by medications (inotropes, vasopressors) and mechanical ventilation.

OVERDOSE/TOXICITY

- **Hemorrhage:** Severe internal hemorrhage may occur (intracranial, retroperitoneal, GI, GU, and respiratory sites). If neurologic status deteriorates or other hemorrhage is present, stop the infusion immediately. If bleeding is outside the cranium, blood transfusions should be given to replace lost red blood cells.
- **Management:** Replace clotting factors with cryoprecipitate and fresh frozen plasma to replace clotting factors depleted by plasmin. Replacing platelets should be considered if bleeding time is abnormal or dilutional thrombocytopenia occurs following massive blood transfusions for bleeding.
- **GI decontamination:** No specific recommendations.

ANTIDOTE/DIALYSIS

- **Antidote:** Consider antifibrinolytic agents (aminocaproic acid [Amicar] or tranexamic acid [Cyklocapron]) or desmopressin if transfusion therapy does not control bleeding.
- **Dialysis:** Tenecteplase is unlikely to be removed by hemodialysis or peritoneal dialysis. No data are available on removal by high-permeability hemodialysis.

tenofovir disoproxil fumarate

See HIV Medications (p. 961)

terazosin hydrochloride

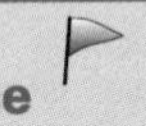

ter-a'-zoe-sin hye-droe-klor'-ide

Classes

Chemical: quinazoline derivative
Therapeutic: antihypertensive, α_1-adrenergic blocker

Pregnancy Category: C

Trade Names

Prescription: Hytrin

CLINICAL PHARMACOLOGY

Mechanism of Action

An antihypertensive and benign prostatic hyperplasia agent that blocks alpha-adrenergic receptors. Produces vasodilation, decreases peripheral resistance, and targets receptors around bladder neck and prostate. **Therapeutic Effect:** In hypertension, decreases BP. In benign prostatic hyperplasia, relaxes smooth muscle and improves urine flow.

PHARMACOKINETICS

Route	Onset	Peak	Duration
PO	15 min	1-2 hr	12-24 hr

Rapidly, completely absorbed from the GI tract. Protein binding: 90%-94%. Metabolized in the liver to active metabolite. Primarily eliminated in feces via biliary system; excreted in urine. Not removed by hemodialysis. **Half-life:** 12 hr.

AVAILABILITY

Capsules: 1 mg, 2 mg, 5 mg, 10 mg.
Tablets: 1 mg, 2 mg, 5 mg, 10 mg.

INDICATIONS AND DOSAGE

Mild to moderate hypertension

PO

Adults, Elderly: Initially, 1 mg at bedtime. Slowly increase dosage to desired levels.

Range: 1-5 mg/day as single or 2 divided doses. Maximum: 20 mg.

Benign prostatic hyperplasia

PO

Adults, Elderly: Initially, 1 mg at bedtime. May increase up to 10 mg/day. Maximum: 20 mg/day.

CONTRAINDICATIONS

Hypersensitivity to terazosin

INTERACTIONS

Drug: Estrogen, NSAIDs, other sympathomimetics: May decrease the effects of terazosin. **Hypotension-producing medications, such as antihypertensives and diuretics:** May increase the effects of terazosin. **Vardenafil:** May increase hypotensive effects. **Herbal: Dong quai, ginseng, garlic, yohimbe:** May decrease the effects of terazosin. **Food:** None known.

DIAGNOSTIC TEST EFFECTS

May decrease blood Hgb and Hct levels, serum albumin level, total serum protein level, and WBC count.

SIDE-EFFECTS

Frequent (9%-5%): Dizziness, headache, unusual tiredness. **Rare (less than 2%):** Peripheral edema, orthostatic hypotension, myalgia, arthralgia, blurred vision, nausea, vomiting, nasal congestion, somnolence

CRITICAL CARE CONSIDERATIONS

ADMINISTRATION/HANDLING

PO ALERT

- Give terazosin without regard to food.
- Tablets may be crushed.
- Administer first dose at bedtime to minimize the risk of fainting due to first-dose syncope.
- If terazosin is discontinued for several days, restart therapy with a 1-mg dose at bedtime.

PRECAUTIONS

HEALTH-RELATED

- Use terazosin cautiously in patients with confirmed or suspected coronary artery disease.
- Prostate cancer should be ruled out before starting terazosin for symptoms of benign prostatic hyperplasia (BPH), which are similar to those of prostate cancer.

AGE-RELATED

- **Children:** Safety and efficacy of terazosin have not been established in children.
- **Elderly:** No age-related precautions have been noted, but elderly may be more sensitive to the drug's hypotensive effects.

PREGNANCY/LACTATION-RELATED

- Pregnancy category C; excretion into breast milk unknown.

MONITORING

- **Baseline assessment:** Assess heart rate and BP immediately before each terazosin dose and every 15-30 min thereafter until BP is stabilized.
- **Lab work:** Baseline CBC with WBC differential and biochemical profile.
- **Labile BP:** Monitor for fluctuations in BP, which can sometimes indicate hypovolemia.
- **First dose syncope:** Give first terazosin dose at bedtime. If initial dose is given during the day, keep recumbent for 3-4 hr. Monitor heart rate frequently because first-dose syncope may be preceded by tachycardia. Assist with ambulation if dizziness occurs.
- **Dysrhythmias:** Assess for tachydysrhythmias if patients are continuously cardiac monitored.
- **Fluid retention:** Assess for peripheral edema and weight gain.
- **Therapeutic effects:** Assess for improvement in voiding if terazosin is used for BPH, and for control of BP if used to manage hypertension.
- **Patient education:** Inform that nasal congestion may occur. Explain the full therapeutic effect of terazosin may not occur for 3-4 wk. Advise to use caution when driving, performing tasks requiring mental alertness, and rising from a sitting or lying position. Instruct to report dizziness or palpitations promptly to a health care provider.

SERIOUS ADVERSE REACTIONS

- **First dose syncope:** Hypotension with sudden loss of consciousness may occur within 30-90 min after administration of initial dose; may be preceded by tachycardia (120-160 beats/min).
- **Hypersensitivity:** Allergic reactions including pruritis, rash, sweating, and anaphylaxis.

OVERDOSE/TOXICITY

- **Hypotension:** Markedly decreased BP, headache, tachycardia, shocklike symptoms, which may lead to symptoms of renal insufficiency (low urine output, nausea, vomiting, elevated BUN and creatinine).

- **Management:** Administer IV fluid bolus; if ineffective, consider use of vasopressors. Tachycardia will resolve with fluid administration if due to relative hypovolemia.
- **GI decontamination:** No specific recommendations.

ANTIDOTE/DIALYSIS

- **Antidote:** No specific recommendations.
- **Dialysis:** Terazosin is not removed by hemodialysis or peritoneal dialysis. No data are available on removal by high-permeability hemodialysis.

terbinafine hydrochloride

ter-bin'-a-feen hye-droe-klor'-ide

Classes

Chemical: allylamine derivative
Therapeutic: antifungal

Pregnancy Category: B

Trade Names

Prescription: Lamisil, Lamisil AT

Do not confuse terbinafine with terbutaline, or Lamisil with Lamictal.

CLINICAL PHARMACOLOGY

Mechanism of Action

A fungicidal antifungal that inhibits the enzyme squalene epoxidase, thereby interfering with fungal biosynthesis. **Therapeutic Effect:** Results in death of fungal cells.

PHARMACOKINETICS

Well absorbed following PO administration. Protein binding: 99%. Metabolized by the liver. Primarily excreted in urine; minimal elimination in feces. **Half-life:** oral—36 hr; topical—22-26 hr.

AVAILABILITY

Tablets (Lamisil): 250 mg.
Cream (Lamisil AT): 1%.
Topical Solution (Lamisil, Lamisil AT): 1%.
Topical Spray (Lamisil AT): 1%.

INDICATIONS AND DOSAGE

Tinea pedis

Topical

Adults, Elderly, Children 12 yr and older: Apply twice daily between toes for 7 days. Apply twice daily on bottom or sides of feet for 2 wk.

Tinea cruris, tinea corporis

Topical

Adults, Elderly, Children 12 yr and older: Apply 1-2 times per day for 7 days.

Onychomycosis

PO

Adults, Elderly, Children 12 yr and older: 250 mg/day for 6 wk (fingernails) or 12 wk (toenails).

Tinea versicolor

Topical Solution

Adults, Elderly: Apply to the affected area twice per day for 7 days.

Systemic mycosis

PO

Adults, Elderly: 250-500 mg/day for up to 16 months.

CONTRAINDICATIONS

Oral: Children younger than 12 yr, preexisting hepatic or renal impairment (creatinine clearance of 50 mL/min or less), hypersensitivity to terbinafine

INTERACTIONS

Drug: **Alcohol, other hepatotoxic medications:** May increase the risk of hepatotoxicity. **Hepatic enzyme inducers, including rifampin:** May increase terbinafine clearance. **Hepatic enzyme inhibitors, including cimetidine:** May decrease terbinafine clearance. **Herbal:** None known. **Food:** None known.

DIAGNOSTIC TEST EFFECTS

May increase AST (SGOT) and ALT (SGPT) levels.

SIDE-EFFECTS

Frequent (13%): **Oral:** Headache. **Occasional (6%-3%):** **Oral:** Diarrhea, rash, dyspepsia, pruritus, taste disturbance, nausea. **Oral:** Abdominal pain, flatulence, urticaria, visual disturbance. **Topical:** Irritation, burning, pruritus, dryness

CRITICAL CARE CONSIDERATIONS

ADMINISTRATION/HANDLING

PO ALERT

- Store terbinafine at controlled room temperature protected from light.

TOPICAL ALERT

- Store cream and solution at controlled room temperature; do not refrigerate.

- Cream and solution are not for ophthalmic, oral, or intravaginal use.
- Therapy should continue until clinical signs and symptoms are significantly improved; treatment should be provided for a minimum of 1 wk and maximum of 4 wk.

PRECAUTIONS

HEALTH-RELATED

- For topical, if irritation develops, treatment should be discontinued and appropriate therapy provided.
- Oral tablets are not recommended for patients with chronic or active liver disease. Terbinafine has not been thoroughly studied in patients with renal impairment (creatinine clearance less than 50 mL/min) and is not recommended for use in this patient population.

AGE-RELATED

- **Children:** Safety and efficacy of terbinafine have not been established in all children for tablets; for topical form, safety and efficacy have not been established for children under 12 yr.
- **Elderly:** No age-related precautions have been noted.

PREGNANCY/LACTATION-RELATED

- Pregnancy category B. It is recommended that treatment of onychomycosis be delayed until after pregnancy. Small amounts of terbinafine are excreted into breast milk when administered orally; not recommended in nursing mothers; avoid application to the breast when breast-feeding.

MONITORING

- **Baseline assessment:** Assess fungal infection and medications/treatments used to manage infection prior to terbinafine.
- **Baseline lab work:** Biochemical profile including renal (BUN, creatinine) and liver (AST [SGOT], ALT [SGPT], alkaline phosphatase, bilirubin) function tests. Monitor hepatic function in patients receiving treatment for longer than 6 wk.
- **Therapeutic response:** Assess for improvement in appearance of affected area.
- **Local reaction:** Discontinue terbinafine if a local reaction occurs such as blistering, burning, irritation, pruritus, oozing, erythema, or edema.
- **Diarrhea:** Assess daily bowel pattern and consistency of stool.
- **Patient education:** Teach patients using topical terbinafine to rub the drug well into the affected and surrounding areas and not to cover the treated area with an occlusive dressing. Advise keeping the affected area clean and dry and to wear light clothing to promote ventilation. Encourage to separate personal items that come in contact with the affected area. Caution not to let topical forms come in contact with eyes, mouth, nose, or other mucous membranes. Instruct to report if diarrhea or skin irritation occurs.

SERIOUS ADVERSE REACTIONS

- **Hypersensitivity:** Rash, pruritis, urticaria, Stevens–Johnson syndrome, toxic epidermal necrolysis, anaphylaxis.
- **Ophthalmic:** Ocular lens and retinal changes have been noted.

OVERDOSE/TOXICITY

- **Hepatotoxicity:** Elevated liver enzymes, cholestatic hepatitis, right upper quadrant pain, nausea, vomiting, liver failure leading to liver transplant, death.
- **Bone marrow suppression:** Severe neutropenia, thrombocytopenia occur rarely.
- **GI decontamination:** No specific recommendations.

ANTIDOTE/DIALYSIS

- **Antidote:** No specific recommendations.
- **Dialysis:** Terbinafine is unlikely to be removed by hemodialysis or peritoneal dialysis. No data are available on removal by high-permeability hemodialysis.

terbutaline sulfate 

ter-byoo'-ta-leen sul'-fate

Classes

Chemical: sympathomimetic amine, β2-adrenergic agonist

Therapeutic: antiasthmatic, bronchodilator, tocolytic

Pregnancy Category: B

Trade Names

Prescription: Brethine, Bricanyl ♣

Do not confuse terbutaline with tolbutamide or terbinafine, or Brethine with Brethaire.

CLINICAL PHARMACOLOGY

Mechanism of Action

An adrenergic agonist that stimulates $beta_2$-adrenergic receptors, resulting in relaxation of uterine and bronchial smooth muscle. **Therapeutic Effect:** Relieves bronchospasm and reduces airway resistance. Also inhibits uterine contractions.

PHARMACOKINETICS

Partially absorbed in GI tract following oral administration. Protein binding: 25%. Metabolized in liver. Excreted in feces and urine. **Half-life:** 11-16 hr.

AVAILABILITY

Tablets: 2.5 mg, 5 mg.
Injection: 1 mg/mL.

INDICATIONS AND DOSAGE

Bronchospasm

PO

Adults, Elderly, Children 15 yr and older: Initially, 2.5 mg 3-4 times per day. Maintenance: 2.5-5 mg 3 times per day every 6 hr while awake. Maximum: 15 mg/day. **Children 12-14 yr:** 2.5 mg 3 times per day. Maximum: 7.5 mg/day. **Children younger than 12 yr:** Initially, 0.05 mg/kg/dose every 8 hr. May increase up to 0.15 mg/kg/dose. Maximum: 5 mg/24 hr or 5 mg/day.

Subcutaneous

Adults, Children 12 yr and older: Initially, 0.25 mg. Repeat in 15-30 min if substantial improvement does not occur. Maximum: 0.5 mg/4 hr. **Children younger than 12 yr:** 0.005-0.01 mg/kg/dose to a maximum of 0.3 mg/dose every 15-20 min for 2 doses.

Preterm labor

PO

Adults: 2.5-10 mg every 4-6 hr.

IV

Adults: 2.5-10 mcg/min. May increase gradually every 15-20 min up to 17.5-30 mcg/min.

CONTRAINDICATIONS

History of hypersensitivity to terbutaline or other sympathomimetics

INTERACTIONS

Drug: **Beta-blockers:** May decrease the effects of beta-blockers. **MAOIs:** May increase the risk of hypertensive crisis. **Tricyclic antidepressants:** May increase cardiovascular effects. **Herbal:** None known. **Food:** None known.

DIAGNOSTIC TEST EFFECTS

May decrease serum potassium level.

SIDE-EFFECTS

Frequent (23%-18%): Tremor, anxiety, nervousness, restlessness. **Occasional (11%-10%):** Somnolence, headache, nausea, heartburn, dizziness. **Rare (3%-1%):** Flushing, asthenia, mouth and throat dryness or irritation (with inhalation therapy)

CRITICAL CARE CONSIDERATIONS

ADMINISTRATION/HANDLING

PO ALERT

- Give terbutaline with food if the patient experiences GI upset.
- Crush tablets as needed.

IV ALERT

- Increase the IV infusion slowly, as prescribed, until contractions stop.

SUBCUTANEOUS ALERT

- Do not use solution if it appears discolored.
- Inject the drug subcutaneously into the lateral deltoid region.

PRECAUTIONS

HEALTH-RELATED

- Use terbutaline cautiously in patients with cardiovascular disorders, hypertension, diabetes mellitus, a history of seizures, or hyperthyroidism.

AGE-RELATED

- **Children:** Safety and efficacy of terbutaline have been established in children 6 yr and older for both tablets and injection.
- **Elderly:** Age-related cardiovascular disorders may prompt cautious use and/or dosage reduction.

PREGNANCY/LACTATION-RELATED

- Pregnancy category B; compatible with breast-feeding.

MONITORING

- **Baseline assessment:** For patients taking terbutaline for preterm labor despite warnings the drug has not been adequately studied to warrant safe use, assess the maternal BP and pulse, duration and frequency of contractions, and the fetal heart rate.
- **Lab work:** Baseline biochemical profile including potassium level; hypokalemia may result from terbutaline administration. Periodically evaluate serum potassium level.
- **Tachycardia:** Monitor heart rate for dysrhythmias.
- **Respiratory distress:** Assess quality and respiratory rate, depth, rhythm, and type. Auscultate breath sounds for rhonchi and wheezing. Monitor pulse oximetry and

obtain ABG levels if respiratory failure is suspected. Observe fingernails and lips for a blue or dusky color in light-skinned patients and grayish color in dark-skinned patients, which may indicate hypoxemia. Observe for clavicular retractions and hand tremor.

- **Bronchospasms:** Offer emotional support to patients taking terbutaline for bronchospasm; these patients are prone to anxiety because of difficulty breathing and the sympathomimetic effects of the drug.
- **Therapeutic effect:** Evaluate for cessation of clavicular retractions, quieter and slower respirations, and a relaxed facial expression.
- **Preterm labor:** When terbutaline is used for preterm labor, monitor the duration and frequency of contractions and diligently monitor the fetal heart rate.
- **Patient education:** Instruct to report promptly chest pain, difficulty breathing, dizziness, flushing, headache, muscle tremors, or palpitations to a health care provider. Inform that terbutaline may cause anxiety, nervousness, and shakiness. Urge reduced consumption of caffeinated products, such as chocolate, cocoa, cola, coffee, and tea.

SERIOUS ADVERSE REACTIONS

- **Hyperglycemia:** May occur in diabetic patients receiving large doses of terbutaline.
- **Hypokalemia:** Beta agonists cause movement of potassium from the bloodstream to inside the cells.

OVERDOSE/TOXICITY

- Too-frequent or excessive use may lead to decreased drug effectiveness and severe, paradoxical bronchoconstriction.
- Excessive sympathomimetic stimulation may cause palpitations, extrasystoles, tachycardia, chest pain, a slight increase in BP followed by a substantial decrease, chills, diaphoresis, and blanching of skin.
- **GI decontamination:** No specific recommendations.

ANTIDOTE/DIALYSIS

- **Antidote:** May consider cautious use of a beta-adrenergic blocking agent (propranolol, metoprolol, esmolol); patients with obstructive lung disease may not tolerate many beta-adrenergic blocking agents.
- **Dialysis:** No data are available on removal of terbutaline by hemodialysis, high-permeability hemodialysis, or peritoneal dialysis.

teriparatide acetate

ter-i-par'-a-tide ass'-e-tate

Classes

Chemical: amino terminal peptide hormone
Therapeutic: synthetic parathyroid hormone

Pregnancy Category: C

Trade Names

Prescription: Forteo

CLINICAL PHARMACOLOGY

Mechanism of Action

A synthetic hormone that acts on bone to mobilize calcium; also acts on kidney to reduce calcium clearance and increase phosphate excretion. **Therapeutic Effect:** Increases the rate at which calcium is released from bone into blood; stimulates new bone formation.

PHARMACOKINETICS

Extensively absorbed following subcutaneous injection. Metabolized in the liver. Excreted in urine. **Half-life:** 1 hr.

AVAILABILITY

Injection: 750 mg in 3-mL prefilled pen delivers 20 mcg/dose.

INDICATIONS AND DOSAGE

Osteoporosis

Subcutaneous

Adults, Elderly: 20 mcg once per day into thigh or abdominal wall.

CONTRAINDICATIONS

Hypersensitivity to teriparatide

INTERACTIONS

Drug: Digoxin: May increase serum digoxin concentration. **Herbal:** None known. **Food:** None known.

DIAGNOSTIC TEST EFFECTS

May increase the serum calcium level.

SIDE-EFFECTS

Occasional (3%-10%): Rhinitis, leg cramps, nausea, dizziness, arthralgia, orthostatic hypotension, tachycardia, vomiting, pharyngitis

CRITICAL CARE CONSIDERATIONS

ADMINISTRATION/HANDLING

SUBCUTANEOUS ALERT

- **Storage:** Keep teriparatide refrigerated, minimizing the time out of the refrigerator. Do not freeze the drug; discard if it

T

becomes frozen. Recap the pen (Forteo) when not in use; protect from light.
- **Administration:** Inject teriparatide into the thigh or abdominal wall.

PRECAUTIONS

HEALTH-RELATED

- Use teriparatide cautiously in patients with bone metastases, a history of skeletal malignancies, or metabolic bone diseases other than osteoporosis and in patients receiving concurrent digoxin therapy.
- Conditions that increase the risk of osteosarcoma (including Paget's disease, unexplained elevations of alkaline phosphatase level, open epiphyses, and prior skeletal radiation therapy, implant therapy), hypercalcemia, hypercalcemic disorders (such as hyperparathyroidism)

AGE-RELATED

- **Children:** Safety and efficacy of teriparatide have not been established in children; teriparatide should not be used in children with open epiphyseal (bone growth) plates.
- **Elderly:** May have increased sensitivity to drug effects; may require a dosage reduction.

PREGNANCY/LACTATION-RELATED

- Pregnancy category C; unknown if excreted in breast milk.

MONITORING

- **Baseline assessment:** Assess history of osteoporosis or other bone disease. Monitor for hypotension and tachycardia.
- **Baseline lab work:** Biochemical profile including serum calcium levels and blood parathyroid hormone level; urinalysis including urine calcium level. Monitor parathyroid hormone level, and urinary and serum calcium levels.
- **Baseline diagnostic tests:** X-rays to assess bone disease. Monitor bone mineral density. Observe for signs and symptoms of hypercalcemia.
- **Patient education:** Instruct to sit or lie down immediately if dizziness or lightheadedness occurs, indicative of hypotension. Instruct to report promptly persistent symptoms of hypercalcemia, including loss of energy or strength, lethargy, constipation, nausea, and vomiting to a health care provider.

SERIOUS ADVERSE REACTIONS

- **Osteosarcoma:** Noted in animal studies when high doses were used; teriparatide should not be used for patients at higher risk of developing a malignant bone tumor.

OVERDOSE/TOXICITY

- **Hypercalcemia:** May lead to lethargy, weakness, constipation, personality changes, hypertension, confusion, paresthesias. Occurs rarely.
- **GI decontamination:** No specific recommendations.

ANTIDOTE/DIALYSIS

- **Antidote:** No specific recommendations.
- **Dialysis:** No data are available on removal of teriparatide by hemodialysis, high-permeability hemodialysis, or peritoneal dialysis.

testosterone

tes-tos'-ter-ohn

DEA Schedule: III

Classes

Chemical: androgen
Therapeutic: androgen, antineoplastic

Pregnancy Category: X

Trade Names

Prescription: Androderm, AndroGel, Andro LA 200, Delatestryl, Depandro 100, Depo-Testosterone, FIRST-Testosterone, FIRST-Testosterone MC, Striant, Testim, Testoderm, Testopel, Testo,Testro AQ, Testro-L.A.

Do not confuse testosterone with testolactone.

CLINICAL PHARMACOLOGY

Mechanism of Action

A primary endogenous androgen that promotes growth and development of male sex organs and maintains secondary sex characteristics in androgen-deficient males. **Therapeutic Effect:** Helps relieve androgen deficiency.

PHARMACOKINETICS

Well absorbed after IM administration. Protein binding: 98%. Undergoes first-pass metabolism in the liver. Primarily excreted in urine. **Half-life:** 10-20 min.

AVAILABILITY

Cypionate injection (Depo-Testosterone): 100 mg/mL, 200 mg/mL.

Ethanate injection (Andro LA 200, Delatestryl, Testro-L.A.): 200 mg/mL.
Propionate injection solution (Depandro 100): 100 mg/mL.
Intramuscular solution: 50 mg/mL (Testro), 100 mg/mL (Testro AQ).
Subcutaneous pellets (Testopel): 75 mg.
Topical gel: 1% 25 mg/2.5 g (AndroGel) 50 mg/5 g (AndroGel, Testim); delivers 50 mg testosterone with 5 mg systemically absorbed.
Topical cream (FIRST-Testosterone MC): 2%.
Topical ointment (FIRST-Testosterone): 2%.
Transdermal patch: 2.5 mg/day (Androderm), 4 mg/day (Testoderm), 5 mg/day (Androderm), 6 mg/day (Testoderm).
Buccal (Striant): 30 mg.

INDICATIONS AND DOSAGE

Male hypogonadism

IM (Cypionate or Enanthate)

Adults: 50-400 mg every 2-4 wk. **Adolescents:** Initially 40-50 mg/m^2/dose monthly until growth rate falls to prepubertal levels; 100 mg/m^2/dose until growth ceases. Maintenance virilizing dose: 100 mg/m^2/dose twice per mo.

Subcutaneous (Pellets)

Adults, adolescents: 150-450 mg every 3-6 mo.

Transdermal (Patch [Testoderm with adhesive])

Adults, Elderly: Start therapy with 6 mg/day patch. Apply patch to scrotal skin.

Transdermal (Patch [Testoderm TTS])

Adults, Elderly: Apply 5 mg TTS patch to arm, back, upper buttocks, abdomen, or thighs every 24 hr.

Transdermal (Patch [Androderm])

Adults, Elderly: Start therapy with 5 mg/day patch or 2-2.5 mg/day patch with 5 mg testosterone absorbed systemically, applied at night. Apply patch to abdomen, back, thighs, or upper arms.

Transdermal (Gel [AndroGel])

Adults, Elderly: Initial dose of 5 g delivers 50 mg testosterone and is applied once daily to the abdomen, shoulders, or upper arms. May increase to 7.5 g, then to 10 g, if necessary.

Transdermal (Gel [Testim])

Adults, Elderly: Initial dose of 5 g delivers 50 mg testosterone with 5 mg testosterone absorbed systemically and is applied once per day to the shoulders or upper arms. May increase to 10 g.

Buccal System (Striant)

Adults, Elderly: 30 mg every 12 hr. Rotate to other side of mouth with each application.

Delayed puberty

IM

Adults: 50-200 mg every 2-4 wk. **Adolescents:** 40-50 mg/m^2/dose every mo for 6 mo.

Subcutaneous (Pellets)

Adults, Adolescents: 150-450 mg every 3-6 mo.

Breast carcinoma

IM (testosterone aqueous)

Adults: 50-100 mg 3 times per wk.

IM (testosterone cypionate or testosterone ethanate)

Adults: 200-400 mg every 2-4 wk.

IM (testosterone propionate)

Adults: 50-100 mg 3 times per wk.

CONTRAINDICATIONS

Breast-feeding, cardiac impairment (systemic use only), hypercalcemia, pregnancy, prostate or breast cancer in males, severe hepatic or renal disease, hypersensitivity to testosterone products or soy products

INTERACTIONS

Drug: Hepatotoxic medications: May increase the risk of hepatotoxicity. **Oral anticoagulants:** May increase the effects of oral anticoagulants. **Herbal:** None known. **Food:** None known.

DIAGNOSTIC TEST EFFECTS

May increase blood Hgb level and Hct, as well as serum LDL, alkaline phosphatase, bilirubin, calcium, potassium, sodium, and AST (SGOT) levels. May decrease serum HDL level.

SIDE-EFFECTS

Frequent: Gynecomastia, acne. **Females:** Hirsutism, amenorrhea or other menstrual irregularities, deepening of voice, clitoral enlargement that may not be reversible when drug is discontinued. **Occasional:** Edema, nausea, insomnia, oligospermia, priapism, male-pattern baldness, bladder irritability, hypercalcemia (in immobilized patients or those with breast cancer), hypercholesterolemia, inflammation and pain at IM injection site. **Transdermal:** Pruritus, erythema, skin irritation. **Rare:** Polycythemia (with high dosage), hypersensitivity

T

CRITICAL CARE CONSIDERATIONS

ADMINISTRATION/HANDLING

IM ALERT

- Do not give testosterone IV.
- **Preparation:** Warming and shaking redissolves crystals that may form in long-acting preparations. A wet needle may cause the solution to become cloudy; this does not affect potency.
- **Administration:** Inject testosterone deep into the gluteal muscle.

TRANSDERMAL PATCH ALERT (TESTODERM, TESTODERM TTS, ANDRODERM)

- **Testoderm:** Apply to clean, dry scrotal skin that has been dry-shaved for optimal skin contact. Apply Testoderm TTS to the back, upper arm, abdomen, or thigh.
- **Androderm:** Apply to clean, dry skin on the back, abdomen, upper arms, or thighs. Do not apply to the scrotum, bony prominences (e.g., shoulder) or oily, damaged, or irritated skin. Do not apply Androderm to the same site for 7 days.

TRANSDERMAL GEL ALERT (ANDROGEL, TESTIM)

- **Sites:** Apply the gel to clean, dry, intact skin of shoulder or upper arm, preferably in the morning. Androgel may also be applied to the abdomen. *Do not apply the gel to the genital area.*
- **Application:** Open the packet, squeeze the entire contents into the palm of the hand, and apply at once to the affected site. Allow the gel to dry.

BUCCAL ALERT (STRIANT)

- **Application:** Remove Striant product before placing a new one. Apply Striant to the gum area above the incisor tooth, alternating sides of the mouth with each application.
- Striant is not affected by consumption of alcohol or food, gum chewing, or tooth brushing.

PRECAUTIONS

HEALTH-RELATED

- Use testosterone cautiously in patients with diabetes and hepatic or renal impairment.

AGE-RELATED

- **Children:** Safety and efficacy of testosterone have not been established in children under 12 yr of age.
- **Elderly:** Testosterone may increase the risk of hyperplasia or stimulate growth of occult prostate carcinoma.

PREGNANCY/LACTATION-RELATED

- Pregnancy category X; excretion into breast milk unknown; contraindicated in nursing mothers.

MONITORING

- **Baseline assessment:** Assess vital signs and weight. If used for male hypogonadism or delayed puberty, assess genitalia. If used for breast cancer, assess for other past/present cancer treatments.
- **Lab work:** CBC with WBC differential and platelet count; biochemical profile including calcium, renal (BUN, creatinine) and liver (AST [SGOT], ALT [SGPT], bilirubin, alkaline phosphatase) function tests, and lipid profile (serum cholesterol, triglycerides). Assess Hgb and Hct, serum cholesterol, electrolyte levels, and liver function periodically when giving high doses.
- **Baseline diagnostic tests:** Wrist x-rays may be ordered to determine bone maturation in children; 12-lead ECG for patients with heart disease for comparison in case of dysrhythmias related to hypercalcemia.
- **Injection site reaction:** Assess injection site for pain, redness, or swelling.
- **Hypertension:** Check BP at least twice per day.
- **Weight gain:** Weigh daily; assess dosage for weekly gains of more than 5 lb. Evaluate intake and output; assess for fluid retention and edema.
- **Insomnia:** Monitor sleep patterns; consider a sedative/hypnotic if needed.
- **Hypercalcemia:** Monitor patients with breast cancer or immobility for hypercalcemia, confusion, irritability, lethargy, and muscle weakness.
- **Malnutrition:** Ensure that adequate calories and protein are consumed.
- **Virilization:** Assess for deepening of the voice or increased facial hair.
- **Patient education:** Instruct to apply the patch to a clean, dry, hairless area of the skin, avoiding bony prominences. Instruct to call the prescriber before taking OTC or other new prescription medications. Advise on how to consume a diet high in calories and protein. Food may be better tolerated with small, frequent meals. Instruct how to perform daily weights and to report a weight gain of 5 lb or more per wk. Inform to report promptly acne, nausea,

T

vomiting, or foot swelling to a health care provider. Tell female patients to report promptly deepening of the voice, hoarseness, and menstrual irregularities. Male patients should report difficulty urinating, frequent erections, and gynecomastia. Stress the importance of regular monitoring tests and visits to the physician.

SERIOUS ADVERSE REACTIONS

- **Hypersensitivity:** Anaphylactic reactions occur rarely.
- **Hypercalcemia:** Occurs more frequently with cancer patients and those who are immobile; may lead to lethargy, weakness, constipation, personality changes, hypertension.
- **Edema:** With or without heart failure may occur in those with cardiac, renal or liver disease; patients may retain sodium, potassium, chloride, calcium, and phosphates.
- **Urethral obstruction:** May occur in those with prostatic hypertrophy.
- **Penile changes:** Priapism, prolonged and painful erections, penile enlargement.

OVERDOSE/TOXICITY

- **Hepatotoxicity:** Peliosis hepatitis (presence of blood-filled cysts in parenchyma of liver), hepatic neoplasms, and hepatocellular carcinoma have been associated with prolonged high-dose therapy.
- **Hematologic:** May suppress clotting factors II, V, VII, and X, leading to bleeding in patients taking anticoagulants; may cause polycythemia.
- **GI decontamination:** No specific recommendations.

ANTIDOTE/DIALYSIS

- **Antidote:** No specific recommendations.
- **Dialysis:** Testosterone is not likely to be removed by peritoneal dialysis. No data are available on removal by hemodialysis or high-permeability hemodialysis.

tetracycline hydrochloride

tet-ra-sye'-kleen high-droe-klor'-ide

Classes

Chemical: tetracycline
Therapeutic: antibiotic

Pregnancy Category: D

Trade Names

Prescription: Achromycin V ♣, Ala-Tet, Apo-Tetra ♣, Novotetra ♣, Panmycin, Sumycin, Tetracon

CLINICAL PHARMACOLOGY

Mechanism of Action

A tetracycline antibiotic that inhibits bacterial protein synthesis by binding to ribosomes. **Therapeutic Effect:** Bacteriostatic.

PHARMACOKINETICS

Readily absorbed from the GI tract. Protein binding: 60%. Widely distributed. Excreted in urine; eliminated in feces through biliary system. Not removed by hemodialysis. **Half-life:** 6-11 hr (increased in impaired renal function).

AVAILABILITY

Capsules: 250 mg (Ala-Tet, Panmycin, Sumycin, Tetracon), 500 mg (Sumycin, Tetracon).
Oral suspension (Sumycin): 125 mg/5 mL.
Tablets (Sumycin): 250 mg, 500 mg.
Topical solution. 2.2 mg/mL.
Topical ointment: 3%.

INDICATIONS AND DOSAGE

Inflammatory acne vulgaris, Lyme disease, mycoplasmal disease, Legionella infections, Rocky Mountain spotted fever, chlamydial infections in patients with gonorrhea

PO

Adults, Elderly: 250-500 mg every 6-12 hr.
Children 8 yr and older: 25-50 mg/kg/day in 4 divided doses. Maximum: 3 g/day.

***Helicobacter pylori* infections**

PO

Adults, Elderly: 500 mg 2-4 times per day (in combination).

Dosage in renal impairment

Dosage interval is modified based on creatinine clearance.

Creatinine Clearance	Dosage Interval
50-80 mL/min	Usual dose every 8-12 hr
10-50 mL/min	Usual dose every 12-24 hr
Less than 10 mL/min	Usual dose every 24 hr

CONTRAINDICATIONS

Children 8 yr and younger, hypersensitivity to tetracycline or sulfites, pregnancy

INTERACTIONS

Drug: Carbamazepine, phenytoin: May decrease tetracycline blood concentration. **Cholestyramine, colestipol:** May decrease tetracycline absorption. **Oral contraceptives:** May decrease the effects of oral contraceptives. **Herbal: St. John's wort:** May increase the risk of photosensitivity. **Food: Dairy products:** Inhibit tetracycline absorption.

DIAGNOSTIC TEST EFFECTS

May increase BUN and serum alkaline phosphatase, amylase, bilirubin, AST (SGOT), and ALT (SGPT) levels.

SIDE-EFFECTS

Frequent: Dizziness, lightheadedness, diarrhea, nausea, vomiting, abdominal cramps, possibly severe photosensitivity. **Topical:** Dry, scaly skin; stinging or burning sensation. **Occasional:** Pigmentation of skin or mucous membranes, rectal or genital pruritus, stomatitis. **Topical:** Pain, redness, swelling, or other skin irritation.

CRITICAL CARE CONSIDERATIONS

ADMINISTRATION/HANDLING

PO ALERT

- Space tetracycline doses evenly around the clock.
- Give tetracycline capsules and tablets with a full glass of water 1 hr before or 2 hr after a meal. Drug is most effective when taken on an empty stomach.

TOPICAL ALERT

- **Preparation:** Cleanse the area gently before application.
- **Application:** Wear gloves during application and apply the drug only to the affected area because tetracycline may stain the skin.

PRECAUTIONS

HEALTH-RELATED

- Use tetracycline cautiously in patients who are unable to avoid sun or ultraviolet light exposure; such exposure may produce a severe photosensitivity reaction.

AGE-RELATED

- **Children:** Tetracycline use is not recommended for children 8 yr and under; may cause permanent discoloration of teeth or enamel hypoplasia; may inhibit skeletal growth.
- **Elderly:** No age-related precautions have been noted.

PREGNANCY/LACTATION-RELATED

- Pregnancy category D (systemic); systemic tetracycline excreted into breast milk in low concentrations. Theoretically, dental staining could occur, but serum levels in infants are undetectable, so it is considered compatible with breast-feeding.

MONITORING

- **Baseline assessment:** Determine history of allergies, especially to tetracyclines or sulfites, before beginning drug therapy.
- **Lab work:** Biochemical profile including renal function studies (BUN, creatinine). Obtain necessary cultures with sensitivity before beginning tetracycline.
- **Diarrhea:** Assess pattern of daily bowel activity and stool consistency.
- **Nausea/vomiting:** Monitor food intake and tolerance.
- **Sensitivity:** Examine skin for a rash or local reaction to topical medication.
- **Superinfection:** Assess for anal or genital pruritus, diarrhea, and stomatitis.
- **Benign increased intracranial pressure:** Monitor BP and LOC.
- **Patient education:** Instruct to take oral tetracycline on an empty stomach 1 hr before or 2 hr after consuming beverages or food. Advise drinking a full glass of water with tetracycline capsules and to avoid bedtime doses. Teach how to space drug doses evenly around the clock and to continue taking tetracycline for the full course of treatment. Instruct to report promptly diarrhea, rash, or any other new symptoms that occur to a health care provider. Discourage from overexposure to the sun or ultraviolet light to prevent photosensitivity reactions. Explain that any other medications, including OTC drugs, should not be taken without first consulting the prescriber. Inform that topical tetracycline may turn skin yellow but that washing removes the solution; fabrics may be stained by heavy topical application. Warn not to apply topical tetracycline to deep or open wounds. Warn to avoid performing tasks that require mental alertness or motor skills until response to the drug is known.

SERIOUS ADVERSE REACTIONS

- **Benign intracranial hypertension:** Confusion, disorientation, decreased level of consciousness.
- **Bulging fontanelles:** Occurs rarely in infants.
- **Photosensitivity:** Sunburn following minimal exposure to sunlight/ultraviolet light.
- **Hypersensitivity:** Patients with a history of allergies are at increased risk for developing a severe hypersensitivity reaction, marked by severe pruritus, angioedema,

bronchospasm, and anaphylaxis. Serum sickness and lupuslike symptoms have been reported. Exfoliative dermatitis occurs rarely.

- **Management of hypersensitivity:** May require treatment with epinephrine and other emergency measures including oxygen, endotracheal intubation, mechanical ventilation, IV fluids, IV antihistamines, corticosteroids, and vasopressors.

OVERDOSE/TOXICITY

- **Nephrotoxicity:** May occur, especially in patients with preexisting renal disease.
- **Superinfections:** Antibiotic-associated colitis and other superinfections, especially fungal, may result from altered bacterial balance.
- **Blood dyscrasias:** Anemia, hemolytic anemia, thrombocytopenia, neutropenia, eosinophilia.
- **GI decontamination:** No specific recommendations.

ANTIDOTE/DIALYSIS

- **Antidote:** No specific recommendations.
- **Dialysis:** Tetracycline is not removed by hemodialysis or peritoneal dialysis. No data are available on removal by high-permeability hemodialysis.

thiamine hydrochloride (vitamin B1)

thye'-a-min hye-droe-klor'-ide

Classes

Chemical: vitamin B complex
Therapeutic: vitamin

Pregnancy Category: A

Trade Names

Prescription: Betaxin ♣, Thiamine
Over the Counter: Thiamilate

CLINICAL PHARMACOLOGY

Mechanism of Action

A water-soluble vitamin that combines with adenosine triphosphate in the liver, kidneys, and leukocytes to form thiamine diphosphate, a coenzyme that is necessary for carbohydrate metabolism. **Therapeutic Effect:** Prevents and reverses thiamine deficiency.

PHARMACOKINETICS

Readily absorbed from the GI tract, primarily in duodenum, after IM administration. Widely distributed. Metabolized in the liver. Primarily excreted in urine.

AVAILABILITY

Tablets: 50 mg, 100 mg, 250 mg, 500 mg.
Injection (Vitamin B1): 100 mg/mL.

INDICATIONS AND DOSAGE

Dietary supplement

PO

Adults, Elderly: 1-2 mg/day. **Children:** 0.5-1 mg/day. **Infants:** 0.3-0.5 mg/day.

Thiamine deficiency

PO

Adults, Elderly: 5-30 mg/day, as a single dose or in 3 divided doses, for 1 mo. **Children:**10-50 mg/day as a single dose or divided doses into 3 doses for 2 wk, then 5-10 mg daily for 1 mo.

Thiamine deficiency in patients who are critically ill or have malabsorption syndrome

IV, IM

Adults, Elderly: 5-100 mg, 3 times per day, then 5-10 mg PO daily for 1 mo. **Children:** 10-25 mg/day, then 5-10 mg PO daily for 1 mo.

Metabolic disorders

PO

Adults, Elderly, Children: 10-20 mg/day; increased up to 4 g/day in divided doses.

CONTRAINDICATIONS

Hypersensitivity to thiamine products

INTERACTIONS

Drug: None known. **Herbal:** None known. **Food:** None known.

DIAGNOSTIC TEST EFFECTS

None known.

IV INCOMPATIBILITIES

Sodium bicarbonate

IV COMPATIBILITIES

Famotidine (Pepcid), multivitamins

SIDE-EFFECTS

Frequent: Pain, induration, and tenderness at IM injection site

CRITICAL CARE CONSIDERATIONS

ADMINISTRATION/HANDLING

IM ALERT

- The IM route is preferred over the IV route.

- IM and IV administration routes are used only in acutely ill patients and those who are unresponsive to the PO route, such as those with malabsorption syndrome.

IV ALERT

- Thiamine may be given by IV push or may be added to most IV solutions to be given as an IV infusion.
- Worsening of Wernicke's encephalopathy (confusion) is possible following glucose administration; administer thiamine before or along with dextrose-containing fluids.
- Single vitamin B_1 deficiency is rare; suspect multiple vitamin deficiencies.

PRECAUTIONS

HEALTH-RELATED

- Use thiamine cautiously in patients with Wernicke's encephalopathy.
- If "wet" beriberi with heart failure is present, symptom is considered an emergency and must be treated with IV thiamine.

AGE-RELATED

- **Children:** No age-related precautions have been noted in children.
- **Elderly:** No age-related precautions have been noted.

PREGNANCY/LACTATION-RELATED

- Pregnancy category A; excreted into breast milk. U.S. recommended daily allowance for thiamine during lactation is 1.5-1.6 mg; supplement women with inadequate intake. Compatible with breastfeeding.

MONITORING

- **Baseline assessment:** Before and during treatment, assess for symptoms of thiamine deficiency including peripheral neuropathy, ataxia, hyporeflexia, muscle weakness, nystagmus, ophthalmoplegia, confusion, peripheral edema, bounding arterial pulse, and tachycardia. Baseline vital signs and weight. Screen for history of alcoholism.
- **Lab work:** Biochemical profile to rule out other causes of symptoms that may mimic thiamine deficiency; CBC with differential. Blood alcohol level in patients suspected of alcohol or drug abuse.
- **Diagnostic tests:** 12-lead ECG to evaluate for dysrhythmias and myocardial ischemia.
- **Cardiac effects of deficiency:** Monitor for worsening of edema, respiratory distress, activity intolerance and tachycardia, which may signal worsening heart failure. Patients may require aggressive management of fluid overload.
- **Hypersensitivity:** If receiving IV thiamine, observe closely for allergic reaction including rash, urticaria, itching, diaphoresis, nausea, and respiratory distress.
- **IM injection site:** Monitor for tenderness and induration of injection sites.
- **Alcoholism:** If alcoholism is suspected, a complete alcohol withdrawal protocol should be initiated, including benzodiazepines (i.e., lorazepam/Ativan), thiamine and other vitamins, and behavioral counseling. Patients who withdraw from alcohol are at high risk for delirium tremens and seizures.
- **Therapeutic effect:** Assess for signs of improvement, including an improved sense of well-being and weight gain; reversal of neurologic symptoms of deficiency (peripheral neuropathy, ataxia, hyporeflexia, muscle weakness, nystagmus, ophthalmoplegia, and confusion) and cardiac symptoms including peripheral edema, bounding arterial pulse, tachycardia, and venous hypertension.
- **Patient education:** Inform that IM injection may cause discomfort. Encourage to consume foods rich in thiamine, including legumes, nuts, organ meats, pork, rice bran, seeds, wheat germ, whole grain and enriched cereals, and yeast. Advise that urine may appear bright yellow during thiamine therapy. Patients with alcohol abuse problems should be advised to seek an outpatient alcohol treatment program including support groups such as Alcoholics Anonymous.

SERIOUS ADVERSE REACTIONS

- **Severe hypersensitivity reaction:** IV administration may result in a rare, severe reaction marked by a feeling of warmth, pruritus, urticaria, weakness, diaphoresis, nausea, restlessness, tightness in throat, angioedema, cyanosis, pulmonary edema, GI tract bleeding, and cardiovascular collapse. May be fatal.

OVERDOSE/TOXICITY

- **Intolerance:** Some patients receiving thiamine develop intolerance over time, especially with repeated IV administration.
- **GI decontamination:** No specific recommendations.

ANTIDOTE/DIALYSIS

- **Antidote:** No specific recommendations.

- **Dialysis:** Thiamine is not removed by hemodialysis and is unlikely to be removed by peritoneal dialysis. No data are available on removal by high-permeability hemodialysis.

thiopental sodium 

thye-oh-pen'-tal soe'-dee-um

DEA Schedule: III

Classes

Chemical: thiobarbiturate
Therapeutic: barbiturate, sedative, hypnotic, anesthesia adjunct

Pregnancy Category: C

Trade Names

Prescription: Pentothal

CLINICAL PHARMACOLOGY

Mechanism of Action

An ultra short-acting IV anesthetic that depresses the CNS. The exact mechanism of action is not fully understood. Therapeutic Effect: Produces hypnosis and anesthesia.

PHARMACOKINETICS

Hypnosis occurs within 30-40 sec of IV injection. Duration is 5-30 min. Protein binding: 80%. Primarily metabolized in liver and to a smaller extent in other tissues. Excreted in urine. Half-life: 3-8 hr.

AVAILABILITY

Powder for injection: 250 mg, 400 mg, 500 mg, 1 g, 2.5 g, 5 g.

INDICATIONS AND DOSAGE

Anesthesia

IV

Adults: 50-75 mg (2-3 mL of a 2.5% solution), slow IV, at intervals of 20-40 sec. Once anesthesia is established, additional injections of 25-100 mg can be given whenever the patient moves. **Children more than 12 yr:** Induction: 3-5 mg/kg. Maintenance: 1 mg/kg as needed. **Children 1-12 yr:** Induction: 5-6 mg/kg. Maintenance: 1 mg/kg as needed. **Infants:** Induction: 5-8 mg/kg. **Neonates:** Induction: 3-4 mg/kg.

Seizures (secondary to anesthesia)

IV

Adults: 75-125 mg (3-5 mL of a 2.5% solution), single dose, as soon as convulsions begin. Convulsions following the use of a local anesthetic may require 125-250 mg of thiopental given over a 10-min period. **Children:** 2-3 mg/kg/dose, repeat as needed.

Raised intracranial pressure (ICP)

IV

Adults: Intermittent bolus injections of 1.5-3.5 mg/kg of body weight may be given to reduce intraoperative elevations of ICP, if adequate ventilation is provided. **Children:** 1.5-5 mg/kg/dose; repeat as needed to control ICP; larger doses (30 mg/kg) to induce coma after hypoxic-ischemic injury does not appear to improve neurologic outcome.

Psychiatric disorders (narcoanalysis, narcosynthesis)

IV

Adults: Premedicate with an anticholinergic agent. Inject thiopental at a slow rate of 100 mg/min (4 mL/min of a 2.5% solution) with the patient counting backward from 100. **Adults:** Alternatively, thiopental may be administered by rapid IV drip (50 mL/min) using a 0.2% concentration in 5% dextrose and water. At this concentration, the rate of administration should not exceed 50 mL/min.

CONTRAINDICATIONS

Absence of suitable veins for intravenous administration, hypersensitivity to thiopental or other barbiturates, *Variegate porphyria* (South African), or acute intermittent porphyria, severe cardiac disease

INTERACTIONS

Drug: **Aminophylline, zimelidine:** May cause thiopental antagonism. **Diazoxide:** May cause hypotension. **Midazolam:** May cause synergistic effects. **Opioid analgesics:** May decrease antinociceptive action. **Probenecid:** May prolong the action of thiopental. Herbal: None known. Food: None known.

DIAGNOSTIC TEST EFFECTS

None known.

SIDE-EFFECTS

Frequency not defined: Prolonged somnolence and recovery, sneezing, coughing, bronchospasm, laryngospasm, shivering, respiratory depression, myocardial depression, cardiac dysrhythmias

CRITICAL CARE CONSIDERATIONS

ADMINISTRATION/HANDLING

IV ALERT

- **Stability:** Use only clear solutions. Use within 24 hr of reconstitution.

- **Reconstitution:** Normal saline, D_5W, or sterile water for injection.
- **For use in anesthesia:** Slow injection is recommended to minimize respiratory depression and the possibility of overdosage.
- **Anesthesia professionals only:** Thiopental should be administered only by professionals specially trained in administration of general anesthetics.
- **For psychiatric disorders:** Have patients begin counting with sequential numbers (1, 2, 3, 4, 5, and so on). Shortly after the counting becomes confused but before falling asleep, discontinue the injection. Allow a return to a semidrowsy state at which conversation is coherent.

PRECAUTIONS

HEALTH-RELATED

- Use thiopental cautiously in patients with severe cardiovascular disease, hypotension or shock, status asthmaticus, and conditions in which the hypnotic effect may be prolonged or potentiated—excessive premedication, Addison's disease, hepatic or renal dysfunction, myxedema, increased blood urea, severe anemia, asthma, myasthenia gravis.

AGE-RELATED

- **Children:** Dosage is based on age and weight.
- **Elderly:** May be more susceptible to age-related adverse effects. Younger patients require much larger doses than do middle-aged or elderly patients.

PREGNANCY/LACTATION-RELATED

- Pregnancy category C; small amounts are excreted in breast milk; breast-feeding should be delayed until drug has cleared the mother's body.

MONITORING

- **Baseline assessment:** Obtain baseline vital signs. Assess for history of severe cardiovascular disease, liver or renal disease, history of neuromuscular disease, asthma, and anemia.
- **Test dose:** A small test dose of thiopental is recommended to assess for unusual sensitivity to thiopental.
- **Lab work:** CBC with differential; baseline biochemical profile including renal (BUN, creatinine) and liver (AST [SGOT], ALT [SGPT], alkaline phosphatase, bilirubin) function studies, urinalysis.
- **Diagnostic tests:** 12-lead ECG to evaluate for myocardial ischemia.
- **Continuous monitoring:** Monitor BP, heart rate, oxygen saturation, and respiratory rate.
- **Dysrhythmias:** Monitor for bradycardia and ventricular dysrhythmias. Myocardial depression is possible.
- **Large veins:** Ensure IV catheter has been placed in a vein rather than an artery. Accidental arterial injection will cause tissue necrosis. Patients who report pain or discomfort upon injection should have the injection discontinued
- **Respiratory depression:** Have resuscitation equipment available at all times and care providers skilled in endotracheal intubation and mechanical ventilation. When used during anesthesia, bronchospasms and laryngeal spasms may be noted during induction.
- **Seizure patients:** Monitor for improvement and control of seizures. Have seizure precautions in place.
- **Neurosurgical patients:** Assess for increased intracranial pressure; drip is titrated to maintain a level of sedation appropriate for lowering ICP.
- **Patient education:** Instruct conscious patients to report promptly chest pain, shortness of breath, or hemoptysis to a health care provider.

SERIOUS ADVERSE REACTIONS

- **Hypersensitivity:** Anaphylactic reactions, immune hemolytic anemia with renal failure, and radial nerve palsy have been reported.
- **Gangrene:** Accidental arterial injection can cause severe pain, arteriospasm with blanching of the arm and the fingers. Appropriate measures must be taken immediately to avoid development of gangrene. If needle is left in place, injection of papaverine and procaine help inhibit arterial spasm, followed by phentolamine throughout the vasospastic area.
- **Shivering:** Twitching face muscles followed by tremors of the body and extremities indicate a thermal reaction due to increased sensitivity to cold. If the room is very cold, likelihood of shivering increases. Patients should be warmed with blankets. *ChlorproMAZINE or methylphenidate may help abate shivering.

OVERDOSE/TOXICITY

- **Overdose:** Respiratory depression, Cheyne-Stokes respirations, apnea, pulmonary edema, cyanosis, tachycardia, delirium, coma, hypotension, hypothermia,

severe CNS depression, flat EEG (reversible unless hypoxic damage has occurred), sluggish or absent reflexes.
- **Management:** Maintain patent airway and support ventilation. Endotracheal intubation and mechanical ventilation may be needed. Support BP with IV fluids, then vasopressors if needed. Keep patients warm. Diuretics may promote elimination of the drug.
- **GI decontamination:** No specific recommendations.

ANTIDOTE/DIALYSIS
- **Antidote:** No specific recommendations.
- **Dialysis:** Thiopental is not removed by hemodialysis and is unlikely to be removed by peritoneal dialysis. No data are available on removal by high-permeability hemodialysis.

thioridazine hydrochloride

See Antipsychotics (p. 934)

thiothixene

See Antipsychotics (p. 934)

tiagabine hydrochloride

tye-ag'-ah-been hye-droe-klor'-ide

Classes
Chemical: nipecotic acid derivative
Therapeutic: anticonvulsant

Pregnancy Category: C

Trade Names
Prescription: Gabitril

CLINICAL PHARMACOLOGY
Mechanism of Action
An anticonvulsant that enhances the activity of gamma-aminobutyric acid, the major inhibitory neurotransmitter in the CNS. **Therapeutic Effect:** Inhibits seizures.

PHARMACOKINETICS
Rapidly and nearly completely absorbed after PO administration. Protein binding: 96%. Metabolized in liver. Eliminated in urine and feces. Not removed by hemodialysis. **Half-life:** 7-9 hr.

AVAILABILITY
Tablets: 2 mg, 4 mg, 6 mg, 8 mg, 10 mg, 12 mg, 16 mg.

INDICATIONS AND DOSAGE
Adjunctive treatment of partial seizures
PO
Adults, Elderly: Initially, 4 mg once per day. May increase by 4-8 mg/day at weekly intervals. Maximum: 56 mg/day in 2-4 divided doses. Range: 32-56 mg/day. **Children 12-18 yr:** Initially, 4 mg once per day. May increase by 4 mg at wk 2 and by 4-8 mg at weekly intervals thereafter. Maximum: 32 mg/day in 2-4 divided doses.

OFF-LABEL USES
Bipolar disorder

CONTRAINDICATIONS
Hypersensitivity to tiagabine

INTERACTIONS
Drug: Cytochrome P4503A4 inducers, including carbamazepine, phenobarbital, phenytoin: May increase tiagabine clearance. **Valproic acid:** May increase the effects of valproic acid by 40%. **Cytochrome P4503A4 enzyme inhibitors:** May decrease tiagabine clearance. **Herbal: Ginkgo biloba:** May increase anticonvulsant effectiveness. **Food:** None known.

DIAGNOSTIC TEST EFFECTS
None known.

SIDE-EFFECTS
Frequent (34%-20%): Dizziness, asthenia, somnolence, nervousness, confusion, headache, infection, tremor, decreased concentration ability. **Occasional:** Nausea, diarrhea, abdominal pain, impaired concentration

CRITICAL CARE CONSIDERATIONS

ADMINISTRATION/HANDLING
PO ALERT
- Tiagabine should be taken with food.
- Store at controlled room temperature; protect from light.

PRECAUTIONS
HEALTH-RELATED
- Use tiagabine cautiously in patients with hepatic impairment and in those who take other CNS depressants concurrently.
- **Cytochrome P450 enzyme metabolism:** Tiagabine is a CYP4503A4 enzyme

inducer and has the potential for drug interactions with other enzyme inducers including cimetidine, theophylline, warfarin, digoxin, ethanol, triazolam, oral contraceptives, and antipyrine.

AGE-RELATED

- **Children:** Safety and efficacy of tiagabine have not been established in children under 12 yr.
- **Elderly:** Tiagabine has not been well studied in patients over 65 yr.

PREGNANCY/LACTATION-RELATED

- Pregnancy category C; unknown if excreted in breast milk.

MONITORING

- **Baseline assessment:** Assess level of consciousness; review the history of the seizure disorder, including the duration, frequency, and intensity of seizures.
- **Lab work:** CBC; biochemical profile including renal (BUN, creatinine) and liver function studies (AST [SGOT], ALT [SGPT], alkaline phosphatase, bilirubin). Plasma levels of tiagabine should be considered when other medications metabolized by the cytochrome P450 pathway are given.
- **Baseline diagnostic tests:** Baseline EEG for patients with history of spike and wave discharges on EEG; exacerbations of these events have been reported when drug is initiated.
- **Seizure precautions:** Observe frequently for a recurrence of seizures. Assess for signs of clinical improvement, such as a decrease in the frequency or intensity of seizures.
- **Dizziness:** Assist with ambulation if dizziness occurs.
- **Patient education:** Instruct to change positions slowly from recumbent to sitting position and to pause before standing to avoid dizziness. Warn to avoid tasks that require mental alertness or motor skills until response to the drug is known. Urge avoidance of alcohol while taking tiagabine. Advise to always carry an identification card or wear an identification bracelet that displays the seizure disorder and anticonvulsant therapy.

SERIOUS ADVERSE REACTIONS

- **Hypersensitivity:** Rash, urticaria, allergic reaction.
- **Cardiovascular:** Hypertension, palpitations, syncope, tachycardia.
- **Metabolic/nutritional:** Weight gain or loss, peripheral edema.
- **Neurologic:** Hallucinations, hyperkinesia, hypotonia, myoclonus, personality disorder.

OVERDOSE/TOXICITY

- Overdose is characterized by agitation, confusion, hostility, and weakness. Full recovery occurs within 24 hr.
- **GI decontamination:** No specific recommendations.

ANTIDOTE/DIALYSIS

- **Antidote:** No specific recommendations.
- **Dialysis:** Tiagabine is not removed by hemodialysis. No data are available on removal by high-permeability hemodialysis or peritoneal dialysis.

ticarcillin disodium/ clavulanate potassium

tye-car-sill'-in/klav'-yoo-lan-ate

Classes

Chemical: penicillin derivative, extended-spectrum
Therapeutic: antibiotic

Pregnancy Category: B

Trade Names

Prescription: Timentin

CLINICAL PHARMACOLOGY

Mechanism of Action

Ticarcillin binds to bacterial cell walls, inhibiting cell wall synthesis. Clavulanate inhibits the action of bacterial beta-lactamase. **Therapeutic Effect:** Ticarcillin is bactericidal in susceptible organisms. Clavulanate protects ticarcillin from enzymatic degradation.

PHARMACOKINETICS

Widely distributed. Protein binding: ticarcillin 45%-60%, clavulanate 9%-30%. Minimally metabolized in the liver. Primarily excreted unchanged in urine. Removed by hemodialysis. **Half-life:** 1-1.2 hr (increased in impaired renal function).

AVAILABILITY

ADD-Vantage vial: 3.1 g.
Powder for injection: 3.1 g.
Premixed solution for infusion: 3.1 g/100 mL.

INDICATIONS AND DOSAGE

Skin and skin structure, bone, joint, and lower respiratory tract infections; septicemia; endometriosis

IV

Adults, Elderly: 3.1 g (3 g ticarcillin) every 4-6 hr. Maximum: 18-24 g/day. **Children 3 mo and older:** 200-300 mg (as ticarcillin) every 4-6 hr.

Urinary tract infections

IV

Adults, Elderly: 3.1 g every 6-8 hr.

Dosage in renal impairment

Dosage interval is modified based on creatinine clearance.

Creatinine Clearance	Dosage Interval
10-30 mL/min	Usual dose every 8 hr
Less than 10 mL/min	Usual dose every 12 hr

CONTRAINDICATIONS

Hypersensitivity to ticarcillin, any penicillin, or clavulanic acid

INTERACTIONS

Drug: Anticoagulants, heparin, NSAIDs, thrombolytics: May increase the risk of hemorrhage with high dosages of ticarcillin. **Probenecid:** May increase ticarcillin blood concentration and risk of toxicity. **Herbal:** None known. **Food:** None known.

DIAGNOSTIC TEST EFFECTS

May increase bleeding time and serum alkaline phosphatase, bilirubin, creatinine, LDH, AST (SGOT), and ALT (SGPT) levels. May decrease serum potassium, sodium, and uric acid levels. May cause a positive Coombs' test.

IV INCOMPATIBILITIES

Amphotericin B complex (Abelcet, AmBisome, Amphotec), vancomycin (Vancocin), total parenteral nutrition (TPN)

IV COMPATIBILITIES

Diltiazem (Cardizem), heparin, insulin, morphine, propofol (Diprivan)

SIDE-EFFECTS

Frequent: Phlebitis or thrombophlebitis (with IV dose), rash, urticaria, pruritus, altered smell or taste. **Occasional:** Nausea, diarrhea, vomiting. **Rare:** Headache, fatigue, hallucinations, bleeding or ecchymosis

CRITICAL CARE CONSIDERATIONS

ADMINISTRATION/HANDLING

IV ALERT

- **Stability:** The solution normally appears colorless to pale yellow; a darker color indicates a loss of potency. Reconstituted IV infusion (piggyback) is stable for 24 hr at room temperature and 3 days if refrigerated. Discard the solution if a precipitate forms.
- **Premixed:** Ticarcillin is available in ready-to-use containers.
- **IV intermittent infusion (piggyback):** Reconstitute each 3.1-g vial with 13 mL sterile water for injection or 0.9% NaCl to provide a concentration of 200 mg ticarcillin and 6.7 mg clavulanic acid per milliliter. Shake the vial to assist reconstitution. Further dilute with 50 to 100 mL D_5W or 0.9% NaCl.
- **Infusion rate:** Infuse the drug over 30 min.
- **Hypersensitivity reactions:** Start the initial dose at a few drops per min, and then increase it slowly to the ordered rate. Stay with patients for the first 10-15 min during the initial dose; then check patients every 10 min during the infusion for signs and symptoms of hypersensitivity or anaphylaxis.

PRECAUTIONS

HEALTH-RELATED

- Use ticarcillin and clavulanate cautiously in patients with renal impairment or a history of allergies, especially to cephalosporins.

AGE-RELATED

- **Children:** Safety and efficacy of ticarcillin have not been established in children under 3 mo. Ticarcillin use in infants may lead to allergic sensitization, candidiasis, diarrhea, and a rash.
- **Elderly:** Age-related renal impairment may require a dosage reduction.

PREGNANCY/LACTATION-RELATED

- Pregnancy category B; excreted into breast milk in low concentrations; compatible with breast-feeding.

MONITORING

- **Baseline assessment:** Determine history of allergies, especially to cephalosporins or penicillins, before beginning drug therapy.

- **Lab work:** CBC with WBC differential; biochemical profile including potassium, liver (AST [SGOT], ALT [SGPT], bilirubin, alkaline phosphatase) and renal function studies (BUN, creatinine). Obtain necessary cultures prior to giving drug, if possible.
- **Penicillin allergy/reaction:** Withhold ticarcillin and promptly notify the physician if patients experience rash or diarrhea. Although a rash is a common side effect of ticarcillin, it may also indicate hypersensitivity.
- **Colitis:** Severe diarrhea with abdominal pain, blood or mucus in stools, and fever may indicate antibiotic-associated colitis.
- **Nausea/vomiting:** Manage with standard measures. Provide IV hydration if severe symptoms occur. Consider use of another antibiotic.
- **Superinfection:** Be alert for superinfection, including anal or genital pruritus, black hairy tongue, diarrhea, increased fever, sore throat, ulceration or changes of oral mucosa, and vomiting.
- **Evenly spaced dosing:** Administer doses evenly around the clock.
- **Offensive drug odor/taste:** Provide with mouth care and sugarless gum or hard candy to offset ticarcillin's bad taste and smell.
- **IV site reactions:** Evaluate for signs of phlebitis, such as heat, pain, and red streaking over the vein.
- **Renal insufficiency:** Monitor intake and output, renal function test results, and urinalysis results.
- **Thrombocytopenia:** Assess for ecchymosis and overt bleeding.
- **Patient education:** Instruct to report immediately pain, redness, or swelling at the infusion site, or severe diarrhea, a rash, itching, or any other unusual signs or symptoms to a health care provider or the prescriber.

SERIOUS ADVERSE REACTIONS

- **Superinfections:** Antibiotic-associated colitis and other superinfections may result from bacterial imbalance.
- **Hypersensitivity reactions:** Including anaphylaxis, skin rashes, urticaria, and drug fever.
- **Hematologic:** Anemia, hemolytic anemia, thrombocytopenia, leukopenia, agranulocytosis, eosinophilia, thrombocytopenic purpura.
- **Hypokalemia:** Disodium formulation of drug may cause low potassium levels.
- **CNS effects:** Reversible hyperactivity, agitation, anxiety, seizures, behavioral changes, dizziness.

OVERDOSE/TOXICITY

- **Overdose:** May produce seizures and other neurologic reactions.
- **Hepatic/liver:** Elevated liver enzymes (AST [SGOT], ALT [SGPT]), confusion, altered behavior.
- **Renal/kidney:** Rare interstitial nephritis is indicative of hypersensitivity.
- **GI decontamination:** No specific recommendations.

ANTIDOTE/DIALYSIS

- **Antidote:** No specific antidote. Discontinuing medication generally resolves adverse effects.
- **Dialysis:** Ticarcillin is removed by hemodialysis and is likely removed by high-permeability hemodialysis. It is not removed by peritoneal dialysis.

ticlopidine hydrochloride 

See Anticoagulants (p. 900)

tigecycline

See Antibiotics (p. 892)

timolol

See Beta-Adrenergic Blockers (p. 943)

tinzaparin sodium 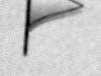

tin-za'-pa-rin soe'-dee-um

Classes

Chemical: heparin derivative, depolymerized; low-molecular weight heparin
Therapeutic: anticoagulant

Pregnancy Category: B

Trade Names

Prescription: Innohep

CLINICAL PHARMACOLOGY

Mechanism of Action

A low-molecular-weight heparin that inhibits factor Xa. Causes less inactivation of thrombin, inhibition of platelets, and bleeding than standard heparin. Does not significantly influence bleeding time, prothrombin time, aPTT. **Therapeutic Effect:** Produces anticoagulation.

PHARMACOKINETICS

Well absorbed after subcutaneous administration. Primarily eliminated in urine. **Half-life:** 3-4 hr.

AVAILABILITY

Injection: 20,000 anti-Xa units/mL.

INDICATIONS AND DOSAGE

Deep vein thrombosis (DVT)

Subcutaneous

Adults, Elderly: 175 anti-Xa units/kg once per day. Continue for at least 6 days and until patient is sufficiently anticoagulated with warfarin (international normalized ratio of 2 or more for 2 consecutive days).

CONTRAINDICATIONS

Active major bleeding; concurrent heparin therapy; hypersensitivity to tinzaparin, heparin, sulfites, benzyl alcohol, or pork products; thrombocytopenia associated with positive in vitro test for antiplatelet antibody

INTERACTIONS

Drug: **Anticoagulants, platelet inhibitors:** May increase the risk of bleeding. **Herbal:** **Ginkgo biloba:** May increase the risk of bleeding. **Food:** None known.

DIAGNOSTIC TEST EFFECTS

Increases (reversible) LDH, serum alkaline phosphatase, AST (SGOT), and ALT (SGPT) levels.

SIDE-EFFECTS

Frequent (16%): Injection site reaction, such as inflammation, oozing, nodules, and skin necrosis. **Rare (less than 2%):** Nausea, asthenia, constipation, epistaxis

CRITICAL CARE CONSIDERATIONS

ADMINISTRATION/HANDLING

SUBCUTANEOUS ALERT

- *Do not mix with other injections or infusions. Do not give IM.*
- **Storage/stability:** Store at room temperature. The parenteral form normally appears clear and colorless to pale yellow.
- **Preparation:** Instruct to lie down before administering by deep subcutaneous injection.

PRECAUTIONS

HEALTH-RELATED

- Use tinzaparin cautiously in the elderly and in patients with conditions associated with increased risk of hemorrhage, history of recent GI ulceration and hemorrhage, history of heparin-induced thrombocytopenia, impaired renal function, or uncontrolled arterial hypertension.

AGE-RELATED

- **Children:** Safety and efficacy of tinzaparin have not been established in children.
- **Elderly:** May be more susceptible to bleeding.

PREGNANCY/LACTATION-RELATED

- Pregnancy category B; low-molecular-weight heparins have been used to prevent and treat thromboembolic disease during pregnancy in lieu of warfarin, which is a known teratogen; excretion into breast milk unknown but thought to be minimal based on pharmacokinetic parameters; use caution in nursing mothers.

MONITORING

- **Baseline assessment:** Assess vital signs and note BP.
- **Lab work:** Assess CBC, including platelet count, prothrombin time, INR; reassess CBC and platelet count periodically throughout therapy.
- **Bleeding:** Assess for bleeding, including bleeding at injection or surgical sites or from gums, blood in stool, bruising, hematuria, and petechiae.
- **DVT prophylaxis:** Perform assessment to determine risk of DVT in all hospitalized patients, especially elderly and those who are not ambulatory.
- **Patient education:** Instruct to administer tinzaparin by subcutaneous route only. Tell about the possibility of a tendency to bleed easily. Suggest the use of an electric razor and a soft toothbrush to prevent bleeding. Instruct to report promptly chest pain; injection site reaction, such as inflammation, nodules, or oozing; numbness, pain, swelling or tingling of joints; or unusual bleeding or bruising to a health care provider.

SERIOUS ADVERSE REACTIONS

- **Thrombocytopenia:** Decreased platelet count occurs in 1% of patients.
- **Liver enzyme elevation:** Serum transaminases (AST [SGOT], ALT [SGPT]) increase to over 3 times the upper limit of normal in 8.8%-13% of patients.
- **Hypersensitivity:** Rash, pruritis, bullous eruptions, anaphylaxis.
- **Spinal hematoma:** Patients with epidural or spinal catheters in place for anesthesia or analgesia are at risk of developing a spinal hematoma that may cause permanent paralysis.

OVERDOSE/TOXICITY

- **Overdose:** May lead to bleeding complications ranging from local ecchymoses to major hemorrhage.
- **GI decontamination:** No specific recommendations.

ANTIDOTE/DIALYSIS

- **Antidote:** Dose of protamine sulfate (1% solution) should be equal to dose of tinzaparin injected. 65% of anti-Xa activity is neutralized with 1 mg. One mg protamine sulfate neutralizes 100 units of tinzaparin. A second dose of 0.5 mg tinzaparin per 1 mg protamine sulfate may be given if aPTT tested 2-4 hr after the initial infusion remains prolonged.
- **Dialysis:** Tinzaparin is unlikely to be removed by hemodialysis. No data are available on removal by high-permeability hemodialysis or peritoneal dialysis.

tiotropium

See Bronchodilators (p. 947)

tirofiban hydrochloride

tye-roe-fye'-ban hye-droe-klor'-ide

Classes

Chemical: glycoprotein (GP) IIb/IIIa inhibitor
Therapeutic: antiplatelet agent

Pregnancy Category: B

Trade Names

Prescription: Aggrastat

Do not confuse Aggrastat with Aggrenox.

CLINICAL PHARMACOLOGY

Mechanism of Action

An antiplatelet and antithrombotic agent that binds to platelet receptor glycoprotein IIb/IIIa, preventing binding of fibrinogen. Therapeutic Effect: Inhibits platelet aggregation and thrombus formation.

PHARMACOKINETICS

Poorly bound to plasma proteins; unbound fraction in plasma: 35%. Limited metabolism. Primarily eliminated in the urine (65%) and, to a lesser amount, in the feces. Removed by hemodialysis. Half-life: 2 hr. Clearance is significantly decreased in severe renal impairment (creatinine clearance less than 30 mL/min).

AVAILABILITY

Injection premix: 12.5 mg/250 mL, 25 mg/500 mL (50 mcg/mL).
Vial: 250 mcg/mL.

INDICATIONS AND DOSAGE

Inhibition of platelet aggregation

IV

Adults, Elderly: Initially, 0.4 mcg/kg/min for 30 min; then continue at 0.1 mcg/kg/min through procedure and for 12-24 hr after procedure.

Severe renal insufficiency (creatinine clearance less than 30 mL/min)

Adults, Elderly: Half the usual rate of infusion.

CONTRAINDICATIONS

Active internal bleeding or a history of bleeding diathesis within previous 30 days, arteriovenous malformation or aneurysm, history of intracranial hemorrhage, history of thrombocytopenia after prior exposure to tirofiban, intracranial neoplasm, major surgical procedure within previous 30 days, severe hypertension, stroke, hypersensitivity to tirofiban

INTERACTIONS

Drug: **Drugs that affect hemostasis (such as aspirin, heparin, NSAIDs, and warfarin):** May increase the risk of bleeding
Herbal: None known. Food: None known.

DIAGNOSTIC TEST EFFECTS

Decreases Hct, Hgb, and platelet count.

IV INCOMPATIBILITIES

Do not mix with other medications.

SIDE-EFFECTS

Occasional (6%-3%): Pelvis pain, bradycardia, dizziness, leg pain. Rare (2%-1%): Edema and swelling, vasovagal reaction, diaphoresis, nausea, fever, headache

CRITICAL CARE CONSIDERATIONS

ADMINISTRATION/HANDLING

IV ALERT

- **Storage:** Store at room temperature and protect from light. Use only clear solution.
- **Stability:** Discard unused solution 24 hr after start of infusion.
- **Injection for solution (250 mcg/mL):** Withdraw and discard 100 mL from a 500-mL bag of 0.9% NaCl or D_5W and replace this volume with 100 mL of tirofiban drawn from two 50-mL vials; (or withdraw and discard 50 mL from a 250-mL bag and replace with 50 mL of tirofiban drawn from one 50-mL vial) to achieve a final concentration of 50 mcg/mL. Mix well before administration.
- **Injection (50 mcg/mL) premix in 500-mL IntraVia container:** Tear off the dust cover to open the IntraVia container. Check the container for leaks by squeezing the inner bag firmly; if a leak is found or if the solution is not clear, discard the solution. Do not add other drugs or remove injection premix solution (50 mcg/mL) directly from the bag with a syringe. Do not use plastic containers in series connections; may result in air embolism caused by drawing air from the first container that holds no solution.
- **Loading dose:** Give 0.4 mcg/kg/min for 30 min. For maintenance infusion, give 0.1 mcg/kg/min.
- **Heparin:** Heparin and tirofiban can be administered through the same IV line.

TIROFIBAN INFUSION RATE TABLE

Weight (kg)	Loading Dose (mL/hr)	Maintenance Infusion (mL/hr)
46-54	24	6
55-62	28	7
63-70	32	8
71-79	36	9
80-87	40	10
88-95	44	11
96-104	48	12

For renal impaired patients, loading dose and maintenance infusion should be reduced by 50% (half the normal dose should be given)

PRECAUTIONS

HEALTH-RELATED

- Use tirofiban cautiously in patients with hemorrhagic retinopathy, platelet counts less than 150,000/mm^3, or renal impairment.
- Use cautiously in patients who are also receiving drugs affecting hemostasis, such as warfarin. Aspirin and heparin may be used as part of the therapy for myocardial ischemia or infarction.
- In clinical studies, patients received aspirin unless it was contraindicated.
- Tirofiban, eptifibitide, and abciximab can all decrease the incidence of cardiac events associated with acute coronary syndromes; direct comparisons are needed to establish which, if any, is superior; for angioplasty, until more data become available, abciximab appears to be the drug of choice.

AGE-RELATED

- **Children:** Safety and efficacy of tirofiban have not been established in children.
- **Elderly:** Have an increased risk of bleeding; use tirofiban with caution.

PREGNANCY/LACTATION-RELATED

- Pregnancy category B; excretion into breast milk unknown; use caution in nursing mothers.

MONITORING

- **Baseline assessment:** Assess bleeding potential, including history of bleeding, liver disease, blood dyscrasias, thrombocytopenia following prior tirofiban infusion, recent stroke, GI bleeding, cancer, and acute pericarditis as drug is contraindicated. Assess for hypertension because drug is contraindicated in patients with systolic BP more than 180 mmHg and diastolic BP more than 110 mmHg.
- **Lab work:** Assess aPTT, Hct, Hgb, platelet count, and serum creatinine level before tirofiban administration, within 6 hr after the loading dose, and then at least daily during therapy. If the platelet count is less than 90,000/mm^3, obtain additional platelet counts routinely to avoid thrombocytopenia. If thrombocytopenia develops, discontinue tirofiban and heparin.
- **Diagnostic tests:** 12-lead ECG to evaluate for myocardial ischemia and dysrhythmias.
- **Anticoagulation:** Monitor aPTT 6 hr after the beginning of the weight-based heparin infusion. Adjust heparin dosage to maintain aPTT at approximately 2 times control.
- **Bleeding:** Closely monitor for bleeding, particularly at other arterial and venous puncture sites, all invasive sites, in urine,

stool, secretions, emesis, and for neurologic changes that may indicate intracranial bleeding. During infusion, avoid placement of invasive devices including endotracheal tube, nasogastric (NG) tube and urinary catheter, if possible. Do not manipulate devices already in place. When bleeding cannot be controlled with pressure, discontinue infusion.

- **Severe bleeding:** Most major bleeding occurs at arterial access site for cardiac catheterization; before pulling femoral artery sheath, discontinue heparin for 3-4 hr and document activated clotting time (ACT) less than 180 sec or aPTT less than 45 sec; achieve sheath hemostasis at least 4 hr before discharge. Avoid NG tube and urinary catheter use, if possible. Maintain patients on complete bed rest, with the head of the bed elevated at 30 degrees.
- **Surgery:** Tirofiban should be discontinued before any surgical procedure.
- **Other medications:** Do not administer additional drugs which may facilitate bleeding unless absolutely necessary. Aspirin is routinely given for patients with acute coronary syndromes in keeping with Advanced Cardiac Life Support (ACLS) guidelines.
- **Patient education:** Inform that it may take longer to stop bleeding during tirofiban therapy. Instruct to report unusual bleeding from invasive sites, chest pain, or dyspnea, back pain, flank pain, rectal pressure, or bladder pressure promptly to a health care provider. Advise to notify the dentist and other physicians of tirofiban therapy before surgery or invasive procedures are scheduled or new drugs are prescribed. Remind about the need to use an electric razor and soft toothbrush to prevent bleeding during infusion. Advise to report black or red stool, dark or red urine, or red-speckled mucus from cough. Advise female patients that menstrual flow may be heavier than usual during infusion.

T

SERIOUS ADVERSE REACTIONS

- Thrombocytopenia occurs rarely.
- **Bleeding:** Signs and symptoms of overdose include generally minor mucocutaneous bleeding and bleeding at the femoral artery access site.

OVERDOSE/TOXICITY

- **Overdose:** Bleeding leading to hypovolemic/hemorrhagic shock, which can compromise coronary circulation leading to chest discomfort and acute MI.
- **GI decontamination:** No specific recommendations.

ANTIDOTE/DIALYSIS

- **Antidote:** No specific antidote. Tirofiban should be discontinued immediately if bleeding occurs; platelet inhibition should reverse quickly. Platelet transfusion may be required in thrombocytopenic patients.
- **Dialysis:** Tirofiban is removed by hemodialysis and is likely to be removed by high-permeability hemodialysis. No data are available on removal by peritoneal dialysis.

tizanidine hydrochloride

tye-zan'-i-deen hye-droe-klor'-ide

Classes

Chemical: imidazoline derivative
Therapeutic: skeletal muscle relaxant

Pregnancy Category: C

Trade Names

Prescription: Zanaflex

CLINICAL PHARMACOLOGY

Mechanism of Action

A skeletal muscle relaxant that increases presynaptic inhibition of spinal motor neurons mediated by alpha$_2$-adrenergic agonists, reducing facilitation to postsynaptic motor neurons. **Therapeutic Effect:** Reduces muscle spasticity.

PHARMACOKINETICS

Route	Onset	Peak	Duration
PO	N/A	1-2 hr	3-6 hr

Well absorbed following PO administration. Protein binding: 30%. Extensive first-pass metabolism. Metabolized in the liver. Partially excreted in urine; minimal elimination in feces. **Half-life:** 2 hr.

AVAILABILITY

Capsules: 2 mg, 4 mg, 6 mg

INDICATIONS AND DOSAGE

Muscle spasticity

PO

Adults, Elderly: Initially 2-4 mg, gradually increased in 2- to 4-mg increments and repeated every 6-8 hr. Maximum: 3 doses/ day or 36 mg/24 hr.

OFF-LABEL USES

Low back pain, spasticity associated with multiple sclerosis or spinal cord injury, tension headaches, trigeminal neuralgia

CONTRAINDICATIONS

Hypersensitivity to tizanidine, concurrent use of ciprofloxacin or fluvoxamine

INTERACTIONS

Drug: Alcohol, other CNS depressants: May increase CNS depressant effects. **Antihypertensives:** May increase tizanidine's hypotensive potential. **Oral contraceptives:** May reduce tizanidine clearance. **Phenytoin:** May increase serum levels and risk of toxicity of phenytoin. **Ciprofloxacin, fluvoxamine:** May increase risk of hypotension; tizanidine levels are increased. **Herbal:** None known. **Food:** None known.

DIAGNOSTIC TEST EFFECTS

May increase serum alkaline phosphatase, AST (SGOT), and ALT (SGPT) levels.

SIDE-EFFECTS

Frequent (49%-16%): Dry mouth, somnolence, asthenia, hypotension (16%-33%). **Occasional (15%-4%):** Dizziness, urinary tract infection, constipation. **Rare (3%):** Nervousness, amblyopia, pharyngitis, rhinitis, vomiting, urinary frequency

CRITICAL CARE CONSIDERATIONS

ADMINISTRATION/HANDLING

PO ALERT

- **Food:** Significant differences in plasma concentration and drug peak are seen between capsules versus tablets when given with food. In a fasting state, capsules and tablets perform equally. Tablets given with food increase plasma concentration by 30% and time to peak is increased to 1 hr, 25 min. Capsules given with food decrease plasma concentration by 20% and time to peak increases to 2-3 hr. When each is administered with food, the amount absorbed from the capsule is about 80% of what is absorbed from the tablet but the extent of the absorption of both forms is higher when given with food.
- **Capsules:** Sprinkling the contents of an open capsule on applesauce or other food results in a 15%-20% increase in plasma concentration and peak occurring in 15 min less time than when capsules are given intact.
- **Long term use dosage:** Clinical experience with long-term use of 8-16 mg single doses or daily total doses 24-36 mg is limited.
- **Reduced drug clearance:** Clearance of tizanidine is reduced by approximately 50% in women taking oral contraceptives and renal impaired patients. Individual doses should be reduced.

PRECAUTIONS

HEALTH-RELATED

- Use tizanidine cautiously in patients with hypotension or cardiac, hepatic, or renal disease. Drug is an alpha-2 adrenergic agonist which reduces BP up to 20% in the first hr; may be associated with bradycardia, orthostatic hypotension, lightheadedness, dizziness, and syncope. Drug has caused hepatocellular injury, severe sedation, hallucinations, and psychosis.
- **Oral contraceptives:** Use with caution in women taking oral contraceptives because drug clearance is reduced by 50%.

AGE-RELATED

- **Children:** Safety and efficacy of tizanidine have not been established in children.
- **Elderly:** Age-related renal impairment may warrant cautious use.

PREGNANCY/LACTATION-RELATED

- Pregnancy category C; lipid soluble, may pass into breast milk

MONITORING

- **Baseline assessment:** Assess vital signs before drug administration because BP is likely to decrease by 20% when drug is given. Record the duration, location, onset, and type of muscle spasm. Examine for immobility, stiffness, and swelling.
- **Lab work:** Basline biochemical profile including renal (BUN, creatinine) and liver (AST [SGOT], ALT [SGPT], alkaline phosphatase, bilirubin) function tests. Perform periodic liver and renal function tests for patients on long-term therapy.
- **Diagnostic tests:** Baseline 12-lead ECG to evaluate for heart disease. Note baseline heart rate, ST segments, and QT interval.
- **Continuous ECG:** Monitor for prolongation of the QT interval, bradycardia, and changes in ST segment related to hypotension for critically ill patients.
- **Dizziness:** Assist with ambulation because orthostatic hypotension is likely.

- **Therapeutic response:** Evaluate for decreased stiffness, tenderness, and intensity of skeletal muscle pain and improved mobility.
- **Patient education:** Inform that tizanidine may cause low BP, impaired coordination, and sedation. Warn to avoid tasks that require mental alertness or motor skills until response to the drug is known. Instruct to change positions slowly to help prevent dizziness. Inform about the differences in drug action when using with and without food.

SERIOUS ADVERSE REACTIONS

- **Hypotension:** Reduction in either diastolic or systolic BP may be associated with bradycardia, orthostatic hypotension, and rarely, syncope. The risk of hypotension increases as dosage increases; BP generally decreases within 1 hr after administration.
- **Abrupt withdrawal:** If tizanidine needs to be discontinued, dose should be decreased slowly to avoid rebound hypertension, tachycardia, and muscle hypertonia.
- **Extreme sedation:** 10% of patients reported sedation that interfered with daily activities. Sedation generally peaked following the first wk of dose titration and remained stable throughout the maintenance phase during studies.
- **Hallucinations/psychosis:** Hallucinations, delusions, and rare psychosis have been reported.
- **Management:** Reduce or discontinue medication.

OVERDOSE/TOXICITY

- **Hepatotoxicity:** Hepatocellular injury may result, reflected by greater than 3 times high normal increased serum transaminases (AST [SGOT], ALT [SGPT]), alkaline phosphatase, and bilrubin with nausea, vomiting, anorexia, and jaundice. Rare instances of hepatic necrosis, encephalopathy, coma, and death have occurred.
- **Hypotension:** Extreme hypotension with bradycardia, prolonged QT syndrome leading to end-organ damage and arrest may occur with overdose if patients do not receive treatment in a timely manner.
- **Overdose:** Severe toxicity (poisoning from imidazoline derivatives) has resulted from ingestion of very small amounts especially in small children. Clinical presentation is generally cyclical coma/respiratory depression, alternating with agitation.
- **Management:** Discontinue tizanidine and observe closely for rebound hypertension, bradycardia, and hypertonia. Ensure patent airway and adequate ventilation. If prolonged QT syndrome is present, avoid antidysrhythmic agents that may further prolong the QT interval. Avoid atropine unless bradycardia has resulted in hypotension. High dose IV naloxone has been used for respiratory depression that is unresponsive to physical stimulation/reminding patients to keep breathing, but patients should be intubated and provided with mechanical ventilation as soon as possible if deemed appropriate.
- **GI decontamination:** No specific recommendations.

ANTIDOTE/DIALYSIS

- **Antidote:** No specific recommendations.
- **Dialysis:** No data are available on removal of tizanidine by hemodialysis, high-permeability hemodialysis, or peritoneal dialysis.

tobramycin sulfate

toe-bra-mye'-sin sul'-fate

Classes

Chemical: aminoglycoside
Therapeutic: antibiotic

Pregnancy Category: D (injection, inhalation), B (ophthalmic)

Trade Names

Prescription: AK-Tob, Nebcin, Nebcin Pediatric, PMS-Tobramycin, TOBI, Tobrex

Combinations

Prescription: Ophthalmic: with dexamethasone (Tobradex); with loteprednol (Zylet)

CLINICAL PHARMACOLOGY

Mechanism of Action

An aminoglycoside antibiotic that irreversibly binds to protein on bacterial ribosomes. **Therapeutic Effect:** Interferes with protein synthesis of susceptible microorganisms.

PHARMACOKINETICS

Rapid, complete absorption after IM administration. Protein binding: less than 30%. Widely distributed (does not cross the blood-brain barrier); low concentrations in cerebrospinal fluid (CSF). Excreted unchanged in urine. Removed by hemodialysis. **Half-life:** 2-4 hr (increased in impaired

T

renal function and neonates; decreased in cystic fibrosis and febrile or burn patients).

AVAILABILITY

Injection solution: 10 mg/mL (Nebcin Pediatric), 40 mg/mL (Nebcin).
Injection powder for reconstitution (Nebcin): 1.2 g.
Ophthalmic ointment (Tobrex): 0.3%.
Ophthalmic solution (AK-Tob, Tobrex): 0.3%.
Nebulization solution (TOBI): 60 mg/mL.

INDICATIONS AND DOSAGE

Usual parenteral dosage

IV

Adults, Elderly: 3-6 mg/kg/day (using ideal body weight) in 3 divided doses. Once daily dosing: 4-7 mg/kg every 24 hr. **Children 7 days and older:** 6-7.5 mg/kg/day every 8-12 hr. **Children younger than 7 days:** 2.5-4 mg/kg/day every 12 hr.

Superficial eye infections, including blepharitis, conjunctivitis, keratitis, and corneal ulcers

Ophthalmic Ointment

Adults, Elderly: Apply a 0.5-inch ribbon to conjunctiva every 8-12 hr (every 3-4 hr for severe infections).

Ophthalmic Solution

Adults, Elderly: Usual dosage, 1-2 drops in affected eye every 4 hr (2 drops/hr for severe infections).

Bronchopulmonary infections in patients with cystic fibrosis

Inhalation Solution

Adults: Usual dosage, 60-80 mg 3 times per day for 28 days, then off for 28 days. **Children:** 40-80 mg 2-3 times per day.

Dosage in renal impairment

Dosage and frequency are modified based on the degree of renal impairment and the serum drug concentration. After a loading dose of 1-2 mg/kg, the maintenance dose and frequency are based on serum creatinine levels and creatinine clearance.

CONTRAINDICATIONS

Hypersensitivity to tobramycin or other aminoglycosides (cross-sensitivity) and their components

INTERACTIONS

Drug: Nephrotoxic medications, other aminoglycosides, ototoxic medications: May increase the risk of nephrotoxicity and ototoxicity. **Neuromuscular blockers:** May increase neuromuscular blockade. **Herbal:** None known. **Food:** None known.

DIAGNOSTIC TEST EFFECTS

May increase serum bilirubin, BUN, serum creatinine, serum LDH, AST (SGOT), and ALT (SGPT) levels. May decrease serum calcium, magnesium, potassium, and sodium concentrations. Therapeutic peak serum level is 5-20 mcg/mL; therapeutic trough serum level is 0.5-2 mcg/mL. Toxic peak serum level is greater than 20 mcg/mL; toxic trough serum level is greater than 2 mcg/mL.

IV INCOMPATIBILITIES

Amphotericin B complex (Abelcet, AmBisome, Amphotec), heparin, hetastarch (Hespan), indomethacin (Indocin), propofol (Diprivan), sargramostim (Leukine, Prokine)

IV COMPATIBILITIES

Amiodarone (Cordarone), calcium gluconate, diltiazem (Cardizem), furosemide (Lasix), hydromorphone (Dilaudid), insulin, magnesium sulfate, midazolam (Versed), morphine, theophylline, total parenteral nutrition (TPN)

SIDE-EFFECTS

Occasional: IM: Pain, induration. **IV:** Phlebitis, thrombophlebitis. **Topical:** Hypersensitivity reaction (fever, pruritus, rash, urticaria). **Ophthalmic:** Tearing, itching, redness, eyelid swelling. **Rare:** Hypotension, nausea, vomiting

CRITICAL CARE CONSIDERATIONS

ADMINISTRATION/HANDLING

DOSAGE ALERT

- **Toxicity:** Monitor peak and trough serum drug levels to ensure that the desired blood concentrations are maintained and to minimize the risk of toxicity. Carefully coordinate drawing of peak and trough drug levels with administration times. Risk of toxicity increases with higher dosages, prolonged therapy, and when the solution is applied directly to the mucosa.
- **Evenly spaced doses:** Space parenteral doses evenly around the clock. Dosages are based on ideal body weight.

IV ALERT

- **Storage:** Store vials at room temperature.
- **Stability:** Solutions may be discolored by light or air, but discoloration does not affect drug potency.

T

- **Dilution:** Dilute with 50-200 mL of D_5W or 0.9% NaCl. The amount of diluent for infant and children dosages depends on individual needs.
- **Infusion rate:** Infuse over 20-60 min.

OPHTHALMIC ALERT

- **Administration:** Pull the lower eyelid out until a pocket is formed between the eye and lower lid. Hold the dropper above the pocket and place the correct number of drops (or one quarter to one half inch of ointment) into the pocket; close the eye gently.
- **Following administration of solution:** Apply digital pressure to the lacrimal sac for 1-2 min to minimize drainage into the nose and throat to reduce risk of systemic effects.
- **Following administration of ointment:** Close the eye for 1-2 min. Roll the eyeball to increase drug contact with the eye. Use a tissue to remove excess solution or ointment around the eye.

PRECAUTIONS

HEALTH-RELATED

- Use tobramycin cautiously in patients who are also on neuromuscular blockers, those with impaired renal function or auditory or vestibular impairment.
- Aminoglycosides such as tobramycin should not be given with potent diuretics (ethacrynic acid or furosemide) to avoid increasing the concentration of tobramycin in the tissues, which may lead to toxicity.

AGE-RELATED

- **Children:** Immature renal function in neonates and premature infants may increase the risk of toxicity.
- **Elderly:** Age-related renal impairment may require a dosage reduction.

PREGNANCY/LACTATION-RELATED

- Pregnancy category D (B, ophthalmic form). Excreted into breast milk; given poor oral absorption, toxicity is minimal, limited to modification of bowel flora and interference with interpretation of culture results if fever workup required.

MONITORING

- **Baseline assessment:** Assess for and correct dehydration if necessary before beginning parenteral tobramycin therapy. Determine history of allergies, especially to aminoglycosides, sulfites, and parabens (for topical and ophthalmic routes), and establish baseline hearing acuity before beginning therapy.
- **Lab work:** CBC including WBC differential and platelet count. Biochemical profile including renal function studies (BUN, creatinine); urinalysis. Obtain necessary cultures before first dose, if possible.
- **Renal support:** Monitor intake and output and urinalysis results. To maintain adequate hydration, provide IV fluids and/or encourage patients to drink fluids. Monitor urinalysis results for casts, RBCs, WBCs, and decreased specific gravity.
- **Drug levels:** Monitor peak and trough serum drug levels. Therapeutic peak serum level is 5-10 mcg/mL with conventional dosing, 15-20 mcg/mL with once-daily dosing; therapeutic trough level is 0.5 to 2 mcg/mL with conventional dosing, less than 0.5 mcg/mL with once-daily dosing. Toxic peak level is greater than 20 mcg/mL; toxic trough level is greater than 2 mcg/mL.
- **Toxicity:** Assess for ototoxic and neurotoxic side effects.
- **Neuromuscular blockade:** Avoid concurrent use, if possible, to avoid potentiating neuromuscular blockade, causing severe respiratory depression.
- **Respiratory distress:** In patients with neuromuscular disorders, assess the respiratory response frequently.
- **Phlebitis:** Evaluate the IV infusion site for heat, pain, and red streaking over the vein.
- **IM injection site:** Assess for pain and induration.
- **Early hypersensitivity:** Inspect the skin for rash.
- **Superinfection:** Assess the mouth for white patches on the mucous membranes or tongue and for severe mouth or tongue soreness; assess for severe anal or genital pruritus or discharge with all forms of tobramycin.
- **Possible *Clostridium difficile* colitis:** Assess pattern of daily bowel activity and stool consistency. Although mild GI effects may be tolerable, severe symptoms including abdominal pain or cramping and moderate to severe diarrhea may indicate the onset of antibiotic-associated colitis.
- **Hand-washing:** If *C. difficile* (antibiotic-associated) colitis develops, wash hands with antibacterial soap. Alcohol-based foam is ineffective against *C. difficile* spores.

- **Skin:** Assess skin for dryness, irritation, and rash with topical application.
- **Ophthalmic:** Assess for itching, redness, eyelid swelling, and tearing of the eyes.
- **Evenly space doses:** Space doses evenly around the clock. If tobramycin is used outside the hospital, instruct to continue taking tobramycin for the full course of treatment.
- **Patient education:** Instruct to report promptly any balance, hearing, urinary, or vision problems to a health care provider, even after therapy is completed. Inform those using ophthalmic tobramycin that irritation, redness, blurred vision, or tearing may occur briefly after application.

SERIOUS ADVERSE REACTIONS

- **Hypersensitivity:** Patients with a history of allergies, especially to other aminoglycosides, are at increased risk for developing a severe hypersensitivity reaction, marked by severe pruritus, angioedema, bronchospasm, and anaphylaxis.
- **Management of hypersensitivity:** May require treatment with epinephrine and other emergency measures including oxygen, endotracheal intubation, mechanical ventilation, IV fluids, IV antihistamines, corticosteroids, and vasopressors.
- **Respiratory depression:** May potentiate neuromuscular blocking agents (tubocurarine, mivacurium), including drugs not primarily used for neuromuscular blockade (streptomycin, kanamycin), to cause severe respiratory depression.
- **Superinfections:** Antibiotic-associated colitis (pseudomembranous colitis, *C. difficile*–associated diarrhea [CDAD]) and other superinfections may result from altered bacterial balance.
- **Management of pseudomembraneous colitis (CDAD):** Fluids, electrolytes, protein supplements, oral vancomycin (Vancocin), or IV metronidazole (Flagyl).

OVERDOSE/TOXICITY

- **Nephrotoxicity:** Increased BUN and serum creatinine levels with decreased creatinine clearance may be reversible if tobramycin is stopped at the first sign of nephrotoxic symptoms.
- **Irreversible ototoxicity:** Tinnitus, dizziness, ringing or roaring in the ears, and hearing loss.
- **Neurotoxicity:** Headache, dizziness, lethargy, tremor, and visual disturbances occur occasionally.
- **GI decontamination:** No specific recommendations.

ANTIDOTE/DIALYSIS

- **Antidote:** No specific recommendations.
- **Dialysis:** Tobramycin is removed by hemodialysis and peritoneal dialysis and is likely to be removed by high-permeability hemodialysis.

tocainide

See Antidysrhythmics (p. 919)

*TOLAZemide

See Antidiabetics (p. 911)

*TOLBUTamide

See Antidiabetics (p. 911)

tolcapone

tole'-ka-pone

Classes

Chemical: catechol-o-methyltransferase (COMT) inhibitor, nitrocatechol
Therapeutic: antiparkinson's agent

Pregnancy Category: C

Trade Names

Prescription: Tasmar

CLINICAL PHARMACOLOGY

Mechanism of Action

An antiparkinson agent that inhibits the enzyme catechol-*O*-methyltransferase (COMT), potentiating dopamine activity and increasing the duration of action of levodopa. **Therapeutic Effect:** Relieves signs and symptoms of Parkinson's disease.

PHARMACOKINETICS

Rapidly absorbed after PO administration. Protein binding: 99%. Metabolized in the liver. Eliminated primarily in urine (60%) and, to a lesser extent, in feces (40%). **Half-life:** 2-3 hr.

AVAILABILITY

Tablets: 100 mg, 200 mg.

INDICATIONS AND DOSAGE

Adjunctive treatment of Parkinson's disease

PO

Adults, Elderly: Initially, 100-200 mg 3 times per day concomitantly with each dose of carbidopa and levodopa. Maximum: 600 mg/day.

Dosage in hepatic impairment

Patients with moderate to severe cirrhosis should not receive more than 200 mg tolcapone 3 times per day.

CONTRAINDICATIONS

Hypersensitivity to tolcapone

INTERACTIONS

Drug: Levodopa: Increases the duration of action of this drug. **MAOIs:** May decrease catecholamine metabolism. **Herbal:** None known. **Food: All foods:** Decrease tolcapone bioavailability by 10%-20% if given within 1 hr before or 2 hr after drug administration.

DIAGNOSTIC TEST EFFECTS

May increase AST (SGOT) and ALT (SGPT) levels.

SIDE-EFFECTS

Alert: Frequency of side effects increases with dosage. The following effects are based on a 200-mg dose. **Frequent (35%-16%):** Nausea, insomnia, somnolence, anorexia, diarrhea, muscle cramps, orthostatic hypotension, excessive dreaming. **Occasional (11%-4%):** Headache, vomiting, confusion, hallucinations, constipation, diaphoresis, bright yellow urine, dry eyes, abdominal pain, dizziness, flatulence. **Rare (3%-2%):** Dyspepsia, neck pain, hypotension, fatigue, chest discomfort

CRITICAL CARE CONSIDERATIONS

ADMINISTRATION/HANDLING

PO ALERT

- Give tolcapone without regard to food.
- Always administer tolcapone with carbidopa and levodopa.
- Discontinue tolcapone if ALT (SGOT) and AST (SGPT) levels exceed the upper limits of normal or patients develop signs and symptoms of hepatic failure.

PRECAUTIONS

HEALTH-RELATED

- Use tolcapone cautiously in patients with baseline hypotension, severe hepatic or renal impairment, history of hallucinations, or orthostatic hypotension.

AGE-RELATED

- **Children:** Tolcapone is not used in children.
- **Elderly:** Are at increased risk for hallucinations.

PREGNANCY/LACTATION-RELATED

- Pregnancy category C; use caution in nursing mothers.

MONITORING

- **Baseline assessment:** Assess symptoms of Parkinson's disease with current medication regime.
- **Lab work:** Baseline biochemical profile including liver (AST [SGOT], ALT [SGPT], bilirubin, alkaline phosphatase), and renal (BUN, creatinine) function tests. Liver enzyme levels every 2 wk for the first yr, every 4 wk for the next 6 mo, and every 8 wk thereafter.
- **Hallucinations:** Reduce the levodopa dosage if hallucinations are experienced. Hallucinations are usually accompanied by confusion and, to a lesser extent, insomnia.
- **Dizziness:** Assist with ambulation if dizziness occurs.
- **Therapeutic effect:** Assess for relief of symptoms, such as improvement of mask-like facial expression, muscular rigidity, shuffling gait, and resting tremors of the hands and head. Discontinue if no benefit is apparent after 3 wk.
- **Patient education:** Advise to take tolcapone with food if nauseous. Inform that dizziness, drowsiness, and nausea may occur initially but will diminish or disappear with continued treatment. Inform that orthostatic hypotension commonly occurs during initial therapy but that changing positions slowly can help prevent or minimize this effect. Warn to avoid tasks that require mental alertness or motor skills until response to the drug is known. Inform that hallucinations occur more often in elderly patients, typically within the first 2 wk of therapy. Explain that urine may turn bright yellow. Instruct to report promptly dark urine, falls, fatigue, itching, loss of appetite, persistent nausea, yellowing of the skin and sclera of the eyes, or

abnormal contractions of the head, neck, or trunk to the prescriber. Caution female patients to report promptly if they are pregnant or plan to become pregnant. Instruct to report frequent falls.

SERIOUS ADVERSE REACTIONS

- Upper respiratory and urinary tract infections occur in 7%-5% of patients.
- Too-rapid withdrawal from therapy may produce withdrawal-emergent hyperpyrexia, characterized by fever, muscular rigidity, and altered LOC.
- Dyskinesia and dystonia occur frequently.

OVERDOSE/TOXICITY

- There are no reported cases of overdose with tolcapone. Highly dosed patients resolved symptoms during studies when medication dosage was significantly reduced or medication was discontinued. Coadministration of tolcapone with an MAOI could theoretically result in central and peripheral catecholamine excess, which may present as sympathomimetic poisoning syndrome.
- **GI decontamination:** No specific recommendations.

ANTIDOTE/DIALYSIS

- **Antidote:** No specific recommendations.
- **Dialysis:** Tolcapone is unlikely to be removed by hemodialysis, high-permeability hemodialysis, or peritoneal dialysis.

tolmetin

See NSAIDs and Cox-2 Inhibitors (p. 976)

topiramate

toe-pyre'-a-mate

Classes

Chemical: sulfamate-substituted monosaccharide derivative
Therapeutic: anticonvulsant

Pregnancy Category: C

Trade Names

Prescription: Topamax

Do not confuse topiramate or Topamax with Tegretol, Tegretol XR, or Toprol XL.

CLINICAL PHARMACOLOGY

Mechanism of Action

An anticonvulsant that blocks repetitive, sustained firing of neurons by enhancing the ability of gamma-aminobutyric acid to induce an influx of chloride ions into the neurons; may also block sodium channels. **Therapeutic Effect:** Decreases seizure activity.

PHARMACOKINETICS

Rapidly absorbed after PO administration. Protein binding: 13%-17%. Not extensively metabolized. Primarily excreted unchanged in urine. Removed by hemodialysis. **Half-life:** 21 hr.

AVAILABILITY

Capsules (Sprinkle): 15 mg, 25 mg.
Tablets: 25 mg, 50 mg, 100 mg, 200 mg.

INDICATIONS AND DOSAGE

Adjunctive treatment of partial seizures, Lennox-Gastaut syndrome, tonic-clonic seizures

PO

Adults, Elderly, Children older than 17 yr: Initially 25-50 mg for 1 wk. May increase by 25-50 mg/day at weekly intervals. Maximum: 1600 mg/day. **Children 2-16 yr:** Initially 1-3 mg/kg/day to maximum of 25 mg. May increase by 1-3 mg/kg/day at weekly intervals. Maintenance: 5-9 mg/kg/day in 2 divided doses.

Monotherapy with partial, tonic-clonic seizures

PO

Adults, Elderly, Children 10 yr and older: Initially 25 mg twice per day. Increase by 50 mg at weekly intervals up to 400 mg/day according to the following schedule:
Wk 1, 25 mg twice per day
Wk 2, 50 mg twice per day
Wk 3, 75 mg twice per day
Wk 4, 100 mg twice per day
Wk 5, 150 mg twice per day
Wk 6, 200 mg twice per day

Migraine prevention

PO

Adults, Elderly: Initially, 25 mg/day. May increase by 25 mg/day at 7-day intervals up to a total daily dose of 100 mg/day in 2 divided doses.

Dosage in renal impairment

Expect to reduce drug dosage by 50% in patients with tonic-clonic seizures who have a creatinine clearance of less than 70 mL/min.

OFF-LABEL USES

Treatment of alcohol dependence

CONTRAINDICATIONS

Bipolar disorder, hypersensitivity to topiramate

INTERACTIONS

Drug: **Alcohol, other CNS depressants:** May increase CNS depression. **Carbamazepine, phenytoin, valproic acid:** May decrease topiramate blood concentration. **Carbonic anhydrase inhibitors:** May increase the risk of renal calculi. **Oral contraceptives:** May decrease the effectiveness of oral contraceptives. **Herbal:** None known. **Food:** None known.

DIAGNOSTIC TEST EFFECTS

None known.

SIDE-EFFECTS

Frequent (30%-10%): Somnolence, dizziness, ataxia, nervousness, nystagmus, diplopia, paresthesia, nausea, tremor. **Occasional (9%-3%):** Confusion, breast pain, dysmenorrhea, dyspepsia, depression, asthenia, pharyngitis, weight loss, anorexia, rash, musculoskeletal pain, abdominal pain, difficulty with coordination, sinusitis, agitation, flulike symptoms. **Rare (3%-2%):** Mood disturbances, such as irritability and depression; dry mouth; aggressive behavior

CRITICAL CARE CONSIDERATIONS

ADMINISTRATION/HANDLING

PO ALERT

- Give topiramate without regard to food.
- Do not break tablets because they have a bitter taste.
- Capsules may be swallowed whole or contents sprinkled on a teaspoonful of soft food and swallowed immediately. They should not be chewed.

PRECAUTIONS

HEALTH-RELATED

- Use topiramate cautiously in patients with impaired hepatic or renal function, predisposition to renal calculi, or hypersensitivity to topiramate.

AGE-RELATED

- **Children:** No age-related precautions have been noted in children over 2 yr. During clinical trials, 10 sudden unexplained deaths in epilepsy were reported in pediatric patients.
- **Elderly:** Age-related renal impairment may require dosage reduction.

PREGNANCY/LACTATION-RELATED

- Pregnancy category C; unknown if distributed in breast milk.

MONITORING

- **Baseline assessment:** Assess mentation and review history of the seizure disorder, including the duration, frequency, and intensity of seizures. Determine pregnancy, sensitivity to topiramate, or use of other anticonvulsants, especially carbamazepine, carbonic anhydrase inhibitors, phenytoin, or valproic acid.
- **Lab work:** Baseline biochemical profile including renal (BUN, creatinine) and liver (AST [SGOT], ALT [SGPT], alkaline phosphatase, bilirubin) function tests. Monitor renal function studies.
- **Seizure control:** Institute seizure precautions, and observe frequently for recurrence of seizure activity. Provide with a quiet, dark environment.
- **Therapeutic effect:** Assess for a decrease in the frequency and intensity of seizures.
- **Dizziness:** Assist with ambulation because orthostatic hypotension is likely.
- **Patient education:** Instruct not to break tablets to avoid their bitter taste. Caution against abruptly discontinuing topiramate because this may precipitate seizures. Explain that strict maintenance of drug therapy is essential for seizure control. Because topiramate may cause dizziness, drowsiness, or impaired thinking, warn to avoid tasks that require mental alertness or motor skills until response to the drug is known. Explain that drowsiness usually diminishes with continued therapy. Urge avoidance of alcohol and other CNS depressants while on topiramate therapy. Recommend drinking plenty of fluids to decrease the risk of kidney stones. Instruct to report promptly blurred vision or other visual changes to a health care provider. Female patients taking oral contraceptives should use additional or alternative means of contraception because topiramate decreases oral contraceptive effectiveness. Advise carrying an identification card or wearing a medical identification bracelet that displays the seizure disorder and anticonvulsant therapy.

SERIOUS ADVERSE REACTIONS

- **Kidney stones:** Incidence of kidney stones is 2-4 times greater than when topiramate is not used in both adults and

T

children. Symptoms include severe flank pain, nausea, and vomiting. Hydration can help reduce incidence of stones.
- **Withdrawal of antiepileptic drugs:** Topiramate should be withdrawn gradually to avoid potential of increased frequency of seizures.

OVERDOSE/TOXICITY
- **Acute myopia and secondary angle closure glaucoma:** Acute onset of decreased visual acuity, and/or ocular pain. Symptoms generally occur within 1 mo of initiating topiramate.
- **Cognitive/neuropsychiatric events:** Psychomotor slowing, impaired concentration, language problems (such as word-finding difficulties), and memory disturbances occur occasionally. These reactions are generally mild to moderate but may be severe enough to require discontinuation of drug therapy.
- **GI decontamination:** No specific recommendations.

ANTIDOTE/DIALYSIS
- **Antidote:** No specific recommendations.
- **Dialysis:** Topiramate is removed by hemodialysis and is likely removed by high-permeability hemodialysis. No data are available on removal by peritoneal dialysis.

torsemide
See Diuretics (p. 956)

tramadol hydrochloride
trah'-ma-doll hye-droe-klor'-ide

Classes
Chemical: cyclohexanol derivative
Therapeutic: centrally acting synthetic analgesic

Pregnancy Category: C

Combinations
Prescription: with acetaminophen (Ultracet)

Trade Names
Prescription: Ultram

Do not confuse tramadol with Toradol, or Ultram with Ultane.

CLINICAL PHARMACOLOGY
Mechanism of Action
An analgesic that binds weakly to mu-opioid receptors and inhibits reuptake of norepinephrine and serotonin. Reduces the intensity of pain stimuli reaching sensory nerve endings. **Therapeutic Effect:** Alters the perception of and emotional response to pain.

PHARMACOKINETICS

Route	Onset	Peak	Duration
PO	Less than 1 hr	2-3 hr	4-6 hr

Rapidly and almost completely absorbed after PO administration. Protein binding: 20%. Extensively metabolized in the liver to active metabolite (reduced in patients with advanced cirrhosis). Primarily excreted in urine. **Half-life:** 6-7 hr.

AVAILABILITY
Tablets: 50 mg.
Orally disintegrating tablets: 50 mg.
Extended-release tablets: 100 mg, 200 mg, 300 mg.

INDICATIONS AND DOSAGE
Moderate to moderately severe pain
PO (Immediate Release, Orally Disintegrating)
Adults, Elderly: 50-100 mg every 4-6 hr. Maximum: 400 mg/day for patients 75 yr and younger; 300 mg/day for patients older than 75 yr.
PO (Extended Release)
Adults, Elderly: 100-300 mg once daily.
Dosage in renal impairment
For patients with creatinine clearance of less than 30 mL/min, increase dosing interval to every 12 hr. Maximum: 200 mg/day.
Dosage in hepatic impairment
Dosage is decreased to 50 mg every 12 hr.

CONTRAINDICATIONS
Acute alcohol intoxication; concurrent use of centrally acting analgesics, hypnotics, opioids, or psychotropic drugs, hypersensitivity to tramadol or opioids

INTERACTIONS
Drug: Alcohol, other CNS depressants: May increase CNS or respiratory depression and hypotension. **Carbamazepine:** Decreases tramadol blood concentration. **MAOIs:** May increase tramadol blood concentration and increase the risk of seizures. **Selective serotonin reuptake inhibitors, tricyclic**

antidepressants, opioids, neuroleptics: May increase the risk of seizures. **Herbal:** None known. **Food:** None known.

DIAGNOSTIC TEST EFFECTS

May increase serum creatinine, AST (SGOT), and ALT (SGPT) hepatic levels. May decrease blood Hgb level. May cause proteinuria.

SIDE-EFFECTS

Frequent (25%-15%): Dizziness or vertigo, nausea, constipation, headache, somnolence. **Occasional (10%-5%):** Vomiting, pruritus, CNS stimulation (such as nervousness, anxiety, agitation, tremor, euphoria, mood swings, and hallucinations), asthenia, diaphoresis, dyspepsia, dry mouth, diarrhea. **Rare (less than 5%):** Malaise, vasodilation, anorexia, flatulence, rash, blurred vision, urine retention or urinary frequency, menopausal symptoms

CRITICAL CARE CONSIDERATIONS

ADMINISTRATION/HANDLING

PO ALERT

- Give tramadol without regard to food.
- Dialysis patients may receive their regular dose on the day of dialysis.

PRECAUTIONS

HEALTH-RELATED

- Use tramadol extremely cautiously in patients with acute alcoholism, advanced cirrhosis, anoxia, CNS depression, epilepsy, those taking CNS depressants or MAOIs, respiratory depression, or shock.
- Use the drug cautiously in patients with acute abdominal conditions, hepatic or renal impairment, increased intracranial pressure, opioid dependence, or sensitivity to opioids.

AGE-RELATED

- **Children:** Safety and efficacy of tramadol have not been established in children.
- **Elderly:** Age-related renal impairment may require a dosage reduction.

PREGNANCY/LACTATION-RELATED

- Pregnancy category C; small amounts excreted into breast milk.

MONITORING

- **Baseline assessment:** Assess the duration, location, onset, and type of pain. Determine medication history, especially use of carbamazepine, CNS depressants, and MAOIs. Review the medical history, especially for seizures.
- **Lab work:** CBC and baseline biochemical profile including liver (AST [SGOT], ALT [SGPT], alkaline phosphatase, bilirubin) and renal (BUN, creatinine) function studies.
- **Pain control:** Tramadol's analgesic effect is reduced if patients experience full pain before the next dose. Instruct to report as soon as pain increases. Assess for clinical improvement, and record the onset of pain relief.
- **Anemia:** Monitor hemoglobin and assess for hypotension and tachycardia.
- **Dizziness:** Assist with ambulation if dizziness occurs.
- **Dry mouth:** Offer sips of tepid water to relieve dry mouth.
- **Nausea:** Offer cola and dry crackers to relieve nausea.
- **Constipation:** Assess pattern of daily bowel activity and stool consistency.
- **Urinary retention:** Palpate the bladder to assess for urinary retention.
- **Patient education:** Inform that tramadol use may cause dependence. Urge to avoid alcohol and OTC drugs such as analgesics and sedatives during tramadol therapy. Inform that tramadol may cause blurred vision, dizziness, and drowsiness. Warn to avoid tasks requiring mental alertness or motor skills until response to the drug is known. Instruct to report promptly chest pain, difficulty breathing, excessive sedation, muscle weakness, palpitations, seizures, severe constipation, or tremors to a health care provider.

SERIOUS ADVERSE REACTIONS

- **Seizures:** Have been reported in patients receiving normal doses of tramadol. Concomitant use of tramadol increases seizure risk in patients taking selective serotonin reuptake inhibitors, tricyclic antidepressants, opioids, and MAOIs. Those with epilepsy, history of seizures, and with increased risk of seizures (head trauma, withdrawal, CNS infection) are more likely to seize when using tramadol.
- **Hypersensitivity:** Rash, urticaria, serious and rarely fatal anaphylactic reactions.
- **Opioid dependence:** Use of tramadol may prompt renewed dependence, so treatment with tramadol is not recommended in these patients.

OVERDOSE/TOXICITY
- **Overdose:** Results in respiratory depression and seizures.
- Tramadol may have a prolonged duration of action and cumulative effect in patients with hepatic or renal impairment.
- **GI decontamination:** No specific recommendations.

ANTIDOTE/DIALYSIS
- **Antidote:** No specific recommendations.
- **Dialysis:** Tramadol is removed by high-permeability hemodialysis but is not removed by hemodialysis. No data are available on removal by peritoneal dialysis.

trandolapril

See ACE Inhibitors (p. 883)

tranylcypromine sulfate

tran-ill-sip'-roe-meen sul'-fate

Classes
Chemical: cyclopropylamine, substituted; nonhydrazine derivative
Therapeutic: antidepressant, monoamine oxidase inhibitor (MAOI)

Pregnancy Category: C

Trade Names
Prescription: Parnate

CLINICAL PHARMACOLOGY

Mechanism of Action
An MAOI that inhibits the activity of the enzyme monoamine oxidase at CNS storage sites, leading to increased levels of the neurotransmitters epinephrine, norepinephrine, serotonin, and dopamine at neuronal receptor sites. **Therapeutic Effect:** Relieves depression.

PHARMACOKINETICS
Well absorbed from GI tract. Metabolized in the liver. Primarily excreted in urine. **Half-life:** 1.5-3.5 hr.

AVAILABILITY
Tablets: 10 mg.

INDICATIONS AND DOSAGE
Depression refractory to or intolerant of other therapy
PO
Adults, Elderly: Initially, 10 mg twice per day. May increase by 10 mg/day at 1- to 3-wk intervals up to 60 mg/day in divided doses.

OFF-LABEL USES
Posttraumatic stress disorder

CONTRAINDICATIONS
Heart failure, children younger than 16 yr, pheochromocytoma, severe hepatic or renal impairment, uncontrolled hypertension, hypersensitivity to tranylcypromine

INTERACTIONS
Drug: Alcohol, other CNS depressants: May increase CNS depressant effects. ***BusPIRone:** May increase BP. **Caffeine-containing medications:** May increase the risk of cardiac dysrhythmias and hypertension. **Carbamazepine, cyclobenzaprine, maprotiline, other MAOIs:** May precipitate hypertensive crisis. ***DOPamine, tryptophan:** May cause sudden, severe hypertension. **Fluoxetine, trazodone, tricyclic antidepressants:** May cause serotonin syndrome and neuroleptic malignant syndrome. **Insulin, oral antidiabetics:** May increase the effects of these drugs. **Meperidine, other opioid analgesics:** May produce diaphoresis, immediate excitation, rigidity, and severe hypertension or hypotension, sometimes leading to severe respiratory distress, vascular collapse, seizures, coma, and death. **Herbal:** None known. **Food: Caffeine, chocolate, tyramine-containing foods (such as aged cheese):** May cause sudden, severe hypertension.

DIAGNOSTIC TEST EFFECTS
None known.

SIDE-EFFECTS
Frequent: Orthostatic hypotension, restlessness, GI upset, insomnia, dizziness, lethargy, weakness, dry mouth, peripheral edema. **Occasional:** Flushing, diaphoresis, rash, urinary frequency, increased appetite, transient impotence. **Rare:** Visual disturbances

CRITICAL CARE CONSIDERATIONS

ADMINISTRATION/HANDLING

GENERAL ALERT
- Make sure at least 14 days elapse between the use of tranylcypromine and a selective serotonin reuptake inhibitor.
- Avoid foods with high tyramine content such as pickled herring, liver, dry sausage

(salami, pepperoni, Lebanon bologna), fava or other broad bean pods, cheese (may have cottage and cream cheeses), yogurt, beer, wine, excessive chocolate and caffeine, products containing brewer's yeast.

PRECAUTIONS

HEALTH-RELATED

- Use tranylcypromine cautiously within several hr of ingestion of a contraindicated substance, such as tyramine-containing foods (avocados, bananas, broad beans, figs, papayas, raisins, sour cream, soy sauce, beer, wine, yeast extracts, meat tenderizers, and smoked or pickled meats).
- Use tranylcypromine cautiously in patients with cardiac dysrhythmias, frequent or severe headaches, hypertension, and suicidal tendencies.

AGE-RELATED

- **Children:** Safety and efficacy of tranylcypromine have not been established for children under 16 yr.
- **Elderly:** Age-related organ impairment may warrant a dosage reduction. Elderly experience a higher level of morbidity after hypertensive crisis or malignant hyperthermia.

PREGNANCY/LACTATION-RELATED

- Pregnancy category C; excreted into breast milk.

MONITORING

- **Baseline assessment:** Assess BP and heart rate. Establish history of hypertension, heart disease, and liver disease. Ensure that patients understand it is necessary to avoid a number of foods and OTC medications while taking tranylcypromine. Assess for sensitivity to tranylcypromine. Determine current medical conditions, especially alcoholism, dysrhythmias, cardiovascular disease, congestive heart failure, hypertension, pheochromocytoma, and suicidal tendencies.
- **Baseline medication history:** Ask patients if they take CNS depressants, meperidine, and other antidepressants (other MAOIs or dibenzazepine-related and other tricyclic drugs), *busPIRone, *buPROPrion, or dextromethorphan. Tranylcypromine should not be used within 14 days of taking selective serotonin reuptake inhibitors.
- **Lab work:** Biochemical profile including renal (BUN, creatinine) and liver (AST [SGOT], ALT [SGPT], alkaline phosphatase, GGT, bilirubin) function tests. Perform periodically throughout therapy.
- **Baseline diagnostic tests:** 12-lead ECG to assess for myocardial ischemia; chest x-ray to evaluate for heart failure.
- **Myocardial ischemia:** Continuous ECG monitoring should be used for the critically ill. Symptoms of myocardial ischemia including angina can be suppressed by MAOIs.
- **Ongoing monitoring:** Monitor BP, heart rate, diet, and weight.
- **Therapeutic effect:** Assess for improved appearance, behavior, level of interest, mood, and sleep pattern.
- **Suicidal patients:** Closely supervise suicidal patients during early therapy. As depression lessens, energy level improves, increasing the suicide potential.
- **Hypertensive crisis:** Monitor for occipital headache radiating frontally and neck stiffness or soreness, which may be the first symptoms of an impending hypertensive crisis. If hypertensive crisis occurs, administer phentolamine 5-10 mg IV. Discontinue tranylcypromine immediately if patients experience frequent headaches or palpitations.
- **Patient education:** Instruct to take the second daily dose no later than 4 PM to avoid insomnia. Depression may start to lift during the first wk of therapy; tranylcypromine's full therapeutic effect may require 3 wk of therapy. Instruct to report promptly headache or neck soreness or stiffness to a health care provider. Instruct to change positions slowly and pause momentarily before standing to avoid dizziness. Warn not to use alcohol. Urge to avoid foods that require bacteria or molds for their preparation or preservation (such as yogurt and aged cheese); foods containing tyramine (including avocados, bananas, broad beans, figs, papayas, raisins, sour cream, soy sauce, beer, wine, yeast extracts, meat tenderizers, and smoked or pickled meats); and excessive amounts of caffeine-containing foods or beverages (such as chocolate, coffee, and tea). Caution to avoid using OTC preparations for colds, hay fever, and weight reduction such as cold and cough medications, nasal decongestants including nose drops and spray, sinus medications, asthma inhalants, appetite suppressants, "high-energy" formulas used for fatigue and weight loss, L-tryptophan-containing formulas.

SERIOUS ADVERSE REACTIONS

- **Hypertensive crisis:** Severe hypertension, occipital headache radiating frontally, neck stiffness or soreness, nausea, vomiting, diaphoresis, fever or chilliness, clammy skin, dilated pupils, palpitations, tachycardia or bradycardia, and constricting chest pain. May lead to intracranial bleeding/hemorrhagic stroke.
- **Malignant hyperthermia:** Increased end tidal CO_2 requiring large volume minute ventilation to control with muscle rigidity, myoglobinuria, rhabdomyolysis, followed by fever (a late sign of malignant hyperthermia). Hyperkalemia, hypercalcemia, and hypocalcemia may lead to dysrhythmias.
- **Hypoglycemia:** May be seen in diabetics using oral hypoglycemic agents.
- **Seizures:** More likely in patients with history of seizures or epilepsy who have been taking medication; tranylcypromine lowers the seizure threshold.
- **Tyramine reaction:** Reaction is variable, but a hallmark sign is occipital or temporal headache associated with hypertension, palpitations, neck stiffness, diaphoresis, excitation, and chest discomfort. Rare fatalities have been reported from intracranial hemorrhage or myocardial infarction.
- **Management:** For hypertension associated with crisis and tyramine reaction, administer phentolamine 5-10 mg IV. Avoid beta-blockers, which may worsen hypertension.

OVERDOSE/TOXICITY

- **MAOI overdose:** The difference between a therapeutic dose and lethal dose is less with MAOIs than with other antidepressants; less than twice the therapeutic dose may be toxic. Furthermore, the symptoms of toxicity are delayed far beyond the normal observation period for patients taking other antidepressants.
- **Overdose symptoms:** May be nonspecific. There is no typical presentation or progression of symptoms. There may be a latent period followed by rapid deterioration with life-threatening symptoms.
- **Initial/mild toxicity:** Initial symptoms include headache, agitation, irritability, tremor, nausea, and palpitations. Patients may experience tachycardia, hyperreflexia, drowsiness, hyperactivity, mydriasis, fasciculations, hyperventilation, flushing, and nystagmus with mild toxicity.
- **Moderate toxicity:** Muscle rigidity, opisthotonos, marked hyperthermia, diaphoresis, hypertension, chest pain, diarrhea, hallucinations, confusion, combativeness, and "ping-pong gaze" with bilateral horizontal eye movements.
- **Severe toxicity:** Bradycardia, hypotension, respiratory failure, cardiac arrest, seizures. Hyperkalemia, metabolic acidosis, and rhabdomyolysis are possible. Hypotension is resistant to management.
- **Management:** No well-controlled studies on management of overdose. Provide supportive care. Onset is gradual and may be delayed to 24 hr following ingestion. Provide patent airway and support ventilation.
- **GI decontamination:** Syrup of ipecac is contraindicated. Activated charcoal should be administered in a single dose. Gastric lavage may be attempted if patients present within 1 hr of ingestion.

ANTIDOTE/DIALYSIS

- **Antidote:** No specific recommendations.
- **Dialysis:** No data are available on removal of tranylcypromine by hemodialysis, high-permeability hemodialysis, or peritoneal dialysis. One source stated that hemodialysis, hemoperfusion, and peritoneal dialysis have no established role in management of MAOI overdose.

trastuzumab 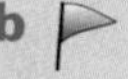

tras-too'-zoo-mab

Classes

Chemical: humanized monoclonal antibody
Therapeutic: anticancer therapy, chemotherapy adjunct for HER-2 positive cancer

Pregnancy Category: B

Trade Names

Prescription: Herceptin

CLINICAL PHARMACOLOGY

Mechanism of Action

Binds to the HER-2 protein, which is overexpressed in 25%-30% of primary breast cancers, thereby inhibiting proliferation of tumor cells. **Therapeutic Effect:** Inhibits the growth of tumor cells and mediates antibody-dependent cellular cytotoxicity.

PHARMACOKINETICS

Half-life: 5.8 days (range: 1-32 days).

AVAILABILITY

Injection, powder for reconstitution: 440 mg.

T

INDICATIONS AND DOSAGE

Breast cancer

IV

Adults, Elderly: Initially, 4 mg/kg as a 90-min infusion, then 2 mg/kg weekly as a 30-min infusion.

CONTRAINDICATIONS

Hypersensitivity to trastuzumab or Chinese hamster ovary cell proteins

INTERACTIONS

Drug: **Cyclophosphamide, *DOXOrubicin, epirubicin:** May increase the risk of cardiac dysfunction. **Herbal:** None known. **Food:** None known.

DIAGNOSTIC TEST EFFECTS

None known.

IV INCOMPATIBILITIES

Do not mix trastuzumab with any other medications or with D_5W.

SIDE-EFFECTS

Frequent (greater than 20%): Pain, asthenia, fever, chills, headache, abdominal pain, back pain, infection, nausea, diarrhea, vomiting, cough, dyspnea. **Occasional (15%-5%):** Tachycardia, heart failure, flulike symptoms, anorexia, edema, bone pain, arthralgia, insomnia, dizziness, paresthesia, depression, rhinitis, pharyngitis, sinusitis. **Rare (less than 5%):** Allergic reaction, anemia, leukopenia, neuropathy, herpes simplex

CRITICAL CARE CONSIDERATIONS

ADMINISTRATION/HANDLING

IV ALERT

- **Storage:** Refrigerate unopened vials.
- **Intermittent infusion (piggyback) only:** Do not give trastuzumab by IV push or IV bolus. *Do not use dextrose solutions for reconstitution.*
- **Reconstitution:** Reconstitute vial with 20 mL bacteriostatic water for injection (with benzyl alcohol) to yield a concentration of 21 mg/mL. Inject water slowly into lyophilized cake; swirl, rather than shake the solution to mix. If patients are hypersensitive to benzyl alcohol, use sterile water for injection. The reconstituted IV solution normally appears colorless to pale yellow.
- **Stability:** After reconstitution with bacteriostatic water for injection (with benzyl alcohol), the solution is stable for 28 days if refrigerated. After reconstitution of the vial with sterile water for injection without a preservative, use the solution immediately; discard unused portions.
- **Dilution:** Add the calculated dose from the vial to an IV solution of 250 mL 0.9% NaCl. *(Do not use D_5W.)* Gently mix contents in bag. IV solution reconstituted in 0.9% NaCl is stable for up to 24 hr if refrigerated.
- **Loading dose:** Give loading dose (4 mg/kg) over 90 min.
- **Maintenance infusion:** Give maintenance infusion (2 mg/kg) over 30 min weekly.
- **Paclitaxel combination therapy:** Trastuzumab is sometimes given in combination with paclitaxel (Taxol).

PRECAUTIONS

HEALTH-RELATED

- Use trastuzumab cautiously in patients with heart or lung disease, especially those who have previously received cardiotoxic drug therapy or radiation therapy to the chest wall.
- **Hypersensitivity:** Use very cautiously in those with a known hypersensitivity to trastuzumab because they may have repeat episodes despite use of antihistamines and corticosteroids.

AGE-RELATED

- **Children:** Safety and efficacy of trastuzumab have not been established in children.
- **Elderly:** Age-related cardiac dysfunction may require cautious use. Elderly have developed heart failure more often than younger patient populations.

PREGNANCY/LACTATION-RELATED

- Pregnancy category B; discontinue breastfeeding during trastuzumab therapy and for 6 mo after the last dose.

MONITORING

- **Baseline assessment:** Assess for history of heart disease. Assess vital signs before and during therapy.
- **Lab work:** CBC with differential before and periodically during therapy.
- **Baseline diagnostic tests:** Obtain 12-lead ECG and echocardiogram or multigated acquisition (MUGA) scan to evaluate left ventricular function before starting therapy.
- **Heart failure:** Frequently monitor chest discomfort, dyspnea, dyspnea when lying flat, cough, activity intolerance, dependent

edema, weakness or extreme fatigue, which may indicate deteriorating cardiac function. Auscultate lung fields for crackles and heart sounds for S3 and S4.
- **Acute respiratory distress syndrome (ARDS):** Monitor for progressive dyspnea with hypoxemia and/or retention of carbon dioxide. Differential diagnosis must be made between heart failure and ARDS using chest x-rays, pulmonary and cardiac function testing.
- **Weakness:** Assess for asthenia, and assist with ambulation if needed.
- **Infusion reaction:** Monitor for abdominal pain, back pain, chills, and fever, nausea and vomiting, especially during loading dose.
- **Nausea/vomiting:** Administer antiemetics to treat nausea or vomiting.
- **Diarrhea:** Assess pattern of daily bowel activity and stool consistency.
- **Patient education:** Urge to avoid receiving vaccinations and coming in contact with crowds, people with known infections, and anyone who has recently received an oral polio vaccine.

SERIOUS ADVERSE REACTIONS
- **Infusion reaction:** Chills, fever, abdominal and back pain occur in 40% of patients during the first infusion. Asthenia (weakness), dyspnea, bronchospasms, dizziness, headache, hypotension, pain (sometimes at tumor site), rash, nausea, and vomiting also sometimes occur. Recurrence of this reaction after the first infusion is uncommon.
- **Hypersensitivity reaction:** Anaphylaxis, angioedema, urticaria, and severe bronchospasms may occur during and after the infusion. Patients may experience an infusion reaction, followed by hypersensitivity.
- **Management:** *DiphenhydrAMINE (Benadryl), acetaminophen (Tylenol), and meperidine (Demerol) may be used, along with supportive care to maintain patent airway, ventilation, and BP, and to control nausea and vomiting.

OVERDOSE/TOXICITY
- **Cardiotoxicity:** Cardiomyopathy, ventricular dysfunction, and heart failure occur rarely. Mural thrombus formation has led to stroke. May be fatal.
- **Pulmonary toxicity:** ARDS. May be fatal.
- **Hematologic:** Pancytopenia may occur.
- **GI decontamination:** No specific recommendations.

ANTIDOTE/DIALYSIS
- **Antidote:** No specific recommendations.
- **Dialysis:** Trastuzumab is unlikely to be removed by hemodialysis, high-permeability hemodialysis, or peritoneal dialysis.

trazodone hydrochloride

tra'-zoe-done high-droe-klor'-ide

Classes
Chemical: triazolopyridine derivative
Therapeutic: antidepressant

Pregnancy Category: C

Trade Names
Prescription: Desyrel, Desyrel Dividose

Do not confuse Desyrel with Delsym or Zestril.

CLINICAL PHARMACOLOGY
Mechanism of Action
An antidepressant that blocks the reuptake of serotonin at neuronal presynaptic membranes, increasing its availability at postsynaptic receptor sites. **Therapeutic Effect:** Relieves depression.

PHARMACOKINETICS
Well absorbed from the GI tract. Protein binding: 85%-95%. Metabolized in the liver. Primarily excreted in urine. **Half-life:** 5-9 hr.

AVAILABILITY
Tablets: 50 mg (Desyrel), 100 mg (Desyrel), 150 mg (Desyrel Dividose), 300 mg (Desyrel Dividose).

INDICATIONS AND DOSAGE
Depression
PO
Adults: Initially, 150 mg/day in equally divided doses. Increase by 50 mg/day at 3- to 4-day intervals until therapeutic response is achieved. Maximum: 600 mg/day. **Elderly:** Initially, 25-50 mg at bedtime. May increase by 25-50 mg every 3-7 days. Range: 75-150 mg/day. **Children 6-18 yr:** Initially, 1.5-2 mg/kg/day in divided doses. May increase gradually to 6 mg/kg/day in 3 divided doses.

OFF-LABEL USES
Treatment of neurogenic pain

CONTRAINDICATIONS
Hypersensitivity to trazodone

INTERACTIONS

Drug: Alcohol, CNS depression-producing medications: May increase CNS depression. **Antihypertensives:** May increase the effects of antihypertensives. **Digoxin, phenytoin:** May increase the blood concentration of these drugs. **Indinavir, ketoconazole, ritonavir:** May increase the blood concentration and toxicity of trazodone. **Herbal: St. John's wort:** May increase the adverse effects of trazodone. **Food:** None known.

DIAGNOSTIC TEST EFFECTS

May decrease serum WBC and neutrophil counts.

SIDE-EFFECTS

Frequent (9%-3%): Somnolence, dry mouth, lightheadedness, dizziness, headache, blurred vision, nausea, vomiting. **Occasional (3%-1%):** Nervousness, fatigue, constipation, generalized aches and pains, mild hypotension. **Rare:** Photosensitivity reaction

CRITICAL CARE CONSIDERATIONS

ADMINISTRATION/HANDLING

PO ALERT

- Give trazodone shortly after a meal or snack to reduce risk of dizziness or lightheadedness.
- Crush tablets as needed.

PRECAUTIONS

HEALTH-RELATED

- Use trazodone cautiously in patients with dysrhythmias or cardiac disease.

AGE-RELATED

- **Children:** Safety and efficacy of trazodone have not been established in children under 6 yr.
- **Elderly:** Lower dosages are recommended; elderly are more likely to experience hypotensive or sedative effects.

PREGNANCY/LACTATION-RELATED

- Pregnancy category C; excreted into human breast milk; effects on nursing infant unknown but of possible concern.

MONITORING

- **Baseline assessment:** Assess level of depression, or how much mood interferes with activities of daily living including appetite/eating, sleeping, level of agitation or retardation, interest level in activities, energy level, libido, feelings about self-worth, concentration, and presence of suicidal ideation.
- **Lab work:** CBC with WBC differential; biochemical profile including liver (AST [SGOT], ALT [SGPT], bilirubin, alkaline phosphatase) and renal (BUN, creatinine) function tests before and periodically during long-term therapy. Monitor serum neutrophil and WBC counts. Discontinue trazodone if these counts drop.
- **Suicidal patients:** Closely supervise suicidal patients during early therapy. As depression lessens, energy level generally improves, increasing the suicide potential.
- **Therapeutic effect:** Assess appearance, behavior, level of interest, mood, and sleep pattern before and during therapy.
- **Dysrhythmias:** Monitor ECG continuously for dysrhythmias, including prolongation of the QT interval, sinus bradycardia, heart block, and ventricular irritability. Torsades de pointes is possible with toxicity.
- **Dizziness:** Assist with ambulation if dizziness or lightheadedness are experienced.
- **Patient education:** Advise taking trazodone after a meal or snack to help prevent dizziness and lightheadedness and to take trazodone at bedtime if drowsy while taking the drug. Explain that a tolerance to the anticholinergic and sedative effects generally is developed early in therapy. Caution against abruptly discontinuing the drug. Instruct to change positions slowly to avoid hypotension. Warn to avoid tasks that require mental alertness or motor skills until response to the drug is known. Instruct male patients to report immediately a painful, prolonged penile erection to the prescriber. Inform that trazodone may cause photosensitivity to sunlight. Instruct to report promptly if visual disturbances occur to a health care provider. Urge avoidance of alcohol while taking trazodone. Suggest sips of tepid water to relieve dry mouth.

SERIOUS ADVERSE REACTIONS

- **Sexual dysfunction:** Priapism, diminished or improved libido, retrograde ejaculation, and impotence occur rarely.

OVERDOSE/TOXICITY

- **Cardiotoxicity:** Trazodone appears to be less cardiotoxic than other antidepressants, although dysrhythmias may occur in patients with preexisting cardiac disease. Prolonged QT syndrome may be seen. With higher doses, overdose or toxicity: sinus arrest, sinus bradycardia, atrioventricular blocks, complete heart block, ventricular beats, and torsades de pointes may be seen.

- **Overdose:** Ataxia, drowsiness, dizziness, dry mouth, nausea, vomiting, hypotension; rarely produces coma and seizures if trazodone is the only drug ingested. There is no established toxic dose for trazodone.
- **Management:** IV fluid infusion to manage hypotension before using vasopressors, if needed. Patients who have ingested multiple substances including alcohol have a higher incidence of coma, seizures, and respiratory arrest, requiring endotracheal intubation and mechanical ventilation.
- **GI decontamination:** Activated charcoal may be used if patients present within a few hr of ingestion. Early lavage may also be attempted before charcoal, but neither has been proven to be beneficial in improving outcomes.

ANTIDOTE/DIALYSIS

- **Antidote:** No specific recommendations.
- **Dialysis:** Trazodone is unlikely to be removed by hemodialysis or peritoneal dialysis. No data are available on removal by high-permeability hemodialysis.

treprostinil sodium

treh-pros'-tin-il soe'-dee-um

Classes

Chemical: prostacyclin analog
Therapeutic: vasodilator

Pregnancy Category: B

Trade Names

Prescription: Remodulin

CLINICAL PHARMACOLOGY

Mechanism of Action

An antiplatelet that directly dilates pulmonary and systemic arterial vascular beds, inhibiting platelet aggregation. **Therapeutic Effect:** Reduces symptoms of pulmonary arterial hypertension associated with exercise.

PHARMACOKINETICS

Rapidly, completely absorbed after subcutaneous infusion; 91% bound to plasma protein. Metabolized by the liver. Excreted mainly in the urine with a lesser amount eliminated in the feces. **Half-life:** 2-4 hr.

AVAILABILITY

Injection: 1 mg/mL, 2.5 mg/mL, 5 mg/mL, 10 mg/mL.

INDICATIONS AND DOSAGE

Pulmonary arterial hypertension

Continuous subcutaneous infusion, IV infusion

Adults, Elderly: Initially, 1.25 ng/kg/min. Reduce infusion rate to 0.625 ng/kg/min if initial dose cannot be tolerated. Increase infusion rate in increments of no more than 1.25 ng/kg/min per wk for the first 4 wk and then no more than 2.5 ng/kg/min per wk for the duration of infusion.

Hepatic impairment (mild to moderate)

Adults, Elderly: Decrease the initial dose to 0.625 ng/kg/min based on ideal body weight and increase cautiously.

CONTRAINDICATIONS

Hypersensitivity to treprostinil

INTERACTIONS

Drug: Anticoagulants, aspirin, heparin, thrombolytics: May increase the risk of bleeding. **Drugs that alter BP, including antihypertensive agents, diuretics, vasodilators:** Reduced BP caused by treprostinil may be exacerbated by these drugs. **Herbal:** None known. **Food:** None known.

DIAGNOSTIC TEST EFFECTS

None known.

SIDE-EFFECTS

Frequent: Infusion site pain, erythema, induration, rash. **Occasional:** Headache, diarrhea, jaw pain, vasodilation, nausea. **Rare:** Dizziness, hypotension, pruritus, edema.

CRITICAL CARE CONSIDERATIONS

ADMINISTRATION/HANDLING

SUBCUTANEOUS ALERT

- **Storage:** Store at room temperature and administer without further dilution.
- **Stability:** Do not use a single vial for longer than 14 days after initial use.
- **Continuous infusion:** Give via a subcutaneous catheter, using an infusion pump designed for subcutaneous drug delivery.
- **Infusion rate:** Calculate using following formula: Infusion rate (mL/hr) = Dose

T

(ng/kg/min) multiplied by weight (kg) multiplied by (0.00006/treprostinil dosage strength concentration [mg/mL]).

- **Backup pump:** To avoid potential interruptions in drug delivery, provide access to a backup infusion pump and spare subcutaneous infusion sets.
- **Rebound pulmonary hypertension:** Avoid ANY interruption in the IV infusion; a short break in infusion may result in rebounding pulmonary hypertension.
- **Skilled providers:** Treprostinil should only be used by physicians and nurses skilled in identifying and managing pulmonary hypertension.

PRECAUTIONS

HEALTH-RELATED

- Use treprostinil cautiously in elderly patients over 65 yr with liver or renal impairment.

AGE-RELATED

- **Children:** Safety and efficacy of treprostinil have not been established in children.
- **Elderly:** Age-related decreased cardiac, hepatic, and renal function as well as concurrent disease or other drug therapy may require dosage reduction.

PREGNANCY/LACTATION-RELATED

- Pregnancy category B; excretion into human breast milk unknown; use caution in nursing mothers.

MONITORING

- **Baseline assessment:** Assess vital signs (especially blood pressure) and perform a cardiopulmonary assessment. Note pulse oximetry reading (SpO_2). Assess for dependent edema and ascites.
- **Lab work:** Baseline biochemical profile including renal (BUN, creatinine) and liver (AST [SGOT], ALT [SGPT], alkaline phosphatase, bilirubin) function tests.
- **Diagnostic tests:** 12-lead ECG to evaluate extent of myocardial ischemia; echocardiogram to assess ventricular wall motion, heart valve function, pulmonary artery pressures, and cardiac output.
- **Hemodynamic monitoring:** Monitor pulmonary artery pressures when drug is initiated using a pulmonary artery catheter. If SVO_2 catheter can be used, a more precise assessment of oxygenation can be done.
- **Therapeutic effect:** Monitor liver enzymes (AST [SGOT], ALT [SGPT], alkaline phosphatase, bilirubin) periodically. If enzymes are elevated, discontinue captopril.
- **Hypotension and tachycardia:** Decreased pulmonary artery pressures (pulmonary artery [PA] systolic, diastolic, and mean pressures), improved oxygen saturation, improved activity tolerance. If SVO_2 catheter is used, oxygen consumption should decrease while SVO_2 reading increases, reflecting that oxygen supply is better meeting oxygen demand. Assess for decreased chest discomfort, less dyspnea, less fatigue; decreased PA pressures, pulmonary vascular resistance, and improved pulmonary function.
- **Dosage adjustment BP monitoring:** Monitor standing and supine BP frequently for hypotension for several hr after a dosage adjustment. Assess for syncope.
- **Acute dose ranging:** Observe continuous ECG monitoring and check frequently vital signs until response to the drug is known. Asymptomatic increases may be seen in pulmonary artery pressures with an increased cardiac output; dosage adjustment may be warranted if PA pressure increase is observed.
- **Insertion site:** Monitor subcutaneous catheter site for redness, induration, and pain. Severe reactions may warrant discontinuation of treprostinil.
- **Patient education:** Show how to administer treprostinil via a self-inserted subcutaneous catheter using an ambulatory pump. Teach how to care for the subcutaneous catheter and troubleshoot infusion pump problems. Instruct to report promptly signs of increased PA pressure, such as dyspnea, cough, or chest pain to a health care provider. Stress that immediate access to a backup pump is necessary to avoid interruption in drug therapy if one pump malfunctions. Rebound pulmonary hypertension can be severe and could be fatal if left unmanaged.

SERIOUS ADVERSE REACTIONS

- **Abrupt withdrawal/sudden large dosage reductions:** May result in worsening of pulmonary arterial hypertension symptoms or rebound pulmonary hypertension.

OVERDOSE/TOXICITY

- **Hepatic insufficiency:** Clearance of treprostinil is reduced by up to 80% in liver-impaired patients, compared with healthy adults. Patients with pulmonary hypertension often have portopulmonary hypertension, which leads to liver dysfunction.

T

- **Overdose:** Hypotension, respiratory distress, hypoxemia, respiratory failure/arrest, death.
- **Management:** Intubation, mechanical ventilation using modes to enhance diffusion of oxygen. Consider use of an alternate agent such as epoprostenol (Flolan) IV or use continuous nebulization. Consider use of nitric oxide. Hypotension may be managed by IV fluid infusion if patients can tolerate volume or by vasopressors. Hypotension will occur with epoprostenol IV but is generally mild with epoprostenol continuous nebulization.
- **GI decontamination:** No specific recommendations.

ANTIDOTE/DIALYSIS

- **Antidote:** No specific recommendations.
- **Dialysis:** Treprostinil is unlikely to be removed using hemodialysis, high-permeability hemodialysis, or peritoneal dialysis.

triamcinolone/ triamcinolone acetonide/ triamcinolone diacetate/ triamcinolone hexacetonide

trye-am-sin'-oh-lone

Classes

Chemical: glucocorticoid, synthetic
Therapeutic: corticosteroid, inhaled; corticosteroid, systemic; corticosteroid, topical

Pregnancy Category: C, D (1st trimester)

Trade Names

Prescription: (Triamcinolone) Aristocort; (Triamcinolone acetonide) Acetocot, Aristocort, Aristocort Forte, Aristospan Injection, Azmacort, Clinacort, Clinalog, Kenalog, Kenalog-10, Kenalog-40, Ken-Jec 40, Nasacort AQ, Triam-A, Triamcot, Triam-Forte, Triamonide 40, Triderm, Tri-Nasal, U-Tri-Lone; (Tiamcinolone diacetate) Amcort, Aristocort Intralesional; (Triamcinolone hexacetonide) Aristospan

Do not confuse triamcinolone with Triaminicin or Triaminicol.

CLINICAL PHARMACOLOGY

Mechanism of Action

An adrenocortical steroid that inhibits accumulation of inflammatory cells at inflammation sites, phagocytosis, lysosomal enzyme release and synthesis, and release of mediators of inflammation. **Therapeutic Effect:** Prevents or suppresses cell-mediated immune reactions. Decreases or prevents tissue response to inflammatory process.

PHARMACOKINETICS

Minimal absorption following nasal and topical administration. Moderate absorption from the lungs and GI tract following administration of inhaled form. Rapidly and almost completely absorbed following PO administration. Metabolized in liver. Excreted in urine. **Half-life:** Unknown.

AVAILABILITY

Oral (topical paste [Kenalog in Orabase]): 0.1% or 5 g.
Tablets (Aristocort): 4 mg, 8 mg.
Inhalation (oral [Azmacort]): 100 mcg/inhalation.
Nasal spray: 50 mcg/inhalation (Tri-Nasal), 55 mcg/inhalation (Nasacort AQ).
Cream: 0.025% (Aristocort A), 0.05% (Aristocort A), 0.1% (Aristocort A, Kenalog, Triderm).
Ointment (Aristocort A, Kenalog): 0.025%, 0.1%.
Injection (acetonide): 10 mg/mL (Kenalog-10), 40 mg/mL (Acetocot, Clinalog, Kenalog-40, Ken-Jec 40, Triam-A, Triamcot, Triamonide 40, U-Tri-Lone).
Injection (diacetate): 25 mg/mL (Aristocort), 40 mg/mL (Aristocort Forte, Clinacort, Triam-Forte).
Injection (hexacetonide [Aristospan Injection]): 5 mg/mL, 20 mg/mL.

INDICATIONS AND DOSAGE

Immunosuppression, relief of acute inflammation

PO

Adults, Elderly: 4-60 mg/day.

IM (triamcinolone acetonide)

Adults, Elderly: Initially, 2.5-60 mg/day.

IM (triamcinolone diacetate)

Adults, Elderly: 40 mg/wk.

IM (triamcinolone hexacetonide)

Adults, Elderly: Initially, 2.5-40 mg up to 100 mg; 2-20 mg.

Intraarticular, Intralesional

Adults, Elderly: 5-40 mg.

Control of bronchial asthma

Inhalation

Adults, Elderly: 2 inhalations 3-4 times per day. **Children 6-12 yr:** 1-2 inhalations 3-4 times per day. Maximum: 12 inhalations/day.

Rhinitis
Intranasal
Adults, Elderly, Children 6 yr and older: Initially, 2 sprays (55 mcg/spray) in each nostril once daily. Maintenance: 1 spray in each nostril once daily.
Relief of inflammation or pruritus associated with corticoid-responsive dermatoses
Topical
Adults, Elderly: 2-4 times per day. May give 1-2 times per day or as intermittent therapy.

CONTRAINDICATIONS

Administration of live virus vaccines, especially smallpox vaccine; hypersensitivity to corticosteroids or tartrazine; IM injection or oral inhalation in children younger than 6 yr; peptic ulcer disease (except life-threatening situations); systemic fungal infection; hypersensitivity to triamcinolone products. **Topical:** Marked circulation impairment

INTERACTIONS

Drug: Amphotericin: May increase hypokalemia. **Digoxin:** May increase the risk of digoxin toxicity caused by hypokalemia. **Diuretics, insulin, oral hypoglycemics, potassium supplements:** May decrease the effects of these drugs. **Hepatic enzyme inducers:** May decrease the effects of triamcinolone. **Live-virus vaccines:** May decrease antibody response to vaccine, increase vaccine side effects, and potentiate virus replication. **Herbal:** None known. **Food:** None known.

DIAGNOSTIC TEST EFFECTS

May increase blood glucose and serum lipid, amylase, and sodium levels. May decrease serum calcium, potassium, and thyroxine levels.

SIDE-EFFECTS

Frequent: Insomnia, dry mouth, heartburn, nervousness, abdominal distention, diaphoresis, acne, mood swings, increased appetite, facial flushing, delayed wound healing, increased susceptibility to infection, diarrhea, or constipation. **Occasional:** Headache, edema, change in skin color, frequent urination. **Rare:** Tachycardia, allergic reaction (including rash and hives), mental changes, hallucinations, depression. **Topical:** Allergic contact dermatitis

CRITICAL CARE CONSIDERATIONS

ADMINISTRATION/HANDLING

PO ALERT

- Give triamcinolone with food or milk.
- Give single doses before 9 AM; give multiple doses at evenly spaced intervals.

IV ALERT

- Do not give triamcinolone IV.

IM ALERT

- Give deep IM injection into gluteus maximus.

INHALATION ALERT

- **Administration:** Shake container well. Exhale completely. Place mouthpiece fully into the mouth and, while holding the inhaler upright, inhale deeply and slowly while pressing the top of the canister. Hold the breath as long as possible before slowly exhaling. Wait 1 min between inhalations when multiple inhalations have been ordered to allow for deeper bronchial penetration. Rinse the mouth with water immediately after inhalations to prevent thrush.

TOPICAL ALERT

- Gently cleanse area before applying triamcinolone. Apply sparingly and rub into area thoroughly.
- Use occlusive dressings only as ordered.

PRECAUTIONS

HEALTH-RELATED

- Use triamcinolone cautiously in patients with heart failure, cirrhosis, diabetes mellitus, history of tuberculosis (it may reactivate disease), hypertension, hypothyroidism, nonspecific ulcerative colitis, psychosis, myasthenia gravis, ocular herpes simplex, osteoporosis, peptic ulcer disease, thromboembolic disorders, ocular herpes simplex, or renal insufficiency.
- Discontinue prolonged therapy slowly.

AGE-RELATED

- **Children:** Monitor growth and development of children receiving long-term steroid therapy. Growth may be suppressed.
- **Elderly:** No special dosage precautions; all patients on prolonged therapy may develop subcapsular cataracts and glaucoma and are at higher risk for ocular infections.

PREGNANCY/LACTATION-RELATED

- Pregnancy category C (D if used in first trimester); excreted in breast milk and could interfere with infant's growth and endogenous corticosteroid production.

MONITORING

- **Baseline assessment:** Vital signs including BP, height, and body weight. Determine hypersensitivity to corticosteroids or tartrazine (Kenacort). Monitor growth rate in children.
- **Baseline lab work:** Biochemical profile including blood glucose and serum electrolyte levels. Check for blood coagulability and evidence of thromboembolism. If digoxin is being taken, draw serum digoxin levels.
- **Diabetes mellitus:** Determine whether diabetes mellitus is present; increase antidiabetic drug regimen because of raised blood glucose level. Diagnostic tests: Evaluate results of tuberculosis skin test, x-rays, and ECG.
- **Live virus vaccines:** Patients taking triamcinolone should never be given live virus vaccines (e.g., smallpox vaccine).
- **Weight gain/BP elevation:** Monitor for salt- and retention-induced weight gain, edema, and increase in BP.
- **Hypokalemia:** Monitor ECG for dysrhythmias induced by increased potassium excretion such as premature ventricular beats and ventricular and supraventricular tachycardias.
- **Electrolyte imbalance:** Monitor for hypocalcemia (muscle twitching, cramps, and positive Chvostek's or Trousseau's signs), or hypokalemia (ECG changes, nausea and vomiting, irritability, weakness and muscle cramps, numbness, and tingling, especially in lower extremities).
- **Adrenal insufficiency:** Wean triamcinolone slowly when discontinuing either short or long-term therapy to avoid adrenal insufficiency.
- **Sleep disturbance and emotional lability:** Assess sleep pattern and emotional status, since triamcinolone may cause sleeplessness, euphoria, high energy, or labile emotional state. Inform that triamcinolone may cause mood swings.
- **Immunosuppression:** Assess the mouth daily for candidal infection (white patches, painful mucous membranes, and tongue). Be alert to signs and symptoms of infection such as fever, pharyngitis, and vague symptoms.
- **Fluid retention:** Monitor BP and intake and output. Record weight daily. Assess for edema.
- **Hyperglycemia:** Consider placing on point of care glucose readings before meals and at bedtime to assess for increasing blood glucose level.
- **Patient education:** Instruct to report promptly fever, muscle aches, sore throat, and sudden weight gain or swelling to a health care provider. Urge avoidance of alcohol and limiting caffeine intake during triamcinolone therapy. Caution against abruptly discontinuing the drug without first discussing with the prescriber. Warn to avoid exposure to chicken pox or measles and that they should NOT be vaccinated for smallpox or receive any live-virus vaccinations. Explain that steroids often cause mood swings, ranging from euphoria to depression. Instruct to report promptly difficulty breathing, muscle weakness, sudden weight gain, or facial edema occurring while taking oral triamcinolone to a health care provider. Instruct to take the drug with food or after meals. Explain that oral triamcinolone may cause dry mouth. Instruct not to use inhaled triamcinolone for acute asthma attacks. Teach to rinse the mouth after drug administration to decrease the risk of mouth soreness. Inform to report promptly stomatitis to a health care provider. Instruct patients to promptly report unusual cough or spasm or persistent nasal bleeding, burning, or infection that occurs while taking nasal triamcinolone to a health care provider.

SERIOUS ADVERSE REACTIONS

- **Anaphylaxis:** Occurs rarely with parenteral administration.
- **Blindness:** Has occurred rarely after intralesional injection around face and head.
- **Hyperglycemia:** Blood glucose increases to 180-200 mg/dL on random glucose samples indicate development of hyperglycemia and requires management.
- **Hypokalemia:** ECG changes, irritability, muscle cramps and weakness, nausea and vomiting, and numbness and tingling in the lower extremities.
- **Long-term therapy:** May cause hypocalcemia, hypokalemia, muscle wasting (especially in the arms and legs), osteoporosis, spontaneous fractures, impaired wound healing, development of cushingoid state, amenorrhea, cataracts,

glaucoma, peptic ulcer disease, and heart failure.
- **Pediatric patients:** Growth suppression.
- **Abrupt withdrawal after long-term therapy:** May cause anorexia, nausea, fever, headache, severe or sudden joint pain, rebound inflammation, fatigue, weakness, lethargy, dizziness, and orthostatic hypotension.
- **Sudden discontinuation:** May be fatal.
- **Hypersensitivity:** Anaphylactoid reactions have been reported.
- **Negative nitrogen balance:** Due to protein catabolism.
- **Severe infection:** Patients who have underlying infection or acquire a significant infection may develop fatal septic shock.

OVERDOSE/TOXICITY
- **Severe behavioral changes:** Extreme euphoria, personality changes, severe depression, frank psychosis (more likely in patients with mental health history).
- **Fluid and electrolyte disturbances:** Significant weight gain (over 15 lb), sodium retention, potassium loss, hypokalemia, fluid retention, pitting edema, heart failure, difficulty breathing, hypertension.
- **GI bleeding:** Hematemesis, bloody stools, ulcerative esophagitis, expectoration of blood.
- **Musculoskeletal:** Muscle weakness, steroid myopathy, vertebral compression fractures, aseptic necrosis of femoral and humeral heads, long bone fractures.
- **Dermatologic:** Impaired wound healing, thin fragile skin, petechiae, and ecchymosis.
- **Neurologic:** Seizures, increased intracranial pressure with papilledema.
- **Ophthalmic:** Posterior subcapsular cataracts, increased intraocular pressure, glaucoma.
- **GI decontamination:** No specific recommendations.

ANTIDOTE/DIALYSIS
- **Antidote:** No specific recommendations.
- **Dialysis:** Triamcinolone is unlikely to be removed by hemodialysis or peritoneal dialysis. No data are available on removal by high-permeability hemodialysis.

triamterene
See Diuretics (p. 956)

triazolam ⚑
try-ay'-zoe-lam

DEA Schedule: IV

Classes
Chemical: benzodiazepine
Therapeutic: hypnotic

Pregnancy Category: X

Trade Names
Prescription: Apo-Triazo ♣, Halcion

Do not confuse Halcion with Haldol or Healon.

CLINICAL PHARMACOLOGY
Mechanism of Action
A benzodiazepine that enhances the action of the inhibitory neurotransmitter gamma-aminobutyric acid, resulting in CNS depression. **Therapeutic Effect:** Induces sleep.

PHARMACOKINETICS
Rapidly and completely absorbed from GI tract. Protein binding: 89%-94%. Metabolized in the liver. Primarily excreted in urine. **Half-life:** 1.5-5.5 hr.

AVAILABILITY
Tablets: 0.125 mg, 0.25 mg.

INDICATIONS AND DOSAGE
Insomnia
PO
Adults, Children 18 yr and older: 0.125-0.5 mg at bedtime. **Elderly:** 0.0625-0.125 mg at bedtime.

CONTRAINDICATIONS
Angle-closure glaucoma; CNS depression; hypersensitivity to triazolam or other benzodiazepines; pregnancy or breast-feeding; severe, uncontrolled pain; sleep apnea

INTERACTIONS
Drug: Alcohol, other CNS depressants: May increase CNS depression. **Fluvoxamine, itraconazole, ketoconazole, nefazodone:** May inhibit metabolism and increase serum concentrations of triazolam. **Herbal: Kava kava, valerian:** May increase CNS depression. **Food: Grapefruit, grapefruit juice:** May alter the absorption of triazolam.

DIAGNOSTIC TEST EFFECTS
None known.

SIDE-EFFECTS

Frequent: Somnolence, sedation, dry mouth, headache, dizziness, nervousness, lightheadedness, incoordination, nausea, rebound insomnia (may occur for 1-2 nights after drug is discontinued). **Occasional:** Euphoria, tachycardia, abdominal cramps, visual disturbances. **Rare:** Paradoxic CNS excitement or restlessness (particularly in elderly or debilitated patients)

CRITICAL CARE CONSIDERATIONS

ADMINISTRATION/HANDLING

PO ALERT

- Give triazolam without regard to food.
- Crush tablets as needed.
- Do not administer triazolam with grapefruit juice.

PRECAUTIONS

HEALTH-RELATED

- Use triazolam cautiously in patients with a potential for drug abuse.
- **Cytochrome P450 enzyme metabolism:** Drugs that inhibit the CYP3A liver enzyme pathway should not be used with triazolam as clearance of the drug will be reduced. Drugs include ketoconazole, itraconazole, nefazodone, cimetidine, and erythromycin. Potential for numerous other drug interactions exists.

AGE-RELATED

- **Children:** Safety and efficacy of triazolam have not been established in children.
- **Elderly:** Age-related organ impairment may warrant a dosage reduction. Elderly are more susceptible to oversedation, dizziness, and impaired coordination.

PREGNANCY/LACTATION-RELATED

- Pregnancy category X (according to manufacturer). No congenital anomalies have been attributed to use during human pregnancies. Other benzodiazepines have been suspected of producing fetal malformations after first-trimester exposure. Not recommended for breast-feeding women.

MONITORING

- **Baseline assessment:** Determine pregnancy before beginning triazolam therapy. Assess pattern of sleep disturbance. Assess vital signs immediately before administering triazolam.
- **Lab work:** Biochemical profile including liver (AST [SGOT], ALT [SGPT], alkaline phosphatase, bilirubin) and renal (BUN, creatinine) function tests. Monitor hepatic function of patients on long-term therapy.
- **Sleep promotion:** Raise top bed rails if triazolam has not been taken before and provide a call bell. Provide a quiet environment conducive to sleep. If possible, offer a back rub and low lighting.
- **Respiratory status:** Assess for patent airway, respiratory rate, and oxygen saturation (pulse oximetry) to detect apnea and respiratory depression. Critically ill patients and others who are intubated and mechanically ventilated are better protected from respiratory compromise.
- **Chest discomfort:** Monitor cardiovascular status if history of heart disease is present.
- **Paradoxic reactions:** Assess elderly or debilitated patients for stimulation, mania, agitation, hallucinations, delusions, falling, muscle rigidity, and syncope, particularly during early therapy.
- **Therapeutic response:** Evaluate for a decrease in the number of nocturnal awakenings and a longer duration of sleep.
- **Patient education:** Inform that triazolam may cause prolonged drowsiness. Warn to avoid activities requiring mental alertness or motor skills until response to the drug is known. Urge avoidance of alcohol and other CNS depressants during therapy. Inform that triazolam may cause dry mouth and physical or psychologic dependence; patients may experience disturbed sleep patterns for 1-2 nights after discontinuing triazolam. Patients should refrain from consuming grapefruit or grapefruit juice during triazolam therapy because grapefruit decreases absorption. Smoking reduces the drug's effectiveness. Provide with information about smoking cessation. Instruct to discuss plans for pregnancy with the prescriber prior to pregnancy, and to report promptly pregnancy to a health care provider.

SERIOUS ADVERSE REACTIONS

- **Abrupt or too rapid withdrawal:** May result in pronounced restlessness, irritability, insomnia, hand tremor, abdominal or muscle cramps, diaphoresis, vomiting, and seizures.
- **Paradoxic reactions:** Some patients are intolerant of benzodiazepines and respond to the drug with cerebral hypoxia, agitation,

involuntary movements, hyperactivity, and combativeness.

OVERDOSE/TOXICITY

- **Overdose:** Somnolence, confusion, diminished reflexes, respiratory depression, hypotension, and coma.
- **Management:** Ensure patent airway with endotracheal intubation if necessary, along with mechanical ventilation. Support BP with fluids and vasopressors if needed. Administer benzodiazepine antidote flumazenil. Forced diuresis and osmotic diuretics (e.g., mannitol) may facilitate elimination.
- **GI decontamination:** No specific recommendations.

ANTIDOTE/DIALYSIS

- **Antidote:** Cautiously use flumazenil (Romazicon) 0.2 mg (2 mL) over 30 sec; may repeat after 30 sec with 0.3 mg (3 mL) over 30 sec. Further doses may be given up to 0.5 mg (5 mL) up to a total of 3 mg (30 mL). Flumazenil reverses CNS depressive effects. Naloxone (Narcan) should be considered in addition to flumazenil if patients have significant respiratory depression.
- **Dialysis:** Triazolam is not removed by hemodialysis and is unlikely to be removed by peritoneal dialysis. No data are available on removal using high-permeability hemodialysis.

trichlormethazide

See Diuretics (p. 956)

trifluoperazine hydrochloride

See Antipsychotics (p. 934)

trimethobenzamide hydrochloride

trye-meth-oh-ben′-za-mide high-droe-klor′-ide

Classes

Chemical: ethanolamine derivative
Therapeutic: antiemetic

Pregnancy Category: C

Trade Names

Prescription: Benzacot, Benzocaine-Trimethobenzamide Adult, Benzocaine-Trimethobenzamide Pediatric, Navogan, Tebamide, Tebamide Pediatric, Tigan, Tigan Adult, Tigan Pediatric

CLINICAL PHARMACOLOGY

Mechanism of Action

An anticholinergic that acts at the chemoreceptor trigger zone in the medulla oblongata. **Therapeutic Effect:** Relieves nausea and vomiting.

PHARMACOKINETICS

Route	Onset	Peak	Duration
PO	10-40 min	N/A	3-4 hr
IM	15-30 min	N/A	2-3 hr

Partially absorbed from the GI tract. Distributed primarily to the liver. Metabolic fate unknown. Excreted in urine. **Half-life:** 7-9 hr.

AVAILABILITY

Capsules (Tigan): 250 mg, 300 mg.
Injection (Benzacot, Tigan): 100 mg/mL.
Suppositories: 100 mg (Benzocaine-Trimethobenzamide Pediatric, Navogan, Tebamide, Tebamide Pediatric, Tigan Pediatric), 200 mg (Benzocaine-Trimethobenzamide Adult, Tebamide, Tigan Adult, Tigan Pediatric).

INDICATIONS AND DOSAGE

Nausea and vomiting

PO

Adults, Elderly: 300 mg 3-4 times per day. **Children weighing 30-100 lb:** 100-200 mg 3-4 times per day.

IM

Adults, Elderly: 200 mg 3-4 times per day.

Rectal

Adults, Elderly: 200 mg 3-4 times per day. **Children weighing less than 30 lb:** 100 mg 3-4 times per day. **Children weighing 30-90 lb:** 100-200 mg 3-4 times per day.

CONTRAINDICATIONS

Hypersensitivity to trimethobenzamide, benzocaine, or similar local anesthetics; use of parenteral form in children or suppositories in premature infants or neonates

INTERACTIONS

Drug: CNS depressants: May increase CNS depression. **Herbal:** None known. **Food:** None known.

DIAGNOSTIC TEST EFFECTS

None known.

SIDE-EFFECTS

Frequent: Somnolence. **Occasional:** Blurred vision, diarrhea, dizziness, headache, muscle cramps. **Rare:** Rash, seizures, depression, opisthotonos, parkinsonian syndrome, Reye's syndrome (marked by vomiting, seizures)

CRITICAL CARE CONSIDERATIONS

ADMINISTRATION/HANDLING

PO ALERT

- Give trimethobenzamide without regard to food.
- Swallow capsules intact; do not crush, open, or break capsules.

IM ALERT

- Inject trimethobenzamide deep into a large muscle mass, usually the upper outer gluteus maximus.
- **Not for IV use:** Do not administer trimethobenzamide by the IV route because it produces severe hypotension.

RECTAL ALERT

- If the suppository is too soft, refrigerate it for 30 min or run cold water over the foil wrapper.
- Moisten the suppository with cold water before inserting it well into the rectum.

PRECAUTIONS

HEALTH-RELATED

- Use trimethobenzamide cautiously in debilitated or elderly patients and in patients with dehydration, electrolyte imbalances, high fever, or liver disease.
- **Reye's syndrome:** Antiemetics are not recommended for uncomplicated vomiting in children because there is suspicion that centrally acting antiemetics given during a viral illness may contribute to development of Reye's syndrome. Drugs with hepatotoxic potential negatively affect the outcome of Reye's syndrome; trimethobenzamide has hepatotoxic potential and should not be given to children suspected of having Reye's syndrome.

AGE-RELATED

- **Children:** Do not administer the parenteral (injectable) form to children or the suppositories to neonates. No other age-related precautions have been noted.
- **Elderly:** Patients over 60 yr are at increased risk for developing agitation, disorientation, confusion, and psychotic-like symptoms.

PREGNANCY/LACTATION-RELATED

- Pregnancy category C; has been used to treat nausea and vomiting during pregnancy.

MONITORING

- **Baseline assessment:** Assess patients who have severe vomiting for dehydration, electrolyte imbalance, and alkalosis.
- **Lab work:** Baseline biochemical profile to assess for electrolyte imbalance and liver function (AST [SGOT], ALT [SGPT], alkaline phosphatase, bilirubin) tests. Monitor serum electrolyte levels and acid-base balance in patients with severe vomiting.
- **Hypotension:** Monitor for decreasing BP especially in elderly patients who are at an increased risk for hypotension.
- **Paradoxic reactions:** Assess children closely for restlessness, agitation, and tremors.
- **Dehydration:** Measure intake and output; assess any vomitus. Provide IV fluids for those who are unable to tolerate PO fluids or who are already dehydrated. Assess mucous membranes and skin turgor to evaluate hydration status.
- **Extrapyramidal symptoms:** Assess for involuntary muscle movements in the trunk, neck, or extremities, gait changes, and tremors, which may indicate a hypersensitivity reaction.
- **Patient education:** Tell that relief from nausea or vomiting generally occurs within 30 min of drug administration. Inform that trimethobenzamide causes drowsiness, so tasks that require mental alertness or motor skills should be avoided until response to the drug is known. Instruct to report promptly headache, visual disturbances, restlessness, or involuntary muscle movements to a health care provider. Teach other methods of relieving nausea and vomiting, including lying quietly and avoiding strong odors.

SERIOUS ADVERSE REACTIONS

- **Hypersensitivity reaction:** Extrapyramidal symptoms such as muscle rigidity and allergic skin reactions occur rarely.
- **Extrapyramidal symptoms:** Symptoms are dose-related and divided into three categories: akathisia (including inability to sit still, tapping of feet); parkinsonian symptoms (such as masklike face, tremors, shuffling gait, hypersalivation);

and acute dystonias (including torticollis, opisthotonos, and oculogyric crisis). A dystonic reaction may also produce diaphoresis and pallor.
- **Paradoxic reactions:** Seen more commonly in children; marked by restlessness, insomnia, euphoria, nervousness, and tremor.

OVERDOSE/TOXICITY
- **Overdose:** CNS depression including sedation, apnea, cardiovascular collapse, and death or severe paradoxic reactions, including hallucinations, tremor, and seizures.
- **Hepatotoxicity:** Jaundice and elevated serum transaminases (AST [SGOT], ALT [SGPT]).
- **GI decontamination:** No specific recommendations.

ANTIDOTE/DIALYSIS
- **Antidote:** No specific recommendations.
- **Dialysis:** No data are available on removal of trimethobenzamide by hemodialysis, high-permeability hemodialysis, or peritoneal dialysis.

trimethoprim

trye-meth'-oh-prim

Classes
Chemical: folate-antagonist, synthetic
Therapeutic: antibiotic

Pregnancy Category: C

Trade Names
Prescription: Primsol, Proloprim, Trimpex

Combinations
Prescription: with sulfamethoxazole (see co-trimoxazole monograph); with polymixin B sulfate (Polytrim Ophthalmic)

CLINICAL PHARMACOLOGY
Mechanism of Action
A folate antagonist that blocks bacterial biosynthesis of nucleic acids and proteins by interfering with the metabolism of folinic acid. **Therapeutic Effect:** Bacteriostatic.

PHARMACOKINETICS
Rapidly and completely absorbed from the GI tract. Protein binding: 42%-46%. Widely distributed, including to cerebrospinal fluid. Metabolized in the liver. Primarily excreted in urine. **Half-life:** 8-10 hr (increased in impaired renal function and newborns; decreased in children).

AVAILABILITY
Oral Solution (Primsol): 50 mg/5 mL.
Tablets (Trimpex, Proloprim): 100 mg, 200 mg.

INDICATIONS AND DOSAGE
Acute, uncomplicated urinary tract infections (UTIs)
PO

Adults, Elderly, Children 12 yr and older: 100 mg every 12 hr or 200 mg once per day for 10 days. **Children younger than 2 mo:** 4-6 mg/kg/day in 2 divided doses for 10 days.

Dosage in renal impairment
Dosage and frequency are modified based on creatinine clearance.

Creatinine Clearance	Dosage Interval
Greater than 30 mL/min	No change
15-29 mL/min	50 mg every 12 hr

OFF-LABEL USES
Prevention of bacterial UTIs, treatment of pneumonia caused by *Pneumocystis carinii*

CONTRAINDICATIONS
Infants younger than 2 mo, megaloblastic anemia due to folic acid deficiency, hypersensitivity to trimethoprim

INTERACTIONS
Drug: Folate antagonists (including methotrexate): May increase the risk of megaloblastic anemia. **Herbal:** None known. **Food:** None known.

DIAGNOSTIC TEST EFFECTS
May increase BUN and serum bilirubin, creatinine, AST (SGOT), and ALT (SGPT) levels.

SIDE-EFFECTS
Occasional: Nausea, vomiting, diarrhea, decreased appetite, abdominal cramps, headache. **Rare:** Hypersensitivity reaction (pruritus, rash), methemoglobinemia (bluish fingernails, lips, or skin; fever; pale skin; sore throat; unusual tiredness), photosensitivity

CRITICAL CARE CONSIDERATIONS

ADMINISTRATION/HANDLING

PO ALERT
- Space doses evenly around the clock to maintain a constant drug level in urine.

- Give trimethoprim without regard to food (or with food if stomach upset occurs).

PRECAUTIONS

HEALTH-RELATED

- Use trimethoprim cautiously in patients with impaired hepatic or renal function or folic acid deficiency.

AGE-RELATED

- **Children:** Safety and efficacy of trimethoprim have not been established in children.
- **Elderly:** May have an increased incidence of hematologic toxicity.

PREGNANCY/LACTATION-RELATED

- Pregnancy category C. Because trimethoprim is a folate antagonist, caution should be used during the first trimester. Excreted into breast milk in low concentrations; compatible with breast-feeding.

MONITORING

- **Baseline assessment:** Assess for symptoms of infection and history of renal or liver dysfunction or anemia.
- **Lab work:** Baseline CBC with differential; biochemical profile with renal (BUN, creatinine) and liver (AST [SGOT], ALT [SGPT], bilirubin, alkaline phosphatase) function studies. Monitor serum hematology reports and liver or renal function test results.
- **Allergic reaction:** Examine skin for rash.
- **Nausea/vomiting:** Evaluate the food tolerance of patients.
- **Hematologic toxicity:** Observe for bleeding, ecchymosis, fever, malaise, pallor, and sore throat.
- **Patient education:** Instruct to space drug doses evenly around the clock and to complete the full course of trimethoprim therapy, which usually lasts 10-14 days. Advise taking trimethoprim with food if stomach upset occurs. Urge avoidance of sun and ultraviolet light and to use sunscreen and wear protective clothing when outdoors. Warn to immediately report bleeding, bruising, skin discoloration, fever, pallor, rash, sore throat, and tiredness to a health care provider.

SERIOUS ADVERSE REACTIONS

- **Hypersensitivity:** Stevens–Johnson syndrome, erythema multiforme, exfoliative dermatitis, and anaphylaxis occur rarely.

OVERDOSE/TOXICITY

- **Hematologic toxicity:** Thrombocytopenia, neutropenia, leukopenia, megaloblastic anemia are more likely to occur in elderly, debilitated, or alcoholic patients, in patients with impaired renal function, and in those receiving prolonged high dosage.
- **GI decontamination:** No specific recommendations.

ANTIDOTE/DIALYSIS

- **Antidote:** No specific recommendations.
- **Dialysis:** Trimethoprim is removed by hemodialysis and is likely to be removed by high-permeability hemodialysis. It is not removed by peritoneal dialysis.

triprolidine

See Antihistamines (p. 925)

ursodiol

er-soe-dye'-ol

Classes
Chemical: ursodeoxycholic acid
Therapeutic: cholelitholytic

Pregnancy Category: B

Trade Names
Prescription: Actigall, Urso

CLINICAL PHARMACOLOGY

Mechanism of Action

A gallstone solubilizing agent that suppresses hepatic synthesis and secretion of cholesterol; inhibits intestinal absorption of cholesterol. **Therapeutic Effect:** Changes the bile of patients with gallstones from precipitating (capable of forming crystals) to cholesterol solubilizing (capable of being dissolved).

PHARMACOKINETICS

Absorbed from the small bowel following PO administration. Protein binding: 70%. Metabolized in colon. Primarily excreted in feces; small amount eliminated in urine. **Half-life:** 3.5-5.8 days.

AVAILABILITY

Capsules (Actigall): 300 mg.
Tablets (Urso): 250 mg.

INDICATIONS AND DOSAGE

Dissolution of radiolucent, noncalcified gallstones when cholecystectomy is not recommended; treatment of biliary cirrhosis

PO

Adults, Elderly: 8-10 mg/kg/day in 2-3 divided doses. Treatment may require months. Obtain ultrasound image of gallbladder at 6-mo intervals for first yr. If gallstones have dissolved, continue therapy and repeat ultrasound within 1-3 mo.

Prevention of gallstones

PO

Adults, Elderly: 300 mg twice per day.

OFF-LABEL USES

Prophylaxis of liver transplant rejection, treatment of alcoholic cirrhosis, biliary atresia, chronic hepatitis, gallstone formation, sclerosing cholangitis

CONTRAINDICATIONS

Allergy to bile acids, calcified cholesterol stones, chronic hepatic disease, radiolucent bile pigment stones, radiopaque stones, hypersensitivity to ursodiol

INTERACTIONS

Drug: Aluminum-containing antacids, cholestyramine: May decrease the absorption and effects of ursodiol. **Estrogens, oral contraceptives:** May decrease the effects of ursodiol. **Herbal:** None known. **Food:** None known.

DIAGNOSTIC TEST EFFECTS

May alter liver function test results.

SIDE-EFFECTS

Frequent (up to 26%): Headache, dizziness, constipation

CRITICAL CARE CONSIDERATIONS

ADMINISTRATION/HANDLING

PO ALERT

- Administer ursodiol with meals or a snack because the drug dissolves more readily in the presence of bile acid and pancreatic juice.

PRECAUTIONS

HEALTH-RELATED

- Ursodiol should be used cautiously in patients with liver disease but may actually improve liver enzyme levels.
- Gallbladder stone dissolution requires months of therapy and is not always fully effective; and stones may recur within 5 yr of treatment.

AGE-RELATED

- **Children:** Safety and efficacy of ursodiol have not been established in children.
- **Elderly:** No age-related precautions have been noted.

PREGNANCY/LACTATION-RELATED

- Pregnancy category B; excretion into breast milk unknown.

MONITORING

- **Baseline assessment:** Patients should be carefully selected for ursodiol therapy because gallstones may not dissolve for months after initiating therapy.
- **Lab work:** Baseline biochemical profile including renal (BUN, creatinine) and liver (alkaline phosphatase, bilirubin, AST [SGOT], and ALT [SGPT]) function tests before the start of ursodiol therapy, 1 and 3 mo after therapy begins, and every 6 mo thereafter, to assess hepatic function.

- **Cholecystitis:** Assess for abdominal pain, especially right upper quadrant pain, nausea, and vomiting.
- **Patient education:** Explain that ursodiol therapy requires months of use to be effective. Instruct to avoid taking antacids within hours of taking ursodiol.

SERIOUS ADVERSE REACTIONS

- None of significance.

OVERDOSE/TOXICITY

- No cases of toxicity have been reported.
- **GI decontamination:** No specific recommendations.

ANTIDOTE/DIALYSIS

- **Antidote:** No specific recommendations.
- **Dialysis:** Ursodiol is unlikely to be removed by hemodialysis or peritoneal dialysis. No data are available on removal by high-permeability hemodialysis.

valacyclovir hydrochloride

val-a-sye'-kloh-vir hye-droe-klor'-ide

Classes

Chemical: acyclic purine nucleoside analog, acyclovir derivative
Therapeutic: antiviral

Pregnancy Category: B

Trade Names

Prescription: Valtrex

CLINICAL PHARMACOLOGY

Mechanism of Action

A virustatic antiviral that is converted to acyclovir triphosphate, becoming part of the viral DNA chain. Therapeutic Effect: Interferes with DNA synthesis and replication of herpes simplex virus and varicella-zoster virus.

PHARMACOKINETICS

Rapidly absorbed after PO administration. Protein binding: 13%-18%. Rapidly converted by hydrolysis to the active compound acyclovir. Widely distributed to tissues and body fluids (including cerebrospinal fluid [CSF]). Primarily eliminated in urine. Removed by hemodialysis. Half-life: 2.5-3.3 hr (increased in impaired renal function).

AVAILABILITY

Caplets: 500 mg, 1000 mg.

INDICATIONS AND DOSAGE

Herpes zoster (shingles)

PO

Adults, Elderly: 1 g 3 times per day for 7 days.

Herpes simplex (cold sores)

PO

Adults, Elderly: 2 g twice per day for 1 day.

Initial episode of genital herpes

PO

Adults, Elderly: 1 g twice per day for 10 days.

Recurrent episodes of genital herpes

PO

Adults, Elderly: 500 mg twice per day for 3 days.

Prevention of genital herpes

PO

Adults, Elderly: 500-1000 mg/day.

Dosage in renal impairment

Dosage and frequency are modified based on creatinine clearance.

Creatinine Clearance	Herpes Zoster	Genital Herpes (initial episode)	Genital Herpes (recurrent)
50 mL/min or higher	1 g every 8 hr	1 g every 12 hr	500 mg every 12 hr
30-49 mL/min	1 g every 12 hr	1 g every 12 hr	500 mg every 12 hr
10-29 mL/min	1 g every 24 hr	1 g every 24 hr	500 mg every 24 hr
Less than 10 mL/min	500 mg every 24 hr	500 mg every 24 hr	500 mg every 24 hr

OFF-LABEL USES

To reduce the risk of heterosexual transmission of genital herpes

CONTRAINDICATIONS

Hypersensitivity to or intolerance of acyclovir, valacyclovir, or their components

INTERACTIONS

Drug: **Cimetidine, probenecid:** May increase acyclovir blood concentration. Herbal: None known. Food: None known.

DIAGNOSTIC TEST EFFECTS

None known.

SIDE-EFFECTS

Frequent: **Herpes zoster (17%-10%):** Nausea, headache. **Genital herpes (17%):** Headache. Occasional: **Herpes zoster (7%-3%):** Vomiting, diarrhea, constipation (50 yr or older), asthenia, dizziness (50 yr and older). **Genital herpes (8%-3%):** Nausea, diarrhea, dizziness. Rare: **Herpes zoster (3%-1%):** Abdominal pain, anorexia. **Genital herpes (3%-1%):** Asthenia, abdominal pain

CRITICAL CARE CONSIDERATIONS

ADMINISTRATION/HANDLING

GENERAL ALERT

- Be aware that valacyclovir therapy for shingles is most effective when started within 48 hr of the onset of the herpes zoster rash.

PO ALERT

- Give valacyclovir without regard to food.
- Do not crush or break tablets.

PRECAUTIONS

HEALTH-RELATED

- Use valacyclovir cautiously in patients with diabetes mellitus or hepatic impairment.
- Use valacyclovir cautiously in patients with advanced HIV infection, fluid or electrolyte

V

imbalances, neurologic abnormalities, or renal or hepatic impairment; in dehydrated patients; in those who have had a bone marrow or kidney transplant; and in those using nephrotoxic agents concurrently.

AGE-RELATED

- **Children:** Safety and efficacy of valacyclovir have not been established in children.
- **Elderly:** Age-related renal impairment may require a dosage reduction.

PREGNANCY/LACTATION-RELATED

- Pregnancy category B; excreted as acyclovir into breast milk; safety not established but should be compatible with breast-feeding.

MONITORING

- **Baseline assessment:** Determine history of allergies, particularly to acyclovir or valacyclovir, before beginning drug therapy. Assess medical history, especially in those with advanced HIV infection, hepatic or renal impairment, and in those who have had a bone marrow or kidney transplant.
- **Lab work:** Baseline CBC with differential; biochemical profile with renal (BUN, creatinine) and liver (AST [SGOT], ALT [SGPT], alkaline phosphatase, bilirubin) function studies. Obtain tissue cultures from herpes simplex and herpes zoster patients before giving the first dose of valacyclovir. Therapy may proceed before test results are known. Monitor CBC, liver and renal function, and urinalysis results.
- **Lesions:** Evaluate for appearance and patterning of cutaneous lesions.
- **Herpes zoster patients:** Follow current Centers for Disease Control guidelines for isolation of patients. Keep fingernails short and hands clean to prevent injury from patients scratching lesions and spreading lesions to new sites.
- **Pain:** Provide analgesics and comfort measures for herpes zoster patients. Herpes zoster is especially exhausting for the elderly.
- **Hydration:** Provide with adequate fluids to help renal clearance of valacyclovir.
- **Patient education:** Encourage to drink adequate fluids. Teach about starting valacyclovir treatment at the first sign of a recurrent episode of genital herpes or herpes zoster. Explain that treatment is most effective when started within 48 hr after prodromal symptoms first appear. Caution not to touch lesions to avoid spreading the infection to new sites. Advise genital herpes patients to follow prescription instructions carefully on how to take valacyclovir and to continue taking the drug for the full course of treatment. Warn genital herpes patients to avoid sexual intercourse while lesions are present or, if prodromal symptoms are present, to prevent infecting partners. Instruct to report if lesions do not improve or if they recur. Urge female patients with genital herpes to have a Pap test at least annually because of the increased risk of cervical cancer associated with genital herpes. Inform that valacyclovir treats but does not cure genital herpes.

SERIOUS ADVERSE REACTIONS

- **Thrombotic thrombocytopenic purpura/hemolytic uremic syndrome (TTP/HUS):** Has occurred in patients with advanced HIV disease, in allogenic bone marrow transplant patients, and renal transplant recipient patients receiving doses of 8 g daily.
- **Hypersensitivity:** Rash, pruritis, erythema multiforme, photosensitivity, angioedema, dyspnea, urticaria, anaphylaxis.
- **Hepatobiliary:** Hepatitis, elevated liver enzymes.

OVERDOSE/TOXICITY

- **Nephrotoxicity:** Elevated BUN, creatinine, nausea, vomiting, back or flank pain, abdominal pain, oliguria, anuria, hematuria.
- **Neurotoxicity:** CNS symptoms, including confusion, agitation, hallucinations, delirium, encephalopathy, are seen more commonly in the elderly.
- **Hematologic:** Thrombocytopenia, aplastic anemia, vasculitis.
- **GI decontamination:** No specific recommendations.

ANTIDOTE/DIALYSIS

- **Antidote:** No specific recommendations.
- **Dialysis:** Valacyclovir is removed by hemodialysis, and is likely to be removed by high-permeability hemodialysis. It is not removed by peritoneal dialysis.

valganciclovir hydrochloride

See Antivirals (p. 937)

V

valproic acid/valproate sodium/divalproex sodium

val-proe'-ik

Classes

Chemical: carboxylic acid derivative
Therapeutic: anticonvulsant

Pregnancy Category: D

Trade Names

Prescription: (valproic acid) Depakene; (valproate sodium) Depakene syrup; (divalproex sodium) Depacon, Depakote, Depakote ER, Depakote Sprinkle

CLINICAL PHARMACOLOGY

Mechanism of Action

An anticonvulsant, antimanic, and antimigraine agent that directly increases concentration of the inhibitory neurotransmitter gamma-aminobutyric acid. **Therapeutic Effect:** Reduces seizure activity.

PHARMACOKINETICS

Well absorbed from the GI tract. Protein binding: 80%-90%. Metabolized in the liver. Primarily excreted in urine. Not removed by hemodialysis. **Half-life:** 6-16 hr (may be increased in hepatic impairment, the elderly, and children younger than 18 mo).

AVAILABILITY

Capsules (Depakene): 250 mg.
Syrup (Depakene): 250 mg/5 mL.
Tablets (delayed release [Depakote]): 125 mg, 250 mg, 500 mg.
Tablets (extended release [Depakote ER]): 250 mg, 500 mg.
Capsule sprinkles (Depakote Sprinkle): 125 mg.
Injection (Depacon): 100 mg/mL.

INDICATIONS AND DOSAGE

Seizures (epilepsy)

PO

Adults, Elderly, Children 10 yr and older: Initially, 10-15 mg/kg/day in 1-3 divided doses. May increase by 5-10 mg/kg/day at weekly intervals up to 30-60 mg/kg/day. Usual adult dosage: 1000-2500 mg/day.

IV

Adults, Elderly, Children: Same as oral dose but given every 6 hr.

Manic episodes

PO

Adults, Elderly: Initially, 750 mg/day in divided doses. Maximum: 60 mg/kg/day.

PO (Extended Release)

Adults, Elderly: 25 mg/kg/day once daily. Maximum: 60 mg/kg/day.

Prevention of migraine headaches

PO (Extended Release)

Adults, Elderly: Initially, 500 mg/day for 7 days. May increase up to 1000 mg/day.

PO (Delayed Release)

Adults, Elderly: Initially, 250 mg twice per day. May increase up to 1000 mg/day.

OFF-LABEL USES

Prevention of migraine; treatment of behavior disorders in Alzheimer's disease; bipolar disorder; chorea, myoclonic, simple partial, and tonic-clonic seizures; organic brain syndrome; schizophrenia; status epilepticus; tardive dyskinesia

CONTRAINDICATIONS

Active hepatic disease, urea cycle disorders, hypersensitivity to valproic acid; not recommended for prevention of seizures following head trauma

INTERACTIONS

Drug: Alcohol, other CNS depressants: May increase CNS depressant effects. **Amitriptyline, primidone:** May increase the blood concentration of these drugs. **Anticoagulants, heparin, platelet aggregation inhibitors, thrombolytics:** May increase the risk of bleeding. **Carbamazepine:** May decrease valproic acid blood concentration. **Hepatotoxic medications:** May increase the risk of hepatotoxicity. **Phenytoin:** May increase the risk of phenytoin toxicity and decrease the effects of valproic acid. **Herbal:** None known. **Food:** None known.

DIAGNOSTIC TEST EFFECTS

May increase serum LDH, bilirubin, AST (SGOT), and ALT (SGPT) levels. Therapeutic serum level is 50-100 mcg/mL; toxic serum level is greater than 100 mcg/mL. May cause false elevation of urine ketones.

IV INCOMPATIBILITIES

Do not mix valproic acid with any other medications.

SIDE-EFFECTS

Frequent: Epilepsy: Abdominal pain, irregular menses, diarrhea, transient alopecia, indigestion, nausea, vomiting, tremors, weight gain or loss. **Mania (22%-19%):** Nausea, somnolence. **Occasional: Epilepsy:** Constipation, dizziness, drowsiness, headache, skin rash, unusual excitement, restlessness. **Mania (12%-6%):** Asthenia, abdominal pain, dyspepsia (heartburn, indigestion,

V

epigastric distress), rash. **Rare: Epilepsy:** Mood changes, diplopia, nystagmus, spots before eyes, unusual bleeding or ecchymosis

CRITICAL CARE CONSIDERATIONS

ADMINISTRATION/HANDLING

PO ALERT

- Give delayed-release or extended-release tablets whole.
- Give valproic acid without regard to food, but do not administer with carbonated drinks. Capsule contents may be sprinkled on applesauce and given immediately; however, do not break, chew, or crush sprinkle beads.
- Regular-release and delayed-release formulations are given in 2-4 divided doses daily; extended-release formulations are given once per day.

IV ALERT

- **Storage:** Store vials at room temperature.
- **Stability:** Diluted solutions are stable for 24 hr. Discard unused portion.
- **Dilution:** Dilute each single dose with at least 50 mL D_5W, 0.9% NaCl, or lactated Ringer's solution.
- **IV intermittent infusion:** Infuse over 5-10 min. Do not exceed an infusion rate of 3 mg/kg/min (5-min infusion) or 1.5 mg/kg/min (10-min infusion). Too-rapid infusion increases the likelihood of side effects.

PRECAUTIONS

HEALTH-RELATED

- Use valproic acid cautiously in patients with bleeding abnormalities or a history of hepatic disease.

AGE-RELATED

- **Children:** Children under 2 yr are at increased risk for hepatotoxicity.
- **Elderly:** Lower dosages are recommended, although no age-related precautions have been noted for elderly.

PREGNANCY/LACTATION-RELATED

- Pregnancy category D. Teratogenic; increased risk of neural tube defects (1%-2% when used between days 17-30 after fertilization); compatible with breast-feeding.

MONITORING

- **Baseline assessment:** Assess seizure patients' LOC and review history of the seizure disorder (duration, frequency, and intensity of seizures). Assess manic patients' appearance, behavior, emotional status, response to environment, speech pattern, and thought content. For migraine management, determine the duration, location, onset, and precipitating factors of migraine headaches.
- **Lab work:** For seizure patients, obtain a CBC and platelet count before beginning valproic acid therapy, 2 wk later, and again 2 wk after the maintenance dose has been established. Monitor CBC and biochemical profile including liver function tests (alkaline phosphatase, ammonia, bilirubin, AST [SGOT], and ALT [SGPT] levels).
- **Seizure precautions:** Initiate precautions and provide patients with a dark, quiet environment. Monitor seizure patients for evidence of clinical improvement, such as a decrease in the frequency or intensity of seizures.
- **Mania:** Assess for improvement in manic patients' appearance, behavior, emotional status, response to environment, speech pattern, and thought content; improved ability to concentrate, increased interest in surroundings, and a relaxed facial expression.
- **Migraine headaches:** Evaluate for relief of migraine headache and associated symptoms, such as nausea, vomiting, phonophobia, and photophobia.
- **Thrombocytopenia:** Assess seizure patients' skin for ecchymosis and petechiae, and observe frequently for recurrence of seizure activity.
- **Drug levels:** Monitor valproic acid serum levels. Therapeutic serum drug level is 50-100 mcg/mL. Toxic drug level is greater than 100 mcg/mL.
- **Patient education:** Caution against abruptly discontinuing valproic acid after long-term use because this may precipitate seizures. Explain that strict maintenance of drug therapy is essential for seizure control. Instruct to report promptly abdominal pain, altered mental status, bleeding, easy bruising, lethargy, loss of appetite, nausea, vomiting, weakness, or yellowing of skin to a health care provider. Warn to avoid tasks that require mental alertness or motor skills until response to the drug is known. Inform that drowsiness usually disappears with continued therapy. Urge avoidance of alcohol while taking valproic acid. Recommend carrying an

identification card or wearing an identification bracelet that displays the seizure disorder and anticonvulsant therapy.

SERIOUS ADVERSE REACTIONS

- **Thrombocytopenia:** Greater incidence of low platelets was seen with higher doses of valproic acid.
- **Somnolence in elderly:** Incidence may be higher in those with poor nutritional intake, malnutrition, and those who experienced weight loss.
- **Posttraumatic seizures:** One study revealed the mortality rate of head trauma patients managed with valproic acid may have been higher than head trauma patients managed with a different anticonvulsant to control seizures.

OVERDOSE/TOXICITY

- **Hepatotoxicity:** May occur, particularly in the first 6 months of valproic acid therapy. It may be preceded by loss of seizure control, malaise, weakness, lethargy, anorexia, and vomiting rather than abnormal serum liver function test results. May be fatal.
- **Pancreatitis:** Cases of life-threatening pancreatitis have been reported in children and adults. Some cases of hemorrhagic pancreatitis progressed rapidly from initial mild symptoms to death. Cases occurred both shortly after initiating therapy and after years of use.
- **GI decontamination:** No specific recommendations.

ANTIDOTE/DIALYSIS

- **Antidote:** No specific recommendations.
- **Dialysis:** Valproic acid is not removed by hemodialysis or peritoneal dialysis. No data are available on removal by high-permeability hemodialysis.

valsartan

val-sar'-tan

V

Classes

Chemical: angiotensin II receptor antagonist

Therapeutic: antihypertensive

Pregnancy Category: C (1st trimester), D (2nd and 3rd trimester)

Trade Names

Prescription: Diovan

Combinations

Prescription: with hydrochlorothiazide (Diovan HCT)

Do not confuse valsartan with Valstan.

CLINICAL PHARMACOLOGY

Mechanism of Action

An angiotensin II receptor, type AT_1, antagonist that blocks vasoconstrictor and aldosterone-secreting effects of angiotensin II, inhibiting the binding of angiotensin II to the AT_1 receptors. **Therapeutic Effect:** Causes vasodilation, decreases peripheral resistance, and decreases BP.

PHARMACOKINETICS

Poorly absorbed after PO administration. Food decreases peak plasma concentration. Protein binding: 95%. Metabolized in the liver. Recovered primarily in feces and, to a lesser extent, in urine. Not removed by hemodialysis. **Half-life:** 6 hr.

AVAILABILITY

Tablets: 40 mg, 80 mg, 160 mg, 320 mg.

INDICATIONS AND DOSAGE

Hypertension

PO

Adults, Elderly: Initially, 80-160 mg/day in patients who are not volume depleted. May increase up to a maximum: 320 mg/day.

Heart failure

PO

Adults, Elderly: Initially, 40 mg twice per day. May increase up to 160 mg twice per day. Maximum: 320 mg/day.

Post–heart attack

PO

Adults, Elderly: Initially, 20 mg twice per day. May increase within 7 days to 40 mg twice per day. May further increase up to target dose of 160 mg twice per day.

OFF-LABEL USES

Diabetic nephropathy

CONTRAINDICATIONS

Bilateral renal artery stenosis, biliary cirrhosis or obstruction, hypoaldosteronism, severe hepatic impairment, hypersensitivity to valsartan

INTERACTIONS

Drug: Diuretics: Produce additive hypotensive effects. **Herbal:** None known. **Food:**

All foods: Decrease peak plasma concentration of valsartan.

DIAGNOSTIC TEST EFFECTS

May increase AST (SGOT), ALT (SGPT), and serum bilirubin, creatinine, and potassium levels. May decrease blood Hgb and Hct levels.

SIDE-EFFECTS

Rare (2%-1%): Insomnia, fatigue, heartburn, abdominal pain, dizziness, headache, diarrhea, nausea, vomiting, arthralgia, edema

CRITICAL CARE CONSIDERATIONS

ADMINISTRATION/HANDLING

PO ALERT

- Give valsartan without regard to meals.
- Valsartan may be given concurrently with other antihypertensives. If BP is not controlled by valsartan alone, a diuretic may be added.

PRECAUTIONS

HEALTH-RELATED

- Use valsartan cautiously in patients also receiving potassium-sparing diuretics or potassium supplements.
- Use cautiously in patients with coronary artery disease, mild to moderate hepatic impairment, or unilateral renal artery stenosis. For patients with severe heart failure, monitor for impaired renal function.

AGE-RELATED

- **Children:** Safety and efficacy of valsartan have not been established in children.
- **Elderly:** No age-related precautions have been noted.

PREGNANCY/LACTATION-RELATED

- Pregnancy category C, first trimester—category D, second and third trimesters. Drugs acting directly on the renin-angiotensin-aldosterone system are documented to cause fetal harm (hypotension, oligohydramnios, neonatal anemia, hyperkalemia, neonatal skull hypoplasia, anuria, and renal failure); neonatal limb contractures, craniofacial deformities, and hypoplastic lung development; unknown if distributed in breast milk.

MONITORING

- **Baseline assessment:** Assess heart rate and BP immediately before each valsartan dose and regularly throughout therapy. Be alert to fluctuations in heart rate and BP. Determine if patients are pregnant. Assess the medication history, especially for diuretics. Determine history of hepatic or renal impairment, renal artery stenosis, or severe heart failure.
- **Lab work:** Baseline and periodic ongoing measurement of CBC; biochemical profile with renal (BUN, creatinine) and liver (AST [SGOT], ALT [SGPT], alkaline phosphatase, bilirubin) function tests.
- **Hypotension:** If an excessive reduction in BP occurs, place in the supine position with feet slightly elevated. Offer fluids frequently to maintain hydration, which helps prevent hypotension.
- **Cardiac ischemia:** Monitor ECG continuously for ST segment depression or elevation in patients new to valsartan with history of chest discomfort or MI.
- **Dependent edema:** Examine for edema of extremities, ankles, and sacrum.
- **Fluid retention:** Auscultate the lungs for rales. Monitor intake and output and daily weights. Edema and fluid retention may indicate worsening heart failure or renal insufficiency.
- **Fall prevention:** Assist with ambulation if dizziness occurs.
- **Cough:** Assess cough. If persistent and severe, discontinuation of therapy may be warranted.
- **Hydration:** Offer fluids frequently or administer IV fluids to maintain hydration. Hypotension is common in volume-depleted patients.
- **Surgery/anesthesia:** If patients become hypotensive during a procedure, the blocked angiotensin II impairs BP compensation, prompting the need for correction of hypovolemia with IV fluid boluses.
- **Upper respiratory tract infection:** Assess for nasal congestion, cough, itching eyes.
- **Patient education:** Advise female patients of the consequences of second- and third-trimester exposure to valsartan. Stress to female patients that they should immediately report plans to become pregnant or pregnancy to the prescriber. Instruct to report promptly infections, including fever and sore throat, to a health care provider. Explain that valsartan must be taken throughout life to control hypertension. Caution against exercising outside during hot weather because of the risks of dehydration and hypotension.

V

SERIOUS ADVERSE REACTIONS

- **Excessive hypotension:** May occur in patients with heart failure and severe salt and volume depletion.
- **Angioedema:** Swelling of face and lips; when involving the tongue, lips, and larynx, may require subcutaneous epinephrine 1:1000 solution (0.3-0.5 mL) with possible endotracheal intubation to maintain patent airway.
- **Hyperkalemia:** Occurs rarely and may be associated with renal insufficiency.

OVERDOSE/TOXICITY

- **Hepatotoxicity:** Elevated liver enzymes (AST [SGOT], ALT [SGPT], alkaline phosphatase, bilirubin).
- **Cardiovascular:** Overdosage may manifest as hypotension and tachycardia due to vasodilation. Bradycardia occurs less often.
- **GI decontamination:** No specific recommendations.

ANTIDOTE/DIALYSIS

- **Antidote:** No specific recommendations.
- **Dialysis:** Valsartan is not removed by hemodialysis and is unlikely to be removed by peritoneal dialysis. No data are available on removal by high-permeability hemodialysis.

vancomycin hydrochloride

van-koe-mye'-sin high-droe-klor'-ide

Classes

Chemical: tricyclic glycopeptide derivative
Therapeutic: antibiotic

Pregnancy Category: C (oral), B (IV)

Trade Names

Prescription: Lyphocin, Vancocin, Vancocin HC1, Vancocin HCl Pulvules

CLINICAL PHARMACOLOGY

Mechanism of Action

A tricyclic glycopeptide antibiotic that binds to bacterial cell walls, altering cell membrane permeability and inhibiting RNA synthesis. **Therapeutic Effect:** Bactericidal.

PHARMACOKINETICS

PO: Not absorbed from the GI tract. Primarily eliminated in feces. **Parenteral:** Widely distributed. Protein binding: 55%. Primarily excreted unchanged in urine. **Half-life:** 4-11 hr (increased in impaired renal function).

AVAILABILITY

Capsules (Vancocin HCl Pulvules): 125 mg, 250 mg.
Powder for oral suspension (Vancocin): 1 g (provides 250 mg/5 mL after mixing).
Powder for injection (Lyphocin, Vancocin HCl): 500 mg, 1 g, 5 g, 10 g.
Infusion (premix [Vancocin HCl]): 500 mg/100 mL, 1 g/200 mL.

INDICATIONS AND DOSAGE

Treatment of bone, respiratory tract, skin and soft-tissue infections, endocarditis, peritonitis, and septicemia; prevention of bacterial endocarditis in those at risk (if penicillin is contraindicated) when undergoing biliary, dental, GI, GU, or respiratory surgery or invasive procedures

IV

Adults, Elderly: 500 mg every 6 hr or 1 g every 12 hr. **Children older than 1 mo:** 40 mg/kg/day in divided doses every 6-8 hr. Maximum: 3-4 g/day. **Neonates:** Initially 15 mg/kg, then 10 mg/kg every 8-12 hr.

Staphylococcal enterocolitis, antibiotic-associated pseudomembranous colitis caused by *Clostridium difficile*

PO

Adults, Elderly: 125 mg 4 times per day for 7-10 days. **Children:** 40 mg/kg/day in 3-4 divided doses for 7-10 days. Maximum: 2 g/day.

Dosage in renal impairment

After a loading dose, subsequent dosages and frequency are modified based on creatinine clearance, the severity of the infection, and the serum concentration of the drug.

OFF-LABEL USES

Treatment of brain abscess, perioperative infections, staphylococcal or streptococcal meningitis

CONTRAINDICATIONS

Hypersensitivity to vancomycin

INTERACTIONS

Drug: Aminoglycosides, amphotericin B, aspirin, bumetanide, carmustine, cisplatin, *cycloSPORINE, ethacrynic acid, furosemide, streptozocin: May increase the risk of ototoxicity and nephrotoxicity of parenteral vancomycin. **Cholestyramine, colestipol:** May decrease the effects of oral vancomycin. **Herbal:** None known. **Food:** None known.

DIAGNOSTIC TEST EFFECTS

May increase BUN level. Therapeutic peak serum level is 20-40 mcg/mL; therapeutic trough serum level is 5-20 mcg/mL. Toxic peak serum level is greater than 40 mcg/mL; toxic trough serum level is greater than 20 mcg/mL. Trough level of 15-20 mcg/mL is acceptable for pneumonia.

IV INCOMPATIBILITIES

Albumin, amphotericin B complex (Abelcet, AmBisome, Amphotec), aztreonam (Azactam), cefazolin (Ancef), cefepime (Maxipime), cefotaxime (Claforan), cefotetan (Cefotan), cefoxitin (Mefoxin), ceftazidime (Fortaz), ceftriaxone (Rocephin), cefuroxime (Zinacef), foscarnet (Foscavir), heparin, idarubicin (Idamycin), nafcillin (Nafcil), piperacillin and tazobactam (Zosyn), ticarcillin and clavulanate (Timentin)

IV COMPATIBILITIES

Amiodarone (Cordarone), calcium gluconate, diltiazem (Cardizem), hydromorphone (Dilaudid), insulin, lorazepam (Ativan), magnesium sulfate, midazolam (Versed), morphine, potassium chloride, propofol (Diprivan), total parenteral nutrition (TPN)

SIDE-EFFECTS

Frequent: PO: Bitter or unpleasant taste, nausea, vomiting, mouth irritation (with oral solution). **Rare: Parenteral:** Phlebitis, thrombophlebitis, or pain at peripheral IV site; dizziness; vertigo; tinnitus; chills; fever; rash; necrosis with extravasation. **PO:** Rash.

CRITICAL CARE CONSIDERATIONS

ADMINISTRATION/HANDLING

PO ALERT

- Oral vancomycin is usually not given for systemic infections because it is poorly absorbed from the GI tract; however, patients with colitis (especially pseudomembranous colitis) are sometimes effectively treated using oral therapy.
- **Reconstitution:** Reconstitute powder for oral solution as appropriate and administer orally or by nasogastric tube. Do not use powder for oral solution for IV administration.
- **Stability:** The refrigerated oral solution is stable for 2 wk.

IV ALERT

- **Not for IV push:** Give vancomycin by intermittent IV infusion (piggyback) or continuous IV infusion. Do not give by IV push because this may result in exaggerated hypotension.
- **Intermittent IV infusion (piggyback):** Reconstitute each 500-mg or 1-g vial with 10 mL or 20 mL, respectively, of sterile water for injection to provide a concentration of 50 mg/mL. Further dilute to a final concentration of no more than 5 mg/mL. Discard the solution if a precipitate forms. Administer the solution over 60 min or more. Monitor BP closely during the infusion.
- **Stability after reconstitution:** IV solution may be refrigerated and should be used within 14 days.
- **ADD-Vantage vials:** Should not be used in neonates, infants, and children requiring less than a 500-mg dose.

PRECAUTIONS

HEALTH-RELATED

- Use vancomycin cautiously in patients with preexisting hearing impairment or renal dysfunction and in patients taking other ototoxic or nephrotoxic medications concurrently.

AGE-RELATED

- **Children:** Close monitoring of serum drug levels is recommended in premature neonates and young infants.
- **Elderly:** Age-related renal impairment may increase the risk of ototoxicity and nephrotoxicity in the elderly. Dosage reduction is recommended.

PREGNANCY/LACTATION-RELATED

- Pregnancy category C (oral), B (IV); excreted into breast milk, milk level 4 hr after steady-state dose, 12.7 mcg/mL (similar to mother's trough level); poorly absorbed orally, systemic absorption not expected. Problems limited to modification of bowel flora, allergic sensitization, and interference with interpretation of culture results during evaluation of febrile illness.

MONITORING

- **Baseline assessment:** Assess for ototoxic and nephrotoxic properties of other medications patients may be taking; do not administer vancomycin concurrently with other ototoxic and nephrotoxic medications. If concurrent use is necessary, administer the drugs cautiously.
- **Lab work:** CBC with WBC differential; biochemical profile with renal (BUN, creatinine) and liver (AST [SGOT], ALT [SGPT], bilirubin, alkaline phosphatase)

function tests. Obtain culture and sensitivity tests before giving the first dose of vancomycin. Therapy may begin before test results are known.

- **Renal dysfunction:** Monitor intake and output and renal function test results.
- **Allergic reaction:** Assess the skin for rash.
- **Ototoxicity:** Evaluate balance and hearing acuity (eighth cranial nerve).
- **Phlebitis:** Evaluate the IV infusion site for heat, pain, and red streaking over the vein.
- **Drug levels:** Assess vancomycin levels. Therapeutic peak serum level is 20-40 mcg/mL, and the trough level is 5-20 mcg/mL. Toxic peak serum level is greater than 40 mcg/mL, and the trough level is greater than 20 mcg/mL.
- **Superinfection:** Assess the mouth for white patches on the mucous membranes or tongue, for severe mouth or tongue soreness and for severe anal or genital pruritus or discharge with all forms of vancomycin.
- **Possible *Clostridium difficile* (CDAD) colitis:** Assess pattern of daily bowel activity and stool consistency. Although mild GI effects may be tolerable, severe symptoms including abdominal pain or cramping and moderate to severe diarrhea may indicate the onset of antibiotic-associated colitis. Vancomycin is used to manage colitis in some patients.
- **Hand washing:** If *C. difficile* (antibiotic-associated) colitis develops, wash hands with antibacterial soap. Alcohol-based foam is ineffective against *C. difficile* spores.
- **Patient education:** Advise to space drug doses evenly around the clock and to continue vancomycin therapy for the full course of treatment. Instruct to report promptly a rash, tinnitus, or symptoms of nephrotoxicity to a health care provider. Inform that laboratory tests are an important part of the therapy regimen.

SERIOUS ADVERSE REACTIONS

- **Red-neck syndrome:** Redness on face, neck, arms, and back; chills; fever; tachycardia; nausea or vomiting; pruritus; rash; unpleasant taste may result from too-rapid injection.
- **Hypersensitivity:** Severe pruritus, angioedema, bronchospasm, and anaphylaxis.
- **Management of hypersensitivity:** May require treatment with epinephrine and other emergency measures including oxygen, endotracheal intubation, mechanical ventilation, IV fluids, IV antihistamines, corticosteroids, and vasopressors.

OVERDOSE/TOXICITY

- **Ototoxicity:** Temporary or permanent hearing loss may occur.
- **Nephrotoxicity:** Increased BUN and creatinine, decreased urine output, anuria, possible hyperkalemia, fluid overload indicative of acute renal failure.
- **Superinfections:** Antibiotic-associated colitis (pseudomembranous colitis, *C. difficile*–associated disease [CDAD]) and other superinfections may result from altered bacterial balance.
- **Management of pseudomembranous colitis (CDAD):** Fluids, electrolytes, protein supplements, oral vancomycin (Vancocin) or IV metronidazole (Flagyl).
- **GI decontamination:** No specific recommendations.

ANTIDOTE/DIALYSIS

- **Antidote:** No specific recommendations.
- **Dialysis:** Vancomycin is removed by high-permeability hemodialysis but is not removed by standard hemodialysis or peritoneal dialysis.

vasopressin

vay-soe-press'-in

Classes

Chemical: arginine vasopressin
Therapeutic: antidiuretic, hemostatic

Pregnancy Category: C

Trade Names

Prescription: Pitressin, Pressyn AR ♣

Do not confuse Pitressin with Pitocin.

CLINICAL PHARMACOLOGY

Mechanism of Action

A posterior pituitary hormone that increases reabsorption of water by the renal tubules. Increases water permeability at the distal tubule and collecting duct. Directly stimulates smooth muscle in the GI tract. **Therapeutic Effect:** Causes peristalsis and vasoconstriction.

PHARMACOKINETICS

Route	Onset	Peak	Duration
IV	N/A	N/A	0.5-1 hr
IM, Subcutaneous	1-2 hr	N/A	2-8 hr

Distributed throughout extracellular fluid. Metabolized in the liver and kidney. Primarily excreted in urine. **Half-life:** 10–20 min.

AVAILABILITY

Injection: 20 units/mL.

INDICATIONS AND DOSAGE

Cardiac arrest

IV

Adults, Elderly: 40 units as a one-time bolus.

Diabetes insipidus

IV Infusion

Adults, Children: 0.5 mUnits/kg/hr (or 0.0005 units/kg/hr). May double dose every 30 min. Maximum: 10 mUnits/kg/hr (or 0.01 units/kg/hr).

IM, Subcutaneous

Adults, Elderly: 5-10 units 2-4 times per day. Range: 5-60 unit/day. **Children:** 2.5-10 units, 2-4 times per day.

Abdominal distention, intestinal paresis

IM

Adults, Elderly: Initially 5 units. Subsequent doses, 10 units every 3-4 hr.

GI hemorrhage

IV Infusion

Adults, Elderly: Initially 0.2-0.4 unit/min progressively increased to 0.9 unit/min. **Children:** 0.002-0.005 unit/kg/min. Titrate as needed. Maximum: 0.01 unit/kg/min.

Vasodilatory shock

IV

Adults, Elderly: Initially, 0.04 unit/min. Do not titrate.

OFF-LABEL USES

Adjunct in treatment of acute, massive hemorrhage

CONTRAINDICATIONS

Hypersensitivity to vasopressin preparations

INTERACTIONS

Drug: Alcohol, demeclocycline, lithium, norepinephrine: May decrease the effects of vasopressin. **Carbamazepine, *chlorproPAMIDE, clofibrate:** May increase the effects of vasopressin. **Herbal:** None known. **Food:** None known.

DIAGNOSTIC TEST EFFECTS

None known.

IV INCOMPATIBILITIES

Amphotericin B complex (Abelcet, AmBisome, Amphotec), diazepam (Valium), etomidate (Amidate), furosemide (Lasix), thiopentothal

IV COMPATIBILITIES

*DOBUTamine (Dobutrex), *DOPamine (Intropin), heparin, lorazepam (Ativan), midazolam (Versed), milrinone (Primacor), verapamil (Calan, Isoptin)

SIDE-EFFECTS

Frequent: Pain at injection site (with vasopressin tannate). **Occasional:** Abdominal cramps, nausea, vomiting, diarrhea, dizziness, diaphoresis, pale skin, circumoral pallor, tremors, headache, eructation, flatulence. **Rare:** Chest pain; confusion; allergic reaction, including rash or hives, pruritus, wheezing or difficulty breathing, facial and peripheral edema; sterile abscess (with vasopressin tannate)

CRITICAL CARE CONSIDERATIONS

ADMINISTRATION/HANDLING

IV ALERT

- **Storage:** Store vasopressin at room temperature.
- **Dilution:** Dilute with D_5W or 0.9% NaCl to concentration of 0.1-1.0 unit/mL.
- **Administration:** Give as IV infusion, unless managing a cardiac arrest due to ventricular fibrillation, wherein full strength drug can be given undiluted IV push.

IM, SUBCUTANEOUS ALERT

- Give with 1-2 glasses of water to reduce side effects.
- Used primarily to manage diabetes insipidus.

INTRANASAL ALERT

- May administer intranasally on cotton pledgets, or by nasal spray; individualize dosage.
- Used to manage diabetes insipidus.

PRECAUTIONS

HEALTH-RELATED

- Use vasopressin cautiously in patients with arteriosclerosis, asthma, cardiac disease, goiter with cardiac complications, migraine, nephritis, renal disease, seizures, or vascular disease.

AGE-RELATED

- Vasopressin should be used cautiously in children and the elderly because of the risk of water intoxication and hyponatremia in these age-groups.

PREGNANCY/LACTATION-RELATED

- Pregnancy category C; breast-feeding reported without complications.

MONITORING

- **Baseline assessment:** Vital signs (note BP and heart rate), urine specific gravity, and

V

weight. If vasopressin is being used to manage hypotension in the intensive care unit, another vasopressor should be used for primary BP support. Vasopressin is used to augment efforts to raise BP with pressor amines, rather than to increase BP as a sole agent. If drug is used to manage ventricular fibrillation during cardiac arrest, vasopressin should be used as the initial drug, rather than beginning drug treatment with epinephrine.

- **Lab work:** Baseline biochemical profile to establish serum electrolyte levels. Monitor serum electrolyte levels and urine specific gravity.
- **Water intoxication:** Monitor fluid intake and output closely, and restrict intake to prevent water intoxication (somnolence, headache, and listlessness). Weigh daily. Patients should have a Foley catheter in place for accurate measurement of urine output.
- **Injection site:** Evaluate site for abscess, erythema, and pain.
- **Side effects:** A reduced dosage may be required depending on side effects.
- **Allergic reaction:** If allergic symptoms or chest pain occurs, withhold the medication.
- **Dysrhythmias:** Continuous ECG monitoring should be used to assess for ST changes and ventricular dysrhythmias.
- **Hypotension:** If vasopressin is used to augment vasopressors, monitor BP response to titration of the vasopressors and then the vasopressin. Vasopressin should be used to try to reduce the dose of vasopressors but should not be used outside the narrow therapeutic window to avoid severe splanchnic vasoconstriction.
- **Patient education:** Warn to report chest pain, headache, shortness of breath, or other symptoms. Stress the importance of monitoring fluid intake and output. Urge avoidance of alcohol during vasopressin therapy.

SERIOUS ADVERSE REACTIONS

- **Hypersensitivity:** Rash, urticaria, anaphylaxis.
- **Acute myocardial infarction:** High doses may lead to coronary arterial vasoconstriction, which may cause myocardial ischemia or infarction, especially in patients with heart disease.

OVERDOSE/TOXICITY

- **Water intoxication:** Retention of high amounts of water results from high doses of vasopressin (which is antidiuretic hormone). The elderly and very young are at higher risk for water intoxication. Symptoms include drowsiness, low energy level, and headache, which may progress to coma and seizures.
- **Splanchnic vasoconstriction:** Vasopressin is a potent vasoconstrictor of intraabdominal blood vessels. High doses used for prolonged periods of time can lead to loss of circulation to abdominal organs, resulting in multiple organ dysfunction syndrome.
- **Management:** Dose of vasopressin should be reduced. If patients have water intoxication, use of a loop diuretic (furosemide, bumetanide) may help to eliminate extra water if urine output does not increase from solely reducing the dose of vasopressin.
- **GI decontamination:** No specific recommendations.

ANTIDOTE/DIALYSIS

- **Antidote:** No specific recommendations.
- **Dialysis:** No data are available on removal of vasopressin by hemodialysis, high-permeability hemodialysis, or peritoneal dialysis.

vecuronium bromide 

vek-yoo-roe'-nee-am broe'-mide

Classes

Chemical: nondepolarizing neuromuscular blocking agent

Therapeutic: skeletal muscle relaxant, paralytic agent, anesthesia adjunct

Pregnancy Category: C

Trade Names

Prescription: Norcuron

CLINICAL PHARMACOLOGY

Mechanism of Action

A nondepolarizing skeletal muscle relaxant that blocks acetylcholine from binding to receptors on motor endplate. **Therapeutic Effect:** Produces skeletal muscle relaxation; inhibits depolarization.

PHARMACOKINETICS

Onset of action is dose dependent and occurs within 2.5-3.0 min. Duration of action is 25-30 min. Protein binding: 60%-80%. Metabolized in liver. Primarily excreted in bile; minimal elimination in urine. **Half-life:** 65-75 min.

AVAILABILITY

Powder for injection: 10 mg, 20 mg (Norcuron).

INDICATIONS AND DOSAGE

Adjunct to general anesthesia; to facilitate endotracheal intubation and to provide skeletal muscle relaxation during surgery or mechanical ventilation

IV

Adults, Elderly, Children older than 10 yr: Initially, 0.08-0.10 mg/kg given as a bolus injection. The first maintenance dose is generally required within 25 to 40 min. The suggested maintenance dose is 0.01-0.015 mg/kg. Subsequent maintenance doses, if required, may be administered at approximately 12- to 15-min intervals. After the bolus dose is given, a continuous infusion may be initiated approximately 20-40 min later. An initial rate of 1 mcg/kg/min is recommended, with the rate of the infusion adjusted thereafter to maintain a 90% suppression of the twitch response. Average infusion rates may range from 0.8 to 1.2 mcg/kg/min.

Children between the ages of 1 and 10 yr: May require a slightly higher initial dose than adults. **Infants, 7 week to 1 yr:** Infants may take about 1.5 times longer to recover compared with adults. 0.08-0.1 mg/kg per dose. Maintenance: 0.05-0.1 mg/kg every 60 min as needed.

CONTRAINDICATIONS

Hypersensitivity to vecuronium or any component of the formulation

INTERACTIONS

Drug: **Isoflurane, halothane, aminoglycosides, polymyxins, lithium, magnesium salts, procainamide, and quinidine:** May enhance neuromuscular blockade, which may lead to respiratory depression and paralysis. **Muscle relaxants:** May block the effects of vecuronium. **Succinylcholine:** May accelerate the onset and/or increase the depth of neuromuscular blockade induced by vecuronium. Herbal: **St. John's wort:** May increase the risk of cardiovascular collapse and/or delay emergence from anesthesia. Food: None known.

DIAGNOSTIC TEST EFFECTS

None known.

IV INCOMPATIBILITIES

None known.

SIDE-EFFECTS

Frequency not defined: Flushing, bradycardia, allergic reactions, rash, urticaria, reaction at injection site, inadequate or prolonged block, hypotension, tachycardia

CRITICAL CARE CONSIDERATIONS

ADMINISTRATION/HANDLING

IV ALERT

- **Storage:** Store vials of powder for injection at room temperature.
- **Dilution:** Infusion solutions of vecuronium bromide can be prepared by mixing vecuronium bromide with an appropriate infusion solution such as D_5W, 0.9% NaCl, D_5NS, or lactated Ringer's solution.
- **Stability:** Use within 24 hr of mixing the solutions. Unused portions should be discarded.
- **Administration:** Do not administer before patent airway, manual or mechanical ventilation have been secured and unconsciousness has been induced. Repeated administration of maintenance doses of vecuronium bromide has little or no cumulative effect on the duration of neuromuscular blockade; repeat doses can be administered at relatively regular intervals.
- **Skilled providers:** Vecuronium should be administered by adequately trained individuals familiar with its actions, characteristics, and hazards.
- **Not for IM use:** Do not give vecuronium as IM injection due to tissue irritation.

PRECAUTIONS

HEALTH-RELATED

- Use cautiously in patients with electrolyte disturbances, hypothermia, myasthenia gravis, Eaton-Lambert syndrome, amyotrophic lateral sclerosis, respiratory acidosis, severe obesity, dystrophia myotonica, or impaired renal or hepatic impairment.

AGE-RELATED

- **Children:** No age-related precautions have been noted. Vecuronium reconstituted with bacteriostatic water for injection should not be administered to newborns because it contains benzyl alcohol.
- **Elderly:** No age-related precautions have been noted.

PREGNANCY/LACTATION-RELATED

- Pregnancy category C; not recommended for use in breast-feeding mothers.

MONITORING

- **Baseline assessment:** Assess heart rate and BP. Ensure patients have been appropriately sedated and pain has been managed.

- **Baseline and ongoing lab work:** Biochemical profile with renal (BUN, creatinine) and liver (AST [SGOT], ALT [SGPT], alkaline phosphatase, bilirubin) studies.
- **Sedation and analgesia:** Patients undergoing neuromuscular blockade with vecuronium should be sedated and have appropriate pain management provided because patients are unable to express anxiety and discomfort during neuromuscular blockade. Vecuronium produces apnea and paralysis.
- **Ongoing assessment:** Monitor heart rate, BP, and respiratory rate. Try to assess level of pain. Assess renal and liver function in ICU patients.
- **Sedation and neuromuscular blockade:** Monitor the degree of neuromuscular blockade using "train of four" technique with a peripheral nerve stimulator and sedation with a bispectral (BIS) brain wave analysis device. Adjust vecuronium and other medications to keep patients still, well ventilated, and as comfortable as possible. Because patients are totally dependent on health care providers to anticipate all needs and provide all care, most patients would rather not have awareness of the neuromuscular blockade experience.
- **Provide mechanical ventilation:** Assess ventilation status using lung assessment, vital signs, pulse oximetry, and end tidal CO_2 monitoring.
- **Weaning neuromuscular blockade:** Sedation with propofol (Diprivan), benzodiazepine infusion (lorazepam/Ativan) or morphine may provide enough relaxation to be able to wean vecuronium without compromising critically ill patients' ventilatory status. Confirm recovery with 5-sec head lift and grip strength once vecuronium is weaned.
- **Patient education:** Explain that patients will be unable to speak, open eyes, or move when full neuromuscular blockade is in place. When weaning vecuronium, explain it will be difficult to talk due to head and neck muscle blockade.

SERIOUS ADVERSE REACTIONS

- Dysrhythmias, edema, and hypotension may occur.
- Anaphylaxis and hypersensitivity reactions have been reported.

OVERDOSE/TOXICITY

- **Malignant hyperthermia:** A potentially fatal hypermetabolic state of skeletal muscle may occur rarely, but literature is conflicted about whether the muscle rigidity reaction is truly malignant hyperthermia due to vecuronium versus another element of general anesthesia. Potent inhalational anesthetics and succinylcholine cause malignant hyperthermia. Nondepolarizing neuromuscular blocking agents such as vecuronium are not proven to cause malignant hyperthermia.
- **Symptoms:** Prolonged apnea, respiratory depression, inability to maintain patent airway or to move extremities, speak, or open eyes. May occur more often when agents that potentiate vecuronium are given concomitantly. Seizures have been reported in critically-ill patients, but cause may be multifactorial. Cardiovascular collapse occurs rarely.
- **Management:** Continue to keep patients endotracheally intubated and mechanically ventilated until fully able to maintain breathing and respiration effectively. Antidote may be administered if needed. Resuscitate per Advanced Cardiac Life Support (ACLS) guidelines for cardiac arrest.
- **GI decontamination:** No specific recommendations.

ANTIDOTE/DIALYSIS

- **Antidote:** Edrophonium (Enlon) or neostigmine (Prostigmin) given with atropine reverses muscle relaxation in most patients but may aggravate severe overdosage. Ensure patients are endotracheally intubated and mechanical or manual ventilation is in place.
- **Dialysis:** Vecuronium is unlikely to be removed by hemodialysis or peritoneal dialysis. No data are available on removal by high-permeability hemodialysis.

venlafaxine hydrochloride

ven-la-fax'-een hye-droe-klor'-ide

Classes

Chemical: phenethylamine derivative
Therapeutic: antidepressant

Pregnancy Category: C

Trade Names

Prescription: Effexor, Effexor XR

V

CLINICAL PHARMACOLOGY

Mechanism of Action

A phenethylamine derivative that potentiates CNS neurotransmitter activity by inhibiting the reuptake of serotonin, norepinephrine and, to a lesser degree, dopamine. **Therapeutic Effect:** Relieves depression.

PHARMACOKINETICS

Well absorbed from the GI tract. Protein binding: 25%-30%. Metabolized in the liver to active metabolite. Primarily excreted in urine. Not removed by hemodialysis. **Half-life:** 3-7 hr; metabolite, 9-13 hr (increased in hepatic or renal impairment).

AVAILABILITY

Capsules (extended release [Effexor XL]): 37.5 mg, 75 mg, 150 mg.
Tablets (Effexor): 25 mg, 37.5 mg, 50 mg, 75 mg, 100 mg.

INDICATIONS AND DOSAGE

Depression

PO

Adults, Elderly: Initially 75 mg/day in 2-3 divided doses with food. May increase by 75 mg/day at intervals of 4 days or longer. Maximum: 375 mg/day in 3 divided doses.

PO (Extended Release)

Adults, Elderly: 75 mg/day as a single dose with food. May increase by 75 mg/day at intervals of 4 days or longer. Maximum: 225 mg/day.

Social anxiety disorder, generalized anxiety disorder

PO (Extended Release)

Adults, Elderly: Initially, 37.5-75 mg/day. May increase by 75 mg/day at 4-day intervals up to 225 mg/day.

Panic disorder

PO (Extended Release)

Adults, Elderly: Initially 37.5 mg/day. May increase to 75 mg after 7 days followed by increases of 75 mg/day at 7-day intervals up to 225 mg/day.

Dosage in renal and hepatic impairment

Expect to decrease venlafaxine dosage by 50% in patients with moderate hepatic impairment, 25% in patients with mild to moderate renal impairment, creatinine clearance less than 70 mL/min, and 50% in patients on dialysis (withhold dose until completion of dialysis).

OFF-LABEL USES

Prevention of relapses of depression; treatment of attention-deficit hyperactivity disorder, autism, chronic fatigue syndrome, obsessive-compulsive disorder

CONTRAINDICATIONS

Use within 14 days of MAOIs, hypersensitivity to venlafaxine

INTERACTIONS

Drug: Cytochrome P450 2D6 inhibitors: May increase the levels/effects of venlafaxine. Example inhibitors include *chlorproMAZINE, delavirdine, fluoxetine, miconazole, paroxetine, pergolide, quinidine, quinine, ritonavir, and ropinirole. **Cytochrome P450 3A4 inducers:** May decrease the levels and effects of venlafaxine. Example inducers include aminoglutethimide, carbamazepine, nafcillin, nevirapine, phenobarbital, phenytoin, and rifamycins. **Cytochrome P450 3A4 inhibitors:** May increase the levels and effects of venlafaxine. Example inhibitors include azole antifungals, clarithromycin, diclofenac, doxycycline, erythromycin, imatinib, isoniazid, nefazodone, nicardipine, propofol, protease inhibitors, quinidine, telithromycin, and verapamil. **MAOIs:** May cause neuroleptic malignant syndrome, autonomic instability (including rapid fluctuations of vital signs), extreme agitation, hyperthermia, mental status changes, myoclonus, rigidity, and coma. **Nefazadone:** May increase the risk of serotonin syndrome. **Herbal: St. John's wort:** May increase the sedative-hypnotic effect of venlafaxine. **Food:** None known.

DIAGNOSTIC TEST EFFECTS

May increase BUN level and serum alkaline phosphatase, bilirubin, cholesterol, uric acid, AST (SGOT), and ALT (SGPT) levels. May decrease serum phosphate and sodium levels. May alter blood glucose and serum potassium levels.

SIDE-EFFECTS

Frequent (34%-11%): Nausea (21%-31%), somnolence (12%-23%), headache (25%-34%), dry mouth (12%-22%), dizziness (11%-20%), insomnia (15%-23%). **Occasional:** Constipation, diaphoresis, nervousness, asthenia, ejaculatory disturbance, anorexia. **Rare:** Anxiety, blurred vision, diarrhea, vomiting, tremor, abnormal dreams, impotence

CRITICAL CARE CONSIDERATIONS

ADMINISTRATION/HANDLING

PO ALERT

- Administer venlafaxine with food or milk if patients experience GI distress.

- Crush scored tablets if needed. Do not break, open, or crush extended-release capsules.
- When discontinuing venlafaxine, taper the dosage slowly over 2 wk.
- **MAOIs:** Allow at least 14 days to elapse before switching patients from an MAOI to venlafaxine and at least 7 days to elapse before switching patients from venlafaxine to an MAOI.

PRECAUTIONS

HEALTH-RELATED

- Use venlafaxine cautiously in suicidal patients and patients with abnormal platelet function, heart failure, volume depletion, hyperthyroidism, mania, angle-closure glaucoma, hepatic or renal impairment, or seizure disorder.

AGE-RELATED

- **Children:** Safety and efficacy of venlafaxine have not been established in children.
- **Elderly:** No age-related precautions have been noted.

PREGNANCY/LACTATION-RELATED

- Pregnancy category C; unknown if distributed in breast milk.

MONITORING

- **Baseline assessment:** Obtain baseline vital signs and weight. Assess appearance, behavior, level of interest, mood, and sleep pattern. Monitor BP and weight.
- **Lab work:** Biochemical profile including renal (BUN, creatinine) and liver (AST [SGOT], ALT [SGPT], alkaline phosphatase, bilirubin) function tests.
- **Suicidal patients:** Closely supervise suicidal patients during early therapy. As depression lessens, energy level improves, increasing the suicide potential.
- **Therapeutic effect:** Assess appearance, behavior, level of interest, mood, and sleep patterns for evidence of a therapeutic response.
- **Weight changes:** Monitor weight. Nausea and vomiting may lead to weight loss, increased appetite may lead to weight gain.
- **Patient education:** Instruct to take venlafaxine with food to minimize GI distress. Caution against abruptly discontinuing the drug or decreasing or increasing the dosage. Warn to avoid tasks that require mental alertness or motor skills until response to the drug is known. Instruct female patients to report if they are breast-feeding, pregnant, or planning to become pregnant. Urge avoidance of alcohol while taking venlafaxine. Caution to get up slowly to avoid possibility of orthostatic hypotension.

SERIOUS ADVERSE REACTIONS

- **Mild hypertension:** A sustained increase in diastolic BP of 10-15 mmHg occurs occasionally.

OVERDOSE/TOXICITY

- **Overdose:** CNS depression, seizures, sinus tachycardia; may have widening of the QRS complex; has an active metabolite. May produce mild to moderate hypertension at therapeutic doses.
- **Management:** There are no established guidelines for venlafaxine overdose. Patients should be observed for at least 8 hr. Patients should be monitored for toxicity with continuous ECG monitoring and have IV lines in place, as occurrence is sometimes precipitous. Benzodiazepines should be used to manage seizures. Sodium bicarbonate should be considered for QRS widening of over 100 msec. Most cases resolve in 36 hr with supportive care alone.
- **GI decontamination:** Charcoal should be given if patients present within 2 hr of ingestion.

ANTIDOTE/DIALYSIS

- **Antidote:** No specific recommendations.
- **Dialysis:** Venlafaxine is not removed by hemodialysis and is unlikely to be removed by peritoneal dialysis. No data are available on removal by high-permeability hemodialysis.

verapamil hydrochloride

ver-ap′-a-mill hye-droe-klor′-ide

Classes

Chemical: phenylalkylamine

Therapeutic: antianginal; antidysrhythmic, class IV; antihypertensive; calcium channel blocker

Pregnancy Category: C

Combinations

Prescription: with trandolapril (Tarka)

Trade Names

Prescription: Apo-Verap ♣, Calan, Calan SR, Covera-HS, Isoptin, Isoptin I.V., Isoptin SR, Novo-Veramil ♣, Verelan, Verelan PM

Do not confuse Isoptin with Intropin, or Verelan with Virilon, Vivarin, or Voltaren.

V

CLINICAL PHARMACOLOGY

Mechanism of Action

A calcium channel blocker and antianginal, antidysrhythmic, and antihypertensive agent that inhibits calcium ion entry across cardiac and vascular smooth-muscle cell membranes. This action causes the dilation of coronary arteries, peripheral arteries, and arterioles. **Therapeutic Effect:** Decreases heart rate and myocardial contractility and slows sinoatrial (SA) and atrioventricular (AV) conduction. Decreases total peripheral vascular resistance by vasodilation.

PHARMACOKINETICS

Route	Onset	Peak	Duration
PO	30 min	1-2 hr	6-8 hr
PO (extended release)	30 min	N/A	N/A
IV	1-2 min	3-5 min	10-20 min

Well absorbed from the GI tract. Protein binding: 90% (60% in neonates.) Undergoes first-pass metabolism in the liver to active metabolite. Primarily excreted in urine. Not removed by hemodialysis. **Half-life:** 2-8 hr.

AVAILABILITY

Caplet (Calan SR): 120 mg, 180 mg, 240 mg.
Capsules (extended release [Verelan PM]): 100 mg, 200 mg, 300 mg.
Capsules (sustained release [Verelan]): 120 mg, 180 mg, 240 mg, 360 mg.
Tablets (Calan): 40 mg, 80 mg, 120 mg.
Tablets (extended release [Covera-HS]): 180 mg, 240 mg.
Tablets (sustained release [Isoptin SR]): 120 mg, 180 mg, 240 mg.
Injection: 2.5 mg/mL.

INDICATIONS AND DOSAGE

Supraventricular tachydysrhythmias (SVT)

IV

Adults, Elderly: Initially, 2.5-5 mg over 2 min. May give 5-10 mg 30 min after initial dose. Maximum initial dose: 20 mg. **Children 1 to 15 yr:** 0.1-0.3 mg/kg over 2 min. Maximum initial dose: 5 mg. May repeat in 15 min. Maximum second dose: 10 mg. **Children younger than 1 yr:** 0.1-0.2 mg/kg over 2 min. May repeat 30 min after initial dose.

Dysrhythmias, including prevention of recurrent paroxysmal supraventricular tachycardia and control of ventricular resting rate in chronic atrial fibrillation or flutter (with digoxin)

PO

Adults, Elderly: 240-480 mg/day in 3-4 divided doses.

Vasospastic angina (Prinzmetal's variant), unstable (crescendo or preinfarction) angina, chronic stable (effort-associated) angina

PO

Adults: Initially, 80-120 mg 3 times per day. For elderly patients and those with hepatic dysfunction, 40 mg 3 times per day. Titrate to optimal dose. Maintenance: 240-480 mg/day in 3-4 divided doses.

Hypertension

PO (Immediate Release)

Adults, Elderly: 80 mg 3 times per day. Range: 80-320 mg/day in 2 divided doses.

PO (Sustained Release)

Adults, Elderly: 120-240 mg/day. Range: 120-360 mg/day as single dose or in 2 divided doses.

PO (Extended Release [Covera-HS])

Adults, Elderly: 120-360 mg once daily at bedtime.

PO (Extended Release [Verelan PM])

Adults, Elderly: 200-400 mg once daily at bedtime.

OFF-LABEL USES

Treatment of bipolar disorder, hypertrophic cardiomyopathy, vascular headaches

CONTRAINDICATIONS

Atrial fibrillation or flutter and an accessory bypass tract, cardiogenic shock, second and third degree AV heart block, hypotension, sick sinus syndrome, sinus bradycardia, ventricular tachycardia, hypersensitivity to verapamil

INTERACTIONS

Drug: Beta blockers: May have additive effect. **Carbamazepine, quinidine, theophylline:** May increase verapamil blood concentration and risk of toxicity. **Digoxin:** May increase digoxin blood concentration. **Disopyramide:** May increase negative inotropic effect. **Procainamide, quinidine:** May increase risk of QT-interval prolongation. **Herbal:** None known. **Food: Grapefruit, grapefruit juice:** May increase verapamil blood concentration.

DIAGNOSTIC TEST EFFECTS

ECG waveform may show increased PR interval. Therapeutic serum level is 0.08-0.3 mcg/mL.

IV INCOMPATIBILITIES

Amphotericin B complex (Abelcet, AmBisome, Amphotec), nafcillin (Nafcil), propofol (Diprivan), sodium bicarbonate

IV COMPATIBILITIES

Amiodarone (Cordarone), calcium chloride, calcium gluconate, dexamethasone (Decadron), digoxin (Lanoxin), *DOBUTamine (Dobutrex), *DOPamine (Intropin), furosemide (Lasix), heparin, hydromorphone (Dilaudid), lidocaine, magnesium sulfate, metoclopramide (Reglan), milrinone (Primacor), morphine, multivitamins, nitroglycerin, norepinephrine (Levophed), potassium chloride, potassium phosphate, procainamide (Pronestyl), propranolol (Inderal)

SIDE-EFFECTS

Frequent (12%-42%): Constipation, gingival hyperplasia. **Occasional (4%-2%):** Dizziness, lightheadedness, headache, asthenia (loss of strength, energy), nausea, peripheral edema, hypotension. **Rare (less than 1%):** Bradycardia, dermatitis or rash

CRITICAL CARE CONSIDERATIONS

ADMINISTRATION/HANDLING

PO ALERT

- Give tablets that are not sustained release with or without food. Sustained-release tablets should be given on an empty stomach.
- Verapamil should not be given with grapefruit juice.
- Sustained-release capsules should be swallowed whole. For those with difficulty swallowing, capsule may be opened with contents sprinkled on food, but patients should not chew the contents. Food, with pellets intact, must be swallowed without chewing.

IV ALERT

- **Storage:** May be stored at controlled room temperature. Do not use if discolored or particulate matter is present.
- **Stability:** After dilution, solution is stable for 24 hr.
- **IV push:** May be given undiluted in tubing containing D_5W, NS or Ringer's solution for infusion. Give a single dose over at least 2 min in adults and children; give over 3 min in the elderly.
- **IV infusion dilution:** For off-label use, dilute 100 mg (40 mL) in 60 mL D_5W to equal 1 mg/mL (total volume is 100 mL). More diluent may be used to reduce concentration. Rate may be constant (5-10 mg/hr) or may be titrated to heart rate.

PRECAUTIONS

HEALTH-RELATED

- Use with extreme caution in patients with hypertrophic cardiomyopathy.
- Use verapamil cautiously in patients with heart failure, liver or renal disease, sick sinus syndrome, and in those receiving beta-adrenergic blockers or digoxin.
- Accurate pretreatment diagnosis differentiating wide complex supraventricular from ventricular tachycardia is imperative. Verapamil is ineffective against ventricular tachycardia and may cause progression to ventricular fibrillation.
- **Anesthesia induction:** Verapamil may precipitate respiratory muscle failure in patients with neuromuscular diseases or prompt increased intracranial pressure in patients with brain tumors located above the tentorium. Drug potentiates nondepolarizing muscle relaxants (vecuronium, pancuronium, cisatracurium).

AGE-RELATED

- **Children:** No age-related precautions have been noted in children. Children under 6 mo may not respond to treatment with verapamil. Severe hemodynamic effects have been reported in infants and neonates (bradycardia, hypotension, accelerated ventricular response in atrial fibrillation or flutter).
- **Elderly:** Age-related renal impairment may require cautious use. IV drug should be administered more slowly in elderly, as drug may have an increased hypotensive effect.

PREGNANCY/LACTATION-RELATED

- Pregnancy category C; excreted in breast milk (approximately 25% of maternal serum); compatible with breast-feeding.

MONITORING

- **Baseline assessment:** Assess heart rate, BP and LOC; if chest discomfort occurs, concurrent nitroglycerin therapy may be used for relief of anginal pain.
- **Chest discomfort assessment:** Note onset, type (sharp, dull, or squeezing), radiation, location, intensity, and duration of anginal pain and its precipitating factors, such as exertion and emotional stress.
- **Baseline lab work:** Assess liver and renal function test results.
- **Diagnostic tests:** Baseline 12-lead ECG to evaluate heart rhythm and to evaluate for myocardial ischemia.

- **Cardiac:** Assess heart rate, BP, and ECG tracing immediately before verapamil administration. Continuous ECG monitoring should be in place. Observe for extreme bradycardia, heart block (possibly second or third degree), PR interval prolongation, and rapid ventricular rates.
- **Hypotension:** BP should be monitored every 5-10 min.
- **Dizziness:** Assist with ambulation if dizziness occurs.
- **Neuromuscular blockade:** Monitor patients on nondepolarizing neuromuscular blocking agents (vecuronium/Norcuron, pancuronium/Pavulon, cisatracurium/Nimbex) carefully, as verapamil potentiates the effects of blockade. Dosage of blocking agent may need to be decreased.
- **Side effects:** Assess for muscle weakness or headache.
- **Patient education:** Caution against abruptly discontinuing verapamil. Instruct to rise slowly from a lying to a sitting position and wait momentarily before standing to avoid dizziness from the hypotensive effect. Warn to avoid tasks that require mental alertness or motor skills until response to the drug is known. Instruct to report constipation, irregular heartbeat, nausea, pronounced dizziness, or shortness of breath.

SERIOUS ADVERSE REACTIONS

- **Abrupt withdrawal:** May manifest accelerated heart rate, which may lead to chest discomfort. Some patients receive verapamil for refractory angina and may experience severe angina and/or acute myocardial infarction if verapamil is discontinued. Recent studies reveal drug may inhibit platelet aggregation, which inhibits thrombus formation.
- **Dysrhythmias:** Heart failure and second- or third-degree AV block occur more often if patients receive other medications that effect conduction through the AV junction, such as beta-adrenergic blockers or digoxin.

OVERDOSE/TOXICITY

- **Overdose:** Nausea, somnolence, confusion, slurred speech; profound bradycardia, hypotension, heart failure, increased ventricular response in atrial fibrillation or flutter, ventricular tachycardia, ventricular fibrillation, second- or third-degree heart block or asystole may ensue. Manage dysrhythmias per Advanced Cardiac Life Support (ACLS) guidelines; consider use of calcium chloride and/or glucagon.
- **GI decontamination:** No specific recommendations.

ANTIDOTE/DIALYSIS

- **Antidote:** Calcium chloride may be helpful in reversing undesirable effects of verapamil. Glucagon may also be effective during toxicity. Depending on situation, maintain IV fluids as appropriate. Rapid ventricular response may respond to cardioversion. Refer to ACLS guidelines for management of specific tachycardias.
- **Dialysis:** Verapamil is not removed by hemodialysis or peritoneal dialysis. No data are available regarding removal using high-permeability hemodialysis.

vitamin K

vye'-ta-min K

Classes

Chemical: naphthoquinone derivative
Therapeutic: antihemorrhagic, vitamin

Pregnancy Category: C

Trade Names

Prescription: AquaMEPHYTON, Mephyton, Vitamin K_1, Phytonadione

Do not confuse Mephyton with melphalan or mephenytoin.

CLINICAL PHARMACOLOGY

Mechanism of Action

A fat-soluble vitamin that promotes hepatic formation of coagulation factors II, VII, IX, and X. **Therapeutic Effect:** Essential for normal clotting of blood.

PHARMACOKINETICS

Readily absorbed from the GI tract (duodenum) after IM or subcutaneous administration. Metabolized in the liver. Excreted in urine; eliminated by biliary system. **Onset of action:** with PO form, 6-10 hr; with parenteral form, hemorrhage controlled in 1-2 hr and prothrombin time returns to normal in 12-14 hr (IV) or 24-48 hr (PO).

AVAILABILITY

Tablets (Mephyton): 5 mg.
Injection (AquaMEPHYTON, Vitamin K_1): 1 mg/0.5 mL, 10 mg/mL.

INDICATIONS AND DOSAGE

Oral anticoagulant overdose

PO, IV, Subcutaneous

Adults, Elderly: 2.5-10 mg/dose. May repeat in 12-48 hr if given orally and in 6-8 hr if given by IV or subcutaneous route. **Children:** 0.5-5 mg depending on need for further anticoagulation and severity of bleeding.

Vitamin K deficiency

PO

Adults, Elderly: 2.5-25 mg/24 hr. **Children:** 2.5-5 mg/24 hr.

IV, IM, Subcutaneous

Adults, Elderly: 10 mg/dose. **Children:** 1-2 mg/dose.

Hemorrhagic disease of newborn

IM, Subcutaneous

Neonate: Treatment: 1-2 mg/dose/day. Prophylaxis: 0.5-1.0 mg within 1 hr of birth; may repeat in 6-8 hr if necessary.

CONTRAINDICATIONS

Hypersensitivity to vitamin K or any component of the product

INTERACTIONS

Drug: Broad-spectrum antibiotics, high-dose salicylates: May increase vitamin K requirements. **Cholestyramine, colestipol, mineral oil, sucralfate:** May decrease the absorption of vitamin K. **Oral anticoagulants:** May decrease the effects of these drugs. **Herbal:** None known. **Food:** None known.

DIAGNOSTIC TEST EFFECTS

None known.

IV INCOMPATIBILITIES

No known incompatibilities for Y-site administration.

IV COMPATIBILITIES

Heparin, potassium chloride

SIDE-EFFECTS

Occasional: Pain, soreness, and swelling at IM injection site; pruritic erythema (with repeated injections); facial flushing; unusual taste

CRITICAL CARE CONSIDERATIONS

ADMINISTRATION/HANDLING

PO ALERT

- Scored tablets may be crushed.
- Oral and subcutaneous routes of administration are less likely to produce side effects than the IM and IV routes.

IV ALERT

- **Emergency use:** IV route should be used only for bleeding emergencies.
- **Storage:** Store vials at room temperature.
- **Dilution:** Vitamin K may be diluted with preservative-free 0.9% NaCl or D_5W immediately before use. Do not use other diluents. Discard unused portions.
- **IV infusion:** IV doses should be diluted and infused slowly over 20-30 min; Administer by slow IV at rate of 1 mg/min.
- **Hypersensitivity:** Monitor for hypersensitivity or anaphylactic reaction during and immediately after IV administration.

IM, SUBCUTANEOUS ALERT

- Subcutaneous route is preferred. IM or IV administration is restricted to emergency situations. Subcutaneous administration produces fewer side effects than IM or IV route.
- **Administration:** Inject the drug into the anterolateral aspect of the thigh or the deltoid region.

PRECAUTIONS

HEALTH-RELATED

- **Discontinue medications that promote bleeding:** As an alternative to giving vitamin K, medications that interfere with coagulation may be discontinued to reduce the possibility of bleeding.
- **Use with warfarin or dicumarol-related bleeding:** Phytonadione is ineffective in controlling bleeding related to heparin.

AGE-RELATED

- **Children:** No age-related precautions have been noted in children. Drug is used prophylactically for HDN (hemorrhagic disease of the newborn).
- **Elderly:** No age-related precautions have been noted.

PREGNANCY/LACTATION-RELATED

- Pregnancy category C. Oral supplementation of women on anticonvulsants during last 2 wk of pregnancy has been done to prevent HDN, but effectiveness is unproven; compatible with breast-feeding.

MONITORING

- **Baseline assessment:** Before and during treatment, assess for bleeding (signs of vitamin K deficiency) including hematuria and increased bruising and petechiae.
- **Lab work:** CBC with differential, biochemical profile including liver (AST [SGOT], ALT [SGPT], alkaline phosphatase, GGT, bilirubin) and coagulation

studies (prothrombin time/international normalized ratios [INR], aPTT and bleeding time). Routinely monitor prothrombin time and INR in patients taking anticoagulants. Assess Hct, platelet count, and stool and urine specimens for occult blood.
- **Bleeding:** Examine skin for ecchymosis and petechiae; gums for erythema and gingival bleeding; for hematuria, excessive bleeding from minor wounds, and increased menstrual flow.
- **Internal bleeding:** Monitor for abdominal or back pain, hypotension, tachycardia, and severe headache which may indicate hemorrhage.
- **Patient education:** Inform that parenteral administration may cause discomfort. Instruct about bleeding and to promptly report black or red stool, coffee-ground vomitus, red or dark urine, or red-speckled mucus from a cough to a health care provider. Caution against taking other medications, including OTC preparations, before discussing with a health care provider to avoid decreasing platelet aggregation. Instruct to use an electric razor and soft toothbrush. Encourage consumption of foods rich in vitamin K, including milk, egg yolks, leafy green vegetables, meat, tomatoes, and vegetable oil.

SERIOUS ADVERSE REACTIONS
- **Newborns (especially premature infants):** May develop hyperbilirubinemia, jaundice, hemolytic anemia, kernicterus, hemoglobinuria, leading to brain damage and death.
- **Severe hypersensitivity reaction:** Cramp-like pain, chest pain, dyspnea, facial flushing, dizziness, rapid or weak pulse, rash, diaphoresis, hypotension progressing to shock, cardiac arrest occurs rarely just after IV administration.

OVERDOSE/TOXICITY
- **Overdose:** Possible hypercoagulability, leading to abnormal clotting throughout the body; may prompt vessel occlusion leading to stroke, acute MI, or acute ischemia of limbs or abdominal organs.
- **Management:** Effects may be reversed by warfarin or heparin administration. Supportive care for affected organs should be provided. If patients experience acute lack of perfusion managed with thrombolysis, fibrinolytic therapy may be considered.
- **GI decontamination:** No specific recommendations.

ANTIDOTE/DIALYSIS
- **Antidote:** Warfarin or heparin IV administration.
- **Dialysis:** No data are available on removal of vitamin K (phytonadione) by hemodialysis, high-permeability hemodialysis, or peritoneal dialysis.

voriconazole

vohr-ih-kon'-uh-zole

Classes
Chemical: triazole derivative
Therapeutic: antifungal

Pregnancy Category: D

Trade Names
Prescription: Vfend

CLINICAL PHARMACOLOGY
Mechanism of Action
A triazole derivative that inhibits the synthesis of ergosterol, a vital component of fungal cell wall formation. **Therapeutic Effect:** Damages fungal cell wall membrane.

PHARMACOKINETICS
Rapidly and completely absorbed after PO administration. Widely distributed. Protein binding: 98%. Metabolized in the liver. Primarily excreted as a metabolite in urine. **Half-life:** 6 hr.

AVAILABILITY
Tablets: 50 mg, 200 mg.
Injection powder for reconstitution: 200 mg.
Powder for oral suspension: 200 mg/5 mL.

INDICATIONS AND DOSAGE
Invasive aspergillosis, other serious fungal infections caused by *Scedosporium apiospermum* and *Fusarium* species
PO

Adults, Elderly weighing 40 kg and more: Initially, 400 mg every 12 hr for 2 doses on day 1. Maintenance: 200 mg every 12 hr (may increase to 200 mg every 12 hr). **Adults, Elderly weighing less than 40 kg:** Initially, 200 mg every 12 hr for 2 doses on day 1. Maintenance: 100 mg every 12 hr (may increase to 150 mg every 12 hr).

Usual parenteral dosage
IV

Adults, Elderly, Children: Initially, 6 mg/kg/dose every 12 hr for 2 doses, then 4

V

mg/kg/dose every 12 hr (may decrease to 3 mg/kg/dose if patient is unable to tolerate 4 mg/kg/dose).

Candidemia in nonneutropenic patients

PO

Adults, Elderly: 200 mg every 12 hr.

IV

Adults, Elderly: Initially, 6 mg/kg/dose every 12 hr for 2 doses, then 3-4 mg/kg/dose every 12 hr.

Esophageal candidiasis

PO

Adults, Elderly weighing 40 kg and more: 200 mg every 12 hr for minimum of 14 days, then at least 7 days following resolution of symptoms. **Adults, Elderly weighing less than 40 kg:** 100 mg every 12 hr for minimum 14 days, then at least 7 days following resolution of symptoms.

CONTRAINDICATIONS

Concurrent administration of carbamazepine; ergot alkaloids; pimozide or quinidine (may cause prolonged QT interval or torsades de pointes); rifabutin; rifampin; sirolimus; hypersensitivity to voriconazole

INTERACTIONS

Drug: Busulfan, methadone, omeprazole, oral contraceptives, phenytoin, quinidine, rifabutin, sirolimus, vinca alkaloids, warfarin: May increase serum levels/effects of these drugs. **Efavirenz, ritonavir:** May decrease voriconazole serum levels/effects. **Oral contraceptives:** May increase voriconazole serum levels/effects. **QTc-prolonging agents:** Risk of dysrhythmia (torsade de pointes) may be increased. **Cytochrome P450 2C9 inducers:** May decrease the levels/effects of voriconazole. Example inducers include carbamazepine, phenobarbital, phenytoin, rifampin, rifapentine, and secobarbital. **Cytochrome P450 2C19 inducers:** May decrease the levels/effects of voriconazole. Example inducers include aminoglutethimide, carbamazepine, phenytoin, and rifampin. **Cytochrome P450 3A4 substrates:** Voriconazole may increase the levels/effects of CYP3A4 substrates. Example substrates include benzodiazepines, calcium channel blockers, *cycloSPORINE, mirtazapine, nateglinide, nefazodone, sildenafil (and other PDE-5 inhibitors), tacrolimus, and venlafaxine. Selected benzodiazepines (midazolam and triazolam), cisapride, ergot alkaloids, selected hydroxymethylglutanyl-CoA reductase inhibitors (lovastatin and simvastatin), and pimozide are generally contraindicated with strong CYP3A4 inhibitors. **Herbal:** None known. **Food:** None known.

DIAGNOSTIC TEST EFFECTS

May increase serum alkaline phosphatase and ALT (SGPT) levels.

IV INCOMPATIBILITIES

Total parenteral nutrition (TPN)

SIDE-EFFECTS

Frequent (20%-5%): Abnormal vision, fever, nausea, rash, vomiting. **Occasional (5%-2%):** Headache, chills, hallucinations, photophobia, tachycardia, hypertension

CRITICAL CARE CONSIDERATIONS

ADMINISTRATION/HANDLING

PO ALERT

- Give voriconazole 1 hr before or after a meal.

IV ALERT

- **Storage:** Store the powder for injection at room temperature.
- **Reconstituted solution:** Reconstitute a 200-mg vial with 19 mL of sterile water for injection to provide a concentration of 10 mg/mL. Further dilute the drug with 0.9% NaCl or D_5W to provide a concentration of 5 mg/mL or less. Use the reconstituted solution immediately. Do not use the reconstituted solution after 24 hr when refrigerated.
- **IV infusion:** Infuse the drug over 1 to 2 hr at a concentration of 5 mg/mL or less.

PRECAUTIONS

HEALTH-RELATED

- Use voriconazole cautiously in patients with a hypersensitivity to other antifungals or impaired renal or hepatic function.
- **Cytochrome P450 enzyme inhibitor:** Voriconazole interacts with drugs that inhibit cytochrome P450 2C19, CYP 2C9, and to a lesser extent, CYP 3A4 enzyme systems, which prompts the need to adjust dosage of voriconazole or the other medications. There are an extensive number of drug interactions.

AGE-RELATED

- **Children:** Safety and efficacy of voriconazole have not been established in children under 12 yr.
- **Elderly:** No age-related precautions have been noted.

PREGNANCY/LACTATION-RELATED

- Pregnancy category D; breast milk excretion unknown.

MONITORING

- **Baseline assessment:** Assess history of infection. Obtain vital signs. Describe symptoms of the fungal infection.
- **Baseline lab work:** CBC with WBC differential and platelet count. Biochemical profile including liver enzymes (AST [SGOT], ALT [SGPT], alkaline phosphatase) and renal function tests (BUN, creatinine). Perform a culture or histologic test for accurate diagnosis of the causative organism.
- **Hepatotoxicity:** Monitor for dark urine, pale stools, jaundice, fatigue, and GI effects (anorexia, nausea, vomiting) unrelieved by giving drug with food.
- **Vision changes:** Monitor visual function, including color perception, visual acuity, and visual field, if drug therapy lasts longer than 28 days.
- **Patient education:** Instruct to take voriconazole at least 1 hr before or after a meal. Caution to avoid driving at night because voriconazole may cause visual changes, such as blurred vision or photophobia. Advise avoidance of direct sunlight and to avoid performing hazardous tasks if visual changes occur. Inform female patients that voriconazole may have detrimental effects on a fetus. Explain importance of using effective contraception to avoid becoming pregnant while taking voriconazole.

SERIOUS ADVERSE REACTIONS

- **Hypersensitivity:** Rash, urticaria, Stevens-Johnson syndrome.
- **Galactose intolerance:** Voriconazole tablets contain lactose and should not be given to patients with hereditary galactose intolerance.

OVERDOSE/TOXICITY

- **Hepatotoxicity:** Clinical hepatitis, cholestasis, fulminant hepatic failure with fatalies, occurs rarely.
- **GI decontamination:** No specific recommendations.

ANTIDOTE/DIALYSIS

- **Antidote:** No specific recommendations.
- **Dialysis:** Voriconazole is not removed by hemodialysis and is unlikely to be removed by peritoneal dialysis. No data are available on removal by high-permeability hemodialysis.

V

warfarin sodium

war'-far-in soe'-dee-um

Classes
Chemical: coumarin derivative
Therapeutic: anticoagulant

Pregnancy Category: X

Trade Names
Prescription: Coumadin, Jantoven

Do not confuse Coumadin with Kemadrin.

CLINICAL PHARMACOLOGY
Mechanism of Action
A coumarin derivative that interferes with hepatic synthesis of vitamin K-dependent clotting factors, resulting in depletion of coagulation factors II, VII, IX, and X. **Therapeutic Effect:** Prevents further extension of formed existing clot; prevents new clot formation or secondary thromboembolic complications.

PHARMACOKINETICS

Route	Onset	Peak	Duration
PO	1.5-3 days	5-7 days	N/A

Well absorbed from the GI tract. Metabolized in the liver. Primarily excreted in urine. Not removed by hemodialysis. **Half-life:** 1.5-2.5 days.

AVAILABILITY
Tablets (Coumadin, Jantoven): 1 mg, 2 mg, 2.5 mg, 3 mg, 4 mg, 5 mg, 6 mg, 7.5 mg, 10 mg.

INDICATIONS AND DOSAGE
Anticoagulant
PO
Adults, Elderly: Initially, 5-10 mg/day for 2-5 days; then adjust based on international normalized ratios (INR). Maintenance: 2-10 mg/day. **Children:** Initially 0.1-0.2 mg/kg (maximum 10 mg). Maintenance: 0.05-0.34 mg/kg/day.

Usual elderly dosage (maintenance)
PO, IV
Elderly: 2-5 mg/day.

OFF-LABEL USES
Prevention of MI, recurrent cerebral embolism; treatment adjunct in transient ischemic attacks

CONTRAINDICATIONS
Neurosurgical procedures, open wounds, pregnancy, severe hypertension, severe hepatic or renal damage, spinal puncture, uncontrolled bleeding, ulcers, hypersensitivity to warfarin

INTERACTIONS
Drug: **Amiodarone:** Increases warfarin effects; dose of warfarin should be decreased by 30%-50%. **Acetaminophen, allopurinol, amiodarone, anabolic steroids, androgens, aspirin, cefamandole, cefoperazone, chloral hydrate, chloramphenicol, cimetidine, clofibrate, danazol, dextrothyroxine, diflunisal, disulfiram, erythromycin, fenoprofen, gemfibrozil, indomethacin, methimazole, metronidazole, oral hypoglycemics, phenytoin, plicamycin, propylthiouracil, quinidine, salicylates, sulfinpyrazone, sulfonamides, sulindac:** Warfarin increases the effects of these drugs. **Celecoxib, metronidazole:** May increase warfarin's anticoagulant effect and increase INR. **Alcohol:** May enhance warfarin's anticoagulant effect. **Azole antifungals:** May increase warfarin's anticoagulant effect and increase INR. **Barbiturates, carbamazepine, cholestyramine, colestipol, estramustine, estrogens, griseofulvin, primidone, rifampin, vitamin K:** Warfarin decreases the effects of these drugs. **Herbal:** **American ginseng, St. John's wort:** May decrease the effectiveness of warfarin. **Feverfew, garlic, ginkgo biloba, ginseng, glucosamine-chondroitin:** May increase the risk of bleeding. **Food:** None known.

DIAGNOSTIC TEST EFFECTS
None known.

SIDE-EFFECTS
Occasional: GI distress, such as nausea, anorexia, abdominal cramps, diarrhea. **Rare:** Hypersensitivity reaction, including dermatitis and urticaria, especially in those sensitive to aspirin

CRITICAL CARE CONSIDERATIONS

ADMINISTRATION/HANDLING
DOSAGE ALERT
- Warfarin dosage is highly individualized and is based on prothrombin time and INR.

PO ALERT
- Crush scored tablets as needed.
- Give warfarin without regard to food. If GI upset occurs, give with food.

W

IV ALERT

- **Storage:** Store at room temperature and protect from light. Do not refrigerate.
- **Reconstitution:** Add 2.7 mL sterile water for injection to 5-mg vial to produce 2 mg of warfarin per mL of solution.
- **Stability:** Use reconstituted solution within 4 hr; discard unused portion.

PRECAUTIONS

HEALTH-RELATED

- Use warfarin cautiously in patients at risk for hemorrhage and in those with active tuberculosis, diabetes, gangrene, heparin-induced thrombocytopenia, and necrosis.

AGE-RELATED

- **Children:** Are more susceptible to the effects of warfarin.
- **Elderly:** Have an increased risk of hemorrhage; a lower drug dosage is recommended. Less warfarin is required to provide successful anticoagulation in patients over 60 yr.

PREGNANCY/LACTATION-RELATED

- Pregnancy category X. Use in first trimester carries significant risk to the fetus. Exposure in the gestational wk 6-9 may produce a pattern of defects termed the fetal warfarin syndrome with an incidence up to 25% in some series. Compatible with breast-feeding for normal, full-term infants.

MONITORING

- **Baseline assessment:** Cross-check warfarin dosage with another nurse before administering. Assess for history of bleeding, use of other medications, herbal remedies, overall state of health, and dietary habits. There are numerous factors that can alter the INR, which indicates increased chance of bleeding when high, decreased chance of bleeding when low. Low INR (less than 2.5) may indicate anticoagulation is ineffective.
- **Lab work:** Baseline CBC with differential and platelet count; baseline biochemical profile including liver function tests (AST [SGOT], ALT [SGPT], alkaline phosphatase, bilirubin). Urinalysis to test for blood in urine and stool samples for occult blood. Determine the INR before administration and daily after therapy begins. When INR is stabilized, follow with INR determinations every 4-6 wk. Monitor the INR diligently. Whole blood clotting and bleeding times are insufficient measurements of effective therapy.
- **Bleeding:** Evaluate for abdominal or back pain (retroperitoneal bleeding), a decrease in BP, increase in heart rate, and severe headache (stroke) which can indicate hemorrhage. Determine the amount of menstrual discharge and monitor for any increase. Assess the gums for erythema and gingival bleeding, skin for ecchymosis and petechiae, and urine for hematuria. Examine for excessive bleeding from minor cuts or scratches.
- **Thrombophlebitis:** Assess the area of peripheral thrombus (if present) for color and temperature. Check peripheral pulses. Be alert for pulmonary embolization if patients have a blood clot in the legs.
- **DVT prophylaxis:** Before clot formation, hospitalized patients should be considered for deep vein thrombosis (DVT) prophylaxis using other medications (enoxaparin/Lovenox), sequential compression stockings, or other measures suggested by current DVT prophylaxis recommendations.
- **Atrial fibrillation:** Continuously monitor ECG to assess for control of atrial fibrillation, if present. Many patients on coumadin are being managed to prevent intracardiac atrial clot formation secondary to fibrillation.
- **Drug interactions:** Numerous drugs interact with warfarin. A pharmacist should be consulted to review all medications to ensure that drugs are appropriately reconciled during hospitalization and upon discharge.
- **Postsurgical patients:** Patients who have undergone major abdominal surgery or orthopedic surgery are high risk for clot formation in the abdominal cavity or in the area of the joint operated on but are unable to have clot prophylaxis in the early postoperative period due to increased risk for bleeding at the surgical site.
- **Patient education:** Instruct to take warfarin exactly as prescribed. Caution against taking or discontinuing other medications without discussing with the prescriber beforehand. Urge avoidance of alcohol, drastic dietary changes, and salicylates, which may promote bleeding. Warn not to change from one brand of warfarin to another. Explain about consulting the prescriber, surgeon, and dentist about modifying/holding warfarin dose before having dental work or surgery. Explain that urine may become red-orange. Teach to use an

electric razor and soft toothbrush to prevent bleeding during warfarin therapy. Advise not to take other medications, including OTC drugs, without prior discussion with the prescriber. Instruct to report promptly black stool, bleeding; brown, dark, or red urine; coffee-ground vomitus; or red-speckled mucus from cough.

SERIOUS ADVERSE REACTIONS

- **Necrosis:** Tissue necrosis resulting from local thrombosis may affect any part of the body and has been reported in the breast, limbs, and penis. Usually appears within the first few days of starting the medication. Warfarin should be discontinued. Heparin or alternate anticoagulant may be used.
- **Plaque microembolization:** "Purple toes syndrome" is a sign that peripheral tissue necrosis has ensued because of release of atheromatous plaque emboli, which is sometimes enhanced by anticoagulation therapy. Usually occurs within 3-10 wk of initiating therapy.

OVERDOSE/TOXICITY

- **Bleeding:** Local ecchymoses to major hemorrhage may occur. Warfarin should be discontinued immediately and vitamin K or phytonadione administered. Mild hemorrhage: 2.5-10 mg PO, IM, or IV. Severe hemorrhage: 10-15 mg IV and repeated every 4 hr, as necessary.
- **Hepatotoxicity:** Elevated liver enzymes, jaundice, right upper quadrant pain, nausea and vomiting.
- **GI decontamination:** No specific recommendations.

ANTIDOTE/DIALYSIS

- **Antidote:** Phytonadione (vitamin K, Aquamephyton) is most often given subcutaneously, but may be given IV. Fresh frozen plasma and Factor IX complex (not purified Factor IX, which may actually increase INR) may help control bleeding.
- **Dialysis:** Warfarin is not removed by hemodialysis or peritoneal dialysis. No data are available on removal by high-permeability hemodialysis.

zalcitabine

See HIV Medications (p. 961)

zaleplon

zal'-e-plon

Classes
Chemical: pyrazolopyrimidine derivative
Therapeutic: sedative/hypnotic

Pregnancy Category: C

Trade Names
Prescription: Sonata, Starnoc ♣

CLINICAL PHARMACOLOGY

Mechanism of Action

A nonbenzodiazepine that enhances the action of the inhibitory neurotransmitter gamma-aminobutyric acid. **Therapeutic Effect:** Induces sleep.

PHARMACOKINETICS

Rapidly and almost completely absorbed following PO administration. Protein binding: 60%. Metabolized in the liver. Primarily excreted in urine. Partially eliminated in feces. **Half-life:** 1 hr.

AVAILABILITY

Capsules: 5 mg, 10 mg.

INDICATIONS AND DOSAGE

Insomnia

PO

Adults: 10 mg at bedtime. Range: 5-20 mg.
Elderly: 5 mg at bedtime.

CONTRAINDICATIONS

Severe hepatic impairment, hypersensitivity to zaleplon

INTERACTIONS

Drug: Alcohol, other CNS depressants: May increase CNS depression. **Cimetidine:** May increase the effect of zaleplon. **Rifampin:** Decreases the zaleplon blood concentration. **Herbal:** None known. **Food: High-fat, heavy meals:** May delay onset of sleep by approximately 2 hr.

DIAGNOSTIC TEST EFFECTS

None known.

SIDE-EFFECTS

Expected: Somnolence, sedation, mild rebound insomnia (on first night after drug is discontinued). **Frequent (28%-7%):** Nausea, headache, myalgia, dizziness. **Occasional (5%-3%):** Abdominal pain, asthenia, dyspepsia, eye pain, paresthesia. **Rare (2%):** Tremors, amnesia, hyperacusis (acute sense of hearing), fever, dysmenorrhea

CRITICAL CARE CONSIDERATIONS

ADMINISTRATION/HANDLING

PO ALERT

- Zaleplon capsules may be opened and contents mixed with food.
- Avoid giving zaleplon with or immediately after a high-fat meal to avoid delayed absorption.

PRECAUTIONS

HEALTH-RELATED

- Use zaleplon cautiously in patients with mild to moderate hepatic impairment, signs or symptoms of depression, or a hypersensitivity to aspirin (may cause an allergic-type reaction).
- **Cytochrome P450 enzyme metabolism:** Drugs that induce CYP3A4 may reduce effectiveness of zaleplon. Drugs which inhibit the enzyme may not affect zaleplon.

AGE-RELATED

- **Children:** Safety and efficacy of zaleplon have not been established in children.
- **Elderly:** Are more likely to have sensitivity to sedative/hypnotic affects; a dosage reduction may be warranted.

PREGNANCY/LACTATION-RELATED

- Pregnancy category C; small amount excreted in breast milk, with highest excreted amount during a feeding 1 hr after zaleplon administration.

MONITORING

- **Baseline assessment:** Assess history of sleep disorder. Assess sleep pattern, including the time needed to fall asleep and the number of nocturnal awakenings. Discuss level of anxiety to determine if other strategies may be added to promote sleep.
- **Lab work:** Biochemical profile including liver function studies (AST [SGOT], ALT [SGPT], alkaline phosphatase, bilirubin).
- **Fall prevention:** Raise the upper bed rails and provide a call light immediately after drug administration.
- **Sleep environment:** Provide an environment conducive to sleep, such as a back rub, a quiet environment, and low lighting.

- **Patient education:** Instruct to take zaleplon right before bedtime but not immediately after a high-fat or heavy meal. Caution not to exceed the prescribed drug dosage. Urge avoidance of alcohol and other CNS depressants during therapy. Warn to avoid activities requiring mental alertness or motor skills until response to the drug is known. Inform that sleep may be disturbed for 1-2 nights after discontinuing the drug.

SERIOUS ADVERSE REACTIONS

- **Cognitive deficits:** Zaleplon may produce altered concentration, behavior changes, and impaired memory.
- **CNS effects:** Taking zaleplon while still performing daily activities (before bedtime) may result in adverse central nervous system effects, such as hallucinations, impaired coordination, dizziness, and light-headedness.

OVERDOSE/TOXICITY

- Overdose results in somnolence, confusion, diminished reflexes, and coma.
- **GI decontamination:** No specific recommendations.

ANTIDOTE/DIALYSIS

- **Antidote:** No specific recommendations.
- **Dialysis:** No data is available on removal of zaleplon by hemodialysis, high-permeability hemodialysis, or peritoneal dialysis.

zanamivir

See Antivirals (p. 937)

ziconotide

See Analgesics, Miscellaneous (p. 888)

zidovudine

zye-doe'-vyoo-deen

Classes

Chemical: nucleoside analog
Therapeutic: antiretroviral

Pregnancy Category: C

Trade Names

Prescription: Apo-Zidovudine ♣, Novo-AZT ♣, Retrovir

Combinations

Prescription: with lamivudine (Combivir)

Do not confuse Retrovir with ritonavir.

CLINICAL PHARMACOLOGY

Mechanism of Action

A nucleoside reverse transcriptase inhibitor that interferes with viral RNA-dependent DNA polymerase, an enzyme necessary for viral HIV replication. **Therapeutic Effect:** Interferes with HIV replication, slowing the progression of HIV infection.

PHARMACOKINETICS

Rapidly and completely absorbed from the GI tract. Protein binding: 25%-38%. Undergoes first-pass metabolism in the liver. Crosses the blood-brain barrier and is widely distributed, including to cerebrospinal fluid (CSF). Primarily excreted in urine. **Half-life:** 0.5-3 hr (increased in impaired renal function).

AVAILABILITY

Capsules (Retrovir): 100 mg.
Syrup (Retrovir): 50 mg/5 mL.
Tablets (Retrovir): 300 mg.
Injection (Retrovir): 10 mg/mL.

INDICATIONS AND DOSAGE

HIV infection

PO

Adults, Elderly, Children older than 12 yr: 200 mg every 8 hr or 300 mg every 12 hr. **Children 12 yr and younger:** 160 mg/m^2/dose every 8 hr. Range: 90-180 mg/m^2/dose every 6-8 hr. Maximum: 200 mg every 8 hr. **Neonates:** 2 mg/kg/dose every 6 hr.

IV

Adults, Elderly, Children older than 12 yr: 1-2 mg/kg/dose every 4 hr. **Children 12 yr and younger:** 120 mg/m^2/dose every 6 hr. **Neonates:** 1.5 mg/kg/dose every 6 hr.

OFF-LABEL USES

Prophylaxis in health care workers at risk of acquiring HIV after occupational exposure

CONTRAINDICATIONS

Life-threatening allergic reactions to zidovudine or its components

INTERACTIONS

Drug: Bone marrow depressants, ganciclovir: May increase myelosuppression. **Clarithromycin:** May decrease zidovudine blood concentration. **Probenecid:** May increase zidovudine blood concentrations and the risk of zidovudine toxicity. **Ribavirin:** May increase the risk of pancreatitis, hepatic decompensation. **Stavudine:** May decrease the activity of zidovudine. **Valproic acid:** May increase zidovudine toxicity. **Herbal:** None known. **Food:** None known.

DIAGNOSTIC TEST EFFECTS
May increase mean corpuscular volume.

IV INCOMPATIBILITIES
None known.

IV COMPATIBILITIES
Dexamethasone (Decadron), *DOBUTamine (Dobutrex), *DOPamine (Intropin), heparin, lorazepam (Ativan), morphine, potassium chloride

SIDE-EFFECTS
Expected (46%-42%): Nausea, headache. **Frequent (20%-16%):** Abdominal pain, asthenia, rash, fever, acne. **Occasional (12%-8%):** Diarrhea, anorexia, malaise, myalgia, somnolence. **Rare (6%-5%):** Dizziness, paresthesia, vomiting, insomnia, dyspnea, altered taste

CRITICAL CARE CONSIDERATIONS

ADMINISTRATION/HANDLING

PO ALERT
- Keep capsules in a cool, dry place, and protect them from light.
- Give zidovudine without regard to food.
- Space doses evenly around the clock. Keep patients in an upright position when giving the drug to prevent esophageal ulceration.

IV ALERT
- **Dilution:** Zidovudine must be diluted before administration. Remove a calculated dose from the vial and add it to D_5W to provide a concentration no greater than 4 mg/mL.
- **Stability after dilution:** IV solution remains stable for 24 hr at room temperature or 48 hr if refrigerated. Use the solution within 8 hr if stored at room temperature or within 24 hr if refrigerated. Do not use the solution if it contains particulate matter or becomes discolored.
- **IV intermittent infusion:** Infuse zidovudine over 1 hr.

PRECAUTIONS

HEALTH-RELATED
- Use zidovudine cautiously in patients with bone marrow depression or renal or hepatic dysfunction.

AGE-RELATED
- **Children:** No age-related precautions have been noted in children.
- **Elderly:** Effects of zidovudine on elderly are unknown.

PREGNANCY/LACTATION-RELATED
- Pregnancy category C. Indicated for pregnant women at more than 14 wk gestation for prevention of maternal-fetus HIV transmission. Excreted in breast milk; breast-feeding by mothers who are HIV-positive is not recommended.

MONITORING
- **Baseline assessment:** Assess for current drugs used to manage HIV.
- **Lab work:** Obtain specimens for viral diagnostic tests before starting zidovudine therapy. Therapy may begin before results are obtained. Baseline CBC with WBC differential. Biochemical profile including renal (BUN, creatinine) and liver function studies (AST [SGOT], ALT [SGPT], alkaline phosphatase, bilirubin). Monitor CD4+ cell count, CBC, Hgb and HIV RNA plasma levels, mean corpuscular volume, and reticulocyte count. All patients with HIV should be tested for chronic hepatitis B before beginning antiretroviral therapy.
- **Toxicity:** Patients should not receive drugs that are cytotoxic, myelosuppressive, or nephrotoxic because they may increase the risk of zidovudine toxicity.
- **Side effects:** Check for bleeding, dizziness, headache, and insomnia.
- **Diarrhea/constipation:** Assess pattern of daily bowel activity and stool consistency. Monitor intake and output to evaluate for dehydration.
- **Nausea/vomiting:** Assess tolerance for adequate food and fluids.
- **Skin changes:** Evaluate skin for acne or a rash.
- **Bleeding:** Assess for bleeding from invasive sites, gums, from small cuts, in stool, urine, and other secretions.
- **Opportunistic infections:** Assess for symptoms of possible opportunistic infections, such as chills, cough, fever, and myalgia.
- **Patient education:** Instruct to space zidovudine doses evenly around the clock. Explain that blood tests are an essential part of therapy because of the bleeding potential. Instruct patients to immediately report bleeding from the gums, nose, or rectum to the prescriber. Suggest dental

work be done before therapy or postpone it until blood counts return to normal, which may be weeks after therapy has stopped. Caution not to take any other medications without the prescriber's prior approval. Instruct to report promptly difficulty breathing, headache, inability to sleep, muscle weakness, a rash, signs of infection, or unusual bleeding to a health care provider. Explain that zidovudine does not cure HIV infection or AIDS but acts to reduce symptoms and slow or arrest disease progression. Advise that zidovudine does not reduce the risk of transmitting HIV or AIDS to others. Offer emotional support to the patient.

SERIOUS ADVERSE REACTIONS

- **Anemia and granulocytopenia:** Occurs most commonly after 4-6 wk of therapy; both effects are more likely to occur in patients who have a low Hgb level or granulocyte count before beginning therapy.

OVERDOSE/TOXICITY

- **Bleeding:** Patients are at risk for minor to major bleeding if bone marrow is suppressed and pancytopenia develops.
- **Neurotoxicity:** Ataxia, fatigue, lethargy, nystagmus, and seizures may occur.
- **Myopathy and myositis:** Muscle pain, weakness.
- **Lactic acidosis/severe hepatomegaly with steatosis:** More commonly seen in women who are obese. Elevated liver enzymes, hepatitis, jaundice, abdominal pain with acidosis related to elevated lactate level.
- **GI decontamination:** No specific recommendations.

ANTIDOTE/DIALYSIS

- **Antidote:** No specific recommendations.
- **Dialysis:** Zidovudine (Retrovir) is not removed by hemodialysis or peritoneal dialysis. No data are available on removal by high-permeability hemodialysis. Glucuronide zidovudine (GZDV), an active metabolite, is removed by hemodialysis and peritoneal dialysis and is likely to be removed by high-permeability hemodialysis.

zinc oxide/zinc sulfate

zink ox'-eyed/zink' sul'-fate

Classes

Chemical: divalent cation

Therapeutic: chelating agent, ophthalmic astringent, trace element

Pregnancy Category: C

Trade Names

Prescription: (zinc oxide) Balmex, Desitin; (zinc sulfate) Orazinc

CLINICAL PHARMACOLOGY

Mechanism of Action

A mineral that acts as a cofactor for enzymes that are important for protein and carbohydrate metabolism. **Therapeutic Effect:** Zinc oxide acts as a mild astringent and skin protectant. Zinc sulfate helps maintain normal growth and tissue repair as well as skin hydration.

PHARMACOKINETICS

Poorly absorbed from GI tract (20%-30%). Zinc is stored primarily in the skeletal muscle and bone. About 90% is eliminated by the intestines; 20% in the urine.

AVAILABILITY

Zinc Oxide

Ointment: 10%, 20%, 40%.

Zinc Sulfate

Capsules: 110 mg, 220 mg.

Tablets: 110 mg.

Injection: 1 mg/mL.

INDICATIONS AND DOSAGE

Mild skin irritations and abrasions (such as chapped skin, diaper rash)

Topical (zinc oxide)

Adults, Elderly, Children: Apply as needed.

Treatment and prevention of zinc deficiency, wound healing

PO (zinc sulfate)

Adults, Elderly: 220 mg 3 times per day.

OFF-LABEL USES

Zinc sulfate: Wilson's disease

CONTRAINDICATIONS

Hypersensitivity to zinc preparations

INTERACTIONS

Drug: **H_2-blockers (such as famotidine):** May decrease zinc absorption. **Quinolones (such as ciprofloxacin, tetracycline):** May decrease the absorption of these drugs. **Herbal:** None known. **Food:** **Coffee, dairy products:** May decrease zinc sulfate (capsules, tablets) absorption.

DIAGNOSTIC TEST EFFECTS

None known.

SIDE-EFFECTS

Frequency not defined: Nausea, vomiting, epigastric discomfort

CRITICAL CARE CONSIDERATIONS

ADMINISTRATION/HANDLING

PO ALERT

- Take zinc sulfate with food.

TOPICAL ALERT

- Apply zinc oxide after cleaning and drying the affected area.
- Zinc oxide is for external use only. Avoid use in the eyes.

PRECAUTIONS

HEALTH-RELATED

- Excessive zinc intake can cause impaired leukocyte function, a reduction in HDL levels, and vomiting. If used orally, dose should fulfill the minimum daily requirement.

AGE-RELATED

- **Children:** No age-related precautions have been noted.
- **Elderly:** No age-related precautions have been noted.

PREGNANCY/LACTATION-RELATED

- Pregnancy category C (in doses not exceeding recommended daily allowance). For zinc acetate, zinc has appeared in breast milk and zinc-induced copper deficiency may occur; nursing not recommended.

MONITORING

- **Baseline assessment:** Assess the skin for signs of infection before applying topical zinc. If taking by mouth, assess for zinc deficiency (decreased weight, low sperm count, impaired wound healing, alopecia, hypogonadism, tremors, impaired resistance to infection).
- **Therapeutic effect:** Monitor skin integrity for improvement.
- **Patient education:** Explain that coffee and dairy products may decrease the absorption of oral zinc sulfate capsules and tablets. If nausea occurs, instruct to take zinc sulfate with food. Instruct to report if the skin condition fails to improve after 7 days of treatment.

SERIOUS ADVERSE REACTIONS

- Impaired leukocyte function, a reduction in HDL levels, and vomiting.

OVERDOSE/TOXICITY

- **Toxicity:** Cough, chest discomfort, gastrointestinal irritation, tachycardia, hypertension, nausea, vomiting, diarrhea, metallic taste in the mouth.
- **GI decontamination:** No specific recommendations.

ANTIDOTE/DIALYSIS

- **Antidote:** No specific recommendations.
- **Dialysis:** No data are available on removal of zinc by hemodialysis, high-permeability hemodialysis, or peritoneal dialysis.

ziprasidone

zi-pray'-si-done

Classes

Chemical: benzisothiazole derivative
Therapeutic: antipsychotic

Pregnancy Category: C

Trade Names

Prescription: Geodon

CLINICAL PHARMACOLOGY

Mechanism of Action

A piperazine derivative that antagonizes alpha-adrenergic, dopamine, histamine, and serotonin receptors; also inhibits reuptake of serotonin and norepinephrine. **Therapeutic Effect:** Diminishes symptoms of schizophrenia and depression.

PHARMACOKINETICS

Well absorbed after PO administration. Food increases bioavailability. Protein binding: 99%. Extensively metabolized in the liver. Not removed by hemodialysis. **Half-life:** 7 hr.

AVAILABILITY

Capsules: 20 mg, 40 mg, 60 mg, 80 mg.
Injection: 20 mg/mL.

INDICATIONS AND DOSAGE

Schizophrenia

PO

Adults, Elderly: Initially, 20 mg twice per day with food. Titrate at intervals of no less than 2 days. Maximum: 80 mg twice per day.

IM

Adults, Elderly: 10 mg every 2 hr or 20 mg every 4 hr. Maximum: 40 mg/day.

Mania in bipolar disorder

PO

Adults, Elderly: Initially, 40 mg twice per day. May increase to 60-80 mg twice per day on second day of treatment. Range: 40-80 mg twice per day.

OFF-LABEL USES

Tourette's syndrome

CONTRAINDICATIONS

Conditions prolonging the QT interval including history (or current) prolonged QT, congenital long QT syndrome, recent myocardial infarction, history of dysrhythmias, uncompensated heart failure. Concurrent use of other QTc-prolonging agents including amiodarone, arsenic trioxide, bretylium, *chlorproMAZINE, cisapride, class Ia antidysrhythmics (quinidine, procainamide), dofetilide, dolasetron, droperidol, halofantrine, ibutilide, levomethadyl, mefloquine, mesoridazine, pentamidine, pimozide, probucol, some quinolone antibiotics (moxifloxacin, sparfloxacin, gatifloxacin), sotalol, tacrolimus, and thioridazine. Hypersensitivity to ziprasidone.

INTERACTIONS

Drug: **Alcohol, other CNS depressants:** May increase CNS depression. **Carbamazepine:** May decrease ziprasidone blood concentration. **Ketoconazole:** May increase ziprasidone blood concentration. **QT interval prolonging drugs:** May increase the risk for lethal dysrhythmias; use is contraindicated. **Herbal:** None known. **Food:** **All foods:** Enhance the bioavailability of ziprasidone.

DIAGNOSTIC TEST EFFECTS

May prolong the QT interval.

SIDE-EFFECTS

Frequent (30%-16%): Headache, somnolence, dizziness. **Occasional:** Rash, orthostatic hypotension, weight gain, restlessness, constipation, dyspepsia. **Rare:** Hyperglycemia, priapism

CRITICAL CARE CONSIDERATIONS

ADMINISTRATION/HANDLING

PO ALERT

- Give ziprasidone with food to increase its bioavailability.

IM ALERT

- **Storage:** Store vials at room temperature, and protect from light.
- **Reconstitution:** Reconstitute each vial with 1.2 mL sterile water for injection to provide a concentration of 20 mg/mL.
- **Stability of reconstituted solution:** 24 hr at room temperature or 7 days refrigerated.

PRECAUTIONS

HEALTH-RELATED

- Use ziprasidone cautiously in patients with bradycardia, hypokalemia, hypomagnesemia, and patients with a history of prolonged QT syndrome because they may be at greater risk for developing torsades de pointes or atypical ventricular tachycardia. Patients should not receive additional medications that prolong the QT interval when taking ziprasidone.

AGE-RELATED

- **Children:** Safety and efficacy of ziprasidone have not been established in children.
- **Elderly:** No age-related precautions have been noted.

PREGNANCY/LACTATION-RELATED

- Pregnancy category C. Animal, not human, studies demonstrated developmental toxicity, including possible teratogenic effects at doses similar to human therapeutic doses. Breast milk excretion is unknown.

MONITORING

- **Baseline assessment:** Assess appearance, behavior, emotional status, response to environment, speech pattern, and thought content.
- **Lab work:** Biochemical profile including magnesium and potassium levels before beginning therapy and routinely thereafter.
- **Baseline diagnostic tests:** 12-lead ECG to assess for prolonged QT interval before beginning treatment.
- **Suicidal patients:** Closely supervise suicidal patients during early therapy. As depression lessens, energy level improves, which increases the suicide potential.
- **Rash:** Observe skin for rash and urticaria; may be severe.
- **Therapeutic response:** Assess for greater interest in surroundings, improved self-care and ability to concentrate, and relaxed facial expression.
- **Patient education:** Instruct to take ziprasidone with food to increase its effectiveness.

Warn to avoid tasks requiring mental alertness or motor skills until response to the drug is known.

SERIOUS ADVERSE REACTIONS

- **Seizures:** Conditions that lower the seizure threshold may be more prevalent in patients over 65 yr.
- **Cognitive impairment:** Somnolence, impaired ability to concentrate, impaired motor skills.
- **Priapism:** Painful erection lasting more than 4 hr occurs very rarely.
- **Dysphagia:** Swallowing dysfunction that may lead to aspiration pneumonia. Seen more commonly in the elderly.

OVERDOSE/TOXICITY

- **Prolongation of QT interval:** May produce torsades de pointes, a form of ventricular tachycardia. Patients with bradycardia, hypokalemia, or hypomagnesemia are at increased risk.
- **Neuroleptic malignant syndrome:** Hyperpyrexia, muscle rigidity, altered mental status, irregular pulse, labile BP, tachycardia, diaphoresis, dysrhythmias.
- **Tardive dyskinesia:** Potentially irreversible involuntary, dyskinetic muscle movements.
- **GI decontamination:** No specific recommendations.

ANTIDOTE/DIALYSIS

- **Antidote:** No specific recommendations.
- **Dialysis:** Ziprasidone is not removed by hemodialysis and is unlikely to be removed by peritoneal dialysis. No data are available on removal by high-permeability hemodialysis.

zolmitriptan

zohl-mi-trip'-tan

Classes

Chemical: serotonin derivative
Therapeutic: antimigraine agent

Pregnancy Category: C

Trade Names

Prescription: Zomig, Zomig Rapimelt ♣, Zomig-ZMT

CLINICAL PHARMACOLOGY

Mechanism of Action

A serotonin receptor agonist that binds selectively to vascular receptors, producing a vasoconstrictive effect on cranial blood vessels. **Therapeutic Effect:** Relieves migraine headache.

PHARMACOKINETICS

Rapidly but incompletely absorbed after PO administration. Protein binding: 25%. Undergoes first-pass metabolism in the liver to active metabolite. Eliminated primarily in urine (60%) and, to a lesser extent, in feces (30%). **Half-life:** 3 hr.

AVAILABILITY

Tablets (Zomig): 2.5 mg, 5 mg.
Tablets (Orally-Disintegrating [Zomig-ZMT]): 2.5 mg, 5 mg.
Nasal Spray (Zomig): 5 mg/0.1 mL.

INDICATIONS AND DOSAGE

Acute migraine attack

PO

Adults, Elderly, Children older than 18 yr: Initially, 2.5 mg or less. If headache returns, may repeat dose in 2 hr. Maximum: 10 mg/24 hr.

Intranasal

Adults, Elderly: 5 mg. May repeat in 2 hr. Maximum: 10 mg/24 hr.

CONTRAINDICATIONS

Dysrhythmias associated with conduction disorders, basilar or hemiplegic migraine, coronary artery disease, ischemic heart disease (including angina pectoris, history of MI, silent ischemia, and Prinzmetal's angina), uncontrolled hypertension, use within 24 hr of ergotamine-containing preparations or another serotonin receptor agonist, use within 14 days of MAOIs, Wolff-Parkinson-White syndrome, hypersensitivity to zolmitriptan

INTERACTIONS

Drug: Ergotamine-containing medications: May produce a vasospastic reaction. **Fluoxetine, fluvoxamine, paroxetine, sertraline:** May produce hyperreflexia, incoordination, and weakness. **MAOIs:** May dramatically increase plasma concentration of zolmitriptan. **Oral contraceptives:** Decrease zolmitriptan clearance and volume of distribution. **Herbal:** None known. **Food:** None known.

DIAGNOSTIC TEST EFFECTS

None known.

SIDE-EFFECTS

Frequent (8%-6%): Oral: Dizziness; tingling; neck, throat, or jaw pressure; somnolence. **Nasal:** Altered taste, paresthesia.

Occasional (5%-3%): Oral: Warm or hot sensation, asthenia, chest pressure. **Nasal:** Nausea, somnolence, nasal discomfort, dizziness, asthenia, dry mouth. **Rare (2%-1%):** Diaphoresis, myalgia, paresthesia

CRITICAL CARE CONSIDERATIONS

ADMINISTRATION/HANDLING

PO ALERT

- Give zolmitriptan without regard to food.

NASAL ALERT

- **Preparation:** Blow the nose gently to clear nasal passages. With the head upright, close one of the nostrils with an index finger and breathe gently through the mouth. Insert the nozzle about a half inch into the open nostril.
- **Administration:** Close the mouth, then take a breath through the nose while depressing the plunger and releasing the spray. Remove the nozzle from the nose, and gently breathe in through the nose and out through the mouth for 15-20 sec. Do not breathe in deeply.

PRECAUTIONS

HEALTH-RELATED

- Use zolmitriptan cautiously in patients with controlled hypertension, a history of cerebrovascular accident, mild to moderate hepatic or renal impairment, or cardiovascular risk factors.

AGE-RELATED

- **Children:** Safety and efficacy of zolmitriptan have not been established in children under 12 yr.
- **Elderly:** No age-related precautions have been noted.

PREGNANCY/LACTATION-RELATED

- Pregnancy category C; excretion into breast milk unknown. Use caution in nursing mothers.

MONITORING

- **Baseline assessment:** Determine history of hepatic or renal impairment, MAOI use, and peripheral vascular or coronary artery disease. Determine the onset, location, and duration of migraines and possible precipitating factors. Determine pregnancy or pregnancy plans. Assess the onset, location, and duration of migraines and possible precipitating factors. Obtain a baseline BP for evidence of uncontrolled hypertension: a contraindication.
- **Lab work:** Biochemical profile including renal (BUN, creatinine) and liver (AST [SGOT], ALT [SGPT], alkaline phosphatase, bilirubin) function tests.
- **Diagnostic tests:** 12-lead ECG to evaluate for myocardial ischemia/coronary artery disease.
- **Dizziness:** Monitor for dizziness.
- **Environment:** Have patients lie in a dark, quiet room until headache subsides.
- **Vomiting:** Migraine headaches may induce sudden onset, projectile vomiting. Have personal protective equipment readily available.
- **Potential for dysrhythmias:** Monitor ECG rhythm continuously if used while patients are in a critical care unit.
- **Potential for cardiovascular crisis:** Monitor for changes in neurologic status, for chest discomfort, severe abdominal pain, low urine output, and limb ischemia. Vasospasms may be severe and create end-organ ischemia and peripheral ischemia leading to tissue damage.
- **Therapeutic effect:** Assess for relief of migraines and associated symptoms, including nausea and vomiting, photophobia, and phonophobia (sound sensitivity).
- **Patient education:** Instruct to take a single dose of zolmitriptan as soon as migraine symptoms appear. Explain that zolmitriptan is intended to relieve migraines, not to prevent them or reduce the number of attacks. Advise to avoid tasks that require mental alertness or motor skills until response to the drug is known. Instruct to promptly report blood in urine or stool, chest pain, palpitations, easy bruising, numbness or pain in the arms or legs, throat tightness, or swelling of the eyelids, face, or lips. Advise to lie down in a dark, quiet room for additional benefit after taking zolmitriptan.

SERIOUS ADVERSE REACTIONS

- **Cardiovascular instability:** Hypertension, chest discomfort, angina, dyspnea, and ventricular dysrhythmias.
- **Peripheral vascular ischemia:** Various organs may be affected secondary to the vasoconstriction created by zolmitriptan, so a wide range of symptoms for organ ischemia is possible, including blood in urine or stool, chest pain, palpitations, easy bruising, numbness or pain in the arms or legs.

OVERDOSE/TOXICITY

- **Cardiovascular crisis:** Coronary artery vasospasm, acute MI, cerebral vasospasm, CVA/stroke. Vasospasm-related reactions and intracranial hemorrhage occur rarely but are more common in patients with cardiovascular risk factors (hypertension, diabetes, strong family history of coronary artery disease, obesity, smokers, males over 40 yr and postmenopausal women).
- **Ophthalmic disturbances:** May bind to the melanin in the eye causing visual impairment or corneal opacities.
- **Death:** Significant cardiovascular events have resulted in death.
- **GI decontamination:** No specific recommendations.

ANTIDOTE/DIALYSIS

- **Antidote:** No specific recommendations.
- **Dialysis:** No data are available on removal of zolmitriptan by hemodialysis, high-permeability hemodialysis, or peritoneal dialysis.

zolpidem tartrate 

zole-pi'-dem tar'-trate

DEA Schedule: IV

Classes
Chemical: imidazopyridine derivative
Therapeutic: hypnotic

Pregnancy Category: C

Trade Names
Prescription: Ambien, Ambien CR

Do not confuse Ambien with Amen.

CLINICAL PHARMACOLOGY

Mechanism of Action
A nonbenzodiazepine that enhances the action of the inhibitory neurotransmitter gamma-aminobutyric acid. **Therapeutic Effect:** Induces sleep and improves sleep quality.

PHARMACOKINETICS

Route	Onset	Peak	Duration
PO	30 min	N/A	6-8 hr

Rapidly absorbed from the GI tract. Protein binding: 92%. Metabolized in the liver; excreted in urine. Not removed by hemodialysis. **Half-life:** 3 hr (increased in hepatic impairment).

AVAILABILITY

Tablets (Ambien): 5 mg, 10 mg.
Tablets (extended release [Ambien CR]): 6.25 mg, 12.5 mg.

INDICATIONS AND DOSAGE

Insomnia
PO
Adults: 10 mg at bedtime. **Elderly, debilitated:** 5 mg at bedtime.
PO (Extended Release)
Adults: 12.5 mg. **Elderly, debilitated:** 6.25 mg.

CONTRAINDICATIONS

Hypersensitivity to zolpidem

INTERACTIONS

Drug: **Alcohol, other CNS depressants:** May increase CNS depression. **Herbal:** None known. **Food:** None known.

DIAGNOSTIC TEST EFFECTS

None known.

SIDE-EFFECTS

Frequent (more than 10%): Headache, dizziness **Rare (less than 2%):** Nausea, diarrhea, muscle pain

CRITICAL CARE CONSIDERATIONS

ADMINISTRATION/HANDLING

PO ALERT
- For faster sleep onset, give zolpidem on an empty stomach.

PRECAUTIONS

HEALTH-RELATED
- Use zolpidem cautiously in patients with depression, hepatic impairment, or a history of drug dependence.

AGE-RELATED
- **Children:** Safety and efficacy of zolpidem have not been established in children.
- **Elderly:** Age-related hepatic impairment and an increased susceptibility to falls or confusion may require a dosage adjustment.

PREGNANCY/LACTATION-RELATED
- Pregnancy category C; excreted into breast milk in small amounts.

MONITORING

- **Baseline assessment:** Assess BP, heart and respiratory rates, rhythm, and degree

Z

of chest rise immediately before administering zolpidem. Assess sleep pattern, including time needed to fall asleep and number of nocturnal awakenings. Discuss level of anxiety to determine if other strategies may be added to promote sleep.
- **Lab work:** Biochemical profile including liver function studies (AST [SGOT], ALT [SGPT], alkaline phosphatase, bilirubin).
- **Fall prevention:** Raise the upper bed rails and provide a call light immediately after drug administration.
- **Sleep environment:** Provide an environment conducive to sleep such as a back rub, a quiet environment, and low lighting.
- **Respiratory status:** Assess for effective breathing without distress.
- **Paradoxic reactions:** Assess for paradoxic CNS reactions (increased agitation), particularly early in therapy.
- **Therapeutic response:** Evaluate for a decrease in the number of nocturnal awakenings and an increased duration of sleep.
- **Patient education:** Caution against abruptly stopping zolpidem after long-term use. Inform that drug dependence or tolerance may occur with prolonged use of high doses. Urge avoidance of alcohol during zolpidem therapy. Warn to avoid activities requiring mental alertness or motor skills until response to the drug is known.

SERIOUS ADVERSE REACTIONS
- **Abrupt withdrawal after long-term use:** Asthenia, facial flushing, diaphoresis, vomiting, and tremor.
- **Drug tolerance or dependence:** May occur with prolonged, high-dose therapy.
- **Cognitive deficits:** Zolpidem may produce altered concentration, behavior changes, and impaired memory.
- **CNS effects:** Taking zolpidem while still performing daily activities (before bedtime) may result in adverse CNS effects, such as hallucinations, impaired coordination, dizziness, and light-headedness.

OVERDOSE/TOXICITY
- **Overdose:** Symptoms range from mildly altered sensorium to coma. Severe ataxia, bradycardia, altered vision (such as diplopia), severe drowsiness, nausea and vomiting, difficulty breathing, and unconsciousness have been reported.
- **Management:** Ensure patent airway with endotracheal intubation if necessary, along with mechanical ventilation. Support blood pressure with fluids and vasopressors if needed. Administer benzodiazepine antidote flumazenil. Forced diuresis and osmotic diuretics (e.g., mannitol) may facilitate elimination.
- **GI decontamination:** No specific recommendations.

ANTIDOTE/DIALYSIS
- **Antidote:** Cautiously use flumazenil (Romazicon) 0.2 mg (2 mL) over 30 sec; may repeat after 30 sec with 0.3 mg (3 mL) over 30 sec. Further doses may be given up to 0.5 mg (5 mL) up to a total of 3 mg (30 mL). Flumazenil reverses CNS depressive effects. Naloxone (Narcan) should be considered in addition to flumazenil if patients have significant respiratory depression.
- **Dialysis:** Zolpidem is not removed by hemodialysis and is unlikely to be removed by peritoneal dialysis. No data are available on removal by high-permeability hemodialysis.

zonisamide

zoh-nis′-a-mide

Classes
Chemical: sulfonamide derivative
Therapeutic: anticonvulsant

Pregnancy Category: C

Trade Names
Prescription: Zonegran

CLINICAL PHARMACOLOGY
Mechanism of Action
A succinimide that may stabilize neuronal membranes and suppress neuronal hypersynchronization by blocking sodium and calcium channels. **Therapeutic Effect:** Reduces seizure activity.

PHARMACOKINETICS
Well absorbed after PO administration. Extensively bound to RBCs. Protein binding: 40%. Primarily excreted in urine. **Half-life:** 63 hr (plasma), 105 hr (RBCs).

AVAILABILITY
Capsules: 25 mg, 50 mg, 100 mg.

INDICATIONS AND DOSAGE
Partial seizures
PO

Adults, Elderly, Children older than 16 yr: Initially, 100 mg/day for 2 wk. May increase by 100 mg/day at intervals of 2 wk or longer. Range: 100-600 mg/day.

OFF-LABEL USES

Treatment of binge eating disorder, bipolar disorder, obesity

CONTRAINDICATIONS

Allergy to zonisamide or other sulfonamides

INTERACTIONS

Drug: Alcohol, other CNS depressants: May increase zonisamide's sedative effect. **Carbamazepine, phenobarbital, phenytoin, valproic acid:** May increase the metabolism and decrease the effect of zonisamide. **Herbal:** None known. **Food:** None known.

DIAGNOSTIC TEST EFFECTS

May increase BUN and serum creatinine levels.

SIDE-EFFECTS

Frequent (17%-9%): Somnolence, dizziness, anorexia, headache, agitation, irritability, nausea. **Occasional (8%-5%):** Fatigue, ataxia, confusion, depression, impaired memory or concentration, insomnia, abdominal pain, diplopia, diarrhea, speech difficulty. **Rare (4%-3%):** Paresthesia, nystagmus, anxiety, rash, dyspepsia, weight loss

CRITICAL CARE CONSIDERATIONS

ADMINISTRATION/HANDLING

PO ALERT

- Give zonisamide without regard to food.
- Swallow capsules whole.
- Do not give zonisamide to patients allergic to sulfonamides.

PRECAUTIONS

HEALTH-RELATED

- Use zonisamide cautiously in patients with renal impairment.

AGE-RELATED

- **Children:** Safety and efficacy of zonisamide have not been established in children under 16 yr.
- **Elderly:** Lower dosages are recommended, although no age-related precautions have been noted.

PREGNANCY/LACTATION-RELATED

- Pregnancy category C. Teratogenic, embryolethal in animals; no adequate and well-controlled studies in pregnant women. Breast milk excretion in women unknown.

MONITORING

- **Baseline assessment:** Assess seizure patients' level of consciousness; review history of the seizure disorder, including the duration, frequency, and intensity of seizures.
- **Lab work:** CBC with differential; biochemical profile including renal (BUN, creatinine) and liver (AST [SGOT], ALT [SGPT], alkaline phosphatase, bilirubin) function tests before and periodically during therapy.
- **Seizure precautions:** Initiate precautions and provide a dark, quiet environment. If a seizure occurs, note duration, frequency, and intensity. Monitor for clinical improvement, such as a decrease in the frequency or intensity of seizures.
- **Dizziness:** Assist with ambulation if dizziness occurs.
- **Decreased sweating:** Monitor pediatric patients for decreased sweating, as this may be a sign of oligohydrosis, which will render patients unable to effectively cool their body, resulting in hyperthermia.
- **CNS depression:** Assess for fatigue, somnolence, difficulty speaking or thinking. Drowsiness may be severe and render patients unable to perform activities of daily living as usual.
- **Patient education:** Caution against abruptly discontinuing zonisamide after long-term use because this may precipitate seizures. Explain that strict maintenance of drug therapy is essential for seizure control. Instruct to report promptly abdominal or back pain, blood in urine, easy bruising, fever, rash, sore throat, or ulcers in the mouth. Warn to avoid tasks that require mental alertness or motor skills until response to the drug is known. Urge avoidance of alcohol and CNS depressants while taking zonisamide. Advise carrying an identification card or wearing an identification bracelet that displays the seizure disorder and anticonvulsant therapy.

SERIOUS ADVERSE REACTIONS

- **Hypersensitivity:** Fatal allergic reactions have rarely occurred in patients who are allergic to sulfonamides including Stevens–Johnson syndrome, toxic epidermal necrolysis, fulminant hepatic necrosis, agranulocytosis, aplastic anemia, and other blood dyscrasias.
- **Serious skin reactions:** Mild rash may be the first sign of development of Stevens-

Johnson syndrome and toxic epidermal necrolysis.
- **Oligohydrosis:** Decreased sweating with an elevation in body temperature has been seen primarily in pediatric patients and has led to heat stroke requiring hospitalization.
- **Kidney stones:** Flank pain, hematuria, which may possibly be avoided by increasing fluid intake to increase urine output.

OVERDOSE/TOXICITY
- **Overdose:** Bradycardia, hypotension, respiratory depression, and coma.
- **Hematologic toxicity:** Aplastic anemia and agranulocytosis.
- **Nephrotoxicity:** Elevated BUN and creatinine, oliguria, nausea, abdominal pain.
- **GI decontamination:** No specific recommendations.

ANTIDOTE/DIALYSIS
- **Antidote:** No specific recommendations.
- **Dialysis:** No data are available on removal of zonisamide by hemodialysis, peritoneal dialysis, or high-permeability hemodialysis.

ACE INHIBITORS

Uses
Treatment of hypertension, adjunctive therapy for congestive heart failure.

Action
Antihypertensive: Exact mechanism unknown. May be related to competitive inhibition of angiotensin I converting enzyme (ACE) activity causing decreased conversion of angiotensin I to angiotensin II, a potent vasoconstrictor. Reduces peripheral arterial resistance.

Congestive heart failure: Decreases peripheral vascular resistance (afterload) and pulmonary capillary wedge pressure (preload); improves cardiac output and exercise tolerance. ACE inhibitor side effects include: cough, dizziness; may cause rapid increase in K^+ or creatinine; watch for signs of angioedema.
Note: ACE inhibitors may cause severe fetal damage or fetal death if used in the second or third trimester of pregnancy.

ACE Inhibitors

Generic Name	Brand Name	Route	Usual Adult Dose	Available Dosage Forms	Comments
Benazepril*	Lotensin	PO	10-40 mg/day	T: 5, 10, 20, 40 mg	
Captopril†*	Capoten	PO	12.5-50 mg	T: 12.5, 25, 50, 100 mg	Give 1 hr before meals or 2 hr after. Increase dose at 1-2 wk intervals.
Enalapril†*	Vasotec	PO	2.5-40 mg/day	T: 2.5, 5, 10, 20 mg	Give 1 hr before meals or 2 hr after. Increase dose at 1-2 wk intervals.
Enalaprilat	Vasotec IV	IV	0.625-1.25 mg every 6 hr	I: 1.25 mg	Infuse over 5 min. Enalaprilat is an active metabolite of enalapril.
Fosinopril†	Monopril	PO	10-80 mg daily	T: 10, 20, 40 mg	
Lisinopril†	Prinivil, Zestril	PO	10-40 mg daily	T: 2.5, 5, 10, 20, 30, 40 mg	
Moexipril*	Univasc	PO	7.5-30 mg/day	T: 7.5, 15 mg	Give 1 hr before meals or 2 hr after. Increase dose at 1-2 wk intervals.
Perindopril*	Aceon	PO	4-8 mg/day	T: 2, 4, 8 mg	
Quinapril†	Accupril	PO	10-40 mg daily	T: 5, 10, 20, 40 mg	
Ramipril	Altace	PO	2.5-20 mg/day	C: 1.25, 2.5, 5, 10 mg	Increase dose at 1-3 wk intervals.
Trandolapril*	Mavik	PO	1-4 mg/day	T: 1, 2, 4 mg	African American patients often need higher doses than other patients (e.g., 2 mg versus 1 mg). Make dose adjustments at less than 1 wk intervals.

*Daily dose can be given as a single dose or divided doses.
†Generic available for one or more dosage forms.
C, capsules; I, injection; T, tablets

ACID SECRETION INHIBITORS

Histamine H_2 Receptor Blockers

Uses

Short-term treatment of duodenal ulcers (DU) and active benign gastric ulcers (GU); maintenance therapy of DU, pathologic hypersecretory conditions (e.g., Zollinger-Ellison syndrome), and gastroesophageal reflux disease (GERD); and prevention of upper GI bleeding in critically ill patients.

Action

Inhibit gastric acid secretion by interfering with histamine at the histamine H_2 receptors in parietal cells. Also inhibit acid secretion caused by gastrin. Inhibition occurs with basal (fasting), nocturnal, food-stimulated, or fundic distention secretion. H_2 antagonists decrease both the volume and H_2 concentration of gastric juices.

Generic Name	Brand Name	Adult Oral Dosage Range	Available Oral Dosage Forms	Dose Adjustment in Renal Dysfunction	Drug Interactions/Comments
Cimetidine*	Tagamet	200-400 mg once daily-four times daily; 800 mg once daily-twice daily; dose varies depending on indication	T: 100, 200, 300, 400, 800 mg O Sol: 300 mg/5 mL I: 150 mg/mL	Yes (CRCL less than 30 mL/min)	Alcohol, amiodarone, antacids, benzodiazepines (except lorazepam, oxazepam, temazepam), caffeine, calcium channel blockers, carbamazepine, carmustine, cefuroxime, cefpodoxime, chloroquine, cigarette smoking, clozapine, digoxin, flecainide, fluconazole, fluorouracil, glipizide, glyburide, indomethacin, iron salts, itraconazole, ketoconazole, labetalol, lidocaine, lomustine, melphalan, meperidine (and other narcotic analgesics), metoprolol, metronidazole, moricizine, pentoxifylline, phenytoin, praziquantel, procainamide, propafenone, propranolol, quinidine, quinine, succinylcholine, sulfonylureas, tacrine, tetracyclines, theophylline, tocainide, triamterene, tricyclic antidepressants, valproic acid, warfarin May be given with meals. May give antacids for pain.

Famotidine*	Pepcid	20-40 mg twice daily or every night; dose varies depending on indication	T: 10, 20, 40 mg T (OD): 20, 40 mg T (Chew)/G: 10 mg I: 10 mg/mL IV minibag: 20 mg/50 mL P for O Sus: 40 mg/5 mL (reconstituted)	Yes (CRCL less than 50 mL/min)	Alcohol, cefpodoxime, cefuroxime, dihydropyridine calcium channel blockers, glipizide, glyburide, itraconazole, ketoconazole, quinolone antibiotics, tolbutamide Oral suspension should be discarded 30 days after mixing.
Nizatidine*	Axid	150 mg twice daily or every night, 300 mg every night; dose varies depending on indication	C: 150, 300 mg O Sol: 15 mg/mL	Yes (CRCL less than 50 mL/min)	Alcohol, cefpodoxime, cefuroxime, dihydropyridine calcium channel blockers, glipizide, glyburide, itraconazole, ketoconazole, quinolone antibiotics, salicylates, tolbutamide
Ranitidine*	Zantac	150 mg twice daily or four times daily; 300 mg once daily; 75 mg once daily-twice daily (OTC); dose varies depending on indication	T: 75, 150, 300 mg T(E): 25, 150 mg S: 75 mg/5 mL I: 1, 25 mg/mL	Yes (CRCL less than 50 mL/min)	Alcohol, cefpodoxime, cefuroxime, dihydropyridine calcium channel blockers, diazepam, glipizide, glyburide, itraconazole, ketoconazole, procainamide, quinolone antibiotics, sulfonylureas, theophylline, warfarin

*Generic available for one or more dosage forms.
C, capsule; Chew, chewable; E, effervescent; G, gelcap; I, injection; OD, orally disintegrating; O Sol, oral solution; O Sus, oral suspension; P, powder; S, syrup; T, tablet

Proton Pump Inhibitors

Uses

Treatment of various gastric disorders, including gastric and duodenal ulcers, GERD, pathologic hypersecretory conditions.

Action

Suppress gastric acid secretion by specific inhibition of the hydrogen-potassium-adenosine triphosphatase (H^+/K^+ ATPase) enzyme system, which transports the acid at the gastric parietal cells. These agents do not have anticholinergic or histamine receptor antagonistic properties.

Generic Name	Trade Name	Adult Dosage Range*	Available Dosage Forms†	Nonprescription (OTC) Strength and Dosage Forms	Dose Adjustment in Renal Dysfunction	Drug Interactions/Comments‡
Esomeprazole	Nexium	20-40 mg daily before eating	C (DR): 20, 40 mg IV: 20 mg/ 40 mg powder	N/A	No	Digoxin, itraconazole, ketoconazole, sucralfate, enteric coated aspirin, iron salts, cyanocobalamin
Lansoprazole	Prevacid	15-30 mg once daily or twice daily on empty stomach	C (DR): 15, 30 mg G (EC DR for oral suspension): 15, 30 mg T (OD): 15 mg IV: 30 mg vials	N/A	No	Same as esomeprazole

Omeprazole[§]	Prilosec	20-40 mg once daily or twice daily before eating	C (DR): 10, 20, 40 mg P for oral suspension: 20, 40 mg	C (DR): 20 mg (Prilosec OTC)	No	Same as esomeprazole plus benzodiazepines, cilostazol, citalopram, clarithromycin, cyclosporine, disulfiram, methotrexate, phenytoin, sulfonylureas, theophylline, warfarin
Pantoprazole	Protonix, Protonix IV	40-240 mg/day	T: 20, 40 mg I: 40 mg/vial	N/A	No	Same as esomeprazole
Rabeprazole	Aciphex	20-100 mg once daily; 60 mg twice daily	T: 20 mg	N/A	No	Same as esomeprazole

*Doses vary depending on indication.
†All oral forms are delayed release.
‡Generic available for one or more dosage forms.
§Do not open the capsules or crush the tablets.
C, capsule; DR, delayed release; EC, enteric-coated; G, granules; I, injection; OD, orally disintegrating; P, powder; T, tablet

References for Acid Secretion Inhibitor tables:

1. Ellsworth, Allan J et al: *Mosby's Medical Drug Reference*. Mosby, St. Louis, 2003
2. Website: U.S. Food and Drug Administration. Online. Internet. 2003. Available: *http://www.fda.gov/cder*

ANALGESICS, MISCELLANEOUS

Name	Usual Adult Dose	Maximum Adult Daily Dose	Prescription Strength	Nonprescription Strength	Comments
Acetaminophen* (Tylenol, Panadol, Tempra, Liquiprin)	325-650 mg every 4-6 hr	4000 mg	N/A	T: 160, 325, 500, 650 mg T (chewable): 80 mg D: 80 mg/0.8 mL, 80 mg/1.66 mL, 100 mg/mL E: 80, 125, 160 mg/5 mL L: 160 mg/5 mL, 500 mg/15 mL RS: 80, 120, 125, 300, 325, 650 mg	Hepatotoxicity if overdosed and in persons with cirrhosis (limit dose to 2000 mg/day in cirrhotics); commonly combined with other drugs.
Clonidine (Duraclon)	Epidural: start at 30 mcg/h; titrate	Limited experience with doses greater than 40 mcg/h	I: 100 mcg/mL	N/A	More likely to be effective against neuropathic cancer pain than somatic or visceral pain.
Tramadol* (Ultram)	25-100 mg every 4-6 hr; reduce in elderly, renal impairment, cirrhosis	400 mg/day	T: 50 mg	N/A	Max daily dose: 400 mg; U.S. clinical trials demonstrate a lesser degree of tolerance and withdrawal effects compared with classic opiates; not recommended for pregnant or nursing women; increased risk of seizures in patients receiving tricyclic antidepressants; contraindicated with current MAOI use.
Ziconotide (Prialt)	2.4-19.2 mcg/day titrated 2-3 times weekly	19.2 mcg/day	I for intrathecal use: 25, 100 mcg/mL	N/A	Indicated for severe chronic pain refractory to all other systemic agents. Psychiatric symptoms may occur. Not for use in patients with history of psychosis. Side effects include dizziness, nausea, confusion, headache, somnolence.

*Generic available for one or more dosage forms.
C, capsules; D, drops; E, elixir; I, injection; L, liquid; RS, rectal suppository; T, tablets

ANGIOTENSIN II RECEPTOR ANTAGONISTS

Uses
Treatment of hypertension alone or in combination with other antihypertensives.

Action
Angiotensin II receptor antagonists (AIIRA) block vasoconstrictor and aldosterone-secreting effects on angiotensin II by selectively blocking the binding of angiotensin II to AT_1 receptors in vascular smooth muscle and adrenal gland, causing vasodilation and a decrease in aldosterone effects.

Angiotensin II Receptor Antagonists

Generic Name	Brand Name	Usual Adult Dose	Available Dosage Forms	Adverse Effects/ Comments
Candesartan cilexetil	Atacand	4-32 mg daily	T: 4, 8, 16, 32 mg	Hypotension, hyperkalemia, increased serum creatinine, dizziness Approved for heart failure
Eprosartan mesylate	Teveten	400-800 mg/day, divided in 1 or 2 doses	T: 300, 400, 600 mg	Hypotension, hyperkalemia, increased serum creatinine, dizziness, upper respiratory tract infection
Irbesartan	Avapro	150-300 mg daily	T: 75, 150, 300 mg	Same as eprosartan mesylate
Losartan potassium	Cozaar	25-100 mg/day divided in 1-2 doses	T: 25, 50, 100 mg	Hypotension, hyperkalemia, increased serum creatinine, dizziness, chest pain, fatigue, anemia, cough
Olmesartan medoxomil	Benicar	20-40 mg daily	T: 5, 20, 40 mg	Hypotension, hyperkalemia, increased serum creatinine, dizziness
Telmisartan	Micardis	20-80 mg daily	T: 20, 40, 80 mg	Same as olmesartan medoxomil
Valsartan	Diovan	80-320 mg daily	T: 40, 80, 160, 320 mg	Hypotension, hyperkalemia, increased serum creatinine, dizziness, diarrhea. Also approved for heart failure.

T, tablets

ANTIANXIETY AGENTS

Action

Benzodiazepines are the largest and most frequently prescribed group of antianxiety agents. The exact mechanism is unknown but they may increase the inhibiting effect of gamma-aminobutyric acid (GABA), which inhibits nerve impulse transmission by binding to specific benzodiazepine receptors in various areas of the central nervous system (CNS).

Alert: Refer to individual entries of nonbenzodiazepine drugs for more information on uses and actions.

Antianxiety Agents

Name	Availability	Uses	Dosage Range (per day)	Side Effects/Notes
Benzodiazepines				
Alprazolam (Xanax)	T: 0.25, 0.5, 1, 2 mg ODT: 0.25, 0.5, 1, 2 mg S: 1 mg/mL ER: 0.5, 1, 2, 3	Anxiety, panic disorder	0.75-10 mg	Drowsiness, weakness or fatigue, ataxia, slurred speech, confusion, lack of coordination, impaired memory, paradoxic agitation, dizziness, nausea
Chlordiazepoxide (Librium, Libritabs)	C: 5, 10, 25 mg I: 100 mg	Anxiety, alcohol withdrawal	5-300 mg	Same as alprazolam Parenteral form not available.
Clonazepam	T: 0.5, 1, 2 mg ODT: 0.125, 0.25, 0.5, 1, 2 mg	Panic disorder, seizure	0.25-4 mg	Same as alprazolam
Clorazepate (Tranxene)	C: 3.75, 7.5, 15 mg SD: 11.25, 22.5 mg	Anxiety, alcohol withdrawal, anticonvulsant	7.5-90 mg Once daily for SD forms only	Same as alprazolam Do not use SD form for initial therapy
Diazepam (Valium)	T: 2.5, 5, 10 mg S: 5 mg/5 mL, 5 mg/mL I: 5 mg/mL	Anxiety, alcohol withdrawal, anticonvulsant, muscle relaxant, preoperative	2-40 mg	Same as alprazolam

Lorazepam (Ativan)	T: 0.5, 1, 2 mg S: 2 mg/mL I: 2 mg/mL, 4 mg/mL	Anxiety, alcohol withdrawal, status epilepticus	0.5-10 mg	Same as alprazolam Total daily dose can go much higher if used for conscious sedation in ICU.
Oxazepam (Serax)	C: 10, 15, 30 mg T: 10, 15, 30 mg	Anxiety, alcohol withdrawal	30-120 mg	Same as alprazolam
Nonbenzodiazepines				
Buspirone (BuSpar)	T: 5, 7.5, 10, 15, 30 mg	Anxiety	7.5-60 mg	Dizziness, lightheadedness, headache, nausea, restlessness
Hydroxyzine (Atarax, Vistaril)	T: 10, 25, 50, 100 mg C: 25, 50, 100 mg S: 10 mg/5 mL OS: 25 mg/5 mL I: 25, 50 mg/mL	Anxiety, rhinitis, pruritus, sedation, urticaria, nausea or vomiting	100-400 mg	Drowsiness; dry mouth, nose, and throat Injection by deep IM administration only
Meprobamate (Miltown)	T: 200, 400 mg	Anxiety	1.2-2.4 mg/day	Drowsiness, ataxia, nausea, vomiting, palpitations, tachycardia Can be addictive

C, capsules; ER, extended release; I,injection; ODT, orally disintegrating tablets; OS, oral suspension; S, syrup; SD, single dose; T, tablets

ANTIBIOTICS

Uses

Cephalosporins: Broad-spectrum antibiotics, which, like penicillins, may be used in a number of diseases, including respiratory diseases, skin and soft tissue infection, bone/joint infections, GU infections, prophylactically in some surgical procedures.

First-generation cephalosporins have good activity against gram-positive organisms and moderate activity against gram-negative organisms, including *Escherichia coli, Klebsiella pneumoniae,* and *Proteus mirabilis*.

Second-generation cephalosporins have increased activity against gram-negative organisms.

Third-generation cephalosporins are less active against gram-positive organisms but more active against the *Enterobacteriaceae,* with some activity against *Pseudomonas aeruginosa.*

Fourth-generation cephalosporins have good activity against gram-positive organisms (e.g., *Staphylococcus aureus*) and gram-negative organisms (e.g., *Pseudomonas aeruginosa*).

Macrolides/Ketolides: Macrolides act primarily against gram-positive microorganisms and gram-negative cocci. Azithromycin and clarithromycin appear to be more potent than erythromycin. Macrolides are used in the treatment of pharyngitis/tonsillitis, sinusitis, chronic bronchitis, pneumonia, uncomplicated skin/skin structure infections.

Penicillins: Penicillins may be used to treat a large number of infections, including pneumonia and other respiratory diseases, UTIs, septicemia, meningitis, intraabdominal infections, gonorrhea, syphilis, and bone/joint infection. Penicillins are classified based on an antimicrobial spectrum:

Natural penicillins are very active against gram-positive cocci but ineffective against most strains of *Staphylococcus aureus* (inactivated by enzyme penicillinase).

Penicillinase-resistant penicillins are effective against penicillinase-producing *Staphylococcus aureus* but are less effective against gram-positive cocci than the natural penicillins.

Broad-spectrum penicillins are effective against gram-positive cocci and some gram-negative bacteria (e.g., *Haemophilus influenzae, Escherichia coli, Proteus mirabilis*).

Extended-spectrum penicillins are effective against *Pseudomonas aeruginosa, Enterobacter, Proteus* species, *Klebsiella,* and some other gram-negative microorganisms.

Actions

Cephalosporins: Inhibit cell wall synthesis or activate enzymes that disrupt the cell wall, causing cell lysis and cell death. May be bacteriostatic or bactericidal. Most effective against rapidly dividing cells.

Macrolides/Ketolides: Bacteriostatic or bactericidal. Reversibly bind to the P site of the 50S ribosomal subunit of susceptible organisms, inhibiting RNA-dependent protein synthesis.

Penicillins: Inhibit cell wall synthesis or activate enzymes, which disrupt the bacterial cell wall, causing cell lysis and cell death. May be bacteriostatic or bactericidal. Most effective against bacteria undergoing active growth and division.

Aminoglycosides

Name	Availability	Dosage Range	Side Effects
Amikacin (Amikin)	I: 250 mg/mL, 50 mg/mL	A: 15 mg/kg/day C: 15 mg/kg/day	Nephrotoxicity, neurotoxicity, ototoxicity (both auditory and vestibular), hypersensitivity (skin itching, redness, rash, swelling)
Gentamicin (Garamycin)	I: 40 mg/mL, 10 mg/mL	A: 3-5 mg/kg/day C: 6-7.5 mg/kg/day	Same as amikacin
Neomycin	T: 500 mg	A: 1 g for 3 doses as preop	Nausea, vomiting, diarrhea
Netilmicin (Netromycin)	I: 100 mg/mL	A: 3-6.5 mg/kg/day C: 5.5-8 mg/kg/day	Same as amikacin
Streptomycin	I: 1 g	A: 15 mg/kg/day in divided doses C: 20-40 mg/kg/day in divided doses Max: 1 g	Same as amikacin Peripheral neuritis (numbness), optic neuritis (any vision loss)
Tobramycin (Nebcin)	I: 40 mg/mL, 10 mg/mL	A: 3-5 mg/kg/day C: 6-7.5 mg/kg/day	Same as amikacin

Carbapenems

Name	Availability	Dosage Range	Side Effects/Comments
Ertapenem (Invanz)	IV: 1 g	1 g daily	Reduce to 500 mg/day in advanced renal insufficiency and SSRD.
Imipenem-cilastatin (Primaxin)	IV: 250, 500, 750 mg	A: 250 mg-1 g every 6 hr C (greater than or equal to 3 mo): 15-25 mg/kg every 6 hr C (4 wk-3 mo): 25 mg/kg every 6 hr C (1 wk-4 wk): 25 mg/kg every 8 hr C (less than 1 wk): 25 mg/kg every 12 hr	Reduce dose in renal failure CNS side effects (seizures)
Meropenem (Merrem)	IV: 500 mg, 1 g	A: 500 mg-2 g every 8 hr C: 20-40 mg/kg every 8 hr C (greater than 50 kg): 1-2 g every 8 hr	Diarrhea Reduce dose in renal failure

Cephalosporins

Name	Availability	Dosage Range	Dosing Interval	Adjust for Renal Insufficiency	Side Effects/Comments
First-Generation					
Cefadroxil (Duricef)	C: 500 mg T: 1 g S: 125/5 mL, 250 mg/5 mL, 500 mg/5 mL	A: 1-2 g/day C: 30 mg/kg/day	Every 12-24 hr	Yes	Abdominal cramps/pain, fever, nausea, vomiting, diarrhea, headaches, oral/vaginal candidiasis
Cefazolin (Ancef, Kefzol)	I: 500 mg, 1 g, multidose	A: 0.75-6 g/day C: 25-100 mg/kg/day	Every 6-8 hr	Yes	Same as cefadroxil
Cephalexin (Keftab, Keflex)	C: 250, 500 mg T: 250, 500 mg, 1 g Powder for S: 125 mg/5 mL, 250 mg/5 mL	A: 1-4 g/day C: 25-100 mg/kg/day	Every 6 hr	Yes	Same as cefadroxil
Cephradine (Velosef)	C: 250, 500 mg S: 125 mg/5 mL, 250 mg/5 mL I: 250, 500 mg, 1 g, 2 g	A: 1-4 g C: 50-100 mg/kg/day	Every 6-12 hr	Yes	Same as cefadroxil
Second-Generation					
Cefaclor (Ceclor)	C: 250, 500 mg T (ER): 375, 500 mg S: 125 mg/5 mL, 187 mg/5 mL, 250 mg/5 mL, 375 mg/5 mL	A: 250-500 mg every 8 hr C: 20-40 mg/kg/day	Every 8-2 hr	Yes (severe only)	Same as cefadroxil May have serum sickness-like reaction Give tablets with food
Cefamandole (Mandol)	I: 1, 2 g	A: 500 mg-2 g every 4-8 hr; max 12 g/day C: 50-150 mg/kg/day in doses divided every 4-8 hr	Every 4-8 hr	Yes	
Cefmetazole (Zefazone)	I: 1, 2 g	A: 4-8 g	Every 6-12 hr	Yes	Same as cefadroxil
Cefotetan (Cefotan)	I: 0.25, 0.5, 1, 2 g, multidose vial	A: 1-6 g/day		Yes	Same as cefadroxil May cause unusual bleeding/ecchymoses

Cefoxitin (Mefoxin)	I: 1, 2 g, multidose vial	A: 3-12 g/day	Every 6-8 hr	Yes	Same as cefadroxil
Cefpodoxime (Vantin)	T: 100, 200 mg S: 50 mg/5 mL, 100 mg/5 mL	A: 200-800 mg/day C: 10 mg/kg/day	12 hr	Yes	Same as cefadroxil Give tablets with food
Cefprozil (Cefzil)	T: 250, 500 mg S: 125 mg/5 mL, 250 mg/5 mL	A: 0.5-1 g/day C: 30 mg/kg/day	Every 12-24 hr	Yes	Same as cefadroxil
Cefuroxime (Ceftin, Kefurox, Zinacef)	T: 125, 250, 500 mg S: 125 mg/5 mL, 250 mg/5 mL I: 750 mg, 1.5 g, multidose vial	A (PO): 0.25-1 g/day (IM/IV): 2.25-9 g/day C (PO): 250-500 mg/day; 20-30 mg/kg/day (IM/IV): 50-100 mg/kg/day	PO: every 12 hr IV: every 8 hr	Yes	Same as cefadroxil
Loracarbef (Lorabid)	C: 200, 400 mg S: 100 mg/5 mL, 200 mg/5 mL	A: 200-800 mg/day C: 15-30 mg/kg/day	12 hr	Yes	Same as cefadroxil, plus rhinitis Administer on an empty stomach
Third-Generation					
Cefdinir (Omnicef)	C: 300 mg S: 125 mg/5 mL, 250 mg/5 mL	A: 600 mg/day C: 14 mg/kg/day	Every 12-24 hr	Yes	Same as cefadroxil
Cefditoren (Spectracef)	T: 200 mg	A: 400-800 mg/day	Every 12 hr	Yes	Same as cefadroxil
Cefixime (Suprax)	T: 400 mg Powder for OS: 100 mg/5 mL	A: 400 mg daily or 200 mg every 12 hr C (less than or equal to 50 kg or less than or equal to 12 yr): 8 mg/kg/day in single or divided dose	Every 12-24 hr	Yes	Same as cefadroxil
Cefoperazone (Cefobid)	I: 1, 2 g, multidose vial	A: 2-4 g/day in divided doses For serious infections or less sensitive organisms, may give up to 16 g either as continuous drip or in 3-4 doses of no more than 4 g each	Every 12 hr	No	Same as cefadroxil
Cefotaxime (Claforan)	I: 500 mg, 1 g, 2 g, multidose vial	A: 2-12 g/day C: 100-200 mg/kg/day	Every 4-12 hr	Yes	Same as cefadroxil
Ceftazidime (Fortaz, Tazicef, Tazidime)	I: 500 mg, 1 g, 2 g, multidose vial	A: 0.5-6 g/day C: 90-150 mg/kg/day up to 6 g/day	Every 8-12 hr	Yes	Same as cefadroxil

Continued

Cephalosporins—cont'd

Name	Availability	Dosage Range	Dosing Interval	Adjust for Renal Insufficiency	Side Effects/Comments
Ceftibuten (Cedax)	C: 400 mg S: 90 mg/5 mL, 180 mg/5 mL	A: 400 mg/day C: 9 mg/kg/day	24 hr	Yes	Same as cefadroxil Administer on an empty stomach
Ceftizoxime (Cefizox)	I: 500 mg, 1 g, 2 g, multidose vial	A: 1-12 g/day C: 150-200 mg/kg/day	Every 6-12 hr	Yes	Same as cefadroxil
Ceftriaxone (Rocephin)	I: 250, 500 mg, 1 g, 2 g, multidose vial	A: 1-4 g/day C: 50-100 mg/kg/day	Every 12-24 hr	No	Same as cefadroxil
Fourth-Generation					
Cefepime (Maxipime)	I: 500 mg, 1 g, 2 g	A: 1-6 g/day	Every 8-12 hr	Yes	Same as cefadroxil

Fluoroquinolones/Quinolones

Name	Availability	Dosage Range (Adults)	Side Effects
Ciprofloxacin (Cipro)	T: 100, 250, 500, 750 mg T (ER): 500 mg/1 g S: 5 g/100 mL, 10 g/100 mL I: 200, 400 mg	PO: 250-750 mg every 12 hr IV: 200-400 mg every 12 hr	Dizziness, headaches, nervousness, drowsiness, insomnia, abdominal pain, nausea, diarrhea, vomiting, phlebitis (parenteral)
Cinoxacin (Cinobac)	C: 250, 500 mg	500 mg twice daily or 250 mg four times daily	Same as ciprofloxacin
Gatifloxacin (Tequin)	T: 200, 400 mg S: 200 mg/5 mL I: 200, 400 mg	200-400 mg every 12 hr	Same as ciprofloxacin
Gemifloxacin (Factive)	T: 320 mg	320 mg/day	Same as ciprofloxacin
Levofloxacin (Levaquin)	T: 250, 500, 750 mg S: 25 mg/mL I: 250, 500, 750 mg	PO/IV: 250-750 mg/day as single dose	Same as ciprofloxacin
Lomefloxacin (Maxaquin)	T: 400 mg	400 mg/day	Same as ciprofloxacin

Moxifloxacin (Avelox)	T: 400 mg I: 400 mg	400 mg/day	Same as ciprofloxacin; may prolong QT interval
Nalidixic acid (NegGram)	T: 500 mg	1 g four times daily	Same as ciprofloxacin
Norfloxacin (Noroxin)	T: 400 mg	400 mg every 12 hr	Same as ciprofloxacin
Ofloxacin (Floxin)	T: 200, 300, 400 mg I: 200, 400 mg	200-400 mg every 12 hr	Same as ciprofloxacin
Sparfloxacin (Zagam)	T: 200 mg	200 mg/day	Same as ciprofloxacin

Macrolides/Ketolides

Name	Availability	Dosage Range	Side Effects/Comments
Azithromycin (Zithromax) (Zmax)	T: 250, 500, 600 mg S: 100 mg/5 mL, 167 mg/5 mL, 200 mg/5 mL, 1 g packet I: 500 mg	A (PO): 500 mg once, then 250 mg days 2-5 (IV): 500 mg/day; some indications 1-2 g as single dose C (PO): 10 mg/kg once, then 5 mg/kg/day on days 2-5, or 30 mg/kg as single dose	PO: Nausea, diarrhea, vomiting, abdominal pain IV: Pain, redness, swelling at injection site
Clarithromycin (Biaxin)	T: 250, 500 mg T (XL): 500, 1000 mg S: 125 mg/5 mL, 250 mg/5 mL	A: 250-500 mg every 12 hr C: 7.5 mg/kg every 12 hr	Headaches, loss of taste, nausea, vomiting, diarrhea, abdominal pain/discomfort
Erythromycin (Ery-Tab, PCE, Eryc, EES, EryPed, Erythrocin)	T: 200, 250, 333, 400, 500 mg C: 250 mg S: 125 mg/5 mL, 200 mg/5 mL, 250 mg/5 mL, 400 mg/5 mL, 100 mg/2.5 mL I: 500 mg, 1 g	A (PO): 250-500 mg every 6 hr C (PO): 30-50 mg/kg/day A, C (IV): 15-20 mg/kg/day Max: 4 g/day	PO: Nausea, vomiting, diarrhea, abdominal pain IV: Inflammation, phlebitis at injection site
Telithromycin (Ketek)	T: 400 mg	A: 800 mg daily as a single dose	Nausea, diarrhea Many drug interactions due to being a strong inhibitor of the cytochrome P450 3A4 system

Glycyclines

Name	Availability	Dosage Range	Side Effects/Comments
Tigecycline (Tygacil)	I: 50 mg	A: 100 mg loading dose, then 50 mg every 12 hr	Nausea, vomiting, diarrhea, tooth discoloration Reduce dose in hepatic impairment

Penicillins

Name	Availability	Dosage Range	Side Effects/Comments
Natural			
Penicillin G benzathine (Bicillin)	I: 600,000 units, 1.2 million units, 2.4 million units	A: 1.2 million units/day C: 0.3-1.2 million units/day (IM only)	Mild diarrhea, nausea, vomiting, headaches, sore mouth/tongue, vaginal itching/discharge, allergic reaction (including anaphylaxis, skin rash, hives, itching)
Penicillin G potassium (Pfizerpen)	I: 1, 2, 3, 5 million-unit vials, 20 mg multidose vial	A: 2-24 million units/day C: 100-300,000 units/kg/day	Same as penicillin G benzathine
Penicillin G procaine (Wycillin)	I: 600,000 units, 1.2 million units, 2.4 million units	A, C: 0.6-1.2 million units/day (IM only)	Same as penicillin G benzathine; increased risk of mental disturbances
Penicillin V potassium (V-Cillin-K)	T: 250, 500 mg S: 125 mg/5 mL, 250 mg/5 mL	A: 0.5-2 g/day C: 25-50 mg/kg/day	Same as penicillin G benzathine
Penicillinase-Resistant			
Dicloxacillin (Dynapen, Pathocil)	C: 250, 500 mg OS: 62.5 mg/15 mL	A: 125-250 mg every 6 hr C: 12.5-25 mg/kg/day divided by 6	Same as penicillin G benzathine; increased risk of hepatic toxicity
Nafcillin (Unipen)	I: 1, 2 g	IV: 2-6 g/day Max: 12 g/day	Same as penicillin G benzathine; increased risk of interstitial nephritis
Oxacillin (Bactocill)	S: 250 mg/5 mL I: 500 mg, 1 g, 2 g, 10 g C: 250, 500 mL	A (PO/IV): 2-6 g/day C (PO/IV): 50-100 mg/kg/day	Same as penicillin G benzathine; increased risk of hepatic toxicity, interstitial nephritis

Broad-Spectrum			
Amoxicillin (Amoxil, Trimox)	T: 500, 875 mg T (chewable): 125, 200, 250, 400 mg T (OS): 200 mg/400 mg C: 250, 500 mg S: 50 mg/mL, 125 mg/5 mL, 250 mg/5 mL, 200 mg/5 mL, 400 mg/5 mL	A: 0.75-1.5 g/day C: 20-40 mg/kg/day	Same as penicillin G benzathine
Amoxicillin/clavulanate (Augmentin)	T: 250, 500, 875 mg T (chewable): 125, 200, 250, 400 mg T (ER): 1000 mg S: 125 mg/5 mL, 200 mg/5 mL, 250 mg/5 mL, 400 mg/5 mL, 600 mg/5 mL	A: 0.75-1.5 g/day C: 20-45 mg/kg/day	Same as penicillin G benzathine
Ampicillin (Principen)	C: 250, 500 mg S: 125 mg/5 mL, 250 mg/5 mL I: 250 mg, 500 mg, 1 g, 2 g	A: 1-12 g/day C: 50-200 mg/kg/day Dosed every 3-6 hr	Same as penicillin G benzathine
Ampicillin/sulbactam (Unasyn)	I: 1.5 g, 3 g, 15 g multidose vial	A: 6-12 g/day C: 300 mg/kg/day	Same as penicillin G benzathine
Extended-Spectrum			
Carbenicillin (Geocillin, Carbapen)	T: 382 mg, 500 g I: 1, 5 g	A: 1-2 tabs 4 times/day, 200 mg/kg/day IV, IM	Same as penicillin G benzathine
Piperacillin/tazobactam (Zosyn)	I: 2.25, 3.375, 4.5 g 40.5 g multidose vial	A: 2.25-4.5 g every 6-8 hr	Same as penicillin G benzathine
Ticarcillin/clavulanate (Timentin)	I: 3.1 g	A: 3.1 g every 4-6 hr C: 200-300 mg/kg/day	Same as penicillin G benzathine

A, adults; C, capsules; C (dosage), children; ER, extended release; I, injection; OS, oral suspension; S, suspension; T, tablets; XL, long acting.

ANTICOAGULANTS/ANTIPLATELETS/THROMBOLYTICS

Uses

Treatment and prevention of venous thromboembolism, acute MI, acute cerebral embolism; reduce risk of acute MI; reduce total mortality in patients with unstable angina; prevent occlusion of saphenous grafts following open heart surgery; prevent embolism in select patients with atrial fibrillation, prosthetic heart valves, valvular heart disease, cardiomyopathy. Heparin also used for acute/chronic consumption coagulopathies (disseminated intravascular coagulation).

Action

Anticoagulants: Inhibit blood coagulation by preventing the formation of new clots and extension of existing ones *but do not dissolve formed clots.* Anticoagulants are subdivided into two common classes: *Heparin:* Indirectly interferes with blood coagulation by blocking the conversion of prothrombin to thrombin and fibrinogen to fibrin. *Coumarin:* Acts indirectly to prevent synthesis in the liver of vitamin K-dependent clotting factors.

Antiplatelets: Interfere with platelet aggregation. Effects are irreversible for life of platelet. Medications in this group act by different mechanisms and are used in combinations to provide desired effect.

Thrombolytics: Act directly or indirectly on fibrinolytic system to dissolve clots (converting plasminogen to plasmin, an enzyme that digests fibrin clots).

Anticoagulants/Antiplatelets/Thrombolytics

Name	Availability	Uses	Side Effects/Comments
Anticoagulants			
Antithrombin III (Thrombate III)	I: 500, 1000 units	Thromboembolism in patients with antithrombin III deficiency	Dizziness, chest pressure, nausea, taste disturbances
Argatroban	I: 100 mg/mL	Prevent/treat VTE in patients with HIT or at risk for HIT undergoing PCI	Bleeding
Bivalirudin (Angiomax)	I: 250-mg vials	Patients with unstable angina undergoing PTCA	Bleeding
Dalteparin (Fragmin)	I: 2500, 5000, 7500, 10,000, 25,000 units/mL	Hip surgery; abdominal surgery; unstable angina or non-Q-wave myocardial infarction, VTE prophylaxis	Bleeding, hematoma
Desirudin (Iprivask)	I: 15-mg vials	Prevent VTE in patients undergoing hip replacement surgery	Bleeding, hematoma

Enoxaparin (Lovenox)	I: 30, 40, 60, 80, 100, 120, 150, 300 mg/3 mL	Hip surgery; knee surgery; abdominal surgery; unstable angina or non-Q-wave myocardial infarction; acute illness	Bleeding, thrombocytopenia, hematoma
Fondaparinux (Arixtra)	I: 2.5, 5, 7.5, 10 mg	Hip surgery; knee surgery; PE/DVT treatment (with warfarin)	Bleeding, thrombocytopenia, hematoma
Heparin	I: 1000, 2500, 5000, 7500, 10,000, 20,000 units/mL	Prevent/treat VTE; prevent clotting in surgery, dialysis, IV lines; coagulopathies, PE, stroke, AMI, ACS	Bleeding, thrombocytopenia, skin rash
Lepirudin (Refludan)	I: 50-mg vials	Prevent VTE in patients with HIT; unstable angina; non-ST-elevated myocardial infarction, PCI	Bleeding
Tinzaparin (Innohep)	I: 20,000 units/mL vials	Treatment of VTE (with warfarin); prophylaxis of VTE in surgery	Bleeding, thrombocytopenia
Warfarin (Coumadin)	PO: 1, 2, 2.5, 3, 4, 5, 6, 7.5, 10 mg I: 5 mg	Prevent/treat VTE in patients; prevent systemic embolism in patients with heart valve replacement, heart valve disease, myocardial infarction, atrial fibrillation	Bleeding, skin necrosis
Antiplatelets			
Abciximab (ReoPro)	I: 2 mg/mL	Adjunct to PCI to prevent acute cardiac ischemic complications (with heparin and aspirin)	Bleeding, hypotension, nausea, vomiting, back pain, allergic reactions, thrombocytopenia
Anagrelide (Agrylin)	PO: 0.5, 1 mg	Thrombocythemia	Abdominal pain, diarrhea, edema, headache, palpitations
Aspirin	PO: 81, 165, 325, 500, 650 mg	TIA in males; myocardial infarction prophylaxis; cardiac vascular disease	Tinnitus, dizziness, hypersensitivity, dyspepsia, minor bleeding, gastrointestinal ulceration
Cilostazol (Pletal)	T: 50, 100 mg	Intermittent claudication	Headache Do *not* use in heart failure
Clopidogrel (Plavix)	PO: 75 mg	Reduce risk in patients with unstable angina, non-Q-wave myocardial infarction recent myocardial infarction, CVA; post-PCI	Bleeding Stop 5 days before major surgery
Dextran 40 and Dextran 70	IV: 10% infusion in D5W or NS	VTE/PE prophylaxis, especially when volume expansion is desirable	Hypersensitivity reactions, nausea, vomiting, headache, dyspnea, fever
Dipyridamole (Persantine)	PO: 25, 50, 75 mg	Prevent postoperative thromboembolic complications following cardiac valve replacement	Dizziness, gastrointestinal distress
Dipyridamole/Aspirin (Aggrenox)	200 mg/25 mg ER	Aggrenox twice daily for secondary stroke prevention	See individual agents for side effects

Continued

Anticoagulants/Antiplatelets/Thrombolytics—cont'd

Name	Availability	Uses	Side Effects/Comments
Eptifibatide (Integrilin)	I: 0.75 mg/mL, 2 mg/mL	Treatment of acute coronary syndrome, PCI	Bleeding, hypotension
Ticlopidine (Ticlid)	PO: 250 mg	Reduce risk stroke in patients with CVA precursors, TIA	Neutropenia, agranulocytosis, thrombocytopenia, aplastic anemia, increased serum cholesterol/triglycerides, rash, diarrhea, nausea, vomiting, gastrointestinal pain
Tirofiban (Aggrastat)	I: 50 mcg/mL, 250 mcg/mL	Treatment of acute coronary syndrome	Bleeding, thrombocytopenia
Thrombolytics			
Alteplase (Activase, Cathflo)	I: 2, 50, 100 mg	Acute myocardial infarction, acute ischemic stroke, pulmonary embolism, catheter clearance	Bleeding, dysrhythmias
Reteplase (Retavase)	I: 10.4 units	Acute myocardial infarction	Bleeding, dysrhythmias
Streptokinase	I: 25,000, 750,000, 1.5 million units	Myocardial infarction; venous thromboembolism; arterial thromboembolism	Bleeding, dysrhythmias, hypersensitivity reaction
Tenecteplase (TNKase)	I: 50 mg	Acute myocardial infarction	Bleeding, dysrhythmias

ACS, acute coronary syndrome; AMI, acute myocardial infarction; CVA, cerebrovascular attack; D5W, dextrose 5% in water solution for injection; DVT, deep vein thrombosis; ER, extended release; HIT, heparin-induced thrombocytopenia; I, injection; IV, intravenous; NS, normal saline for injection; PCI, percutaneous coronary intervention; PE, pulmonary embolism; PO, oral; PTCA, percutaneous transluminal coronary angioplasty; T, tablets; TIA, transient ischemic attack; VTE, venous thromboembolism

ANTICONVULSANTS

Uses
Anticonvulsants are used to treat seizures. Seizures can be divided into two broad categories: partial seizures and generalized seizures. Partial seizures begin focally in the cerebral cortex, undergoing limited spread. Simple partial seizures do not involve loss of consciousness but may evolve secondarily into generalized seizures. Complex partial seizures involve impairment of consciousness. Generalized seizures may be convulsive or nonconvulsive and usually produce immediate loss of consciousness.

Action
Anticonvulsants can prevent or reduce excessive discharge of neurons with seizure foci or decrease the spread of excitation from seizure foci to normal neurons. The exact mechanism is unknown but may be due to (1) suppressing sodium influx; (2) suppressing calcium influx; or (3) increasing the action of GABA, which inhibits neurotransmitters throughout the brain.

Anticonvulsants

Name	Availability	Uses	Dosage Range	Side Effects/Comments
Carbamazepine (Tegretol)	S: 100 mg/5 mL T (chewable): 100 mg T: 200, 300, 400 mg T (ER): 100, 200, 400 mg C (ER): 200, 300 mg	Complex partial, tonic-clonic, mixed seizures; trigeminal neuralgia	A: 800-1200 mg/day C (6-12 yr): 400-800 mg/day C (less than 6 yr): 10-20 mg/kg/day; Max 35 mg/kg/day	Dizziness, diplopia, leukopenia, somnolence, nausea Many drug interactions exist because it increases hepatic metabolism of cytochrome P450 drugs
Clonazepam (Klonopin)	T: 0.5, 1, 2 mg T (OD): 0.125, 0.25, 0.5, 1, 2 mg	Akinetic, myoclonic, absence seizures	A: 1.5-20 mg/day	CNS depression, sedation, ataxia, confusion, depression
Diazepam (Valium)	T: 2, 5, 10 mg OS: 1 mg/mL, 5 mg/mL I: 5 mg/mL R: 2.5, 5, 10, 15, 20 mg	Adjunctive therapy status epilepticus	A (PO): 4-40 mg/day A (IM/IV): 5-30 mg C (PO): 3-10 mg/day C (IM/IV): 1-10 mg	CNS depression, sedation, confusion, depression, respiratory depression
Ethosuximide (Zarontin)	C: 250 mg Syrup: 250 mg/5 mL	Absence seizures	A, C (greater than or equal to 6 yr): 500 mg/day C (3-6 yr): 250 mg/day initially, 20 mg/kg/day	Drowsiness, ataxia, dizziness, blood dyscrasias

Continued

Anticonvulsants—cont'd

Name	Availability	Uses	Dosage Range	Side Effects/Comments
Ethotoin (Peganone)	T: 250, 500 mg	Tonic-clonic, psychomotor seizures, status epilepticus	A: 2-3 mg/day C: 500 mg-1 g/day	Nystagmus, ataxia, hypertrichosis, gingival hyperplasia, rashes, osteomalacia, lymphadenopathy, hypotension with rapid IV administration (give less than 50 mg/min)
Felbamate (Felbatol)	T: 400, 600 mg S: 600 mg/5 mL	Partial seizures with and without generalization	1200 mg/day initially; 1200-3600/day maintenance (divided three times daily-four times daily)	Insomnia, dyspepsia, vomiting Warning: Aplastic anemia and hepatic failure have been associated with felbamate. Risk assessment is important.
Fosphenytoin (Cerebyx)	I: 50 mg PE/mL	Status epilepticus, seizures occurring during neurosurgery	A: 15-20 mg PE/kg bolus, then 4-6 mg PE/kg/day maintenance	Burning, itching, paraesthesia, nystagmus, ataxia Can give up to 150 PE/min
Gabapentin (Neurontin)	C: 100, 300, 400 mg T: 600, 700 mg OS: 250 mg/5 mL	Partial seizures with and without secondary generalization	A: 900-1800 mg/day	CNS depression, fatigue, somnolence, dizziness, ataxia
Lamotrigine (Lamictal)	T: 25, 100, 150, 200 mg T (chewable): 2, 5, 25 mg	Partial seizures	A: 100-500 mg/day	Dizziness, ataxia, diplopia, nausea, rash (can be serious), insomnia and somnolence
Levetiracetam (Keppra)	T: 250, 500, 750 mg Syrup: 100 mg/mL IV: 100 mg/mL	Partial seizures	A: 500 mg twice daily initially; increase by 1000 mg/day every 2 wk; max dose 3000 mg/day C (4-15 yr): 10 mg/kg PO; increase by 20 mg/kg every 2 wk; max 60 mg/kg/day (in 2 divided doses)	Dizziness, somnolence, asthenia
Lorazepam (Ativan)	T: 0.5, 1, 2, 2.5 mg (not used for status epilepticus) I: 2 mg/mL, 4 mg/mL	Status epilepticus	A: 4 mg over 2 min; repeat every 10-15 min; may give deep IM if IV route not available C: 0.05 mg/kg repeated × 2 at 15-20 min intervals; use in children under 18 yr not established	CNS depression, sedation, confusion, depression, respiratory depression
Mephenytoin (Mesantoin)	T: 100 mg	Tonic-clonic, psychomotor, focal, Jacksonian seizures	A: 50-100 mg/day initially; increase by 50-100 mg every wk; maintenance range 200-600 mg/day up to 800 mg C: 100-400 mg/day	

Methsuximide (Celontin)	C: 150, 300 mg	Absence seizures	A: 300 mg/day initially; increase by 300 mg every wk to final range of 1200 mg/day	Drowsiness, ataxia, dizziness, blood dyscrasias Use when seizures are refractory to other drugs
Oxcarbazepine (Trileptal)	T: 150, 300, 600 mg S: 300 mg/5 mL	Partial seizures	A: 900-1800 mg/day	Somnolence, dizziness, diplopia
Phenobarbital	T: 30, 60, 100 mg I: 65 mg, 130 mg	Tonic-clonic, partial seizures; status epilepticus	A (PO): 100-300 mg/day A (IM/IV): 200-600 mg C (PO): 3-5 mg/kg/day C (IM/IV): 100-400 mg	CNS depression, sedation, paradoxic excitement and hyperactivity, rash
Phensuximide (Milontin)	C: 500 mg	Absence seizures	1-3 g/day	Drowsiness, ataxia, dizziness, blood dyscrasias
Phenytoin (Dilantin)	C: 100 mg C (ER): 30, 100 mg T (chewable): 50 mg S: 125 mg/5 mL I: 50 mg/mL	Tonic-clonic, psychomotor seizures, status epilepticus	A (PO): 300-600 mg/day A (IV): 150-250 mg C (PO): 4-8 mg/kg/day C (IV): 10-15 mg/kg	Nystagmus, ataxia, hypertrichosis, gingival hyperplasia, rashes, osteomalacia, lymphadenopathy, hypotension with rapid IV administration (give less than or equal to 50 mg/min)
Pregabalin (Lyrica)	C: 25, 50, 75, 100, 150, 200, 225, 300 mg	Partial onset seizures	150 mg/day initially; max 600 mg/day divided into 2-3 doses	Dizziness, somnolence
Primidone (Mysoline)	T: 50, 250 mg S: 250 mg/5 mL	Complex, partial, akinetic, tonic-clonic seizures	A: 750-2000 mg/day C: 10-25 mg/kg/day	CNS depression, sedation, paradoxic excitement and hyperactivity, rash, dizziness, ataxia
Tiagabine (Gabitril)	T: 2, 4, 12, 16, 20 mg	Partial seizures	A: 4 mg up to 56 mg initially C: 4 mg up to 32 mg initially	Dizziness, asthenia, nervousness, anxiety, tremors, abdominal pain, irritability, slowed thinking
Topiramate (Topamax)	T: 25, 50, 100, 200 mg C (sprinkle): 15, 25 mg	Partial, generalized tonic-clonic seizures	A: 25-400 mg/day C: 1-9 mg/kg/day	Impaired concentration, speech impairment, fatigue, ataxia
Valproic acid (Depakene, Depakote)	C: 250 mg S: 250 mg/5 mL Sprinkles: 125 mg T: 125, 250, 500 mg T (ER): 250, 500 mg I: 100 mg/mL	Complex partial, absence seizures	A, C: 15-60 mg/kg/day	Nausea, vomiting, tremors, thrombocytopenia, hair loss, hepatic dysfunction
Zonisamide (Zonegran)	C: 25, 50 100 mg	Partial seizures	A: 100-400 mg/day; max 600 mg/day C: 4-8 mg/kg/day; max 12 mg/kg/day	Somnolence, dizziness, anorexia, headaches, nausea Because of long half-life, increase dose every 2 wk while titrating up and taper slowly off when discontinuing

A, adults; C, capsules; C (dosage), children; ER, extended release; I, injection; OD, orally disintegrating; OS, oral solution; PE, phenytoin equivalents; R, rectal; S, suspension; T, tablets

ANTIDEPRESSANTS

Uses

Used primarily for the treatment of depression. Imipramine is also used for childhood enuresis. Clomipramine is used only for obsessive-compulsive disorder (OCD). Monoamine oxidase inhibitors (MAOIs) are rarely used as initial therapy except in patients unresponsive to other therapy or when other therapy is contraindicated.

Action

Antidepressants are classified as tricyclics, MAOIs, or second-generation antidepressants (further subdivided into selective serotonin reuptake inhibitors [SSRIs] and atypical antidepressants). Depression may be due to reduced functioning of monoamine neurotransmitters (e.g., norepinephrine, serotonin [5-HT], dopamine) in the CNS (decreased amount and/or decreased effects at the receptor sites). Antidepressants block metabolism, increase amount/effects of monoamine neurotransmitters, and act at receptor sites (change responsiveness/sensitivities of both presynaptic and postsynaptic receptor sites).

Antidepressants

Generic Name	Brand Name	Adult Therapeutic Dose Range	Available Dosage Forms	Relative Sedation Effect	Relative Anticholinergic Effect	Relative Orthostatic Hypotension	Comments/Other Uses
Tetracyclics							
Maprotiline*	Ludiomil	25-225 mg/day in single or divided doses	T: 25, 50, 75 mg	2+	2+	1+	Increased risk of seizures. Separate from MAOIs × 14 days. Alcohol may potentiate CNS effects. Contraindicated in narrow-angle glaucoma.
Mirtazapine*	Remeron, Remeron SolTab	15-45 mg/day	T: 7.5, 15, 30, 45 mg T (OD): 15, 30, 45 mg	3+	2+	2+	Separate from MAOIs × 14 days. Alcohol may potentiate CNS effects. Contraindicated in narrow-angle glaucoma.
Triazolopyridines							
Trazodone*	Desyrel	150-600 mg/day	T: 50, 100, 150, 300 mg	4+	1+	2+	Not for use during recovery phase of myocardial infarction. Priapism has occurred.
Tricyclics[†]							
Amitriptyline*	Elavil	25-300 mg/day in 3 doses per day less than 100 mg/day doses as single dose at bedtime	T: 10, 25, 50, 75, 100, 150 mg	4+	4+	2+	Use lower doses in outpatients (less than or equal to 150 mg/day)

Amoxapine*	Asendin	100-300 mg/day in 2-3 doses per day	T: 25, 50, 100, 150 mg	2+	3+	1+	Dopamine-blocking effects (tardive dyskinesia). Max. daily dose = 400 mg (outpatients), 600 mg (inpatients)
Clomipramine*	Anafranil	25-250 mg/day in divided doses with meals	C: 25, 50, 75 mg	3+	3+	2+	Increased risk of seizures; indicated for obsessive-compulsive disorder only. GI side effects; take with food.
Desipramine*	Norpramin	100-300 mg/day	T: 10, 25, 50, 75, 100, 150 mg	1+	1+	1+	Metabolite of imipramine
Doxepin*	Sinequan	25-300 mg/day	C: 10, 25, 50, 75, 100, 150 mg OC: 10 mg/mL	3+	2+	2+	Potent antihistamine
Imipramine hydrochloride*	Tofranil	50-300 mg/day	T: 10, 25, 50 mg	2+	2+	3+	
Imipramine pamoate	Tofranil-PM	75-300 mg/day at bedtime	C: 75, 100, 125, 150 mg	2+	2+	3+	
Nortriptyline*	Pamelor, Aventyl	75-150 mg/day at bedtime	C: 10, 25, 50, 75 mg OS: 10 mg/5 mL	2+	2+	1+	Metabolite of amitriptyline; entire daily dose may be given at bedtime
Protriptyline*	Vivactil	15-60 mg/day	T: 5, 10 mg	1+	3+	1+	
Trimipramine	Surmontil	50-300 mg/day at bedtime	C: 25, 50, 100 mg	3+	2+	2+	

Continued

Antidepressants—cont'd

Tetracyclics

Generic Name	Brand Name	Adult Therapeutic Dose Range	Available Dosage Forms	Relative Sedation Effect	Relative Anticholinergic Effect	Relative Orthostatic Hypotension	Comments/Other Uses
Monoamine Oxidase Inhibitors							
Isocarboxazid	Marplan	10-60 mg/day divided in 2-4 doses	T: 10 mg	1+	1+	2+	Avoid tyramine-containing foods and certain OTC drug products, including dextromethorphan, and sympathomimetics such as pseudoephedrine (e.g., Sudafed) and phenylephrine (e.g., Neo-Synephrine). Usually reserved for patients who are intolerant of other antidepressant classes. Drug interaction: trazodone, SSRIs, venlafaxine-increases risk of serotonin syndrome (hypertension, hyperthermia, tachycardia, death). Many other drug interactions also. See individual drug monographs.
Phenelzine	Nardil	15-90 mg/day	T: 15 mg	1+	1+	1+	Same as isocarboxazid.
Tranylcypromine	Parnate	20-60 mg/day divided in 2-4 doses	T: 10 mg	1+	1+	0	Same as isocarboxazid.
Selective Serotonin Reuptake Inhibitors‡							
Citalopram*	Celexa	20-40 mg/day; max 60 mg/day	T: 10, 20, 40 mg OS: 10 mg/5 mL	0-1+	0-1+	0-1+	Also used for panic disorder, anxiety.
Escitalopram oxalate	Lexapro	10-20 mg/day	T: 5, 10, 20 mg OS: 5 mg/5 mL	0-1+	0-1+	0-1+	Active metabolite of citalopram. Also used for panic disorder.

Fluoxetine*	Prozac, Prozac Weekly, Sarafem	10-80 mg/day 1-2 times per day, 90 mg every wk	C: 10, 20, 40 mg T: 10, 20 mg C (DR): 90 mg (for weekly dosing) OL: 20 mg/5 mL	0	0-1+	0-1+	Doses taken later than noon may cause insomnia; Sarafem is indicated for premenstrual dysphoric disorder (PMDD). Also used for bulimia nervosa, obsessive-compulsive disorder, panic disorder, posttraumatic stress disorder (PTSD), Raynaud's, and generalized anxiety disorder (GAD).
Fluvoxamine*	Luvox	50-300 mg/day at bedtime	T: 25, 50, 100 mg	1+	0-1+	0	Primary indication is OCD.
Paroxetine*	Paxil, Paxil CR	10-60 mg/day	T: 10, 20, 30, 40 mg T (CR): 12.5, 25, 37.5 mg OS: 10 mg/5 mL	1+	0	0	Also used for GAD, OCD, PTSD, PMDD, hot flashes, panic disorder, and diabetic neuropathy.
Sertraline	Zoloft	25-200 mg/day	T: 25, 50, 100 mg OS concentrated: 20 mg/mL	0	0	0	Also used for OCD, PTSD, PMDD, panic disorder, and social anxiety disorder.

Antidepressants—cont'd

Atypical					
Bupropion*	Wellbutrin	150-450 mg/day	T: 75, 100 mg T (24-hr ER): 150, 300 mg SR (12-hr): 100, 150, 200 mg	Depression, neuropathic pain, attention deficit/hyperactivity disorder	Insomnia, irritability, seizures, agitation
Duloxetine*	Cymbalta	40-60 mg/day	C: 20, 30, 60 mg	Depression, neuropathic pain	Nausea, dry mouth, constipation, decreased appetite, fatigue, diaphoresis
Mirtazapine*	Remeron	15-45 mg/day	T: 15, 30, 45 mg	Depression	Sedation, dry mouth, weight gain, agranulocytosis, hepatic toxicity
Nefazodone*	Serzone	200-600 mg/day	T: 50, 100, 150, 200, 250 mg	Depression	Sedation, orthostatic hypotension, nausea; life-threatening liver failure rarely occurs
Venlafaxine	Effexor	75-375 mg/day	T: 25, 37.5, 50, 75, 100 mg T (ER): 37.5, 75, 150 mg	Depression, anxiety	Increased BP, agitation, sedation, insomnia, nausea

*Generic available for one or more dosage forms.

†General Information:

1. Separate from MAOI therapy by at least 14 days.
2. Alcohol may increase CNS effects.
3. Grapefruit juice may decrease metabolic clearance.
4. Contraindicated in narrow-angle glaucoma or active cardiac disease.

‡General Information:

1. MAOIs, hypericum (St. John's wort) may potentiate serotonergic effects.
2. Alcohol may potentiate CNS effects.

C, capsules; CR, controlled release; DR, delayed release; ER, extended release; OC, oral concentrate; OD, orally disintegrating; OL, oral liquid; OS, oral solution/suspension; SR, sustained release; T, tablets.

ANTIDIABETICS

Uses
Insulin: Treatment of insulin-dependent diabetes (type 1) and non-insulin-dependent diabetes (type 2). Also used in acute situations such as ketoacidosis, severe infections, and major surgery in otherwise non-insulin-dependent diabetics. Administered to patients receiving parenteral nutrition. Drug of choice during pregnancy.

Sulfonylureas: Control hyperglycemia in type 2 diabetes not controlled by weight and diet alone. Chlorpropamide also used in adjunctive treatment of neurogenic diabetes insipidus.

Alpha-glucosidase inhibitors: Adjunct to diet to lower blood glucose in patients with type 2 diabetes mellitus whose hyperglycemia cannot be managed by diet alone.

Biguanides: Adjunct to diet to lower blood glucose in patients with type 2 diabetes mellitus whose hyperglycemia cannot be managed by diet alone.

Thiazolinediones: Adjunct in patients with type 2 diabetes currently on insulin therapy.

Action
Insulin: A hormone synthesized and secreted by beta cells of Langerhans' islet in the pancreas. Controls storage and utilization of glucose, amino acids, and fatty acids by activated transport systems/enzymes. Inhibits breakdown of glycogen, fat, protein. Insulin lowers blood glucose by inhibiting glycogenolysis and gluconeogenesis in liver; stimulates glucose uptake by muscle, adipose tissue. Activity of insulin is initiated by binding to cell surface receptors.

Sulfonylureas: Stimulate release of insulin from beta cells; increase sensitivity of insulin to peripheral tissue. Endogenous insulin must be present for oral hypoglycemics to be effective.

Alpha-glucosidase inhibitors: Work locally in small intestine, slowing carbohydrate breakdown and glucose absorption.

Biguanides: Decrease hepatic glucose output; enhance peripheral glucose uptake.

Thiazolinediones: Decrease insulin resistance.

Insulin

Name	Onset (hr)	Peak Effect (hr)	Duration (hr)	Route of Administration	Comments
Insulin aspart (Novolog)	¼	1-3	3-5	Subcutaneous	Compatible with recombinant human NPH insulin Side effects include hypoglycemia, weight gain, lipodystrophy, local skin reactions.
Insulin glargine (Lantus)	1	5	24	Subcutaneous	Not compatible with other insulins. Side effects same as insulin aspart.
Insulin glulisine (Apidra)				Subcutaneous, pump	Faster onset and shorter duration than regular insulin. May be used in insulin pump. May be mixed with NPH insulin. Draw insulin glulisine into syringe first.

Continued

Insulin—cont'd

Name	Onset (hr)	Peak Effect (hr)	Duration (hr)	Route of Administration	Comments
Insulin lispro (Humalog)	¼	1	3-6.5	Subcutaneous	Recombinant human insulin analog; compatible with Ultralente and NPH Side effects same as insulin aspart.
Regular insulin (subcutaneous)	½-1	1-5	6-10	Subcutaneous	Clear solution; compatible with all other insulins; draw regular into syringe first; inject regular/lente mixtures immediately to avoid potency loss due to chemical binding. Side effects same as insulin aspart.
Regular insulin (IV)	⅙-½	¼-½	½-1	IV, IM	Clear solution; compatible with all other insulins; draw regular into syringe first; inject regular/lente mixtures immediately to avoid potency loss due to chemical binding.
Isophane insulin suspension (NPH insulin)	1-2	6-14	16-24	Subcutaneous	Compatible with regular
Lente insulin	1-3	5-14	16-24	Subcutaneous	Compatible with regular
Ultralente insulin	4-8	8-20	24-28	Subcutaneous	Compatible with regular
Insulin detemir (Levemir)	Given 1-2 times daily for basal insulin requirements. If once daily, give in the evening.				
50/50 insulin	½-1	4-8	24	Subcutaneous	50% Isophane insulin suspension (NPH) and 50% regular insulin
70/30 insulin	½-1	4-8	24	Subcutaneous	70% Isophane insulin suspension (NPH) and 30% regular insulin

Notes:

1. Most insulin types are available as beef, pork, or human types. Onset of action is faster and duration of action is shorter with human insulin preparations.
2. Insulin is available in U-100 (100 units per mL) and U-500 (500 units per mL) forms. Duration of action of U-500 forms is longer than that of U-100 forms.

References:

1. Ellsworth, Allan J et al: *Mosby's Medical Drug Reference.* Mosby, St. Louis, 2003
2. *U.S. Food and Drug Administration.* Online. Internet. May 2003. Available http://www.fda.gov/
3. *Centers for Disease Control and Prevention.* Online. Internet. May 2003. Available http://www.cdc.gov/
4. *National Guideline Clearinghouse* [documents produced by the Agency for Healthcare Policy and Research (AHCPR) in partnership with the American Medical Association (AMA) and the American Association of Health Plans (AAHP)]. Online. Internet. May 2003. Available http://www.guideline.gov

Oral Hypoglycemic Agents

Sulfonylureas

Generic Name	Brand Name	Initial Dose	Maintenance Dose	Available Dosage Forms	Administration/Comments
					Side effects of first and second generation sulfonylureas include hypoglycemia, weight gain, GI disturbances, cholestasis, rash, and weight gain.
First Generation					
Acetohexamide*	Dymelor	250-1500 mg/day	Same	T: 250, 500 mg	Doses greater than 1500 mg/day are not recommended. Take doses less than 1500 mg/day before breakfast. At 1500 mg/day, divide dose twice daily.
Chlorpropamide*	Diabinese	250 mg daily (100-125 mg daily for elderly)	100-500 mg daily	T: 100, 250 mg	Avoid doses greater than 750 mg/day (500 mg/day in elderly).
Tolazamide*	Tolinase	100-250 mg daily	100-1000 mg daily (give twice daily if greater than 500 mg required)	T: 100, 250, 500 mg	Take with breakfast or first main meal. Max. daily dose = 1000 mg. Titrate dose to patient response. Divide doses greater than 500 mg twice daily.
Tolbutamide*	Orinase	1000-2000 mg daily in divided doses	250-3000 mg daily in divided doses	T: 500 mg	Dose may be taken in the morning or in divided doses. Max. daily dose = 3000 g. Doses greater than 2000 mg are seldom needed.
Second Generation					
Glimepiride	Amaryl	1-2 mg daily	1-8 mg daily	T: 1, 2, 4 mg	Take with breakfast or first main meal. Max. daily dose = 8 mg.
Glipizide*	Glucotrol, Glucotrol XL	5 mg daily	2.5-40 mg daily (divide doses if greater than 15 mg required)	T: 5, 10 mg T (ER): 2.5, 5, 10 mg	Take 30 min before breakfast. Advantages: no renal elimination and few drug interactions. Use with caution in hepatic disease.
Glyburide*	Diabeta, Micronase	1.25-5 mg daily	1.25-20 mg daily	T: 1.25, 2.5, 3, 5, 6 mg	Single dose or in divided doses. Max. daily dose = 20 mg/day.
	Glynase PresTab	0.75-3 mg daily	0.75-12 mg daily	T (M): 1.5, 3, 4.5, 6 mg	Micronized tablets are scored and can be broken in half. Max. daily dose of micronized form = 12 mg/day. Micronized tablets allow faster absorption and smaller doses.

Oral Hypoglycemic Agents—cont'd

Alpha-Glucosidase Inhibitors

Generic Name	Brand Name	Initial Dose	Maintenance Dose	Available Dosage Forms	Administration/Comments
Acarbose	Precose	25 mg three times daily with meals	50-100 mg three times daily with meals	T: 25, 50, 100 mg	Monotherapy or in combination with sulfonylureas. Take with first bite of each main meal. Contraindicated in bowel disease. Side effects include flatulence and diarrhea.
Miglitol	Glyset	25 mg three times daily	50-100 mg three times daily	T: 25, 50, 100 mg	Same as above. No dose adjustment needed in hepatic impairment. Side effects same as above, plus rash.

Biguanides

Generic Name	Brand Name	Initial Dose	Maintenance Dose	Available Dosage Forms	Administration/Comments
Metformin*	Glucophage	500 mg twice daily, or 850 mg daily	Up to 2550 mg daily in 2-3 divided doses	T: 500, 850, 1000 mg OS: 500 mg/ 5 mL	Twice daily dosing with AM and PM meals; single daily dosing with AM meal. Max. daily dose = 2550 mg. As monotherapy or in combination with sulfonylureas. Contraindicated in patients with subnormal renal function (creatinine greater than 1.5 in men or 1.4 in women) for age due to increased risk of lactic acidosis. Side effects include nausea, vomiting, diarrhea, anorexia.
	Glucophage XR	500 mg once daily with evening meal	Up to 2000 mg once daily with evening meal	T (ER): 500, 750, 1000 mg	If 2000 mg once daily not effective, may try 1000 mg twice daily. If this is not effective, switch to immediate-release regimen described above, up to a maximum daily dose of 2550 mg.

Thiazolidinediones

Generic Name	Brand Name	Initial Dose	Maintenance Dose	Available Dosage Forms	Administration/Comments
Pioglitazone	Actos	15-30 mg daily	Up to 45 mg daily	T: 15, 30, 45 mg	May take without regard to meals. Monotherapy or in combination with metformin or sulfonylureas.
Rosiglitazone	Avandia	4 mg daily	Up to 8 mg daily	T: 2, 4, 8 mg	No dose change needed for elderly. No dose change needed when used as monotherapy with renally impaired patients. May take without regard to meals as either a single AM dose or in divided AM and PM doses. Monotherapy or in combination with metformin or sulfonylureas.

Meglitinides

Generic Name	Brand Name	Initial Dose	Maintenance Dose	Available Dosage Forms	Administration/Comments
Nateglinide	Starlix	60-120 mg three times daily 1-30 min before meals.	Same	T: 60, 120 mg	Monotherapy or in combination with metformin. Should not be used with glyburide or other sulfonylureas, nor is it indicated for patients who fail treatment with these agents. No dosage adjustment required in even severe renal dysfunction or in mild hepatic dysfunction. The 60-mg dose is intended for patients near their goal HbA_{1C}. Side effects include hypoglycemia, weight gain.
Repaglinide	Prandin	0.5-2 mg three times daily before meals	0.5-4 mg twice daily, three times daily, or four times daily depending on changes in patient's meal pattern	T: 0.5, 1, 2 mg	Take 15 min before a meal. Max. daily dose of 16 mg. Side effects same as for nateglinide.

Oral Hypoglycemic Agents—cont'd

Miscellaneous Agents

Generic Name	Brand Name	Initial Dose	Maintenance Dose	Available Dosage Forms	Administration/Comments
Exenatide	Byetta	5 mcg twice daily subcutaneously 60 min before meals	10 mcg	I (subcutaneous): 5 or 10 mcg/dose in prefilled pens	Used as an adjunct to oral therapy in type II diabetes. Watch for hypoglycemia. Nausea is the main side effect.
Pramlintide acetate	Symlin	60-120 mcg subcutaneously before big meals	Same	Solution for I: 0.6 mg/mL in 5-mL vials	Insulin doses should be decreased as needed. Useful in type 1 and 2 diabetes; lower doses are used in type 1. Nausea is the main side effect.

Combination Products

Generic Name	Brand Name	Initial Dose	Maintenance Dose	Available Dosage Forms	Administration/Comments
*GlyBURIDE/ metformin	Glucovance	1.25 mg/250 mg once daily or twice daily with meals	2.5 mg/500 mg or 5 mg/500 mg twice daily with meals	T: glyburide/metformin, 1.25/ 250, 2.5/500, 5/500 mg	Maximum daily dose: glyburide/ metformin 20/2000 mg
*GlipiZIDE/ metformin	Metaglip	2.5 mg/250 mg once daily to 2.5 mg/500 mg twice daily	Up to 20 mg/2000 mg/day in divided doses	T: glipizide/metformin, 2.5/250, 2.5/500, 5/500 mg	Give with meals

*Generic available for one or more dosage forms.

References:

1. Website: U.S. Food and Drug Administration. Online. Internet. 2003. Available: http://www.fda.gov/cder
2. Micromedex.com

ER, extended release; I, injection; M, micronized; OS, oral solution; T, tablet

ANTIDIARRHEALS

Uses
Acute diarrhea, chronic diarrhea of inflammatory bowel disease, reduction of fluid from ileostomies.

Action
Systemic agents: Act at smooth muscle receptors (enteric), disrupting peristaltic movements, decreasing GI motility, increasing transit time of intestinal contents.

Local agents: Adsorb toxic substances and fluids to large surface areas of particles in the preparation. Some of these agents coat and protect irritated intestinal walls. May have local antiinflammatory action.

Antidiarrheals

Name	Availability	Type	Dosage Range
Bismuth subsalicylate (Pepto-Bismol)	T: 262 mg C: 262 mg L: 130 mg/15 mL, 262 mg/15 mL, 524 mg/15 mL	Local	A: 2 tabs or 30 mL C (9-12 yr): 1 tabs or 15 mL C (6-8 yr): ⅔ tabs or 10 mL C (3-5 yr): ⅓ tabs or 5 mL
Cholestyramine (Questran)	Powder packets: 4 g	Local	*Specific for antibiotic-associated diarrhea and pseudomembranous colitis* A: 4 g 3-4 times/day C: 400 mg-1.3 g 3-4 times/day
Difenoxin (with atropine) (Motofen)	T: 1 mg difenoxin/0.025 mg atropine	Systemic	2 tablets initially, then 1-2 tablets every 3-4 hr as needed; max. 8 tabs/day Not recommended for children less than 2 yr
Diphenoxylate (with atropine) (Lomotil)	T: 2.5 mg diphenoxylate/0.25 mg atropine L: 2.5 mg/5 mL diphenoxylate/0.25 mg/5 mL atropine	Systemic	A: 5 mg 4 times/day as needed C: 0.3-0.4 mg/kg/day in 4 divided doses (L); max. 8 tabs/day
Kaolin (with pectin) (Kaopectate)	S	Local	A: 60-120 mL after each bowel movement C (6-12 yr): 30-60 mL C (3-5 yr): 15-30 mL
Loperamide (Imodium)	C: 2 mg T: 2 mg L: 1 mg/5 mL, 1 mg/mL	Systemic	A: Initially, 4 mg (Max.: 16 mg/day) C (9-12 yr): 2 mg 3 times/day C (6-8 yr): 2 mg 2 times/day C (2-5 yr): 1 mg 3 times/day (L)

A, adults; C, capsules; C (dosage), children; L, liquid; S, suspension; T, tablets

ANTIDOTES

Uses
To reverse or treat accidental or intentional drug/poison overdoses.

Antidotes

Name	Availability	Dosage Range	Side Effects	Drug/Poison Reversed
Acetylcysteine (Mucomyst, Acetadote)	OS: 10%, 20% I: 20%	I: 150 mg/kg over 15 min, then 50 mg/kg over 4 hr, then 100 mg/kg over 16 hr PO: 140 mg/kg once, then 70 mg/kg every 4 hr × 17 doses	Pruritus, rash, urticaria, vomiting	Acetaminophen
Digoxin immune fab (Digibind, Digifab)	I: Digibind: 38 mg/vial I: Digifab: 40 mg/vial	Individualized based on digoxin level/amount ingested	Hypokalemia, rapid ventricular response in atrial fibrillation controlled by digoxin Note: Digoxin levels cannot be accurately measured after giving digoxin immune fab.	Digoxin, digitoxin
Flumazenil (Romazicon)	I: 0.1 mg/mL	0.2 mg over 15 sec; repeat in 45 sec up to a max of 1 mg based on symptomatic improvement	Dizziness, agitation, tremors, seizures	Benzodiazepines
Fomepizole (Antizol)	I: 1 g/mL	15 mg/kg, then 10 mg/kg every 12 hr for 4 doses, then 15 mg/kg every 12 hr until ethylene glycol/methanol levels are undetectable. All doses over 30 min.	Headache, nausea, dizziness, drowsiness	Ethylene glycol, methanol
Nalmefene (Revex)	I: 100 mcg/mL, 1 mg/mL	IV/IM/Subcutaneous: Titrated individually	Nausea, vomiting, tachycardia, hypertension	Opiate analgesics (i.e., morphine)
Naloxone (Narcan)	I: 0.02 mg/mL, 0.4 mg/mL, 1 mg/mL	IV/IM/Subcutaneous (A): 0.4-2 mg, may repeat at 2- to 3-min intervals IV/IM/Subcutaneous (C): 0.01 mg/kg, may give subsequent doses of 0.1 mg/kg	Same as for nalmefene	Opiate analgesics (i.e., morphine)
Naltrexone (Depade, ReVia)	T: 50 mg	PO: 50 mg/day or 100 mg every other day or 150 mg every third day	Abdominal pain, anxiety, diarrhea, tachycardia, diaphoresis, loss of appetite, nausea; hepatic failure at large doses, contraindicated in hepatitis	For chronic use in alcohol and narcotic addiction
Sodium nitrate	I: 30 mg/mL	A: 2.5-5 mL/min × 10 mL C: 6-8 mL/m^2 up to 10 mL Follow with sodium thiosulfate	Hypotension	Adjunct cyanide (along with sodium thiosulfate)
Sodium thiosulfate	I: 10%, 25%	A: 12.5 g IV over 10 min C: 7 g/m^2; max 12.5 g		Cyanide

A, adults; C, children; I, injection; OS, oral solution; PO, oral.

ANTIDYSRHYTHMICS

Uses
Prevention and treatment of cardiac dysrhythmias, such as premature ventricular contractions, ventricular tachycardia, premature atrial contractions, paroxysmal atrial tachycardia, atrial fibrillation and flutter.

Action
The antidysrhythmics are divided into four classes based on their effects on certain ion channels and/or receptors located on the myocardial cell membrane. Class I is further divided into three subclasses (1A, 1B, 1C) based on electrophysiologic effects.*Class I:* Block cardiac sodium channels and slow conduction velocity, prolonging refractoriness and decreasing automaticity of sodium-dependent tissue.

Class 1A: Block sodium and potassium channels.

Class 1B: Shorten the repolarization phase.

Class 1C: No effect on repolarization phase, but slow conduction velocity.

Class II: Slow the sinus and atrioventricular (AV) nodal conduction.

Class III: Block cardiac potassium channels, prolonging the repolarization phase of electrical cells.

Class IV: Inhibit the influx of calcium through its channels, causing slower conduction through the sinus and AV nodes.

Antidysrhythmics

Name	Availability	Uses	Dosage Range	Side Effects
Class 1A				
Disopyramide (Norpace SR, Norpace CR)	C: 100, 150 mg C (ER): 100, 150 mg	AF, WPW, PSVT, PVCs, VT	400-800 mg/day	Dry mouth, blurred vision, urinary retention, CHF, proarrhythmia
Procainamide (Pronestyl, Procan-SR)	T: 250, 375, 500 mg C: 250, 375, 500 mg T (SR): 250, 500, 750, 1000 mg I: 100 mg/mL, 500 mg/mL	AF, WPW, PVCs, VT	A (PO): 25-500 mg every 3 hr; (ER): 250-750 mg every 6 hr	Hypotension, fever, agranulocytosis, SLE, headaches, proarrhythmia

Continued

Antidysrhythmics—cont'd

Name	Availability	Uses	Dosage Range	Side Effects
Quinidine (Quinidex, Quinaglute)	T: 200, 300 mg T (ER): 300, 324 mg I: 80 mg/mL	AF, WPW, PVCs, VT	A: 200-600 mg every 2-4 hr (ER): 300-600 mg every 8 hr	Diarrhea, hypotension, nausea, vomiting, cinchonism, fever, thrombocytopenia, proarrhythmia
Class 1B				
Lidocaine (Xylocaine)	I: 300 mg for IM IV infusion: 2 mg/mL, 4 mg/mL	PVCs, VT, VF	IV: 50-100 mg bolus, then 1-4 mg/min infusion	Drowsiness, agitation, muscle twitching, seizures, paresthesias, proarrhythmia. Central nervous system toxicity more likely in elderly or hepatic patients.
Mexiletine (Mexitil)	C: 150, 200, 250 mg	PVCs, VT, VF	A: 600-1200 mg/day	Drowsiness, agitation, muscle twitching, seizures, paresthesias, proarrhythmia, nausea, vomiting
Tocainide (Tonocard)	T: 400, 600 mg	PVCs, VT, VF	A: 1200-1800 mg/day	Drowsiness, agitation, muscle twitching, seizures, paresthesias, proarrhythmia, nausea, vomiting, diarrhea, agranulocytosis
Class 1C				
Flecainide (Tambocor)	T: 50, 100, 150 mg	AF, PSVT, life-threatening ventricular dysrhythmias	A: 200-400 mg/day	Dizziness, tremors, lightheadedness, flushing, blurred vision, metallic taste, proarrhythmia
Moricizine (Ethmozine)	T: 200, 250, 300 mg	Life-threatening ventricular dysrhythmias	A: 600-900 mg/day	Nausea, dizziness, perioral numbness, euphoria
Propafenone (Rythmol)	T: 150, 225, 300 mg C (SR): 225, 325, 425 mg	PAF, WPW, life-threatening ventricular dysrhythmias	A: 450-900 mg/day every 8 hr for non-SR; every 12 hr for SR	Dizziness, blurred vision, altered taste, nausea, exacerbation of asthma, proarrhythmia
Class II (Beta-Blockers)				
Acebutolol (Sectral)	C: 200, 400 mg	AF, atrial flutter, PSVT, PVCs	A: 600-1200 mg/day	Bradycardia, hypotension, depression, nightmares, fatigue, sexual dysfunction
Esmolol (Brevibloc)	I: 10 mg/mL, 250 mg/mL	AF, atrial flutter, PSVT, PVCs	A: 50-200 mcg/kg/min	Hypotension
Propranolol (Inderal)	T: 10, 20 mg	AF, atrial flutter, PSVT, PVCs	A: 10-30 mg 3-4 times/day	Bradycardia, hypotension, depression, nightmares, fatigue, sexual dysfunction

Class III				
Amiodarone (Cordarone, Pacerone)	T: 200, 400 mg I: 50 mg/mL	AF, PAF, PSVT, life-threatening ventricular dysrhythmias	A (PO): 800-1600 mg/day for 1-3 wk, then 200-400 mg/day (IV): 150 mg bolus, then IV infusion 60 mg/hr 300 mg IV push if patient is pulseless	Blurred vision, photosensitivity (skin), constipation, ataxia, proarrhythmia, pulmonary, liver, thyroid toxicities
Dofetilide (Tikosyn)	C: 125 mcg, 250 mcg, 500 mcg	AF, atrial flutter	A: Individualized 125-500 mcg every 12 hr based on patient's renal function	Torsades de pointes, hypotension
Ibutilide (Corvert)	I: 0.1 mg/mL in 10-mL vials	AF, atrial flutter	A (greater than 60 kg): 1 mg over 10 min; (less than 60 kg): 0.01 mg/kg over 10 min Repeat in 10 min if no response	Torsades de pointes, heart block
Sotalol (Betapace)	T: 80, 120, 160, 240 mg	AF, PAF, PSVT, life-threatening ventricular dysrhythmias	A: 160-640 mg/day	Fatigue, dizziness, dyspnea, bradycardia, proarrhythmia
Class IV (Calcium Channel Blockers)				
Diltiazem (Cardizem)	I: 25-mg/mL vials Infusion: 1 mg/mL	AF, atrial flutter, PSVT	A (IV): 20-25 mg bolus, then infusion of 5-15 mg/hr	Hypotension, bradycardia, dizziness, headache
Verapamil (Isoptin)	I: 5 mg/2 mL	AF, atrial flutter, PSVT	A (IV): 5-10 mg	Hypotension, bradycardia, dizziness, headache, constipation

A, adults; AF, atrial fibrillation; C, capsules; CHF, congestive heart failure; CR, controlled release; ER, extended release; I, injection; PAF, paroxysmal atrial fibrillation; PSVT, paroxysmal supraventricular tachycardia; PVCs, premature ventricular contractions; SLE, systemic lupus erythematosus; SR, sustained release; T, tablets; VF, ventricular fibrillation; VT, ventricular tachycardia; WPW, Wolff-Parkinson-White syndrome

ANTIFUNGALS

Name	Adult Dose Ranges	Available Dosage Forms	Common Indications	Comments
Amphotericin B desoxycholate (Fungizone)	IV: 0.25-1.5 mg/kg/day for 4-12 wk	Powder for I: 50 mg	Aspergillosis, blastomycosis, candidiasis, coccidioidomycosis, cryptococcosis, histoplasmosis, mucormycosis, rhinocerebral phycomycosis, sporotrichosis	Used as bladder irrigation; causes multiple electrolyte abnormalities (hypokalemia, renal tubular acidosis, hypomagnesemia, azotemia); give 1 mg test dose prior to giving full dose; cholesteryl and liposomal formulations (e.g., AmBisome, Amphotec) are used in renally impaired patients or in cases of unacceptable toxicity resulting from requisite antifungal dosages of the deoxycholate form (e.g., Fungizone). Only use for serious, invasive, potentially fatal fungal infections.
Amphotericin B, lipid based (Abelcet, Amphotec, AmBisome)	IV: 3-5 mg/kg/day; infusion rates vary depending on the brand used	Suspension for I: 100 mg/ 20 mL Powder for I: 50, 100 mg	Same as amphotericin B desoxycholate. Only use for serious, invasive, potentially fatal fungal infections.	May be used as a bladder irrigator; causes multiple electrolyte abnormalities (hypokalemia, renal tubular acidosis, hypomagnesemia, azotemia); give 1 mg test dose prior to giving full dose; cholesteryl and liposomal formulations (e.g., AmBisome, Amphotec) are used in renally impaired patients or in cases of unacceptable toxicity resulting from requisite antifungal dosages of the deoxycholate form (e.g., Fungizone).
Anidulafungin (Eraxis)	IV: 100-200 mg IV load and then 50-100 mg day	IV: 50 mg per vial	Candidiasis, systemic, esophageal, intraabdominal, and peritoneal	Hepatic dysfunction, significant worsening hepatic failure, hepatitis, or clinically significant hepatic abnormalities have rarely occurred.
Caspofungin acetate (Cancidas)	IV: 70 mg loading dose, then 50 mg daily	Powder for I: 50, 70 mg	Aspergillosis, candidemia, or other candidal infections, empiric fungal infections	Avoid in combination with cyclosporine if possible. Adjust dose downward for hepatic impairment.

Fluconazole (Diflucan)	PO or IV: 50-400 mg daily	T: 50, 100, 150, 200 mg Powder for OS: 10 and 40 mg/mL I: 2 mg/mL	Candidiasis, cryptococcal meningitis	Increases serum rifabutin levels and toxicity; increases effect of cyclosporine, warfarin, sulfonylureas, statins, theophylline, phenytoin, and other drugs metabolized by the CYP450 3A4 enzymes. Single dose treatment for vaginal infection (150 mg).
Flucytosine (Ancobon)	PO: 12.5-37.5 mg/kg every 6 hr	C: 250, 500 mg	Candidiasis, cryptococcosis	Usually used in combination with amphotericin B (allows lower dose of amphotericin B); converted to fluorouracil in fungal cell; monitor renal function.
Griseofulvin* *Microsize:* Fulvicin U/F, Grifulvin V, Grisactin *Ultramicrosize:* Fulvicin P/G, Gris-PEG, Grisactin Ultra	PO: 500 mg once daily-twice daily PO: 330 mg daily-twice daily	*Microsize:* T: 250, 500 mg C: 250 mg OS: 125 mg *Ultramicrosize:* T: 125, 165, 250, 330 mg	Dermatophytes	Cytochrome P450 inducer; absorption enhanced when taken with fatty foods; ultramicrosize is absorbed better than microsize.
Itraconazole (Sporanox)	PO: 100-200 mg daily-twice daily IV: 200 twice daily × 4 doses followed by 200 mg daily	C: 100 mg OS: 50 mg/5 mL I: 10 mg/mL	Aspergillosis, blastomycosis, candidiasis, chromomycosis, cryptococcosis, dermatomycosis, histoplasmosis, onychomycosis, paracoccidioidomycosis, sporotrichosis	Cytochrome P450 3A inhibitor affects metabolism of cyclosporine, warfarin, sulfonylureas, dofetilide, and many others; can precipitate or worsen CHF; take capsules after a full meal. Do not use if creatinine clearance is less than 30 mL/min.
Ketoconazole (Nizoral)	PO: 200-400 mg daily	T: 200 mg	Blastomycosis, candidiasis, chromomycosis, coccidioidomycosis dermatophytes, histoplasmosis, paracoccidioidomycosis	Cytochrome P450 3A similar to itraconazole; requires acid pH for absorption; don't take with antacids; can cause liver damage, reduces testosterone synthesis (gynecomastia); available in topical form.
Micafungin (Mycamin)	50-150 mg/day	IV powder for I: 50 mg	Esophageal candidiasis, prophylaxis of candidal infections in hematopoietic stem cell transplantation	Watch for hypersensitivity reactions/hepatic or renal dysfunction

Continued

Antifungals—cont'd

Name	Adult Dose Ranges	Available Dosage Forms	Common Indications	Comments
Terbinafine (Lamisil)	PO: 250 mg daily × 6-12 wk	T: 250 mg	Onychomycosis	Hepatic clearance increased by rifampin, decreased by cimetidine; reported to cause liver failure
Voriconazole (Vfend)	IV loading dose: 6 mg/kg every 12 hr × 2 doses, then 4 mg/kg every 12 hr. Infuse over 1-2 hr. May switch to oral, 100-200 mg every 12 hr	T: 50, 200 mg Powder for OS: 40 mg/mL Powder for I: 200 mg	Infections due to *Aspergillus candida* in non-neutropenic patients, *Fusarium*, *Scedosporium apiospermum*	Oral doses should be taken either 1 hr before or 1 hr after a meal. May cause vision changes and photosensitivity. Many drug interactions.

C, capsules; I, injection; OS, oral suspension; T, tablets

ANTIHISTAMINES

Uses

Symptomatic relief of upper respiratory allergic disorders. Allergic reactions associated with other drugs respond to antihistamines, as do blood transfusion reactions. Used as a second-choice drug in treatment of angioneurotic edema. Effective in treatment of acute urticaria and other dermatologic conditions. May also be used for preoperative sedation, Parkinson's disease, and motion sickness.

Action

Antihistamines (H_1 antagonists) inhibit vasoconstrictor effects and vasodilator effects on endothelial cells of histamine. They block increased capillary permeability, formation of edema/wheal caused by histamine. Many antihistamines can bind to receptors in CNS, causing primarily depression (decreased alertness, slowed reaction times, somnolence) but also stimulation (restlessness, nervousness, inability to sleep). Some may counter motion sickness.

Antihistamines

Name	Availability	Dosage Range	Side Effects/Notes
Azatadine (Optimine)	T: 1 mg	A: 1-2 mg every 12 hr C: 0.05 mg/kg/day	Dry mouth, urinary retention, blurred vision, sedation, dizziness, paradoxic excitement
Brompheniramine (Dimetane)	T: 4 mg T (chewable): 12 mg T (SR): 4, 6 mg S: 2 mg/5 mL	A: 4-8 mg every 4-6 hr or T (SR): 8-12 mg every 12-24 hr C: 0.5 mg/kg/day	Dry mouth, urinary retention, blurred vision, sedation
Carbinoxamine (Histex)	T: 4 mg T (SR): 8 mg L: 1.5 mg/5 mL, 4 mg/5 mL	A: 4-8 mg 3-4 times/day C (6 yr and older): 4-6 mg 3-4 times/day C (3-6 yr): 2-4 mg 3-4 times/day C (1-3 yr): 2 mg 3-4 times/day Give SR dosage forms twice daily	Same as azatadine
Cetirizine (Zyrtec)	T: 5, 10 mg T (chewable): 5, 10 mg S: 5 mg/5 mL	A: 5-10 mg/day C (6-12 yr): 5-10 mg/day C (2-5 yr): 2.5-5 mg/day	Minimal CNS and anticholinergic side effects
Chlorpheniramine (Chlor-Trimeton)	T: 4 mg T (chewable): 2 mg T (SR): 8, 12, 16 mg S: 2 mg/5 mL	A: 2-4 mg every 4-6 hr or SR: 8-12 mg every 12-24 hr C: 0.35 mg/kg/day	Same as brompheniramine

Continued

Antihistamines—cont'd

Name	Availability	Dosage Range	Side Effects/Notes
Clemastine (Tavist)	T: 1.34, 2.68 mg S: 0.67 mg/5 mL	A: 1.34-2.68 mg every 8-12 hr C (6-12 yr): 0.67-1.34 mg every 8-12 hr	Same as azatadine
Cyproheptadine (Periactin)	T: 4 mg S: 2 mg/5 mL	A: 4 mg every 8 hr C: 0.25 mg/kg/day	Same as azatadine
Desloratadine (Clarinex)	T: 5 mg T (OD): 5 mg S: 2.5 mg/15 mL	A: 5 mg daily	If patient is renally/hepatically impaired, decrease dose to every other day
Dexchlorpheniramine (Polaramine)	T: 2 mg T (SR): 4, 6 mg S: 2 mg/5 mL	A: 2 mg every 4-6 hr C: 0.5-1 mg every 4-6 hr	Same as brompheniramine
Dimenhydrinate (Dramamine)	T: 50 mg L: 12.5 mg/5 mL	A: 50-100 mg every 4-6 hr C: 12.5-50 mg every 6-8 hr	Same as azatadine
Diphenhydramine (Benadryl)	T: 25, 50 mg T (chewable): 12.5/25 mg T (OD): 12.5 mg C: 25, 50 mg L: 6.25 mg/5 mL, 12.5 mg/5 mL I: 50 mg/mL	A: 25-50 mg every 6-8 hr C: (6-11 yr): 12.5-25 mg every 4-6 hr C: (2-5 yr): 6.25 mg every 4-6 hr	Same as azatadine
Fexofenadine (Allegra)	T: 30, 60, 180 mg C: 60 mg	A: 60 mg every 12 hr or 180 mg/day C (6-11 yr): 30 mg every 12 hr	Same as cetirizine 60 mg once daily for patients with renal impairment
Hydroxyzine (Atarax, Vistaril)	T: 10, 25, 50, 100 mg C: 25, 50, 100 mg S: 10 mg/5 mL, 25 mg/5 mL I: 25-50 mg/mL	A: 25 mg every 6-8 hr C: 2 mg/kg/day in divided doses	Same as azatadine
Loratadine (Claritin)	T: 10 mg T (OD): 10 mg S: 1 mg/mL	A: 10 mg/day C (6-12 yr): 10 mg/day	Same as cetirizine Take on an empty stomach For patients with renal or hepatic impairment, give every other day
Phenindamine (Nolahist)	T: 25 mg	A: 25 mg every 4-6 hr; max 150 mg/day C (6-12 yr): 12.5 mg every 4-6 hr; max 75 mg/day	Same as azatadine, less sedation

Promethazine (Phenergan)	T: 12.5, 25, 50 mg S: 6.25 mg/5 mL, 25 mg/5 mL I: 25, 50 mg Suppositories: 12.5, 25, 50 mg	A: 25 mg at bedtime or 12.5 mg every 8 hr C: 0.5 mg/kg at bedtime or 0.1 mg/kg every 6-8 hr	Same as azatadine
Triprolidine (Zymine)	L: 1.25 mg/5 mL	A: 10 mL every 4-6 hr; max 40 mL/24 hr C (6-12 yr): 5 mL every 4-6 hr; max 20 mL/24 hr C (4-6 yr): 3.75 mL every 4-6 hr; max 15 mL/24 hr C (2-4 yr): 2.5 mL every 4-6 hr; max 10 mL/24 hr C (4 mo-2 yr): 1.25 mL every 4-6 hr; max 5 mL/24 hr	Blurred vision, sedation, slight dry mouth, slight urinary retention

A, adults; C, capsules; C (dosage), children; I, injection; L, liquid; OD, orally disintegrating; S, syrup; SR, sustained release; T, tablets

ANTIHYPERLIPIDEMICS

Uses
Cholesterol management.

Action
Bile acid sequestrants: Bind bile acids in the intestine, prevent active transport and reabsorption, and enhance bile acid excretion. Depletion of hepatic bile acid results in the increased conversion of cholesterol to bile acids.

HMG-CoA reductase inhibitors (statins): Inhibit HMG-CoA reductase, the last regulated step in the synthesis of cholesterol. Cholesterol synthesis in the liver is reduced.

Niacin (nicotinic acid): Reduces hepatic synthesis of triglycerides and secretion of very low-density lipoproteins (VLDL) by inhibiting the mobilization of free fatty acids from peripheral tissues.

Fibric acid: Increases the oxidation of fatty acids in the liver, resulting in reduced secretion of triglyceride-rich lipoproteins and increases lipoprotein lipase activity and fatty acid uptake.

Antihyperlipidemics

Generic Name	Brand Name	Available Dosage Forms	Usual Adult Dose	Side Effects/Comments
Bile Acid Binding Resins (Sequestrants) *Class side effects: GI effects (constipation, nausea and vomiting, heartburn, stomach pain, etc.), elevated triglycerides*				
Colesevelam*	Welchol	T: 625 mg	Monotherapy: 3 tabs twice daily or 6 tabs daily, with food (max: 7 tabs/day) Combo w/ statins: 4-6 tabs daily (max: 6 tabs/day)	May be taken concurrently with HMG-CoA reductase inhibitor therapy. Take with food. Take other medications 1 hr before or 2 hr after this medication. Report skeletal muscle pain and weakness.
Cholestyramine[†]*	Questran, Questran Light, Prevalite	P (for oral suspension): 4 g	4-24 g/day in divided doses (max: 6 times/day)	Take other medications 1 hr before or 4-6 hr after this medication.
Colestipol*	Colestid	G: 5 g packet T: 1 g	G: 5-30 g/day in 2-4 divided doses T: 2-16 g/day	Take other medications 1 hr before or 4 hr after this medication.

HMG-CoA Reductase Inhibitors (Statins)[‡] *Class side effects: headache, GI effects, abnormal liver function tests, monitor for signs/symptoms of rhabdomyolysis/myopathy*				
Atorvastatin	Lipitor	T: 10, 20, 40, 80 mg	10-80 mg daily	May take without regard to meals or time of day.
Fluvastatin	Lescol, Lescol XL	C: 20, 40 mg T (ER): 80 mg	20-80 mg in single or divided doses	May take without regard to meals, preferably in the evening.
Lovastatin[†]	Mevacor, Altocor	T: 10, 20, 40 mg T (ER): 10, 20, 40, 60 mg	10-80 mg daily (max: 80 mg/day, ER 60 mg/day)	Take with evening meal.
Pravastatin*	Pravachol	T: 10, 20, 40, 80 mg	10-80 mg daily	May take without regard to meals, preferably in the evening.
Rosuvastatin	Crestor	T: 5, 10, 20, 40 mg	5-40 mg daily	May take without regard to meals or time of day.
Simvastatin	Zocor	T: 5, 10, 20, 40, 80 mg	5-80 mg daily in the evening	May take without regard to meals, preferably in the evening.
Nicotinic Acid Derivatives *Class side effects: edema, flushing, dermatologic changes, GI effects, abnormal liver function tests, dizziness, elevated glucose, monitor for signs/symptoms of rhabdomyolysis/myopathy when used with statins*				
Niacin (nicotinic acid)[†]	Niaspan, Niacor	T: 50, 100, 250, 500 mg T (ER): 500, 750, 1000 mg T (CR): 250, 500, 750 mg T (TR): 250, 500, 750, 1000 mg C (TR): 250 mg C (ER): 125, 250, 400, 500 mg	1.5-6 g/day three times daily with or after meals (start at 100-250 mg/day and titrate gradually) ER: 375 mg-2 g at bedtime with gradual titration	Taking 325 mg aspirin 30 min before niacin reduces flushing. Take with food.

Continued

Antihyperlipidemics—cont'd

Generic Name	Brand Name	Available Dosage Forms	Usual Adult Dose	Side Effects/Comments
Fibric Acid Derivatives *Class side effects: GI effects, abnormal liver function tests, monitor for signs/symptoms of rhabdomyolysis/myopathy when used with statins*				
Fenofibrate†	Tricor	C: 48, 145 mg. Generics come in other strengths	48-145 mg/day	Increased absorption when taken with food.
Gemfibrozil†	Lopid	T: 600 mg	600 mg twice daily 30 min before AM and PM meals	
Other Lipid-Lowering Agents				
Ezetimibe	Zetia	T: 10 mg	10 mg/day	May be taken with or without food.
Niacin/lovastatin	Advicor	T: (niacin/lovastatin) 500/20, 750/20, 1000/20 mg	500 mg (niacin content) to 2000 mg at bedtime	Niacin portion is extended release. Taking 325 mg aspirin 30 min before niacin reduces flushing. Do not increase niacin content by greater than 500 mg/4 wk. Take with food. Do not crush or chew.
Simvastatin/ezetimibe	Vytorin	T: (ezetimibe/simvastatin) 10/10, 10/20, 10/40, 10/80 mg	10/10 mg-10/80 mg daily	May be taken with or without food.

*Generic available for one or more dosage forms.

†Daily dose can be given as a single dose or divided doses.

‡General statement: All HMG-CoA reductase inhibitors are contraindicated in pregnancy and in severe renal or hepatic disease. Significant drug interactions are possible with several drug categories, including other antihyperlipidemic agents, antacids, amiodarone, verapamil, anti-HIV drugs, rifampin, cyclosporine, macrolide antibiotics, azole antifungals, warfarin, cimetidine, and diltiazem. An unusual but severe adverse reaction, which may be potentiated by drug interactions, is a breakdown of muscle tissue known as rhabdomyolysis. Symptoms include unexplained muscular discomfort and dark urine, signifying myoglobinuria. Advise patients to report any such symptoms immediately.

C, capsules; CR, controlled release; ER, extended release; G, granules; GI, gastrointestinal; P, powder; T, tablets; TR, timed release

References:

1. *Dorland's Illustrated Medical Dictionary* 30th edition. WB Saunders, Philadelphia, 2003.
2. Website: *US Food and Drug Administration*. Online. Internet. 2003. Available: http://www.fda.gov/cder
3. Micromedex.
4. Lexi-Complete.

ANTIHYPERTENSIVES, MISCELLANEOUS

Uses
Treatment of mild to severe hypertension.

Action
Many groups of medications are used in the treatment of hypertension. In addition to the alpha-adrenergic central agonists, peripheral antagonists, and vasodilators listed in the following table, refer to the classifications of diuretics, beta-adrenergic blockers, calcium channel blockers, and ACE inhibitors or to individual drug monographs.

Alpha-agonists (central action): Stimulate alpha$_2$-adrenergic receptors in the cardiovascular centers of the CNS, reducing sympathetic outflow and producing an antihypertensive effect.

Alpha-antagonists (peripheral action): Block alpha$_1$-adrenergic receptors in arterioles and veins, inhibiting vasoconstriction and decreasing peripheral vascular resistance, causing a fall in BP.

Vasodilators: Directly relax arteriolar smooth muscle, decreasing vascular resistance. Exact mechanism unknown.

Antihypertensive side effects include drowsiness, dizziness, dry mouth, constipation, nasal congestion, and weakness.

Antihypertensives, Miscellaneous

Generic Name	Brand Name	Route	Usual Adult Dose	Available Dosage Forms	Side Effects/Comments
Alpha-2 Receptor Agonists					
Clonidine*	Catapres	PO	0.2–2.4 mg/day in divided doses	T: 0.1, 0.2, 0.3 mg	Raise dose at weekly intervals until the desired effect. Give majority of daily dose at bedtime to minimize sedation. Gradual withdrawal over 1 wk (PO).
	Catapres-TTS	Transdermal	Initial: 0.1-mg patch Maintenance: 0.1–0.3 mg weekly	P: 0.1, 0. 2. 0.3 mg/ 24 hr	Apply a new patch every 7 days. Allow 2–3 days to see therapeutic effect. Less side effects associated with patch.
Guanabenz*†	Wytensin	PO	8–30 mg/day	T: 4, 8 mg	May cause rebound if discontinued abruptly. May also cause orthostatic hypotension and xerostomia.
Guanfacine*	Tenex	PO	1–2 mg at bedtime	T: 1, 2 mg	Rebound may occur 2–4 days after last dose. May also cause orthostatic hypotension and xerostomia.

Continued

Antihypertensives, Miscellaneous—cont'd

Generic Name	Brand Name	Route	Usual Adult Dose	Available Dosage Forms	Side Effects/Comments
Methyldopa*	Aldomet	PO	Initial: 250 mg twice daily-three times daily × 2 days Maintenance: 250–1000 mg/day in 2 divided doses	T: 250, 500 mg	Transient sedation and depression is common for first 72 hr. May also cause peripheral edema.
Methyldopate	Aldomet	IV	250–1000 mg every 6–8 hr (max: 1 g every 6 hr)	I: 50 mg/mL	Switch to PO once control is established; PO dose is same as IV. Infuse over 30 min. May also cause impaired memory and depression.
Alpha-1 Receptor Blockers[‡]					
Alfuzosin	Uroxatral	PO	2.5–20 mg twice daily has been used for hypertension	T (ER): 10 mg	Primary use of agent is for benign prostatic hyperplasia (BPH).
Doxazosin*	Cardura	PO	Initial: 1 mg daily Maintenance: 1–18 mg/day	T: 1, 2, 4, 8 mg	Orthostatic hypotension and syncope (especially with first dose or rapid dose increase), dizziness, headache May be used to treat BPH
Prazosin*	Minipress	PO	Initial: 1 mg twice daily-three times daily Maintenance: Up to 20 mg/day in divided doses	C: 1, 2, 5 mg	Same as doxazosin
Terazosin*	Hytrin	PO	Initial: 1 mg at bedtime Maintenance: 1–20 mg/day	T: 1, 2, 5, 10 mg C: 1, 2, 5, 10 mg	Same as doxazosin May be used to treat BPH

Vasodilators

Hydralazine*	Apresoline	PO, IV, IM	PO, initial: 10 mg every 4 days × 2–4 days. Increase by 10–25 mg/dose every 2–5 days. Maintenance: Titrate up to 300 mg/day in divided doses if necessary. IM, IV: 10–20 mg/dose every 4–6 hr as needed (max: 40 mg/dose)	T: 10, 25, 50, 100 mg I: 20 mg/mL	Tablets are absorbed better with food. IV injection over 1 min Side effects include weight gain, swelling, dizziness, GI problems, tachycardia Note the product BiDil combines hydralazine with isosorbide dinitrate (37.5 and 20 mg) for three times daily use in African-Americans with heart failure
Minoxidil*	Loniten	PO	Initial: 5 mg daily Maintenance: 2.5–10 mg/day in divided doses. Max: 100 mg/day	T: 2.5, 10 mg	Increase dose gradually every 3 days. Side effects include congestive heart failure, edema, tachycardia

*Generic available for one or more dosage forms.
†Daily dose can be given as a single dose or divided into two equal doses.
‡Note: Tanzulosin (Flomax) is also in this class, but it used exclusively for BPH and other urinary system indications.
C, capsules; ER, extended release; I, injection; P, powder; T, tablets

References:
1. Ellsworth, Allan J et al: *Mosby's Medical Drug Reference.* Mosby, St. Louis, 2003.
2. Website: U.S. Food and Drug Administration. Online. Internet. 2003. Available: http://www.fda.gov/cder
3. Micromedex
4. Lexi-Complete

ANTIPSYCHOTICS

Uses
Antipsychotics are primarily used in managing psychotic illness (especially in patients with increased psychomotor activity). They are also used to treat the manic phase of bipolar disorder, behavioral problems in children, nausea and vomiting, intractable hiccups, anxiety and agitation, as adjunct in treatment of tetanus, and to potentiate effects of narcotics.

Action
Effects of these agents occur at all levels of the CNS. Antipsychotic mechanism is unknown but it may antagonize dopamine action as a neurotransmitter in basal ganglia and limbic system. Antipsychotics may block postsynaptic dopamine receptors, inhibit dopamine release, and increase dopamine turnover. These medications can be divided into the phenothiazines and nonphenothiazines (miscellaneous). In addition to their use in symptomatic treatment of psychiatric illness, some have antiemetic, antinausea, antihistamine, anticholinergic, and/or sedative effects.

Antipsychotics

Name	Availability	Dosage	Relative Side Effects Profile				Notes
			EPS	Anticholinergic	Sedation	Hypotension	
Aripiprazole (Abilify)	T: 5, 10, 15, 20, 30 mg OS: 1 mg/mL	15-30 mg/day	Low	Low	Low	Low	
Chlorpromazine (Thorazine)	T: 10, 25, 50, 100, 200 mg OC: 30 mg/mL, 100 mg/mL I: 25 mg/mL RS: 100 mg	25-1000 mg/day	Moderate	Moderate	High	High	Also useful for intractable hiccups
Clozapine (Clozaril)	T: 25, 100 mg T (OD): 12.5, 25, 100 mg	75-900 mg/day	Rare	High	High	High	Due to risk of agranulocytosis and circulatory collapse, reserve as last agent or for recurrent suicidal behavior. Also may cause seizures and myocarditis.
Fluphenazine (Prolixin)	T: 1, 2.5, 5, 10 mg I (decanoate): 25 mg/mL E: 2.5 mg/5 mL	PO: 2-40 mg/day I: 12.5-75 mg every 2 wk (as decanoate)	High	Low	Low	Low	

Haloperidol (Haldol)	T: 0.5, 1, 2, 5, 10, 20 mg I: 5 mg/mL I (decanoate): 50, 100 mg/mL OC: 2 mg/mL	PO: 2-100 mg/day I: 2.5 mg every 1-4 hr I (decanoate): individual monthly doses	High	Low	Low	Low	Also used for Tourette disorder and hyperactivity
Lithium	T: 300 mg T (ER): 300, 450 mg C: 150, 300, 600 mg S: equivalent of 300 mg lithium carbonate/ 5 mL	600-1800 mg/day	Rare	Rare	Rare	Rare	Monitor serum levels for toxicity
Loxapine (Loxitane)	C: 5, 10, 25, 50 mg	20-250 mg/day	High	Low	Moderate	Moderate	
Mesoridazine (Serentil)	T: 10, 25, 50, 100 mg I: 25 mg/mL OC: 25 mg/mL	100-400 mg/day	Low	High	High	High	May prolong QT interval and lead to possible dysrhythmias
Molindone (Moban)	OS: 20 mg/mL T: 5, 10, 25, 50, 100 mg	50-225 mg/day	Moderate	Low	Low	Low	
Olanzapine (Zyprexa)	T: 2.5, 5, 7.5, 10, 15, 20 mg DT: 5, 10, 15, 20 mg I: 10 mg	10-20 mg/day	Low	Low	Moderate	Low	IM only for injections up to 30 mg (10 mg every 2 hr × 3). May be associated with orthostatic hypotension.
Perphenazine	T: 2, 4, 8, 16 mg OC: 16 mg/ 5 mL	16-64 mg/day	Moderate	Low	Moderate	Low	Also used for severe nausea and vomiting
Pimozide (Orap)	T: 1, 2 mg	1-10 mg/day	High	Moderate	Low	Low	Also used for Tourette disorder

Continued

Antipsychotics—cont'd

Name	Availability	Dosage	Relative Side Effects Profile				Notes
			EPS	Anticholinergic	Sedation	Hypotension	
Prochlorperazine (Compazine)	T: 5, 10 mg C (SR): 10, 15 mg S: 5 mg/5 mL I: 5 mg/mL RS: 2.5, 5, 25 mg	15-150 mg/day	Moderate	Low	Moderate	Low	Also used for severe nausea and vomiting, anxiety
Quetiapine (Seroquel)	T: 25, 100, 200 300 mg	100-800 mg/day	Rare	Low	Moderate	Moderate	
Risperidone (Risperdal)	T: 0.25, 0.5, 1, 2, 3, 4 mg DT: 0.5, 1, 2 mg OC: 1 mg/mL I: 25, 37.5, 50 mg	2-6 mg/day IM: 25-50 mg every 2 wk	Low	Low	Low	Moderate	
Thioridazine (Mellaril)	T: 10, 15, 25, 50, 100, 150, 200 mg	50-800 mg/day	Low	High	High	High	May prolong QT interval and cause dysrhythmias
Thiothixene (Navane)	C: 1, 2, 5, 10, 20 mg	5-60 mg/day	High	Low	Low	Low	Also used for nonpsychotic anxiety
Trifluoperazine (Stelazine)	T: 1, 2, 5, 10 mg	5-80 mg/day	High	Low	Low	Low	
Ziprasidone (Geodon)	C: 20, 40, 60, 80 mg I: 20 mg	40-160 mg/day IM: 10-40 mg/day	Low	Low	Low to moderate	Low to moderate	Note many contraindicated drug interactions per package insert

C, capsules; DT, disintegrating tablets; E, elixer; EPS, extrapyramidal symptoms; ER, extended release; I, injection; OC, oral concentrate; OD, orally disintegrating; OS, oral solution; RS, rectal suppository; S, syrup; SR, sustained release; T, tablets

ANTIVIRALS

Uses

Antiviral drugs are used for managing viral infections. These drugs target specific viruses, similar to how antibiotics are used to treat specific bacteria. The antiviral drugs available cover the following types of virus: *herpes virus,* including herpes simplex (HSV), herpes zoster, herpes genitalis, and varicella; *cytomegalovirus (CMV),* present in immunosuppressed patients; *respiratory syncytial virus (RSV)* in infants; *hepatitis C;* and *influenza A* and *B virus.*

Antiviral therapy is generally effective only when initiated within 48 hours of the onset of the infection. Drugs used for influenza may be used throughout the influenza season to manage high-risk patients or within 48 hours of suspected exposure. Drugs for management of herpes should be initiated at the first sign of an outbreak. Anticytomegalovirus medications are used for maintenance therapy after initial treatment to prevent reinfection in immunosuppressed patients.

Actions

The mechanism of action of antiviral medications is to inactivate the enzymes needed for viral replication. This reduces the rate of viral growth but does not destroy or inactivate the viral load already present. Many viruses have evolved specific enzymatic systems to replicate viral nucleic acids at the expense of cellular molecules. Viral gene expression is less amenable to treatment than genome replication because viruses are more heavily dependent on cellular processes involved with transcription, mRNA splicing, cytoplasmic export, and translation than with replication. For the majority of viruses, these processes are not well understood.

The majority of these drugs act as polymerase substrate, such as the nucleoside analogues including acyclovir, ganciclovir, valganciclovir and valacyclovir. Other mechanisms of action include triazole carboxamides such as ribavirin, which prompt mutation of RNA; tricyclic amines such as amantadine and rimantadine, which prompt matrix protein agglutination; and neuraminic acid mimetics, such as oseltamivir and zanamivir, which inhibit the enzyme neuraminidase.

Name and Availability	Indications and Dosage	Side Effects and Drug Interactions	Notes
Acyclovir (Zovirax, Avirax ♣) C: 200 mg T: 400 mg, 800 mg I: 50 mg/mL (solution) OS: 200 mg/5 mL Topical cream: 5% Topical ointment: 5%	*Genital herpes (initial):* PO: 200 mg every 4 hr, 5 times daily IV: 5 mg/kg every 8 hr for 5 days *Genital herpes (recurrent):* PO: 200 mg every 4 hr, 5 times daily for 5 days or 400 mg twice daily. *Herpes simplex (mucocutaneous):* IV: 5-10 mg/kg every 8 hr for 7 days *Herpes simplex (neonatal):* IV: 10 mg/kg every 8 hr for 10 days *Herpes simplex (encephalitis):* IV: 10-20 mg/kg every 8 hr for 10 days	*IV:* Phlebitis or IV site inflammation, nausea and vomiting, pruritus, rash, urticaria; rarely, confusion, seizure, tremors *Oral:* Malaise, nausea; rarely diarrhea, vomiting, headache, rash *Topical:* Burning, stinging, pruritus; rarely rash *Serious reactions:* Renal failure has occurred with high doses or too-rapid parenteral administration. *IV drug incompatibilities:* Aztreonam, cefepime, diltiazem, dobutamine, dopamine, levofloxacin, meropenem, ondansetron, piperacillin, tazobactam	For recurrent genital herpes, dosage and length of therapy varies based on number of episodes per yr. For other conditions, age affects dosage. *Renal impairment:* Dosage is modified based on severity of both renal failure and infection. *Off-label uses:* Herpes simplex ocular infections, infectious mononucleosis *Contraindications:* Use in neonates when solution has been reconstituted using benzyl alcohol; hypersensitivity to acyclovir

Continued

Antivirals—cont'd

Name and Availability	Indications and Dosage	Side Effects and Drug Interactions	Notes
	Herpes zoster (Varicella): IV: 10-20 mg/kg every 8 hr for 7 days *Herpes zoster (shingles):* PO: 800 mg every 4 hr, 5 times daily for 7 days Topical: 3-6 times daily for 7 days to affected area *Varicella (chicken pox):* PO: 20 mg/kg up to 800 mg, 4 times daily for 5 days; less than 2 yr old: 80 mg/kg/day	*Interactions*: Nephrotoxic medications such as aminoglycosides may increase nephrotoxicity of acyclovir. Probenecid may increase half life of acyclovir.	*Precautions:* Use cautiously in patients with dehydration, fluid and electrolyte imbalances, neurologic abnormalities, renal and liver impairment, and if the patient is concurrently receiving other nephrotoxic drugs. *Drug should be infused over at least 1 hr to avoid damage to the kidneys.*
Adefovir dipivoxil (Hepsera) T: 10 mg	*Chronic hepatitis B with normal kidneys:* 10 mg once daily *Chronic hepatitis B with renal impairment:* Creatinine clearance 20-49 mL/min: 10 mg once every 48 hr Creatinine clearance 10-19 mL/min: 10 mg once every 72 hr On hemodialysis: 10 mg weekly following hemodialysis	Weakness, asthenia, headache, abdominal pain, nausea, flatulence; rarely, diarrhea, dyspepsia *Interactions:* Ibuprofen increases adefovir plasma concentration. *Serious reactions:* Nephrotoxicity is a treatment limiting toxicity; rare lactic acidosis and severe hepatomegaly.	Age and degree of renal impairment affects dosage. *Precautions:* Use with caution in renal impaired patients, those at risk for hepatic disease, and elderly; lactic acidosis and hepatomegaly are seen more often in females *Contraindications:* Hypersensitivity to adefovir
Amantadine hydrochloride (Symmetryl, Edantadine ✱ PMS-Amantadine ✱) C: 100 mg S: 50 mg/5 mL T: 100 mg	*Prevention and treatment of symptoms of influenza A virus:* A: 100-200 mg daily C: 5 mg/kg/day up to 150-200 mg/day *Parkinson's disease to prevent extrapyramidal symptoms:* 100 mg twice daily; may increase to 3 times daily: Renal Impairment Dose: Creatinine clearance 30-50 mL/min: 200 mg first day, 100 mg daily thereafter Creatinine clearance 15-29 mL/min: 200 mg first day, 100 mg every other day thereafter Creatinine clearance less than 15 mL/min: 200 mg weekly	Nausea, dizziness, poor concentration, insomnia, nervousness, orthostatic hypotension, anorexia, headache, livedo reticularis (reddish blue, weblike skin rash), blurred vision, urinary retention, dry mouth or nose; rare vomiting, irritation, eye swelling, rash *Interactions:* Alcohol may increase CNS effects. Anticholinergics, antihistamines, phenothiazines, tricyclic antidepressants may increase anticholinergic effects of amantadine; hydrochlorothiazide, triamterene increase amantadine blood level	Age and degree of renal impairment affect dosage. Children under 10 yr and elderly over 64 yr should receive lower daily doses. *Serious reactions*: Heart failure, leucopenia, neutropenia, hyperexcitability, seizures, and ventricular dysrhythmias *Precautions:* Use cautiously in patients with cerebrovascular disease, heart failure, seizures, hepatic or renal dysfunction, orthostatic hypotension, peripheral edema, recurrent eczema, or those receiving CNS stimulants *Contraindications:* Hypersensitivity to amantadine

Cidofovir (Vistide) I: 75 mg/mL (5 mL ampules)	*CMV retinitis (HIV positive patients in combination with probenecid):* IV: 5 mg/kg at a constant rate over 1 hr weekly for 2 wk during induction; precede dose by 3 hr with probenecid 2 g orally and 1 L normal saline infusion; then give 1 g 1 hr following cidofovir infusion. IV maintenance infusion: 5 mg/kg at a constant rate over 1 hr every 2 wk Renal impairment induction/maintenance: IV, creatinine clearance 41-55 mL/min: 2 mg/kg IV, creatinine clearance 30-40 mL/min: 1.5 mg/kg IV, creatinine clearance 20-29 mL/min: 1 mg/kg IV, creatinine clearance less than 19 mL/min: 0.5 mg/kg	Nausea, vomiting, fever, weakness, rash, diarrhea, headache, alopecia, chills, anorexia, dyspnea, abdominal pain *Serious reactions:* Proteinuria, nephrotoxicity, neutropenia, elevated creatinine, infection, anemia, decreased intraocular pressure, pneumonia; concurrent use of probenecid may produce a hypersensitivity reaction; rare acute renal failure *Interactions:* Nephrotoxic medications (aminoglycosides, amphotericin B, foscarnet, pentamidine) increase the risk of nephrotoxicity	Age and degree of renal impairment affects dosage. *Off-label uses:* Treatment of ganciclovir-resistant CMV, adenovirus; acyclovir-resistant herpes simplex or varicella zoster virus *Contraindications:* Direct intraocular injection, history of clinically severe hypersensitivity to cidofovir, probenecid, or other sulfa-containing drugs, renal impairment
Famciclovir (Famvir) T: 125 mg, 250 mg, 500 mg	*Herpes zoster:* 500 mg every 8 hr for 7 days *Recurrent genital herpes:* 125 mg twice daily for 5 days *Suppression of recurrent genital herpes:* 250 mg twice daily for up to 1 yr *Recurrent herpes simplex:* 500 mg twice daily for 7 days Renal Impairment Dose: *Herpes zoster:* Creatinine clearance 40-59 mL/min: 500 mg every 12 hr Creatinine clearance 20-39 mL/min: 500 mg every 24 hr Creatinine clearance less than 20 mL/min: 250 mg every 24 hr *Genital herpes:* Creatinine clearance 40-59 mL/min: 125 mg every 12 hr Creatinine clearance 0-39 mL/min: 125 mg every 24 hr	Headache, nausea, dizziness, somnolence, numbness in feet, diarrhea, vomiting, constipation, anorexia, fatigue, fever, pharyngitis, sinusitis, pruritus; rare insomnia, abdominal pain, dyspepsia, flatulence, back pain, arthralgia *Serious reactions:* None *Interactions:* None	Dosage is affected by level of renal impairment *Contraindications:* Hypersensitivity to famciclovir *Precautions:* Use cautiously in patients with hepatic or renal impairment.

Continued

Antivirals—cont'd

Name and Availability	Indications and Dosage	Side Effects and Drug Interactions	Notes
Fomivirsen (Vitravene) I: 6.6 mg/mL (intravitreal)	*CMV retinitis:* 330 mg (0.05 mL) every other wk for 2 doses, then 330 mg every 4 wk	Fever, headache, nausea, diarrhea, vomiting, uveitis, anemia, abdominal pain, abnormal vision, chest pain, confusion, dizziness, depression, neuropathy, anorexia, weight loss, cough, liver enzyme elevation *Interactions:* None	Safety and efficacy not established for children. *Serious reactions:* Thrombocytopenia *Contraindications:* Hypersensitivity to fomivirsen *Precautions:* Use with caution in liver-impaired patients.
Foscarnet sodium (Foscavir) I: 24 mg/mL	*CMV retinitis:* IV, initially: 60 mg/kg every 8 hr or 100 mg/kg every 12 hr for 2-3 wk IV, maintenance: 90-120 mg/kg once daily *Herpes infection:* IV: 40 mg/kg every 8-12 hr for 2-3 wk or until healed *Drug should be infused over at least 1 hr to avoid damage to the kidneys.*	Fever, nausea, vomiting, diarrhea, anorexia, painful injection site, rigors, malaise, headache, paresthesia, dizziness, rash, diaphoresis, pain in abdomen, chest or back, dry mouth, flushing *Interactions:* Use of other nephrotoxic medications increases nephrotoxicity; use of pentamidine causes hypocalcemia, hypomagnesemia; use of zidovudine causes anemia	Dosage is less in renal-impaired patients; refer to manufacturer's package insert to adjust dose *Contraindications:* Hypersensitivity to foscarnet *Precautions:* Use with caution in renal-impaired patients. *Serious reactions:* Nephrotoxicity, seizures, life-threatening electrolyte imbalances
Ganciclovir sodium (Cytovene, Vitrasert) C: 250 mg, 500 mg (Cytovene) P: 500 mg (Cytovene) for injection Implant: 4.5 mg (Vitrasert)	*CMV retinitis:* IV: 10 mg/kg/day in divided doses every 12 hr for 14-21 days, then 5 mg/kg once daily *CMV prevention in organ transplant patients:* IV: 10 mg/kg/day in divided doses every 12 hr for 7-14 days, then 5 mg/kg once daily *Other CMV infections:* IV: 10 mg/kg/day in divided doses every 12 hr for 14-21 days, then 5 mg/kg once daily C (Maintenance): 30 mg/kg every 8 hr A (Maintenance): 1000 mg three times daily *Intravitreal implant:* One implant every 6-9 mo plus oral ganciclovir	Diarrhea, fever, nausea, abdominal pain, vomiting, diaphoresis, infection, paresthesia, flatulence, pruritis, headache, stomatitis, dyspepsia, phlebitis *Serious reactions:* Hematologic toxicity, including anemia and leukopenia, is common; intraocular insertion can result in loss of vision or decreased vision, or vitreal hemorrhage; GI bleeding occurs rarely. *Interactions:* Bone marrow depressants may increase hematologic toxicity; use of imipenem and cilastin may increase risk of seizures; use of zidovudine may increase risk of hepatotoxicity	Age and renal status affect dosing; refer to manufacturer's package insert to adjust dose. *Off label uses:* Treatment of CMV infections of liver, lungs, and GI tract *Precautions:* Use cautiously in children; long-term safety has not been determined since drug has adverse effects on reproduction and is carcinogenic *Contraindications:* Absolute neutrophil count of less than 500/mm^3, platelet count less than 25,000/mm^3, hypersensitivity to acyclovir or ganciclovir, patients with congenital or neonatal CMV disease

Oseltamivir (Tamiflu) C: 75 mg OS: 12 mg/mL	*Influenza:* A: 75 mg twice daily for 5 days C: 30-60 mg twice daily for 5 days *Prevention of influenza:* 75 mg once daily *Renal impaired:* 75 mg once daily for 1-6 wk	Nausea, vomiting, diarrhea, abdominal pain, bronchitis, dizziness, headache, cough, insomnia, fatigue, vertigo *Interactions:* None	Dosage is decreased for children of lower weights and for those with renal impairment; see manufacturer's package insert for instructions *Contraindications*: Hypersensitivity to oseltamivir
Ribavirin (Cepegus, Rebetol, Virazole) C: 200 mg (Rebetol) T: 200, 400, 600 mg (Rebetol) P: 6 g (Virazole) for reconstitution (aerosol) OS: 40 mg/mL (Rebetol)	*Chronic hepatitis C:* A: Combined with use of interferon alfa-2b: 1000-1200 mg/day in 2 divided doses C: 200-400 mg twice daily Combined with use of peginterferon alfa-2b: 800-1200 mg/day in 2 divided doses *Respiratory syncytial virus (RSV) infection:* 20 mg/mL over 12-18 hr aerosolized for 3-7 days	Dizziness, headache, fatigue, fever, insomnia, emotional lability, impaired concentration, alopecia, rash, pruritus, nausea, vomiting, anemia, bone pain, hemolysis, arthralgia, muscular pain, malaise *Serious reactions:* Cardiac or respiratory arrest, pneumonia. *Interactions:* Nucleoside analogues may increase risk of lactic acidosis	Dosage is decreased for children of lower weights. Tablets and capsules may require different doses. *Off-label uses:* Treatment of influenza A or B or West Nile virus *Contraindications*: Women of childbearing age who do not use contraception *Precautions:* Use with caution in elderly, those with heart or lung disease, or psychiatric disorders
Rimantadine hydrochloride (Flumadine) S: 50 mg/5 mL T: 100 mg	*Influenza A virus:* 100 mg twice daily for 7 days *Prevention of influenza A virus:* A: 100 mg twice daily for 10 days to 8 weeks C: 5 mg/kg up to 150 mg once daily	Insomnia, nausea, nervousness, impaired concentration, dizziness, vomiting, anorexia, abdominal pain, weakness *Serious reactions:* None *Interactions:* Aspirin and acetominophen decrease rimantadine blood levels; anticholinergics, CNS stimulants may increase rimantadine side effects; use of cimetidine may increase rimantadine blood level	Dosage may be decreased for elderly, nursing home patients, and those with hepatic or renal impairment *Contraindications:* Hypersensitivity to amatadine or rimantadine *Precautions:* Use with caution in patients with recurrent eczema, liver or renal impairment, seizures, psychosis
Valacyclovir (Valtrex) Caplets: 500 mg, 1000 mg	*Herpes zoster (shingles):* 1 g three times daily for 7 days *Herpes simplex (cold sores):* 2 g twice daily for 1 day *Genital herpes:* Initial: 1 g twice daily for 10 days Recurrent: 500 mg twice daily for 3 days Prevention: 500-1000 mg daily Renal insufficiency:	Nausea, headache, vomiting, diarrhea, constipation, weakness, dizziness; rare abdominal pain, anorexia *Serious reactions:* None *Interactions:* Cimetidine and probenecid may increase acyclovir blood level	Dosage is decreased for renal insufficiency. Safety of this drug has not been established in children. *Contraindications:* Hypersensitivity to acyclovir, valacyclovir *Precautions:* Use with caution in patients with advanced HIV, neurologic abnormalities, hepatic or renal disease, fluid and electrolyte imbalance,

Continued

Antivirals—cont'd

Name and Availability	Indications and Dosage	Side Effects and Drug Interactions	Notes
	Genital herpes: Creatinine clearance more than 50 mL/min: 1 g every 8 hr Creatinine clearance 30-49 mL/min: 1 g every 12 hr Creatinine clearance 10-29 mL/min: 1 g every 24 hr Creatinine clearance less than 10 mL/min: 500 mg daily *Herpes zoster:* Creatinine clearance more than 50 mL/min: 500 mg every 12 hr Creatinine clearance 30-49 mL/min: 500 mg every 12 hr Creatinine clearance 0-29 mL/min: 500 mg daily		dehydrated patients, bone marrow or renal transplant patients, and those using other nephrotoxic drugs
Valganciclovir hydrochloride (Valcyte) T: 450 mg	*CMV retinitis:* Initial: 900 mg twice daily for 21 days, then 900 mg daily for maintenance *Prevention of CMV post-transplant:* 900 mg daily for up to 100 days post-transplant Renal insufficiency: Creatinine clearance at least 60 mL/min: 900 mg twice daily for induction, 900 daily for maintenance Creatinine clearance 40-59 mL/min: 450 mg twice daily for induction, 450 mg daily for maintenance Creatinine clearance 25-39 mL/min: 450 mg daily for induction, 450 mg every 2 days for maintenance Creatinine clearance 10-24 mL/min: 500 mg every 2 days for induction, 500 mg twice weekly for maintenance	Diarrhea, neutropenia, thrombocytopenia, anemia, headache, nausea; rare insomnia, vomiting, abdominal pain, fever *Serious reactions:* Hematologic toxicity with bone marrow suppression, retinal detachment, acute renal failure, infertility and decreased sperm count *Interactions:* Use of other nephrotoxic drugs may increase renal toxicity; use of bone marrow-suppressing drugs increases hematologic toxicity; use of imipenem, cilastatin increases risk of seizures; use of probenecid decreases clearance of valganciclovir; use of zidovudine increases risk of hematologic toxicity	Dosage is decreased for renal insufficiency for advanced age. *Contraindications:* Hypersensitivity to acyclovir, ganciclovir, or valganciclovir *Precautions:* Use with extreme caution in children, with long-term risk of reproductive toxicity and carcinogenicity; use cautiously with patients with bone marrow suppression with cytopenias, or history of cytopenic reactions to other drugs; and with renal-impaired patients or elderly with increased probability of renal impairment
Zanamivir (Relenza) P: 5 mg (blister) for inhalation	*Influenza virus:* 2 inhalations (one 5 mg blister per inhalation) every 12 hr for 5 days *Prevention of influenza:* 2 inhalations daily throughout the exposure period	Diarrhea, sinusitis, nausea, bronchitis, cough, dizziness, headache; rare: malaise, fatigue, fever, abdominal pain, myalgia, arthalgia, urticaria *Serious reactions:* Neutropenia, bronchospasms in COPD or asthmatic patients *Interactions:* None	Safety has not been established for children under 7 yr. *Precautions:* Use with caution in COPD or asthmatic patients. *Contraindications:* Hypersensitivity to zanamivir

A, adults; C, capsules; C (dosage), children; I, injection; P, powder; OS, oral suspension; S, syrup; T, tablets.

BETA-ADRENERGIC BLOCKERS

Uses
Management of hypertension, angina pectoris, dysrhythmias, hypertrophic subaortic stenosis, migraine headaches, and glaucoma; prevention of myocardial infarction.

Action
Beta adrenergic blockers competitively block $beta_1$-adrenergic receptors, which are located primarily in myocardium, and $beta_2$-adrenergic receptors, which are located primarily in bronchial and vascular smooth muscle. By occupying beta receptor sites, these agents prevent naturally occurring or administered epinephrine/norepinephrine from exerting their effects. The results are basically opposite to those of sympathetic stimulation.
Effects of $beta_1$-blockade include slowing heart rate, decreasing cardiac output and contractility; effects of $beta_2$ blockade include bronchoconstriction, increased airway resistance in patients with asthma or chronic obstructive pulmonary disease (COPD). Beta blockers can affect cardiac rhythm/automaticity (decrease sinus rate, SA/AV conduction; increase refractory period in AV node). Beta blockers can decrease systolic and diastolic BP; the exact mechanism is unknown, but they may block peripheral receptors, decrease sympathetic outflow from CNS, or decrease renin release from kidney. All beta blockers mask tachycardia that occurs with hypoglycemia. When applied to the eye, they reduce intraocular pressure and aqueous production.

Beta-Adrenergic Blockers

Generic Name	Brand Name	Adrenergic Receptor Blocking Activity	Route	Usual Adult Dose	Available Dosage Forms	Adverse Effects	Comments
Acebutolol*†	Sectral	β_1	PO	200-400 mg twice daily, max 1200 mg/day divided in 2 doses	C: 200, 400 mg	Bradydysrhythmia, chest pain, edema, heart failure, hypotension, myalgia, dizziness, headache, insomnia, vertigo, dyspnea, fatigue	Discontinue over 2 wk
Atenolol*†	Tenormin	β_1	PO, IV	PO: 50-100 mg daily; IV: 5 mg IV over 5 min; give 2nd dose in 10 min then begin PO therapy	T: 25, 50, 100 mg I: 5 mg/ 10 mL	Bradydysrhythmia, hypotension, dizziness, fatigue, insomnia, depression	Discontinue over 2 wk, IV use for acute myocardial infarction
Betaxolol†	Kerlone	β_1	PO	10-40 mg daily	T: 10, 20 mg	Bradydysrhythmia, chest pain, arthralgia, asthenia, dizziness, headache, insomnia, fatigue	Consider 5 mg starting dose for elderly patients; discontinue over 2 wk

Continued

Beta-Adrenergic Blockers—cont'd

Generic Name	Brand Name	Adrenergic Receptor Blocking Activity	Route	Usual Adult Dose	Available Dosage Forms	Adverse Effects	Comments
Bisoprolol[†]	Zebeta	β_1	PO	2.5-20 mg daily, max 40 mg/day	T: 5, 10 mg	Bradydysrhythmia, dizziness, headache, dyssomnia, respiratory infection, fatigue	Discontinue over 2 wk
Carteolol	Cartrol	β_1, β_2	PO	2.5-10 daily, max 60 mg/day	T: 2.5, 5 mg	Edema, abdominal pain, diarrhea, nausea, asthenia, dizziness, insomnia, somnolence, tremor, anxiety	Discontinue over 2 wk
Carvedilol	Coreg	β_1, β_2, α_1	PO	6.25-25 mg twice daily	T: 3.125, 6.25, 12.5, 25 mg	Bradydysrhythmia, edema, hypotension, hyperglycemia, dizziness, fatigue	Discontinue over 2 wk
Carvedilol phosphate	Coreg CR	β_1, β_2, α	PO	10-80 mg once daily	C: 10, 20, 40, 80 mg	Same as carvedilol	Ratio: 10 mg Coreg CR = 3.125 mg Coreg twice daily, etc.
Esmolol[†]	Brevibloc	β_1	IV	*Intraoperative tachydysrhythmia:* 80 mg IV bolus over 30 sec followed by 150 mcg/kg/min IV infusion; may titrate up to 300 mcg/kg/min *Postoperative tachydysrhythmia:* 500 mcg/kg/min IV bolus over 1 min followed by sequential step-up in infusion rate 50, 100, 150, 200, 250, 300 mcg/kg/min over 4 min; repeat bolus before each sequential step up in infusion rate	I: 10, 20, 250 mg/mL	Bradydysrhythmia, chest pain, hypotension, injection site pain, nausea	Indicated for supraventricular arrhythmia
Labetalol	Normodyne, Trandate	β_1, β_2, α_1	PO, IV	PO: 100-400 mg twice daily, increase in increment of 100 mg twice daily every 2-3 days; IV: 20 mg over 2 min, titrating up to 40-80 mg every 10 min, max dose 300 mg	T: 100, 200, 300 mg I: 5 mg/mL	Lightheadedness, orthostatic hypotension, pruritus, rash, dizziness, fatigue, nausea	Discontinue over 2 wk

Metoprolol*†	Lopressor	β_1	PO, IV	PO: 50-450 mg/day divided in 1 or 2 doses; IV: 3 boluses of 5 mg each at 2 min intervals, 15 min after full IV dose start 50 mg PO every 6 hr for 48 hr	T: 25, 50, 100 mg I: 1 mg/mL		IV for acute myocardial infarction, allow 1-2 wk to achieve optimum effect, discontinue over 2 wk
Metoprolol, long-acting†	Toprol XL	β_1	PO	25-400 mg daily	T (ER): 25, 50, 100, 200 mg	Pruritus, rash, diarrhea, dizziness, fatigue, depression	Allow 1-2 wk to achieve optimal effect, use same total daily dose when switching to immediate-release tablets, discontinue over 2 wk
Nadolol*	Corgard	β_1, β_2	PO	40-320 mg daily, increase in 40-80 mg increments at 1-3 wk intervals	T: 20, 40, 80, 120, 160 mg	Bradydysrhythmia, hypotension, dizziness, fatigue	Discontinue over 2 wk
Penbutolol	Levatol	β_1, β_2	PO	20-40 mg daily	T: 20 mg	Flatulence, stomach cramps, dizziness, fatigue	Discontinue over 2 wk
Pindolol*	Visken	β_1, β_2	PO	10-60 mg/day divided in 2-3 doses, increase in 10 mg/day increments at 3-4 wk intervals	T: 5, 10 mg	Edema, abdominal discomfort, nausea, increased liver enzymes, arthralgia, myalgia, dizziness, insomnia, nervousness, fatigue	Discontinue over 2 wk
Propranolol*	Inderal, Inderal LA	β_1, β_2	PO, IV	Immediate release: 80-240 mg/day in 2-3 divided doses Long acting: 80-160 mg daily IV: 1-3 mg IV, may repeat after 2 min, additional doses not in less than 4 hr	T: 10, 20, 40, 60, 80, 90 mg C (ER): 60, 80, 120, 160 mg S: 20 mg/5 mL, 40 mg/5 mL, 80 mg/mL I: 1 mg/mL	Atrioventricular block, bradydysrhythmia, cold extremities, urticaria sleepiness, impaired cognition, insomnia, paresthesia, depression, psychotic disorder, dyspnea, wheezing	IV use reserved for life-threatening dysrhythmias or dysrhythmias occurring under general anesthesia

Continued

Beta-Adrenergic Blockers—cont'd

Generic Name	Brand Name	Adrenergic Receptor Blocking Activity	Route	Usual Adult Dose	Available Dosage Forms	Adverse Effects	Comments
Sotalol*	Betapace, Betapace AF	β_1, β_2 Also has class III antidysrhythmic activity and primary use of drug is in atrial dysrhythmias	PO	160-320 mg/day in divided doses	T: 80, 120, 160, 240 mg	Abnormal ECG, bradydysrhythmia, chest pain, congestive heart failure, edema, hypotension, syncope, asthenia, dizziness, headache, dyspnea, fatigue	If QT interval prolongs to greater than 500 msec, the dose should be reduced or discontinued
Timolol*	Blocadren	β_1, β_2	PO	5-20 mg twice daily, max 60 mg/day	T: 5, 10, 20 mg	Bradydysrhythmia, depression, hallucinations, fatigue	Discontinue over 2 wk

*Generic available for one or more dosage forms.

†β_1 blockers also block β_2 receptors in high doses.

C, capsules; ER, extended release; I, injection; S, solution; T, tablets

BRONCHODILATORS

Uses
Relief of bronchospasm occuring during anesthesia and in bronchial asthma, bronchitis, emphysema.

Action
Inhaled corticosteroids: Exact mechanism unknown. May act as antiinflammatories, decrease mucous secretion.

Beta$_2$-adrenergic agonists: Stimulate beta-receptors in lung, relax bronchial smooth muscle, increase vital capacity, decrease airway resistance.

Anticholinergics: Inhibit cholinergic receptors on bronchial smooth muscle (block acetylcholine action).

Leukotriene modifiers: Decrease effect of leukotrienes, which increase migration of eosinophils, producing mucous/edema of airway wall, causing bronchoconstriction.

Methylxanthines: Directly relax smooth muscle of bronchial airway, pulmonary blood vessels (relieve bronchospasm, increase vital capacity). Increase cyclic 3,5-adenosinc monophosphate.

Bronchodilators

Name	Availability	Dosage Range	Side Effects
Anticholinergics			
Ipratropium (Atrovent)	Neb: 0.02% MDI: 18 mcg/actuation Nasal: 0.03%, 0.06%	A (Neb): 0.02% every 3-4 hr A (MDI): 2 puffs 4 times per day A (Nasal): 2 sprays 2-4 times per day	Palpitations, nervousness, dizziness, headaches, pain, nausea, dry mucous membranes, dyspnea
Tiotropium (Spiriva)	Inhalation powder: 18 mcg	A: Once per day	Dry mouth, tachycardia, constipation, blurred vision, urinary difficulty/retention, upper respiratory tract infections
Beta-Agonists			
Albuterol* (Proventil, Ventolin, Volmax)	T: 2, 4 mg T (SR): 4, 8 mg S: 2 mg/5 mL MDI: 90 mcg/actuation Neb: 0.83% unit dose 3-mL vials; 0.5% in 0.5-mL vials and 20-mL vials with dropper; 0.63-mg/3-mL and 1.25-mg/3-mL unit dose vials	A, C (MDI): 2 puffs every 4-6 hr as needed A, C (Rotacaps): 1-2 caps every 4-6 hr as needed A (Neb): 2.5 mg every 4-6 hr as needed C (Neb): 0.1-0.15 mg/kg every 4-6 hr as needed A [T (SR)]: 4-8 mg every 12 hr C [T (SR)]: 4 mg every 12 hr	Tremors, tachycardia, palpitations, hypokalemia

Continued

Bronchodilators—cont'd

Name	Availability	Dosage Range	Side Effects
Bitolterol (Tornalate)	Sol for inhalation: 0.2%	A: 0.5-1.5 mg three times daily-four times daily	Same as albuterol
Epinephrine* (MicroNephrin, Primatene Mist)	Aerosol: 200 mcg/actuation Sol for inhalation: 10 mg/mL (1:100)	A: 1-2 inhalations every 3-4 hr (max 12 per day)	Same as albuterol
Formoterol (Foradil)	C (inhalation): 12 mcg	A: 1 capsule every 12 hr	Same as albuterol
Isoetharine*	Sol for inhalation: 1%	A: 4 inhalations every 4 hr	Same as albuterol
Isoproterenol	I: 0.02 mg/mL Sol for inhalation: 0.25, 0.5, 1%	A: 0.01-0.02 mg IV push as needed for bronchospasm during anesthesia, inhalations via nebulizer up to 5 times daily	Tachycardia
Levalbuterol (Xopenex)	Neb: 0.63 mg/3 mL, 1.25 mg/3 mL	A: 0.63-1.25 mg every 6-8 hr as needed C (6-11 yr): 0.31-0.63 3 times/day	Same as albuterol
Metaproterenol (Alupent, Metaprel)	MDI: 0.65 mg/actuation Neb: 0.4%, 0.6%, 5% S: 10 mg/5 mL T: 10, 20 mg	A: 2-3 inhalations every 2-3 hr Max 12 inhalations/day Not recommended for children less than 2 yr (use nebulizer)	Same as albuterol
Piruterol (Maxair)	MDI: 0.2 mg/actuation	A, C: 2 puffs every 4-6 hr as needed	Same as albuterol
Salmeterol (Serevent)	Discus (powder for inhalation): Unit dosed 50 µg/inhalation	A, C: 1 inhalation every 12 hr	Same as albuterol
Terbutaline (Brethine, Bricanyl)	MDI: 0.2 mg/actuation I: 1 mg/mL T: 2.5, 5 mg	A: 2.5 mg 3-4 times/day A (MDI): 2 puffs every 4-6 hr C: 0.05 mg/kg/dose 3 times/day	Same as albuterol
Inhaled Antiinflammatory Agents			
Beclomethasone (Beclovent, Vanceril, Qvar)	MDI: 40, 80 mcg/actuation	1-2 inhalations 2-4 times/day A: Max 320 mcg twice daily C (5-11 yr): Max 80 mcg twice daily	Oropharyngeal candidiasis, dysphonia, hoarseness, cough
Budesonide (Pulmicort)	MDI: 200 mcg/metered dose Neb: 0.25 mg/2 mL, 0.5 mg/2 mL	MDI (A): 1-4 inhalations 2 times/day C (older than 6 yr): 1-2 inhalations 2 times/day	Same as beclomethasone

Cromolyn (Intal)	MDI: 800 mcg/actuation Neb: 20 mg/2 mL	MDI (C [older than 5 yr]): 2 inhalations up to 4 times/day Neb (C [older than 2 yr]): 20 mg 4 times/day	Cough, urticaria, bronchospasm
Flunisolide (AeroBid)	MDI: 250 mcg/actuation	A: 2-4 inhalations 2 times/day C (6-15 yr): 1-2 inhalations 2 times/day	Same as beclomethasone
Fluticasone (Flovent)	MDI: 44, 110, 220 mcg/actuation Rotadisk/Discus: 50, 100, 250 mcg/actuation	MDI (A, C [older than 12 yr]): 2 inhalations 2 times/day Rotadisk/Discus (A, C [older than 4 yr]): 1 inhalation 2 times/day	Same as beclomethasone
Nedocromil (Tilade)	MDI: 1.75 mg/actuation	A, C (older than 6 yr): 2 inhalations 4 times/day	Altered taste, headaches, nausea
Triamcinolone (Azmacort)	MDI: 100 mcg/actuation	A: 2 inhalations 3-4 times/day or 4-8 inhalations 2 times/day C: 1-2 inhalations 3-4 times/day or 2-6 inhalations 2 times/day	Same as beclomethasone
Mometasone (Asmanex)	MDI: 220 mcg/actuation	1-2 inhalations daily in the evening; max of 4	Same as beclomethasone
Leukotriene Modifiers			
Montelukast (Singulair)	T: 10 mg T (chewable): 4, 5 mg G: 4 mg pkt	A: 10 mg/day C (6-14 yr): 5 mg/day C (2-5 yr): 4 mg/day	Dyspepsia, increased hepatic function tests
Zafirlukast (Accolate)	T: 10, 20 mg	A, C (greater than or equal to 12 yr): 20 mg 2 times/day C (5-11 yr): 10 mg 2 times/day	Same as montelukast
Zileuton (Zyflo)	T: 600 mg T (SR): 600 mg	A: 600 mg 4 times daily with meals and at bedtime SR: 1200 mg twice daily	Liver enzyme elevation, dyspepsia
Monoclonal Antibodies			
Omalizumab (Xolair)	Powder for I: 202.5 mg (150 mg/1.2 mL after reconstitution)	A: 150-375 mg subcutaneous every 2-4 weeks for moderate to severe persistent asthma	Injection site reaction, infection, anaphylaxis

*Generic available for one or more dosage forms
A, adults; C, capsule; C (dosage) children; G, granules; I, injection; MDI, metered-dose inhaler; Neb, nebulization; S, syrup; Sol, solution; SR, sustained release; T, tablet

CALCIUM CHANNEL BLOCKERS

Uses
Treatment of essential hypertension, treatment of and prophylaxis of angina pectoris (including vasospastic, chronic stable, unstable), prevention/control of supraventricular tachydysrhythmias, prevention of neurologic damage due to subarachnoid hemorrhage.

Action
Calcium channel blockers inhibit the flow of extracellular CA^{2+} ions across cell membranes of cardiac cells, vascular tissue. They relax arterial smooth muscle, depress the rate of sinus node pacemaker, slow AV conduction, decrease heart rate, produce negative inotropic effect (rarely seen clinically due to reflex response). Calcium channel blockers decrease coronary vascular resistance, increase coronary blood flow, reduce myocardial oxygen demand. Degree of action varies with individual agent.

Calcium Channel Blockers (CCBs)

Generic Name	Brand Name	Usual Adult Dose	Available Dosage Forms	Adverse Effects	Comments
Amlodipine	Norvasc	Initial: 5 mg once daily; liver disease, start at 2.5 mg/day Maintenance: 5-10 mg once daily	T: 2.5, 5, 10 mg	Palpitations, peripheral edema, flushing, dizziness, headache, fatigue	Dihydropyridine class, titrate over 7-14 days
Diltiazem hydrochloride	Cardizem, Cardizem CD, Cardizem LA, Cardizem SR, Cartia XT, Dilacor XR, Dilt-CD, Dilt-XR	T: Initial: 30 mg four times daily in the morning and at bedtime Maintenance: increase dose at 1-2 day intervals to 180-360 mg in 3 or 4 divided doses T (ER) (Cardizem LA): 120-540 mg daily, max 540 mg/day C (ER) (Dilacor XR): 120-360 mg daily, max 540 mg/day C (SR) (Cardizem SR): 60-180 mg twice daily, max 360 mg/day	T: 30, 60, 90, 120 mg C (ER): 240 mg C (ER 12-hr): 60, 90, 120 mg C (ER 24-hr): 120, 180, 240, 300, 360, 420 mg T (ER): 120, 180, 240, 300, 360, 420 mg IV P for Sol: 25,	Atrioventricular block, bradydysrhythmia, congestive heart failure, peripheral edema, syncope, drug-induced gingival hyperplasia, dizziness, headache	Non-dihydropyridine class

		IV: Initial: bolus of 0.25 mg/kg given over 2 min; second dose of 0.35 mg/kg over 2 min may be necessary. Maintenance: continuous infusion of 5-15 mg/hr	100 mg IV Sol: 5 mg/mL		
Felodipine	Plendil	2.5-10 mg daily	T (ER): 2.5, 5, 10 mg	Peripheral edema, flushing, drug-induced gingival hyperplasia, dizziness, headache	Dihydropyridine class, allow at least 2 wk between dosage changes
Isradipine	DynaCirc, DynaCirc CR	Immediate: 2.5-10 mg twice daily CR: 5-10 mg twice daily	C: 2.5, 5 mg T (CR): 5, 10 mg	Peripheral edema, flushing, drug-induced gingival hyperplasia, dizziness, headache	Dihydropyridine class, maximum response may require 2-4 wk
Nicardipine hydrochloride*	Cardene, Cardene SR, Cardene IV	C: Initial: 20 mg three times daily Maintenance: 20-40 mg three times daily; allow at least 3 days between dosage increases SR: Initial: 30 mg twice daily Maintenance: 30-60 mg twice daily IV: Infuse at rate comparable to oral dosing: 20 mg PO every 8 hr = 0.5 mg/hr IV, 30 mg PO every 8 hr = 1.2 mg/hr IV, 40 mg PO every 8 hr = 2.2 mg/hr IV	C: 20, 30 mg C (SR): 30, 45, 60 mg I: 2.5 mg/mL	Hypotension, peripheral edema, tachydysrhythmia, drug-induced gingival hyperplasia, dizziness, headache	Dihydropyridine class, only immediate-release capsules are used for angina
Nifedipine*	Adalat, Adalat CC, Afeditab CR, Nifediac CC, Nifedical XL, Procardia, Procardia XL	C: Initial: 10 mg three times daily Maintenance: 10 mg three times daily to 30 mg three times daily-four times daily SR: Initial: 30-60 mg daily Maintenance: 30-90 mg daily	C: 10, 20 mg T (SR): 30, 60, 90 mg	Palpitations, peripheral edema, flushing, constipation, heartburn, nausea, dizziness, headache	Dihydropyridine class, no rebound effects if abruptly discontinued; avoid sublingual use or chronic use of immediate release dosage form
Nimodipine	Nimotop	60 mg every 4 hr for 21 days, start treatment within 96 hr of subarachnoid hemorrhage (SAH)	C: 30 mg	Decreased BP (not hypotension), diarrhea, nausea, stomach cramps	Dihydropyridine class, only approved use is SAH

Continued

Calcium Channel Blockers—cont'd

Generic Name	Brand Name	Usual Adult Dose	Available Dosage Forms	Adverse Effects	Comments
Nisoldipine	Sular	Initial: 20 mg once daily, adjust by adding 10 mg/wk Maintenance: 20-40 mg once daily; max 60 mg/day	T (ER): 10, 20, 30, 40 mg		Dihydropyridine class, avoid grapefruit or grapefruit juice before or after doses
Verapamil hydrochloride*	Calan, Calan SR, Isoptin, Isoptin SR, Verelan, Verelan PM	T (IR): 80-480 mg/day divided in 3 doses C (ER): 200-400 mg daily T (ER): 180-480 mg every evening C (SR): 240-480 mg every morning T (SR): 240 mg every morning-240 mg twice daily	T: 40, 80, 120 mg C (ER): 100, 120, 180, 200, 240, 300 mg T (ER): 120, 180, 240 mg C (SR): 120, 180, 240, 360 mg T (SR): 120, 180, 240 mg I: 2.5 mg/mL		Non-dihydropyridine class, sustained-release capsules may be emptied and sprinkled over applesauce, avoid grapefruit juice

*Generic available for one or more dosage forms

C, capsules; CR, controlled release; ER, extended release; I, injection; IV, intravenous; P, powder; SR, sustained release; T, tablets

CORTICOSTEROIDS

Uses
Replacement therapy in adrenal insufficiency, including Addison's disease. Symptomatic treatment of multiorgan disease/conditions. Rheumatoid arthritis, osteoarthritis, severe psoriasis, ulcerative colitis, lupus erythematosus, anaphylactic shock, acute exacerbation of asthma, status asthmaticus, organ transplant.

Action
Suppress migration of polymorphonuclear leukocytes (PML) and reverse increased capillary permeability by their antiinflammatory effect. Suppress immune system by decreasing activity of lymphatic system.

Corticosteroids

Name	Relative Dose for Equivalent Glucocorticoid Effect (Systemic)	Availability	Route of Administration	Side Effects/Comments
Beclomethasone (Beclovent, Beconase, Vanceril)	–	Inhalation: 40, 80 mcg Nasal: 42 mcg/spray	Inhalation, intranasal	Inhalation: Cough dry mouth/throat, headaches, throat irritation Nasal: Headaches, sore throat, intranasal ulceration
Betamethasone (Celestone, Diprosone)	0.8 mg	I: 4 mg/mL I (long-acting): 6 mg/mL* S: 0.6 mg/5 mL	IV, intralesional, intraarticular	Nausea, vomiting, increased appetite, weight gain, insomnia
Budesonide (Rhinocort, Pulmicort)	–	Inhalation: 200 mcg/dose Inhalation suspension: 0.25 mg/2 mL, 0.5 mg/2 mL Nasal: 32 mcg/spray C: 3 mg	Intranasal, inhalation, PO	Nasal: Headaches, sore throat, intranasal ulceration PO: same as betamethasone
Cortisone (Cortone)	25 mg	T: 5, 10, 25 mg	PO	Same as betamethasone

Continued

Corticosteroids—cont'd

Name	Relative Dose for Equivalent Glucocorticoid Effect (Systemic)	Availability	Route of Administration	Side Effects/Comments
Dexamethasone (Decadron)	0.8 mg	T: 0.25, 0.5, 0.75, 1, 1.5, 2, 4, 6 mg OS: 0.5 mg/5 mL, 1 mg/mL I: 4 mg/mL I (dexamethasone acetate) (long-acting): 8, 16 mg/mL I (dexamethasone sodium phosphate): 4, 10, 20, 24 mg/mL	PO, parenteral	Same as betamethasone
Fludrocortisone (Florinel)	–	T: 0.1 mg	PO	Same as betamethasone Used as a mineralocorticoid
Flunisolide (AeroBid, Nasalide)	–	Inhalation: 250 mcg/spray Nasal: 25 mcg/spray	Inhalation, intranasal	Same as beclomethasone
Fluticasone (Flonase, Flovent)	–	Inhalation: 44 mcg, 110 mg/220 mcg P for inhalation: 50, 100, 200 mcg/actuation Nasal: 50 mg	Inhalation, intranasal	Same as beclomethasone
Hydrocortisone (Cortef, Solu-Cortef, others)	20 mg	T: 5, 10, 25 mg I: 100, 250, 500 mg, 1 g OS: 10 mg/5 mL I (hydrocortisone acetate) (long-acting): 25 mg/50 mg/mL I (hydrocortisone sodium phosphate): 50 mg/mL I (hydrocortisone sodium succinate): 100, 250, 500, 1000 mg/vial	PO, parenteral	Same as betamethasone
Mometasone	–	P for inhalation: 220 mcg/actuation Nasal spray: 50 mcg/actuation	Inhalation, intranasal	Same as betamethasone

Methylprednisolone (Medrol, Solu-Medrol, Depo-Medrol)	4 mg	T: 2, 4, 8, 16, 24, 32 mg I: 40, 125, 500 mg, 1 g, 2 g I (methylprednisolone acetate) (long acting): 20, 40, 80 mg/mL I (methylprednisolone sodium succinate): 40, 125, 500, 1000, 2000 mg/vial	PO, parenteral	Same as betamethasone
Prednisolone (Prelone)	5 mg	T (disintegrating): 5, 10, 15, 30 mg OS: 5 mg/5 mL, 6.7 mg/mL, 15 mg/5 mL OL (prednisolone sodium phosphate): 5 mg/5 mL I (prednisolone acetate) (long-acting): 25, 50 mg/mL I (prednisolone tebutate) (long-acting): 20 mg/mL I (prednisolone sodium phosphate) (long-acting): 20 mg/mL	PO	Same as betamethasone

*Betamethasone long-acting is 3 mg betamethasone acetate and 3 mg betamethasone sodium phosphate.
C, capsules; I, injection; OS, oral suspension; OL, oral liquid; P, powder; S, syrup; T, tablets

DIURETICS

Uses

Thiazides: Management of edema resulting from a number of causes (e.g., congestive heart failure [CHF], hepatic cirrhosis); hypertension either alone or in combination with other antihypertensives.

Loop: Management of edema associated with CHF, cirrhosis of the liver, and renal disease. Furosemide used in treatment of hypertension alone or in combination with other antihypertensives.

Potassium-sparing: Adjunctive treatment with thiazides, loop diuretics in treatment of CHF and hypertension.

Action

Diuretics act to increase the excretion of water/sodium and other electrolytes via the kidneys. Exact mechanism of antihypertensive effect unknown; may be due to reduced plasma volume or decreased peripheral vascular resistance. Subclassifications of diuretics are based on their mechanism and site of action.

Thiazides: Act at the cortical diluting segment of nephron, block reabsorption of Na, Cl, and water; promote excretion of Na, Cl, K, and water.

Loop: Act primarily at the thick ascending limb of Henle's loop to inhibit Na, Cl, and water absorption.

Potassium-sparing: Spironolactone blocks aldosterone action on distal nephron (causes K retention, Na excretion). Triamterene, amiloride act on distal nephron, decreasing Na reuptake, reducing K secretion.

Diuretics

Generic Name	Brand Name	Usual Adult Dose	Available Dosage Forms	Adverse Effects	Comments
Thiazides					
Bendroflumethiazide	Aprinox	2.5-15 mg daily	T: 5, 10 mg	Hypotension, vasculitis, photosensitivity, ecchymosis, spasticity, dizziness, headache, vertigo, blurred vision	
Chlorothiazide	Diuril	T: 0.5-1 g/day in 1-2 divided doses IV: 0.5-1 g/day in 1-2 divided doses	T: 250, 500 mg OS: 250 mg/5 mL IV: 500 mg	Hypotension, alopecia, photosensitivity, hyperglycemia, hyperuricemia, spasticity, dizziness, headache, blurred vision, xanthopsia, impotence	
Chlorthalidone	Hygroton, Thalitone	15-50 mg daily	T: 15, 25, 50, 100 mg	Hypotension, vasculitis, photosensitivity, abnormal electrolytes, hyperglycemia, hyperuricemia, spasticity, dizziness, headache, paresthesia, blurred vision, xanthopsia, impotence	Take in the morning with food

Hydrochlorothiazide	Aquazide H, Hydrocot, Hydrodiuril, Microzide, Zide	12.5-100 mg daily	C: 12.5 mg T: 25, 50, 100 mg OS: 50 mg/5 mL	Hypotension, vasculitis, photosensitivity, abnormal electrolytes, hyperglycemia, hyperuricemia, spasticity, dizziness, headache, paresthesia, blurred vision, xanthopsia, impotence	Allow 2-3 wk to achieve optimum antihypertensive effect, monitor serum potassium
Hydroflumethiazide	Saluron, Aldactide	50-200 mg/ day in 2 divided doses	T: 25, 50 mg		
Indapamide	Lozol	1.25-5 mg daily	T: 1.25, 2.5 mg	Orthostatic hypotension, vasculitis, flushing, abnormal electrolytes, hyperuricemia, dizziness, fatigue, headache, paresthesia	
Methyclothiazide	Aquatensen, Enduron	2.5-5 mg daily	T: 2.5, 5 mg	Hypotension, photosensitivity, abnormal electrolytes, hyperglycemia, hyperuricemia, purpuric disorder, spasticity, dizziness, headache, paresthesia, glycosuria	
Metolazone	Mykrox, Zaroxolyn	Mykrox: 0.5-1 mg daily Zaroxolyn: 2.5-20 mg daily	T: 0.5, 2.5, 5, 10 mg	Chest pain, orthostatic hypotension, syncope, abnormal electrolytes, hyperuricemia, dizziness, headache, depression, impotence	
Polythiazide	Renese	2-4 mg daily	T: 1, 2, 4 mg	Hypotension, vasculitis, photosensitivity, abnormal electrolytes, hyperglycemia, hyperuricemia, spasticity, dizziness, headache, paresthesia, glycosuria	
Quinethazone	Hydromox	25-200 mg/ day	T: 50 mg	Orthostatic hypotension, phototoxicity, purpura, hyperglycemia, abnormal electrolytes, hyperuricemia	
Trichlormethiazide	Diurese, Metahydrin, Naqua, Naquival	1-4 mg/day in 1-2 divided doses	T: 2, 4 mg	Cardiac dysrhythmia, hypotension, photosensitivity, hyperglycemia, abnormal electrolytes	

Continued

Diuretics—cont'd

Generic Name	Brand Name	Usual Adult Dose	Available Dosage Forms	Adverse Effects	Comments
Loop *(Class side effects: hyperuricemia, hypokalemia, orthostatic hypotension; allow 3-4 wk for maximum effect; best if given in the morning)*					
Bumetanide	Bumex	PO: 0.5-2 mg daily (max: 10 mg/day) IV/IM: 0.5-1 mg	T: 0.5, 1, 2 mg I: 0.25 mg/mL	Orthostatic hypotension	Give IV over 1-2 min; can give a 2nd and 3rd dose at 2-3 hr intervals (max: 10 mg/day).
Ethacrynic acid	Edecrin	PO: Initial: 12.5-25 mg daily Maintenance: 50-200 mg daily IV: 0.5-1 mg/kg (max: 100 mg/dose)	T: 25, 50 mg I: 50 mg	Orthostatic hypotension	Adjust in 25-50 mg increments.
Furosemide[*,†]	Lasix	PO: 80 mg daily	T: 20, 40, 80 mg I: 10 mg/mL S: 40 mg/5, 10 mg/mL	Orthostatic hypotension	
Torsemide[†]	Demadex	PO: 5-10 mg daily	T: 5, 10, 20, 100 mg IV: 10 mg/mL	Constipation, dizziness, headache, abdominal discomfort	Titrate as needed. May give with or without food. PO and IV are equivalent doses, therefore may switch.

Potassium-Sparing
(Class side effects: hyperkalemia, GI problems, orthostatic hypotension, photosensitivity)

Amiloride†	Midamor	PO: 5-20 mg/day	T: 5 mg	Hyperkalemia	Give with food.
Spironolactone†*	Aldactone	PO: 50-100 mg/day (max: 400 mg/day)	T: 25, 50, 100 mg	Hyperkalemia, nausea, vomiting, abdominal cramps, diarrhea	Continue for 2 wk before adjusting dose. Give with food.
Triamterene†	Dyrenium	PO: 100 mg twice daily (max: 300 mg/day)	C: 50, 100 mg	Hyperkalemia	Give after meals.

*Generic available for one or more dosage forms.
†Daily dose can be given as a single dose or divided doses.
C, capsule; GI, gastrointestinal; I, injection; IV, intravenous; OS, oral solution; S, solution; T, tablet

References for antihypertensive tables:

1. Ellsworth, Allan J et al: *Mosby's Medical Drug Reference.* Mosby, St. Louis, 2003.
2. Website: U.S. Food and Drug Administration. Online. Internet. 2003. Available: *http://www.fda.gov/cder*
3. Micromedex
4. Lexi-Complete

HEMATINIC IRON PREPARATIONS

Uses
Prevention or treatment of iron deficiency resulting from improper diet, pregnancy, impaired absorption, or prolonged blood loss.

Action
Iron supplements are provided to ensure adequate supplies for the formation of hemoglobin, which is needed for erythropoiesis and O_2 transport.

Hematinic (Iron) Preparations

Name	Availability	Elemental Iron (%)	Side Effects
Ferrous fumarate (Femiron, Feostat)	T: 90, 324, 350 mg T (TR): 150 mg	33	Constipation, nausea, vomiting, diarrhea, abdominal pain/cramps
Ferrous gluconate (Fergon)	T: 225, 300, 324, 325 mg	12	Same as ferrous fumarate
Ferrous sulphate (Fer-In-Sol)	T: 325 mg E: 220 mg/5 mL D: 75 mg/0.6 mL	20	Same as ferrous fumarate
Ferrous sulphate exsiccated (Slow-Fe, Feosol)	T: 200, 300 mg T (SR): 160 mg C (ER): 160 mg	30	Same as ferrous fumarate
Iron dextran (Infed)	I (IV): 50 mg iron/mL (as dextran)		Dysrhythmias, convulsions, dizziness, rash Due to high risk of anaphylactic reaction, a test dose must be given and the possibility of oral supplementation ruled out. Resuscitation equipment should be available.
Iron sucrose (Venofen)	I: 20 mg elemental iron/mL		Cramps, hypotension, diarrhea, nausea, vomiting, headache
Polysaccharide iron complex (Niferex, Nu Iron)	C: 60, 150 mg E: 100 mg/5 mL		
Sodium ferric gluconate complex (Ferrlecit)	I: 62.5 mg/5 mL elemental iron		Hypotension, hypersensitivity, cramps, nausea, vomiting

C, caplets; D, drops; E, elixir; ER, extended release; I, injection; S, suspension; SR, sustained release; T, tablets; TR, timed release

HIV MEDICATIONS (ANTIRETROVIRALS)

Uses
Antiretroviral agents are used in the treatment of HIV infection.

Action
There are currently five classes of antiretroviral agents used in the treatment of HIV.

Protease inhibitors (PIs) bind to the active site of HIV-1 protease and prevent the processing of viral gag and gag-pol polyprotein precursors, resulting in immature, noninfectious viral particles.

Nucleoside reverse transcriptase inhibitors (NRTIs) compete with natural substrates for formation of proviral DNA by reverse transcriptase, inhibiting viral replication.

Nucleotide reverse transcriptase inhibitors (NtRTIs) inhibit reverse transcriptase by competing with the natural substrate deoxyadenosine triphosphate and by DNA chain termination.

Nonnucleoside reverse transcriptase inhibitors (NNRTIs) directly bind to reverse transcriptase and block the RNA-dependent and DNA-dependent DNA polymerase activities by causing a disruption of the enzyme's catalytic site.

Fusion inhibitors interfere with the entry of HIV-1 into cells by inhibiting fusion of viral and cellular membranes.

HIV Medications

Name and Dosage Forms	Dose	Side Effects/Drug Interactions	Notes
Protease Inhibitors (PIs)			
Atazanavir (Reyataz) 100-, 150-, and 200-mg capsules	PI naive patients: 400 mg daily. PI experienced patients: 300 mg plus 100 mg Norvir daily	Increased bilirubin, abnormal electrocardiogram results, increased glucose, lipodystrophy, and increased bleeding in patients with hemophilia. Contraindicated with ergot derivatives, cisapride, pimozide, triazolam, and midazolam. Inhibits CYP3A4, 1A2, 2C9, and UGT1A1 metabolic pathways and can cause toxicity of applicable drugs.	Increased bilirubin is not clinically significant but may cause cosmetic concerns. Take with food.

Continued

HIV Medications—cont'd

Name and Dosage Forms	Dose	Side Effects/Drug Interactions	Notes
Darunavir ethanolate (Prezista) 300-mg tablets	600 mg with ritonavir 100 mg twice daily with food	Nausea, diarrhea, stomach discomfort, headache, increased cholesterol, increased triglycerides, lipodystrophy, increased glucose, increased liver enzyme levels, inflammation of the nose and throat, and increased bleeding in patients with hemophilia. See ritonavir for drug interactions.	Darunavir and ritonavir should be taken with food, although the type and amount of food does not matter. If taken with didanosine (Videx or Videx EC), darunavir and ritonavin should be taken at least 2 hr before or 1 hr after taking didanosine.
Fosamprenavir (Lexiva) * 700-mg tablets	PI naive patients: 1400 mg twice daily *or* 1400 mg plus 200 mg Norvir capsules once daily. PI experienced patients: one 700 mg tablet plus one 100 mg Norvir capsule twice daily	Skin rash, nausea, diarrhea, stomach discomfort, headache, increased cholesterol, increased triglycerides, lipodystrophy, increased glucose, increased liver enzyme levels, and increased bleeding in patients with hemophilia Contraindicated with ergot derivatives, pimozide, midazolam, cisapride, and triazolam. Use caution with CYP3A4 drugs.	Use caution in patients with known sulfonamide allergies. May take without regard to meals.
Indinavir (Crixivan) 100-, 200-, 333-, and 400-mg capsules	800 mg every 8 hr with water or another liquid. Reduce dose if given with delavirdine, itraconazole, or ketoconazole. Increase if given with rifabutin. Often used in combination with Norvir; may reduce dose. Separate from didanosine by 1 hr. Reduce in hepatic patients.	Kidney stones, nausea, vomiting, diarrhea, increased cholesterol, increased triglycerides, increased glucose, lipodystrophy, increased bilirubin (not harmful), increased bleeding in patients with hemophilia. ***Others:*** headache, weakness, blurred vision, dizziness, rash, metallic taste, low platelet count, hair loss, anemia. ***Contraindicated drugs:*** amiodarone, ergot derivatives, pimozide, triazolam, midazolam, and cisapride. Reacts with CYP3A4 drugs. Do not use with St. John's wort.	Without ritonavir: Take on an empty stomach (no food 2 hr before or 1 hr after dosing), or with a light, low-fat snack. With ritonavir: Take with or without food. Drink at least 48 oz (six 8-oz glasses or about 1.5 liters) of water daily to prevent kidney stones.
Lopinavir/ritonavir (Kaletra) 200-mg/50-mg tablets and 80-mg/20-mg/mL oral solution	2 tablets twice daily *or*, if starting therapy for the first time, 4 tablets once daily	Nausea, diarrhea, stomach discomfort, weakness, increased cholesterol, increased triglycerides, lipodystrophy, increased glucose, increased liver enzyme levels, and increased bleeding in patients with hemophilia. ***Contraindicated:*** same drugs as ritonavir. Use caution with rifampin, St. John's wort, lovastatin, simvastatin, sildenafil, tadalafil, vardenafil, and many others.	Take oral solution with food but tablets may be taken with or without food.

Nelfinavir mesylate (Viracept) 250-mg and 625-mg tablets or 50-mg/g powder	1250 mg twice daily or 750 mg three times daily	Diarrhea, increased cholesterol, increased triglycerides, lipodystrophy, increased glucose, increased liver enzyme levels, increased bleeding in patients with hemophilia, increased liver enzymes. ***Contraindicated:*** amiodarone, quinidine, St. John's wort, ergot derivatives, rifampin, pimozide, triazolam, midazolam, lovastatin, cisapride, and simvastatin. Reacts with CYP3A4 drugs.	Take with a meal or light snack. If trouble swallowing the pills, powder formulation can be dissolved in water, milk, soy milk, or dietary supplement. Rinse glass with water and swallow afterward to ensure entire dose is consumed. Do not mix with juice or acidic food. After mixing, refrigerate.
Ritonavir (Norvir) 100-mg gelatin caps or 80-mg/mL oral solution	300 mg twice daily initially, increasing by 100 mg twice daily every 2-3 days until receiving 600 mg twice daily. See saquinavir dosing for combination.	Nausea, diarrhea, stomach discomfort, numbness or tingling around the mouth and in the limbs (paresthesias), increased cholesterol, increased triglycerides, lipodystrophy, hepatitis, weakness, increased glucose, increased liver enzyme levels, and increased bleeding in patients with hemophilia. ***Contraindicated:*** alfuzosin, cisapride, most antidysrhythmics, voriconazole, astemizole, ergot derivatives, pimozide, triazolam, and midazolam. Reacts with CYP3A drugs.	Take with food. High-fat snacks may reduce side effects. Capsules and oral solution may be stored at room temperature, but should be refrigerated in hot weather. Solution can be mixed with chocolate syrup, chocolate ice cream, or an oral diet supplement for palatability.
Saquinavir mesylate (Invirase) 200-mg caps, 500-mg tablets	Invirase (usually used in combination with ritonavir): two 500-mg Invirase tablets plus one 100-mg ritonavir capsule twice daily Without ritonavir: 1200 mg three times daily	Nausea, diarrhea, stomach discomfort, headache, increased cholesterol, increased triglycerides, lipodystrophy, increased glucose, increased liver enzyme levels, and increased bleeding in patients with hemophilia. ***Contraindicated:*** most antidysrhythmics, St. John's wort, ergot derivatives, rifampin, pimozide, triazolam, midazolam, lovastatin, cisapride, and simvastatin. Reacts with CYP3A4 drugs.	Invirase and ritonavir should be taken with food, preferably a full nutritious meal (e.g., breakfast and dinner), or within 2 hr after a meal.

Continued

HIV Medications—cont'd

Name and Dosage Forms	Dose	Side Effects/Drug Interactions	Notes
Tipranavir (Aptivus) 250-mg capsules	500 mg coadministered with ritonavir 200 mg twice daily	***Special warnings:*** Hepatitis (extra care needed for HIV-positive people with hepatitis B or hepatitis C). Rash, increased cholesterol, increased triglycerides, lipodystrophy, increased bleeding in patients with hemophilia. See ritonavir for drug interactions.	Aptivus and ritonavir should be taken with food, preferably a full nutritious meal (e.g., breakfast and dinner). Aptivus/ritonavir should not be taken with other protease inhibitors. Take at least 2 hr before or 2 hr after didanosine (Videx).
Nucleoside/Nucleotide Reverse Transcriptase Inhibitors (NRTIs)			
Abacavir (Ziagen) 300-mg tablets or 20-mg/mL oral solution	300 mg twice daily or 600 mg once daily, always in combination with other agents. Reduce dose with hepatic impairment	GI pain, nausea and vomiting, diarrhea, anxiety, headache, malaise fatigue	***Box warning:*** severe allergic reactions (symptoms include fever; rash; severe nausea, diarrhea, abdominal pain; sore throat; cough; and shortness of breath). Lactic acidosis and hepatomegaly with steatosis have occurred. May take with or without food.
Didanosine (ddl) (Videx) 25-, 50-, 100-, 150-, and 200-mg buffered tablets; 100-, 167-, and 250-mg powder packets Videx EC: 125-, 200-, 250-, and 400-mg capsules	2 100-mg tablets twice daily (preferred) or 2 200-mg tablets once daily. Reduced dosing for patients weighing less than 60 kg. Videx EC: 1 400-mg capsule once daily. For patients weighing less than 60 kg, the dose is 1 250-mg capsule once daily. Only use this dosage form when once daily dosing is required by patient.	Numbness, tingling, or pain in the hands or feet (peripheral neuropathy); retinal changes and optic neuritis, nausea; diarrhea. Drug interactions include allopurinol, ganciclovir, methadone, antacids, antifungal agents, fluoroquinolones, and stavudine (see notes).	Pancreatitis, sometimes fatal, has occurred. Lactic acidosis and hepatomegaly with steatosis have occurred. Only use with stavudine in pregnant women if benefit outweighs risk of lactic acidosis. Administer on empty stomach. 2-4 of the buffered tablets must be taken per dose for adequate buffering without GI side effects. May take same time as all NRTIs. The buffered versions of Videx should not be taken at the same time as any of the PI's—take 2 hr before or 2 hr after Videx. The NNRTIs nevirapine and efavirenz can be taken at the same time as Videx; the NNRTI delavirdine should be taken at least 1 hr before or 1 hr after Videx. Videx EC should be taken at least 2 hr before or 2 hr after tipranavir. Avoid alcohol.

Emtricitabine (Emtriva) 200-mg tablets or 10-mg/mL oral solution	200-mg capsule or 240-mg of oral solution once daily. Reduce in renal impairment.	Headache, nausea and vomiting, rash—usually well tolerated. No known drug interactions.	***Box warning:*** lactic acidosis and hepatomegaly with steatosis have occurred. Emtricitabine is not FDA indicated for hepatitis B; monitor hepatic function closely when discontinued in patients with hepatitis B comorbidity. May take without regard to food.
Lamivudine (3TC) (Epivir) 150-, 300-mg tablets or 10-mg/mL oral solution	300 mg daily in one or two doses. Administer with or without food. Give with other antiretrovirals, and reduce dose in renal dysfunction.	Nasal problems, dizziness, depression, headache.	***Box warning:*** lactic acidosis and hepatomegaly with steatosis have occurred. The product Epivir-HBV is FDA indicated for chronic hepatitis B. The dose is lower for this indication and it is important to know this lest HIV resistance emerge. Box warning for severe hepatomegaly with steatosis and lactic acidosis.
Stavudine (d4T) (Zerit) 15-, 20-, 30-, and 40-mg capsules Zerit XR: 37.5-, 50-, 75-, and 100-mg extended-release capsules	Zerit: 40 mg every 12 hr if weighing more than 60 kg, 30 mg every 12 hr if weighing less than 60 kg. Reduced dosing in renal impairment. Zerit XR: 100 mg daily if weighing more than 60 kg, 75 mg daily if weighing less than 60 kg. Has not been studied in renal impairment.	Numbness, tingling, or pain in the hands or feet (peripheral neuropathy); lipodystrophy; muscular weakness (rare); increased cholesterol and triglycerides. Drug interactions with didanosine, hydroxyurea, doxorubicin, ribavirin, methadone, and zidovudine.	Box warning for severe hepatomegaly with steatosis and lactic acidosis. Use cautiously, if at all, with didanosine in pregnant women. Pancreatitis is also more common with the combination. Do not take with zidovudine or zidovudine/lamivudine.
Telbivudine (Tyzeka) 600-mg tablets	600 mg once daily, with or without food	Generally well tolerated. Caution in combination with drugs that reduce renal function	Box warning for severe hepatomegaly with steatosis and lactic acidosis. Monitor hepatic function closely when discontinued in patients with hepatitis B comorbidity. Adjust dose in renal dysfunction.
Tenofovir disoproxil fumarate (PMPA) (Viread) 300-mg tablets	One 300-mg tablet once daily, with or without food	Nausea, vomiting, diarrhea, flatulence, and kidney problems. Use cautiously with drugs that reduce renal function.	Box warning for severe hepatomegaly with steatosis and lactic acidosis. Monitor hepatic function closely when discontinued in patients with hepatitis B comorbidity. Adjust dose in renal dysfunction.

Continued

HIV Medications—cont'd

Name and Dosage Forms	Dose	Side Effects/Drug Interactions	Notes
Zalcitabine (ddC) (Hivid) 0.375- and 0.75-mg tablets	0.75-mg every 8 hr in combination with other antiretrovirals. Reduce with impaired renal function.	Headache, nausea and vomiting, abdominal pain, fever, fatigue, hematologic toxicities. ***Drug interactions:*** amphotericin B antacids, cimetidine, doxorubicin, probenecid, other antiretrovirals, or drugs that may cause peripheral neuropathy or pancreatitis.	Box warning for peripheral neuropathy and pancreatitis as well as hepatomegaly with steatosis and lactic acidosis. Rare cases of liver failure with zalcitabine and hepatitis B. Use in combination with didanosine not recommended.
Zidovudine (AZT) (Retrovir) 10-mg/mL IV solution, 100-mg capsules, 300-mg tablets, 50-mg/5-mL oral solution	300 mg twice daily. Take without regard to meals, reduce dose in severe renal or hepatic insufficiency. See monograph for complete dosing and other information.	Constipation, loss of appetite, nausea, vomiting, asthenia, headache, insomnia, malaise, lactic acidosis, anemia, neutropenia, hepatomegaly, steatosis of liver, myopathy. Interactions with ganciclovir, dapsone, pyrazinamide, others.	***Box warning:*** zidovudine has been associated with hematologic toxicity, including neutropenia and severe anemia, particularly in patients with advanced HIV disease. Prolonged use of zidovudine has been associated with symptomatic myopathy. Lactic acidosis and severe hepatomegaly with steatosis, including fatal cases, have been reported with the use of nucleoside analogues alone or in combination, including zidovudine and other antiretrovirals.
Non-Nucleoside Reverse Transcriptase Inhibitors (NNRTIs)			
Delavirdine (Rescriptor) 100- and 200-mg tablets	400 mg three times daily in combination with other antiretroviral agents.	Rash, increased liver enzymes, nausea and vomiting, and headaches. Increases blood levels of all available PIs; doses may need to be reduced. Can increase levels of cisapride, benzodiazepines, rifabutin, clarithromycin, dapsone, calcium channel blockers such as nifedipine, ergot derivatives, quinidine, and sildenafil as well. Do not take buffered Videx (didanosine) tablets or anything containing an antacid within 1 hr of a dose of delavirdine.	May take without regard to food. Patients with achlorhydria should take with an acidic beverage.

Efavirenz (Sustiva) 50-, 100-, 200-mg capsules or 600-mg tablets	600 mg once daily. For combination use.	Rash; central nervous system symptoms, such as drowsiness, insomnia, confusion, inability to concentrate, dizziness, and vivid dreams; increased liver enzymes; false-positive drug testing (marijuana); and birth defects if taken during pregnancy. Contraindicated: ergot, midazolam, triazolam, and cisapride. Induces CYP3A4, thereby reducing levels of drugs metabolized by this pathway, including PIs.	It is recommended that efavirenz be taken on an empty stomach. Dose should be taken at bedtime to minimize dizziness, drowsiness and impaired concentration. Avoid alcohol.
Nevirapine (Viramune) 200-mg tablets or 50-mg/5-mL oral suspension	One 200 mg tablet per day for 14 days, then one 200 mg tablet, twice daily. Used in combination with other antiretrovirals.	Nevirapine induces CYP3A4 enzyme system; reducing levels of oral contraceptives, clarithromycin, efavirenz, ketoconazole, methadone, and PIs warfarin and zidovudine. Numerous other potential drug interactions exist via this mechanism. Side effects include rash, somnolence, arthralgias and hematologic disorders; see box warning.	***Box warning:*** severe life-threatening liver failure, especially in women with CD4 counts greater than 250. Severe, sometimes fatal skin reactions/rash (especially in the first 6 wk). Monitor patients closely for these for the first 18 wk of therapy.
Fusion Inhibitors (inhibit fusion of HIV and CD4+ cells)			
Enfuvirtide (Fuzeon) Powder for subcutaneous injection 108 mg, or about 90 mg/mL when reconstituted	90 mg subcutaneously twice daily into upper arm, anterior thigh, or abdomen. For use with other antiretrovirals in patients showing HIV replication despite ongoing antiretroviral therapy.	Skin reactions at the injection site are common and can include itching, swelling, redness, pain or tenderness, hardened skin, or bumps. Increased risk of bacterial pneumonia; serious allergic reaction (rare).	More information is available at www.fuzeon.com or 1-877-4fuzeon.
Combination Products			
Lamivudine 150 mg and zidovudine 300 mg (Combivir)			
Abacavir 300 mg, lamivudine 150 mg, zidovudine 300 mg (Trizivir)			
Emtricitabine 200 mg and tenofovir disoproxil fumarate 300 mg (Truvada)			
Abacavir 600 mg and lamivudine 300 mg (Epzicom)			
Efavirenz 600 mg, emtricitabine 200 mg and tenofovir disoproxil fumarate 300 mg (Atripla)			

*Fosamprenavir has largely replaced **amprenavir,** its active metabolite, which is still available under the brand name **Agenerase.**

IMMUNOLOGICS

Uses

Suppression of immune system responses, resulting in reduction of inflammation, improvement in inflammation-related disease states, and improved survival of both short- and long-term allografts.

Actions

Adalimumab: Binds specifically to tumor necrosis factor (TNF)-alpha and blocks its interaction with the p55 and p75 cell surface TNF receptors. It will also lyse surface TNF-expressing cells in vitro in the presence of complement. It will not bind or inactiviate TNF-alpha.

Alefacept: Interferes with lymphocyte activation by specifically binding to the lymphocyte antigen, CD2, and inhibiting LFA-3/CD2 interaction. Also causes a reduction in subsets of CD2+ T lymphocytes, resulting in a reduction in circulating total CD4+ and CD8+ T lymphocyte counts.

Anakinra: Competitively inhibits IL-1 from binding to the interleukin-1 type I receptor (IL-1RI).

Azathioprine: Antagonizes purine metabolism and may inhibit synthesis of DNA, RNA, and proteins; may also interfere with cellular metabolism and inhibit mitosis.

Basiliximab: An interleukin-2 (IL-2) receptor antagonist inhibiting IL-2 binding; this prevents activation of lymphocytes and the response of the immune system to antigens is impaired.

Cyclosporine: Inhibits production and release of IL-2.

Daclizumab: An IL-2 receptor antagonist inhibiting IL-2 binding.

Efalizumab: Binds to CD11a, the alpha subunit of leukocyte function antigen-1 (LFA-1), which inhibits the binding of LFA-1 to intercellular adhesion molecule-1 (ICAM-1), thereby inhibiting the adhesion of leukocytes to other cell types.

Etanercept: Specifically binds TNF-alpha and TNF-beta receptors.

Glatiramer: Believed to modify immune processes or functions which are thought to be liable for multiple sclerosis pathogenesis.

Interferon alfa-2a: Has antiproliferative action against tumor cells, inhibits virus replication, and modulates host immune response.

Interferon alfa-2b: Secretes proteins in response to viral infection through binding at specific membrane receptors on the cell surface. Binding results in induction of certain enzymes, suppression of cell proliferation, enhancement of the phagocytic activity of macrophages, augmentation of specific cytotoxicity of lymphocytes for target cells, and inhibition of virus replication in virus-infected cells.

Interferon alfa-n3: Induces protein synthesis by binding to specific membrane receptors, which leads to inhibition of virus replication and suppression of cell proliferation.

Interferon alfacon-1: Possesses antiviral, antiproliferative, and immunomodulatory activities.

Interferon beta 1a: Binds to specific receptors on the surface of human cells, which initiates a complex cascade of intracellular events that leads to the expression of numerous interferon-induced gene products and markers that mediate antiviral, antiproliferative, and immunomodulatory activities in response to viral infection and other biologic inducers.

Interferon beta-1b: Exerts its effects through its interactions with specific cell receptors found on the surface of human cells, which induces the expression of a number of interferon-induced gene products that mediate antiviral, antiproliferative, and immunomodulatory activities in response to viral infection and other biologic inducers.

Interferon gamma-1b: Stimulates natural killer (NK) cells, improves oxidative metabolism of macrophages, creates antibody dependent cellular cytotoxicity (ADCC), and causes the expression of major histocompatibility antigens and Fc receptors.

Lymphocyte immune globulin, antithymocyte globulin: May involve elimination of antigen-reactive T lymphocytes (killer cells) in peripheral blood or alteration of T-cell function.

Muromonab CD3: Reacts with a T3 (CD3) molecule that is linked to an antigen receptor on the surface membrane of human T lymphocytes and thereby blocks both the generation and function of the T cells in response to antigenic challenge.

Mycophenolate: A prodrug that reversibly binds and inhibits inosine monophosphate dehydrogenase (IMPD), resulting in inhibition of purine nucleotide synthesis, inhibiting DNA and RNA synthesis and subsequent synthesis of T and B cells.

Peginterferon alfa-2a: Binds to specific receptors on the cell surface and initiates intracellular signalling via a complex cascade of protein-protein interactions, leading to rapid activation of gene transcription. Its effects include inhibition of viral replication in infected cells, inhibition of cell proliferation, and immunomodulation

Peginterferon alfa-2b: Binds to specific membrane receptors on the cell surface, which raises concentrations of effector proteins, raises body temperature, and causes reversible decreases in leukocyte and platelet counts.

Sirolimus: Inhibits IL-2-stimulated T-lymphocyte activation and proliferation, which may occur through formation of a complex.

Tacrolimus: Inhibits IL-2-stimulated T-lymphocyte activation and proliferation, which may occur through formation of a complex.

Thalidomide: Its effects are thought to cause disruption of neural crest development, inhibition of angiogenesis, and down-regulation of adhesion receptors on early limb-bud cells and on cells of the heart in embryos.

Immunologics

Name	Availability	Dosage	Side Effects/Comments
Adalimumab (Humira)	I: 40 mg/0.8 mL	RA, psoriatic arthritis, AS: 40 mg subcutaneously every other wk Maintenance: 40 mg subcutaneously every other wk beginning wk 4	Warning: Hepatitis B reactivation, tuberculosis, invasive fungal infections, and other opportunistic infections have been observed. Hypertension, injection site reaction, rash, antibody development to adalimumab, antinuclear antibody positive, headache
Alefacept (Amevive)	I: 15 mg/0.5 mL (IM), 7.5 mg/0.5 mL (IV)	Psoriasis: 15 mg every wk IM × 12 wk or 7.5 mg IV bolus every wk × 12 wk. May repeat course after 12 wk.	Serious: Liver damage, malignancies, opportunistic infection Other: Injection site reaction (IM), pain, inflammation, bleeding, pruritus, shivering, nausea, myalgia, dizziness, pharyngitis, lymphocytopenia
Anakinra (Kineret)	I: 100 mg/0.67 mL	RA: 100 mg subcutaneously daily	Injection site reaction, infection, headaches

Continued

Immunologics—cont'd

Name	Availability	Dosage	Side Effects/Comments
Antithymocyte globulin (rabbit) (Thymoglobulin)	I: 25 mg	Acute renal TP rejection: 1.5 mg/kg/day times 7 days over 6 hr. May give another 7 days if indicated.	Thrombocytopenia, leukopenia, infection, secondary malignancy Fever/chills, headache, hypertension, abdominal pain
Azathioprine (Imuran)	T: 25, 50, 75, 100 mg I: 100-mg/vial	TP initial: 3-5 mg/kg/day Maintenance: 1-2 mg/kg/day Also used in RA, severe recurrent aphthous stomatitis, Crohn's disease, and ulcerative colitis.	Warning: Increased risk of neoplasia, serious infections, hematologic disorders (leukopenia, thrombocytopenia, anemia) Nausea, vomiting, diarrhea, rash, fever, malaise, myalgias Use with caution in patients with liver disease, renal impairment; monitor hematologic function closely
Basiliximab (Simulect)	I: 20 mg	TP: 20 mg for 2 doses post transplant on days 0 (2 hr prior to surgery) and 4. Avoid reexposure to drug.	Abdominal pain, asthenia, cough, dizziness, dyspnea, dysuria, edema, hypertension, infection, tremors, headache, opportunistic infections
Cyclosporine (Neoral, Sandimmune)	C: 25, 50, 100 mg S: 100 mg/mL I: 50 mg/mL	TP: 7-10 mg/kg/day. Also used for Crohn's disease, ulcerative colitis, psoriasis, and RA at lower doses.	Hypertension, hyperkalemia, nephrotoxicity, coarsening of facial features, hirsutism, gingival hyperplasia, nausea, vomiting, diarrhea, hepatic toxicity, hyperuricemia, hypertriglycerides/cholesterol, tremors, paresthesia, seizures, risk of infection/malignancy Note: Different brands are NOT interchangeable; has many important drug interactions
Daclizumab (Zenapax)	I: 25 mg/5 mL	TP: 1 mg/kg (max: 100 mg) on transplant day 0, then every 2 wk × 4 more doses. Also used in graft versus host disease.	Dyspnea, fever, hypertension, nausea, peripheral edema, tachycardia, tremors, vomiting, weakness, wound infection
Efalizumab (Raptiva)	I: 125 mg	Psoriasis: 0.7 mg/kg once subcutaneously Maintenance: 1 mg/kg/wk subcutaneously (do not exceed 200 mg)	Acne, leukocytosis, lymphocytosis, back pain, headache, influenza-like illness or symptoms, infectious gastroenteritis, infectious disease, arthritis, nausea, first dose reaction
Etanercept (Enbrel)	I: 25 mg, 50 mg/0.5 mL	RA, AS, and psoriatic arthritis: 50 mg subcutaneously every wk, or two 25 mg doses on the same day or 3-4 days apart Plaque psoriasis: Initial: 50 mg subcutaneously twice weekly for 3 mo Maintenance: 50 mg every wk	Neutropenia, pancytopenia, thrombocytopenia, abdominal pain, vomiting, demyelinating disease of central nervous system, cough, rhinitis, upper respiratory infection, anemia, aplastic anemia, leukopenia Use with caution in hepatic failure; do not use with active infections
Glatiramer (Copaxone)	I: 20 mg	Multiple sclerosis: 20 mg subcutaneously every day	Transient chest pain, palpitations, vasodilatation, facial edema, injection site reaction, pain, edema, nausea, arthralgia, increased muscle tone, asthenia, tremor, anxiety, hypertension, transient raised eosinophil, lymphadenopathy, transient dyspnea

Interferon alfa-2a (Roferon-A)	I: 9 million units, 6 million units, 3 million units	Chronic hepatitis C: 3 million units 3 times weekly × 12 mo Hairy cell leukemia: 3 million units daily × 16-24 wk then 3 million units 3 times per wk for up to 6-24 mo AIDS-related Kaposi's sarcoma: 36 million units daily × 10-12 wk, then 36 million units 3 times per wk pH-positive chronic myelogenous leukemia in chronic phase: 9 million units daily	Warning: Alpha interferons, including interferon alfa-2a, recombinant, cause or aggravate fatal or life-threatening neuropsychiatric, autoimmune, ischemic, and infectious disorders. Injection site reaction, diarrhea, loss of appetite, nausea, vomiting, altered mental status, dizziness, headache, memory impairment, depression, fever, chills, fatigue, myalgia, thrombocytopenia, increased liver enzymes, autoimmune disease, vasculitis, Raynaud's phenomenon, rheumatoid arthritis, lupus
Interferon alfa-2b (Intron A)	I: 3, 5, 6, 10, 18, 25, 50 million units	AIDS-related Kaposi's sarcoma: 30 million units/m^2 IM/subcutaneous 3 times per wk Condyloma acuminatum, when external surfaces of the genital and perianal areas are involved: 1 million units intralesionally 3 times per wk on alternate days for 3 wk; up to 5 lesions at one time Follicular lymphoma: Initial treatment in conjunction with anthracycline-containing combination chemotherapy: 5 million units subcutaneously 3 times per wk for up to 18 mo Hairy cell leukemia: 2 million units/m^2 IM/subcutaneous 3 times per wk for up to 6 mo Hepatitis C, chronic, in patients with compensated liver disease: 3 million units IM/subcutaneous 3 times per wk for 18-24 mo Malignant melanoma: (adjuvant): Initial: 20 million units/m^2 IV 5 days per wk for 4 wk Maintenance: 10 million units/m^2 subcutaneously 3 times per wk for 48 wk Renal cell carcinoma: 5-20 million units/day Type B viral hepatitis, chronic, in patients with compensated liver disease: 5 million units IM/subcutaneous daily, OR 10 million units IM/subcutaneous 3 times per wk for 16 wk	Warning: Alpha interferons, including interferon alfa-2b, cause or aggravate fatal or life-threatening neuropsychiatric, autoimmune, ischemic, and infectious disorders. Patients should be monitored closely with periodic clinical and laboratory evaluations. In many, but not all, cases these disorders resolve after stopping interferon alfa-2b therapy. Loss of appetite, nausea, vomiting, sarcoidosis, depression, fever, chills, headache, fatigue, myalgia, pancreatitis, neutropenia, thrombocytopenia, hepatotoxicity, increased liver enzymes, cotton wool spot, nephrotic syndrome, renal failure, pneumonia

Continued

Immunologics—cont'd

Name	Availability	Dosage	Side Effects/Comments
Interferon alfa-n3 (Alferon-N)	I: 5 million units/mL	Condylomata acuminata: 0.05 mL (250,000 units)/wart twice weekly for up to 8 wk; max: 0.5 mL/treatment session. Must wait at least 3 mo before repeating.	Pruritus, diarrhea, loss of appetite, nausea, vomiting, dizziness, influenza-like illness, myalgias, fever, headache, neutropenia, thrombocytopenia
Interferon alfacon-1 (Infergen)	I: 30 mcg/mL	9 mcg subcutaneously 3 times weekly for 24 wk, at least 48 hr between injections. Relapse or non-responders: 15 mcg subcutaneously 3 times per wk for 6 mo	Warning: Alpha interferons, including interferon alfacon-1, cause or aggravate fatal or life-threatening neuropsychiatric, autoimmune, ischemic, and infectious disorders. Use with caution in autoimmune disorders and in patients with myelosuppression. Diarrhea, loss of appetite, nausea, mild to moderate depression, influenza-like illness, headache, fatigue, fever, myalgia, rigors, hypertension, palpitations, tachydysrhythmia, disorder of thyroid gland
Interferon beta-1a (Avonex, Rebif)	I: (Avonex) 30 mcg/0.5 mL; (Rebif) 8.8 mcg/0.2 mL, 22 mcg/0.5 mL, 44 mcg/ 0.5 mL	Multiple sclerosis (Avonex): 30 mcg every wk IM (Rebif): titrate up to 22 or 44 mcg 3 times per wk subcutaneously	Headache, influenza-like illness, fever, chills, myalgia, anemia, leukopenia, thrombocytopenia, increased liver enzymes, injury of liver, seizure, psychiatric events Caution in hepatic patients, preexisting cardiovascular disease, pulmonary disease, seizure disorders, myelosuppression, or renal impairment Flu-like adverse effects are common; may want to use antipyretics/analgesics with administration
Interferon beta-1b (Betaseron)	I: 0.3 mg	Multiple sclerosis (relapsing-remitting): Initial: 0.0625 mg subcutaneously every other day, increase by 25% every 1 to 2 wk Maintenance: 0.25 mg subcutaneously every other day	Injection site pain, skin reaction, sweating symptom, myasthenia, lymphopenia, headache, influenza-like illness, fever, chills, myalgia, flu-like syndrome, injection site reactions, psychiatric disturbances. Cautions same as for interferon beta 1b.
Interferon gamma-1b (Actimmune)	I: 2 million units (100 mcg)/0.5 mL	Chronic granulomatous disease or severe, malignant osteoporosis C: greater than 1 yr: (subcutaneous) BSA per greater than 0.5 m^2: 50 mcg/m^2 (1 million units/m^2) 3 times per wk; BSA less than or equal to 0.5 m^2: 1.5 mcg/kg/dose 3 times per wk	Injection site pain, rash, nausea, vomiting, arthralgia, myalgia, headache, fatigue, fever, influenza-like illness, leukopenia, thrombocytopenia Patients with preexisting cardiac disease, seizure disorders, CNS disturbances, or myelosuppression should be carefully monitored.

Lymphocyte immune globulin, antithymocyte globulin (equine) (Atgam)	I: 50 mg/mL	15 mg/kg/day over 4 hr × 14 days, then every other day × 14 days for acute renal allograft rejection Aplastic anemia protocol: (IV) 10-20 mg/kg/day for 8-14 days, then give every other day for 7 more doses for a total of 21 doses in 28 days Premedication with diphenhydramine, hydrocortisone, and is recommended prior to first dose	Skin test to determine if allergic Phlebitis/thrombosis can occur; use a central line Fever, chills, dermatologic reactions, thrombocytopenia, arthralgias, chest/back pain
Muromonab CD3 (OKT3)	I: 5 mg/5 mL	A: Treatment of acute allograft rejection or acute graft-versus-host disease: 5 mg/day IV for 10-14 days for acute rejection. Premedicating with methylprednisolone recommended	Anaphylaxis, pulmonary edema, shock, arrest, seizures, cytokine release syndrome, fever, headache, pyrexia, chills, tachycardia, diarrhea, nausea and vomiting
Mycophenolate (CellCept, Myfortic)	C: 250 mg T: 500 mg T (DR): 180, 360 mg I: 500 mg S: 200 mg/mL	Renal TP: 1 g 2 times/day PO or IV Myfortic: (oral) 720 mg twice daily (1440 mg/day) Cardiac TP: 1.5 g twice daily IV or PO Hepatic TP: 1.5 g twice daily PO, 1 g twice daily IV Myasthenia gravis (unlabeled use): Oral (CellCept): 1 g twice daily (range 1-3 g/day) Pediatric dosing available Adjust in renal dysfunction	Diarrhea, vomiting, leukopenia, neutropenia, hypertension hypotension, peripheral edema, edema, tachycardia, pain, headache, insomnia, fever, dizziness, anxiety, rash, hyperglycemia, hypercholesterolemia, hypokalemia, hypocalcemia, hypomagnesemia, hyperkalemia, abdominal pain, nausea, anorexia, hypochromic anemia, thrombocytopenia, liver function tests abnormal, ascites, back pain, weakness, tremor, paresthesia, dyspnea, respiratory tract infection, cough, lung disorder
Peginterferon alfa-2a (Pegasys)	I: 180 mcg/mL, 180 mcg/ 0.5 mL	Chronic hepatitis C (monoinfection or coinfection with HIV): Subcutaneous: (monotherapy) 180 mcg once weekly for 48 wk; (combination therapy with ribavirin) recommended dosage 180 mcg once per wk with ribavirin (Copegus) Duration of therapy: Monoinfection (based on genotype): Genotype 1,4: 48 wk; genotype 2,3: 24 wk Duration of therapy: Coinfection: 48 wk Chronic hepatitis B: Subcutaneous: 180 mcg once weekly for 48 wk	Warning: Alpha interferons, including peginterferon alfa-2a, may cause or aggravate fatal or life-threatening neuropsychiatric, autoimmune, ischemic, and infectious disorders. Patients should be monitored closely with periodic clinical and laboratory evaluations. Therapy should be withdrawn in patients with persistently severe or worsening signs or symptoms of these conditions. In many, but not all cases, these disorders resolve after stopping peginterferon alfa-2a therapy. Injection site reaction, disorder of eye region, influenza-like illness, colitis, pancreatitis, autoimmune thrombocytopenia, myelosuppression, headache, fatigue, pyrexia, insomnia, depression, dizziness, irritability/anxiety/nervousness, alopecia, pruritus, dermatitis, nausea/vomiting, abnormal liver function tests, weakness, myalgia, rigors, arthralgia

Continued

Immunologics—cont'd

Name	Availability	Dosage	Side Effects/Comments
Peginterferon alfa-2b (Peg-Intron, Peg Intron RP)	I: 50 mcg, 80 mcg, 120 mcg, 150 mcg	Chronic hepatitis C: (monotherapy) 1 mcg/kg/wk subcutaneous for 1 yr; (combination therapy) 1.5 mcg/kg/wk subcutaneous for 1 yr with ribavirin 800 mg/day Do not use with creatinine clearances of less than 50 mL/min	Warning: Alpha interferons, including peginterferon alfa-2b, may cause or aggravate fatal or life-threatening neuropsychiatric, autoimmune, ischemic, and infectious disorders. Patients should be monitored closely with periodic clinical and laboratory evaluations. In many, but not all, cases these disorders resolve after stopping peginterferon alfa-2b therapy. Adverse reactions similar to peginterferon alfa-2a without as frequent an incidence of LFT abnormalities
Sirolimus (Rapamune)	S: 1 mg/mL T: 1, 2 mg	TP: 2-10 mg/day Dosages of approximately ⅓ the usual should be used in hepatic impairment with extra monitoring	Dyspnea, leukopenia, thrombocytopenia, hyperlipidemia, abdominal pain, acne, arthralgia, fever, diarrhea, constipation, headaches, vomiting, weight gain Hemolytic uremic syndrome/thrombotic microangiopathy has been reported with the combination cyclosporine/sirolimus immunosuppressive regimen
Tacrolimus (Prograf)	C: 0.5, 1, 5 mg I: 5 mg/mL	TP: PO: 0.075-0.2 mg/kg/day (IV dose is approximately ⅓ of oral dose, given as a continuous infusion) Monitor closely in renal and hepatic impairment: dosage adjustments may be needed.	Nephrotoxicity, neurotoxicity, hyperglycemia, photophobia, infections, hypertension, hyperlipidemia, chest pain, hypertension, pericardial effusion (heart transplant), dizziness, headache, insomnia, tremor (headache and tremor are associated with high whole blood concentrations and may respond to decreased dosage), pruritus, rash, diabetes mellitus, hyperglycemia, hyper-/hypokalemia, hyperlipemia, hypomagnesemia, hypophosphatemia, abdominal pain, constipation, diarrhea, dyspepsia, nausea, vomiting, anemia, leukocytosis, leukopenia, thrombocytopenia, ascites, arthralgia, back pain, paresthesia, tremor, weakness, abnormal kidney function, increased BUN, increased creatinine, oliguria, atelectasis, bronchitis, dyspnea, increased cough, pleural effusion
Thalidomide (Thalomid)	C: 50, 100, 200 mg	Aphthous ulceration: HIV infection: ulcer of esophagus: 200 mg orally once daily at bedtime Behet's syndrome: Doses range from 50 mg to 400 mg orally daily	Warning: Severe, life-threatening human birth defects: If thalidomide is taken during pregnancy, it can cause severe birth defects or death to a fetus. Thalidomide should never be used by women who are pregnant or who could become

	Cachexia associated with AIDS: 100 mg orally every 6 hr Erythema nodosum leprosum: Initial, 100-300 mg orally once daily at bedtime; max. 400 mg/day (may be given in divided doses) Erythema nodosum leprosum; Prophylaxis: Minimum dose necessary should be used to control erythema nodosum leprosum (ENL); attempt to taper every 3-6 mo in decrements of 50 mg every 2 to 4 wk Multiple myeloma: 200 mg once daily (with dexamethasone 40 mg daily on days 1-4, 9-12, and 17-20 of a 28-day treatment cycle) Graft versus host reactions: (oral) 100-1600 mg/day; usual initial dose: 200 mg 4 times a day for use up to 700 days	pregnant while taking the drug. Even a single dose (one 50, 100, or 200 mg capsule) taken by a pregnant woman can cause severe birth defects. Because of this toxicity and in an effort to make the chance of fetal exposure to thalidomide as negligible as possible, thalidomide is approved for marketing only under a special restricted distribution program approved by the Food and Drug Administration (FDA). This program is called the System for Thalidomide Education and Prescribing Safety (S.T.E.P.S.). Under this restricted distribution program, only prescribers and pharmacists registered with the program are allowed to prescribe and dispense the product. In addition, patients must be advised of, agree to, and comply with the requirements of the S.T.E.P.S. program in order to receive the product Other side effects/adverse drug reactions: edema, thrombosis/embolism, hypotension, fatigue, somnolence, dizziness, sensory neuropathy, confusion, anxiety/agitation, fever, motor neuropathy, headache, rash, dry skin, acne, hypocalcemia, constipation, anorexia, nausea, weight loss, weight gain, diarrhea, oral moniliasis, leukopenia, neutropenia, anemia, lymphadenopathy, hepatic impairment, muscle weakness, tremor, weakness, myalgias, paresthesia, arthralgia, hematuria, dyspnea, diaphoresis

A, adults; AS, ankylosing spondylitis; C, capsules; C (dosage) children; DR, delayed release; I, injection; RA, rheumatoid arthritis; S, oral solution or suspension; T, tablets; TP, transplant

NSAIDS AND COX-2 INHIBITORS

Uses

Provide symptomatic relief from pain/inflammation in the treatment of musculoskeletal disorders (e.g., rheumatoid arthritis, osteoarthritis, ankylosing spondylitis), analgesic for low to moderate pain, reduction in fever (many agents not suited for routine/prolonged therapy due to toxicity). By virtue of its action on platelet function, aspirin is used in treatment or prophylaxis of diseases associated with hypercoagulability (reduces risk of stroke/heart attack).

Action

Exact mechanism for antiinflammatory, analgesic, antipyretic effects unknown. Inhibition of enzyme cyclo-oxygenase, the enzyme responsible for prostaglandin synthesis, appears to be a major mechanism of action. May inhibit other mediators of inflammation (e.g., leukotrienes). Direct action on hypothalamus heat-regulating center may contribute to antipyretic effect.

Box Warning

NSAIDs

These agents may increase the risk of cardiovascular (CV) events, including MI and stroke. The risk increases with duration of use and in patients with CV disease or other risk factors. These agents are contraindicated for treatment of perioperative pain in coronary artery bypass graft surgery. These agents cause increased risk of gastrointestinal adverse effects, including bleeding, ulceration, and peforation of the stomach or intestines, especially in the elderly.

NSAIDs and Cox-2 Inhibitors*

Drug Name	Usual Adult Dose	Maximum Adult Daily Dose	Prescription Strength	Nonprescription Strength	Comments
Celecoxib (Celebrex)	Osteoarthritis: 100 mg twice daily or 200 mg once daily Rheumatoid arthritis: 100 to 200 mg twice daily Pain or dysmenorrhea: 400 mg (initial), 200 mg twice daily if needed	400 mg	C: 50, 100, 200, 400 mg	N/A	Decrease dose 50% in moderate liver impairment Note: COX-2 inhibitor
Diclofenac Potassium[†] (immediate release) (Cataflam)	50 mg twice daily-four times daily	200 mg	T: 50 mg	N/A	

Diclofenac Sodium[†] (delayed release, extended release) (Voltaren, Voltaren XR)	50 mg twice daily-four times daily; 75-100 mg twice daily; 100 mg daily (extended release)	225 mg	T (DR): 25, 50, 75 mg T (ER): 100 mg	N/A	
Diclofenac sodium/ misoprostol (Arthrotec)	50 mg (diclofenac) twice daily-three times daily	225 mg/day (diclofenac)	T: 50 mg diclofenac/ 200 mcg misoprostol T: 75 mg diclofenac/ 200 mcg misoprostol	N/A	Swallow tablets whole
Diclofenac Epolamine (Flector)	1 patch every 12 hr applied to painful area	180 mg	patch	N/A	Topical use only to intact skin
Etodolac[†] (Lodine, Lodine XL)	200-600 mg every 6-8 hr (maximum: 1200 mg/day)	1200 mg	T: 400, 500 mg C: 200, 300 mg T (ER): 400, 500, 600 mg	N/A	Antacids reduce peak concentration by 20%
Fenoprofen[†] (Nalfon)	200-600 mg every 6-8 hr	3200 mg	C: 200, 300 mg T: 600 mg	N/A	Highly protein-bound (to albumin); greater renal toxicity
Flurbiprofen[†] (Ansaid)	50-100 mg twice daily-four times daily	300 mg	T: 50, 100 mg	N/A	May cause CNS stimulation
Ibuprofen[†] (Motrin, Rufen; OTC: Advil, Nuprin, Motrin IB, Midol Cramp formula)	A: 400-800 mg every 6-8 hr C: 20-40 mg/kg/day for juvenile arthritis C (6-12 yr) for pain/fever: 5-10 mg/kg every 6-8 hr; max 40 mg/kg/day	3200 mg	T: 400, 600, 800 mg	T: 100, 200 mg T (chewable): 50, 100 mg C: 200 mg S: 100 mg/ 2.5 mL, 100 mg/ 5 mL D: 40 mg/mL	Also approved for primary dysmenorrhea; available in combination with hydrocodone (Vicoprofen)

Continued

NSAIDs and Cox-2 Inhibitors*—cont'd

Drug Name	Usual Adult Dose	Maximum Adult Daily Dose	Prescription Strength	Nonprescription Strength	Comments
Indomethacin[†] (Indocin, Indocin SR)	25-50 mg twice daily-three times daily or 75 mg once daily-twice daily (sustained release)	200 mg	C: 25, 50 mg C (SR): 75 mg S: 25 mg/ 5 mL RS: 50 mg	N/A	Do not crush the sustained-release form
Ketoprofen[†] (Orudis, Oruvail, Orudis KT)	50-75 mg every 6-8 hr	300 mg or 200 mg for sustained release	C: 50, 75 mg C (SR): 100, 150, 200 mg	12.5 mg (Orudis KT)	High rate of dyspepsia (11%)
Ketorolac tromethamine[†] (Toradol)	PO: 10 mg every 4-6 hr IM/IV: 30 or 60 mg initially, then 15-30 mg every 6 hr	PO: 40 mg IM/IV: 150 mg 1st day, then 120 mg daily; use no more than 5 days	T: 10 mg I: 15, 30 mg/ mL	N/A	Total duration of treatment should not exceed 5 days; 30 mg IM/IV equal to 6-12 mg morphine sulfate; oral form is indicated only as continuation of parenteral ketorolac, short-term; switch to another analgesic ASAP Reduce dose in elderly, renal, or patients who weigh less than 50 kg. Can cause peptic ulcers and GI bleeding. Contraindications: labor, delivery, and lactation; intrathecal or epidural administration. Contraindicated with other NSAIDs.
Meclofenamate sodium[†] (Meclomen)	50-100 mg every 6 hr	400 mg	C: 50, 100 mg	N/A	High rate of diarrhea (10%-33%); also indicated to treat excessive menstrual bleeding
Mefenamic acid (Ponstel)	500 mg, then 250 mg every 6 hr	1000 mg	C: 250 mg	N/A	Also approved for primary dysmenorrhea
Meloxicam (Mobic)	7.5-15 mg once daily	15 mg	T: 7.5, 15 mg OS: 7.5 mg/ 5 mL	N/A	"Preferential" COX-2 activity; less selective than others in the class
Nabumetone (Relafen)	500-750 mg twice daily; 1000-2000 mg daily	2000 mg	T: 500, 750 mg	N/A	High rate of diarrhea (14%); metabolized to active agent
Naproxen[†] (Naproxen, EC-Naprosyn)	250-500 mg every 8-12 hr, or 250 mg every 6-8 hr; or 1000 mg daily (delayed-release tablets)	1250 mg (first 24 hr then 1000 mg thereafter)	T: 250, 375, 500 mg T (DR): 375, 500 mg S: 125 mg/ 5 mL	N/A	Approved for acute gout; may increase effect of protein-bound drugs such as phenytoin, sulfonylureas, and warfarin; available in daily dosage form

Naproxen sodium† (Anaprox, Anaprox DS, Naprelan)	275-550 mg every 8-12 hr, or 1000 mg daily (controlled-release tablets)	1375 mg (first 24 hr then 1100 mg thereafter); 600 mg/day unless directed for OTC	T: 250, 500 mg T (CR): 375, 500 mg	T: 220 mg (Aleve)	Approved for acute gout; may increase effect of protein-bound drugs such as phenytoin, sulfonylureas, and warfarin
Naproxen/ Lansoprazole (Prevacid NapraPAC)	Naproxen 375-500 mg twice daily/Lansoprazole 15 mg daily	Naproxen 1000 mg/ Lansoprazole 15 mg	Naproxen 375 mg/ lansoprazole 15 mg; Naproxen 500 mg/ lansoprazole 15 mg	N/A	Provided on blister cards containing 2 naproxen tablets and 1 lansoprazole capsule
Oxaprozin (Daypro)	600-1200 mg daily	1800 mg	C/T: 600 mg	N/A	
Piroxicam† (Feldene)	10-20 mg daily	20 mg	C: 10, 20 mg	N/A	High rate of dyspepsia (20%); may increase effect of protein-bound drugs such as phenytoin, sulfonylureas, and warfarin; 7-12 days required for steady-state blood levels
Sulindac† (Clinoril)	150-200 mg every 12 hr	400 mg	T: 150, 200 mg	N/A	Approved for gout; less renal toxicity
Tolmetin† (Tolectin)	400 mg every 6-8 hr, 600 mg every 8 hr	1800 mg	T: 200, 600 mg C: 400 mg	N/A	High rate of nausea (11%)

*GI irritation is a common adverse effect that can occur with all NSAIDs, even the newer agents which have greater receptor selectivity. Taking these medications with food will reduce the likelihood of GI irritation, and is especially recommended for the older, non-cyclo-oxygenase-2 (COX-2) selective agents.

†Generic available for one or more dosage forms.

C, capsules; CR, controlled release; DR, delayed release; ER, extended release; I, injection; OS, oral suspension; RS, rectal suppository; S, suspension; SR, sustained release; T, tablets

OPIOID ANALGESICS

Uses

Relief of moderate to severe pain associated with surgical procedures, MI, burns, cancer, or other conditions. May be used as an adjunct to anesthesia, either as a preoperative medication or intraoperatively as a supplement to anesthesia. Also used for obstetric analgesia. Codeine and hydrocodone have an antitussive effect. Opium tinctures, such as paregoric, are used for severe diarrhea. Methadone relieves severe pain but is used primarily as part of heroin detoxification.

Action

Opioids refer to all drugs having actions similar to morphine and to receptors combining with these agents. Major effects are on the CNS (produce analgesia, drowsiness, mood changes, impaired concentration, analgesia without loss of consciousness, nausea and vomiting) and GI tract (decrease HCl secretion; diminish biliary, pancreatic, and intestinal secretions; diminish propulsive peristalsis). Also affects respiration (depressed) and cardiovascular system (peripheral vasodilation, decrease peripheral resistance, inhibit baroreceptor reflexes).

Opioid Analgesics

Names	Equianalgesic Dose	Analgesic Effect			Dosage Range
		Onset (min)	Peak (min)	Duration (hr)	
Alfentanil	—	Immediate	1.5-2	Less than 10 min	130-245 mcg/kg followed by 0.5-1.5 mcg/kg/min Anesthesia induction is primary use
Buprenorphine* (Buprenex)	I: 0.3 mg	IM: 15 IV: shortened	IM: 60 IV: shortened	IM: greater than 6	IM/IV: 0.3-0.6 every 6 hr (slow IV) Also comes as 2-, 8-mg sublingual tablets.
Butorphanol (Stadol)*	IM: 2 mg IV: —	IM: 10-30 IV: 2-3	IM: 30-60 IV: 30	IM: 3-4 IV: 2-4	IM: 1-4 mg every 3-4 hr IV: 0.5-2 mg every 3-4 hr Also comes as 10 mg/mL nasal spray
Codeine	IM: 120-130 mg PO: 180-200 mg	IM: 10-30 PO: 30-45 IV: 15	IM: 30-60 PO: 60-120	IM/PO: 4-6 IV: 5	IM/PO (A): 15-60 mg every 4-6 hr (C): 0.5 mg/kg every 4-6 hr
Fentanyl (Sublimaze)	IM: 0.1-0.2 mg IV: —	IM: 7-15 IV: 1-2	IM: 20-30 IV: 3-5	IM: 1-2 IV: 0.5-1	IV/IM: 50-100 mcg every 1-2 hr Also given transdermally and transmucosally
Hydrocodone	PO: 30 mg	10-30	30-60	4-6	5-10 mg every 4-6 hr Only available in combination products for pain and cough.

Hydromorphone (Dilaudid)	PO: 7.5 mg IM: 1.5 mg	PO: 30 IM: 15 IV: 10-15	PO: 90-120 IM: 30-60 IV: 15-30	PO: 4-5 IM: 4-5 IV: 4	PO: 1-4 mg every 3-6 hr IM: 1-4 mg every 3-6 hr IV: 0.5-1 mg every 3 hr R: 3 mg every 4-8 hr
Levorphanol (Levo-dromoran)	PO: 4 mg IM: 2 mg	PO: 10-60 IM: —	PO: 90-120 IM: 60	4-5	PO: 2-4 mg every 4 hr IM: 2-3 mg every 4 hr
Meperidine (Demerol)	PO: 300 mg IM/IV: 75 mg	PO: 15 IM: 10-15 IV: 1	PO: 60-90 IM: 30-60 IV: 5-7	2-4	PO, IM (A): 50-150 mg every 3-4 hr (C): 1-1.8 mg/kg every 3-4 hr
Methadone (Dolophine)	PO: 10-20 mg IM: 5-10 mg	PO: 30-60 IM: 10-20 IV: —	PO: 90-120 IM: 60-120 IV: 15-30	PO: 4-6 IM: 4-5 IV: 3-4	IM, PO: 2.5-10 mg every 3-4 hr
Morphine (Roxanol, MS Contin)	PO: 30 mg IM/IV: 10 mg	PO: 30-60 IM: 10-30 IV: —	PO: 90 IM: 30-60 IV: 20	PO: 4 IM/IV: 4-5	PO: 10-30 mg every 4 hr IM: 5-20 mg every 4 hr IV: 0.05-0.1 mg/kg every 4 hr
Nalbuphine* (Nubain)	IM: 10 mg IV: —	IM: 2-15 IV: 2-3	IM: 60 IV: 30	IM: 3-6 IV: 3-4	IM/IV: 10-20 mg every 3-6 hr
Oxycodone (Roxicodone)	PO: 20-30 mg	30	60	3-4	5-15 mg or 5 mL every 4-6 hr (ER): every 12 hr (dose titrated)
Oxymorphone	IM/IV: 1 mg PO: 10 mg	IM/IV: 5-10	—	IM/IV: 3-6	IV: 0.5 mg IM/Subcutaneous: 1-1.5 every 4-6 hr PO: 5-20 mg every 4-6 hr
Pentazocine* (Talwin)	30 mg	Subcutaneous/IM: 15-20 IV: 2-3	Subcutaneous/IM: 15-60 IV: —	Subcutaneous/IM: 4-6 IV: —	IM: 30-60 mg every 3-4 hr; max: 360 mg/day IV: 30 mg every 3-4 hr
Propoxyphene (Darvon)	PO: 65 mg	15-60	60-120	4-6	PO: 100 mg every 4-6 hr
Remifentanil (Ultiva)	—	Immediate	—	—	0.5-1 mcg/kg/min For anesthetic induction
Sufentanil (Sufenta)	—	IV: Immediate Epidural: 10	—	Epidural: 1.7	Epidural: 10-15 mcg Anesthesia induction: 1-8 mcg/kg if used for analgesia; 8-30 mcg/kg for anesthesia dosing

*Mixed opioid agonist-antagonist. They work primarily at the K-opioid receptor and antagonize the receptor. Therefore, they can precipitate withdrawal in patients who are dependant on morphine-like drugs.

A, adults; C, children; ER, extended release; I, injection; R, rectal

SALICYLATES*

Name	Usual Adult Dose	Maximum Adult Daily Dose	Prescription Strength	Nonprescription Strength	Comments
Aspirin† (Empirin, Ecotrin, Halprin, Easprin, Zorprin)	325-975 mg every 4-6 hr	4000 mg	T (EC): 975 mg T (SR): 800 mg	T: 325, 500 mg T (chewable): 81 mg T (gum): 227.5 mg T (EC): 81, 165, 325, 500, 650 mg T (SR): 81, 650 mg L: 870 mg/5 mL RS: 120, 200, 300, 600 mg	Antagonizes effect of probenecid; increases effect of sulfonylureas; reduces renal clearance of methotrexate; often combined with other prescription or nonprescription drugs
Aspirin, buffered† (Ascriptin, Bufferin, Arthritis Pain Formula)	325-975 mg of aspirin every 4-6 hr	4000 mg of aspirin	N/A	T: 325, 500 mg of aspirin with buffers CP: 325, 500 mg of aspirin with buffers T (coated): 325, 500 mg of aspirin with buffers T (E): 325, 500 mg of aspirin with buffers	Antagonizes effect of probenecid; increases effect of sulfonylureas; reduces renal clearance of methotrexate; buffers include aluminum hydroxide, calcium carbonate, magnesium carbonate, magnesium oxide, and magnesium hydroxide. Effervescent tablets contain an acid (e.g., citric acid) and a base (e.g., sodium bicarbonate)
Diflunisal† (also a salicylate) (Dolobid)	250-500 mg every 8-12 hr	1500 mg	T: 250, 500 mg	N/A	Not metabolized to salicylate; increases acetaminophen level by 50% when coadministered
Salsalate† (Salflex, Salsitab, Amigesic)	500-1000 mg every 8 hr, 750-1500 mg every 12 hr	3000 mg	T: 500, 750 mg C: 500 mg	N/A	Antagonizes effect of probenecid; increases effect of sulfonylureas; reduces renal clearance of methotrexate

Choline salicylate† (Arthropan)	870 mg every 3-4 hr	5220 mg; 6960 mg for rheumatoid arthritis	N/A	870 mg/5 mL	Antagonizes effect of probenecid; increases effect of sulfonylureas; reduces renal clearance of methotrexate
Magnesium salicylate† (Magan, Mobidin, Extra Strength Doan's, Momentum Backache)	650 mg every 4 hr or 1090 mg three times daily	4800 mg	T: 545, 600 mg	CP: 467, 500, 580 mg	Sodium-free; possible magnesium toxicity in renal failure
Sodium salicylate†	325-650 mg every 4 hr	3900 mg	N/A	T (EC): 325, 650 mg	Contains 6.25 mEq sodium per gram
Sodium thiosalicylate† (Rexolate)	100 mg/day IM; varies depending on indication	900 mg	I: 50 mg/mL	N/A	IM route is preferred

*GI irritation is a common adverse effect that can occur with all NSAIDs, even the newer agents which have greater receptor selectivity. Taking these medications with food will reduce the likelihood of GI irritation, and is especially recommended for the older, non-cyclo-oxygenase-2 (COX-2) selective agents.

†Generic available for one or more dosage forms.

C, capsule; CP, caplet; E, effervescent; EC, enteric-coated; I, injection; L, liquid; RS, rectal suppository; SR, slow release; T, tablets

TRIPTANS (VASCULAR SEROTONIN AGONISTS)*

Uses
Treatment of migraine and cluster headaches with or without aura in adults 18 yr and older.

Action
Triptans are selective, agonists of the serotonin (5-HT) receptor that inhibit neuropeptide release and vasodilation, causing vasoconstriction.

Generic Name	Brand Name	Adult Dose	Available Dosage Forms	Response Rate (% of patients reporting improvement)	Comments
Almotriptan maleate	Axert	Initially 6.25 or 12.5 mg. May repeat in 2 hr. No more than 2 doses per 24 hr	T: 6.25, 12.5 mg	55%-65% after 2 hr	
Eletriptan hydrochloride	Relpax	Initially 20-40 mg. May repeat in 2 hr. No more than 80 mg/24 hr	T: 20, 40 mg	47%-54% after 2 hr	
Frovatriptan succinate	Frova	Initially 2.5 mg. May repeat in 2 hr. No more than 7.5 mg/24 hr	T: 2.5 mg	37%-46% after 2 hr	
Naratriptan hydrochloride	Amerge	Initially 1 or 2.5 mg. May repeat in 4 hr. No more than 5 mg/24 hr	T: 1, 2.5 mg	50%-66% after 4 hr	Initial dose of 2.5 mg is more effective than 1 mg
Rizatriptan benzoate	Maxalt, Maxalt-MLT	Initially 5 or 10 mg. May repeat in 2 hr. No more than 30 mg/24 hr	T: 5, 10 mg T (OD): 5, 10 mg	60%-77% after 2 hr	
Sumatriptan succinate	Imitrex	Oral: 25-100 mg. May repeat in 2 hr. No more than 200 mg/24 hr Subcutaneous: 6 mg. May repeat in 1 hr. No more than 2 injections per 24 hr Intranasal: 5 to 20 mg. May repeat in 2 hr. No more than 40 mg/24 hr	T: 25, 50, 100 mg Spray (nasal): 5, 20 mg I: 6 mg/ 0.5 mL	T: 52%-62% after 2 hr Spray (nasal): 45%-64% after 2 hr I: 15%-63% after 30 min; 21%-83% after 2 hr	First injection should be given under medical supervision. Needle penetrates ¼ inch (5-6 mm). Give into areas with sufficient subcutaneous tissue.

Zolmitriptan	Zomig, Zomig ZMT	Initially 2.5 mg. May repeat in 2 hr. No more than 10 mg/24 hr	T: 2.5, 5 mg; T (OD): 2.5 mg Spray (nasal): 5 mg	27%-67% after 2 hr

*Triptans are contraindicated in coronary, cerebral, or peripheral vascular disease; uncontrolled hypertension; and concurrent (within 2 wk) use of an MAOI inhibitor or another triptan or ergotamine-containing preparation within 24 hr. Side effects include drowsiness, dizziness, fatigue, and nausea. Atypical sensations, hot flashes, and pain have also been reported. Medication overuse headache is an increased frequency of migraines associated with greater than 6 mo of continuous therapy, and the recommended treatment is withdrawal of the drug.

References:

1. Ellsworth, Allan J et al. *Mosby's Medical Drug Reference.* Mosby, St. Louis, 2003.
2. Website: *U.S. Food and Drug Administration.* Online. Internet. 2003. Available: http://www.fda.gov/cder
3. Micromedex.com

I, injection; OD, orally disintegrating; T, tablets

INDEX

Entries can be identified as followed: generic name, Trade Name, DRUG CATEGORY, *Combination Product*

A

B

C

E

F

G

H

I

J

K

L

M

N

O

P

Q

R

S

T

U

V

W

X

Y

Z

(FIGURE No. 1)

DIRECTIONS:

TARGET BG 90-140 (1 ml = 1 unit)

Columnar Insulin Dosing Chart*

Start infusion using the drip rate (ml/hr) in **COLUMN No.2** for the current Blood Glucose Tier	**Blood Glucose Tiers** (mg/dl)	column **1** (ml/hr)	column **2** (ml/hr)	column **3** (ml/hr)	column **4** (ml/hr)	column **5** (ml/hr)	column **6** (ml/hr)	column **7** (ml/hr)	column **8** (ml/hr)	column **9** (ml/hr)	column **10** (ml/hr)	column **11** (ml/hr)	column **12** (ml/hr)	column **13** (ml/hr)	column **14** (ml/hr)	column **15** (ml/hr)	column **16** (ml/hr)
To determine the new drip rate, compare the current BG Tier to the previous BG Tier. If current BG Tier is lower than the previous BG Tier, **STAY IN THE SAME COLUMN** If current BG Tier has not dropped **MOVE 1 COLUMN TO THE RIGHT** *If over 32 columns are needed: 33 = 32 +1, etc.*	Over 450	4.4	8.8	13.2	17.6	22	**26.4**	**30.8**	**35.2**	**39.6**	**44**	**48.4**	**52.8**	**57.2**	**61.6**	**66**	**70.4**
	385-450	3.6	7.2	10.8	14.4	18	21.6	**25.2**	**28.8**	**32.4**	**36**	**39.6**	**43.2**	**46.8**	**50.4**	**54**	**57.6**
	334-384	3	6	9	12	15	18	21	24	**27**	**30**	**33**	**36**	**39**	**42**	**45**	**48**
	290-333	2.5	5	7.5	10	12.5	15	17.5	20	22.5	**25**	**27.5**	**30**	**32.5**	**35**	**37.5**	**40**
	251-289	2.1	4.2	6.3	8.4	10.5	12.6	14.7	16.8	18.9	21	23.1	**25.2**	**27.3**	**29.4**	**31.5**	**33.6**
	217-250	1.7	3.4	5.1	6.8	8.5	10.2	11.9	13.6	15.3	17	18.7	20.4	22.1	23.8	**25.5**	**27.2**
	188-216	1.4	2.8	4.2	5.6	7	8.4	9.8	11.2	12.6	14	15.4	16.8	18.2	19.6	21	22.4
	163-187	1.2	2.4	3.6	4.8	6	7.2	8.4	9.6	10.8	12	13.2	14.4	15.6	16.8	18	19.2
	151-162	1	2	3	4	5	6	7	8	9	10	11	12	13	14	15	16
	141-150	0.9	1.8	2.7	3.6	4.5	5.4	6.3	7.2	8.1	9	9.9	10.8	11.7	12.6	13.5	14.4
When hourly BG is 90-140, stay in the same column to determine the new drip rate. **Do Not Change Columns**	131-140	0.8	1.6	2.4	3.2	4	4.8	5.6	6.4	7.2	8	8.8	9.6	10.4	11.2	12	12.8
	121-130	0.7	1.4	2.1	2.8	3.5	4.2	4.9	5.6	6.3	7	7.7	8.4	9.1	9.8	10.5	11.2
	111-120	0.6	1.2	1.8	2.4	3	3.6	4.2	4.8	5.4	6	6.6	7.2	7.8	8.4	9	9.6
	106-110	0.5	1	1.5	2	2.5	3	3.5	4	4.5	5	5.5	6	6.5	7	7.5	8
	101-105	**0.4**	0.9	1.3	1.8	2.2	2.7	3.1	3.6	4	4.5	4.9	5.4	5.9	6.4	6.9	7.4
	96-100	**0.4**	0.8	1.2	1.6	2	2.4	2.8	3.2	3.6	4	4.4	4.8	5.2	5.6	6	6.4
	90-95	**0.3**	0.7	1	1.4	1.7	2.1	2.4	2.8	3.2	3.5	3.8	4.1	4.4	4.7	5	5.3
When new BG is less than **90, Move 1 Column To The Left** and refer to Figure No. 2 for D50 treatment.	80-89	**0.3**	0.6	0.9	1.2	1.5	1.8	2.1	2.4	2.7	3	3.3	3.6	3.9	4.2	4.5	4.8
	70-79	**0.2**	0.4	0.6	0.8	1.0	1.2	1.4	1.6	1.8	2	2.2	2.4	2.6	2.8	3.0	3.2
	60-69	**0.1**	**0.2**	**0.3**	0.4	0.5	0.6	0.7	0.8	.9	1	1.1	1.2	1.3	1.4	1.5	1.6
	Under 60	**0**	**0**	0	0	0	0	0	0	0	0	0	0	0	0	0	0

(Figure No.2)

BG	D50W	ACTION
80-89	Do Not Give	If you have not moved 1 column to the left as directed above, do so now
70-79	10 ml IV Push	* If you have not moved 1 column to the left as directed above, do so now * Recheck BG in 15 minutes * Repeat as necessary
60-69	15 ml IV Push	
50-59	20 ml IV Push	* If you have not moved 1 column to the left as directed above, do so now * Recheck BG in 15 minutes * Repeat as necessary * Contact physician if BG is under 60 for 2 consecutive BG measurements
30-49	25 ml IV Push	
Under 30	30 ml IV Push	

NOTIFY PHYSICIAN IF: (Figure No.3)
* BG is less than 60 for 2 consecutive BG measurements
* BG reverts to greater than 200 for 2 consecutive BG measurements
* **If an insulin requirement exceeding 24 units/hour does not result in a lower BG Level or if the drip rate (ml/hr) drops to less than 0.5 units/hr**
* If the K+ level drops to less than 4
* If continuous enteral feeding, TPN, or IV insulin infusion is stopped

*The Columnar Insulin Dosing Chart and Guideline were designed by the Georgia Hospital Association Research and Education Foundation Partnership for Health and Accountability Diabetes Special Interest Group's Pharmacy representative Lawrence Stockton using studies and work of Drs. Davidson, Steed, Bode, White, Skor, and Santiago, Hawkins, Shipp along with the valuable input and insight of the Diabetes SIG expert panel.

 Revised4/06